BOVINE MEDICINE

DISEASES AND HUSBANDRY

OF CATTLE

BOVINE MEDICINE

DISEASES AND HUSBANDRY OF CATTLE

EDITED BY

A.H. ANDREWS
BVetMed, PhD, MRCVS
Department of
Large Animal Medicine and Surgery
Royal Veterinary College
London

WITH

R.W. BLOWEY
BSc, BVSc, MRCVS

H. BOYD
MRCVS, VMD

R.G. EDDY
BVetMed, FRCVS

OXFORD

BLACKWELL SCIENTIFIC PUBLICATIONS

LONDON EDINBURGH BOSTON

MELBOURNE PARIS BERLIN VIENNA

Editorial Offices:
Osney Mead, Oxford OX2 0EL
25 John Street, London WC1N 2BL
23 Ainslie Place, Edinburgh EH3 6AJ
3 Cambridge Center, Cambridge
Massachusetts 02142, USA
54 University Street, Carlton
Victoria 3053, Australia

Other Editorial Offices:
Arnette SA
2, rue Casimir-Delavigne
75006 Paris
France

Blackwell Wissenschaft
Meinekestrasse 4
D-1000 Berlin 15
Germany

Blackwell MZV
Feldgasse 13
A-1238 Wien
Austria

First published 1992

Set by Excel Typesetters Company, Hong Kong
Printed and bound in Great Britain by
William Clowes Ltd, Beccles and London

DISTRIBUTORS

Marston Book Services Ltd
PO Box 87
Oxford OX2 0DT
(*Orders*: Tel. 0865 791155
Fax: 0865 791927
Telex: 837515)

USA
Blackwell Scientific Publications, Inc.
3 Cambridge Center
Cambridge, MA02142
(*Orders*: Tel: 800 759-6102)

Canada
Times Mirror Professional, Ltd.
5240 Finch Avenue East
Scarborough, Ontario M1S 5A2
(*Orders*: Tel: 03 347-0300)

Australia
Blackwell Scientific Publications
(Australia) Pty Ltd
54 University Street
Carlton, Victoria 3053
(*Orders*: Tel: 03 347-0300)

British Library
Cataloguing in Publication Data

Bovine medicine
1. Livestock : Cattle. Diseases
I. Andrews, A. H.
636.20896

ISBN 0-632-03039-9

Library of Congress
Cataloging-in-Publication Data

Bovine medicine: diseases and husbandry of cattle / edited by
A.H. Andrews.
p. cm.
ISBN 0-632-03039-9
1. Cattle—Diseases. 2. Cattle.
I. Andrews, A.H.
SF961.B78 1992
636.2′0896—dc20

Contents

List of Colour Plates

All colour plates appear between pages 506 and 507

List of Contributors

D.M. ALLEN BSc PhD, *North Coach House, Burcott, Wing, Leighton Buzzard, Bedfordshire LU7 0LZ, UK*

E.C. ANDERSON BVM&S PhD MRCVS, *Veterinary Research Laboratory, PO Box 8101, Causeway, Harare, Zimbabwe*

A.H. ANDREWS BVetMed PhD MRCVS, *Department of Large Animal Medicine and Surgery, Royal Veterinary College, Hawkshead House, Hawkshead Lane, North Mymms, Hatfield, Hertfordshire AL9 7TA, UK*

J.D. BAGGOT BSc MVM PhD DSc FACVPT MRCVS, *Irish Equine Centre, Johnstown, Naas, Co Kildare, Eire*

I.D. BAKER BVSc MRCVS, *49 Cambridge Street, Aylesbury, Buckinghamshire HP20 1RP, UK*

R.M. BARLOW DSc DVM&S MRCVS, *Professor, Department of Veterinary Pathology, Royal Veterinary College Hawkshead House, Hawkshead Lane, North Mymms, Hatfield, Hertfordshire AL9 7TA, UK*

F. BASTIDA-CORCVERA DVM, *Department of Clinical Sciences, New York College of Veterinary Medicine, Cornell University, Ithaca, New York 14853, USA*

E.H. BATTEN BSc PhD, *School of Veterinary Sciences, 'Three Stones', Station Road, Flax Bourton, Bristol BS19 3QN, UK*

P.G.C. BEDFORD BVetMed PhD FRCVS DVOphthal, *Department of Small Animal Studies, Royal Veterinary College Hawkshead House, Hawkshead Lane, North Mymms, Hatfield, Hertfordshire AL9 7TA, UK*

R.W. BLOWEY BSc BVSc MRCVS, *Wood Veterinary Group, 124 Stroud Road, Gloucester GL1 5JN, UK*

H. BOYD MRCVS VMD, *65 Antonine Road, Bearsden, Glasgow G61 4DS, UK*

A.J. BRAMLEY BSc PhD, *Department of Animal Sciences, University of Vermont, Carrigan Hall, Burlington, Vermont 05405-0844, USA*

D.M. BROOM BSc PhD, *Department of Clinical Veterinary Medicine, University of Cambridge, Madingley Road, Cambridge CB3 0ES, UK*

N. CRAVEN BVSc BSc PhD MRCVS, *Technical Services, Animal Sciences Division, Europe & Africa, Monsanto PLC, Chineham Court, Chineham, Basingstoke, Hampshire RG24 0UL, UK*

C.E.I. DAY MA VetMB MRCVS, *Chinham House, Stanford-in-the-Vale, Faringdon, Oxfordshire SN7 8NQ*

B. DREW BSc PhD, *Agricultural Development and Advisory Service, Ministry of Agriculture, Fisheries and Food, Block A, Government Buildings, Coley Park, Reading RG1 6DT, UK*

W.P.H. DUFFUS MA BVSc PhD MRCVS, *School of Veterinary Science, University of Bristol, Langford House, Langford, Bristol BS18 7DU, UK*

R.G. EDDY BVetMed FRCVS, *Penmayne, North Wootton, Shepton Mallet, Somerset BA4 4ES, UK*

R.D. FIELDING BSc MSc PhD, *Edinburgh School of Agriculture, West Mains Road, Edinburgh EH9 3JG, UK*

E.P.J. GIBBS BVSc PhD FRCVS, *Department of Infectious Diseases, College of Veterinary Medicine, University of Florida, Gainesville, Florida 32610, USA*

C.J. GILES BVetMed PhD MRCVS, *Animal Health Development Department, Pfizer Ltd, Ramsgate Road, Sandwich, Kent CT13 9NJ, UK*

D. GRAY BVMS MSc MRCVS, *Scottish Agricultural Colleges, Veterinary Investigation Services, Cleeve Gardens, Oakbank Road, Perth PH1 1HF, UK*

G.A. HALL BVSc PhD MRCPath MRCVS, *Agricultural and Food Research Council, Institute of Animal Health, Compton, Newbury, Berkshire RG16 0NN, UK*

P.J. HARTIGAN MA BSc MVM PhD MRCVS, *Department of Physiology, Faculty of Medical Sciences, Trinity College, Dublin 2, Eire*

K.G. HIBBITT BVSc PhD MRCVS, *Whitecleave House, Burrington, Umberleigh, Devon EX37 9JN, UK*

J.E. HILLERTON BSc PhD, *Agricultural and Food Research Council, Institute for Animal Health, Compton, Newbury, Berkshire RG16 0NN, UK*

A.G. HUNTER BVM&S MRCVS DTVM, *Centre for Tropical Veterinary Medicine, Royal (Dick) School of Veterinary Studies, Easter Bush, Roslin, Midlothian EH25 9RG, UK*

J. ISBISTER MRCVS, *East Lodge, Southbar Estate, Inchinnan, Renfrewshire PA4 9ND, UK*

P.S. JARVIS BSc, *Farm Management Services Consultant, Milk Marketing Board, 61 Newbury Lane, Silsoe, Bedfordshire MK45 4EX, UK*

P.W. JONES BSc PhD, *Agricultural and Food Research Council, Compton, Newbury, Berkshire RG16 0NN, UK*

K. KENNY MVB MRCVS, *Department of Clinical Sciences, New York State College of Veterinary Medicine, Cornell University, Ithaca, New York 14853, USA*

R.P. KITCHING BVetMed BSc MSc PhD MRCVS, *Institute for Animal Health, Pirbright Laboratory, Pirbright, Woking, Surrey GU24 0NF, UK*

P. LEES BPharm PhD, *Department of Veterinary Basic Sciences, Royal Veterinary College, Hawkshead House, Hawkshead Lane, North Mymms, Hatfield, Hertfordshire AL9 7TA, UK*

D.N. LOGUE BVM&S PhD FRCVS, *Veterinary Investigation Service, Animal Production Department, The Scottish Agricultural College, Auchincruive, Ayr KA6 5HW, UK*

M.H. LUCAS BVSc(Q) BSc MRCVS DipBact, *Ministry of Agriculture, Fisheries and Food, Central Veterinary Laboratory, New Haw, Weybridge, Surrey KT15 3NB, UK*

R.W. MATTHEWMAN BSc MAgSc PhD, *Centre for Tropical Veterinary Medicine, University of Edinburgh, Royal (Dick) School of Veterinary Studies, Easter Bush, Roslin, Midlothian EH25 9RG, UK*

S.A. MAY MA VetMB PhD DVR CertEo MRCVS *The University of Liverpool, Department of Veterinary Clinical Science, Leahurst, Neston, South Wirral L64 7TE, UK*

J.H. MORGAN MA VetMB PhD MRCVS, *Agricultural and Food Research Council, Compton, Newbury, Berkshire RG16 0NN, UK*

N.L. NORCROSS PhD, *Department of Clinical Sciences, New York College of Veterinary Medicine, Cornell University, Ithaca, New York 14853, USA*

D.J. O'ROURKE MVB MRCVS, *Coopers Pitman-Moore Ltd, Harefield, Uxbridge, Middlesex UB9 6LS, UK*

A.R. PETERS BA DVetMed PhD FRCVS, *Hoechst UK Ltd, Animal Health Division, Walton Manor, Walton, Milton Keynes, Buckinghamshire MK7 7AJ, UK*

D.J. PETERSE PhD, *Gezondheidsdienst voor dieren Noord-Nederland, Morra 2, Postbus 361, 9200 AJ Drachten, Netherlands*

P.J.N. PINSENT BVSc FRCVS, *Saxon Place, Langford, Bristol, Avon BS18 7BP, UK*

A.H. POOLE NDA CDA, *Farm Management Services Information Unit, Milk Marketing Board, Cleeve House, Malvern Road, Lower Wick, Worcester WR2 4NS, UK*

J.H. PRATT BVM&S MRCVS DVSM, *Meat and Livestock Commission, P O Box 44, Winterhill House, Snowdon Drive, Bletchley, Milton Keynes, Buckinghamshire MK7 7AJ, UK*

D.W.B. SAINSBURY MA PhD BSc MRCVS, *Department of Clinical Veterinary Medicine, University of Cambridge, Madingley Road, Cambridge CB3 0ES, UK*

J.K. SHEARER DVM MS, *Department of Preventive Medicine, College of Veterinary Medicine, University of Florida, Box J-136, Health Science Center, Gainesville, Florida 32610, USA*

N.F. SUTTLE PhD, *Animal Diseases Research Association, Moredun Institute, 408 Gilmerton Road, Edinburgh EH17 7JH, UK*

M.A. TAYLOR BVMS PhD MRCVS CIBiol MIBiol, *Central Veterinary Laboratory, New Haw, Weybridge, Surrey KT15 3NB, UK*

S.M. TAYLOR BVM&S PhD MRCVS, *Veterinary Research Laboratory, Stormont, Belfast BT4 3SD, N Ireland, UK*

T. TESOPGONI DVM, *Department of Infectious Diseases, College of Veterinary Medicine, University of Florida, Gainesville, Florida 32610, USA*

L.R. THOMSETT FRCVS DVD, *352 Hempstead Road, Watford, Herts WD1 3NA, UK*

J.W. TYLER DVM MPVM PhD, *Department of Large Animal Surgery and Medicine, College of Veterinary Medicine, Auburn University, Auburn, USA*

A.D. WEAVER BSc DrMedVet PhD FRCVS, *College of Veterinary Medicine, University of Missouri-Columbia, Columbia, Mo 65211, USA*

J.M. WILKINSON BSc PhD CBiol MIBiol, *Chalcombe Agricultural Resources, 13 Highwoods Drive, Marlow Bottom, Marlow, Buckinghamshire SL7 3PU, UK*

B.M. WILLIAMS MRCVS DVSM, *Knightswood, 4 Lincoln Drive, Pyrford, Woking, Surrey GU22 8RL, UK*

G.B. YOUNG PhD MRCVS, *89 Comiston Drive, Edinburgh, Midlothian EH10 5QT, UK*

Preface

Bovine Medicine aims to provide, within the covers of one book, much of the practical information available on cattle disease and production. Such an objective is admirable in sentiment but very difficult to achieve in practice. It involves the concentration of effort by a large number of different, and often very busy, experts into one volume. For the present part it is hoped that what we have produced will not only be a source of information but, in many areas, it will be an enjoyable, educational read. It is hoped that it will be used as a working guide rather than a reference book and that it will be of particular help to those at the 'sharp end' of the veterinary profession, i.e. in practice. Bearing this in mind, this work does not contain every detail concerning each disease, organism or clinical entity.

Inevitably there are some areas of subject-overlap as might be expected with skin conditions and ectoparasites and 'downer cow', etc. Where possible each author has provided his/her own perspective on the subject.

In addition, references have been kept to a minimum to ensure a less disjointed read. In consequence, we would be pleased to receive comments from readers on any deficiencies or difficulties encountered in presentation or content.

It has taken approximately 2 years to complete a work of this magnitude. The continual expansion in veterinary knowledge and expertise may well mean that in certain areas some recent developments have been omitted. Again, we would be pleased for any such deficiencies to be pointed out to us.

There has been considerable recent interest in alternative medicine for animals. Mindful of this, a section is included on the subject to help readers make up their own minds on its relevance to cattle therapy.

I must thank Blackwell Scientific Publications, and particularly Peter Saugman for his patience during the production of this book. Much work has also fallen on my co-editers Hugh Boyd, Roger Blowey and Roger Eddy. However, the book would not have been completed but for the dedicated secretarial and managerial help of Mrs Rosemary Forster.

A.H. Andrews

PART 1
MANAGEMENT

Chapter 1: Calf Rearing

by D.M. ALLEN

Dairy-bred calves for beef rearing are purchased at about two weeks of age. The early weaning system pioneered in Great Britain is used by most rearers in one form or another and is applicable world-wide. Its success is based upon the fact that calves can be weaned from milk replacer after about five weeks, which makes the system convenient and saves feed costs compared with weaning at an older age.

It is essential that dairy farmers give calves colostrum immediately after they are born. The passive immunity conferred on calves by the immune lactoglobulin in colostrum is vital when the calves may have to cope with transference from one farm to another, probably via an auction market. Mortality among calves deprived of colostrum is high. Also, colostrum is a rich feed and is a good source of vitamins A, D and E.

Calf reception

When they arrive at the farm, calves should be given a thorough health inspection and any showing signs of ill health returned to the supplier or isolated. Navels should be dipped in an approved iodine or other disinfectant solution to prevent navel ill and any calves with signs of lice dusted with insecticide powder. A multivitamin injection (vitamins A, D and E) is good value for money.

The calves should then be placed in pens liberally bedded with dry straw and with clean fresh water available. Milk should be withheld for a few hours. If the calves are held in individual pens calf welfare is met by minimum dimensions of 1.5 × 0.75 m up to four weeks and 1.8 × 1.0 m from four to eight weeks.

Calves do not mind cold weather but need good ventilation without draughts. In the coldest weather straw bales can be placed above the rear half of the pens so that the calves have a warm nest. The modern trend in buildings in temperate climates is away from fan ventilation to simple monopitch buildings in which calves can be housed right through to 12 weeks. At weaning the pens are dismantled and the calves left where they are as a rearing group.

Rearing systems

There are several variations of the early weaning system that can be chosen according to farm circumstances. Most common is twice daily feeding of restricted quantities of warm milk replacer from a bucket. A successful variation of this is once daily bucket feeding. If individual penning is inconvenient then consideration can be given to so-called *ad libitum* rearing systems. This may be from a sophisticated machine which reconstitutes warm milk replacer, or it may involve feeding cold acidified milk replacer from a simple plastic container.

Whichever rearing system is adopted scrupulous attention to cleanliness is essential and so is a high standard of individual calf management.

Scouring is a problem of the milk feeding period and causes dehydration, which may be fatal. If salmonella infection is suspected rectal swabs should be taken for laboratory analysis (see p. 189). At the onset of scouring milk feeding should be stopped and proprietary electrolyte solution fed to prevent dehydration. If body temperature is elevated it is advised that veterinary help is sought in case antibiotic treatment is necessary. Usually, scouring stops after about two days and milk feeding can be resumed.

Salmonella infection is an altogether more serious cause of scouring causing ill health and death. Moreover, many *Salmonella* spp. are transmissible to humans, so during an outbreak special attention needs to be paid to personal hygiene. An outbreak of salmonellosis usually occurs in the first two or three weeks but exceptionally can occur later, even beyond the milk feeding period. If salmonellosis is suspected veterinary advice should be sought immediately so that the appropriate antibiotic treatment can be identified and prescribed. Infected calves should be isolated (see p. 190).

Dehorning and castration cause stress so should not be done at the same time, nor should they coincide with the stress of weaning. In a five-week milk feeding period healthy calves can be dehorned after three weeks, using a hot iron or hot air disbudder, with castration after four weeks.

Early weaning: restricted milk, bucket fed

The classic early weaning system pioneered in Britain weans calves off milk replacer after five weeks. Calves are fed warm milk from buckets. There is little difference in calf performance between feeding milk replacer twice or only once daily, but the latter approach reduces labour requirements by one-third. Twice daily feeding is probably best for inexperienced rearers and lightweight calves at least for the first two weeks until the calves are stronger.

The choice of milk replacer is important and it pays to purchase a high-quality product. Good-quality milk replacers are almost invariably based on dried skimmed milk. Severely heat-treated milk powder has poor clotting ability and digestibility thereby predisposing the calf to diarrhoea (scours). To minimize this risk, manufacturers add fat to the powder to comprise 20 per cent of the dry matter because this has been found to reduce the incidence of scouring (see also Chapter 14).

For bucket feeding it is best if the calves are housed in individual pens but, at the cost of extra labour, it is possible to use calf yokes in a group pen.

Purchased calves should be rested for about 3 hours after arrival at the farm. Then they can be fed 1 litre of milk replacer mixed at 150 g milk powder per litre. The amount is increased gradually over a period of 10 days to a daily maximum for Friesian/Holsteins of 2.75 l.

Fresh concentrate should be fed *ad libitum* from a bucket; it should have an overall crude protein of 18 per cent based on products that supply rumen undegradable protein, e.g. fishmeal, soya. Clean water should be available at all times, even though calves consume considerable fluid with the milk diet.

After five weeks, when each calf has been observed to consume 1 kg of concentrate daily, the calves can be weaned abruptly. Any backward calves should be fed milk replacer for a few days longer. At the other extreme, calves that were obviously three weeks old or more at purchase could be weaned earlier than five weeks.

After weaning it is usually necessary to move calves from individual pens to follow-on accommodation. This is a time of stress and in the European winter may precipitate an outbreak of enzootic pneumonia, which causes more ill health and greater mortality than scouring. So it will pay to wait a few days for calves to overcome the immediate stress of weaning before moving them. Also avoid moving the calves during cold damp weather when there is little air movement and in consequence the risk of pneumonia is high. Intensive research has now reached the stage where vaccines that will give some protection against enzootic pneumonia are on the point of commercial production (see Chapter 15).

The early weaning concentrate can be fed right through to the conclusion of the calf rearing period at three months. However, it is more economical and prepares the calf for the subsequent rearing period, if feeds from the next stage are gradually introduced. So for cereal beef production the rolled barley/protein mix can be introduced gradually from eight weeks. For cattle going on to forage-based systems, the forage can be introduced to the diet in increasing quantities from eight weeks with the early weaning concentrate rationed at 2–2.5 kg daily.

Targets for bucket-rearing systems are shown in Table 1.1.

Early weaning: *ad libitum* milk

Feeding milk *ad libitum* to calves housed in groups may be appropriate on farms where the buildings used are not suitable for the erection of individual pens. It may also be useful where calves become available in small numbers over a long period.

The total labour demand in *ad libitum* rearing is for not less than once daily bucket feeding because although mixing feed and cleaning equipment is quicker, handling the calves, especially teaching them to drink, is more time consuming.

It is absolutely essential with group rearing to ensure that each calf learns to suckle the teat and to check carefully for early signs of scouring, which can spread rapidly through the groups of calves. Do not be misled by the rather loose faeces in the early stages of *ad libitum* milk feeding, which are inevitable given the

Table 1.1 Calf rearing targets to three months of age for bucket-rearing systems. Source: Meat and Livestock Commission (MLC)

	Friesian/Holstein Hereford × Friesian	Charolais × Friesian
Feed (kg)		
Milk powder	16	16
Concentrates	170	185
Weight (kg)		
Purchase	45	50
Weaning	70	78
3 months	110	122
Daily gain (kg)		
To weaning	0.7	0.8
5–12 weeks	0.8	0.9
Overall	0.8	0.9

Table 1.2 Calf rearing targets to three months of age for *ad libitum* milk replacer

	Friesian/Holstein Hereford × Friesian	Charolais × Friesian
Feed (kg)		
Milk powder	30	33
Concentrates	160	180
Weight (kg)		
Purchase	45	50
Weaning	75	85
3 months	115	130
Daily gain (kg)		
To weaning	0.8	0.9
5–12 weeks	0.8	0.9
Overall	0.8	0.9

high level of milk intake. It takes experience to spot the difference between this condition and scouring.

With small numbers of calves differing in age it is convenient to erect two or more pens around a single *ad libitum* feeder with one or more teats serving each pen.

COLD ACIDIFIED MILK

Ad libitum rearing has been greatly simplified by the manufacture of acidified milk replacers. They contain small concentrations of organic acids so that mixes can be stored for two or three days without going sour. This means that milk can be mixed in a simple plastic container with milk drawn through plastic tubes, preferably fitted with non-return valves, to teats. The equipment required is both inexpensive and foolproof.

The convenience of the system should not deflect the rearer from the need for a high level of individual calf management. At the start, each calf should be trained to suckle the teat and be given 1 litre of milk replacer. When all the calves have been fed the milk supply should be removed. The procedure should be repeated twice in the next 24 hours. Thereafter the calves can be allowed continuous access to the teats with no more than six calves per teat. Milk intake may be considerably depressed in very cold weather.

Fresh water should always be available and early weaning concentrates should be provided *ad libitum* in a trough placed close to the teats but far enough away to avoid spoilage from spilt milk or saliva. The plastic container, all tubes and teats must be cleaned thoroughly between mixes.

By the third week milk intake will be around 7 l daily and a gradual weaning procedure is followed to limit total consumption of milk replacer to 25–30 kg. Weaning is carried out by denying calves access to teats for progressively longer each day. At first the teats are removed overnight, then mid-morning and so on until weaning finally occurs after five weeks. Concentrate consumption, which is very low in the first three weeks, rises rapidly during the weaning process so that there is no greater check at weaning than in bucket-feeding systems. Postweaning management is the same as for bucket-reared calves.

Targets for the systems are shown in Table 1.2.

AUTOMATIC MACHINES

Highly sophisticated automatic milk feeding machines are available for calf rearing that reconstitute warm milk replacer continuously. The machines can service calves in more than one pen and it is possible to vary the concentration of milk from one pen to another, which is useful during gradual weaning. Some machines have computer control systems and calves fitted with electronic transponders can be individually rationed.

Inevitably, automatic machines are expensive but they save labour by mixing milk little and often. This does not exclude the need for scrupulous cleaning — those parts involved in mixing and dispensing milk must be cleaned daily.

Training the calves to drink is the same as for cold acidified milk. The same gradual weaning procedure can be used also but more commonly gradual weaning is achieved by progressively diluting the milk replacer.

Targets for machine rearing are the same as for cold acidified milk (see Table 1.2). Compared with bucket rearing more than twice as much milk powder is used but concentrate consumption is slightly lower. The higher overall feed cost is offset by the higher calf weight at three months.

Veal production

Veal production is a specialized system of calf rearing designed to produce a white meat that is very popular in continental Europe. Traditionally, calves were fed milk *ad libitum* and slaughtered at 14–16 weeks producing carcasses weighing 100–110 kg. In recent years the feeding period has been extended to 20 weeks or more, despite rapidly declining feed conversion efficiency.

Welfare legislation in Britain now bans the narrow calf crates used in continental veal units, which do not allow the calf to turn round or groom itself. The iron content of milk replacers must be declared and concentrates must be fed from two weeks of age to prevent the anaemia which is a feature of veal calves fed milk without iron supplementation. Eventually, similar legislation will be enacted in continental Europe.

Chapter 2: Beef Finishing Systems

by D.M. ALLEN

The term 'beef finishing systems' has been taken as the title of this chapter in place of the former 'fattening systems' to indicate that rearing cattle for beef is concerned with the production of lean meat not fat. A whole range of beef systems is available for the production of beef from suckler-bred and dairy-bred calves.

Suckler herds on upland farms or rangelands usually sell their calves in the autumn, though spring-born calves may be overwintered for sale in the spring. In Europe, heavy yearling calves from the autumn sales are finished during the ensuing winter for sale at 16–18 months of age. Lighter autumn-born calves and spring-born calves are overwintered in preparation for finishing off grass at 18–20 months or they are grown through the grazing season and finished during their second winter of life.

Under rangeland conditions in the USA the growth performance of the calves is poorer than on grassland farms in Europe and, against a background of plentiful supplies of cheap feed grains, a special approach to beef production has been adopted using beef feedlots. Calves weaned from rangeland herds are taken to farms on better land where they are grown on in 'store' condition until 12–18 months of age when they are transferred to large-scale feedlots for short-term finishing on a high-grain ration.

For dairy-bred calves several beef systems have been developed that vary in grassland utilization, the amount of concentrates fed and the age and weight at which cattle are slaughtered. At one extreme is cereal beef (commonly known as barley beef) in which cattle are housed throughout life and fed an all-concentrate diet for rapid growth to slaughter at 11–13 months of age. At the other extreme are grass/cereal systems in which finishing is either through the winter on silage supplemented with cereals with slaughter at 16–20 months of age, or off grazed grass at 20–24 months of age.

An important point to note is that although there are many beef systems, for most of them slaughter is compressed into the age range 16–24 months, which means that carcasses are in a tighter weight range than might be supposed at first sight.

Finishing suckled calves

Meat and Livestock Commission (MLC) Beefplan results show that buying and selling prices have a crucial effect on average gross margins. Prices for suckled calves and older store cattle are volatile and this, together with the short duration of the finishing period, causes financial margins to fluctuate wildly from one year to the next. One consequence is that finishers become so preoccupied with buying and selling prices that they do not pay sufficient attention to the even more important effect on profitability of the standard of management achieved during the finishing period. Moreover, it is absolutely essential that the finishing enterprise is carefully planned and tightly budgeted.

Table 2.1 Comparative performance of suckler-bred steers slaughtered at EC fat class 4L. Source: MLC

	Sire breed				
	Angus	Charolais	Hereford	Limousin	Simmental
Daily gain (kg)	0.77	0.84	0.78	0.78	0.86
Feeding period (days)	105	148	120	145	145
Slaughter weight (kg)	393	494	410	454	490
Feed (DM)	0.83	1.34	0.95	1.20	1.32
Efficiency (kg feed DM/kg gain)	10.3	10.9	10.1	10.5	10.6

Table 2.2 Comparative carcass quality of suckler-bred steers slaughtered at EC fat class 4L. Source: MLC

	Sire breed				
	Angus	Charolais	Hereford	Limousin	Simmental
Slaughter weight (kg)	393	494	410	454	490
Killing-out (%)	52.5	54.8	52.3	54.7	53.0
Carcass weight (kg)	205	268	214	247	258
Saleable meat (%)	72.5	72.7	71.9	73.3	72.0
High-priced cuts (%)	44.1	44.8	44.1	45.4	44.8

Winter finishing

Choice of breed or cross, the sex of cattle and the feeds used all have an important bearing on the duration of the finishing period and the weight of cattle at slaughter.

Breed choice has a major influence on output and inputs. Results from MLC experiments show that calves by heavy, late maturing sire breeds grow fastest but must be fed longer to reach a specified carcass fatness (Table 2.1). This takes a greater total quantity of feed but with no penalty to feed efficiency. Indeed, Angus and Charolais crosses, which have completely different performance characteristics, are of similar overall feed efficiency.

There is a clear advantage to the continental breed crosses e.g. Charolais and Limousin, in killing-out percentage and they are at the upper end of the range of per cent saleable meat and the proportion of high-priced cuts (Table 2.2).

Two types of finishing ration can support profitable winter finishing. Most profitable is high quality silage supplemented with cereals. Also in some cases arable by-products, in particular straw, supplemented with higher levels of a balanced concentrate can be used profitably for finishing. Results from winter finishing units using silage and recorded by MLC are shown in Table 2.3. They demonstrate that producers within the top third of gross margins owed their success to better cattle performance than average, achieved with similar concentrates but more silage than average.

Table 2.3 Results for winter finishing suckled calves, 1989–90. Source: MLC

	Average	Top third of gross margins
Output (£/head)	174	249
Variable costs (£/head)	131	125
Gross margin/head (£)	43	124
Gross margin/ha (£)	—	—
Feeding period (days)	190	198
Daily gain (kg)	1.04	1.16
Slaughter weight (kg)	496	509
Concentrates (kg)	685	701
Silage (t)	2.0	2.3
Stocking rate (cattle/ha)	—	—

In some countries growth promoting hormone implants are licensed for use and increase the daily gain of steers by up to 20 per cent and heifers by up to 10 per cent. In the EC these useful compounds have been banned for political reasons. One consequence has been an interest in rearing male suckled calves as bulls, a practice already common in France. Bulls grow faster and leaner than steers to higher slaughter weights. Bull

Table 2.4 Bull beef production from suckler-bred cattle. Source: Great Britain Ministry of Agriculture

	Bulls	Steers
Daily gain (kg)	1.89	1.4
Slaughter age (days)	321	355
Slaughter weight (kg)	496	464
Killing-out (%)	56.5	54.4
Carcass weight (kg)	280	253
EC carcass class*	U3	R4L

* Conformation: P (poor), −O, O+, R (average), −U, U+, E (Excellent).
Fat: 1 (lean), 2, 3, 4L (average) 4H, 5L, 5H (fat).

beef production is simplest with the spring-born calf that is weaned in the autumn before behavioural problems are at all troublesome.

Bulls can be finished profitably on silage and cereals, managed at a daily gain of 1.0 kg per day or more. An interesting alternative approach is rapid finishing on a cereal beef concentrate. After weaning at around six months the bulls are gradually introduced to the concentrate diet over a three-week period with a declining allowance of a forage feed such as straw. With Charolais crosses gains of 1.75 kg/day or more can be achieved with a feed efficiency better than 6 kg feed/kg gain. The bulls are slaughtered at about 500 kg liveweight at only 10–12 months of age. Experimental results shown in Table 2.4 show the potential of the system.

Grass finishing

Financial margins for grass finishing are very sensitive to buying and selling prices because store cattle are purchased in the spring when prices are high but finished cattle are sold as prices fall to the seasonal low in the autumn.

Nevertheless, good cattle performance and high stocking rates are still essential ingredients of profitable production. The main skill is balancing the variable supply of grass through the season with the changing needs of the cattle. Probably the best approach is a buffer grazing system where part of the grassland is split off as a buffer area to be conserved as silage if possible but grazed if necessary. Then grazing is managed to maintain the sward at a height of about 6–8 cm (3 in.).

Differences in performance between early and late maturing crosses are very important in grass finishing. For example, whereas early maturing Hereford crosses require a grass finishing period of only four months, late maturing Charolais crosses take five months.

Table 2.5 Overwintering and grass finishing results for steers and heifers, 1986. Source: MLC

	Heifers	Steers
Gross margin/head (£)	79	126
Gross margin/ha (£)	377	441
Grazing gain (kg/day)	0.7	0.8
Slaughter weight (kg)	446	475
Sale price (p/kg)	101	104

Early maturity is an advantage in grass finishing and so heifers that fatten too fast to be grown rapidly on high quality winter finishing rations show to best advantage when grass finished. Even so they are often less profitable than steers because of poorer performance, lower slaughter weight and a poorer sale price (Table 2.5).

Feedlots

Feedlots should be differentiated from other systems of producing beef because of their scale and the fact that feeds are usually purchased rather than being grown on an associated land area.

Beef feedlots account for a high proportion of slaughter cattle in the USA but are also found in Canada and Australia. There is also a rather distinct type of operation in Europe typified by the maize silage feedlots in the Po Valley of northern Italy.

North American feedlots

Spring-born suckled calves from rangeland herds weigh about 180 kg when weaned at six months of age in the autumn. They are then sold to farms on slightly better land where they are grazed in summer and fed hay in winter during a grazing period of between six and twelve months. This is called 'backgrounding' in the USA. Feedlot operators purchase cattle throughout the year for their feedlots. However, some of the cattle in feedlots are not owned by the feedlot operator but are 'custom-fed' for a daily charge. Large feedlots are categorized as those with more than 15 000 cattle and feedlots with 50 000+ cattle are quite common.

The USA feedlots are open-air with at most shading from the sun in hotter climates. In the drier areas wire-fenced enclosures each holding 200 cattle are located on gently sloping land with drainage to a lagoon, the contents of which are pumped onto arable crops. In wetter states, such as Nebraska, earth moving equipment is used to form mounds in each pen so that cattle can lie out of the mud. Surface manure is skimmed off periodically and spread on neighbouring arable land.

At the front of the pen a feed bunker is erected providing 450 mm (18 in.) of trough length per head. Usually the cattle are fed three times daily. The pens back onto a handling race.

Cattle entering the feedlots are weighed, tagged, dosed for worms, vaccinated against pneumonia and soil-borne diseases, dipped against external parasites and implanted with a hormonal growth promoter (see Chapter 57).

Some feedlots use maize silage as a source of roughage, others chopped alfalfa hay. The cattle are fed a 75 per cent roughage diet for up to three weeks before being fed a changeover ration with 50 per cent roughage for one week and then the 'hot' ration with only 15–25 per cent roughage.

A protein/mineral/vitamin premix is purchased in bulk from a local feed mill. The most commonly used grain is maize, which is steam-rolled at the feedlot and incorporated into a complete ration including the protein premix and roughage, and is usually still warm when fed.

The performance targets for feedlot steers are a daily gain of 1.25 kg wth 8.4 kg feed DM/kg gain. The feeding period is about five months and cattle are usually marketed on an all-out basis.

By its very nature, feedlot beef production is highly sensitive to cattle and feed prices and volatile margins are a feature of the USA feedlots.

Maize silage feedlots

The maize silage feedlots of the Po Valley in Italy are smaller than their USA counterparts, ranging from a few hundred to a few thousand cattle, and feed diets in which silage forms a much higher proportion of the ration. Moreover, the feeding period is much longer and many of the cattle are dairy bred rather than suckler bred. Somewhat similar, but smaller, maize silage beeflots have been developed in France and Germany.

Dairy beef systems

Dairy beef systems have developed rapidly during the last 30 years and there are several methods of production using calves born at various times of the year. Notably, cereal beef production takes place in buildings and permits production throughout the year. More recently, grass silage beef production has also developed as an indoor system and, for the first time, makes year-round production possible from a grass-based system.

Cereal beef

Commonly known as barley beef, cereal beef uses an all-concentrate diet fed to housed cattle, mainly bulls, which are slaughtered at 11–13 months of age. Because of the high concentrate diet and young age at slaughter the carcasses have a marble-white fat cover and are popular with some supermarkets.

High rates of gain are essential for profitable production so bull beef is the rule. Feed additives such as monensin sodium improve feed efficiency. During the course of the production cycle the protein content of the concentrate is reduced from 18 per cent in calfhood to 12 per cent in the finishing ration. After six months of age part of the protein can be supplied by urea.

Recorded results in Table 2.6 are mainly for Friesian/Holstein bulls slaughtered at 440–460 kg liveweight. Continental breed × Friesian cattle are leaner and can be taken to 500 kg. However, beyond these weights feed efficiency soon deteriorates to a point where profitability is reduced.

Maize silage beef

Reference has already been made to the use of maize silage as a forage in the feedlots of USA and Europe. In Europe, maize is already the most important arable forage crop and the development by plant breeders of earlier maturing varieties continues to increase the climatic range in which the crop can be grown.

Maize is a high-energy feed but in many of the continental Europe feedlots it is still supplemented by high levels of maize grain. In fact, comparatively low levels of concentrate supplementation are sufficient to

Table 2.6 Cereal beef results, 1989. Source: MLC

	Average	Top third of gross margins
Gross margin/head (£)	105	166
Feeding period (days)	344	361
Daily gain (kg)	1.23	1.24
Slaughter weight (kg)	476	496
Finishing concentrates (kg)	1966	1981
Feed efficiency (kg feed/kg gain)	4.65	4.42

Table 2.7 Production standards for dairy-bred cattle in maize silage beef. Source: MLC

	Friesian/ Holstein	Limousin × Friesian	Charolais × Friesian
Reared calf (kg)	110	110	115
Feeding period (weeks)	47	49	49
Daily gain (kg)	1.1	1.1	1.2
Protein concentrate (kg)	500	450	500
Rolled barley (kg)	100	90	100
Maize silage (t)	6.2	5.7	6.5
Slaughter weight (kg)	475	490	530
Carcass weight (kg)	250	270	290
Typical EC carcass class*	O+3	R/−U3	R/−U3

* Conformation: P (poor), −O, O+, R (average), −U, U+, E (Excellent).
Fat: 1 (lean), 2, 3, 4L (average), 4H, 5L, 5H (fat).

support gains of 1.1–1.2 kg daily. However, with late maturing bulls it may be necessary to increase the level of concentrates in the last three months to produce the level of fat cover on the carcass demanded by the meat trade.

The important thing to remember is that maize is short of protein and the concentrate needs to be formulated with this in mind. A simple but effective feeding system is to introduce maize silage into the diet by three months of age and supplement it throughout the feeding period with a flat-rate allowance of 1.5 kg of a 35 per cent crude protein concentrate. This satisfies the high protein requirement of young cattle and keeps in step with declining protein requirements as they get older. Production standards for various types of dairy-bred calves are shown in Table 2.7.

Grass silage beef

Grass silage beef is a recent development by researchers of a forage-based system in which cattle are housed throughout permitting year-round production. It also permits very intensive grassland management, with all the grass made into silage, and high levels of cattle performance harnessing the rapid lean growth of bulls.

From three months of age the cattle are introduced gradually to grass silage supplemented with cereals and, up to 350 kg liveweight, 0.2 kg daily of a high quality protein supplement such as fishmeal to satisfy the requirements of young cattle for rumen undegradable protein. The aim is a daily gain around 1.0 kg.

Grass silage beef depends most for its success on the production of high yields of high quality silage. Then target gains can be achieved with low levels of concentrate supplementation. Before introducing a grass silage beef system careful budgeting is necessary. High stocking rates mean that the working capital investment per hectare is considerable. Also it may be necessary to construct extra silos when changing from a beef system in which cattle graze during summer. On the other hand, continuous production allows 20 per cent more cattle to be produced from a single building than when it is occupied by a single seasonal batch of cattle.

Table 2.8 presents standards for bulls of various breed types. Hereford × Friesians are likely to make a smaller gross margin per head than Friesian/Holsteins because of lower output. However, the higher stocking rate allows Hereford × Friesians to rival the gross margin per hectare of Friesian/Holsteins. Under UK conditions the superior performance of Limousin × and Charolais × Friesians make them worth £60–70/head more as calves than Friesian/Holsteins.

Table 2.8 Performance standards for grass silage beef from three months of age. Source: MLC

	Friesian/Holstein	Hereford × Friesian	Limousin × Friesian	Charolais × Friesian
Reared calf (kg)	110	110	110	115
Feeding period (days)	55	50	57	56
Daily gain (kg)	1.0	1.0	1.0	1.1
Concentrates (t)	1.0	0.7	0.9	1.0
Silage (t)	6.0	4.5	5.5	6.3
Stocking (cattle/ha)	6.0	7.4	6.5	5.7
Slaughter weight (kg)	495	460	510	550
Carcass weight (kg)	260	240	280	300
Typical EC carcass class*	O+3	O+/R3	R/−U3	R/−U3

* Conformation: P (poor), −O, O+, R (average), −U, U+, E (excellent).
Fat: 1 (lean), 2, 3, 4L (average), 4H, 5L, 5H (fat).

Eighteen-month beef

Eighteen-month beef is a forage system that uses dairy-bred calves born in the autumn, are reared through their first winter, grazed from six to twelve months of age and then finished during the second winter on a diet of grass silage and cereals.

Target gains are 0.8 kg/day during the rearing winter aiming at a weight of 180 kg when turned out in the spring. High grazing gains are very important for profitable production and the target gain is at least 0.8 kg/day. On high quality silage supplemented with about 3 kg of rolled barley daily a finishing gain of 0.9 kg/day should be achieved. The overall stocking rate target on grassland is 3.5 Friesian/Holsteins per ha or 4.0 earlier maturing Hereford × Friesians.

Results recorded on farms by MLC show the financial importance of achieving the daily gain and stocking rate targets (Table 2.9).

In Britain, male cattle in the system are usually reared as steers because safety regulations effectively prevent grazing bulls beyond 10 months of age.

On farms seeking to intensify grassland management the tendency in recent years has been for 18-month beef to be replaced by grass silage beef.

Grass beef

The most extensive forage-based dairy beef system is grass beef in which cattle are finished off grass at 20–24 months of age.

Dairy-bred calves born in the autumn or winter are reared through their first winter and then grazed through the summer. The second winter is a store period when the cattle are fed an inexpensive ration designed to support a daily gain of about 0.5 kg. Turned out to grass in the spring the cattle exhibit compensatory growth — a period of especially rapid gains following a period of feed restriction — so that they reach market condition before the end of their second grazing season. (Incidentally this same system of store feeding is also used in winter feeding suckled calves in preparation for grass finishing and in 'backgrounding' cattle for feedlots.)

Table 2.9 Results for 18-month beef, 1990. Source: MLC

	Average	Top third of gross margins
Output (£/head)	336	350
Variable costs (£/head)	210	194
Gross margin/head (£)	126	156
Gross margin/ha (£)	446	579
Daily gain (kg)		
First winter	0.7	0.7
Grazing	0.7	0.7
Second winter	0.9	0.9
Slaughter weight (kg)	488	499
Concentrates (t)	0.9	0.8
Silage (t)	4.5	4.6
Stocking rate (cattle/ha)	3.5	3.7

Table 2.10 Performance targets for grass beef. Source: MLC

	Friesian/ Holstein	Hereford × Friesian
Daily gain (kg)		
Rearing winter	0.7	0.7
First summer	0.7	0.7
Second winter	0.5	0.4
Second summer	1.0	1.0
Overall	0.7	0.7
Slaughter weight (kg)	525	465
Stocking rate (cattle/ha)	2.5	3.0

The calves turned out in the spring are rather young to utilize grass well, especially if they are winter-born. A clever way of providing preferential grazing for the young calves is to adopt a leader/follower system in which the calves graze ahead of the older generation of cattle around a series of small fields or paddocks. The young calves can graze selectively and the older cattle, whose nutritional requirements are less critical, clear up the grass.

In any grass finishing system early maturing cattle are an advantage because they easily reach market condition before the end of the grazing season. Slaughter from mid-season reduces cattle numbers nicely in step with declining cattle production. So the Hereford × Friesian has advantages over late maturing Friesian/Holsteins or Charolais × Friesians, which finish later and may run short of grass.

Performance targets for grass beef are shown in Table 2.10. In practice many farmers carry out only part of the system and so there is a good deal of trading in dairy-bred stores, which are finally slaughtered at 20–24 months of age.

A problem with systems of long duration such as grass beef is the long lead time before any cattle are sold. Usually the third batch of calves is being purchased before the cattle of the first batch are all slaughtered. The consequence is a high working capital requirement per head.

Chapter 3: Suckler Herds

by D.M. ALLEN

On the face of it nothing could be simpler than managing a beef suckler herd. Cows can be kept at low cost and each cow suckles its single calf. In reality high standards of enterprise planning and individual cow management are necessary if the herd is to be profitable. This is as true in extensive rangelands as it is in highly productive grassland.

Suckler cows are usually kept on marginal land or in a low-cost system where winter (or dry season) feeds are scarce. So it is common for calves to be sold at weaning to farmers on better land. Inevitably, this places emphasis on the weight of calf produced per cow bulled as the main profit indicator.

Planning the suckler herd

Fitting the suckler herd into farm resources is of key importance to profitability. Can the herd be integrated with a sheep flock? Are there arable crop residues for cow feeding? Can calves be finished or should they be sold at weaning? Getting the right answers to these questions creates a framework on which profitable production can be built.

A most important choice is season of calving. On rangelands with severe winters or a dry season and in upland and mountain areas, winter- /dry-season feed supplies are scarce and there is no option but to calve at the start of the growing season. On the other hand, on better land in Europe, autumn calving is a realistic option. A greater weight of weaned calf is produced albeit at the expense of higher feed costs.

The availability of housing and labour may also dictate season of calving, regardless of feed availability. Winter housing gives freedom of choice on calving season, and by preventing poaching of land should allow higher stocking rates. But the provision of housing adds fixed costs to the enterprise.

Choice of cow breed

There are great advantages in using crossbred cows because hybrid vigour enhances reproductive efficiency, which increases the number of calves weaned.

In Great Britain, the traditional crossbred cow, typified by the Blue Grey (Shorthorn × Galloway) and Shorthorn × Highland, was bred on upland and mountain farms. Another popular crossbred cow was the Aberdeen Angus × Shorthorn cow imported from Ireland.

During the last two decades these specialist beef cows have been augmented by beef × dairy cows, notably Hereford × Friesian and Aberdeen Angus × Friesian. The Hereford × Friesian produces more milk than the Blue Grey and weans a heavier calf but the Blue Grey has better reproductive efficiency so that, overall, the two types of cow are roughly equal (Table 3.1).

One characteristic shared by the Blue Grey and Hereford × Friesian is medium size. Small and medium size seems to be associated with the highest cow efficiency. Heavy cows, such as Charolais crosses, simply cannot translate enough of their heavier weight into calf weaning weight to rival the efficiency of a lighter breed type.

Table 3.1 Comparative performance of Blue Grey and Hereford × Friesian cows. Source: MLC

	Blue Grey	Hereford × Friesian
Cow weight (kg)	450	500
Assisted calvings (%)	9.0	10.1
Calving percentage	95.6	94.9
Calving interval (days)	369	378
Calf weaning weight (kg)	278	294
Calf weight/cow (kg)	265	269
Calf weight/500 kg cow weight (kg)	29.3	26.9

None the less, many British suckler producers are now trying crossbred cows sired by continental beef breeds, e.g. Limousin × Friesian. They are prepared to trade a theoretical reduction in efficiency (which may not be manifest at farm level) for the improved conformation of the calf, which commands a financial premium in the market place. Much the same is happening in the USA.

It must not be overlooked that in the mountain breeds, where a high proportion of cows must be bred pure to breed sufficient replacements, crossbreeding is not an option. Also, French farmers have rejected crossbred cows and have a substantial suckler herd based on purebred cows such as Charolais, Limousin, etc. Again there is a trade-off — the ability to breed for improved growth and carcass quality at the expense of hybrid vigour in reproductive efficiency. Even in breeds such as Salers, which are commonly crossbred to terminal sires, the cows are bred pure.

Rearing replacement heifers

There should be a planned replacement policy for suckler herds with strict rules on culling of cows in the herd for infertility, unacceptably late calving and culling old cows before they drift into the emaciated body condition associated with old age.

A typical replacement rate in British suckler herds is 16 per cent, which gives cows an average herd life of seven years.

Replacement heifers may be purchased as calves from dairy herds for rearing or, more commonly, purchased as bulling heifers or heifers due to calve. With young calves or bulling heifers it is wise to purchase a surplus of 20 per cent to allow for any which fail to become pregnant.

The management of replacement heifers during rearing needs just the same care as any other branch of cattle production. It is important to achieve the target weights at mating and calving shown in Table 3.2 for heifers calving at two years of age.

Table 3.2 Targets for replacement heifers. Source: MLC

	Hereford × Friesian	Blue Grey
Target weight at mating (kg)	325	280
Target weight at calving (kg)	475	425

It must be remembered that difficult calvings are a much greater problem in heifers than in cows. It is therefore safest to mate heifers to breeds such as Aberdeen Angus and Hereford. Calf performance is moderate but there is likely to be greater lifetime performance.

The heifers should be mated to calve early in the herd calving season so that a slight delay in rebreeding does not lead to a late second calving. Calving at the right time is more important than aiming slavishly to calve at two years of age.

Choice of sire breed

Choice of sire breed and the selection of an individual sire within the chosen breed are, if anything, even more important than the choice of dam breed. This is because the sire has major effects on calf growth. Even at weaning, when maternal effects are at a maximum, sire breed has greater effects on weaning weight than dam breed.

Heavy breeds such as Charolais, Simmental and South Devon produce calves with the highest weaning weights (Table 3.3). These calves also have higher birthweights, which means an inexorable increase in assisted calvings and neonatal calf mortality.

Nevertheless, annual productivity is higher for the heavy sire breeds because higher calf weight more than offsets the extra calf mortality and the inevitable delay in rebreeding after a difficult calving, reflected in a lengthening of the calving interval (Table 3.4).

Suckled calf producers have recognized the overall superiority of the heavy breeds, which have now largely supplanted the native British breeds in commercial suckler herds.

Having selected sire breed it is then important to purchase the best individual bull that can be afforded. One of the common measures of individual bull performance is yearling or 400-day weight. With a heritability of about 0.4 a bull that is 100 kg heavier than his

Table 3.3 Effect of sire breed on calf weaning weights. Source: MLC

	Lowland	Upland	Hill
Hereford 200-day weight (kg)	208	194	184
Difference from Hereford × (kg)			
Charolais	+32	+33	+21
Simmental	+24	+28	+14
South Devon	+23	+27	+16
North Devon	+17	+21	+7
Lincoln Red	+14	+20	+5
Sussex	+7	+13	+2
Limousin	+7	+10	+2
Aberdeen Angus	−14	−12	−8

Table 3.4 Effects of sire breed on annual cow productivity. Source: MLC

Sire breed	Assisted calvings (%)	Calf mortality (%)	Calving interval (days)	Calf weaning weight/cow per year (kg)
Charolais	9.0	4.8	374	208
Simmental	8.9	4.2	374	203
South Devon	8.7	4.0	375	203
North Devon	6.4	2.6	373	200
Limousin	7.4	3.8	375	199
Lincoln Red	6.7	2.0	373	198
Sussex	4.5	1.5	372	196
Hereford	4.0	1.6	372	189
Aberdeen Angus	2.4	1.3	370	179

herd group is likely to sire calves 25 kg heavier than average, worth a tidy sum spread over the bull's lifetime offspring. Note that the measure is '100 kg above his herd group', i.e. relative performance. With bulls from different herds it is not at all clear whether differences in weight between bulls are due to inherited effects or feeding management. Therefore, the practice at sales of simply comparing weights with the breed average is highly misleading.

Now more sophisticated estimates of breeding value are available. These are usually selection indices in which the various measures of performance are combined together into a single index score that describes overall merit. For example, the MLC Beef Index is based on calving difficulty score, birthweight, 200- and 400-day weight, feed intake, muscling score and an ultrasonic estimate of backfat. The objective of the Beef Index is to improve the financial margin between the saleable meat produced and the cost of feed taking account of the cost of calving difficulty. Beef Index scores range from 50 (poor) through 100 (average) to 150 (excellent).

Functional soundness is not included in the score and must be judged independently. This includes sound legs and feet, leading to a good walking action, good jaw structure and a calm temperament. In addition, the testicles should be of normal size because under-developed testicles may be associated with subnormal fertility (see Chapter 35 p. 492).

In his first season a young bull should be given no more than 20–25 cows to serve. The bull should be watched to ensure that he is active and an unusual proportion of returns to service should warn of possible infertility. A mature bull should cope with 20 cows.

Suckler cow management

The key objective in suckler herd management is to achieve a compact calving, ideally six weeks but at the outside no longer than 12 weeks. The advantages of compact calving are that herd rationing meets closely the nutritional needs of individual cows, calvings can be closely supervised to provide assistance when necessary and reduce calf mortality, and much more uniform calf performance is obtained.

In most situations a long drawn-out calving is a sure sign of low conception rate, which nibbles away at profitability. It is not possible through feeding management to make a long drawn-out calving compact. The only strategy that will work is to cull late calving cows. This need not be as expensive as it first seems because, culled at the time of year when cull cow prices are high, the income from cow sales may almost cover the cost of replacement heifers. Even if there is a cost in the year of culling, over a three-year period overall profitability is higher.

Some suckler producers run autumn- and spring-calving herds and switch late calving cows from one to the other. This creates two compact calvings but does not necessarily tackle the cause of late calving.

Once having established a compact calving it is essential to maintain it. Firstly, there must be discipline so that bulls are joined with the herd for a bulling period of only six weeks, certainly no longer than eight weeks. Secondly, pregnancy diagnosis should be introduced as a routine so that barren cows can be identified and culled at the most advantageous time. Thirdly, as mentioned earlier, heifers should be mated to calve early in the period in case there is any delay in rebreeding. And fourthly, a watchful eye is needed for bulls that are lazy or infertile; if necessary use a chin ball marker on the bull or tail paint on the cows to record matings.

All of these actions will be to no avail if the underlying conception rate of the herd is low due to poor nutrition. It is possible that some specific aspect of nutrition is to blame for poor conception but more likely it is the overall nutritional level of the herd that is at fault.

The most sensitive indicator of overall nutrition is the body condition of the cow. A method of condition scoring cows has been developed by which changes in fatness can be monitored. Then feeding can be adjusted to ensure that cows are in the right body condition at the key times in the production cycle (see also Chapter 7 p. 96).

The method of condition scoring (Fig. 3.1) is to grip the loin between the thumb and forefinger. The thumb curls around the ledge formed by the transverse processes of the spine to feel the overlying fat cover. The position for handling is midway between the hip (hook) bone and the last rib, ideally on the left side of the cow.

Body condition is scored on a 6-point scale from 0 (emaciated) to 5 (grossly overfat).

0 Spine prominent and no detectable fat cover over the transverse processes.
1 Spine still prominent but transverse processes no longer sharp.
2 Transverse processes can still be felt but now rounded with a thin covering of fat.
3 Individual transverse processes can now only be detected with firm pressure from the thumb.
4 Transverse processes can hardly be felt even with firm pressure.
5 Transverse processes covered by an obvious thick layer of soft fat.

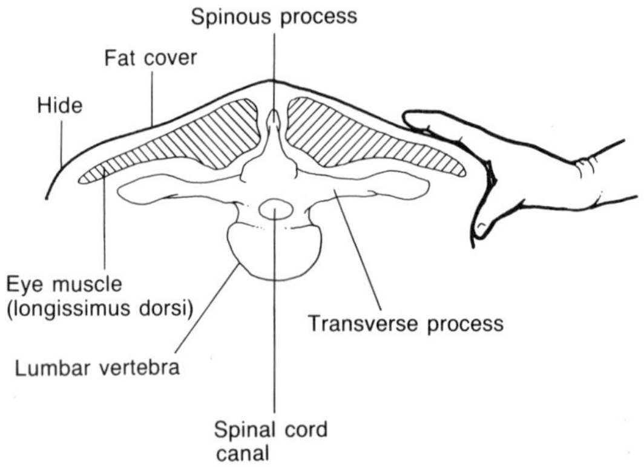

Fig. 3.1 Technique for condition scoring.

Table 3.5 Target body condition scores for suckler cows. Source: MLC

	Autumn-calving cow	Spring-calving cow
Mating	2.5	2–2.5
Mid-pregnancy	2	3
Calving	3	2

* Scores on a scale 0 (emaciated) to 5 (very fat).

The handling technique is soon learned and consistent results can be achieved. The worst mistake is to decide that condition scores can be estimated visually without recourse to handling. Only after considerable handling practice can a skilled herdsman hope to get a general impression of condition from visual inspection.

The only possible confusion is with cows carrying blood of the continental European breeds where the thick muscling may overhang the transverse processes and confuse the handling assessment. If this is the case check condition by handling over the ribs.

It is important to set target condition scores at key points in the production cycle (Table 3.5). Most important of all is the condition score at mating, which should normally be 2.5, possibly 2 when cows are grazing nutritious spring grass. The mid-pregnancy target for the autumn-calving cow is 2 (at turnout in the spring) and for the spring-calving cow 3 when calves are weaned in the autumn. The higher mid-pregnancy target for the spring-calving cow provides adequate body reserves so that part can be used up during the winter while the cow is fed a cheap winter ration. At calving the autumn calver has a target score of 3; much higher than this and there is the risk of a difficult calving. The target calving score for the spring calver is 2, knowing that spring grazing will provide a nutritious diet.

Mid-pregnancy is the best time to check body condition when there is still time to adjust feeding and management so that cows attain the critical calving target.

The autumn calvers at mid pregnancy in the spring should have a condition score of about 2. A score higher than this indicates that winter feeding was overgenerous but much lower than 2 and the cow may not be able to achieve the calving target.

If autumn-calving cows are too thin in the spring it is worth considering early weaning the calves to remove the drain of lactation. Also, grazing management should ensure the highest possible liveweight gains in the cow. If only a proportion of the herd is below target it is a good idea to pick out the poorer cows for preferential treatment.

Spring calvers should easily attain the autumn mid-pregnancy target condition score of 3, unless management is seriously at fault. Any cows that are too thin can be given preferential feeding during the winter.

Suckled calf management

It is a fair assumption that if cow management is good then calf management will be good also. A compact calving means even calf performance and no late-born calves that are poorly grown at weaning. Good control of body condition in the cow, through feeding management, is conducive to good milk yield. However, this is not to say that calf performance takes care of itself.

Scouring can be a problem in the infant calf, especially when spring-calving cows are grazing highly digestible grass that stimulates milk production. If scouring is a persistent problem it is worth considering using one of the antiscour vaccines.

In general, the appetite of the calf is the main determinant of milk yield, though on occasions poor milk potential in the cow will be the overriding factor. If the calf gets off to a poor start, for example, following a difficult calving, there may be a reduction of milk flow that reduces peak yield at the sixth week of lactation.

The appetite of the calf for milk rises quickly during the first month and, although calves pick at solid food from early on, it is milk intake that dominates performance in the first three months. With a Blue Grey cow of moderate milk potential half the daily gain is derived from solid food in the third month. With a higher yielding Hereford × Friesian this balance occurs a month later.

In consequence of these effects milk is the main influence on the performance of the spring-born calf. The nutritional requirement of the calf and seasonal grass growth are well matched. Spring grass supports high milk yields early on but later, as the calf's appetite for solid food comes into play, grass quality and availability decline.

Management of the autumn-born calf is much more difficult because the suckling period is longer and peak milk production must be supported on winter rations. The best approach is to feed the cow well during the first three months to promote high milk yield and to ensure that body condition is right at mating. From then on lower feeding levels can be adopted but calf performance is maintained by introducing creep fed concentrates.

When the autumn-calving herd is turned out in the spring there is a boost to milk production early on but from midsummer creep feed should be reintroduced. Weaning is probably best carried out sooner rather than later so that calves and cows can be managed separately.

All too often weaning takes place on the day of the autumn calf sale but it is far better if there is a gap between weaning and sale so that the calves settle. Probably the best method of weaning is to put the cows and calves in adjacent fields so that suckling is prevented but the calves are in sight and sound of their dams.

In most parts of the world bull calves are castrated by four months of age. This eliminates problems of managing mixed sexes and produces steers for finishing, which is the conventional approach. However, in countries like France and Italy it is the custom to rear bulls entire because they grow faster and are leaner than steers. Obviously, in these countries the management problems have been overcome.

An important prerequisite for bull beef is a compact calving period, with an absolute maximum of 12 weeks, otherwise older bull calves will pester late-calving cows as they come into oestrus.

In autumn-calving herds it becomes necessary to separate cows with bull calves from those with heifers by the time the calves are six months of age, or there is a risk of premature pregnancy. Again the risk is greater if calving is spread over a long period. This problem is least in spring-calving herds where there is no need to split the herd.

Stocking rates

A discussion of stocking rate is hardly relevant in mountain and rangeland herds that graze unimproved pastures. However, in all situations where productive pastures are used stocking rate is a key measure of management efficiency.

In general the level of fertilizer N applied to grassland carrying suckler cows is below the level at which an economic response can be expected. This may be justified if grassland management is aimed at encouraging clover swards. But in many situations stocking rates could be increased by the simple expedient of applying more N fertilizer.

There are two components of high stocking rates. The first is adjusting grazing stocking rates as closely as possible to grassland potential. The secret is to employ high grazing stocking rates early in the season. An area of grassland can be set aside so that part or all

Table 3.6 Performance targets for suckler herds. Source: MLC

	Continental sire breed, e.g. Charolais		British sire breed, e.g. Hereford	
	Autumn calving	Spring calving	Autumn calving	Spring calving
Lowland herds				
Calving period (max. days)	90	85	90	85
Calves weaned/100 cows bulled	92	92	95	95
Calf daily gain (kg)	1.0	1.1	0.9	1.0
Autumn sale weight (kg)	350	280	300	240
Stocking rate (cows/ha)	1.9	2.3	2.0	2.4
Upland herds				
Calving period (max. days)	90	85	90	85
Calves weaned/100 cows bulled	92	92	95	95
Calf daily gain (kg)	1.0	1.1	0.9	1.0
Autumn sale weight (kg)	350	280	300	240
Stocking rate (cows/ha)	1.5	1.9	1.6	2.0
Hill herds				
Calving period (max. days)	100	90	100	90
Calves weaned/100 cows bulled	85	85	90	90
Calf daily gain (kg)	0.9	1.0	0.8	0.9
Autumn sale weight (kg)	310	265	260	220

of it can be grazed if necessary, but preferably it is cut for silage.

The second component of high stocking rate is making high yields of high quality silage and then integrating grazing and conservation. Silage making should use early cutting to ensure that the first-cut silage has high digestibility and a two- or three-cut regimen so that later cuts are also of high digestibility. Silage of this quality will support lactation in the autumn-calved cow with little or no concentrate supplementation. Such silage is actually too high in quality to allow spring-calving cows to consume it *ad libitum* through the winter. A sound policy is to ration silage and feed straw to appetite.

Integrating grazing and conservation provides aftermath grazing so that the grazing area can be expanded during the grazing season to take account of falling grass production but increasing requirements as the calves grow bigger.

Double suckling

In theory double suckling offers a possible increase in suckler herd productivity because it should be possible for the cow to produce sufficient milk for two calves. Inevitably, there is some decline in the growth rate of individual calves but total weaning weight is increased.

Table 3.7 MLC Beefplan suckler herd results, 1989. Source: MLC

	Average	Top third of gross margins/ha
Lowland herds		
Financial		
Output/cow (£)	334	390
Variable costs/cow (£)	120	121
Gross margin/cow (£)	214	269
Gross margin/ha (£)	409	611
Physical		
Calving period (weeks)	12	12
Calves reared per 100 cows	91	92
Calf daily gain (kg)	0.98	1.05
Autumn sale weight (kg)	280	296
Stocking rate (cows/ha)	1.91	2.27
Upland herds		
Financial		
Output/cow (£)	411	443
Variable costs/cow (£)	118	124
Gross margin/cow (£)	293	319
Gross margin/ha (£)	469	641
Physical		
Calving period (weeks)	12	11
Calves reared per 100 cows	92	93
Calf daily gain (kg)	0.93	0.98
Autumn sale weight (kg)	307	321
Stocking rate (cows/ha)	1.60	2.01

In practice, few suckler herd owners persist with double suckling. All too often two moderate calves are produced in place of one good one. Then there is the danger of the purchased calf bringing in *Escherichia coli* and rotavirus scour, which can spread through the herd. Moreover, the purchased calf is often so expensive that the added value is insufficient to justify the effort involved. And finally, there is always a proportion of nervous or bad-tempered cows that refuse to mother the set-on calf. Not surprisingly double suckling is rarely seen in commercial practice.

Suckler herd targets

The objectives of suckler herd management outlined in this chapter have been compiled into a set of suckler herd targets appropriate to European conditions on lowland, upland and hill farms (Table 3.6).

MLC Beefplan results from lowland and upland suckler herds in 1986 show that herds with the top third of gross margins per hectare owed their success to better all-round cow and calf performance achieved at above average stocking rates (Table 3.7).

Chapter 4: Dairy Farming

by A. POOLE AND A.H. ANDREWS

Structure in Europe

Dairy farming in Europe is a very diverse industry ranging from large herds of high-yielding cows in the Netherlands, Denmark and the UK to the small low-yielding herds of Greece, Portugal, Spain and Italy.

Table 4.1 shows the structure of European dairying. Because of the difficulty of obtaining data from some countries the table is based on the information from the most recent year available, in most cases 1990.

Over the past 23 years, to reach this position, each country has expanded herd size and yield per cow to increase total production. Total cow population has not increased to the same extent as the number of dairy producers has been generally declining. Reasons for this have been tied up with national government policy and EC requirements. The common agricultural policy (CAP) set out to increase food production, maintain farm incomes and prevent rural depopulation. This policy encouraged the very small farms of much of Europe to stay in business and expand, while for the larger producers, financial help made dairy farming relatively profitable compared with other sectors of agriculture. Total milk production for the then 10 members of the EC rose from 87.5 million tonnes in 1965 to a peak of 120.7 million tonnes in 1983.

Whilst the CAP was proving very satisfactory for dairy farmers, the financial support they were receiving was increasingly threatening the whole EC budget. Most of this aid was provided through intervention buying of surplus products. In fact sale into intervention became an accepted market rather than the market of last resort.

Self-sufficiency ratios within the EC in 1983 rose to 125 per cent for butterfat (BF) and 116 per cent for solids-not-fat (SNF) (Table 4.1), while the cost of dairy support made up one-quarter of the whole EC agriculture budget. At this stage milk quotas were imposed to control milk production and each member country had to take a cut of varying proportions (Table 4.2).

If national production exceeded the quota allocated then a super-levy was imposed. This super-levy was to

Table 4.1 EEC dairy structure 1983 (pre milk structures). Source: *EEC Dairy Facts and Figures*, 1986 (MMB, Thames Ditton)

	Cows ('000)	Herds ('000)	Average herd size	Yield (l/cow)	Total production ('000 t)	Self-sufficiency	
						BF (%)	SNF (%)
Germany	5451	363	15.3	4650	26007	116	136
France	6506	367	19.8	3950	33337	122	128
Italy	3120	424	7.3	3540	11030	66	63
Netherlands	2333	58	40.8	5330	12550	256	116
Belgium	946	45	21.7	3930	4145	104	116
Luxembourg	70	2	29.7	4274	320		
UK	3257	54	58.2	4906	17680	86	104
Irish Republic	1528	77	19.9	3910	6480	298	175
Denmark	913	35	28.2	5585	5205	212	142
Greece	219	77	3.1	3200	770	–	–
Portugal	369	115	3.2	3021	1115	–	–
Spain	1885	–	–	3382	6375	–	–

Table 4.2 Production and quota ('000 tonnes) for EEC member countries. Source: *EEC Dairy Facts and Figures*, 1990 (MMB)

	Production	Quota	
		1983–84	1991–92
Germany	26429	23792	22927
France	33230	26768	24613
Italy	11310	9914	9221
Netherlands	12782	12197	11213
Belgium	4149	3643	3364
Luxembourg	319	294	272
UK	17878	15950	14789
Irish Republic	6380	5599	5301
Denmark	5361	4933	4525
Greece	765	588	581

be calculated either on a dairy basis or on an on-farm basis. On a dairy basis, if national production and the supplying dairy were both over quota, then levy was imposed on the dairy and hence back to the individual over-quota producers at a rate of 100 per cent of the target price for milk. Alternatively, quota would be applied on an on-farm basis, where provided national production exceeded quota then each farm paid super-levy on excess production above its individual quota at the rate of 75 per cent of the target price for milk. In 1987–88 further changes to the means of determining super-levy liability have been made so that those producers most over quota pay the highest proportion of levy, again provided national quota is exceeded.

Quota has been transferable between individual farmers within a member state either on a sale (attached to land) or lease basis or else on an administratively based system where unused quota reverts to an authority and is re-allocated.

Further regulations in 1987 have imposed a butterfat ceiling on quotas giving a reduction in national quota if the average butterfat percentage for 1985–86 is exceeded. Also in 1987 further quota cuts were announced for both 1987–88 and 1988–89 resulting in a reduction of about 8 per cent. The calculations of any liability for excess production for a farmer is extremely complex. It initially depends on the amount of milk over-quota and from 1987–1988 on the average butterfat content of the milk. Each producer has a butterfat reference figure. If a levy is to be charged then the farmer's production volume will be adjusted up or down by the amount that the butterfat average differs from his/her reference figure. Levys only arise when national production is too high.

Table 4.3 England and Wales dairy structure 1965–1990. Source: *UK Dairy Facts and Figures*, 1986 (FMMB)

	Producers ('000)	Cows (millions)	Herd size	Yield (l/cow)
1965	100.5	2.65	26	3545
1970	80.3	2.71	33	3755
1975	60.3	2.70	46	4070
1980	43.4	2.67	58	4715
1983	39.7	2.74	67	5085
1984	39.3	2.70	67	4950
1986	37.1	2.57	68	4930
1988	33.7	2.38	69	4870
1990	31.5	2.33	70	5020

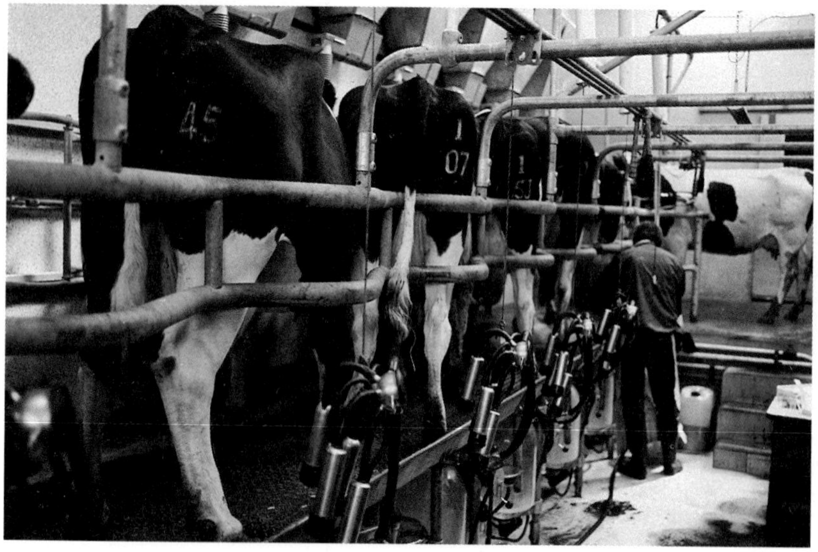

Fig. 4.1 Milking in the herringbone parlour.

For the future it is expected that the quota system will be retained at least until supply and demand are in balance, which, with consumption of dairy products falling, may necessitate further quota restrictions.

Trends of structure in England and Wales

Changes to the structure of dairy farming in England and Wales over the past 25 years have mirrored the European situation with less producers, similar numbers of cows in larger herds, and with a higher yield per cow (Table 4.3).

This has been achieved by the virtual elimination of small herds. In 1990 just over 5 per cent of cows were in herds of less than 30 cows, whereas in 1972 the figure was 20 per cent.

New technology and mechanization have largely contributed to this with 67 per cent of farms milking through a cowshed in 1972 compared with only 28 per cent in 1990. Herringbone parlours, which accounted for only 11 per cent of milking installations in 1972, made up over 45 per cent in 1990 (Fig. 4.1).

The rise in yield has been realized by improved feeding, breeding and management techniques. The breed of cow, 64 per cent Friesian in 1965 moving to over 91 per cent Friesian/Holstein in 1990, will also have made a major contribution.

For the future, providing quota remains transferable, it is likely that these trends will continue. By 1995, Milk Marketing Board (MMB) forecasts indicate that in England and Wales there will be 29 000 producers with 2.1 million cows and an average herd size of almost 73 cows. Yield per cow is also likely to keep rising to almost 5500 l/cows. These figures are all assuming no further quota reductions. If there were to be further cuts then these would have a major influence on these figures. However, the Milk Marketing Board itself is now likely to be markedly changed.

Milk utilization

As milk production has increased over the past 25 years while consumption of liquid milk has slightly reduced, the production of all milk used as liquid milk has declined from 73 to 45 per cent. With quotas now

Table 4.4 Utilization of milk in England and Wales (%). Source: *UK Dairy Facts and Figures*, 1986 (MMB, Thames Ditton)

	Liquid milk	Butter	Cheese	Condensed milk	Cream	Others
1964–65	73	3	11	5	5	3
1969–70	66	10	10	4	7	3
1974–75	62	8	16	4	8	2
1979–80	50	23	15	3	7	2
1982–83	45	31	14	2	6	2
1983–84	45	30	14	2	6	3
1984–85	48	27	15	2	5	3
1987–88	49	23	19	2	3	4
1989–90	51	20	18	2	4	4

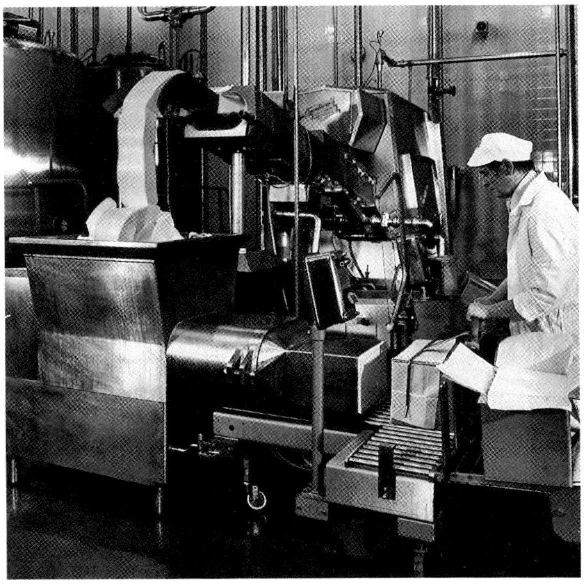

Fig. 4.2 A modern butter-making creamery produces and packs 5 tonnes of butter an hour.

limiting output that percentage is now starting to increase again (Table 4.4).

From being in the position of mainly supplying the liquid market, with Commonwealth countries making up the requirement for butter and cheese, the British dairy industry now manufactures about half the milk. Cheese production has increased as imports have been reduced but the large increase in butter manufacture, from 3 to 30 per cent, has been largely sold into intervention until recently (Fig. 4.2).

With liquid milk realizing the highest return to the producer, the producers of England and Wales are in a more favourable position than the rest of the EC as Table 4.5 shows.

The large quantity of other uses is mainly milk powder and milk fed to livestock, which is prevalent in many countries.

The surplus situation is further exacerbated by the fact that most liquid milk on the Continent is skimmed or semi-skimmed, which releases butterfat for manufacture. This trend is also taking place in the UK with about 20 per cent of liquid milk now being consumed as skimmed or semi-skimmed milk.

Dairy breeds

The principal dairy breeds of England and Wales are shown in Table 4.6.

Every breed will have its enthusiasts but the vast majority of herds are now of the Friesian or Holstein type. These black and white cows are renowned for their high yields of average quality milk and also the good beefing qualities of their offspring.

The Channel Island breeds, Guernseys and Jerseys, are still popular with a minority of breeders. They are docile cows producing lower yields of very high quality 'gold top' milk. This sells at a premium to the liquid milk or cream markets. The beefing qualities of the pure bred calf are low but can make quite an acceptable calf when crossed with one of the continental beef breeds such as Charolais, Limousin, Simmental or Belgian Blue.

The Ayrshire is still regionally very popular in its native Scotland. A smaller cow than the Friesian it produces lower milk yields but of a higher quality. It is a breed renowned for its dairy type but not so suitable for beef.

The Dairy Shorthorn has suffered a demise, from being the major breed prewar it has now slipped almost to insignificance. With good beefing qualities it tended

Table 4.5 Utilization of whole milk, 1984–1989 (%). Source: *EEC dairy facts and figures*, 1986–1990 (MMB)

	Liquid milk		Butter		Cheese		Condensed milk		Cream		Others	
	'84	'89	'84	'89	'84	'89	'84	'89	'84	'89	'84	'89
Germany	13	14	46	34	13	17	4	3	9	13	15	19
France	9	17	38	36	22	28	1	1	4	5	26	13
Italy	29	28	14	14	44	43	–	–	4	5	9	10
Netherlands	6	6	42	36	27	32	8	6	3	4	14	16
Belgium	15	16	55	51	5	7	–	1	5	8	20	17
Luxembourg	11	13	56	53	3	4	–	–	9	13	21	17
UK	41	48	26	20	14	19	2	3	4	3	13	7
Irish Republic	10	11	62	58	9	13	2	2	3	4	14	12
Denmark	8	6	38	37	30	32	–	–	5	8	19	17
Greece	29	30	3	2	47	53	–	–	2	3	19	12

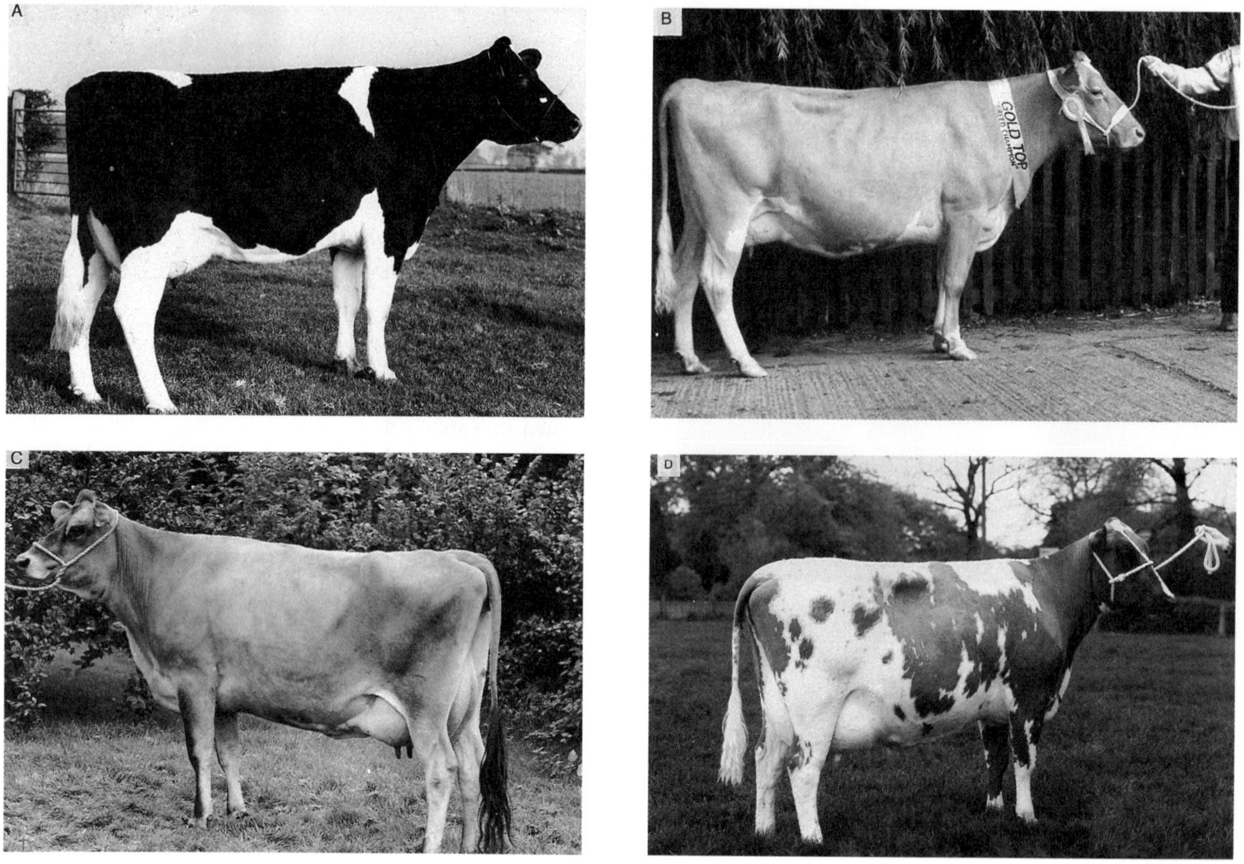

Fig. 4.3 (a) A Friesian cow, (b) a Guernsey cow, (c) a Jersey cow, (d) an Ayrshire cow.

Table 4.6 Dairy herd breed distribution 1985–86. Source, UK: *Dairy facts and figures*, 1986 (FMMB)

	Percentage of national herd	Yield (kg/cow)	Butterfat (%)	Protein (%)
Ayrshire	2.2	5026	3.96	3.34
Friesian	85.8	5556	3.87	3.23
Holstein	3.9	6214	3.84	3.17
Guernsey	1.8	4005	4.67	3.55
Jersey	1.6	3835	5.27	3.80
Dairy Shorthorn	0.5	4996	3.69	3.27
Others and crosses	4.2	5469	3.87	3.23

to fall between two stools, with neither the milk quantity of the Friesian nor the quality of the Channel Island breeds.

The beefing characteristics of the dairy breeds are of importance in England and Wales as 63 per cent of the beef produced originates from the dairy herd as cull cows and pure and crossbred calves (Fig. 4.4).

The Friesian breed has played an important part in this and most farmers breed sufficient of their cows pure to provide heifer replacements for the dairy herd, the remainder being bred to a beef bull to maximize calf returns. Figure 4.5 shows that in most years 60–70 per cent of inseminations have been to a dairy breed with the remainder to beef breeds.

The most numerous breeds of bull used for artificial insemination (AI) are shown in Table 4.7. The dairy inseminations follow the pattern of breed distribution, while with beef the continental breeds are gradually replacing the traditional British beef breed, the Hereford. The Aberdeen Angus continues to enjoy some support mainly because of the ease of calving, particularly when used on maiden heifers or small cows.

Feeding dairy cows (see also Chapter 7)

A vital feature of dairy cow management is correct feeding. Food, either purchased or home produced, accounts for 60 per cent of the variable costs of production so the efficiency of feed use is extremely im-

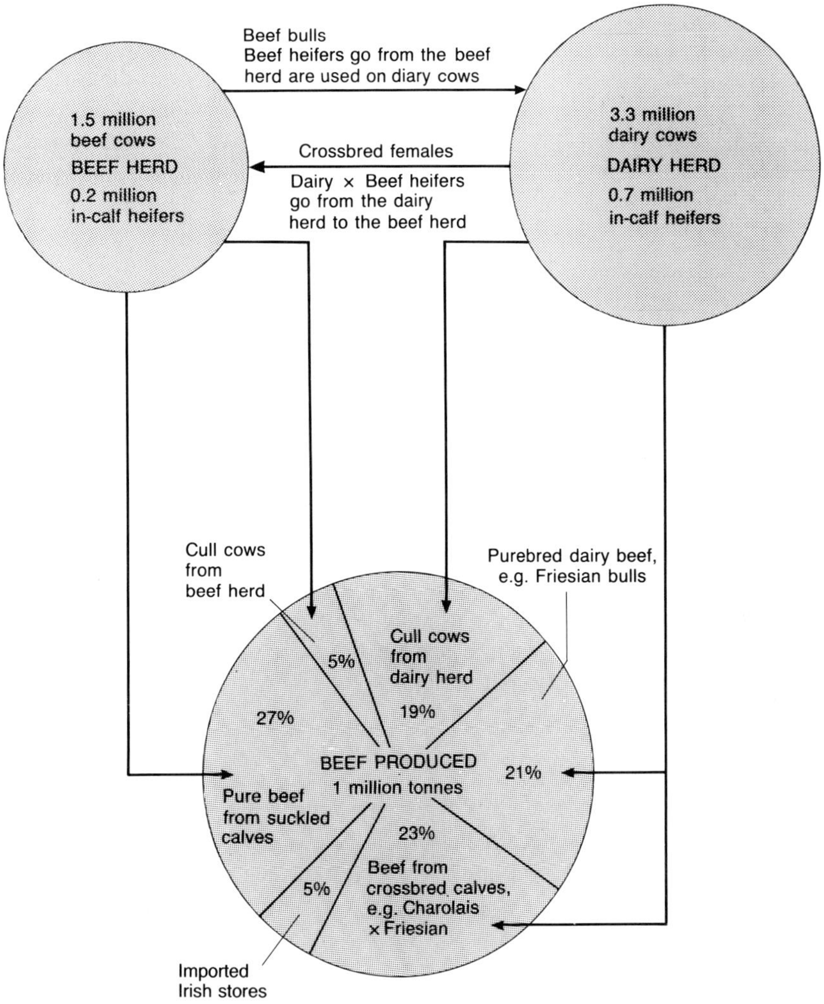

Fig. 4.4 Sources of beef in the UK. Source: MLC (1982).

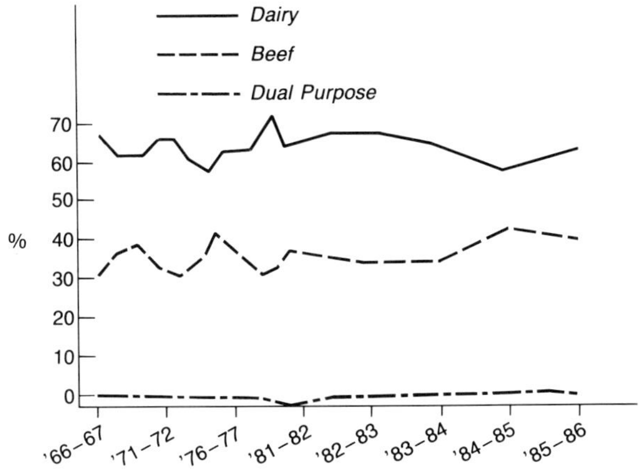

Fig. 4.5 Dairy, dual purpose and beef inseminations as percentages of total inseminations. Source: *Report of Breeding and Production Organization*, MMB (1986).

Table 4.7 AI breed demand in MMB areas, 1986 (%). Source: *Report of the Breeding and Production Organisation*, MMB (1986)

Ayrshire	0.7
Friesian/Holstein	57.8
Guernsey	0.8
Jersey	1.2
Shorthorn	0.2
Total dairy breeds	*60.7*
Aberdeen Angus	2.8
Belgian Blue	1.1
Charolais	7.4
Hereford	12.0
Limousin	12.7
Simmental	1.7
Others	1.6
Total beef breeds	*39.3*

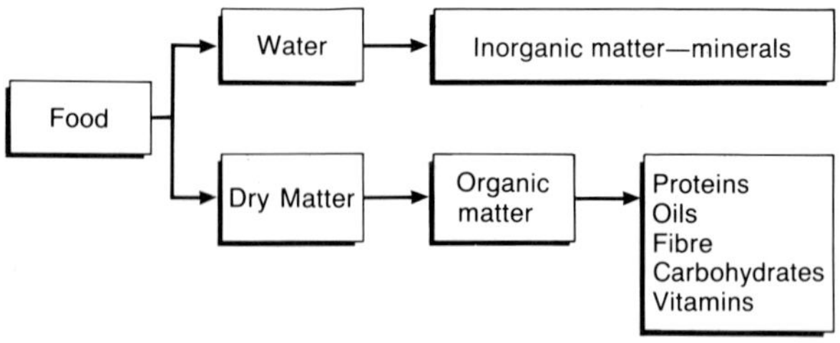

Fig. 4.6 Food components.

portant. The main components of food are shown in Fig. 4.6.

All foods contain water in varying amounts. Dry feeds such as cereals will only have about 14 per cent water while other feeds such as mangels and other root crops will be up to 90 per cent water.

Whilst all cows require water it is the dry matter portion of the total feed that supplies the nutrients for maintenance and production. Apart from the need for minerals and vitamins the main aspects to consider in dairy cow feeding are dry matter intake and energy and protein levels.

Dry matter intake

Dry matter intake (DMI) is affected by the liveweight of the cow, stage of lactation, milk yield, type of feed and frequency of feeding. As a guide for estimating DMI the following equation is used:

$$\text{DMI (kg/day)} = 0.025 \times \text{liveweight (kg)} + 0.1 \times \text{milk yield (kg/day)}.$$

At calving DMI will be 2–3 kg/day lower than calculated but it will then increase to peak at three to five months after calving. After peak, intake declines slowly through lactation and is lower during the dry period.

Dry matter intake can be increased by feeding highly digestible food. Thus cows will eat greater quantities of a 70 per cent digestibility (D) silage than one of 64D. Also, succulent feeds such as brewers grains, kale and roots will considerably enhance intakes in an otherwise dry diet of hay or silage and concentrates. When feeding large quantities of concentrates, splitting the feed into three or four feeds rather than the conventional two in the parlour will also increase intake and reduce rumen acidity.

Energy

An essential component of any feed is the energy level, which is supplied mainly by the oils, carbohydrates and digestible fibre. Energy levels in feeds are measured by metabolizable energy, which is the gross energy less the energy value of the faeces, urine and methane. It is expressed as megajoules (MJ) per kilogram dry matter (DM).

The dairy cow requires energy for maintenance, liveweight gain, fetus growth and production. If energy is in deficit then body fat can be mobilized, causing liveweight loss to make up some or all of the deficit. This will contribute 28 MJ/kg liveweight loss. Estimated requirements are shown in Table 4.8. For example, a 600 kg Friesian cow, producing 20 kg/day of milk, in calf and gaining 0.5 kg/day liveweight would require:

Maintenance	63 MJ
Production (20 × 5.2)	104 MJ
Liveweight gain (0.5 × 34)	17 MJ
Pregnancy	23 MJ
Total energy	*207 MJ/day*

Protein

Protein is required by the dairy cow for both maintenance and production. Unlike energy body tissue cannot be used to make up a shortfall in protein and milk yields will suffer, especially in early lactation, if protein is in deficit. Protein is measured as grams of digestible crude protein (DCP) per kilogram DM.

Table 4.8 Energy requirements of dairy cows

Breed	Liveweight (kg)	Maintenance (MJ/day)	Production (MJ/kg milk)	Liveweight gain (MJ/kg gain)	Pregnancy (MJ/day)
Ayrshire	500	54	5.3	34	23
Friesian	600	63	5.2	34	23
Guernsey	450	49	5.8	34	23
Jersey	350	40	5.9	34	23
Shorthorn	550	59	5.1	34	23

Table 4.9 Digestible crude protein requirements of dairy cows

Breed	Liveweight (kg)	Maintenance (g/day)	Production (g/kg milk)	Pregnancy (g/day)
Ayrshire	500	300	60	150
Friesian	600	350	55	150
Guernsey	450	275	70	150
Jersey	350	225	70	150
Shorthorn	550	325	55	150

Requirements for maintenance and production are shown in Table 4.9.

A refinement of the DCP system divides protein into rumen degradable protein (RDP) and rumen undegradable protein (UDP). A dairy cow has a need for both RDP and UDP and different feeds have a different rating, e.g. silage is about 80 per cent degradable whereas soya is only 60 per cent degradable. Hence, although the protein supplied may be sufficient in terms of DCP it may be deficient in either RDP or UDP. In early lactation on a silage diet, that shortfall will more probably be in UDP, which partially explains the good response to fishmeal (highly undegradable) in fresh calved cows.

Many textbooks have been written on strategies for feeding dairy cows. Broadly speaking the need is to (i) maximize dry matter intake, and (ii) provide the cow's requirement as cheaply as feasible. These two requirements are associated as the higher the DMI then the lower can be the energy concentration in the diet and hence the cheaper it can be produced.

As has been discussed a cow's feed requirement will vary throughout the lactation. In early lactation it will be very difficult to satisfy that requirement within appetite. This will result in a loss of body weight,

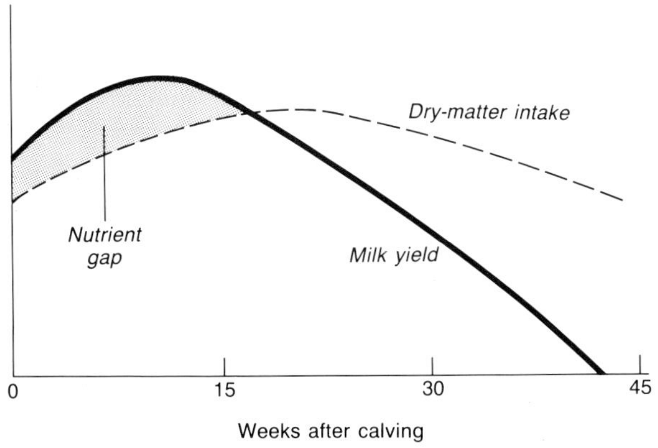

Fig. 4.7 Nutrient gap.

perhaps 0.5 kg or more per day, for the first 90–120 days of lactation. As yield declines and appetite increases then balance should be reached and liveweight loss can be replaced in mid to late lactation (Fig. 4.7). As will be discussed later, a compromise has to be achieved between biological efficiency and economic efficiency.

Very approximately, the most common feeds for dairy cows (grazing grass, silage and concentrates) have a relative cost of 1 : 2 : 3. Therefore, greater profit will be shown as the proportion of grass and silage in the total diet increases provided performance does not suffer (Fig. 4.8).

Although flat rate feeding of concentrates is gaining in popularity, the most common method is 'feeding to yield', whereby concentrates are allocated on an individual basis depending on the yield attained. Then the cow has *ad libitum* access to forage feeds to satisfy appetite. As has been stated, appetite is controlled by DMI so as concentrate consumption increases, forage intake diminishes. Thus concentrates are fed heavily in early lactation and reduced as lactation progresses. This has the effect of limiting forage intake in early lactation as concentrates are normally eaten in preference to forages. Table 4.10 shows the effect of this on the cow's diet.

For correct digestion the dry matter ratio between concentrates and forage should be in the range 70 : 30

Table 4.10 Examples of possible cow diets

Stage of lactation	Early	Mid	Late
Concentrates (kg DM/day)	8	6	2
Silage (kg DM/day)	8	12	12
Total DMI (kg/day)	16	18	14
Energy supplied (MJ/day)	180	195	145
Energy required (MJ/day)	195	186	133

Table 4.11 Mineral requirement of dairy cows

	Ca	P	Mg	Na
Maintenance (g/day)				
Liveweight (kg)				
400	14	19	6	7
500	18	26	8	9
600	21	32	9	10
Production (g/10 kg milk)				
Fat content of milk (%)				
4.0	28	17	6	6
5.0	30	17	6	6

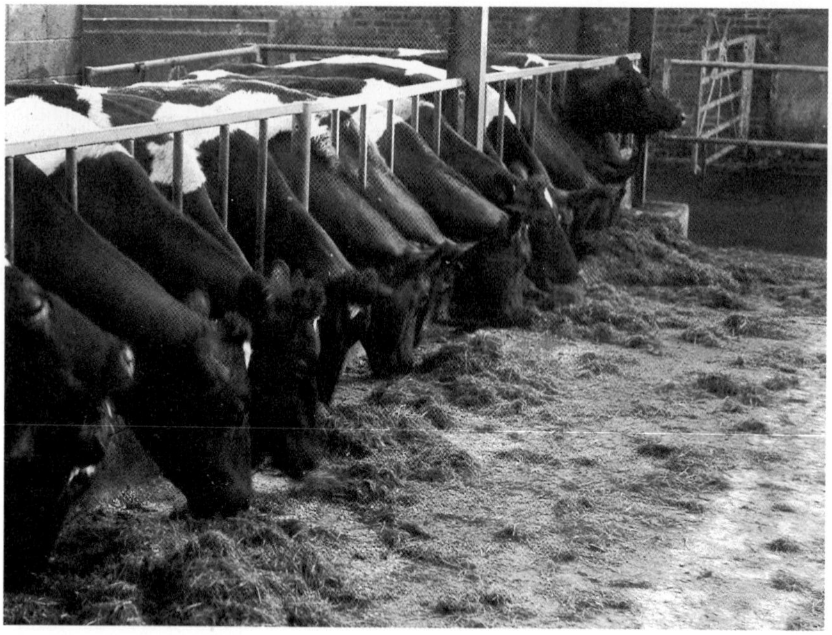

Fig. 4.8 Feeding silage at a barrier.

to 30:70 in early to mid lactation. Any lower and performance will suffer, any higher and digestion will suffer (see pp. 633, 634).

Minerals and vitamins

The requirement for these must be adequately met if the dairy cow is to remain healthy and produce effectively. The major essential elements are calcium, phosphorus, magnesium, sodium, potassium, chlorine and sulphur. Table 4.11 shows the daily requirement for four of these. Apart from the major elements, trace elements include iron, iodine, copper, manganese and zinc.

The main vitamins required are A and D. Dairy concentrates normally contain adequate quantities of minerals and vitamins to balance any deficiencies in the ration. However, farmers mixing their own rations or using extreme feeding techniques such as very low concentrate use, kale or straw feeding, or using high proportions of 'straight' feeds should take advice on mineral and vitamin requirements. It is not sufficient just to offer access to free choice minerals as intake cannot be guaranteed and is very variable.

Grassland farming

Grass and its derivatives, hay and silage, form an important part of dairy farming. The two major aspects to consider are grassland production and grassland utilization.

Grassland production

To get optimum production from grassland the basics must be correct. These include climate and soil type about which little can be done. Grass grows best on a medium loam soil with adequate summer rainfall. These conditions are most often found in the west of England and Wales. Where soil is heavy and waterlogged, then drainage can give good results. Conversely, in dry areas, irrigation has a part to play, although the economics of grassland irrigation in Britain are questionable on all except the driest farms. Soil acidity should be corrected to a pH of 5.5–6.5.

Having achieved as near optimum as possible with the basics the next area to consider is grass varieties. For grazing, most seed mixtures are based on varieties of perennial ryegrass (Fig. 4.9). There are many recommended varieties in the National Institute of Agricultural Botany (NIAB) lists. Timothy is often sown, which adds some palatability and midsummer growth. Older grass varieties such as meadow fescue and cocksfoot are not often sown now. Most mixtures will also include some white clover. This provides nutrients by fixing atmospheric nitrogen and also increases intake by improving the palatability of the sward. But clover is difficult to establish and maintain in grassland receiving high levels of fertilizer nitrogen.

Once established, and with good management, a grazing sward should remain highly productive for 10 years or more. The main enemy to this is grazing in too wet conditions, when treading and poaching will

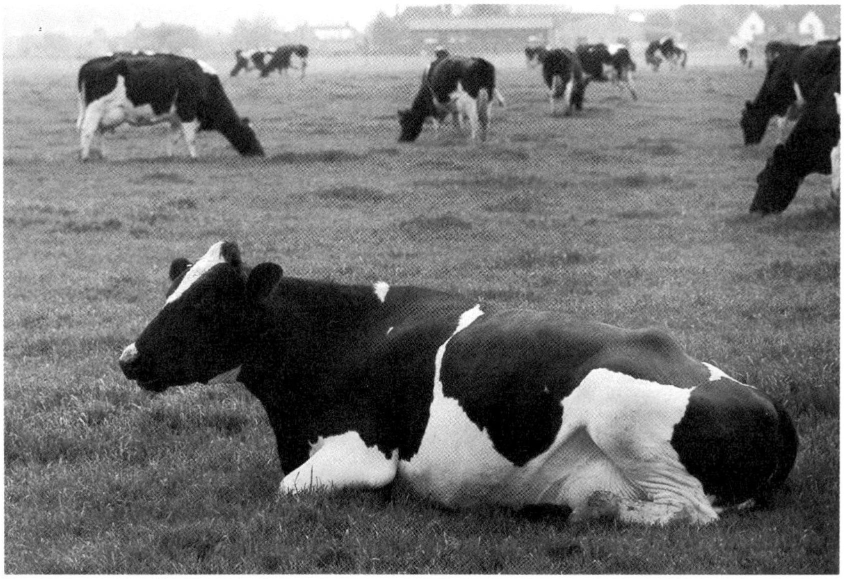

Fig. 4.9 Cow set stocking, grazing a ryegrass sward.

quickly destroy a sward and allow weed grasses to establish. Swards mainly for cutting are usually based on a shorter term perennial ryegrass or Italian ryegrass. These have a more erect growth habit and are easier to cut but are not so persistent. They are often grown as a grass break in an arable rotation for two to three years. Often the species are sown pure. If clover is required then red clover is more suited to a cutting regimen than white clover. In between these extremes are many dual purpose mixtures that are both grazed and cut during a season.

The best time to sow grass is in August–September. This gives it a chance to establish before winter and to be in full production the following spring. A spring reseed in April–May will lose much of the first year's production and can be vulnerable to summer drought.

Having established the grass the fertilizer requirement must be satisfied. Normal recommendations for grazing would be an annual application of 300 kg/ha nitrogen, 40 kg/ha phosphate and 40 kg/ha potash. Under a cutting regimen the nitrogen and potash would be increased to 350 and 150 kg respectively. Whilst phosphate and potash are essential for grass growth the main response is shown to nitrogen. Much trial work has been undertaken showing a good response up to 400 kg/ha, but the average nitrogen use is still under 200 kg/ha (Fig. 4.10). Researchers have defined a target nitrogen use as being the point in the response curve where 10 kg of grass dry matter are produced for each 1 kg of fertilizer nitrogen.

Figure 4.11 shows the target point for five site classes, class 1 being the most suited to grass growth and class 5 the least suitable.

Grassland utilization

Grass growth is uneven through the year with a peak in the spring and then falling away through the growing season (Fig. 4.12). Grass growth will also vary greatly between seasons depending mainly on the summer rainfall. Nor are the animal requirements even over the season. For all these reasons any system for grassland utilization must be flexible and adaptable to cover any situation.

The overall aim is to provide the cow with her maintenance requirement and as much of her production as possible for each day of the year. This will be achieved with an integrated grazing and cutting system whereby in early season about one-third of the grass area is grazed and two-thirds is cut. This is reversed in mid season and then the whole farm is grazed in the autumn.

The most common systems of grazing management are either continuous grazing or rotational grazing with paddocks or strip grazing. There is little to choose between systems in terms of output so choice is down to personal preference and ease of management.

Under any system, cows should be stocked at a heavy density (6–8/ha) in the spring, which will allow a maximum area to be cut without affecting milk production. Maintenance plus 20–25 l/day of milk can easily be obtained from spring grass. For an autumn-calving cow, as grass declines so milk yield declines and there should be no need to introduce supplementary feeding. Spring-calving cows may need supplementary feeding to sustain yields in the summer. This

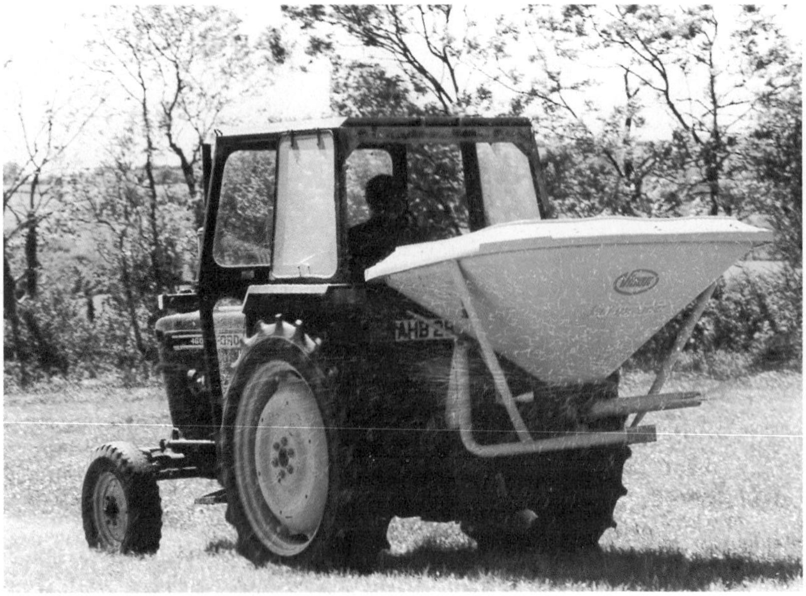

Fig. 4.10 A good response is shown from nitrogen fertilizer.

may be concentrates or forage crops such as rape or stubble turnips.

Efficient conservation is a vital part of grassland management. It both provides a feed for winter use by the cows and also aids grassland management by utilizing grass surplus to the grazing requirement. The main options for conservation are either hay or silage. There is a continuing move away from hay towards silage on dairy farms because:

1 it is more flexible and integrates better with grazing;
2 silage is a better feed for feeding cows;
3 silage can be made in poorer (not poor) weather conditions; and
4 silage can respond to higher levels of fertilizer nitrogen use.

However, silage making does require a higher capital investment in both machinery and storage areas (Fig. 4.13). Much of these criticisms have now been overcome by the use of contractors and with the advent of big bale silage. These have given even the smallest

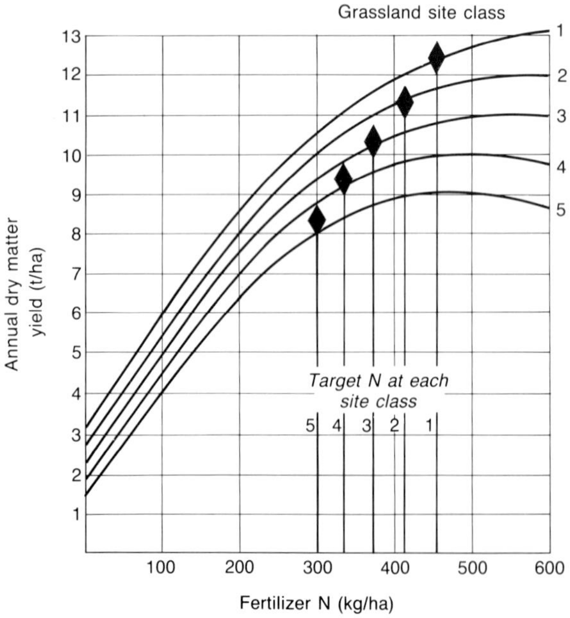

Fig. 4.11 Target nitrogen on five site classes. Source. *Milk from Grass* (GRI and ICI).

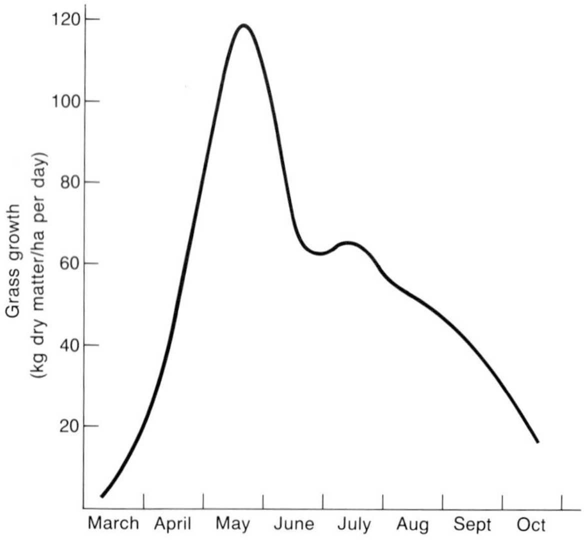

Fig. 4.12 Seasonal pattern of grass growth. Source: *Milk from Grass* (GRI and ICI).

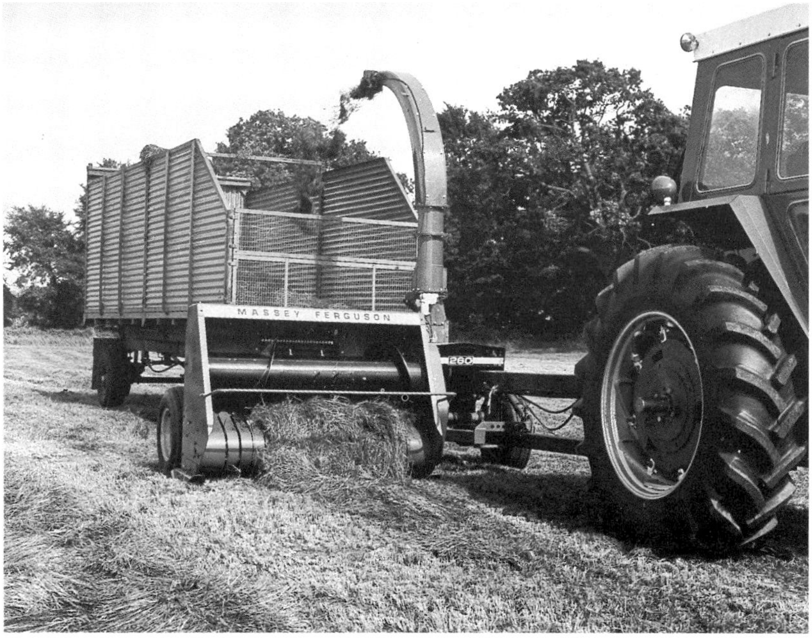

Fig. 4.13 Silage making with a precision chop forage harvester.

dairy farm the opportunity to improve grassland utilization and profitability by changing to silage making.

Whilst grass is the most important forage crop, reference must be made to other forage crops that may have a place on dairy farms by producing heavier yields than grass or producing feed at a season when grass is not available. The most popular forage crops are maize, fodder beet, kale, lucerne, and stubble turnips and rape.

MAIZE

This is increasing in popularity in southern England and is normally made into silage but can be fed green. To be successful it requires high summer temperatures so even in southern England a sheltered field should be used. It produces a similar or heavier yield per hectare than grass and has the advantage of being harvested in one cut. The resultant silage is a very palatable, high energy, low protein feed that improves a winter ration. It is often mixed with grass silage in the proportion 1 : 3 or 4 maize : grass but can successfully be fed on its own.

FODDER BEET

This has about the highest yield of dry matter of any fodder crop. It can be grown successfully anywhere but prefers a heavier soil. It is an arable crop and the farmer needs arable techniques to grow it successfully, especially for establishment, weed control and harvesting. It is harvested in October/November and stored for winter use. It provides a palatable high energy feed, which helps butterfat percentages.

KALE

This is a high protein green feed grown mainly for grazing in the autumn and early winter. It produces a high yield of succulent feed that stimulates milk production. It can be cut and fed to dairy cows in the yards but is more commonly grazed, which means that it should be grown in dry fields with good access. Mud, dirty cows and bad feet can be a problem.

LUCERNE

This is a drought-resistant legume that grows well on light chalky soils. Being a legume it fixes atmospheric nitrogen and hence is cheap to grow. Cut four or five times during the season it provides good yields of high protein silage, but it can be difficult to get a good fermentation in the silage.

STUBBLE TURNIPS AND RAPE

Although these are not the same they are used for the same purpose — to provide a succulent green feed either in the summer or autumn. For summer use they

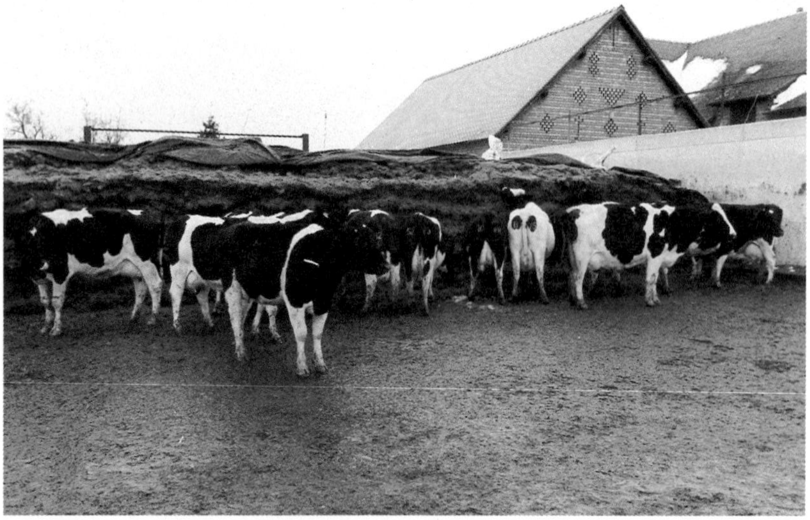

Fig. 4.14 Self-feeding silage.

need sowing in the spring but autumn grazing can be achieved by drilling after harvesting an early cereal crop. They both provide grazing when feed might otherwise be short.

Winter feeding systems

A winter feeding system will be partially dictated by the objectives, high or low milk yields, and by the facilities available.

In all cases the first requirement is to know the quantity of bulk feeds available. Over a 200-day winter a Friesian cow may well consume about 3.5 t of dry matter. If there are 2.2 t of silage dry matter per cow then this will leave 1.3 t to be made up with concentrates or other purchased feed. Provided there are about 1.8 t of forage dry matter for a 200-day winter then a reasonable feeding system can be devised. This equates to about 7 t/cow of fresh weight silage. Anything much less than this will create problems, not so much from the cow's point of view but from the economic side as it will tend to be an unprofitable winter. Anything more than this will be a bonus and an asset to the farm especially if of a high D value.

All feed changes should be done gradually to prevent digestive upsets. Thus silage should be gradually introduced on a limited access basis from calving or by mid-September, whichever is the earlier. The herd should be housed at night by some time in October depending on conditions and then housed continually from mid-October onwards, again depending on weather conditions. Over this period silage consumption will increase and other feeds can be gradually introduced. The same principle applies in the spring, when ideally the herd should be kept inside at night on silage for seven to ten days after turning out with grazing time gradually increased.

Silage will either be self-fed (Fig. 4.14) or fed mechanically behind a barrier or in a trough. Self-feeding works well, provided that the silage quality is even throughout the clamp, that the face is not more than 2 m high and that there is enough space at the face, 24 hour access for at least 250 cm/cow.

To avoid secondary fermentation the silage face needs to move back by at least 150 cm/day. Self-feeding is labour saving and requires no machinery. It is better but not essential to have a roof over the silo and intakes will improve if a light is left on at night. Keep cows back from the silage face with a barrier, either a solid rail or an electric wire. The latter, however, can reduce intake in heifers. To prevent waste the face must be kept tidy and waste silage removed.

Mechanical feeding of silage will either involve putting the silage in a trough or behind a barrier with a tractor and fore-loader/blockcutter or else loading the silage into a forage wagon that will spread it behind the barrier. Many people claim that this will increase intake compared with self-feeding. Two simple barrier designs are shown in Fig. 4.15.

For 24-hour access the herd will need feed space of 250 cm/cow. Again cleanliness is important and waste silage should be removed on a regular basis. It is important to ensure that silage is always available *ad libitum*. Leaving the trough empty for two to three

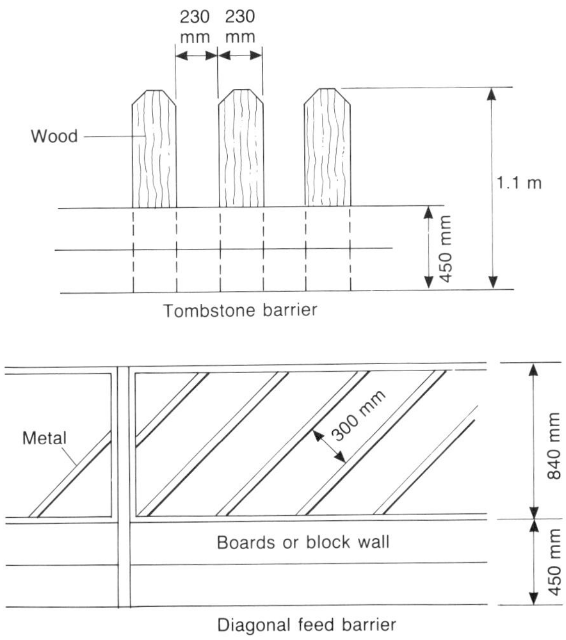

Fig. 4.15 Two types of feed barrier.

hours before feeding will suppress intake. It is a tremendous advantage to a winter feeding system to have a trough or barrier available as almost any feed can be fed behind it, from silage to hay, roots, brewers grains, sugar beet pulp or concentrates. This gives a great flexibility. Where feeds such as dried beet pulp or concentrates are fed it is essential to have at least 600 cm/cow of trough space to ensure a reasonably even intake between cows.

A sophistication of this system is complete diet feeding. Here all the feeds are placed in a mixer wagon, which mixes them together and delivers the diet behind a barrier. Because of the degree of mixing the cow is unable to separate say barley from silage and so eats the whole mixture uniformly. Usually the wagon has weigh cells so giving very accurate measurement of feeds. Use of a feed wagon allows the feeding of a wide range of feeds that may represent a very economical buy but which are normally either difficult to feed or unpalatable, e.g. molasses and rapeseed meal.

Most milking parlours have facilities to feed concentrates and it is usual to feed these twice per day at milking time. A limit to be fed during each milking would be 4–5 kg. If anything above this is needed then an out-of-parlour feed at the barrier is beneficial. This not only splits the feeds, which helps digestion, but also allows a proportion of the concentrate to be replaced with alternative feeds such as cereals, maize gluten or sugar beet pulp.

A sophistication of this system is with computerized out-of-parlour feeders (Fig. 4.16). Each cow has a transponder identifying her to a feeder station. This is then programmed to allow a specified amount of feed per day in a number of feeds. The cow can then eat up to her allowance but no more. Although the capital cost of these installations is high they make for very accurate feeding, based on the sound principle of 'little

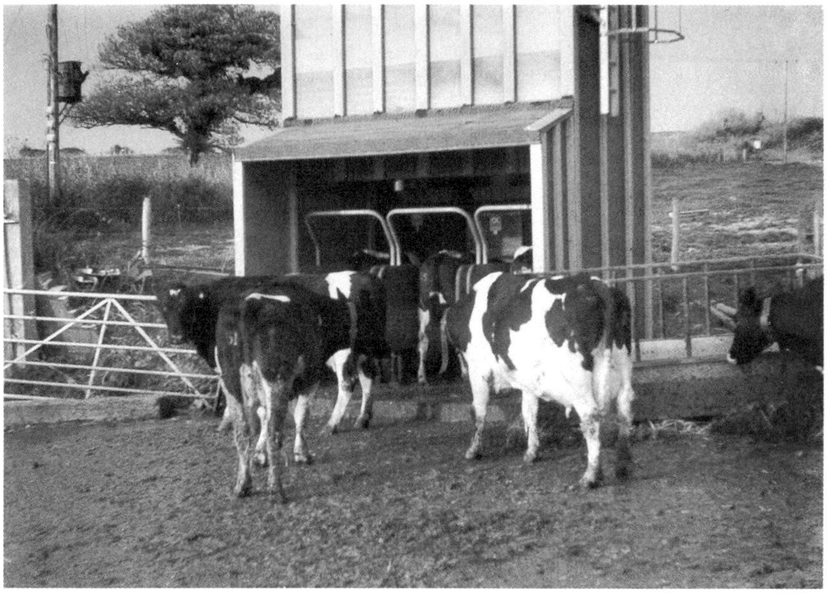

Fig. 4.16 Cows at a computerized out-of-parlour feed station.

and often'. They perhaps demonstrate the way dairying will go in the future. Printouts can be obtained for cows not consuming their allocated amounts.

In all feeding systems water must not be overlooked. With milk being 86 per cent water any shortage of water will quickly limit milk production. A dairy cow will need 60–80 kg of water per day and being creatures of habit tend to all want to drink at the same time. This makes a large reservoir and fast flow of water essential.

Dairy farm buildings

Because of the diverse nature of dairy farming there are almost as many different designs of dairy building units as there are dairy farmers.

However, if starting from scratch the main needs are for a milking parlour and dairy, winter housing and feeding barn, food storage area, calving and isolation boxes, slurry handling area and various collecting yards and access concrete. A typical set of dairy buildings is shown in Fig. 4.17.

Important considerations when designing a dairy unit include the following.

1 Cow-free access for the milk tanker so that collection can be made at any time.
2 Good cow flow so that cows come from the bedded area through the parlour and back with a minimum of narrow passages and sharp corners.
3 Good feeding access so that cows can be fed without having to work amongst them.
4 Access to silage storage areas away from the cows so that silage making can take place while the cows are in the yards or in for milking.
5 Good handling arrangements for veterinary treatment and AI.
6 Adequate slurry storage preferably for a whole winter's slurry.
7 Thought should be given to the way the buildings blend in with the surroundings. Choice of materials and site are important.
8 Adequate loose boxes for calving, sick animals, etc.

Parlour and dairy

This is the key to the whole dairy unit being used twice a day 365 days of the year. Cowsheds are very labour intensive and outdated while rotary parlours have proved unreliable in use and with no benefits over a static parlour. Figure 4.18 shows the most common parlours used, an abreast and a herringbone parlour.

The most simple parlour is the abreast, which is particularly suitable for herds of up to 80 cows with one man milking either with three milking units and six standings or six units and six standings. The cows enter and leave one at a time so a degree of individual treatment for a slow milker or slow eater is possible. The parlour should have a loft above to hold the concentrates, which fall by gravity to the feeder situated between each pair of cows. Milking rate will be about 30–40 cows/hour.

In a herringbone parlour the milker stands in a pit, which removes most of the bending required. The cows come in and out of the parlour in batches and stand at an angle to the pit on either side. They are suitable for any sized herd and one man could comfortably milk 100–120 cows in two hours with a 10 : 10 herringbone, i.e. 10 milking units, 10 standings. For 300 cows or

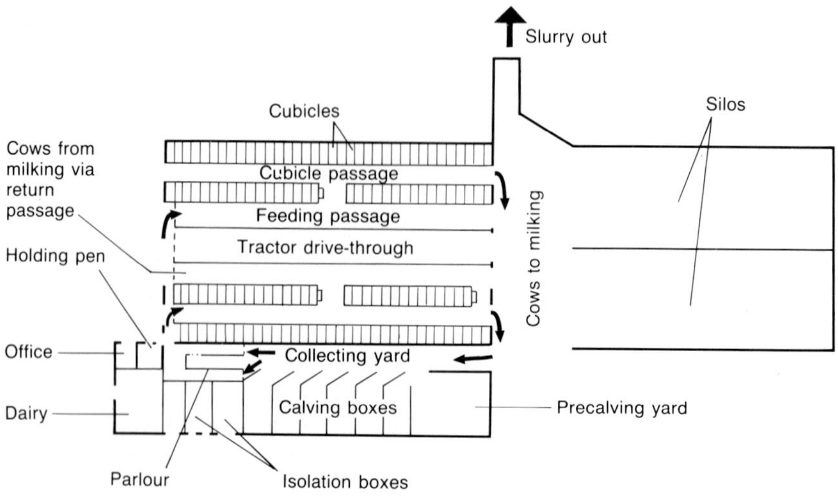

Fig. 4.17 Typical layout of a dairy unit.

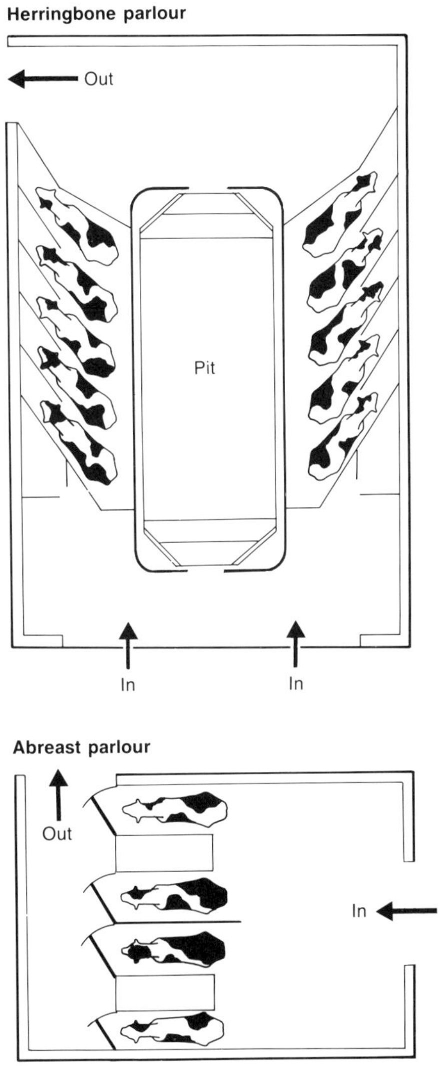

Fig. 4.18 An abreast and a herringbone parlour.

more larger herringbones with two or three milkers are common. A loft above the parlour will hold the concentrates and each standing will have a feeder.

Automatic cluster removers are now available that make it possible for one man to handle more machines without the danger of overmilking.

In any parlour the work routine is to let the cow or group of cows in, feed them, wash the udder, test the foremilk, attach the cluster, remove the cluster, teat dip or spray, transfer the milk and let the cows out.

The dairy should be adjacent to the parlour and will contain some dairy equipment such as the vacuum regulator, milk pump, water heater and washing equipment. The bulk milk tank will also be situated here. The capacity of the bulk tank is important and must

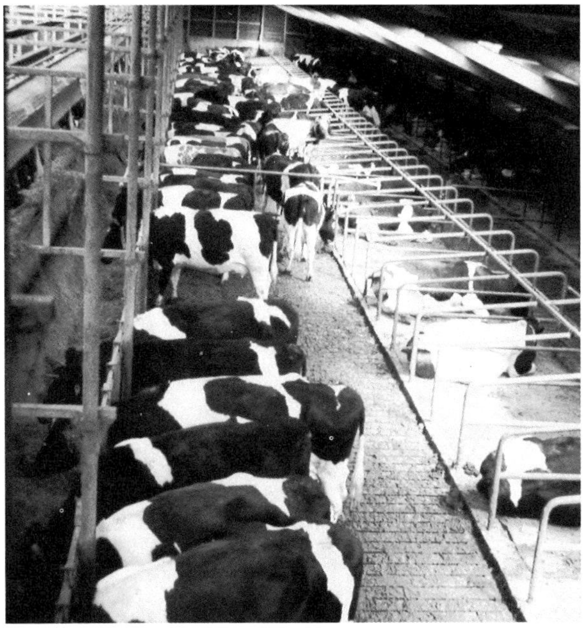

Fig. 4.19 A feed/sleep arrangement with metal cubicles.

be sufficient to hold the likely peak milk production. Except in a herd with a very compact calving pattern about 20 l/cow capacity is normally sufficient.

Both the parlour and dairy must be kept scrupulously clean and in Britain will be inspected regularly by the Ministry of Agriculture. The motors and refrigeration unit should be housed separately in an engine house. It is also useful to have a small area near the parlour where the cowman can keep the records necessary for herd management.

Cow housing and feeding barn

The choice for cow housing will rest between housing in straw yards and cubicles.

Cows often appear more comfortable in a straw yard but if they are to keep clean they need about 6 m^2/cow. They also use a lot of straw over a winter, which creates work to cart in and take out each day. But straw yards do help to alleviate a problem by reducing the volume of slurry produced.

Cubicles have gained in popularity and, well designed, can be a very trouble-free system with a low demand on labour (Fig. 4.19). The main requirement for comfort is to make the cubicle large enough, about 1.2 m wide and 2.2 m long. They can be made of metal or timber and a typical design is shown in Fig. 4.20.

The cubicle should slope from the head to tail end

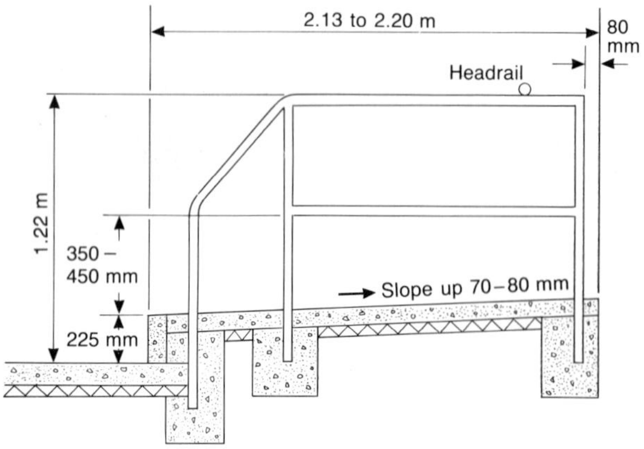

Fig. 4.20 A metal cubicle division.

and the best surface is concrete with chopped straw or sawdust as a bed. A strategically placed headrail is essential to ensure the cow dungs in the scraper passageway. Passageways should be 2.3 m wide to allow for good cow flow and sufficient width for the scraper.

The whole cubicle and scraper passageway can either be situated within an open span building or else can be part of a purpose-built cubicle or kennel type building. For all situations it is important to have a draught-free environment with plenty of ventilation. This is normally achieved by the use of Yorkshire boarding (vertical boarding with gaps to allow free movement of air) or with an open ridge to the building or kennel.

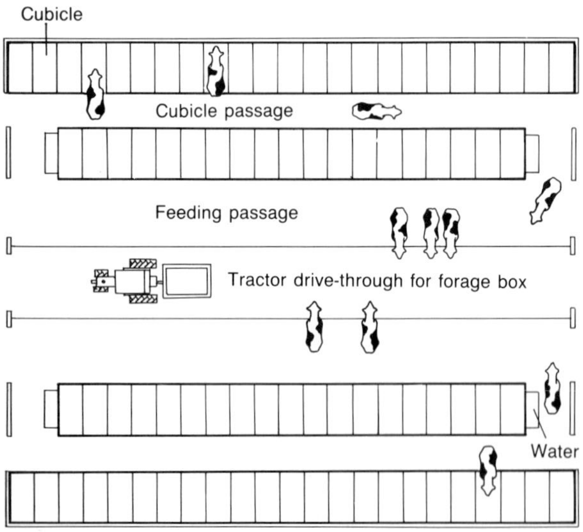

Fig. 4.21 Sleep and feed arrangements.

With either straw yards or cubicle beds, the feeding areas can be either inside or outside the building. An inside area is preferable but will add to the cost. An example of an arrangement with a centre feed passage is shown in Fig. 4.21.

The advantages of this type of arrangement are that the cows can be shut in the feed area while the cubicles are scraped and vice versa. Feed can be put out without driving through the cows and it is also possible to split the whole herd into groups, by milk yield or calving date, which can assist management.

Feed storage area

The major item here is the silage storage facility. This can range from a tower silo to a simple hardcore pad.

Construction of a simple silo is worthwhile to make handling easier and to prevent waste. Clamp silos are the most common and are usually constructed with a concrete base and walls of earth, sleepers or concrete. Safety is essential and in Britain walls must be up to Ministry of Agriculture, Fisheries and Food (MAFF) standards bearing in mind the walls have not only to contain the weight of the silage but also pressure from the tractor when consolidating the clamp. For open silos, guide rails must be provided 900 mm above the wall and for roofed silos sufficient height (5.5 m) must be allowed for tractor clearance. All effluent must be contained in a sealed tank that can be pumped out.

For self-feeding of silage the height of clamp must not be more than 2 m and capacity will need to be about 12–15 m^3 per cow for a winter's storage.

Calving and isolation boxes

These need siting in a convenient position to allow for ease of entry and exit for cows. The area would also probably include a cow handling area where cows can be restrained for veterinary treatment or insemination.

Boxes should be reasonably spacious and must have a tying-up ring or some other method to aid cow restraint. Walls must be rendered so that disinfection can take place. It is also useful to have a water bowl and feed rack, tractor access for cleaning out and, maybe, a milking point so that cows can be milked in the box. Sick cows may die or have to be destroyed in the boxes so good access for the slaughterer's lorry is essential.

For a herd with spread calving pattern, one box for every 20 cows should suffice.

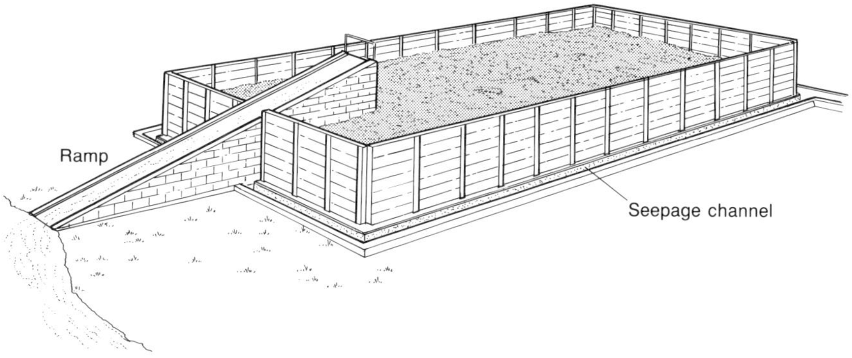

Fig. 4.22 A weepy-walled slurry compound.

Slurry

With more and more farmers using a loose housing and cubicle system, disposal of slurry is becoming an increasing problem. Also, water authorities are rightly demanding more control of pollution. A dairy cow will produce about 7000–8000 l (7–8 m^3) of slurry over a winter. This has quite a high fertilizer value (10 000 l will contain 25 kg N, 10 kg P_2O_5, 45 kg K_2O) but much of this will be lost by leaching if it is spread during the winter when the soil is saturated. Also, the pollution risk is much increased. Therefore, winter storage becomes almost essential. Slurry is usually scraped with a tractor-mounted squeegy to the store. The store must be able to cope with slurry, water, waste feed and bedding. It will reduce the volume considerably if clean water from roofs is diverted to a separate soakaway or drain.

Long-term storage can be provided in a sealed tower or a storage compound. With a slurry tower, the slurry is scraped into a reception pit and then pumped into the sealed tower. This is kept agitated to prevent settling or crusting of material. For emptying, the slurry runs back by gravity to the reception pit and is then pumped into the slurry spreader. It provides a good pollution-free system but is expensive to install and can create problems if management is not good leading to crusting and blockage of pumps.

By contrast the storage compound, although not cheap to construct, provides a simple-to-manage system with very few problems. The compound should be large enough to hold a winter's slurry, have a concrete or hard base to facilitate emptying and a shallow ramp to push the slurry up for filling. Slurry is pushed in all winter and then at a suitable time emptying takes place with a tractor and fore-loader direct into spreaders. A sophistication is a 'weepy wall' silo with walls constructed of timber or concrete sleepers with gaps between the sleepers (Fig. 4.22). This allows water to drain from the slurry, which is collected and spread separately. This considerably reduces the volume of material needing to be stored for the winter and improves the handling of the remaining material.

Herd records

Herd records are essential for management of the herd but they must be simple to keep, understood by the farmer and his staff and of use in the herd management. Before records can be kept, cows must be individually identified. With herds becoming larger and to make identifying cows by relief staff possible, this identification must be permanent and clear.

Freeze branding with liquid nitrogen kills the pigment cells in hair and results in a clear white number on black cows but is not so successful with light coloured cows. Ear tags are also often used and can be very clear if large. However, there is always the possibility of losing tags. With the coming of new technology it is possible that most cow identification in the future will be by transponder, either implanted into the cow or worn on a collar or ear tag.

For short-term cow identification, e.g. for a cow needing treatment, etc., spray cans of different coloured paints or tail tape, sticky coloured tape, can be successfully used.

Many large herds are now starting to use computers for keeping records but this is by no means essential and the capital cost will result in a place for manual recording for many years to come. Records kept will be either physical or financial.

Physical records

The notebook. The herdsman or farmer should always have a notebook in his pocket to record information such as bulling cows when the event is observed, before transferring this to more permanent records.

Cow record cards. This will be the cow's 'log book' and will give a concise picture of each cow's history. It must contain basic details such as name, pedigree number, ear tag number, herd number, date of birth, service dates, calving dates, sex and sire of calf data, production details, health records and details of veterinary treatment. An example is shown in Fig. 4.23.

Breeding records

Apart from information kept on the cow record card a simple breeding record should be kept. This will be used to keep dates of calving, pre-service oestrus, services and identification of sire and expected calving dates. These records should allow the farmer or herdsman quickly to identify any problem cows, such as those not cycling or not holding to service, so that treatment can be carried out before the calving interval slips. These records can be successfully maintained with written entries on a card but often a more visual record is kept. This is usually a rotary board with pins or magnetic blocks of different colours used to identify cows. These are placed on the board to record events so any cow 'out of line' is quickly obvious and can be investigated. If this method is used it is important to have a more permanent back-up in case the pins are all pulled out by a child. Figure 4.24 shows examples of these records.

Milk records

Whilst it is possible to record milk yields from cows personally, most farmers who wish to record milk use National Milk Records operated by the MMB. This scheme supplies a milk recorder to measure the milk

Cow record card

Cow name ________ Pedigree number ________ Ear tag number ________

Sire Date of birth ________

Dam ________

Lactation									
1	Calving date	Sex of calf	Sire	Milk yield	Days	Fat %	Protein %	Lactose %	Date dry
	Service dates				Veterinary treatment				
2	Calving date	Sex of calf	Sire	Milk yield	Days	Fat %	Protein %	Lactose %	Date dry
	Service dates				Veterinary treatment				
3	Calving date	Sex of calf	Sire	Milk yield	Days	Fat %	Protein %	Lactose %	Date dry
	Service dates				Veterinary treatment				

Fig. 4.23 Cow record card.

and take a sample, which is then sent to a laboratory for testing for the percentage of butterfat, protein and lactose. The recorder also enters dates of calving, service, drying off and culling (Fig. 4.25). The results are sent back to the farmer within a week and contain records not only for that month but also on a cumulative basis from the commencement of lactation. At the end of the lactation a cow record card is produced. From the dates provided an action list is produced for the next month with lists of cows due to calve, to dry off, to serve or to pregnancy diagnose.

Milk records are used for pedigree purposes, to provide information to prepare Improved Contemporary Comparisons (ICC) for bulls and to assist with cow selection for breeding purposes.

Apart from this, milk records can be used for management purposes for individually rationing cows or for use in a milk prediction scheme such as Herdwatch.

Financial records

Farmers keep many financial records with varying degrees of sophistication to assist with the management of the herd. Many farmers use a bureau service provided by the firm supplying his feed or use a service such as Milkminder operated by the MMB. All these measure the main output from the dairy herd, milk income, and relate this to the main variable cost of production feed. This then gives a margin over feed analysis expressed on the basis of per herd, per hectare, per cow or per litre.

These services are all computerized and rely on the farmer supplying information monthly on cow numbers, milk quantity and quality, feed used and price, fertilizer used and price, and land area used.

The farmer then has the results returned to him and often has a league table comparing his results with other farmers or comparing his results for this year with the previous year or budget.

Differences between the various schemes are small but some form of financial monitoring provides an essential part of the dairy herd management.

Labour

No dairy system will work efficiently without good labour. In many cases this is supplied by the farmer and

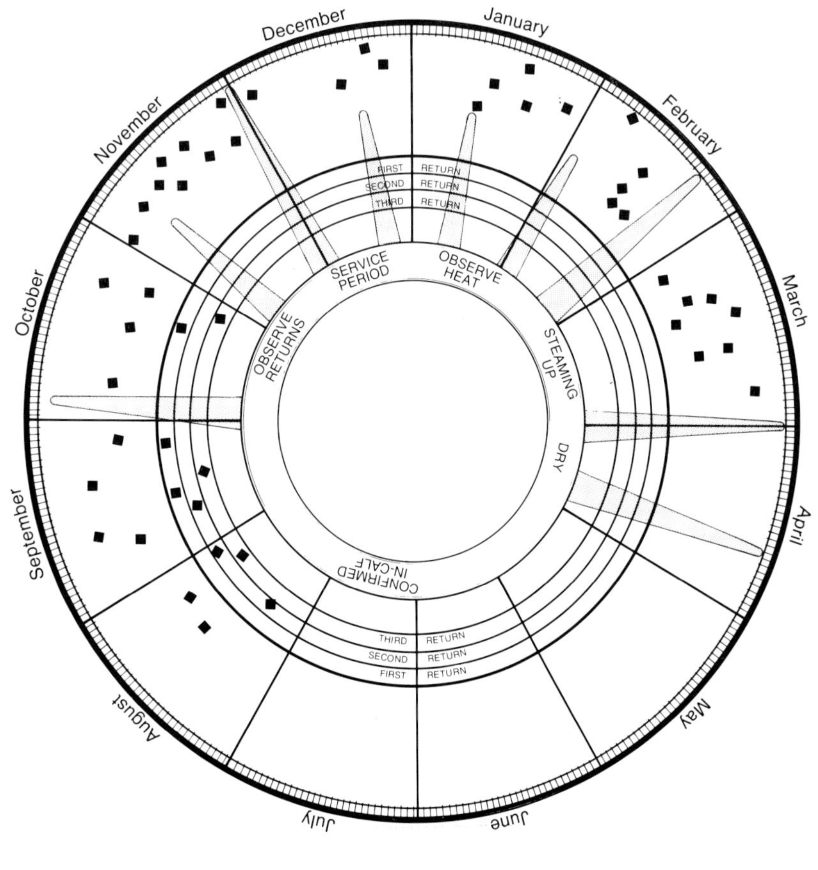

Fig. 4.24 Breeding board.

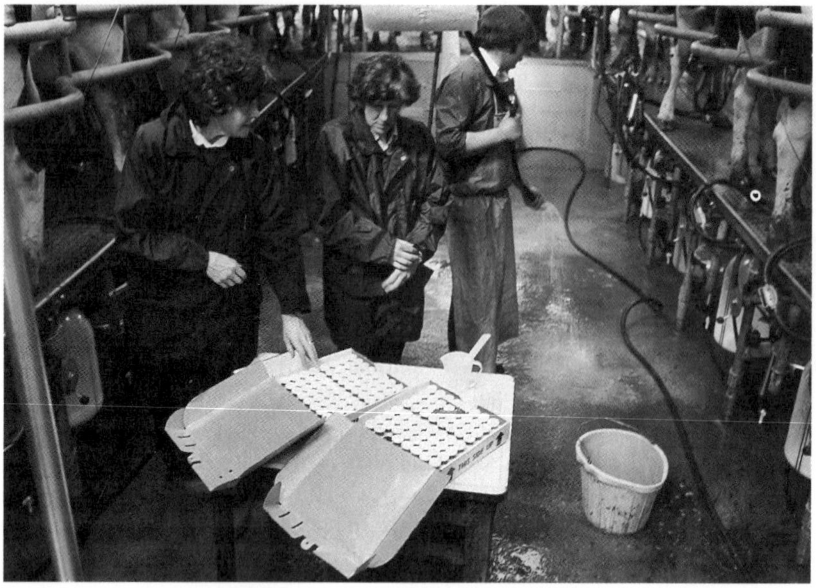

Fig. 4.25 The milk recorder sampling milk in the parlour.

his family but for larger herds employing a herdsman is common. In the milk costs survey for 1986–87, 63 per cent of herds only used family labour. From the same survey there was an average labour use of 35 hours/cow per year. This ranged from 79 hours/cow for herds of below 30 cows to 27 hours/cow for those above 100 cows. About half of this time was spent milking the cows and the other half tending them. Labour costs will vary depending on factors such as herd size, facilities available and type of person employed but will range between £120 and £180/cow.

A herdsman will be one of the most skilled workers employed on the farm. He must enjoy working with cows and be prepared to work the long hours made necessary by milking twice a day, seven days a week. He must be observant to see signs of unhealthy cows, to see cows in oestrus or about to calve and to see signs of under- or overfeeding. He must be capable of keeping records accurately.

He must be clean, to produce high quality milk and to prevent a dirty environment. He must be strong as there is still considerable physical work involved in cow feeding and calving especially. Fortunately, the herdsman's job provides a high degree of job satisfaction and interest for a dedicated man.

Most herdsmen are paid a fixed wage for the job but may also have bonus schemes related to such things as milk yield per cow (less common since quotas), margin over feed costs, calving percentage or calves sold.

Apart from the main herdsman, relief will be needed for weekends, holidays and sickness. Often this relief will be provided by the farmer or another farm worker. Failing this, relief agencies exist which can provide a herdsman often at short notice.

Breeding

The aim of a breeding policy must be to get the cows in calf regularly and to provide sufficient replacements of high genetic potential to maintain the herd size at the optimum level. This will depend on the culling rate, the age at first calving, the breed of sire used and the genetic worth of that sire.

Culling

Studies have shown that the majority of culls are sold for reasons such as poor breeding, mastitis, bad feet, injury, etc (Table 4.12). These might be termed unplanned reasons and will not lead to overall herd improvement.

With good management it should be possible to keep the annual culling rate to 20 per cent. But the national average is about 25 per cent. Also, because so much of that culling is for the unplanned reasons outlined above, the rate of genetic progress is considerably slowed.

Age at first calving (see Chapter 5)

This is very much linked with culing rate. Table 4.13 shows the effect of three culling rates and three differ-

Table 4.12 Reasons for culling (%). Source: Cull cow surveys 1984 (FMS Information Unit. MMB)

Poor yield/quality	12
Poor breeder	21
Bad legs or feet	9
Mastitis	15
Udder/test fault	8
Old age	10
Injury	5
Others	20

Table 4.13 Number of replacement heifers needed per 100 cows

Culling rate (%)	Age at first calving (years)		
	2	2½	3
15	30	38	45
20	40	50	60
25	50	63	75

ent ages of first calving. The number of heifer replacements needed more than doubles between options. Although heifers need a higher plane of nutrition to reach sufficient weight to calve at two years old their lifetime yield will exceed those calving at three years (Table 4.14).

Breed of sire used

Most dairy farmers breed sufficient cows pure to get the desired number of replacements, the remainder being put to a beef sire to maximize the value of the calf. Depending on the factors outlined above this can mean between 40 and 80 per cent of the herd will need to be bred pure.

With the majority of first calf heifers still being bred to a beef bull this gives very limited scope to do other than breed pure with the dairy cows especially if management is below average. However, where choice is available then cows with the highest cow genetic index (CGI) should be used to breed replacements.

Genetic worth of the sire

The choice here will rest between using natural service and AI. The chances of having a high 'ICC' bull available for natural service are very remote, so AI is to be recommended. Also, AI gives choice for traits other than production such as ease of calving, conformation or size. Within the overall traits desired, bulls with the highest ICCs for weight of fat plus protein should be used. Also, it is important to choose bulls with a reliable proof, i.e. with a weighting of +40 or above, with daughters in over 20 herds and with less than 25 per cent of daughters in the two herds with most daughters. A wide selection of bulls are available meeting these requirements (Fig. 4.26) (see also Chapter 10).

Table 4.14 Production associated with age at first calving. Source: Rearing replacements for beef and dairy herds (MLC and MMB)

	Age at first calving (months)				
	23–25	26–28	29–31	32–34	35–37
Herd life (years)	4.0	4.0	3.8	3.8	3.8
Lifetime yield (kg)	18725	18708	17943	17970	17637
Yield/day in herd (kg)	13.1	13.2	13.1	13.1	13.2
Yield/day of life (kg)	8.8	8.4	7.9	7.5	7.3

The other objective of obtaining a calf per year will largely depend on herd management. Very few cows are infertile but many fail to breed regularly. Key management times are as follows:

1 Postcalving: ensure the cow is clean, has no discharges and is cycling regularly.

2 At service: ensure the cow is on a rising plan of nutrition and not losing weight. Oestrous detection is a skill found in a good herdsman. Four observation periods during the day, of at least 20 minutes each will aid oestrous detection. Oestrous detectors such as tail paint, dyes or vasectomized bulls can be used to help detection.

3 Postservice: cows should still be closely observed for repeat heats. Cows apparently in calf should be pregnancy tested at 24 days after service with a milk progesterone test or at seven to nine weeks after service with a veterinary examination.

To achieve a regular 365-day calving interval, first service should be at 50–60 days from calving, which allows time for one repeat service before losing time.

An MMB report on Checkmate, the Board's fertility monitoring service, showed a wide difference between the top and bottom 10 per cent selected on the interval between calving and assumed conception (Table 4.15).

New techniques to improve the rate of genetic progress will doubtless be developed further over the next few years. These mainly revolve around embryo transplants and include possibilities with sexed embryos and super-ovulated cows producing many embryos for non-surgical transplants. As the cost comes down and the success rate improves these techniques will be used on more commercial farms.

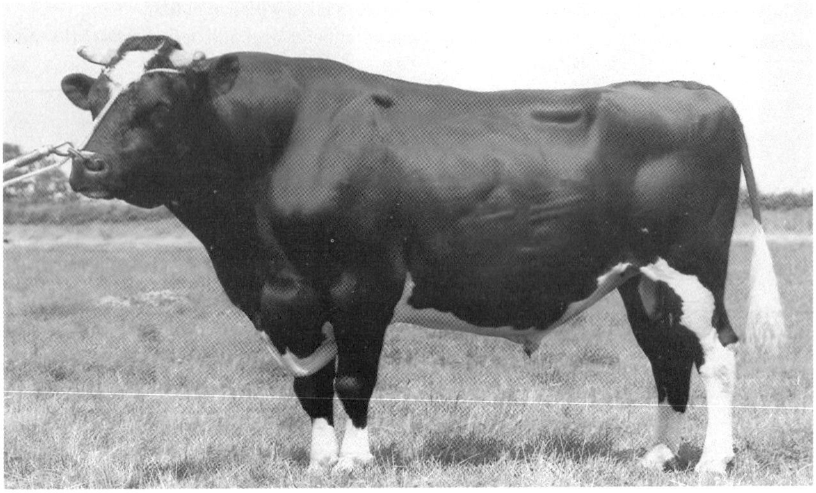

Fig. 4.26 Peckforton Citation River ET — a high ICC Friesian bull.

Health

This subject will be dealt with very fully in the main text of the book. Suffice to say here that cow health is paramount to success in dairying.

Veterinary and medicine charges are between £15–25/cow and are made up of drugs, particularly anthelmintics and antibiotics, and veterinary charges. The main diseases that cause losses to the farmer through loss of production, cost of treatment or even death of the cow are mastitis (see Chapter 21), hypocalcaemia (see p. 577), hypomagnesaemia (see p. 583), lameness (see Chapter 28) and calving problems.

Economics of dairy farming

Measures of efficiency

The overall measure of efficiency on any dairy farm is profit. Profit is calculated by deducting from the whole farm gross margin the overhead costs of the business. The gross margin (GM) is the output of milk, calves and cull cows less the herd replacement charge to give the gross output. From this are deducted the variable costs, of production, purchased feed, forage costs, veterinary costs, and medicine and sundry costs. The overhead costs are paid wages, power and machinery, sundries, property charges, interest and depreciation.

Each year the MMBs farm advisory service, Farm Management Services (FMS) now called Genus Management, produces a report looking at the economics of specialist dairy farms. This analyses the top and bottom 25 per cent of farms selected by profit/ha. The results, highlighting the main differences, are shown in Table 4.16.

For all the major factors the top group out-perform the others showing the enormous range of results found on fairly similar farms. However, on very many farms full records are not available to carry out this type of analysis and simpler records must be used. There are many, such as margin over concentrates, margin over all purchased feed (MOPF) or gross margin, all per litre, per cow or per hectare. Statistical analysis shows none of these measures to be closely correlated to profit. The best measures are those where land area, and hence intensity of farming, are taken into account. Provided the overhead costs are not exceptionally high, then margin over feed/ha will have a large influence on profit.

However, with the quota system now limiting pro-

Table 4.15 Checkmate results. Source: Checkmate report, 1985 (FMS Information Unit, MMB)

	Whole sample	Top 10%	Bottom 10%
Average interval calving: assumed conception (days)	99	81	130
Average interval calving: first service (days)	71	64	80
Services/assumed conception	1.82	1.65	2.22

duction on farms, many people are now saying that margin per quota volume and hence margin per litre has become the most important measure. Tables 4.17–4.19 show that, depending on the criteria chosen, very different methods of production give the best results. These tables are based on the 1986–87 Milkminder report, which analysed data from 2459 herds and Genus Management costed Dairy Farming 1989–90.

A high margin per cow results from a high yield per cow with modest concentrate use. Stocking rate does not change substantially over the range of results. Farms with a high margin per litre had a lower milk yield per cow but with a much lower concentrate usage. Stocking rate also fell so there was little improvement in margin per hectare. Those with a high margin per hectare had a higher yield produced with increased concentrate usage and with a much higher stocking rate. The intensity of farming was much greater.

All these different systems of producing milk can lead to good profits if carried out efficiently. Therefore, depending on the farm situation and the circumstances appertaining, different systems can suit different farms.

A vigorous debate also ensues about the merits of seasonality of calving and its effect on profits. Both spring calving and autumn calving are very defined systems that can be successful and profitable if operated efficiently. Table 4.20 shows the differences between the systems.

A British spring-calving herd (calving February–April) produces a lower yield with less purchased feed than an autumn-calving herd (September–December). This gives a higher margin per litre but lower margin per cow and per hectare.

Both systems can be equally profitable but as the margin per cow is lower for the spring calver then the overhead costs must also be lower to show the same profit.

Thus the level of overhead costs goes a long way to determining the farm system. Where overhead costs are very low (i.e. an owner-occupied farm with no rent, no borrowed money, no paid labour and little machinery), then a very extensive system with low yields and low outputs can be practised and still show a good profit. However, if the overhead costs are high then the farm must be intensively run with high yields and high stocking rates, putting surplus land into arable crops to generate a high gross output. Only then will a satisfactory profit be generated.

There are many ways of making a profit in dairy farming. The skilled operator and the one making the greatest profit will be the one managing the resources of land, labour, capital, stock and quota most efficiently.

Table 4.16 Top and bottom 25% selected by profit/ha, 1990

	Top 25%	Bottom 25%
Herd size	130	110
Yield (l/cow)	5763	6399
Concentrate use (kg/cow)	1603	1605
Stocking rate* (LSU/ha)	2.31	1.81
GM (£/cow)	733	653
Whole farm GM (£/ha)	1439	868
Overhead costs (£/ha)	793	853
Profit/Loss (£/ha)	423	−102

* LSU: livestock stocking units; GM: gross margin

Table 4.17 Analysis by margin over purchased feeds (MOPF) (£/cow)

	MOPF (£/cow)				
	<575	575–625	625–675	675–725	>725
Milk yield (l/cow)	4741	5118	5414	5724	6245
Concentrate use (kg/l)	0.30	0.28	0.27	0.27	0.27
MOPF (p/l)	10.95	11.76	12.02	12.26	12.38
MOPF (£/cow)	519	602	651	702	773
Stocking rate* (LSU/ha)	2.24	2.15	2.18	2.18	2.27
MOPF (£/ha)	1079	1195	1314	1425	1634

* MOPF: margin over purchased feeds; LSU: livestock stocking units.

Table 4.18 Analysis by margin over purchased feeds (MOPF) (p/l)

	MOPF (£/cow)				
	<10.5	10.5–11.1	11.1–11.7	11.7–12.3	>12.3
Milk yield (l/cow)	5730	5677	5621	5494	5270
Concentrate use (kg/l)	0.33	0.29	0.27	0.24	0.21
MOPF (p/l)	9.7	10.8	11.3	11.9	12.6
MOPF (£/cow)	616	663	686	697	700
Stocking rate* (LSU/ha)	2.30	2.24	2.20	2.14	2.11
MOPF (£/ha)	1275	1370	1401	1395	1398

* MOPF: margin over purchased feeds; LSU: livestock stocking units.

Table 4.19 Analysis by margin over purchased feeds (MOPF) (£/ha)

	MOPF (£/ha)				
	<1100	1100–1300	1300–1500	1500–1700	>1700
Milk yield (l/cow)	4975	5309	5538	5821	6172
Concentrate use (kg/l)	0.27	0.26	0.27	0.27	0.29
MOPF (p/l)	11.76	12.09	12.19	12.18	11.83
MOPF (£/cow)	585	642	675	709	730
Stocking rate* (LSU/ha)	1.73	2.02	2.23	2.42	2.80
MOPF (£/ha)	940	1195	1389	1598	1916

* MOPF: margin over purchased feeds; LSU: livestock stocking units.

The future

The future for European dairy farming is intrinsically tied up with political decisions. It is likely that the quota system will remain and may even increase in severity. This will make some farms, mainly the smaller or less efficient farms, unviable. These will then be taken over by the larger more efficient farms who will thus become larger.

The number of cows will reduce nationally but herd size will increase as the number of producers fall. Yield per cow will continue to rise as farmers become more efficient through improved breeding and technology.

There will continue to be a squeeze on dairy farm incomes and it will be difficult for the new entrant to get started. But for those doing the job well there will continue to be satisfactory returns. Whilst political decisions and quotas will close some doors, others will open and there will be good opportunities in dairy farming for many producers.

Table 4.20 Details of spring- and autumn-calving systems

	Spring	Autumn
Yield (l/cow)	5228	5634
Concentrate use (kg/cow)	946	1409
MOPF (p/l)	13.0	12.4
MOPF (£/cow)	678	698
Stocking rate (cows/ha)	2.29	2.30
MOPF (£/ha)	1553	1605

References

Farm Management Services Information (1990). Checkmate report. Milk Marketing Board, Thames Dilton, pp. 1–17.

Federation of United Kingdom Milk Marketing Board (1984) United Kingdom Dairy Facts and Figures, Thames Dilton, pp. 1–200.

Federation of United Kingdom Milk Marketing Board (1990) United Kingdom Dairy Facts and Figures, Thames Dilton, pp. 1–209.

Genus Management (1990) An analysis of Genus Management Costed Dairy Farming 1989–90, Crewe, pp. 1–24.

Milk Marketing Board (1986) EEC Dairy Facts and Figures, Thames Dilton, pp. 1–178.

Milk Marketing Board (1990) EEC Dairy Facts and Figures, Thames Dilton, pp. 1–210.

Chapter 5: Heifer Rearing — 12 Weeks To Calving

by B. DREW

Introduction

Dairy heifer rearing is generally considered to be a non-intensive, low-profit enterprise. Indeed, few farmers would rear heifers at all if it were not for their interest in herd improvement and disease control. However, planned heifer rearing is the starting point for profitable dairying. An increasing number of farmers now realize the importance of this and are adopting more intensive methods, particularly where the land involved could be used for alternative, more profitable, enterprises.

Calving at two years is more profitable than calving at two and a half to three years as little over half the area of land is required, lifetime milk yield is greater and the amount of feed, housing, labour and working capital required for the rearing enterprise are reduced. Despite these obvious advantages, the average age at first calving remains at about 32 months because most farmers prefer to calve heifers at a particular time of year. A policy of calving at two years can only be achieved if the majority of cows calve within a relatively short period or a proportion of herd replacements are taken from heifers.

The management of a dairy heifer between 12 weeks and calving has a considerable effect on her potential for milk yield, fertility, the incidence of dystokia and on longevity. Insufficient growth rates during the rearing period result in the production of small-framed heifers with disappointing milk yields due to their inability to compete with older cows during the first lactation. Poor growth rates at around the time of service result in low pregnancy rates and delayed entry into the herd.

The faster a heifer grows, the more efficient she is in converting feed into liveweight gain. This may suggest that heifers should be fed to grow as rapidly as possible especially during the summer months when grass provides an abundant and relatively inexpensive source of feed. However, high growth rates during the first year result in lower milk yields due to the effect of rapid growth on the relative proportion of fat and milk secretory cells in the developing udder.

The potential of a heifer will only be maximized if she is reared to a plan with careful control over performance at all stages of the rearing period. Target growth rates and intermediate target weights should be set as soon as the predicted date of first calving has been decided. Optimal growth rates will depend on age at calving, estimated mature body size, management after calving and average herd yield.

Dairy heifer rearing is a specific farm enterprise involving capital, land and labour. It should be managed and recorded with the same attention to detail as that given to the other enterprises on the farm with preplanned target rates of growth being achieved throughout the rearing period.

A detailed description of the management and targets required for autumn-born heifers reared to calve at two years is given in this chapter. The pattern of growth and targets for weight-for-age for spring-born heifers calving at two years are similar. There is less pressure to maintain steady weight gains when the aim is to calve at an older age and there are periods when lower growth rates are acceptable.

Age at calving

The younger a heifer is at calving the less land, housing and capital is required during her rearing period but heifers should not calve at less than 23 months because a higher incidence of calving problems can be expected and subsequent milk yields are disappointing. With a high stocking rate of 0.4 ha/livestock unit, the area of land required for each replacement unit is 0.4 ha for heifers calving at two years, 0.5 ha for heifers calving at two and a half years and 0.7 ha for heifers calving at three years. When the stocking rate is 0.5 ha/livestock unit the area required for heifers calving at three years is twice that required for heifers calving at two. The housing and capital required to sustain a two year system is also reduced. For instance, a 100 cow, autumn-calving herd calving at two years needs 40 replacements requiring accommodation for calves and yearling heifers. However, a similar herd calving at three years must maintain 60 heifers and house the third-year heifers during their third winter when space requirements are approaching those of adult cattle.

The first lactation milk yields of heifers calving at two years are likely to be lower than if the age of first calving is delayed. Milk yields of two-year-old calving heifers on the Agricultural Development and Advisory Service's (ADAS) Bridgets Experimental Husbandry Farm averaged 4544 kg milk as compared with a yield of 4980 kg for heifers calving at three years (Furniss *et al.*, 1986). However, when differences in the mean calving interval are taken into account the effect on yield is marginal (Table 5.1). It is known that the average life expectancy of two-year calvers is greater and the lifetime milk production higher than heifers calving at three years. A two-year calver can be expected to survive for 4.0 lactations rather than 3.8 and give 1000 kg more milk than a heifer calving at three (see p. 58).

Table 5.1 Effect of age at calving on first lactation milk yield. Source Furniss *et al.* (1986)

	Age (years)	
	2	3
Milk yield (305 days) (kg)	4544	4980
Calving interval (days)	386	401

There are a few circumstances when it is preferable to adopt a policy of calving heifers at two and a half to three years. Calving at an older age reduces the management pressures imposed by the two-year system and permits the utilization of marginal land unsuitable for cropping. It also enables replacements to be taken from cows of high genetic merit even if they calve later in the season. Calving at three years can only be justified when there is a large area of outlying rough grazing or when heifers are reared for sale.

Month of calving

Most dairy farmers plan to calve their heifers in a batch at one season of the year. Autumn-calving herds find difficulty in maintaining this seasonality in the pattern of calving unless either herd fertility is high or a proportion of the calves reared for replacements are taken from heifers. The optimum month of calving varies with the relative prices of milk and compound feed and with the management pressures from other enterprises. Having established the optimum month of calving for a herd the heifers should be mated to calve at the same time or shortly before the earliest calving cows.

Calving heifers before the cows reduces the stress imposed following introduction to the herd and allows for a longer interval between calving and service. However, some farmers prefer to calve heifers at the same time as the early calving cows as they find that they are then easier to manage in the parlour.

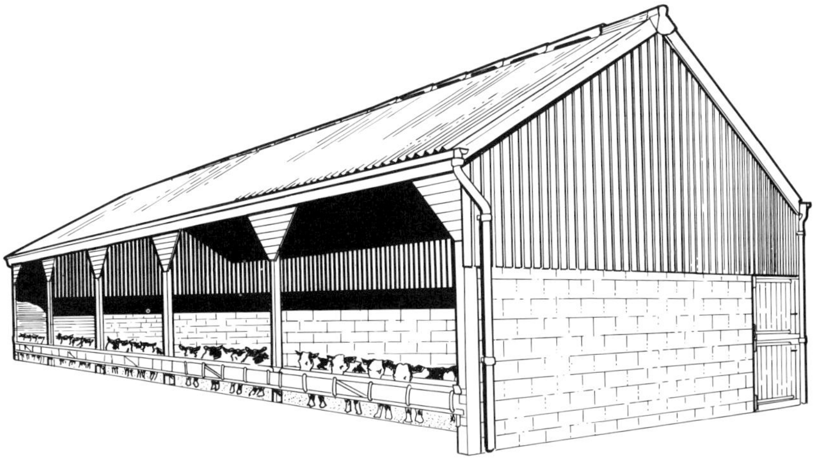

Fig. 5.1 Example of a well-ventilated calf house.

Rearing management, three to six months

Management and housing

Heifers should be housed in semi-covered yards such as that shown in Fig. 5.1. The calves should be given as much fresh air as possible with a draught-free lying area. Autumn-born heifers should be housed throughout the period but spring-born heifers may be turned out towards the end of the period if aftermaths are available.

Feeding

Target growth rates during the first year of life should be based on estimated mature body weight. A steady liveweight gain at a rate equivalent to the estimated mature body weight in g/day is required. Thus a Jersey heifer with a mature weight of 500 kg should be predicted to grow at 500 g/day (0.5 kg) while a Holstein should be expected to grow at 700 g/day (0.7 kg).

It is important to maintain a constant rate of gain. Poor growth rates, whether caused by an inadequate diet, or disease, are likely to lead to compensatory gain at grass, which can have an adverse effect on subsequent milk yield.

From 12 weeks of age, a rearing nut or home mix (16 per cent crude protein (CP)) concentrate should be offered to a maximum of 2.3 kg/day with hay or silage fed to appetite. Silage should be of high quality, fresh and palatable. If the fermentation is good and the quality sufficiently high (over 65D), 50 per cent of compound feed can be replaced by 200–300 g of white fishmeal reducing the cost of the overall ration. Calves should not be given silage that would be unacceptable to cows. Calves fed silage should also be offered clean barley straw and can be expected to take about 5 per cent of their roughage in this form. Regular monthly weighings are essential to monitor progress and adjust nutrition. On infected farms consideration should be given to vaccination against lungworm prior to turnout (see p. 237).

Rearing management, six to twelve months

Management at turnout

Autumn-born heifers should be turned out to pasture when weather and soil conditions permit. After turnout the winter ration should be continued until the forage intake declines, generally within one to two weeks. The compound can then be withdrawn. Spring-born heifers are normally housed until aftermaths become available.

Supplementary feeding

Following withdrawal of compound feed soon after turnout, no supplementary feed should be required until late August or early September. Attention should be given to mineral and trace element supplementation especially in areas of known deficiency (see Chapter 19).

Optimum growth rates

Stocking rates should be adjusted to maintain a steady rate of liveweight gain over the summer. The ideal daily gain remains at the heifer's estimated mature weight

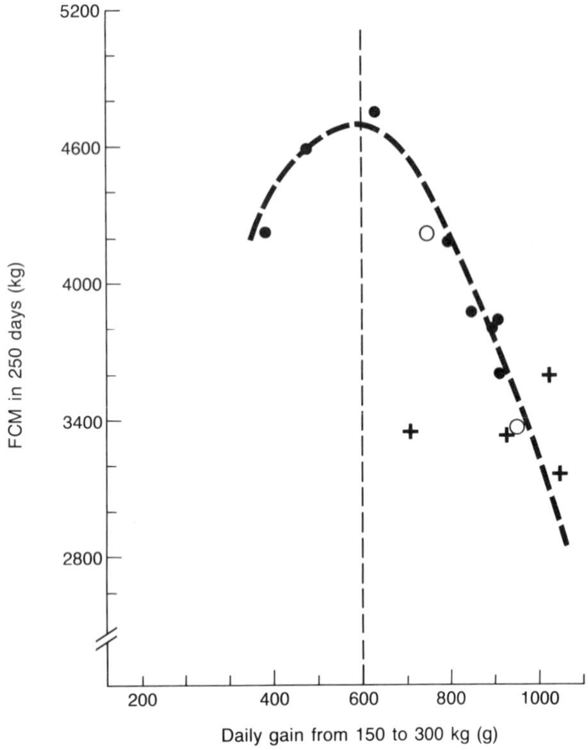

Fig. 5.2 First lactation milk production in relation to early life liveweight gain (after Foldager & Sejrsen, 1982).

(kg) in g/day. During May and June when grass is of high quality it is not unusual for heifers to grow at 0.8–1.0 kg/day unless a tight stocking density is maintained.

It is known that high growth rates in prepubertal heifers are detrimental to milk production (Little & Kay, 1979; Drew & Altman, 1982). A typical relationship between early liveweight gain and the first lactation milk yield of heifers is shown in Fig. 5.2. Mammary growth and development is under hormonal control and serum concentrations of some of the hormones involved are affected by plane of nutrition. It is likely that the negative influence of a high plane of nutrition on mammary growth is caused by changes in the secretion of these hormones. Rapid growth before puberty has been shown to coincide with impaired development of the mammary epithelium, decreased serum growth hormone and elevated serum prolactin concentrations (Foldager & Sejrsen, 1982). After puberty there is little or no effect (Fig 5.3).

Grazing systems

Ideally, calves should be turned out to parasite-free pasture. Up to late June this can be classified as land that falls into one of the following categories: new seeds after an arable rotation; or pasture grazed by sheep only in the previous year and grassland used for conservation only in the previous year. After mid July a

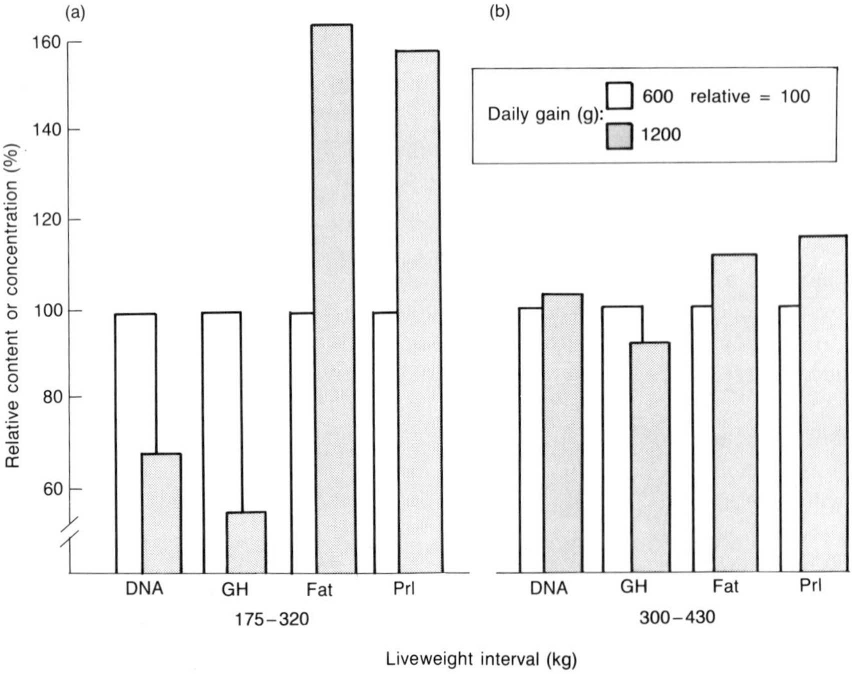

Fig. 5.3 Relative content of DNA and fat in mammary glands and serum growth hormone (GH) and prolactin (Pr1) concentrations in (a) prepubertal and (b) postpubertal heifers raised on two planes of nutrition (after Foldager & Sejrsen, 1982).

pasture can be assumed clean if either it is an aftermath not grazed by cattle earlier in the year, or the pasture has been grazed only by sheep during the first part of the year.

If parasite-free calves are turned out to and remain on a clean pasture it should be safe to graze for the remainder of the season. Unfortunately, in intensive dairy systems it is seldom possible to provide clean grazing as such. On permanent pasture, helminth egg output can be suppressed by anthelmintic treatment. Turnout should be delayed until there is sufficient grass to sustain adequate growth. Calves should be treated 21, 42 and 63 days after turnout (depending on the time of turnout). Further treatment is rarely required.

In continuous grazing systems the stocking rate should be adjusted to match the grass available, aiming for a sward height of 5–6 cm in spring, 7–8 cm in midsummer and 9–10 cm in autumn. A practical system in widespread use involves the use of three-year leys in a silage/grazing regimen. During the early part of the grazing season the calves graze the first-year ley (one-third of the total area). The remaining two-thirds are cut. During July and August the calves are moved to the silage aftermath and the first-year ley is cut. If grass growth declines in September the calves can be allowed access to the total area. If permitted to graze maiden seeds they should be dosed with anthelmintics immediately before being turned in, so that the ley will remain clean for the following year.

The leader/follower system in which calves graze ahead of older cattle has gained in popularity in recent years. Well managed, it is an effective method of maintaining growth rates. The calves should be treated with anthelmintic 21, 42 and possibly 63 days after turnout (see also p. 234).

Autumn management

During the period May–August target liveweight gains should be achieved without difficulty. At the end of this period the heifers should be well grown for their age and breed without any obvious fatness.

Heifers calving at two years require supplementary feeding from late August or early September depending on grass growth, soil and weather conditions. Growth rates decline rapidly from this time and if additional energy is not supplied liveweight gains will be low. A compound feed or home mixed cereal ration supplemented with minerals and vitamins should be fed.

Regular weighings are essential at this time for both autumn- and spring-born heifers programmed for calving at two years. Heifers being reared to calve at three years can be allowed a store period.

Autumn-born heifers should be assessed for size and suitability for service. Actual weights should be compared with targets. If any animal is found to be below target but, with additional feeding, could attain the minimum service weight, she should be housed at the beginning of September and fed an appropriate ration.

Rearing management 12–15 months

Housing and management

Heifers reared for two-year calving should be housed at least six weeks prior to service and given any routine veterinary treatments required during the period. They should be housed in semi-covered yards with a space allowance of 3.3–3.7 m^2/animal.

Feeding for fertility

It is known that the level of nutrition over the service period is important in ensuring high pregnancy rates and entry into the herd at the optimum time. In a study undertaken on six commercial dairy farms, the fertility of heifers fed rations considered to be adequate by the farmers was compared with the fertility of heifers fed the same diets supplemented with cereal (Drew & Pointer, 1977). The supplemented diets were calculated to provide an additional 20 MJ/day metabolizable energy (ME) and were fed for a 12-week period commencing six weeks prior to service. Ovulation was controlled and the heifers were inseminated at a fixed time. Semen and inseminators were used equally over all groups.

The calving rates to fixed time insemination are shown in Table 5.2. There was a wide variation in fertility between farms but on each farm a higher proportion of heifers fed the improved ration calved

Table 5.2 The effect of level of nutrition on the fertility of dairy heifers

Farm	Number of heifers	Percentage calved to the synchronized insemination	
		Control	Supplemented
1	62	40	67
2	58	59	75
3	56	32	59
4	37	67	79
5	78	54	69
6	73	53	67
Mean	61	50.0	68.9

to the synchronized service. The calving rates to first service for the heifers on the farm ration ranged from 32 to 67 per cent and for the supplemented groups from 59 to 79 per cent. In this study, no significant relationship between body condition score and fertility was found. However, other workers have reported a relationship between body condition and fertility with lower pregnancy rates occurring at each end of the score range.

It is likely that change in body condition score has a greater effect on fertility than the actual score at service. Friesian heifers weighing 300 kg require to grow at a rate of 0.7 kg/day in order to maintain body condition. As it has been shown that loss of body condition is associated with low pregnancy rates a ration calculated to provide for maintenance and 0.7 kg/day liveweight gain should be provided to Friesian heifers over the service period. Rations for other breeds should be adjusted according to relative body size.

Attempts to reduce the period of supplementary feeding to three weeks before and after service have been only partially successful. Reducing the period of supplementary feeding to three weeks prior to service should only be considered if Friesian heifers are in condition score 2.5–3.0 (Holstein and Jersey 2.0–2.5), or heifers are to be mated by natural service or observed oestrus artificial insemination (AI) and the reduced period of feeding does not affect the time of housing. The period of supplementary feeding after service should not be shortened as it is likely to increase the incidence of early embryonic loss.

In addition to providing a ration to satisfy the above standards it is important to avoid major changes to the composition of the diet during the 10 days before and after service. Changes in diet are almost always associated with disappointing pregnancy rates.

Stress

Stress, such as that caused by noise, physical trauma, overcrowding or some routine veterinary treatments, can alter the concentration and pattern of secretion of the reproductive hormones and is, therefore, potentially detrimental to fertility. In intensive management systems it is difficult to eliminate the possibility of stress but with careful planning it can be reduced to a level at which pregnancy rates are not likely to be affected.

Housing should be undertaken six weeks prior to service as oestrous behaviour is suppressed during the first oestrous cycle after housing. It is important to ensure that sufficient trough space is provided to avoid competition. There should be an adequate loafing area, the building should be well ventilated and the floor such that animals in oestrus will not slip. If AI is to be used, the handling facilities should be designed to allow for quiet and efficient movement of animals. The heifer should be presented standing at the same level as the inseminator and restrained from sideways movement.

Breeding policy

Traditionally, maiden heifers are mated by natural service. Many farmers consider oestrous detection to be too difficult and time consuming for AI to be practical. This problem increases when groups of heifers graze outlying fields away from satisfactory handling facilities. Synchronization offers a possible solution to this problem but the management standards on farms are often too low for acceptable results to be obtained.

The cost of keeping a bull is often less than AI but the risk of disease and injury are greater. The increased cost of using AI can only be justified if a pure bred sire is used and the female calves reared for herd replacements. Some farmers are reluctant to take replacements from heifers, preferring to use mature cows with a proven record of performance. However, the rate of genetic progress should be greater when replacements are taken from heifers providing a sire of high genetic merit is used.

A study by Furniss *et al.* (1988) of the first lactation and breeding records of 569 heifers calving in a Friesian/Holstein-based herd showed that those heifers born to heifers yielded significantly more milk in 305-day lactation than those from cows (Table 5.3). These findings provide practical evidence in support of the hypothesis illustrated in Fig. 5.4.

Rearing replacements from heifers and the earliest calving cows enables a two-year calving policy to be adopted with herd replacements entering the herd at the optimum time. The management of the heifer rearing enterprise is simplified as it should only be necessary to rear calves born over a six to eight week period.

Table 5.3 The effect of the parity of the dam on early performance

	Dam	
	Heifer	Cow
Weight at first service (kg)	370	360
Weight at calving (kg)	496	503
First lactation yield (305-day) (kg)	4977	4742
Proportion rebred	0.8	0.8

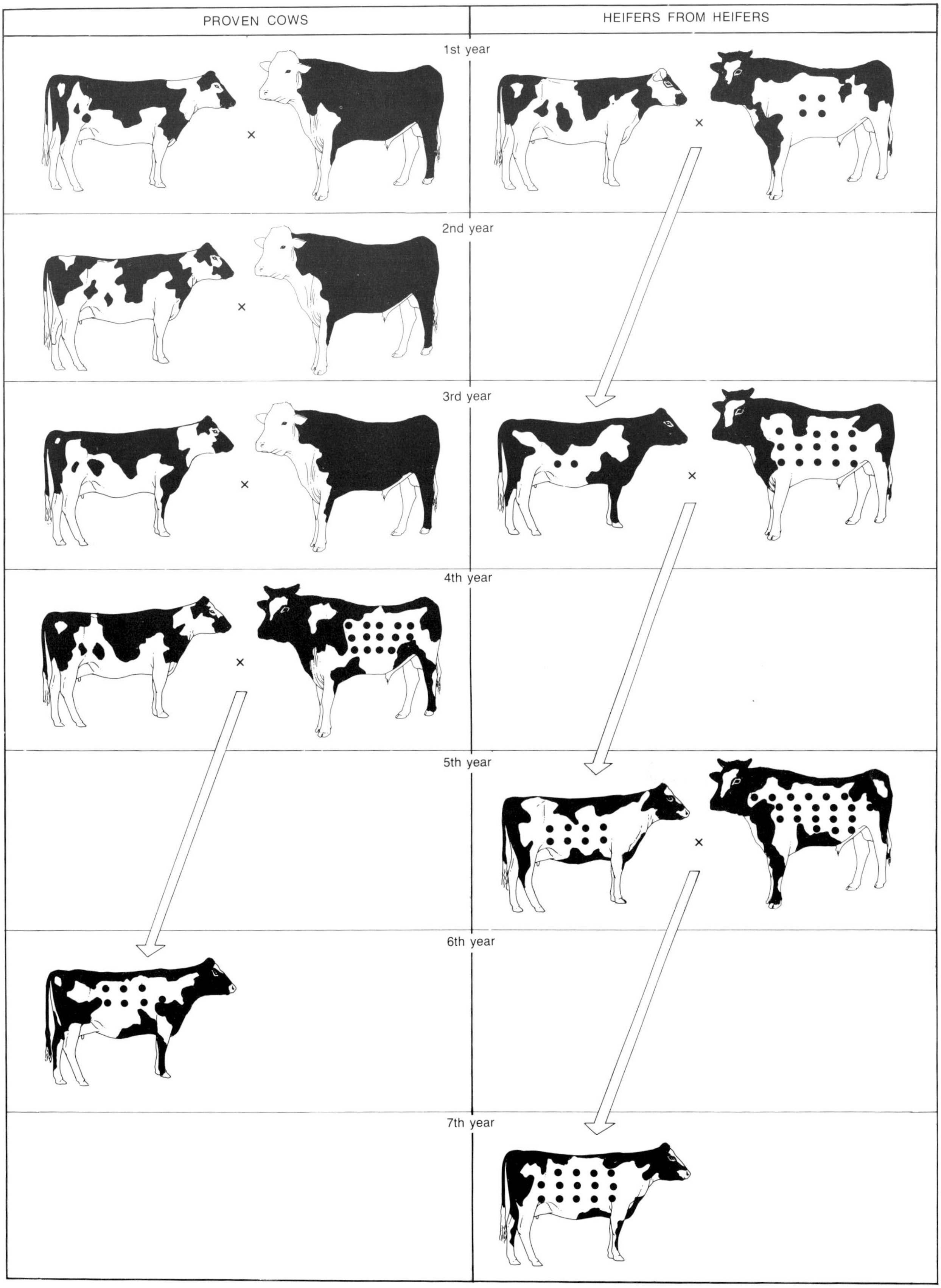

Fig. 5.4 The effect on the rate of genetic improvement of breeding herd replacements from heifers or from proven cows.

It also assists in the maintenance of the optimum calving pattern as the later calving cows can be mated to a beef bull.

The risk of dystokia is a further reason limiting the use of AI on heifers although this is mainly confined to the Friesian/Holstein. For many years it was common practice to use an Aberdeen Angus bull on maiden Friesian heifers. Although calvings to this breed are generally easier than with the Friesian and Hereford, the Angus has changed in recent years becoming larger and easy calvings can no longer always be assumed.

Although the incidence of dystokia is greater with most Hereford bulls than with the majority of Angus, the incidence is generally not unacceptably high. If natural service is to be used, the Hereford has attractions in that the progeny are colour marked and attractive in the market place and the breed is one of the most docile.

The incidence of dystokia, however, need be no greater with a selected AI Friesian bull, than a Hereford bull used in natural service. In a survey of 61 herds recording aspects of rearing and calving experience with heifer calvings, the incidence of dystokia associated with Hereford sires, averaged over all data, was almost identical to that associated with Friesians (Table 5.4). There was no difference between the breed in calf mortality rates.

Sire selection: breeding replacements from heifers

A recent survey of farmers breeding replacements from heifers showed that the main selection criterion was 'ease of calving'. It would appear that it is not unusual for this issue completely to override all the principles taken into account when selecting replacements from cows. Any heifer mated to a pure bred bull is potentially a dam of the next generation. The bull used must be at least as good as those used on the cows and should also be genetically superior to the sire of the heifer to which it is mated. Only by adopting these basic principles can genetic progress be made. When a bull is considered to be of sufficient merit to be a sire of the next generation, attention should be given to the effect that he may have on the incidence of dystokia.

Table 5.4 Effect of breed of sire on dystokia in heifers

Breed of sire (No. of heifers)	Percentage of calvings		
	Unassisted	Assisted	Difficult
Friesian (1181)	63	25	12
Hereford (753)	63	24	13

Reliability of proof

The weighting of a bull gives an indication as to the reliability or accuracy of the proof. The higher the weighting the lower is the statistical error associated with the proof and the less likely it is that the proof will change markedly with the addition of more daughters. A bull should have a weighting of at least 30 before he is considered for widespread use within a herd.

Also associated with reliability of proof is the 'daughter distribution' of a bull. The more herds from which the proof is obtained the greater the probability that the production figures of his daughters relative to those of other bulls will be maintained. On the basis of this criterion a bull should be regarded as having a widespread daughter distribution if the production records of his daughters are obtained from more than 10 herds and less than 25 per cent of the records are obtained from the two herds with a greatest number of daughters.

Selecting for production

The method of sire evaluation used in Britain is 'improved contemporary comparison' (ICC). This represents the mean difference in milk yield between heifer daughters of a sire and their contemporary herdmates adjusted for seasonality of calving, age at calving, the genetic merit of the sires of the contemporaries, the genetic merit of the dams of the contemporaries and the average merit of the group of bulls tested.

Payment is generally based on the weight of milk solids produced and not the liquid milk yield. The ICC for milk fat and milk protein should be used as the basis for selecting bulls. A bull with a higher ICC for milk plus protein than the bull used to sire the heifer should always be used even within a quota regimen as the progeny of such bulls are also more efficient at converting feed into milk.

Selecting for conformation

The main factors to consider are udder shape, teat shape and placement, legs and feet. The greater the number of selection criteria used, the slower will be the rate of genetic progress in any one direction. Conformation score should only be considered if there are particular weaknesses in the herd. The effect of selecting a bull with good conformation but a lower ICC for milk on the rate of genetic progress is illustrated in Table 5.5.

Table 5.5 Accumulating genetic merit

Generation	Herd genetic level	ICC of sire	Breeding value	Progeny merit	Genetic Change
1	0	+20	+40	+20	+20
2	+20	+20	+40	+30	+10
3	+30	+20	+40	+35	+5
4	+35	+5	+10	+22.5	−12.5
5	+22.5	−10	−20	+1.25	−0.25

It can be seen from generation 4 that a plus bull on his ICC figures may not be a 'plus' bull in all herds. If he is mated to heifers genetically superior to himself, the resulting progeny will be poorer than their dams and so the genetic merit of the herd will be reduced. If, after several generations of using genetically superior bulls, a farmer decides to improve conformation and by so doing uses a minus bull, all the progress made can be eliminated by that single mating (generation 5).

Selecting for longevity

Few studies have been undertaken in this country on the relationship between conformation (type), production and longevity. Many studies of these relationships have been undertaken in the USA and show that first lactation yield is the best early indicator of longevity and lifetime yield of dairy cattle. Type scores may add a little to the accuracy of prediction but not nearly as much as is commonly assumed by breeders. To a great extent, longevity in cows depends on the management decisions of the farmer rather than because some cows have an inherent ability to live longer than others.

Selecting for a low incidence of dystokia

The service sire has a considerable effect on dystokia. The results of a detailed analysis of 1485 heifer calvings to six Friesian/Holstein bulls used equally on 58 farms showed that the differences between the bulls used in the percentage of assisted and difficult calvings were statistically highly significant (Table 5.6). However, the effect of the bull was far less marked than the management on the farm on which the heifer calved. Of the 58 farms in the study, 18 reported mean calf mortality rates of 1.3 per cent born dead or died within 24 hours and recorded a low incidence of dystokia with all bulls. Twelve farms reported mean calf mortality rates of 26.9 per cent, which on some farms was associated with a high incidence of dystokia. On the farms with low mortality, none of the bulls were associated with an incidence of dystokia of more than 4 per cent while on the high mortality farms no bulls resulted in an incidence of less than 20 per cent. In this study the bulls used were known to be breed average or less for both dystokia on cows (<2.7 per cent) and gestation length (<281 days).

Table 5.6 The effect of bull on dystokia in heifers

Bull (number of calvings)	Percentage calvings		
	Normal	Assisted	Difficult
1 (236)	52	37	11
2 (231)	70	25	5
3 (249)	79	19	2
4 (221)	71	24	5
5 (261)	79	19	2
6 (263)	63	31	6

In Table 5.6 only bulls 1 and 3 were specifically recommended for ease of calving. This highlights the importance of ensuring that if a recommendation is based on heifer calvings, that the bull has been used on sufficient farms for the data to be reliable.

In general, bulls with short gestation lengths give easier calvings. The mean gestation lengths of bulls in this study ranged from 273 to 279 days. Providing a bull is known to be below breed average for dystokia on cows, he can be considered for use on heifers, especially if the gestation length is also less than the mean for the breed. However, some farmers reported dystokia with bulls that were the easiest calving overall, while other farmers reported that heifers calved without assistance to bulls that caused the most problems generally. In view of the considerable variation between farms and farm/bull interactions it is not possible to be certain whether dystokia will occur on an individual farm. Other factors involved in dystokia are discussed in the section on 'Management at calving' (see p. 58).

Service management

Controlled breeding (see also p. 522)

The introduction of synchronization techniques in the mid 1970s offered farmers a unique opportunity to exploit the use of AI without the time consuming and difficult task of oestrous detection or the need to separate individuals from a group for service. The results of numerous studies have shown that the pregnancy rates following prostaglandin or progestagen treatment are similar to those obtained with untreated controls inseminated at observed oestrus. Despite these findings, the uptake of commercial techniques to control the bovine oestrous cycle have fallen well short of expectations.

There are many reasons why group synchronization of heifers has failed to become a technique in widespread use. Initially, farmer expectation was too high. Many had been accustomed to running heifers with a natural service bull for perhaps nine to twelve weeks. By this time around 90 per cent should have become pregnant even with modest levels of performance. Farmers have, therefore, become used to finding the majority of heifers confirmed in calf when manually examined as a group and tend to expect similar results from a single AI mating.

Compared with natural service the cost of a controlled breeding programme with AI is likely to be at least £20–30 if a double insemination is given. If only 40 per cent of served heifers produce a calf and 50 per cent of those are male the service cost per heifer calf born could easily be in excess of £100.

Although pregnancy rates of 40 per cent are not unusual, the management factors affecting fertility in dairy heifers are generally well understood. Providing the recommendations given in the section 'Rearing management 12–15 months' (see p. 50) are followed pregnancy rates of 60–70 per cent should be achieved. At this level of fertility the use of synchronization becomes more attractive if used only for a proportion of the group.

Of the synchronization techniques currently available, the prostaglandins are usually considered the most appropriate for well-managed dairy heifers. The oestrous response is generally precise and pregnancy rates to fixed time insemination satisfactory. However, a proportion of heifers do not show oestrus within the normal three to five day response period after the second injection (Hafs *et al.*, 1975). This, coupled with the necessity to reduce costs, has led to the development of a number of systems combining the use of prostaglandin with either observed AI, or with AI at a fixed time followed by natural service.

A variation on the double injection, double insemination regimen now in widespread use is a system whereby the heifers are housed or moved to a field adjacent to the handling facilities six weeks before commencement of service. At the same time the heifers are weighed and the diet adjusted to ensure a gain of 0.7 kg/day with adequate mineral supplementation. Any routine veterinary treatments necessary are undertaken and a check made to ensure that the heifers can be clearly and easily identified. After a minimum of four weeks all heifers are injected with prostaglandin and observed closely for standing oestrus. Heifers not inseminated after the first injection are given a second injection and inseminated at a fixed time either once at around 84 hours after treatment, or twice at 72 and 96 hours after injection. Following the synchronized mating the heifers are either observed for repeat AI, or a bull of another breed is turned in as soon as the period of intense oestrous behaviour has subsided, which is usually on the fifth or sixth day after the second injection.

Rearing management, 15–18 months

Housed heifers should be allowed 4.9 m^2/head from this age. The preservice ration should be maintained for at least six weeks. As soon as it is known that pregnancy has been established in the majority of heifers, decisions can be taken on the level of nutrition for the remainder of the period. Their weights should be recorded and compared with target. They should be grouped according to size. Heifers below the target weight for age should continue to receive a ration calculated to provide for maintenance and gain of 0.7–0.8 kg/day. Heifers above their target weight can be allowed to gain at 0.6–0.7 kg/day. It is likely that, at this age the variation in weights of heifers of similar age will be around 80–100 kg. Adjusting feed levels according to size at this time enables the heifer group to become more evenly matched. High-quality silage and barley straw without further supplementation is sufficient for well-grown heifers. Smaller animals require an additional 1.0–1.5 kg of mineralized barley. A mineral mix should be fed to heifers given silage and straw alone.

Rearing management, 18–24 months

Autumn-born heifers should be turned out as soon as soil and weather conditions permit. Nitrogenous fertilizer with phosphate and potash according to soil requirements should be applied. Heavily fertilized pastures should be avoided. The sward height should be maintained at about 6–8 cm. Target stocking rate at this stage should be six to seven animals/ha.

Growth rates in pregnancy

Growth rates between the third to eighth month of pregnancy should be adjusted to ensure adequate calving weights. The target calving weight for a heifer depends on her estimated mature body size and the

Table 5.7 The effect of weight at calving on first lactation yield (305-day milk yield)

Weight of heifer (kg)	Mean herd milk yield (l)			
	<5000	5000–6000	>6000	Mean
<480 (small)	3933 (80)*	4172 (308)	4910 (95)	4278
480–520 (average)	4063 (27)	4388 (259)	5224 (81)	4548
>520 (large)	4337 (12)	4549 (239)	5402 (92)	4770

* Numbers in parentheses represent numbers of animals.

management routine during the first lactation. In management systems where heifers are fed as a heifer group in the first lactation there is obviously less competition than where heifers are competing with older cows.

Two-year calving heifers competing with cows in self-fed silage systems are at the greatest risk as not only are they relatively small in weight and stature but they are also changing their teeth at this time.

In an investigation involving Friesian/Holstein heifers calving at two years, Drew (1988) showed that growth rate during pregnancy has a significant effect on milk production, with the heavier heifers at calving producing the most milk (Table 5.7).

Weight, height and pelvic length at calving were found to affect milk yield. All these relationships were statistically significant and suggest that while rapid growth in the prepubertal heifer is detrimental to milk yield, the converse applies during pregnancy.

The initial results suggested that there is a positive relationship between body condition score and milk yield throughout the condition score range. However, a more detailed analysis showed that when heifers are fed adequately during the first lactation there is no beneficial effect on milk yield of feeding to calve them at body condition scores above 2.5 for Friesians or greater than 2.0 for Holsteins or the Channel Island breeds. This information is reassuring in view of the fact that an increased level of assistance at calving was required when heifers calved in condition scores of 3.0 or more (see p. 16).

To a considerable extent dystokia can be avoided by careful management in the ninth month of pregnancy. Growth rate should be restricted at this time.

Fly prevention

Summer mastitis is a frequent cause of loss in heifers (see Chapter 22). It is most likely to occur between the fifth and eighth month of pregnancy, usually in July, August and September. The incidence of summer mastitis can be reduced by grazing large open fields away from woods and streams and by the use of fly repellent measures. Cypermethrin-impregnated ear tags have proved to be of benefit in preventing disturbance and irritation caused by flies and reducing the incidence of New Forest eye and summer mastitis. The incidence of the latter can also be reduced by regular teat treatment with proprietary fly repellents.

Cubicle training

Some dairy heifers can show clinical signs of laminitis early in their first lactation. This is frequently a stress-related condition associated with changes in the environment, social grouping and feeding, which occur at the time of first calving. It has been shown that housing heifers for a few weeks during a period when cubicles are not occupied by cows has two advantages. Firstly, the heifers become accustomed to using cubicles and are less likely to reject them following introduction into the herd, and secondly, as one of the postparturient stresses is eliminated, the incidence of laminitis and other stress-related metabolic diseases is reduced.

Minerals and trace elements

A detailed description of some of the minerals and trace elements of particular significance to the dairy heifer is given in Chapter 19. In view of the fact that dairy heifers receive relatively little compound feed, deficiencies are more likely than with the milking herd. The advice given regarding minerals such as phosphorus, copper, cobalt, selenium and manganese apply equally to dairy heifers. (see p. 217 and Chapter 19.)

Although iodine deficiency may not be a widespread problem it can be responsible for serious losses on individual farms (see p. 221). If perinatal calf mortality in heifer calvings has exceeded 10 per cent in previous years an investigation into the iodine status of the herd is recommended early in the season and treatment undertaken during the fifth to eighth months of pregnancy.

Magnesium supplementation is normally given to dairy cows prior to calving in order to reduce the incidence of hypocalcaemia. As heifers are less prone to this condition, supplementary magnesium is not always provided (see Chapter 39). Data from ADAS trials suggests that magnesium supplementation in the month prior to calving reduces the incidence of dystokia. As the energy intake should be restricted at this time it is usually most convenient to provide this via the water.

Table 5.8 Effect of weight gain during pregnancy on dystokia

Weight gain (kg/day)	Calf mortality	Percentage calvings		
		Normal	Assisted	Difficult
<0.4 (49)	19	61	35	7
0.41–0.60 (348)	10	74	25	3
0.61–0.80 (854)	11	69	26	5
>8.0 (199)	14	64	28	8

Management factors affecting dystokia and calf mortality

Management at around the time of calving has a major effect on dystokia and calf mortality. Management prior to service and during the first eight months of pregnancy is generally considered to have little effect, although opinion is divided. The results of a large-scale investigation into the factors affecting dystokia showed a tendency for calf mortality and dystokia to be greater at each end of the growth-rate range (Table 5.8).

On the basis of this study, high weight gains during pregnancy should not result in unacceptable levels of dystokia especially if liveweight gain is restricted during the final month of pregnancy. An analysis of the pre-calving weight and height records showed there to be no significant relationships with dystokia.

In order to study the effect of management on the factors affecting calving difficulty and calf mortality, the performance of the 18 farms with calf mortality rates below 5 per cent was compared with the performance of the 12 farms with calf mortality rates over 20 per cent. There was no difference between the groups in the growth rates of the heifers (Table 5.9).

These figures suggest that growth rate of the heifer has little effect on dystokia. Equally, there appeared to be no differences between the groups in the size of the calves born, farmers with both low and high mortality rates recording a similar proportion of small, medium and large calves. The high mortality rate farms assisted a greater proportion of heifers in all of the size group categories and classified 58 per cent of large calves as difficult calvings compared with only 8 per cent of the large calves on the low mortality rate farms.

There is no evidence from these data to suggest that the management of the heifer during pregnancy accounted for the differences obtained. The differences would, therefore, appear to be due mainly to factors relating to the management of the heifer at around the time of calving.

Management prior to calving

Providing weather conditions permit, it is preferable to graze heifers in a field or paddock adjacent to the dairy complex, where the forage is naturally sparse or can be deliberately restricted to ensure that the optimum body condition at calving is achieved. The heifers should have the opportunity for exercise. If possible, they should be grazed as a heifer group. Supplementary magnesium should be provided. The ration fed to the milking herd should be introduced, but restricted to the amount required to acquaint heifers with their post-calving diet.

The group should be observed at least four to five times daily from three weeks prior to the estimated date of the first calving. Care should be taken to adjust the 'due to calve' dates for the gestation length of the bulls used.

Table 5.9 Farms with calf mortality rates below 5 per cent compared with farms with calf mortality rates above 20 per cent

Heifer measurements	Low mortality	High mortality
Number of farms	18	12
Number of heifers	447	212
Average number/farm	25	18
Mean age at calving (days)	731	734
Mean weight at service (kg)	330	323
Mean weight at calving (kg)	504	492
Mean height at service (cm)	117	118
Mean height at calving (cm)	128	127
Mean distance hook to pin at service (cm)	44	43
Mean distance hook to tail head at service (cm)	38	38

Table 5.10 Targets for growth for two-year calving

Months		Target weight (kg)			
		Jersey	Ayrshire/small Friesian	Average Friesian	Holstein
3	Maximum gain mature weight g/day	60	80	85	95
6	Maximum gain mature weight g/day	95	140	150	170
9	Maximum gain mature weight g/day	130	200	210	235
12	Minimum gain 13.5–15 months mature weight g/day	170	260	275	290
15	Feed as required to attain target calving weight	215	290	310	330
18	Feed to gain as required to attain target calving weight	235	340	370	390
21	From month 23 reduce liveweight gain to minimize dystokia (precalving)	290	415	445	470
24	Feed for lactation and continued growth	350	490	510	540
Mature weight		480	600	650	700

Management at calving

Grazed heifers should calve in their allotted field or paddock if possible, housed heifers should calve in buildings with which they are familiar.

There is evidence to suggest that moving a heifer to a calving box increases the risk of dystokia and therefore it is preferable to avoid movement unless this is essential for adequate assistance. The field should be well fenced to avoid the possibility of heifers rolling into positions from where it would be difficult to assist. The herdsman should be trained to recognize fear, abnormal pain or distress and instructed on the correct use of calving aids.

Targets for growth for two-year calving

The targets shown in Table 5.10 refer to heifers calving at two years. The target growth rates for heifers calving at 2.5 or 3.0 years are less as they can grow at a slower rate overall and during growth they can be allowed a store period. The maximum growth rates suggested for the first year and the minimum growth rates during the immediate preservice period apply.

Management during the first lactation

Heifers fed in competition with cows during their first lactation are likely to give less milk in the first lactation and have less chance of surviving to calve for a second time than when fed in a heifer group.

A study involving 179 small-framed Friesian heifers calving at two years, all the progeny of one sire, compared the milk yields and longevity of heifers fed with or without competition during their first lactation.

Table 5.11 The effect of competition on first lactation milk yield and survival rates to the end of the fifth lactation

Weight at service (kg)	Milk yield (kg)	
	Competition	No competition
225–259	2892 (33)*	3852 (37)
260–279	3334 (46)	4070 (73)
280–299	3639 (18)	3992 (52)
300–349	3131 (21)	3857 (32)

* Numbers in parentheses represent survival rate percentage.

The first lactation milk yields and survival rates to the end of the fifth lactation of heifers at a range of service weights are shown in Table 5.1.

On this farm no allowances were made for the size of heifer or the effect of competition on milk yield. A higher percentage of heifers in the group fed with cows were therefore culled on grounds of disappointing milk yields.

In a subsequent study, the lactation records of 1346 cows on 54 farms were examined to determine the extent to which heifers were affected by competition with cows. The farms were allocated to one of three groups according to the method of management during the first lactation.

Group 1: fed as a heifer group throughout the winter period.
Group 2: housed with cows. Fed a complete diet or manger fed.
Group 3: housed with cows. Fed on self-feed silage.

Heifers fed as a heifer group (Group 1) gave more milk than those fed in competition with cows (Table 5.12).

Table 5.12 Mean first lactation milk yields

Group (No.)	305-day yield			Total lactation yield	Lactation length
	Milk	Fat	Protein		
1(207)	5200	209	170	5369	319
2(580)	4504	180	146	4641	308
3(559)	4274	174	140	4358	309

Table 5.13 Mean first lactation yields (kg) as percentage of mature yields

Group	Mean heifer yield	Mean cow yield	Yield difference	Heifer yield as percentage of cow yield
1	5200	6265	−1065	83
2	4504	5630	−1126	80
3	4274	5479	−1205	78

Farmers electing to feed cows in groups are more likely to be aiming for high yields than those where the whole herd is managed as a single unit. When the milk yields are compared with the average herd yield it can be seen that the true effect is some 5 per cent of mature potential (Table 5.13).

Although heifers fed in competition with cows during their first lactation are likely to yield less milk, it is not always possible, feasible or economic to manage, milk, and feed them separately.

The effect of competition can be minimized by ensuring that heifers are well grown prior to calving. Size is important, but not the only factor determining the peck order within a group of cows.

Immediately after calving a heifer is maternally orientated and may be weakened by a prolonged and difficult calving. She is, therefore, least able to establish her place in the peck order. Bullying following introduction to the herd can be reduced by ensuring that the heifer has regained her strength after calving and by allowing her to join the herd in the late afternoon or early evening when there appears to be less aggressive behaviour. Competition for food can be reduced by providing access to 'easy'-feed silage in self-fed systems. It is as well to remember that heifers calving at two years of age are changing their teeth at this time and find difficulty in extracting silage from well-consolidated clamps. The problem is obviously most acute on farms where the width of the silage face is inadequate or where true 24-hour access is not provided. Silage or other forage should be fed in mangers or cut from clamps and fed behind an easy-feed barrier. The newly introduced heifers should be observed carefully to ensure that they are maximizing forage and concentrate intake. Sufficient loafing areas and loose housing or cubicles should be provided for all the cows in the herd. There is a tendency for farmers to provide 5 per cent less cubicles than cows in the group on the assumption that not all the animals will wish to lie down at the same time. Heifers will not always lie in empty cubicles between older cows and therefore it is recommended that one cubicle is provided for each cow and heifer in the group.

Survival rates

On average, cows in Britain fail to survive in the herd for sufficient time to fulfil their mature yield potential. The mean length of herd life is some 3.7 lactations while mature yields are not obtained until the fourth, fifth or even the sixth lactation. It is also estimated that some 40 per cent of all heifer calves born alive fail to calve for a second time. The main reasons for disposal are fertility and low milk production. It is evident that the rate of growth during the rearing period influences milk yield; the level of nutrition at around the time of service affects pregnancy rates and the management of the heifer at calving the incidence of dystokia and calf mortality. It must be emphasized that attention to detail and good management throughout the rearing period has a considerable effect on longevity and overall herd profitability.

References

Drew, S.B. (1988) The influence of management factors during rearing on the subsequent performance of Friesian heifers. *British Cattle Breeders Digest*, **43**, 41–8.

Drew, S.B. & Altman, J.F.B. (1982) The effect of weight at first insemination on the subsequent performance of Friesian dairy heifers. *Animal Production*, **34**, 371.

Drew, S.B. & Pointer, C.G. (1977) The effect of level of nutrition on fertility in Friesian heifers in autumn and early winter. EAAP 28th Annual Meeting Brussels, 22–27 August 1977. Commission on Animal Health and Production Paper 77/8, pp. 1–3.

Foldager, J. & Sejrsen, K. (1982) Nutrition of replacement heifers affect mammary development and their ability to produce milk. World Congress on Diseases of Cattle, The Netherlands, vol. I, p. 45.

Furniss, S.J., Stroud, A., Barrington, H., Kirby, S.P.J., Wray, J.P. & Dakin, P. (1986) The effect of dams's parity on first lactation performance of dairy heifers. *Animal Production*, **42**, 463.

Furniss, S.J., Kirby, S.P.J. & Smith, G. (1988) The effect of dam's parity on the performance of daughters. *British Cattle Breeders Conference Digest*, **43**, 49–50.
Hafs, H.D., Manns, J.G. & Drew, S.B. (1975) The onset of oestrus and fertility of dairy heifers and suckled beef cows treated with prostaglandin. Animal Production, **21**, 13–28.
Little, W. & Kay, R.M. (1979) The effects of rapid rearing and early calving on the subsequent performance of dairy heifers. *Animal Production*, **29**, 131–42.

Chapter 6: Tropical Cattle Management

by R.W. MATTHEWMAN AND R.D. FIELDING

Introduction

In the following sections an overview is given of tropical cattle management and the tropical production systems in which cattle are found. Attention is paid to the main differences between tropical and temperate production systems in order to introduce the unfamiliar reader to these. The majority of tropical cattle are kept in extensive subsistence systems that differ fundamentally in their management objectives from commercial temperate enterprises. Since production systems differ widely, depending on climate and land ownership patterns, no generalizations can be made about management and production. The references cited in the text provide a further introduction to tropical cattle production systems and some of the key issues raised.

Statistics

The major tropical and subtropical areas of Asia, Africa and South America contain approximately 64 per cent of the world's cattle (Table 6.1) and if other tropical areas are taken into account such as Central America then over 66 per cent are found in the tropics. The tropics produce only 30–40 per cent of the world's beef and veal and 20–25 per cent of the world's milk (Tables 6.2 and 6.3).

This discrepancy represents a challenge for those involved in tropical cattle management, since the tropics have many advantages for bovine production. These include: a potential year-round growing season in the absence of very low temperatures; grass species capable of greater energy capture and dry matter yields than temperate grasses; vast land areas unutilized or underutilized; labour availability, much with strong animal keeping traditions; many locally adapted breeds that have been selected for production in the adverse environments.

Counteracting the advantages are several constraints,

Table 6.1 World cattle numbers by continent and level of development (1000 head). Source: Food and Agriculture Organization (1989)

	1979–81	(%)	1988	(%)
World	1 218 135		1 263 584	(+3.7)
Africa	172 094	14.1	181 190	14.3
North and Central America	173 500	14.2	163 643	13.0
South America	239 246	19.7	257 199	20.4
Asia	350 405	28.8	384 057	30.4
Europe	133 353	10.9	124 780	9.9
Oceania	34 789	2.9	32 122	2.5
USSR	114 748	9.4	120 593	9.5
Developed (all)	426 003	35.0	404 797	32.0
Developing (all)	792 132	65.0	858 786	68.0

Table 6.2 World beef and veal production by continent and level of development (1000 t). Source: Food and Agriculture Organization (1989)

	1979–81	(%)	1988	(%)
World	44 078		48 834	(+10.8)
Africa	2 929	6.7	3 265	6.7
North and Central America	12 403	28.1	13 645	27.9
South America	6 854	15.5	6 944	14.2
Asia	2 422	5.5	3 471	7.1
Europe	10 552	23.9	10 753	22.0
Oceania	2 198	5.0	2 156	4.5
USSR	6 720	15.3	8 600	17.6
Developed (all)	31 566	71.6	34 570	70.8
Developing (all)	12 512	28.4	14 264	29.2

Table 6.3 World milk production from cows, by continent and level of development (1000 t, whole, fresh). Source: Food and Agriculture Organization (1989)

	1979–81	(%)	1988	(%)
World	423 053		468 362	(+10.7)
Africa	10 615	2.5	12 523	2.7
North and Central America	76 417	18.1	85 184	18.2
South America	24 082	5.7	29 119	6.2
Asia	32 960	7.8	48 820	10.4
Europe	176 182	41.6	172 557	36.8
Oceania	12 240	2.9	14 209	3.1
USSR	90 557	21.4	105 950	22.6
Developed (all)	354 665	83.8	377 913	80.7
Developing (all)	68 388	16.2	90 449	19.3

which include: long periods without rain when grass growth is impossible; animal diseases, such as trypanosomiasis and those transmitted by ticks; communal grazing systems that inhibit investment and the use of improved management techniques; and a lack of effective local demand and infrastructure to stimulate and support production. These advantages and constraints are discussed in greater detail in the subsequent sections.

The productivity of tropical cattle

The productivity of tropical cattle is often said to be low. This is often untrue when total output is considered. Absolute production levels of milk or meat are low compared with temperate cattle, but capital inputs are also low. Productivity levels as opposed to production levels therefore may be relatively high.

The multiple outputs of tropical cattle systems include milk, meat, draught power, dung and hides (Fig. 6.1). Additional functions include acting as a saving mechanism, as a means of security, as a means of fulfilling social obligations and as a symbol of wealth and status within the community. These outputs are not reflected in commonly used measurements of performance such as offtake, which refer only to animals sold for slaughter and do not indicate the quality or nature of the offtake, i.e. store condition or finished, sex and age. Social offtake, barter offtake, subsistence offtake, increases in herd size and the use of animals for draught power are not reflected in normal offtake measurements. The difference between typical subsistence and

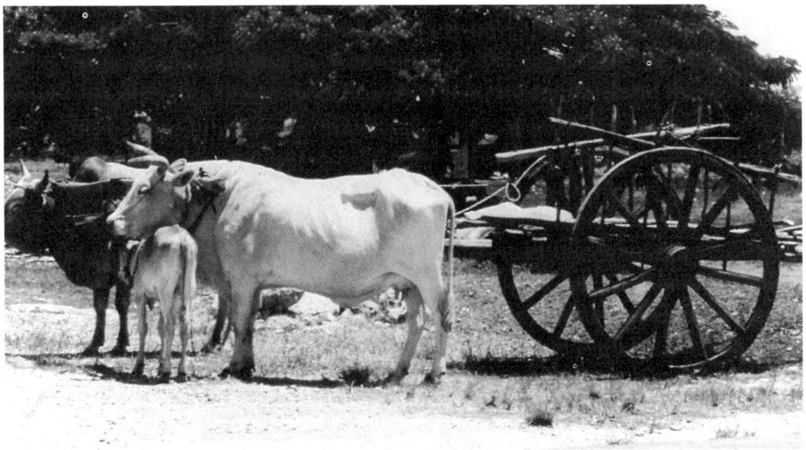

Fig. 6.1 Draught cows in Guadaloup.

ranch offtakes of 8–10 per cent and 18–20 per cent respectively may be explained largely by these differences.

Production strategy

Some workers have argued that the tropics are suited to multipurpose low input/low output systems. The environmental constraints on high producing animals and the lower quality forages and byproducts of the tropics support this. However, specialization is inhibited by multipurpose production. It seems likely that as technology evolves it will promote the type of specialization that has taken place in temperate areas. The speed of this evolution will be determined by our ability to counteract the direct and indirect environmental effects on the production systems, which in turn will require appropriate research and financial investment.

Calf management

In traditional cattle systems, such as pastoralism and settled extensive systems, reproductive cycles follow seasonal climatic variation. The peak of calving often occurs in the early wet season. In Sudan, in southern Darfur, most calvings occur in April, May and June. South of the Equator in Zambia the corresponding peak occurs in October and November. In humid areas where there is less seasonal nutritional stress, calvings occur throughout the year.

Preweaning management

In pastoral systems, young calves are separated from the grazing herd during the day and kept in special calf areas. After evening suckling cows and calves may again be separated. In Nigeria, Fulani pastoralists allow calves to suckle briefly in the morning to induce milk let-down and then tether them until milking is completed. After milking the calves suckle until the herds move off for grazing. Calves seldom receive supplements and may not even receive adequate milk due to overmilking for human consumption. This is typical of pastoralism in Africa and the Middle East.

Calf management inputs in these systems are minimal and this is reflected in the levels of production. In Darfur, Sudan, the average weekly calf gain was found to be 1.8 kg, equivalent to a liveweight of 66 kg at 6 months and 140 kg at 18 months. This is for a small breed, but indicates the relative difference to temperate breeds. Calf mortality rates were reported as approximately 16 per cent up to six months of age for migratory herds as compared with losses of 40 per cent in sedentary herds (Wilson & Clark, 1976). Similar levels are experienced in other migratory systems such as those of the Masai in East Africa and the Fulani in West Africa.

Environmental stress, principally due to high ambient temperatures, is best minimized through correct time of grazing, use or planting of shade trees and provision of simple open houses that offer protection from the direct rays of the sun, but ensure maximum air flow.

As production systems improve indoor rearing systems may be adopted. Semi-intensive and intensive calf rearing systems found in the tropics include the following.

1 Single suckling for beef calves where the objective is to achieve greatest calf growth rates and conversion of milk to meat.

2 Dairy ranching where calves are separated at night and the cows are milked once in the morning and limited or restricted suckling is allowed throughout the day. If management would allow evening milking, suckling all night and separating the cow and calf during the day would be a better option, as carried out by some pastoralists.

In the tropics calves may be reared inside, outside or a combination of both. Calves can be reared outside all year, though a number of disadvantages are associated with outside rearing on grass paddocks.

1 It is difficult to keep grass sufficiently young and nutritious for calves.

2 It is difficult to keep calves free from internal parasites if they are grazing in small enclosed areas.

3 Environmental stress (temperature and radiation) can be high, even if good shading is available.

The combination of poor nutrition, parasites and climatic stress is a major constraint to calf rearing. Adequate nutrition is the key to success and to enabling a stable host–parasite relationship to be established.

For the first two months the calf should ideally be kept in an individual stall measuring about 2 × 1.5 m. In warmer areas, portable calf pens may be used. The most practical indoor system is a shed sited in a gravel or concrete yard where the calves may exercise. The house must provide shelter, be easily cleaned and should keep calves warm in cool weather and cool in warm weather. It may be no more than a simple roof over a concrete base. Slatted-floor houses have advantages, but are more expensive (Fig. 6.2). No walls are necessary in the humid tropics, but adequate overhangs are required in high rainfall areas.

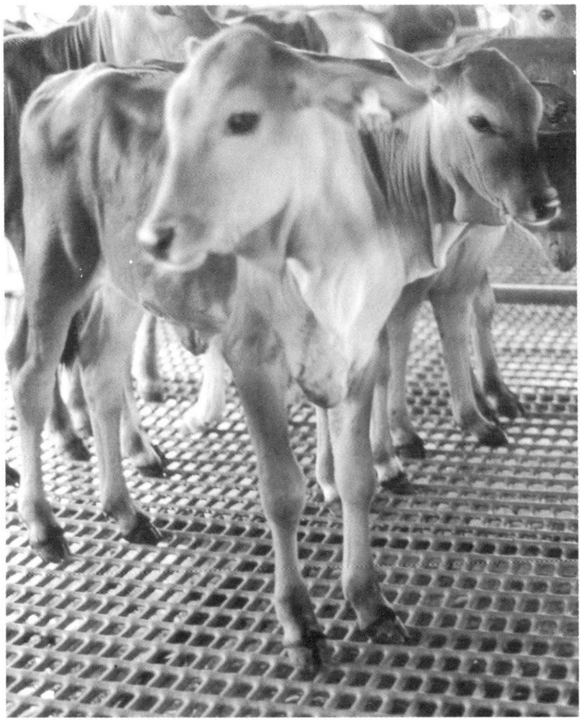

Fig. 6.2 Australian milking Zebu calves in Malaysia.

Brinckman (1971), in Nigeria, found that confined calves performed better than pasture calves and a system of confined management for bucket-fed calves was adopted at Shika Research Station. The calves received whole milk with a mixture of 50 per cent ground guinea corn and 50 per cent groundnut cake from two to three weeks of age. At two months, a zebu calf will eat about 0.5 kg concentrate/day. Older groups (four to six months) received 2.23 kg/head of a 21 per cent crude protein mix of 22 per cent cottonseed cake, 27 per cent groundnut cake and 51 per cent ground guinea corn.

The calf cannot utilize average quality tropical forage successfully until it is four or five months old. Consequently, it is desirable to suckle or bucket feed for as many months as possible and to feed concentrates and high-quality roughage. In intensive systems, the provision of some good quality forage is beneficial to stimulate rumen development.

Major calf diseases in intensive systems include scouring (gastroenteritis) (see Chapter 12), pneumonia (see Chapter 15) and worms (roundworms, threadworms, hookworms, lungworms and tapeworms) (see Chapter 17). In commercial enterprises in Zambia, the mortality rate for female calves was reported by Bessell and Daplyn (1976) to be 19 per cent overall. In suckling systems the mortality was 8 per cent and in bucket-fed systems approximately twice that level. This demonstrates the superiority of suckling. The advantage is due to the avoidance of disease caused by incomplete sterilization of buckets and equipment and suckled calves may receive more milk at more frequent intervals. In herds with many calves to be fed twice a day, maintenance of sanitation is a problem and the incidence of gastrointestinal disorders and indigestion in bucket-fed calves is often high.

Restricted suckling can overcome many problems and is the system commonly practised in pastoral and semi-intensive systems. It is also widely used in the dairy ranching systems of South America. Calves are housed separately, either at night or during the day, and are then allowed to suckle for one minute to achieve let-down before the cows are milked in the morning or evening. The cows are fully milked-out and the calves then run with the cows for the rest of the day or night. When properly managed, restricted suckling systems have several advantages including better calf growth and health, higher milk yields including more saleable milk and reduced mastitis in the cow (Preston, 1977).

Weaning

In many systems calves are naturally weaned when the milk supply from the cows ceases due to the poorer nutrition of the dry season. This leaves calves at varying liveweights and different degrees of readiness for survival during the dry period. Where cows continue to produce milk, the chances of reconception are reduced, often to such an extent that a calving pattern of a calf every two years develops.

In some systems weaning is effected earlier by traditional methods. These may include thorns tied to the calf's head or sacks tied around the cows' udders. Dairy heifers in more intensive systems are best weaned at four to six months of age. Beef calves should have maximum benefit from the cows' milk and hence should be weaned as late as seven months. Heifer calves should be weaned early enough to prevent them conceiving to the bull running with the cows. Avoiding early conception is difficult in many extensive traditional systems, though in many zebu breeds maturity does not occur until a greater age (i.e. 18 months plus) when animals reach 66 per cent of their mature weight.

Postweaning management

Once weaned, calves enter a critical period due to poor nutrition. Reasonable gains can be made in the rainy season, but weight loss occurs in the dry season caused by combined energy and protein deficiencies. Of the two, protein is usually the more important. Levels of nitrogen in dry tropical grasses commonly fall to around 0.5 per cent, equivalent to 3–4 per cent digestible crude protein (DCP) in the dry matter. At this level of protein, grass digestibility is low and intake falls. The calf may enter a negative nitrogen balance as metabolic faecal nitrogen loss exceeds nitrogen intake. Young cattle allowed only poor quality roughages thus tend to develop a 'bloated' appearance and effects on long-term performance can be expected negative.

Breeds differ in their ability to recover from weight loss. These differences include the ability to reduce metabolic rate during feed shortage and the efficiency of water conservation in periods of water shortage. The latter may lead to increases in feed digestibility due to slower rates of passage. The risk with major weight loss, in excess of 15–20 per cent is permanent stunting and increased disease susceptibility.

During normal dry periods deaths are often rare, but once the rains begin, losses may occur due to the stresses of wetting, lower temperatures and highly succulent grasses causing digestive upsets. Weight losses may also occur at this period.

Provided that the dry season weight loss is within the range of tolerance of the breed type, then rearing cattle usually show some degree of compensatory growth during the subsequent rainy season and make rapid gains. Tropical cattle have been naturally selected to cope with recurring periods of undernutrition and then to compensate effectively. This is a characteristic of great importance, which may be threatened by the increased introduction of exotic genes. The physiological mechanisms that allow compensation involve reduced metabolic rate, induced by a period of undernutrition, and increased voluntary food intake during realimentation. The period of realimentation and compensation is determined by the length of the rainy season. This is often short and animals again enter a period of undernutrition resulting in further weight loss. A 'zig-zag' pattern of animal growth thus characterizes many tropical rearing systems. Whilst dry season losses can be avoided by supplementation this is rarely justified economically. Careful recording work in Botswana, for example, has demonstrated that exploiting compensatory growth is normally preferable to supplementation (Anon, 1980).

It is also clear that stunting of young stock is a danger in arid conditions. The younger the stock the more prone they are to the permanent effects of undernutrition. An understanding of compensatory growth is important for reasons of rearing economy and in the management of feeding trials involving measurement of liveweight gain. Animals that are in a compensation phase may give a misleading result if compared with animals not in a compensation phase.

The consequences of the weight gain/weight loss pattern of growing tropical cattle are several and include delayed oestrus, reduced lifetime performance, reduced selection opportunities and also increased susceptibility to disease.

When rearing stock are housed or confined they may still suffer extended periods of poor nutrition when they are fed adult diets, such as sugar-cane tops or other low-quality byproduct feeds. In pastoral systems greater care is normally given to female stock because of their importance in producing calves and milk. Suboptimal management of rearing stock is common in all ruminant systems tropical or temperate. It is unfortunate that the consequences cannot be better quantified to provide arguments for improved treatment of this type of stock.

Onset of puberty

OESTRUS

In heifers, the period between weaning and calving can be divided into two phases: weaning to first service and first service to calving. The aim is to achieve optimum growth with the earliest maturity at the lowest cost. To achieve this small quantities of concentrate or supplement can be a great benefit. A check in growth occurs at weaning, but can be compensated for by the addition of concentrates such as those suggested by Brinkman (1971) (see p. 63).

The onset of oestrus occurs at ill-defined target weights. Under good conditions target weights may be achieved at 13–14 months. Lower nutritive quality of grasses, disease and environmental stresses result in delayed oestrus compared with temperate conditions. Whereas *Bos taurus* reach puberty at 30–40 per cent of mature weight, *B. indicus* reach puberty at 60 per cent of mature weight (Macfarlane and Worrall, 1970).

The size of the young heifer at first service and its rate of growth up to calving have an important effect on milk yield in later lactations. If early calving is combined with underfeeding in the rearing stage, heifers may be permanently stunted and milk production low. Immature heifers may also die at calving due to dystokia.

Once heifers are cycling normally and have achieved

an adequate body weight, mating or service should be timed to ensure calving at the optimum time of the year. This is often assumed to be the beginning of the rains, but it may be better to aim for calving just before the rainy season. This avoids chilling and stress during periods of heavy rain. If some form of shelter is available this consideration will be less important.

SPERM PRODUCTION

The onset of sperm production is not as critical as the onset of oestrus. Where conditions are poor and liveweights low the onset of sperm production is delayed.

Castration is carried out in many traditional cattle systems, but is usually delayed until the animal's potential has been assessed. Inferior animals are castrated in order to stop them mating, but oxen are important in many areas as draught animals.

Monitoring growth

In traditional systems, no monitoring of liveweight occurs, but in more controlled systems an objective of management should be to keep a close check on the development of stock. Young stock should be weighed every two weeks or so, and adult cattle should be weighed once or twice a year. If weighing facilities are not available on the farm, heart-girth measurements can be taken that give good weight correlations. Attention should be paid to the breed for which the weigh-bands have been designed, and if possible the accuracy should be checked against actual weighings and the bands calibrated appropriately. Direct weighing and heart-girths do not always fully define the condition of the animal and condition scoring may be appropriate. Systems of condition scoring for *B. taurus* cattle may not be appropriate for *B. indicus* breeds, and scoring systems designed for tropical cattle should be used (Pullen, 1978; Nicholson and Butterworth, 1985). Pullen suggested a score range of 0–5 from emaciated to fattest while Nicholson and Butterworth suggested a nine-point scoring range.

Adult production

The different tropical cattle production systems are the result of differing levels of dry matter production per unit area available for grazing. This varies from very low levels in the arid areas (<1000 kg/ha per annum) to high levels (>10 000 kg/ha per annum) in the humid areas, reducing again to low levels where intensive crop production limits feed supplies to grazing of roadside verges and intercrop areas.

Grazing utilization is complicated by land ownership, which includes 'ownership' by nation, tribe, group or individual. Most grazing is communal and herders have the right to graze as many animals as they wish. Individual ownership and/or leasing, e.g. Botswana (1975), is increasing and may stimulate intensification and improvement. Much depends on the employment opportunities for those who leave the land when land rights are allocated. Since grazing is crucial in cattle nutrition, the following sections highlight important aspects of grassland production.

Grass production

Grass represents the major link between the sun as the ultimate source of energy and the grazing animal. For the grass, however, the grazing animal can be regarded as a parasite. It is thus important that this relationship is not a destructive one for the grass. Animal productivity depends on a vigorous grass sward and management must safeguard the viability of the herbage above all else.

The factors that determine grassland dry matter production are amount of light, leaf area, efficiency of species, amount of carbon dioxide, temperature, water and nutrients.

In the short term the manager can increase leaf area and nutrient level and in the longer term the species and possibly water, through run-off control. Tropical grasses are physiologically different from temperate grasses. They fix carbon as C_4 rather than C_3 compounds and are regarded as more efficient than temperate grasses. This is partly the result of the structure of tropical grasses, which are taller and more effective in sunlight interception.

Tropical grasses have evolved to survive short rainy season. They grow quickly, reproduce and senesce. Whilst grass breeders have extended the growing period of many species, the short period is still a problem when grazing animals require dry matter throughout the year.

Figure 6.3 illustrates the changes in the nutrient composition of grasses with time.

The fall-off in crude protein (CP) percentages reduces the rate of degradation and rate of passage and thereby dry matter intake. While growing conditions are good in the wet season, CP levels can be as high as 9–10 per cent, but can be as low as 2–3 per cent in the dry season. The aim of the manager is to counteract low dry matter intake by appropriate management measures as discussed below.

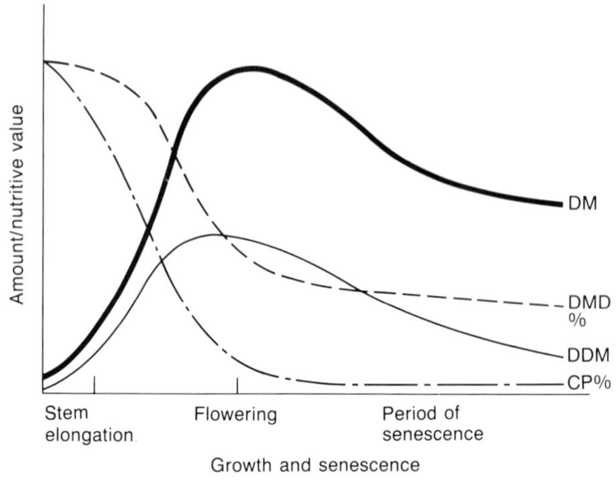

Fig. 6.3 Generalized changes in the amount and nutritive value of herbage during growth and senescence of the herbage. DM, dry matter available for grazing; determined by species and available nutrients; DMD, dry matter digestibility — falls from over 65% to around 40% largely as a result of changes in the crude protein level; DDM, available digestible dry matter — the resultant of DM and DMD; CP, crude protein — falls from over 12% to around 2%.

RANGE MONITORING

The interaction between animals and range is constantly changing and the result may be a long-term improvement or deterioration. A knowledge of the direction of this trend is very important and regular observation (monitoring) should be carried out using the following methods.

Remote sensing. This involves the use of satellites or aircraft to determine land use, land potential and degradation over large areas. Frequency of use is usually three to five years.

Soil and botanical trend monitoring. This involves establishing specific points or transects on the range that can be visited annually to assess the degree of soil erosion and ground cover. The botanical species are identified and the increase or decrease in particular species is recorded.

MANAGEMENT TO MAXIMIZE VOLUNTARY FOOD INTAKE

Maximization of voluntary food intake is the underlying objective in ruminant feeding management. Tropical grasses are less digestible at the same stage of growth than temperate grasses, due to greater lignification. The lower digestibility reduces rate of passage and hence reduces feed intake. Some breeds of tropical cattle may have evolved to cope with poor quality feeds through a greater dry matter intake capacity per unit body weight than temperate cattle (Orskov, 1982).

Management strategies to maximize voluntary intake involve maximizing food production, avoiding food losses and stimulating intake as follows.

1 Provision of adequate water and water harvesting through the use of bunds and micro terraces.
2 Control of grazing time, intensity and frequency to maximize grass production, i.e. maintenance of correct carrying capacity.
3 Inclusion of legumes in the sward or as browse.
4 Fire control to prevent destruction of accumulated standing hay in the dry season and to control bush encroachment.
5 Exclusion of wildlife and non-authorized grazers.
6 Provision of minerals and in the long term, correction of soil mineral deficiencies.
7 Simple rotation and grazing by appropriate herding, or use of fencing under intensive systems.
8 Division of the herd into units of need, i.e. young stock, dry cows, lactating cows.
9 Good herding practices.
10 Routine health maintenance.

Systems of production

Management and production levels are determined by factors such as climate and land tenure. In communally owned dry areas that are marginal or exclude crops, pastoral livestock systems are found with cattle, sheep, goats and camels (Fig. 6.4). In wetter areas small-scale mixed arable systems have developed where sheep and goats are important and where cattle and buffaloes may have a role for milk, meat, dung and draught power. In tropical highland areas milk production is often based on exotic cross cattle. Where land is privately owned, particularly in South America, more intensive dairy farming methods occur in combination with large-scale dairy and beef ranching. Throughout the tropics more intensive systems also operate on parastatal and other similar farms (Fig. 6.5).

PASTORALISM AND SETTLED EXTENSIVE SYSTEMS OF PRODUCTION

Low and often unpredictable rainfall coupled with communal land-use rights have led to migratory and

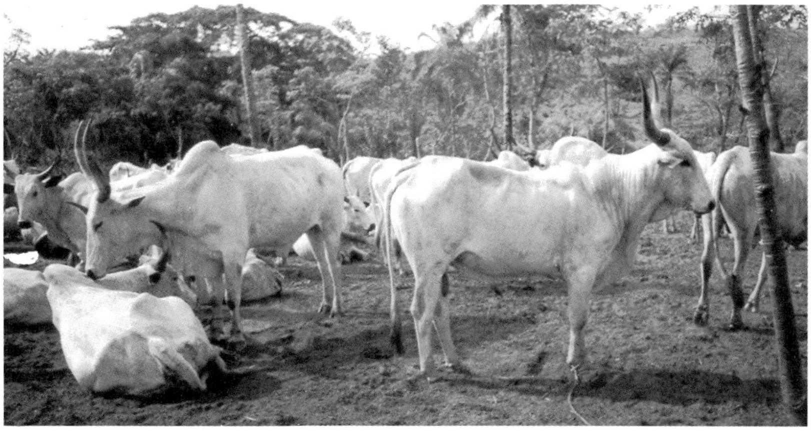

Fig. 6.4 Fulani cattle in Nigeria.

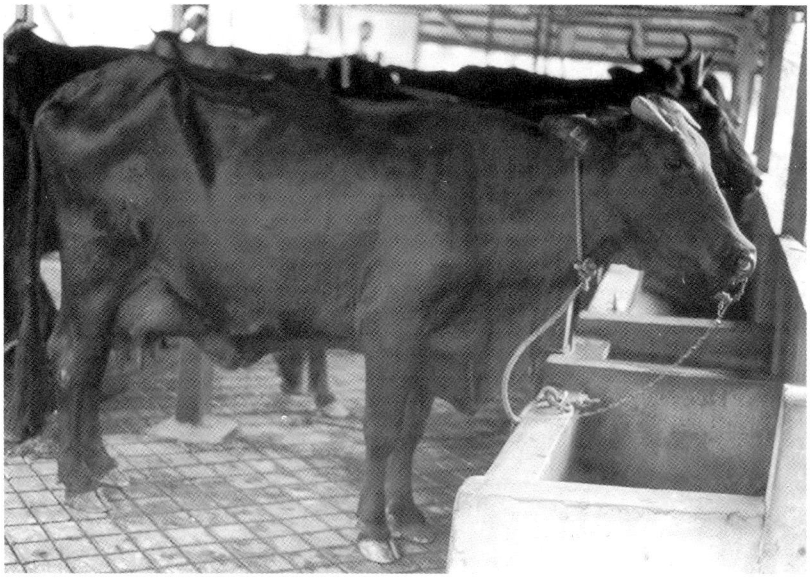

Fig. 6.5 Sahiwal × Friesian cattle in Malaysia.

seasonal patterns of grazing. Such systems are found throughout the Sahel from Mauritania to Sudan and through Ethiopia, Somalia, Kenya, Uganda and Tanzania. Cattle owners include the Fulani (Fulbe), Tuareg, Dinka, Borana, Karamajong and Masai. Pastoralists keep cattle to meet subsistence needs in areas unsuitable for crops. Milk is a major product that provides a daily source of food or tradeable produce and allows herders to exploit more remote drier areas. Due to drought over the past two decades and increased population, these patterns are changing in many areas.

In other areas settled production occurs where cattle are combined with crop production. Cattle are owned by settled village farmers and form part of mixed farming systems. In Nigeria the term 'mixed farming' has been used to denote the use of cattle as draught animals for cultivation. Draught animals are common throughout the tropics and their management is often better than that of cattle which are not used for draught, due to their vital role in the production of subsistence crops such as maize, sorghum, millet or rice.

Most settled farming is subsistence in nature and except where used for draught, livestock form only an adjunct to crop farming. Livestock production in settled systems may be slightly more intensive, but management inputs are often relatively low. Land is seldom individually owned and communal grazing is a major method of feed supply. The management and improvement of communally owned land is limited by the difficulties associated with getting people to cooperate.

Feed inputs are natural pasture, browse, crop residues and supplements. Crop residue grazing is seasonal, but important for extensively managed cattle. Millet and sorghum residues provide early dry-season feed and may be stored in stacks for use in the dry season.

The International Livestock Centre for Africa (ILCA) in Addis Ababa has pioneered over the last few years the concept of fodder banks to improve the nutrition of grazing animals. Fodder banks are fenced areas of high-quality forage that are made available for grazing for only a few hours per day and for only the most needy stock. The establishment of fodder banks has been described by Otsyina *et al.* (1987) using *Stylosanthes* species such as *S. guianensis* cv. Cook and *S. hamata* cv. Verano.

MILK PRODUCTION

Milk is produced under a variety of systems, ranging from one-cow zero-grazed units in Mauritius where cows are fed on sugar-cane tops and roadside grasses, to large-scale extensive dairy ranching in Central and South America, intensive large-scale milk cooperatives in India, and very large, zero-grazed exotic cow units in Saudi Arabia.

Consumers in the tropics accord a high value to milk and are often prepared to pay the required price. The rate of increase in milk production has been considerably greater in tropical countries than in traditional milk producing and exporting nations (FAO, 1989). World milk production grew by only 18 per cent between 1972 and 1982, but grew by 38 per cent in developing nations. Milk production can be an important enterprise in rural development for several reasons:

1 it provides a year-round source of income for the farmer;
2 it contributes to family nutrition;
3 it can utilize crop byproducts;
4 it serves to draw money from urban to rural areas; and
5 it creates rural employment opportunities.

These advantages have led to many development initiatives involving local/exotic crossbreds and sometimes pure exotics. There have been many disasters and failures, but also some major successes as in India with Operation Flood and in Kenya with smallholder milk production schemes.

However, the production of milk in the tropics is constrained by unavailability of feed throughout the year, disease prevalence, unfavourable environments, particularly seasonally, no high temperatures, underdeveloped infrastructure including storage, transport, marketing and processing facilities, low genetic potential of the animals, lack of farmer experience and inadequate training.

Dairy ranching

Tropical South America is a net importer of milk, but considerable quantities are produced from large numbers of low-yielding cows in dual-purpose systems called dairy ranching. Preston (1977) has discussed the merits of appropriate systems for different regions according to local characteristics, and encourages the use of dual-purpose systems. Dairy ranching is an example of such a system that utilizes local and crossbred cows.

In Latin America approximately 3 million km^2 of non-arable land are utilized for stock production (Weniger, 1983). Important tropical savannah regions occur in Colombia, Venezuela, Brazil, Guyana and Bolivia. These regions lie mainly below 2000 m and beef ranching occurs on private land using zebu breeds and their crosses, with the exception of some criollo breeds in Colombia. European breeds are not usually used in the lowland regions, but in highland regions (exceeding 2000 m) conditions permit the use of European breeds in intensive systems.

Sere (1983) has classified milk production systems in tropical South America according to altitude and feeding system adopted. A unique feature of lowland ranching is that beef cattle are also kept for milk production. The traditional system is dual purpose, and is well suited to the region. Depending on the market and feed supply, some cows in the beef herd may be milked. Cows are milked once a day in the rainy season, and the calves are only allowed restricted access to the cow. This is not a new practice, but has spread as the demand for milk has increased in urban centres. The system flourishes where both land and labour are cheap and plentiful, but price is also important. In Nicaragua, 70–80 per cent of lactating beef cows are milked, while in Colombia over 50 per cent of the milk consumed comes from dual-purpose systems.

Smallholder dairying: the Indian model

India is famous for its Anand pattern of dairy development. It is the fourth highest milk producer in the world after the EEC, USSR and USA and since 1950 it has more than doubled output. This has involved the setting up of dairy cooperative societies in which all milk producers are eligible to join. Farmers are usually paid for their milk within 12 hours of delivery to a collection point. Payment is based on quality and quantity.

The societies are formed into milk unions, which provide collection, processing and marketing services and may market livestock feed and provide artificial insemination (AI), veterinary and other services. The productivity of cows is low, but buffaloes can produce up to 2500 kg/lactation (Gupta, 1985).

Semi-intensive and intensive dairy production

In South America, exotic breeds are used in highland areas. Highland areas are found throughout South America and also in Africa on the Jos Plateau in Nigeria, the Kenyan and Ethiopian Highlands and in parts of Tanzania such as Arusha.

Kenya Highlands. It has been estimated that there are 1.48 million commercial dairy cattle in Kenya, which consist of *B. indicus* breeds, *B. taurus* breeds and crosses and grades between the two (Goldson and Ndeda, 1985a,b). Probably two or three times the above figure of zebu animals are also milked in the traditional smallholder sector. Artificial insemination records indicate a general trend in favour of Ayrshire and to a lesser extent Guernsey cattle.

Past grazing systems in Kenya, based on sown leys or indigenous pastures, have given way in suitable areas to more intensive systems of production based on stall feeding and zero grazing. On some farms virtually all feeds, including bulk fodders, are bought in. Probably 80 per cent of smallholder cattle are stall-fed for the greater part of the year. The diet includes Napier grass (*Pennisetum purpureum*) and other fodders including banana stems, maize stover, sweet potato vines and other arable byproducts.

Medium-sized and large-scale dairy units are based on Kikuyu grass (*P. clandestinium*) and star grass (*Cynodam dactylon*) and planted leys of Rhodes grass (*Chloris gayana*), Nandi setaria (*Setaria sphacelata*) and Guinea grass (*Panicum* spp.). Production is based on grass for seven to eight months and then relies on conserved material (silage and hay) or cut fodders (maize and Napier grass) during the dry season.

Artificial insemination is well established in Kenya and 700 000 doses/year are distributed. Pure exotic breeds and high grades are kept in cooler, high potential areas. Crosses are recommended in more marginal areas. The Ayrshire × Sahiwal has been found useful, but others involving Sahiwal, Jersey and Brown Swiss have also been successful (Fig. 6.6).

BEEF PRODUCTION

In Africa and Asia beef has traditionally been a byproduct of milk and draught power production. Governments have often been disappointed with the level of beef production from their traditional herds. This has led to the mounting of many projects aimed at increasing beef production. These have included group ranching schemes as in Kenya and parastatal ranching initiatives as in Uganda and several other countries. Most of these projects have ultimately proved uneconomic, although private commercial ranches have usually been more successful.

Increased beef production from medium to large-

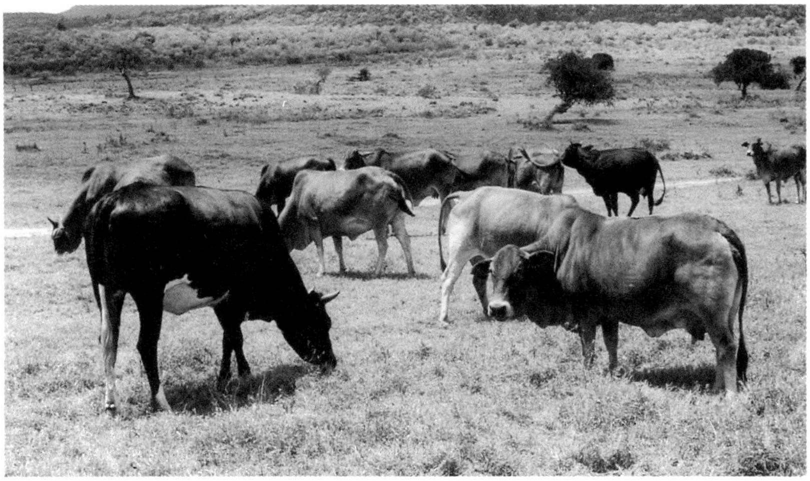

Fig. 6.6 Sahiwal and Sahiwal × Fresian cattle in Kenya.

scale intensive feedlots also has been attempted with the aim of drawing immature stock from the rural areas for finishing to produce improved quality beef. These initiatives have not usually been successful and small-scale finishing schemes will probably prove a more successful form of intensification in the future.

Beef may remain a byproduct of milk and draught power in Africa and Asia for the foreseeable future. It is appropriate therefore to focus research on ways of feeding and managing culled cows and oxen so as to maximize their value as meat animals.

In South America the situation is different and specialized high-quality ranch beef from extensive systems has found a ready market in America, Europe and the Far East for many years.

Management of dairy cows

The general objectives of management can be assumed to be broadly the same for all types of dairy cattle.

Ideally, dairy cows should produce a calf every year, since milk production is usually maximized with a 305-day lactation and yearly calving. Since gestation lengths vary between 275 and 287 days, it is necessary for the cow to conceive again within 80–90 days. First service should be at about 50 days after calving. This is seldom achieved in tropical systems, and calving intervals of up to 500 days occur. The main reason is a delayed return to oestrus due to poor nutrition, suckling and other stresses including those of climate and disease.

Artificial insemination is not widespread in the tropics, but in some countries, such as Kenya and Pakistan, insemination services have been operational for many years. The benefits of genetic improvement from AI are constrained by the problems of detecting oestrus. The achievement of optimum breeding patterns and milk production also depends on the provision of suitable environmental conditions and proper feeding.

A major objective of the management of dairy cows in the tropics should be the reduction or the spread of environmental heat load. This can be achieved in a number of ways.

1 Rations should be provided that do not exceed the optimum metabolizable energy (ME) plus crude protein (CP) concentrations.

2 Where possible animals should be grazed at night.

3 Concentrates should be fed early in the morning and late in the afternoon.

4 Adequate water should be provided.

5 Natural and constructed shade should be provided.

6 Buildings and shelters should be made of appropriate materials.

7 Houses and yards should be sited so as to take full advantage of prevailing winds.

8 Calving should occur in the coolest season, if nutrition allows.

9 Animals should be managed indoors wherever possible, so as to reduce muscular work.

10 Animals should be sprayed with water during the hottest periods to facilitate cooling.

The effect of adverse tropical environmental conditions can be overcome to a large extent if cost is not a constraint. In the Middle East, exotic breeds of dairy cattle are maintained in intensive systems and can achieve high milk yields per year (3000–4000 l). Ansell (1981) considers that the effects of high environmental temperatures can be counterbalanced by the factors listed above.

Tropical dairy houses can assist in this and should combine three essential components: they should be hygienic, airy and shaded so as to provide protection with least risk of disease spread. A number of designs exist that incorporate feeding and milking facilities in the stalls.

FEEDING

Dairy cows require higher levels of feeding than growing or working animals. Energy inputs for lactation may equal or even exceed maintenance requirements, though in the tropics requirements for lactation will not usually exceed maintenance. For a 300 kg cow producing 1000 l in a 300-day lactation, average daily metabolisable energy (ME) requirements will be approximately 30 MJ for maintenance and 15–20 MJ for lactation depending on the butterfat (BF) content of the milk. Such levels of milk production can be achieved by a number of rations and feeds can be combined according to their degradability, ME content and their CP content. Oliver (1971) has listed the combinations of feed-stuffs (wet weights) used in Zimbabwe as examples of the diets that may be effective (Table 6.4).

Other concentrate mixtures can be devised for different tropical regions based on a knowledge of locally available feeds such as groundnut cake, wheat bran, maize, oats/barley, green gram, tapioca, rice bran, urea, molasses and cottonseed.

HEALTH AND HYGIENE

The two prime considerations of dairy cow health are the need to maintain optimum milk production throughout lactation and optimum levels of fertility so that cows produce calves at regular intervals. In

Table 6.4 Diets for dairy cows using combinations of feedstuffs (from Oliver, 1971)

Feedstuff	Diet (kg wet weight)	
	360 kg cow	540 kg cow
	Diet 1	**Diet 2**
Legume hay (average)	1	1.6
Maize silage (average)	11	16
Grass hay (mature)	2	3.9
	Diet 3	**Diet 4**
Legume hay (average)	4	4
Maize silage (average)	18	27
Maintenance + 4 l	(5.0% BF)	(3.5% BF)
	Diet 5	**Diet 6**
Green lucerne (early flower)	11	3
Grass hay (average)	3.5	18
Maize silage (average)	9	4.5
Maintenance + 4 l	(5.0% BF)	(3.5% BF)

addition it is necessary to rear a healthy calf to weaning and to first calving. Attention must be given to a number of disease and general health problems.

Tick-borne infections, trypanosomiasis (Chapter 47), helminths and liver fluke (Chapter 17) are major problems in many areas, as is streptothricosis (see p. 688) in parts of Africa. Exotic animals are particularly susceptible to many of the endemic diseases.

Other conditions can be dealt with routinely by the farm manager. Adequate attention to disease prevention is of primary importance in the tropics, where veterinary services are often unavailable.

In hot climates it is better to milk at the cooler times of day. Milk cooling can present problems where constant electricity supplies are not present. Water supplies to local dairies are often poor and hygiene is therefore neglected. Utensils can be sun-dried to kill bacteria.

Management of beef production

RANCHING

In ranching systems both land and animals are under the control of the same management. This contrasts with pastoral systems where land is communally owned and animals are owned by individuals or groups of individuals.

Ranching can operate throughout a range of intensity levels. Extensive systems may involve a one-herd system with little or no monetary investment other than in the cattle. Intensification may involve one or more of the following stages.

1 Water development, e.g. boreholes or small dams.
2 Routine health care.
3 Mineral supplementation.
4 Construction of handling and dipping facilities.
5 Correct use of fire, e.g. creation of firebreaks.
6 Multiple herd systems, e.g. young stock, steer herds, etc.
7 Protein supplementation.
8 Fencing, e.g. perimeter and paddock.
9 Forage conservation.

The Government, parastatal and commercial companies have often involved themselves in ranching to intensify cattle production away from subsistence systems. The attempts have rarely been successful. The reasons have often been economic, arising from low meat prices and the high costs of intensification, which have rarely been justified.

An important aspect of ranch management is organizing routines. A routine approach means that the important husbandry tasks are designated to be carried out at particular times during the year. All concerned then know what should be done and when it should be carried out. Table 6.5 shows an example of a routine programme for a cattle ranch in East Africa. The programme of activities is determined by seasonal feed availability, which is determined by rainfall variations throughout the year.

SUPPLEMENTATION

Tropical cattle commonly suffer a period of weight loss during the dry season. Compensatory growth can overcome the worst effects, but feed supplementation may be feasible where it can be controlled. The practical approach should include the use of correct stocking rates, fire control, deferred grazing, seasonal control of breeding and tactical marketing. Once supplementation is accepted as a workable option two considerations arise: the nature of the supplement and the stock to be supplemented.

Nature of the supplementation

The supplement should improve the quality of the overall diet rather than act as a substitute for a part of

Table 6.5 Routine management programme for an East African cattle ranch

Month	Approximate monthly rainfall (mm)	Operation
December/January/February	110	Calving; ear tagging, weighing and recording
February	100	Check breeding bulls and cows; cull and replace
March	160	Improved nutrition for breeding bulls and cows (bulls throughout mating season)
March/April/May	140	Brand, castrate, dehorn last year's calves
April/May/June	110	Join breeding bulls to herd of breeding cows Sell marketable stock; steers, surplus heifers, culls
May/June	60	Supplementation of lactating cows Conserve forage
July	10	Remove bulls from breeding herd
July/August/September	10	Wean
August	10	Pregnancy diagnosis; remove non-pregnant stock

Under some circumstances a system with two 70-day breeding seasons at four month intervals can be applied and may improve annual calving percentage and economic returns.

that diet. The effective utilization of nitrogen supplementation in the form of urea mixed in a carrier such as molasses, depends upon there being a deficiency of degradable protein in the rumen. This is not always the case and the response to urea supplementation has not always been as predictable as anticipated.

Other forms of background supplement such as minerals are important over the long term, but have no effect on reducing dry-season weight losses. The possible exception is salt, which may serve to stimulate the intake of poor-quality roughage. In Nigeria, a naturally occurring and renewable mineral supplement known as Kanwa is fed to both settled and transhumant cattle owned by Fulani and agropastoralists. Kanwa contains 1.5 per cent Na, 4.7 per cent K, 23.7 per cent Ca, 0.6 per cent P and trace amounts of Mg, Fe, Mn, Cu, Co and Zn.

Increased attention is being paid to the potential of highly digestible cellulose as a supplement in the form of legume or browse material. Such material can stimulate cellulolytic bacteria and enable an improved utilization of the whole poor-quality diet. The importance of browse has been increasingly recognized as a component of tropical animal feed (Le Houerou, 1980). Browse usually contains over 10 per cent CP/unit DM and can often have as high as 25 per cent CP/unit DM. It thus forms a good supplement to poor-quality roughage.

Other forms of supplement in Nigeria include cottonseed cake, groundnut tops, cow pea, stalks, groundnut cake and also salt, chaff, bran, cut branches and cut grass. In Sudan some livestock owners in the Gezira area provide daily supplement mixtures containing cottonseed cake, groundnut cake, bran and molasses. Where breweries are nearby, brewers' grains may also be available.

Animals to supplement

Not all animals have the same need for supplementation and optimum use of resources can be achieved by identifying an order of priority, e.g. weaned calves, late pregnancy/early lactation cows, breeding heifers. Lowest priority will normally be given to growing steers.

Drought

Drought conditions represent a special case for supplementation where survival is the objective. An early difficulty is establishing that drought, as opposed to a long dry season, exists. When the fact is established a number of options are available: (i) do nothing; (ii) sell some stock and buy feed; (iii) sell all stock and restock later; or (iv) move animals to an area with grazing.

Where supplementation is adopted it is important not to start supplementing too soon, but to allow animals to lose some weight to reduce their maintenance requirements. Bovines have adaptive mechanisms for dealing with drought, one of which involves a reduction in metabolic rate. Such mechanisms should be activated prior to supplementation.

Animals at greatest risk and females required to continue the herd after the drought should be given priority for drought feeding. Once a decision has been taken to provide survival feeding the feedstuff is usually determined by cost and availability. Infrequent feeding of large amounts is probably preferred so as to ensure every targeted animal gets some feed. Survival watering also may be considered during droughts and will be related to feed and distances walked.

FEEDLOTS

Feedlots have been set up in different forms and for a wide variety of reasons; as large- or small-scale units, as commercial or government sponsored ventures to produce export quality carcasses as a means of reducing overgrazing of communal areas. Initial developments tended to follow the large-scale pattern of North American feedlots, but it is now recognized that small-scale projects that demand more labour than capital are often appropriate.

Certain circumstances are required before intensification becomes an economic strategy, as follows.

1 Beef is one of the most expensive meats within the country.
2 Animals are economically available for feeding on a continuing basis.
3 Above average quality feeds are economically available on a continuing basis.
4 Adequate initial funding is available.
5 Infrastructural factors such as transport, communications, husbandry and health services are available and adequate.
6 There is an absence of restrictive factors, e.g. butcher cartels or legal restrictions on export.

A failure to satisfy these requirements has led to the limited success of many feedlots. In 1972, Kenya had facilities to produce 30 000 head/annum, but the sys-

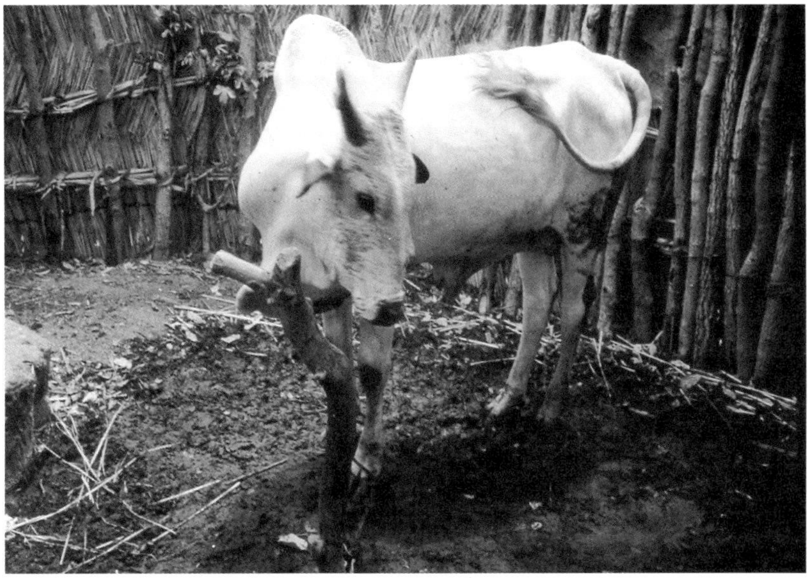

Fig. 6.7 Stall-fed fattening of Fulani cattle in Nigeria.

tem failed when maize prices increased and it proved impossible to maintain quarantine against foot-and-mouth disease.

SMALLHOLDER FATTENING

In Malawi a smallholder fattening project was started in 1957 and has now expanded to other parts of the country. It has proved to have many benefits, as follows.

1 Home-grown beef for the local market saving foreign exchange.

2 A means of saving for farmers, which can be used to invest in crop production.

3 The provision of manure for the maintenance of soil fertility.

4 Stabilization of the farming system by providing an employment opportunity.

The participating farmer must build a suitable stall for one or two animals, and farmers commonly build their stalls together. Farmers receive a credit steer of 260–280 kg with the assistance of the extension services. This is fed on maize stover, groundnut haulms and maize bran during the dry season and cut-and-carry Napier grass (*P. purpureum*) and/or Rhodes grass (*Chloris gayana*) during the rainy season. Average daily gain is about 0.5 kg and with approximately 200 days on feed total gains of 100 kg are achieved producing a final weight of 360–380 kg.

In Nigeria, stall feeding and fattening is also carried out and is a common method of cattle production in the subhumid zone and northern savannah areas (Fig. 6.7). Farmers often keep up to six animals, usually young bulls, for 18–24 months before selling them to urban traders. This method of production has been the subject of a major extension exercise by the National Livestock Projects Department in Nigeria, and has been of some success in Kano State where work bulls after 2–3 years are stall-fattened for 6–8 months and sold to butchers.

References

Anon. (1980) Ten years of animal production and range research in Botswana. Ministry of Agriculture, Private Bag 0033, Gaborone, Botswana, p. 31.

Ansell, R.H. (1981) Extreme heat stress in dairy cattle and its alleviation: a case report. In *Environmental Aspects of Housing for Animal Production* (ed. by J.A. Clarke), pp. 285–306. Butterworths, London.

Bessell, J.E. & Daplyn, M.G. (1976) Dairying in Zambia: The Commercial Sector UNGZAMI Bulletin No. 1. University of Nottingham, Department of Agriculture and Horticulture, pp. 35–58.

Botswana (1975) National Policy on Tribal Grazing Land. Government Paper No. 2 of 1975, pp. 1–18. Gaborone, Botswana.

Brinkman, W.L. (1971) Indoor and outdoor rearing of bucket-fed calves at Shika. *Samara Agricultural Newsletter*, **13**, 139–41.

Food and Agricultural Organization (1989) *Production Yearbook 42*, pp. 244–6, 253–5, 272–4.

Goldson, J.R. & Ndeda, J.O. (1985a) Cattle in Kenya. 1. Milk production. *Span*, **28**, 111–13.

Goldson, J.R. & Ndeda, J.O. (1985b). Cattle in Kenya. 2. Beef production. *Span*, **28**, 113–15.

Gupta, P.R. (1985) *Dairy India*, P.R. Gupta, New Delhi, India, p. 39.

Le Houerou, H.N. (1980) *Browse in Africa: The Current State of Knowledge*, International Livestock Centre for Africa, Addis Ababa, Ethiopia, pp. 3–491.

Macfarlane, J.S. & Worrall, K. (1970) Observations on the occurrence of puberty in *Bos indicus* heifers. *East African Agricultural and Forestry Journal*, **35**, 409–10.

Nicholson, M.J. & Butterworth, M.H. (1985) *A Guide to Condition Scoring of Zebu Cattle*, International Livestock Centre for Africa, Addis Ababa, Ethiopia, pp. 3–30.

Oliver, J. (1971) *An Introduction to Dairying in Zimbabwe*, Department of Agriculture, University of Zimbabwe, Harare, pp. 55–67.

Orskov, E.R. (1982) Voluntary intake of poor quality roughage by ruminants. In *Maximum Livestock Production from Minimum Land, Proceedings of the Third Seminar held in Bangladesh, 15–18 February, 1982*, Bangladesh Agricultural Research Institute, Joydebpur, Bangladesh, pp. 72–6.

Otsyina, R.M., von Kaufman, R.R., Mohamed Saleem, M.A. & Suleiman, H. (1987) *Manual on Fodder Bank Establishment and Management*, International Livestock Centre for Africa, Addis Ababa, Ethiopia, pp. 8–12.

Preston, T.R. (1977) A strategy for cattle production in the tropics. *World Animal Review*, **21**, 1–17.

Pullen, N.B. (1978) Condition scoring of White Fulani Cattle. *Tropical Animal Health and Production*, **10**, 118–20.

Sere, C.R. (1983) Classification of milk production systems in tropical South America: A first approximation. *Tropical Animal Production*, **8**, 99–110.

Weniger, J.H. (1983) Beef and dairy ranching in Latin America. *Animal Research and Development*, **17**, 118–26.

Wilson R.T. & Clark, S.E. (1976) Studies on the livestock of Southern Darfur, Sudan. II. Production traits of cattle. *Tropical Animal Health and Production*, **8**, 47–57.

Chapter 7: Nutrition

by J.M. WILKINSON

Introduction

The bovine animal, along with the other ruminants, depends very heavily on its symbiotic relationship with the microbial population of the rumen. Thus any consideration of the nutrition of the bovine must be focused on the rumen as the most important part of the bovine digestive system. The fermentation in the rumen is geared to the degradation of plant cell walls, of which the most abundant constituent is cellulose. This adaptation to plant cell wall digestion, in addition to cell content degradation places the ruminant and the bovine in an important strategic position relative to other animals.

Van Soest (1982) classified cattle feeding habits as being one of grazing fresh grass, rather than browsing trees and shrubs. Cattle have a greater need for water than other ruminants, possibly because they retain fibre for relatively long periods in the rumen and a high water content, typically around 90 per cent, is essential for optimal bacterial activity.

The bovine is a relatively unselective eater compared with the other ruminants. This may be a disadvantage when tree and shrub leaves are abundant at a time when pasture supply is scarce because of drought. But the bovine can and does browse, and given an excess of food supply over consumption, selective eating does occur.

In temperate regions of the world, a constant supply of feed throughout the year is achieved by preserving excess herbage growth as hay or as silage. This activity, coupled with the production of root crops specifically for use when grass growth is slow or non-existent, has transformed the annual cycle of production from one which was totally dependent on grass growth to one which is not. Thus beef cattle, for example, no longer lose weight in the winter when grass is scarce, but are able to maintain or even increase in weight on a winter diet of hay, silage or stored root crops. The development of the food and drink industry has released a wide range of byproducts, such as bran from flour milling and spent grains from the brewing of beer and the production of spirits, which plays a vital role in the nutrition of the bovine when grazed grass is in short supply.

A remaining challenge in bovine nutrition is to achieve a similar constancy of feed supply to the bovine populations of those areas of the world where drought is common, and where the technology of feed preservation and byproduct utilization is less well developed.

In this chapter, the fermentation in the rumen is described, with particular emphasis on the kinetics of the process and its interaction with feed intake. Requirements for energy and protein are considered. The composition of feeds is outlined, together with technologies for feed preservation and feed processing. Finally, the management of the feeding of the bovine is outlined in relation to maintaining stability in the rumen, maximizing intake, and meeting requirements for high levels of productivity.

Fermentation in the rumen

The bovine animal relies very heavily on the reactions that occur in the rumen for its supply of major nutrients. Thus on a sole diet of grazed grass some 90 per cent of the animal's total energy and protein supply is derived directly from the rumen micro-organisms and the endproducts of their metabolism.

Therefore, the importance of maintaining optimal conditions for fermentation cannot be overstressed; apart from acute disorders such as bloat, the animal's whole digestive economy revolves around the rumen, especially when cellulosic feeds such as grazed herbage, hay or silage form the major part of the diet.

This symbiotic relationship between the micro-organisms of the rumen and the host animal has been crucial to the survival of the bovine, since the animal itself cannot digest cellulose without the help of its microbial population. In the wild, surrounded by foliage and limited supplies of feeds containing starch or sugar, the bovine's fermentation of plant cell wall material secured not only the supply of energy, but also a vital supply of microbial protein. The ruminant has evolved a nutritional niche whereby it is independent of external sources of amino acids and B vitamins — a considerable advantage when grass is the only feed available.

Saliva

Feeds are chewed during eating and also regurgitated during rumination to allow very thorough mastication. Throughout these activities large quantities of saliva are mixed with food. The effect of saliva is to buffer the acids that are produced in the rumen as a result of fermentation. This buffering is vital to the maintenance of the correct type of fermentation, and can even prevent the collapse of normal rumen function in extreme situations.

The principal buffering constituent of saliva is bicarbonate. It has been estimated that a dairy cow may produce up to 3.5 kg/day of bicarbonate. Clearly, the need for adequate buffering is more important if the diet is rapidly fermented than if it is only slowly fermented. Further, if the diet is acidic, as in the case of silage, it is essential that salivary secretion is sufficient to prevent a build-up of excessive acidity in the rumen or in blood.

It follows that feeds which stimulate rumination are more useful to the maintenance of optimal conditions for fermentation in the rumen than those which do not. Unfortunately, rapidly fermented feeds such as molasses and ground cereal grains do not stimulate rumination. At the other extreme, straws are chewed extensively to break down the fibre; they are also fermented relatively slowly in the rumen. Hence a compromise with respect to saliva production is required; fibre is required together with concentrated feed sources in order that saliva output is maintained.

The actions of micro-organisms

The major organisms responsible for digestion in the rumen are anaerobic bacteria and protozoa, though anaerobic fungi are thought to be responsible for much of the initial colonization of feed particles in the rumen. The cellulolytic bacteria adhere to particles of fibrous feeds and secrete enzymes that gradually erode out the

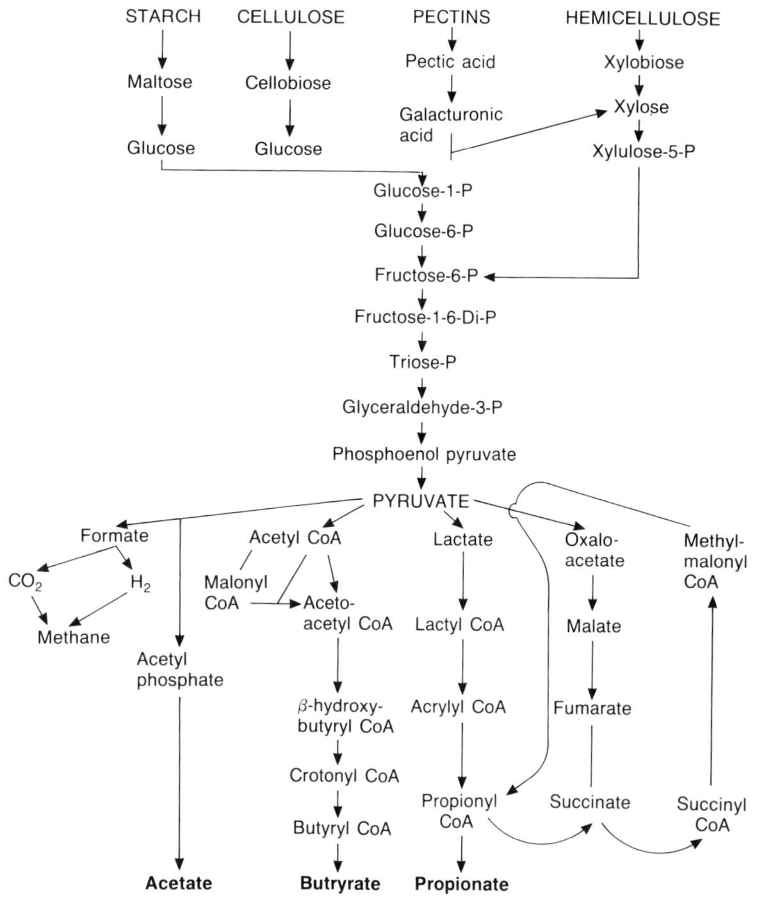

Fig. 7.1 Chemistry of rumen fermentation.

digestible material. Their enzymes break down hemicellulose and cellulose to glucose and fructose. Starch and pectins are also similarly degraded (Fig. 7.1). In the case of cell wall, this erosion continues until lignified tissue is encountered. Lignin, which is cross-linked to cellulose, provides structural strength to the plant; it is also very resistant to bacterial enzymic attack.

The protozoa in the rumen mainly ferment starch and sugar, but they also consume bacteria. The protozoa are thought to be active is assisting the bacterial population in adapting to new feeds.

The endproducts of bacterial digestion are short-chain acids acetic, proprionic and butyric (the volatile fatty acids, VFA), microbial cells (and their constituent protein), and the gases methane and carbon dioxide. Methane comprises the major gaseous energy loss as a result of fermentation. Gas is lost by eructation whilst the VFA are mainly absorbed through the rumen wall.

The common types of rumen micro-organisms and their actions are summarized in Table 7.1.

Fermentation of different types of feed

The fermentation of plant cell walls is optimal at relatively high rumen pH (i.e. around pH 7.0) because the bacteria responsible are sensitive to excess acidity. Their growth is depressed if rumen pH falls below about pH 6.2. The principal endproduct of cellulose fermentation is acetate, an important precursor of milk fat.

Starch and surgar are fermented to give propionic and butyric acids as the main endproducts. The micro-organisms responsible for their fermentation are more tolerant of acidity than those which ferment cell wall. One species of bacteria (*Selenomonas ruminantium*) produces lactic acid, a stronger acid than the VFA. Large amounts of lactic acid can predispose the animal to rumen stasis and to acidosis (see p. 634).

Protein is fermented to yield ammonia, and VFA from the carbon skeletons of amino acids. The ammonia may be used by bacteria to synthesize new protein in their cells, but since bacterial growth is generally

Table 7.1 Common types of rumen micro-organisms and their action

Species	Energy source	Fermentation products	Requirements
Bacteria			
Bacteroides			
amylophilus	Starch	F, A, S	CO_2, NH_3, BrVFA
succinogenes	Cellulose	F, A, S	CO_2, NH_3, BrVFA, SVFA, Vit.
Ruminococcus			
albus	Cellulose, xylan	F, A, E, H_2, CO_2	BrVFA, CO_2, NH_3, Vit.(A)
flavefaciens	Cellulose, xylan	F, A, S, H_2	
Butyrivibrio			
fibrosolvens	Xylan, starch	F, A, B, L, H_2, CO_2	BrVFA, A, CO_2, NH_3, Vit.(A)
Lachnospira			
multiparus	Pectin	F, A, L, E, H_2, CO_2, A, Vit.	
Selenomonas			
ruminantium	Lactate, starch	A, P, L, CO_2, H_2	A(CO_2)
Methanobacterium			
ruminantium	Formate, H_2	Methane	A,BrVFA, Haem, CO_2, NH_3
Protozoa			
Holotrichs			
Isotricha	Starch and sugars	A, B, L, H_2	
Dasytricha	Starch and sugars	A, B, L, H_2	
Entodiniomorphs			
Entodinium	Starch	F, A, P, B, (L)	
Epidinium	Starch, hemicell.	A, B, H_2, (F, P, L)	
Ophryoscolex	Starch	A, B, H_2, (P)	
Diplodinium			
Eudiplodinium		H_2, fatty acids	
Polyplastron			

Symbols: F, formate; A, acetate; P, propionate; B, butyrate; BrVFA, branched-chain VFAs; E, ethanol; L, lactate; S, succinate; SVFA, straight-chain VFAs; Vit., B vitamins.

limited by the energy available from carbohydrate digestion, rather than from protein digestion, ammonia in excess of microbial requirements can easily be produced, especially on high-protein diets. Excess ammonia is converted, at an energy cost, to urea in the liver, and excreted in urine. A deficit of ammonia in the rumen slows down bacterial growth, reduces rate of digestion and depresses feed intake. Thus it is important that the rate of release of ammonia matches as closely as possible the release of energy (Figure 7.2).

Actual and potential digestion

Fibre that has been reduced to particle size at which it can pass out of the rumen, and which has also resisted being digested by microbial activity, is liable to pass on down the tract and out in the faeces. The rate of passage out of the rumen can influence the extent to which fibrous particles are actually digested; the faster the rate of passage, the lower the actual, relative to the potential, digestibility.

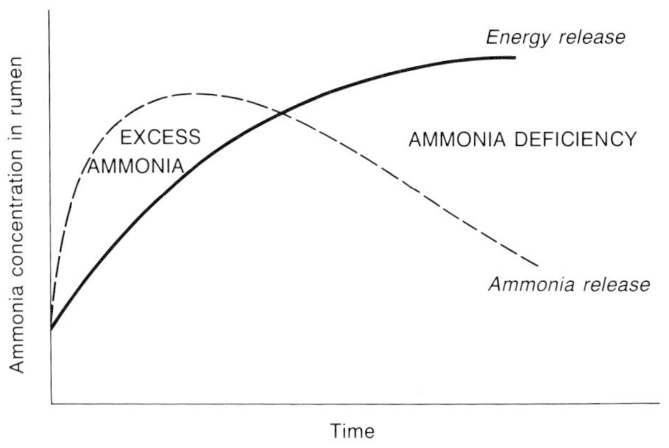

Fig. 7.2 Typical patterns for the rates of release in the rumen of ammonia from the breakdown of protein, and of energy, following a meal. The rate of ammonia release should match as closely as possible that of energy, either by reducing the amount of quickly degraded protein in the diet, or by increasing the quantity of readily-fermentable energy (e.g. starch or sugar) in the diet.

The same concept applies to protein, especially that fraction which is available for microbial fermentation in the rumen (see Table 7.12). Thus a high-yielding dairy cow, given a high-quality diet with a fast rate of passage of feed through the rumen, will have a relatively lower fibre digestibility than a dry cow given less of the same diet, or a diet of lower energy content. But the protein in the diet of the high-yielding cow will have a lower digestibility in the rumen, yield less ammonia, and provide more undegraded protein to the abomasum, than that in the dry cow's diet.

Paradoxically, the lower the actual, relative to potential, digestibility in the rumen, the worse off the animal is with respect to energy, but the better off it is likely to be with respect to protein.

Optimizing digestion in the rumen

It follows from the above discussion that the following principles need to be adopted in order to optimize the fermentation in the rumen.

1 Cell wall is the principal source of digestible energy in the diet of the bovine, and conditions in the rumen should be optimal for its digestion.

2 Sufficient saliva must be produced to maintain rumen pH above 6.5, otherwise cell wall digestion will be reduced.

3 Adequate protein must be supplied to meet the requirements for microbial protein synthesis (see section on protein requirements p. 84).

4 Supplementary energy in the form of starch or sugar must not interfere with the maintenance of the above conditions in the rumen (see section on feeding management, p. 93).

When cell wall digestion is optimized, then feed intake is likely to be maximal, at least with respect to fibrous feeds.

Feed intake

Most diets for cattle are offered in excess of the amount the animal actually consumes, though there are situations where the amount of feed offered each day is restricted intentionally. Two such situations are readily apparent: the dry cow and the suckler cow in late lactation. Both situations require that the animal does not overeat and become excessively fat.

The concept of voluntary feed intake is discussed in this section, i.e. the amount of feed the animal will eat when offered an excess supply so that about 10–15 per cent of the daily amount offered is refused.

Is feed intake under control?

The fact that cattle can become overfat suggests that feed intake is under relatively imprecise control. Equally, sparse availability of range pastures or the provision of very low quality roughages as the sole feeds can lead to inadequate levels of feed intake and chronic undernutrition. The animal can suffer from deprivation because it is unable to ingest, or digest, enough nutrients daily to meet its requirements for maintenance of body weight.

Nevertheless, there is evidence that cattle eat to satisfy their demand for energy to maintain weight and produce tissue growth or milk. The generalized relationship (Fig. 7.3) between the energy content of the

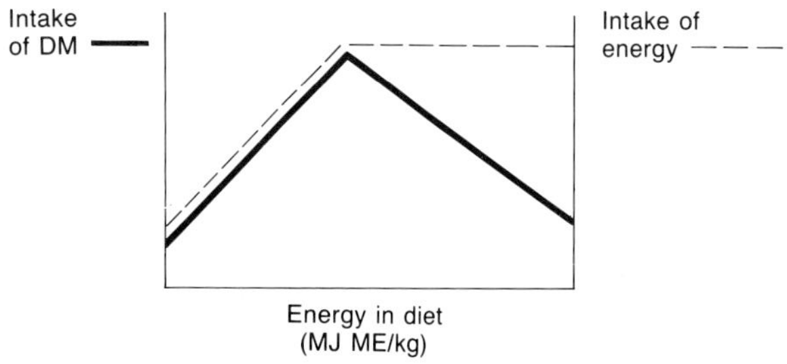

Fig. 7.3 Simplified relationship between the energy content of the diet and feed intake. As the energy content of the diet increases, dry matter intake will increase until it reaches a maximum. If energy content increases further, dry matter intake is reduced because metabolic factors, rather than the bulk, or 'fill', of the diet now control intake.

diet and dry matter intake suggests that signals received by the brain when the animal's energy needs are met, in turn elicit the response to cease eating.

Concentrates

With concentrates, satiety occurs long before the capacity of the rumen is reached. Intake is determined by the animal's capacity to metabolize nutrients. Enhanced metabolism, for example following the administration of somatotrophin, is reflected in increased feed consumption — at least on high-energy diets where physical limitations do not apply.

Roughages

With roughage feeds the volume of the rumen usually restricts intake. Thus intake is proportional to the volume of the rumen — the larger the rumen, the more feed is consumed. Larger animals eat more than smaller animals because their rumen volumes are greater.

Rumen capacity

Animals with large rumen capacities relative to their total body weight will eat more roughages than those with relatively smaller rumen volumes. The implications of this feature are that calves should be reared on diets that encourage rumen development, and cattle should be selected for large rumen capacities.

Digestibility of forages

Digestibility of forage feeds exerts an enormous influence on feed intake (Fig. 7.4). But the relationship between intake and digestibility is imprecise for silages, where the pattern of fermentation in the silo can have an overriding influence on intake.

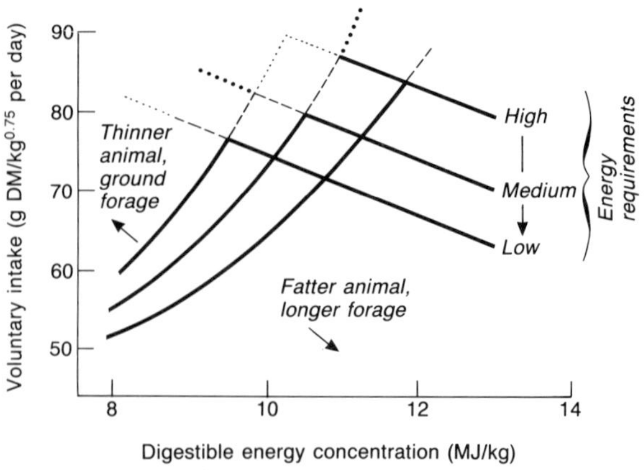

Fig. 7.4 Composite diagram of the relationships between intake and animal and feed factors in ruminants. At any given energy content, intake is higher for cows that have a greater requirement for energy (or potential milk production). Also, intake of dry matter is greater the thinner the cow, and the smaller the particle size of the feed. From Forbes (1938).

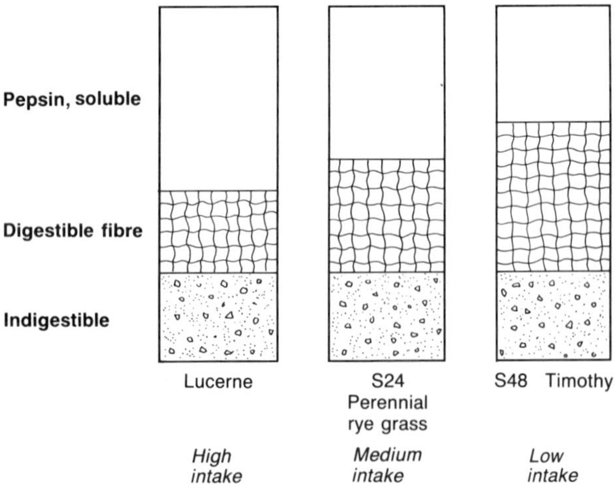

Fig. 7.5 Variations in the ratio of material soluble in acid pepsin (cell contents) to digestible fibre (cell wall) in three forages of same digestibility, but differing in intake. From Osbourn (1967).

Speed of digestion

Speed of digestion also has an important influence on intake, since it determines the length of time the feed remains in the rumen. Legumes are digested at a faster rate than grasses of the same overall digestibility partly because they contain less cell wall than grasses (Fig. 7.5). Also, the structure of the cell walls of legumes enables bacteria to gain access more rapidly than with grasses.

The cell contents of forages are fermented very quickly in the rumen, provided they are released by eating and by rumination. For example, young grass may contain up to 40 per cent of its dry matter in the form of cell contents, principally sugars, and in this regard it is nearer to a concentrate in terms of its speed of digestion in the rumen.

Cell walls are generally fermented at a slower rate than cell contents. The actual rate of cell wall digestion depends on initial particle size, the extent to which it is broken down by rumination, and the extent to which it may be lignified. Three feeds with the same potential digestibility but different speeds of digestion are represented in Fig. 7.6. The feed with the fastest speed of

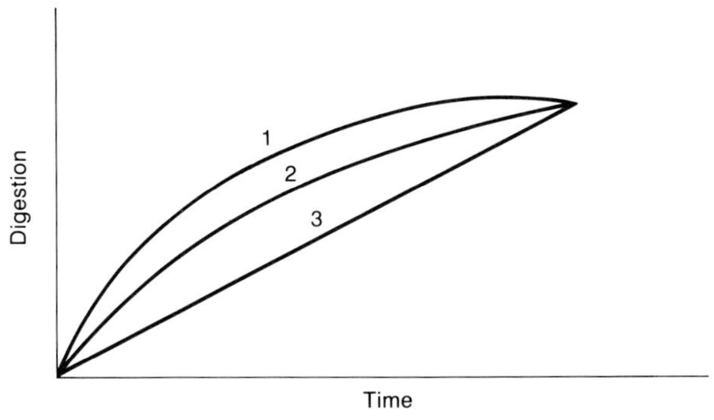

Fig. 7.6 Three feeds with the same potential digestibility but different speeds of digestion. The animal will eat most of feed 1 and least of feed 3. From Orskov (1987).

digestion will be eaten in the greatest amount by the animal.

Grazed pasture

Unlike indoor feeding, grazing animals select what they eat to a considerable extent, particularly when the herbage on offer is heterogeneous and is offered in excess of consumption. Thus a measure of the digestibility of the herbage on offer is of little use as an indicator of intake, since the animal will usually be able to select material of higher digestibility than the average of that on offer.

Herbage intake under grazing is predominantly influenced by the amount on offer. To achieve maximum intake, the amount on offer should exceed that actually consumed by three to four times (Figs 7.7 and 7.8).

Intake is usually expressed relative to liveweight, and it follows that the amount of herbage on offer should be expressed *per kilogram liveweight* rather than *per hectare*. It follows that stocking rate, a commonly used but empirical and inflexible way of describing herbage allowance, should not be expressed as *number* of animals per hectare, but as *kilograms liveweight* per

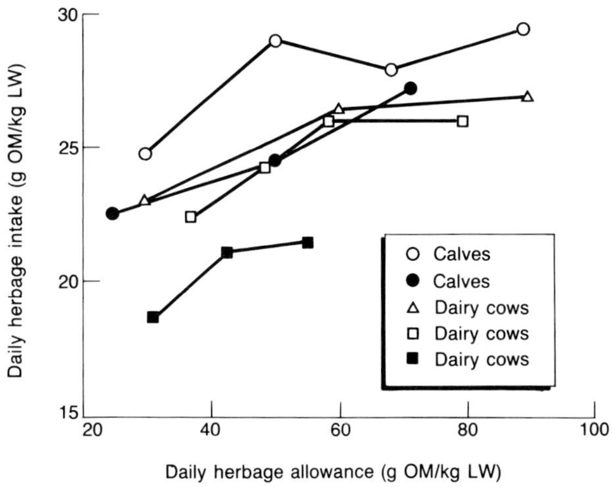

Fig. 7.8 Relationship between daily herbage allowance and herbage intake in cattle. (Data from different studies.) From Hodgson (1975).

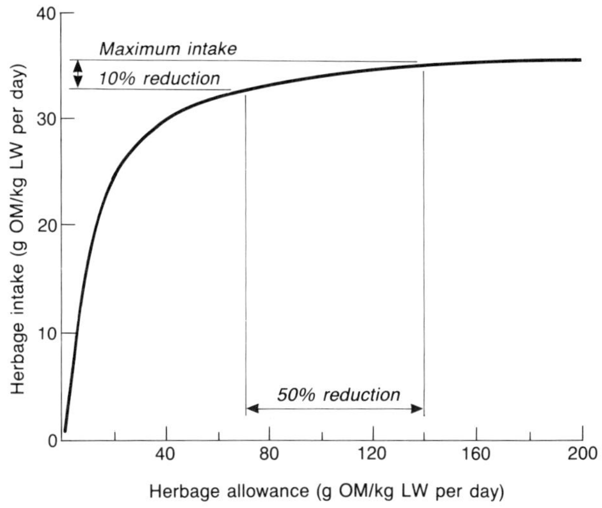

Fig. 7.7 Relationship between daily herbage allowance and herbage intake in grazing lambs. From Hodgson (1975).

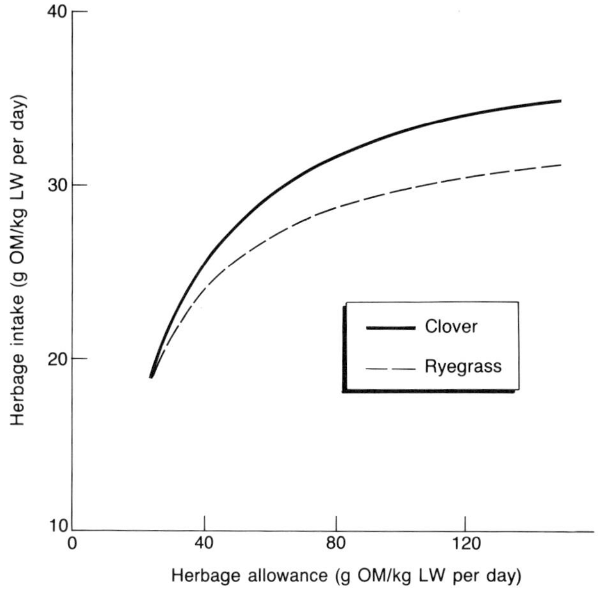

Fig. 7.9 Herbage intake of lambs grazing perennial ryegrass and red clover. From Gibb and Treacher (1978).

Table 7.2 Dry matter intake of growing cattle (kg/day). Source: Agricultural Research Council (ARC) (1980)

Type of diet	Metabolizability of dietary energy (q)*	Liveweight (kg)					
		100	200	300	400	500	600
Coarse	0.4	2.1	3.5	4.8	6.0	7.1	8.1
	0.5	2.4	4.1	5.6	6.9	8.2	9.4
	0.6	2.8	4.7	6.3	7.9	9.3	10.7
	0.7	3.1	5.2	7.1	8.8	10.4	12.0
Fine	0.5	3.0	5.0	6.7	8.4	9.9	11.3
	0.6	2.8	4.7	6.4	7.9	9.4	10.8
	0.7	2.7	4.5	6.1	7.5	8.9	10.2
For each 10% of concentrates in the diet increase intake as follows:							
Increase (kg/day)		0.12	0.20	0.27	0.33	0.39	0.45

* See p. 83.

hectare (see section on feeding management, p. 93).

The relationship between herbage allowance and intake holds for animals in different physiological states, and for legumes as well as grasses (Fig. 7.9).

Probable levels of intake

Probable levels of dry matter intake for growing and lactating cattle are shown in Tables 7.2 and 7.3. The relative intake of cows given the same diet throughout lactation, expressed as a percentage of the mean for the whole lactation, is shown in Table 7.4. The important feature in Table 7.4 is the relatively low intake in the first month of lactation, when the demand for nutrients for milk production is at its highest.

Table 7.3 Probable dry matter intake of cows in mid and late lactation (kg/day). From Ministry of Agriculture, Fisheries and Food (MAFF) (1984)

Liveweight (W) (kg)	Milk yield (Y) (kg/day)							
	5	10	15	20	25	30	35	40
350	9.3	9.8	10.3	10.8	11.3	11.8		
400	10.5	11.0	11.5	12.0	12.5	13.0		
450	11.8	12.3	12.8	13.3	13.8	14.3	14.8	
500	13.0	13.5	14.0	14.5	15.0	15.5	16.0	
550	14.3	14.8	15.3	15.8	16.3	16.8	17.3	17.8
600	15.5	16.0	16.5	17.0	17.5	18.0	18.5	19.0
650	16.8	17.3	17.8	18.3	18.8	19.3	19.8	20.3
700	18.0	18.5	19.0	19.5	20.0	20.5	21.0	21.5

Note: In the first 6 weeks of lactation, reduce these values by 2–3 kg DMI/day.
Based on DMI (kg/day) = $0.025\ W + 0.1\ Y$.

Table 7.4 Relative intake of dairy cows fed on the same diet throughout lactation (daily intake per cent of mean intake for complete lactation). From ARC (1980)

Month	Relative intake	Month	Relative intake
1	81	6	108
2	98	7	101
3	107	8	99
4	108	9	97
5	109	10	93

Energy requirements

The concept of requirements

The concept of requirements for energy (and indeed for protein or for any particular nutrient) is currently undergoing major review. A series of Agricultural and Food Research Council (AFRC) Technical Committees on Responses to Nutrients (TCORN) has been established to review the response of livestock to nutrients, and their reports are awaited.

The major reason for reviewing requirements is that a requirement is only valid with respect to a specified level of output. The defined output may or may not be valid in the first place, or remain valid once established. There is often a need to answer the question 'What if?', thereby begging the question of how the animal might respond to changes in the supply of a particular nutrient, e.g. energy.

The establishment of the TCORN committees represents a major change in attitude in nutritional science, from determining requirements for unit levels of production to describing responses to a range of nutrient inputs.

Requirements and allowances

The notion of requirements takes no account of the variation between animals when kept in groups. Hence, if a group is given enough feed to meet the mean requirement for a given performance, a proportion of the group will be underfed, and a proportion will be overfed. Since underfeeding is considered to be the more serious failure of the system, allowances are made so that only a small proportion of the group remains underfed. If, as is the case with beef cattle, the metabolizable energy system of assessing requirements overpredicts performance, an additional increment (15 per cent) is added on to account for this inaccuracy. The result (Fig. 7.10) is that allowances may exceed requirements by some 30 per cent.

Partition of feed energy

The proportion of the gross energy (GE) of a feed that is absorbed by the animal depends on its digestibility. The amount remaining for metabolism (metabolizable energy, ME) is the digested energy less energy lost as methane or in urine. Further heat losses occur as a result of metabolism; the remaining energy (the net energy) is that which is available to the animal for maintenance of body weight, for weight gain, or for milk production. The partitioning is show diagrammatically in Fig. 7.11.

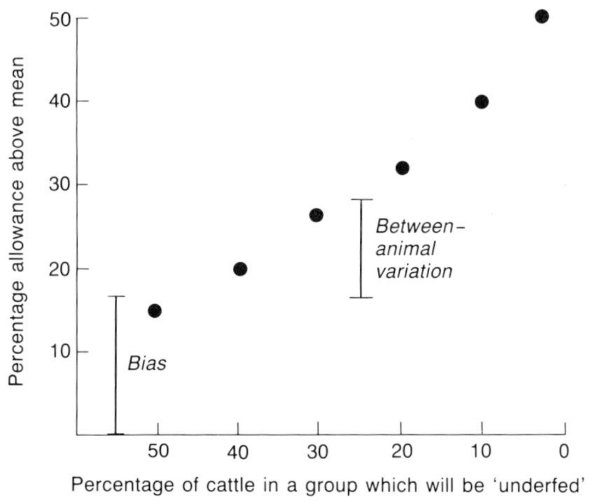

Fig. 7.10 Estimated allowances above mean requirements (ARC, 1980) required to meet the ME needs of a defined proportion of beef cattle in a group. Additional allowance due to bias in the estimate of requirements is shown separately from that due to estimated between-animal variation. Source: *Energy Group Report* (1988) Inter-Departmental Working Party.

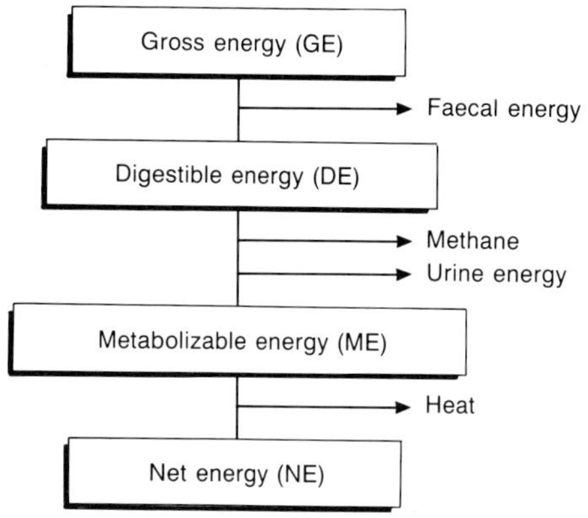

Fig. 7.11 Partition of energy.

In calculating energy requirements, the term 'metabolizability' (q) is used. This is an expression of ME/GE, where GE is usually about 18.4 MJ/kg dry matter (DM) for conventional feeds.

Efficiency of use of ME

The proportion of ME actually used for maintenance and production depends on the efficiency with which it is utilized by the animal (k). This depends on q, the level of feeding above maintenance, and on the productive purpose for which the energy is to be used. Thus for cattle, k for maintenance (k_m) varies as shown in Fig. 7.12.

For lactation (k_l), efficiency is more constant, and a value of 0.62 is used for most normal feeding situations.

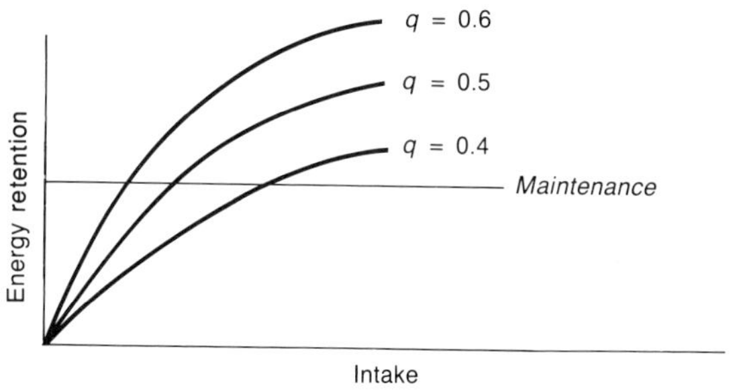

Fig. 7.12 Efficiency of use of ME for maintenance (k_m) is relatively high at 0.7. At twice the maintenance energy intake (common level for growing animals) efficiency of use of ME for growth (k_g) = 0.3 to 0.5 for diets ranging from q = 0.4 to q = 0.6; k_g declines further at higher levels of energy intake and correction must be made for the curvilinear decline.

Requirements

For growing cattle, a variable net energy system has been adopted to take account of the fact that k_m varies with q. The system involves assessing the *animal production level* (APL), which depends on the weight of the animal and the desired level of weight gain, the *net energy allowance* for the particular animal and level of gain, and the *net energy value* of a feed, which depends on its ME content and the particular APL. The relevant information is shown in Tables 7.5, 7.6 and 7.7. For two ingredient rations, a Pearson Square is used to solve the simultaneous equations to derive the amount of each feed required in the diet (see example in Table 7.8).

For lactation the situation is less complex, since k_l is assumed not to vary with q.

A summary of ME requirements for lactation is shown in Table 7.9.

Protein requirements

Traditionally, protein requirements were expressed as *digestible crude protein* (DCP), that is, the proportion of the *crude protein* (CP, or N × 6.25) that is apparently digestible and therefore available to the animal. It is now recognized that DCP is totally inadequate as a system for assessing the protein requirements of ruminants.

The concept of digestible crude protein ignored the fact that a proportion of the digestible protein is degraded to ammonia by the action of the rumen microflora. Some of this ammonia is synthesized into microbial protein in the rumen; the rest is absorbed into the bloodstream, converted to urea in the liver, and excreted in the urine.

Table 7.5 Net energy allowances for maintenance and production (MJ/day). From MAFF (1975)

Liveweight (kg)	Liveweight gain (kg/day)					
	0.25	0.50	0.75	1.00	1.25	1.50
100	14.7	17.4	20.7	24.6		
200	21.6	25.0	29.0	33.9	39.9	
300	28.6	32.6	37.3	43.1	50.2	
400	35.5	40.1	45.6	52.3	65.8	77.0
500	42.4	47.7	53.9	61.5	70.9	82.9

Table 7.6 Values for animal production level (APL). From MAFF (1975)

Liveweight (kg)	Liveweight gain (kg/day)					
	0.25	0.50	0.75	1.00	1.25	1.50
100	1.19	1.40	1.66	1.98		
200	1.15	1.33	1.54	1.79	2.11	
300	1.13	1.29	1.47	1.70	1.97	2.33
400	1.12	1.26	1.43	1.64	1.90	2.22
500	1.11	1.25	1.41	1.60	1.84	2.15

Table 7.7 Net energy values of feeds for maintenance and production. From MAFF (1975)

APL	Energy concentration in feed (MJ ME/kg DM)						
	8	9	10	11	12	13	14
	Net energy value (NE/kg DM)						
1.00	5.8	6.5	7.2	7.9	8.6	9.4	10.1
1.10	5.2	6.0	6.8	7.6	8.3	9.1	9.9
1.15	5.1	5.8	6.6	7.4	8.2	9.0	9.8
1.20	4.9	5.7	6.5	7.3	8.1	8.9	9.8
1.30	4.6	5.4	6.3	7.1	7.9	8.8	9.7
1.40	4.4	5.2	6.1	6.9	7.9	8.8	9.7
1.50	4.2	5.1	5.9	6.8	7.7	8.6	9.5
1.75	3.9	4.8	5.6	6.5	7.4	8.4	9.3
2.00	3.8	4.6	5.4	6.3	7.3	8.2	9.2
2.25	3.6	4.4	5.3	6.2	7.1	8.1	9.1

Table 7.8 Example of feed requirements for a 300 kg steer growing at 0.7 kg/day on silage (ME 10) and barley (ME 13)

1. Dry matter intake (simplified), $0.02\,W = 6$ kg/day
2. Net energy for M + LWG (from Table 7.5), 35.5 MJ/day
3. Animal production level (from Tables 7.6), 1.46
4. Net energy values of feeds (from $\frac{NE_m + NE_p}{ME_{mp}}$ or Table 7.7)

   Silage ME 10 = 5.9 MJ/kg
   Barley ME 13 = 8.6 MJ/kg
5. Energy concentration in ration, $NE_{mp}/DMI = \frac{35.5}{6} = 6.23$ MJ/kg
6. Pearson Square to calculate ration:

```
Barley 8.6        0.3   0.3/2.7 × 6 = 0.67 kg barley DM
             \   /
              6.2
             /   \
Silage 5.9        2.4   2.4/2.7 × 6 = 5.33 kg silage DM
                  ---
                  2.7
```

7. Divide by DM, 0.67/0.85 = 0.8 kg fresh barley
   5.33/0.25 = 21.3 kg fresh silage

Table 7.9 Summary of energy requirements of dairy cows. From MAFF (1975, 1984, 1986a)

Maintenance allowances (ME_m), including activity allowance and safety margin
$ME_m = 8.3 + 0.091W$ (from MAFF, 1975) where W = liveweight (kg)
ME_m = 63–67 MJ for cows 600–650 kg liveweight

Milk production (ME milk)
ME for milk = 5.3 MJ/kg (4% fat, 3.2% protein)
Based on ME milk (MJ/kg) = $[(0.376 \times \%\ \text{fat} + 0.209 \times \%\ \text{protein}) + 0.946] \times 1.694$

Adjustments to allow for weight gain or weight loss
add 34 MJ ME/kg weight gain
deduct 28 MJ ME/kg weight loss

Whilst there are some situations where the animal's requirements can be met entirely by microbial protein, there are others where the animal requires more protein than that supplied by the microbial cells and it is necessary to supply additional dietary protein to the abomasum that has not been broken down *en route* through the rumen.

Thus it became necessary to distinguish between rumen degradable and undegraded protein, both when assessing requirements, and also when assessing the composition of feeds.

The action of the ruminal microbial population

A proportion of the protein in feeds is broken down to amino acids and ammonia by the action of the rumen microbial population. Ammonia, small peptides and amino acids are used to resynthesize microbial protein. Low-producing animals, such as suckler cows, can rely totally on microbial protein to meet their requirements for *tissue protein* (TP). Their diet may contain supplementary *non-protein nitrogen* (NPN), usually in the form of urea, as the sole source of additional N in the diet. On the other hand, high-yielding cows and rapidly growing beef calves have a greater TP requirement than can be met by microbial protein (MP), and extra *undegraded dietary protein* (UDP) is necessary.

The total protein supply to the animal's small intestine is therefore a mixture of MP and UDP.

Degradation of protein in the rumen

The digestion and metabolism of dietary protein in the rumen is shown in simplified form in Fig. 7.13. Dietary

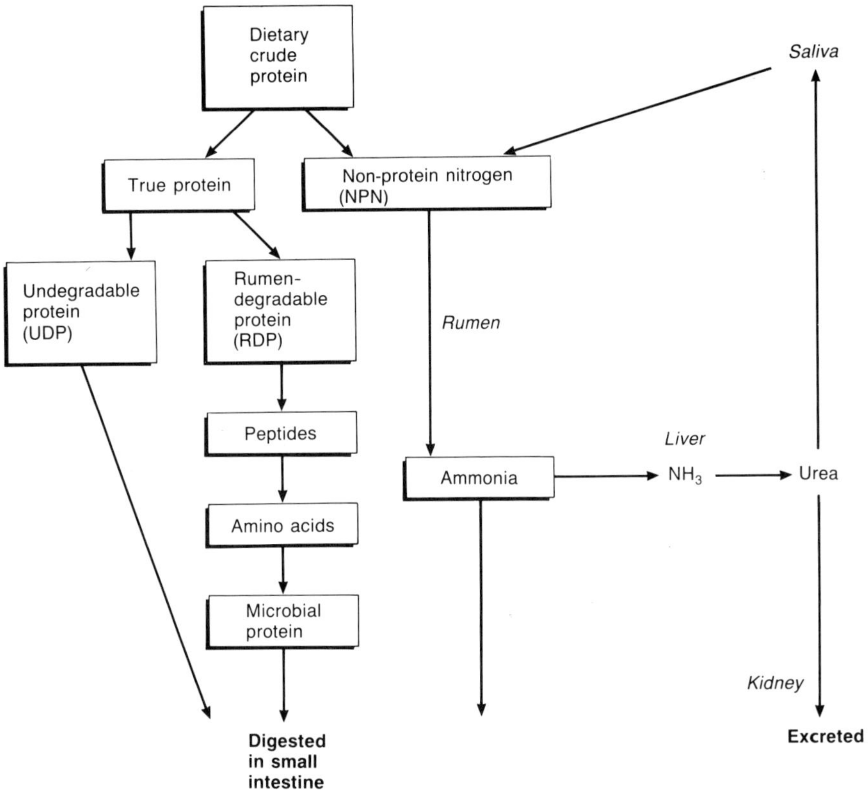

Fig. 7.13 Digestion and metabolism of nitrogenous compounds in the rumen.

Table 7.10 Amino acid composition of bacterial protein and animal proteins (g amino acid/100 g protein)

Amino acid	Microbial protein	Milk	Beef
Isoleucine	5.8	5.6	5.1
Leucine	8.0	10.2	8.0
Lysine	9.2	8.2	9.1
Methionine	2.5	2.9	2.7
Cysteine	1.4	1.0	1.3
Phenylalanine	5.3	5.4	4.5
Tyrosine	4.9	4.5	3.8
Threonine	5.7	5.0	4.6
Tryptophan	1.5	1.4	1.3
Valine	5.8	7.4	5.3
Arginine	5.3	4.0	6.7
Histidine	2.1	3.0	3.7
Alanine	6.8	3.8	6.4
Aspartic acid	11.9	8.5	9.6
Glutamic acid	12.4	23.0	17.3
Glycine	5.4	2.2	5.6
Proline	3.6	9.4	5.1
Serine	4.7	5.9	4.5

crude protein (N × 6.25) contains true protein and NPN. Urea, recycled to the rumen in saliva, is produced in the liver from absorbed ammonia, which is in excess to that used by the microbial population of the rumen to synthesize MP. The amino acid content of MP is very constant, and similar to the required composition of tissue protein (beef) and also of milk (Table 7.10).

The proportion of feed protein degraded in the rumen is known as its *degradability* (dg), or alternatively as the content of *rumen degradable protein* (RDP). The amount of RDP is the dietary nitrogen available for MP synthesis. Approximate dg values for different sources of dietary protein are shown in Table 7.11. The extent of degradation depends not only on the inherent characteristics of the protein source, but also on the time the material is exposed to degradation in the rumen, i.e. on outflow rate. Thus the same protein may have quite different dg values when given with different roughages or other feeds in different production systems (Table 7.12).

Microbial requirements for N

The microbes can use NPN (from feed and saliva) and RDP to produce MP. The yield of MP is almost completely dependent on the amount of energy fermented in the rumen. Since the amount of energy fermented is closely related to the digestibility of the feed, the

Table 7.11 Grouping of dietary protein sources by extent of rumen degradation

Class	Range of degradability	Forages	Cereals	Protein supplements
A	0.7–0.9	Hay Silage Swedes	Barley Wheat	Casein Wheat gluten Groundnut meal Sunflower meal Soya bean meal (uncooked) Rapeseed meal Field bean meal
B	0.5–0.7	Grass Legumes Dried grass	Maize	Soya bean meal (cooked) Lupin meal Coconut meal Cottonseed meal Ground peas Linseed cake
C	0.3–0.5	–	Milo	Meat and bone meal White fishmeal
D	<0.3	–	–	Peruvian fishmeal

Table 7.12 Example of differences in the percentage of RDP and UDP in protein supplements for different feeding systems. From Orskov (1987)

Protein source	Dairy cows		Fattening cattle		Suckler cows	
	RDP	UDP	RDP	UDP	RDP	UDP
Soya bean	50	50	65	35	85	15
Fishmeal	30	70	35	65	40	60

RDP, rumen degradable protein.
UDP, undegradable protein.

microbial requirement for N is also related to diet digestibility, or ME content. Further, since RDP and NPN are similar as far as the microbes are concerned (they both end up as ammonia following degradation by microbial enzyme action), the requirement for N to meet microbial growth is usually expressed as grams of RDP (from whatever source: feed protein or NPN or both) per MJ of ME consumed (or required, or allowed). The RDP requirement of the microbial population is 7.8 g/MJ ME (ARC, 1984).

Two important principles follow from this close association between microbial requirement and ME intake. First, the requirement for RDP is considerably lower with straw than for concentrates because straw is less digestible. If excess RDP is included in the diet it will be wasted and excreted in urine as urea. There will also be the added energy cost of converting excess ammonia to urea in the liver.

Second, if the microbial population is deficient in RDP, the digestibility of the diet is reduced, and feed intake is depressed as a result.

Animal requirements for protein

The requirement of the animal depends on the amount of protein produced in tissue growth or in milk. The young calf has a high rate of lean tissue growth relative to its feed intake. Hence the concentration of protein in its diet needs to be relatively high. The cow in early lactation yields more milk and eats less feed than in midlactation. As a result she requires more protein per unit of feed in early lactation than later on. Energy output in milk is higher than that consumed in the feed because the cow is using stored reserves of body fat. But fat for body reserves yields no microbial protein, and at this early stage of lactation the cow has relatively little stored protein in her body. Thus the requirement for UDP is inversely proportional to the extent to which she is underfed and is in negative energy balance.

If sufficient energy is provided to maintain the animal, then MP produced from RDP is likely to be sufficient to meet the maintenance requirement for TP (ARC, 1980). On the other hand, if the animal is restricted to a submaintenance level of feeding, then it will lose not only body fat but also protein or lean tissue.

Calculating protein requirements

The complete calculation of protein requirements is described in ARC (1984). Essentially, the procedure involves determining RDP requirement, and then converting to *tissue microbial protein* (TMP). This is the tissue protein that has been derived from MP. The difference between MP yield, and TMP is the loss of N due to microbial digestion, the absorption of amino acids therefrom, and the incorporation of those amino acids into tissue or milk. Thus only about 42 per cent of the N synthesized into MP will be used at tissue level to meet requirements (ARC, 1984).

Tissue microbial protein yield is therefore 3.3 g/MJ ME consumed (or required). If total tissue protein (TP) requirement (ARC, 1980) exceeds TMP yield, then the shortfall must be made up by UDP. There are losses in absorption of UDP, and in the conversion of absorbed amino acids from absorbed UDP into TP. These losses are 30 per cent and 25 per cent, respectively.

$$\text{UDP requirement therefore} = \frac{\text{TP} - (3.3 \times \text{ME})}{0.70 \times 0.75}$$

or

$$\text{UDP} = (1.91 \times \text{TP}) - 6.25 \times \text{ME}$$

An example of the calculation of requirements is shown in Table 7.13.

Composition of feeds

Cellulosic and non-cellulosic feeds

Feeds for cattle are best described in terms of the major components that undergo fermentation in the rumen. In other words, the conventional division into concentrates and roughages is only a crude way of distinguishing between feeds that contain mainly non-cellulosic (starch and sugar) or cellulosic (plant cell wall) material.

The division into cellulosic and non-cellulosic feeds is relevant because the two fractions are fermented by different types of bacteria (see section on fermentation

Table 7.13 Simplified example of calculation of protein requirements for lactation (600 kg cow yielding 30 l of milk)

Rumen degradable protein requirement
RDP requirement is linked to ME requirement (Table 7.9)
ME for maintenance = 63 MJ
ME for lactation = 5.3 × 30 = 159 MJ
Total ME requirement = 222 MJ ME/day

Tissue protein requirement
TP for maintenance = 74.8 g
TP for lactation = 32.8 × 30 = 948 g
Total TP requirement = 1059 g TP/day

RDP requirement
RDP = 7.8 × 222 = 1732 g

TMP produced
= 3.3 × 222 = 733 g
As TP requirement is greater than TMP produced, RDP – derived protein will not meet all of TP requirements and so some UDP is required

UDP required: = (1.91 × TP) – (6.25 × ME) = 636 g

Total crude protein requirement
= RDP + UDP = 1732 + 636 = 2368

Degradability (dg) required

$$= \frac{1732}{1732 + 636} = 0.73, \text{ or } 73\%$$

in the rumen, p. 77), and at different rates. Cellulosic feeds are fermented at a slower rate, occupy more space in the rumen, and are usually eaten in smaller quantities (i.e. at a slower rate) than non-cellulosic feeds.

When formulating diets it is useful to recognize the different fermentation patterns of the two types of feed, and their different rates of intake by the animal. With productive cattle it is important to avoid too much of one type, or intake may be depressed — by acidosis if too much non-cellulosic material is eaten, or by a slow fermentation in the rumen and slow outflow rate if too much cellulosic material is eaten.

Feeds are classified into mainly cellulosic and mainly non-cellulosic as shown in Table 7.14. Some forage feeds, which would at first sight be considered cellulosic, are intermediate. High-quality grass, for example, contains less than 50 per cent of the DM as cell wall, or *neutral detergent fibre* (NDF) (MAFF, 1986b); maize silage contains only 39 per cent cell wall, because of its high grain content, and as a result about 25 per cent of the DM is starch. Fodder beet contains 65 per cent of the DM as sugars, but they are contained within cell walls and are released in the rumen for fermentation at a slower rate than, say, the sugar from molasses.

Energy and protein

The two most important nutrients are energy and protein, in that order. Other nutrients, particularly minerals, can limit efficiency of feed use, but in practice if a wide range of raw material feeds are used in the diet the risk of mineral imbalance is low. Most farmers add proprietary mineral supplements to the diets of their cattle. However, particular deficiency situations do arise due to inadequate management, e.g. hypomagnesaemia (see Chapter 19).

Lonsdale (1989) has classified raw material feeds into those that typically have high, medium or low contents of ME, and high, medium or low contents of crude protein. Using this approach a two-way matrix can be constructed (Table 7.15). Within each of the nine categories, feeds are listed in descending order of their typical protein content, and the dg of the protein is also indicated, according to the classification in Table 7.11.

A fuller description of the composition of feeds is described in the UK Ministry of Agriculture, Fisheries and Food's book *Feed Composition* (1986b).

Fresh herbages, silages and hays typically have medium contents of both energy and protein (MAFF, 1986b). The dg of their protein is high (category A, Table 7.11). Straws are low in energy, and for most practical purposes their content of protein is too low to meet microbial requirements for RDP.

Table 7.14 Classification of feeds. Source: MAFF (1986b) and Lonsdale (1989)

Mainly cellulosic (NDF >500 g/kg DM)	Mainly non-cellulosic (NDF <400 g/kg DM)
Straw	Kale
Hay	Very young grass
Grass (except very young grass)	Maize silage
	Fodder beet, root crops
Silage (except maize)	Cereal grains
Brewers' grains	Molasses
Malt distillers draff	Molassed sugar beet pulp
Pectin-extracted fruit	Fishmeal
Coffee grounds	Maize gluten feed
Unmolassed sugar beet pulp	Soya bean meal
Bran	Fat
Wheat feed	Cottonseed cake
	Distillers dark grains
	Citrus pulp
	Legume seeds
	Blood meal

Physical form

There are three easily-recognizable categories for the physical form of feeds: (i) liquids, (ii) moist solids, and (iii) dry solids. Examples of each category are shown in Table 7.16.

Liquids range from very low DM materials such as whey, which has handling characteristics similar to water, to viscous liquids such as molasses, which has a typical DM content of 75 per cent. With the exception of whey, most liquid feeds have been condensed prior to shipment, in an attempt to reduce haulage costs.

Moist solids comprise those which contain fermentable sugars (e.g. fresh grass, molassed sugar beet pulp), and that are usually stored as silage (see section on feed preservation, p. 90), and those which are low in fermentable components (e.g apple pomace), and that benefit from the addition of a preservative.

Dry solids are a common form of feed and include cereal grains and byproducts from the milling industry, hays, straws, blood meals, and residues from oil seed extraction. The DM content of dry solids is usually in the range 83–93 per cent. Higher moisture contents increase the risk of spoilage during storage, and for this reason most manufacturers of dry feeds aim to approach 90 per cent DM if possible. Hays are usually stored at an initial moisture content of around

Table 7.15 Classification of raw materials according to their energy and protein contents. The degradability of the protein is also indicated*. From Lonsdale (1989)

Protein content (g/kg DM)	Metabolizable energy content (MJ/kg DM)		
	High >12.0	Medium 9.0–12.0	Low <9.0
High >200	Blood meal (D) Fishmeal (D) Maize gluten meal (prairie meal) (B) Poultry offal meal (B/C) Meat meal (C) Groundnut cake (A) Soya bean meal (B) Sesame meal (B) Soya beans (whole processed) (C) Condensed corn steep liquor Lupins (sweet) (B) Pot ale syrup (A) Linseed meal (B) Spent wash syrups (A) US corn distillers' dark grains (C) Beans (field) (C) Wheat distillers' dark grains (C) Malt distillers' dark grains (C) Peas (B) Delactosed whey syrup Copra expeller (B) Maize gluten feed (B)	Feather meal (hydrolysed) (D) Meat and bone meal (C) Rapeseed meal (B) Sunflower seed meal (B) Cottonseed cake (B) Safflower meal (A) Malt culms (B) Brussel sprout packhouse waste (A) Malt residual pellets (B) Brewers' grains (B) Palm kernel meal (extr.) (B)	Cotton cake (undec.) (B) Sunflower seed meal (undec.) (B) Safflower meal expeller (A)
Medium 120–200	Maize germ meal (B) Whey (A) Triticale (A) Wheat (A)	Wheat bran (B) Dried forages (grass, lucerne) (B) Wheatfeed (A)	Rice bran (C) Shea nut meal (D) Illipe meal (D)
Low <120	Barley (A) Oats (A) Sugar beet pulp (molassed, dried, pressed, ensiled) (B) Potatoes (A) Maize grain (B) Carrots (A) Citrus pulp (B) Molasses (A) Manioc (B)	Pectin extracted fruit (B) Apple pomace (B)	Oatfeed (C)

* Degradability: category A = 0.71–0.90, B = 0.51–0.70, C = 0.31–0.50, D = <0.31.

Table 7.16 Examples of the physical forms of straights. From Stark & Lonsdale (1989)

Liquid	Moist solid	Dry solid
Condensed corn steep liquor	Apple pomace	Blood meal
Delactosed whey syrup	Brewers' grains	Bran (wheat and rice)
Fresh whey	Brussel sprout packhouse waste	Cereal grains
Molasses	Carrot rejects	Citrus pulp
Pot ale syrup	Maize gluten feed*	Distillers' dark grains
	Pectin-extracted fruit	Dried grass and lucerne
	Potatoes	Fishmeal
	Sugar beet pulp*	Legume seeds
		Maize germ meal
		Maize gluten feed*
		Maize gluten meal
		Malt culms
		Malt residual pellets
		Meat meal
		Oatfeed
		Oilseed residues
		Sugar beet pulp*
		Wheatfeed
		Whole oilseeds

* Available as either a moist or dry solid.

20 per cent, but final moisture content is typically 10 per cent.

Feed preservation

The principle of preservation is to prevent the development of spoilage organisms such as the putrefying bacteria and moulds. These organisms prefer warm temperatures, low levels of acidity (pH 6 to 8), oxygen and water. Hence preservation may be achieved by cooling, preferably freezing, by acidification, by exclusion or removal of oxygen, or by drying.

Drying

Drying is the most effective form of feed preservation. It is also the most costly, and therefore tends to be used with the more valuable feeds (e.g. cereals), and with feeds that are also very prone to deterioration (e.g. blood).

The DM content of cereals is normally increased by drying to 85–86 per cent prior to storage. Hay is dried in the field to about 80 per cent DM, unless it is to be dried artificially in the barn, when it may be harvested in a moist state at between 65 and 75 per cent DM. Drying in the barn proceeds until the safe DM content, more than 80 per cent, has been reached and the crop shows little sign of heating and moulding.

Ensiling

As already discussed, moist solids are often preserved by ensiling but other feeds, such as cereal grains and hays, can be preserved by adding a preservative.

The process of ensilage involves the fermentation of plant sugars to organic acids, principally lactic acid. The acidity thus produced effectively 'pickles' the crop or feed in a stable state in the absence of air.

Fermentation is an anaerobic process. The crop must be completely sealed from the air to facilitate the growth of the desirable anaerobic bacteria that are present on the crop in the field in relatively small numbers. As much air as possible should be removed from the crop at the time of ensiling, so that residual oxygen is exhausted as rapidly as possible. This is achieved by first chopping the crop as it is harvested from the field, by consolidating it once the crop is in the silo, and finally by sealing it completely using a plastic sheet.

Primary and secondary fermentations

It is important to distinguish between primary and secondary fermentations, and to recognize that both are quite distinct from the process of aerobic spoilage that occurs on exposure of silage to the air at the time of feed-out.

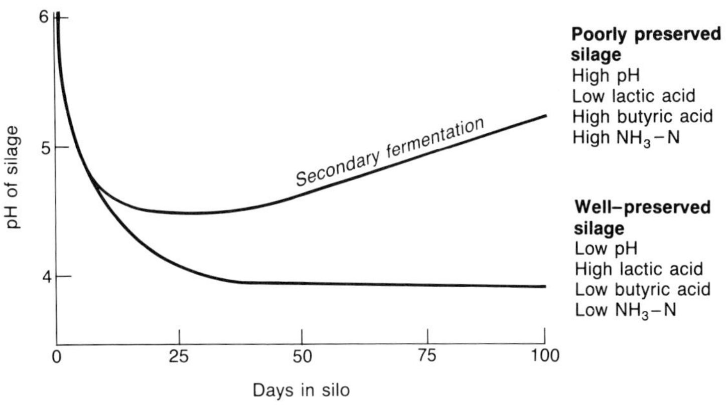

Fig. 7.14 Patterns of fermentation and changes in the pH value of silage as a result of secondary fermentation.

Primary fermentation essentially comprises the conversion by lactic acid bacteria of fermentable sugars (water-soluble carbohydrates, WSC) to lactic and other acids.

Secondary fermentation involves the degradation of lactic and other acids, with the formation of evil-smelling acids like butyric acid. The process can also be accompanied by complete degradation of nitrogenous compounds to ammonia. The main organisms involved in secondary fermentations are the obligate anaerobic clostridial bacteria.

At the point of entry to the silo the pH of the crop is usually about 6.0. The crop is still alive, but consuming the products of photosynthesis (sugars) by respiration and producing carbon dioxide, water and heat. In addition, aerobic bacteria such as the *Enterobacteriaceae* (coliforms) consume sugars to produce acetic acid and degrade protein to ammonia.

As the supply of oxygen is exhausted, the primary fermentation dominates, with lactic acid the predominant product. Acidity increases as the conversion of sugars to acids continues.

Primary fermentation proceeds until either the supply of fermentable substrate is exhausted or the amount of free water (i.e. that not associated with products of fermentation) is reduced to a sufficiently low level to restrict bacterial activity. A stable low pH is reached. The silage contains lactic acid as the main fermentation acid, and the amount of protein completely degraded to ammonia is small (see Fig. 7.14).

However, if the supply of sugar in the crop is low, or its resistance to acidification, or buffering capacity, is relatively high, secondary fermentation may occur during the storage period. In this situation the silage is unstable. Wet crops of low sugar content are particularly prone to secondary fermentation. Typical changes in the content of fermentation acids in silage as a result of secondary fermentation are shown in Fig. 7.15.

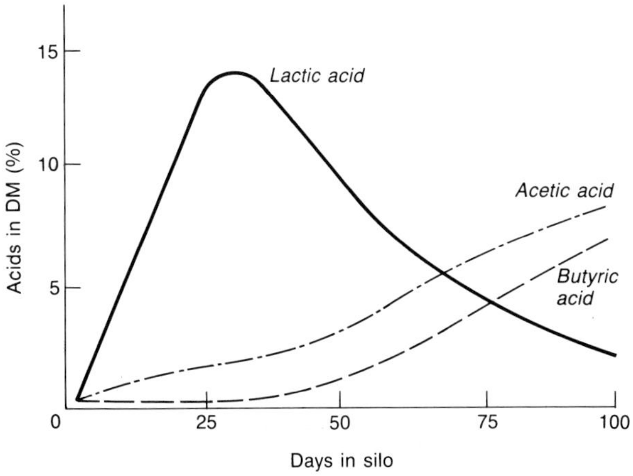

Fig. 7.15 Typical changes in the content of fermentation acids in silage as a result of secondary fermentation.

Some crops, because they contain relatively low contents of WSC, or have relatively high buffering capacities, are more prone than others to secondary fermentations — their 'ensilability' is relatively low. Crops are ranked in order of their ensilability in Table 7.17. Maize combines adequate WSC with low buffering capacity, whilst the legumes, and lucerne in particular, is the reverse.

Wilting in good weather prior to harvest has the effect of concentrating the sugars in the crop, and this is beneficial in terms of reducing the risk of secondary fermentation.

Silages that have undergone secondary fermentations are poorly preserved, but paradoxically they tend to be relatively stable on exposure to air. A major consequence of clostridial activity is an increase in the proportion of nitrogen present as ammonia in the silage

Table 7.17 Crops ranked in order of their 'ensilability'. Source: Wilkinson (1990)

Good	Maize
	Whole crop cereals
	Italian and hybrid ryegrass
	Perennial ryegrass
	Bromegrass
	Timothy/meadow fescue
	Permanent pasture
	Cocksfoot
	Arable silage containing legumes
	Grass/clover
	Red clover
Poor	Lucerne

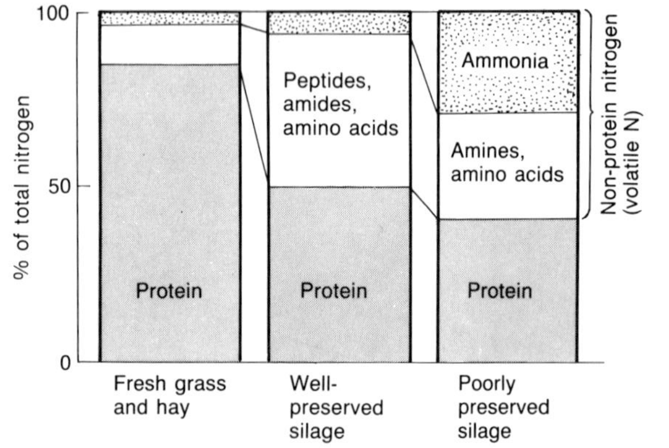

Fig. 7.16 The nitrogenous components of fresh grass, well-preserved silage and poorly preserved silage. From Wilkinson (1985).

(Fig. 7.16). Digestibility and energy value is also reduced due to secondary fermentation; hence losses of nutrients are elevated in poorly preserved silages.

Additives for silage

The main objective in applying an additive at the time of harvest is to prevent the development of clostridiam. The lactic acid bacteria are more tolerant of acid conditions than are the clostridia, so traditionally their growth has been inhibited by direct acidification of the crop with an organic acid such as formic, or an inorganic acid such as sulphuric. The former is relatively more expensive, but it does have a specific antimicrobial action against clostridia, whilst sulphuric acid acts solely through it effect in reducing pH. Some products comprise mixtures of acids, and synergistic properties are claimed for them.

If the pH of the crop can be reduced from 6.0 to about 4.5 by acidification at the time of harvest, then the risk of clostridial growth is very low indeed.

A more recent approach is to accelerate the production of lactic acid by direct inoculation of the crop at harvest. Provided sufficient live bacteria are added (ideally, 1 million colony forming units/g fresh crop), and provided the content of fermentable sugar in the crop is sufficient for their growth, then good preservation quality should be assured. Problems can arise with inoculants if there is insufficient sugar, either because the crop itself is deficient, or because the crop is too wet at the time of ensiling. The most common species of bacteria in inoculants is *Lactobacillus plantarum*.

Enzyme additives, containing hemicellulase and cellulase, are another recent development; the object is to generate extra sugar from cell wall components to ensure sufficient acidification during primary fermentation that clostridia are inhibited.

Products are now available which contain both lactic acid bacteria and enzymes. It is essential, however, to establish that the active ingredients in these biological additives really are active, and have not been destroyed by processing, packaging or storage.

Additives for hay and moist grain

The development of moulds and mycotoxins in moist hay and moist grain may be reduced or prevented by adding an effective preservative at the time of storage. Propionic acid and salts of propionic are effective in reducing mould development in both hay and grain (and also in big bale silage, where moulding due to incomplete sealing is a common problem). Ammonia, preferably in its aqueous form, has also been used successfully as a preservative. In the case of low-quality hay made from mature crops of grass, ammonia can also increase digestibilty and protein value.

Feed processing

Physical processing of roughages

Traditionally, feeds like hays and straws were chopped or ground prior to feeding. There is now increasing evidence to indicate that although these procedures may have been convenient for the processor, they were inconvenient from the point of view of the nutrition of the animal.

With fibrous feeds such as straw, intake is often limited by the speed with which long particles are reduced in size by chewing so that they can pass out of the rumen. Grinding removes this restriction to intake, but a consequence is that particles pass out of the rumen before they are fully digested. The net result is that although dry matter intake is increased, digestibility is reduced and nutrient intake is little changed.

Chopping long forages also reduces the opportunity for the animal to select the best quality material on offer. But if straw is to be used in a complete diet, coarse chopping is a useful way of incorporating the feed uniformly into the total mixture.

Long fibre is essential for milk fat synthesis, and for the maintenance of rumen function on high-concentrate diets. It is therefore important to bear in mind that physical processing of roughages is likely to diminish their particular value with respect to milk quality and the health status of the rumen.

Chemical processing of roughages

The use of alkalis, such as sodium hydroxide, for upgrading straw is not new, but recently, additional benefits from the use of the technique have been recognized.

Essentially, the technique involves adding sodium hydroxide to straw at about 5 per cent by weight. The alkali degrades and swells the plant cell wall material, with a consequent increase in digestibility and intake. The benefits are valuable where straw is plentiful, and where it comprises a high proportion of the total diet, for example, in the case of beef suckler cows.

The residual alkalinity in straw treated with sodium hydroxide can help to reduce the risk of acidosis in high-yielding dairy cows given diets containing large proportions of concentrates, and/or highly acid silages. In these situations, where fibre is needed to maintain milk fat content but the overall energy content is required to be high at the same time, the provision of a source of long fibre of enhanced digestibility is also valuable.

Ammonia (usually added at 3 per cent of straw fresh weight) is a useful alternative alkali to sodium hydroxide. It has the advantage of also contributing nitrogen, a valuable feature if the diet is deficient in rumen degradable nitrogen but a disadvantage if silage of high protein content is the major forage in the diet.

Urea may also be used to upgrade straw, but both the moisture content of the straw and ambient temperature need to be relatively high for the technique to be successful.

The effect of an increase in digestibility of straw on intake can be considerable. Thus a 10 per cent improvement in digestibility can lead to a 50 per cent increase in dry matter intake. Since the feed consumed is more digestible, the increase in ME intake is even greater.

Processing of cereals

Grinding of cereals was until recently considered essential to achieve complete digestion by cattle. A trade-off was accepted between rapid digestion in the rumen and possible acidosis on the one hand, and poor digestibility with undigested grains appearing in the faeces, on the other.

It is now accepted that the passage of a few undigested grains has no measurable effect on digestibility, but that forage digestibility can be reduced when grain is overprocessed.

The need for cereal processing depends on the size of the reticulo-omasal orifice. In the case of sheep and calves less than 150 kg liveweight, it is difficult for whole barley and whole oat grains to pass through the orifice, whilst it is easy in larger cattle.

Thus whole grains may be given to young calves, but some processing is necessary for older cattle. If possible, the extent of processing should be as small as possible: it is sufficient to crack the seed coat. Crimping is better than rolling, but treatment with sodium hydroxide, which has the effect of breaking the seed coat by swelling it, is probably the best method from the animal's point of view. In addition to slowing down the rate of digestion of the starch in the grain, the residual alkali buffers acidity in the rumen.

Feeding management

Successful nutrition of the bovine not only requires an understanding of the principles of nutrient requirement, nutrient supply and animal response; it also involves appropriate management of feed resources. This includes presenting the correct amount of feed to the animal for the appropriate period of time, formulating diets from available resources that meet requirements, taking into account the condition of the animal and the desired direction and rate of change in weight and condition, and budgeting ahead so that rapid changes in diet are avoided and performance targets are achieved.

The importance of selective eating

The need to maintain stability in the rumen has led to the presentation of feeds to the animal over a large proportion of the day. This is particularly so with forages and straws, where rate of intake is relatively

Table 7.18 Effect of amount offered on selection and intake of straw by goats. Source: Wahed & Owen (1986)

	Straw offered (g DM/kg LW/day)		
	18	54	90
Intake of straw (g DM/kg LW/day)	15.5	22.8	26.2
Straw refused (% of offered)	12.5	56.6	70.3
Estimated intake of straw digestible organic matter (g/kg LW/day)	7.2	12.8	14.5

Table 7.19 Target sward surface height for grazing cattle

	Post-grazing height (cm)	
	Rotational grazing	Continuous grazing
Spring (April–June)	8	5
Summer (July and August)	9	7
Autumn (September–November)	10	8
Winter (December and January)	<5	<5

Note: when grazing clean aftermath regrowths, graze to spring sward height.

slow. It is also important that the animal has access to feed for most if not all the time when selectivity is desirable. Thus the presentation to goats of more than four times as much straw as was being consumed, allowing the animals extensive scope for selection amongst what was on offer, was reflected in an increase in intake of straw DM of almost 70 per cent, and an increase in intake of digestible organic matter of 100 per cent (Table 7.18). Whilst goats are more selective eaters than bovines, the principle still applies (see, for example, Fig. 7.8, p. 81).

At pasture, maximum intake is only achieved when herbage is offered in substantial excess (Figs 7.7–7.9). In general, the amount of herbage on offer should be three to four times the amount eaten in order to achieve maximum potential voluntary intake (see section on grazed pasture, p. 81).

Targets for sward surface height at pasture

A simple guide to the amount of herbage on offer is the sward surface height of the grazed pasture. Regular measurement of sward height is now recommended as a tactical aid to pasture management. Targets for sward height for dairy cows and beef cattle are shown in Table 7.19.

It is important to measure sward height in grazed areas, since herbage that is rejected due to contamination by faeces, urine or treading is unlikely to be eaten until the height of herbage in grazed areas is well below that at which intake is restricted below maximum.

Buffer feeding

The concept of buffer feeding was developed as a way of reducing losses in output from grazed pasture, especially when herbage allowance was apparently adequate but intake less than maximal due to poor weather, inadequate grass growth, short day length, or reduced time of access to pasture.

The buffer feed should be less acceptable than the herbage on offer at pasture, otherwise the buffer acts as a substitute rather than a supplement for grazed grass. Typically, silage or hay are used as buffer feeds, offered *ad libitum* at the farm buildings to dairy cows after each milking, or placed in the field for other classes of stock.

Frequency of feeding and feedlot bloat

It is significant that when cereal concentrates are offered *ad libitum*, the animal eats a little at a time. Thus the general practice in feedlots, and in areas of the world where milk is produced from high-concentrate diets, is to allow the animals 24-hour access to all feeds (both concentrate and roughage) to avoid 'feedlot bloat'. This condition is caused by the rapid fermentation of starches and sugars, and can occur as the result of infrequent ingestion of large feeds of concentrates. It can also occur as the result of inadequate long fibre to maintain rumination and saliva production. Essentially, the condition is one of acidosis due to the dominance in the rumen fermentation of lactic acid producing bacteria. Ruminal stasis can occur at low rumen pH (less than pH 5.5), and the inability of the animal to eructate leads to the accumulation of gas and the resultant bloat.

Cattle given *ad libitum* concentrates should therefore also be allowed access to long forage, or a source of roughage such as straw, at about 15 per cent of the total diet dry matter.

Traditionally, dairy cows were given concentrates, usually in the form of milled compounded feeds, in the parlour at milking, and forages *ad libitum* for the rest of the day. With ever-increasing milk yields per cow, the pressure on the available time in the parlour meant that the cow had difficulty consuming a large feed of compounds during the milking period. Further, the rapid fermentation of the two relatively large meals (sometimes as much as 5 kg/meal) meant that rumen pH decreased, fibre digestion slowed down, and forage intake was reduced as a result (see Fig. 7.17). Accordingly, a midday feed of compounds or of byproducts such as dried sugar beet pulp was introduced to reduce the quantity of compound to be fed through the parlour.

Sodium bicarbonate may be a suitable ingredient of the diet when the cow is suffering from acidosis. But the problem with bicarbonate is that it is relatively unpalatable, and large quantities are required to have a significant effect. Thus adding 100–150 g/cow per day is insignificant by comparison with the kilograms of bicarbonate produced in saliva. It is better therefore to include feeds, like hay or straw, that stimulate rumination and salivation.

Out-of-parlour feeders

The advent of computerized cow identification has enabled cows to be rationed accurately in the parlour according to yield, and it was a relatively logical step to introduce out-of-parlour feeders to allow the higher yielding individuals to eat compounds and concentrates during the rest of the day. The nutritional advantages were that higher levels of compounds could be given to those cows that 'deserved' to receive them, and in a relatively large number of meals per day. Feeders could be programmed to deliver equal proportions of the total day's allocation in up to 12 feeds per day; cows not taking their feeds were readily identifiable and could be checked for disease immediately.

Flat-rate feeding

The introduction of milk quotas placed a limit on output, and the emphasis switched to simplifying the day-to-day feeding management of the dairy herd, especially in those herds where the input of concentrate was moderate.

The principle of flat-rate feeding is that all cows receive the same amount of concentrate, irrespective of their actual or potential milk production, together with silage *ad libitum*. The system works best when there is a compact calving pattern, with most cows at the same stage of lactation, and when the input of concentrates is relatively low. Silage quality should be relatively high, and if necessary the level of concentrate should be reduced when the herd is in late lactation to prevent cows becoming overfat.

In practice, higher yielding cows in the herd eat more silage, and it is important that the silage is on offer *ad libitum* otherwise these animals are underfed. Peak lactation yields tend to be lower than in herds given concentrates to yield, but the rate of decline in yield postpeak tends also to be slower than in herds fed to yield, giving a flatter lactation curve for flat-rate feeding.

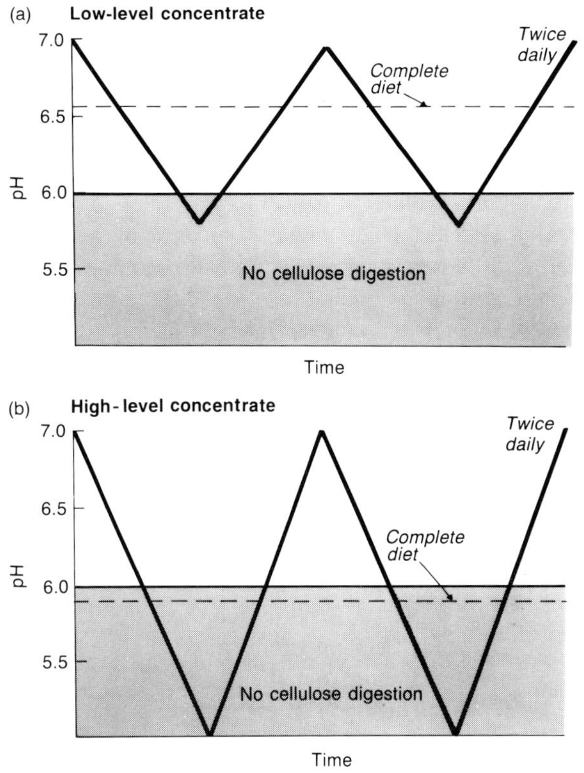

Fig. 7.17 It is important to prevent the pH of the rumen from falling below 6.0 for long periods of time, otherwise cellulose digestion will be greatly reduced. The problem is less at low levels of concentrate feeding (a) than at high levels (b). From Orskov (1987)

Complete diets

The main principle of complete diet feeding is that the animal receives slowly and rapidly fermented feeds in an intimate mix, thus balancing the inflow to the rumen of feeds with widely differing rates of fermentation, and (hopefully) thereby maintaining stable conditions in the rumen.

However, with high proportions of concentrates in the mix, the level of acidity in the rumen may be so high that fibre digestion is permanently depressed (Fig. 7.17). In this situation, the proportion of propionate in the rumen VFAs is elevated, and as a result cows tend to gain in weight, and produce milk of relatively low fat content. Overfat cows with fatty livers were a feature of early mismanagement of herds given complete diets.

Thus provided cows in late lactation and dry cows are not given the same high-energy mix as higher yielding animals, complete diets offer a logical approach to feeding management. Byproducts can be incorporated into complete diets with greater ease than in other feeding systems. Higher intakes are usually achieved than with separate feeding, and milk compositional quality is often improved as a result of the higher energy status of the animal and improved fibre digestion in the rumen.

Diet formulation

Diets are formulated to meet calculated requirements for major nutrients (see sections on energy and protein requirements), taking account also of the needs of the animal for macro- and microelements. Recent research in the USA indicates that formulations for lactation should also take account of dry matter content and the content of neutral detergent fibre (cell wall) in the total diet. The dry matter content of the whole diet should be between 50 and 65 per cent for maximum intake, whilst the content of NDF should be between 35 and 45 per cent for maximal output of milk of the desired quality, particularly with respect to fat content. Constraints in diet formulation programmes now include dry matter and NDF in addition to conventional prediction equations for voluntary intake and nutrient requirements.

Condition score

Condition scoring cows is relatively easy; there is no fleece to hide the animal's fatness (or thinness). The essential area for physical examination is the top of the loin, halfway between the last rib and the hip bone, and the tail head (Fig. 3.1, p. 16) and is further described in Chapter 3.

With practice, visual scoring is possible taking into account the visibility of the ribs and the amount of fat at the tail head. Cows in condition score 1 have no fat at the tail head, and their ribs are prominent. The ribs are visible in condition score 2 but not in condition score 3 and above. As condition score rises above 2, the amount of fat visible at the tail head increases.

Target condition scores for cows at different stages of the production cycle are shown in Table 7.20.

Regular condition scoring helps to identify overthin cows that require preferential treatment (extra feed) and overfat cows, especially those in late pregnancy, that are at risk of dystokia and need slimming down prior to calving. Scoring in early lactation to monitor the effectiveness of nutrient inputs to achieve weight gain at mating is an essential part of successful rebreeding. Economies may also be made in high-energy feeds at times when the whole herd is scored as being slightly overfat.

Table 7.20 Target condition scores for cows. Source: Fuller (1988)

Stage of reproductive cycle	Target condition score	
	Autumn-calving cows	Spring-calving cows
At calving	3	2.5
At mating	2.5	2
Mid-pregnancy	2	3

Table 7.21 Feed budget for a dairy herd of 100 cows, average milk yield 5500 l/cow, calving September to November. Anticipated silage available is 10 t fresh weight/cow of 10.5 MJ ME/kg DM

Grazing
- Turnout to mid May: 5 cows/ha
- Mid May to mid August: 3.5 cows/ha
- Mid August to housing: 2.5 cows/ha

Concentrates
- Winter period: 1.1 t/cow
- Rest of year: 0.1 t/cow

Feed budgeting

Feed budgeting is the extension of daily diet formulation to annual feed planning. Future levels of output are set and a feeding policy is developed which takes into account the home-produced feeds available, or likely to become available during the year, and the type and quantity of purchased feeds required to meet the target level of output. A buying strategy is developed to meet the projected requirements.

Simplified examples of feed budgets for grazing and winter feeding are shown in Tables 7.21–7.23 for dairy cows, suckler cows and growing beef cattle, respectively.

References

Agricultural Research Council (1980) *The Nutrient Requirements of Ruminant Livestock*. Commonwealth Agricultural Bureaux, Farnham Royal, Bucks, pp. 1–347.

Agricultural Research Council (1984) *The Nutrient Requirements*

Table 7.22 Feed budget for suckler cows (t fresh weight/cow and calf per annum). Silage and other feeds 25 per cent DM

Grazing
Hill pastures and semi-arid lowlands: 0.5–1.0 cows/ha
Upland pastures: 1.2–1.8 cows/ha
Lowland temperate pastures: 1.5–2.1 cows/ha
Winter feeding

	Autumn calving	Spring calving
Lowland herds		
Concentrates	0.4	0.2
Silage	3.5	2.5
Straw	1.0	0.8
Other feeds (wet byproducts)	0.3	0.4
Upland herds		
Concentrates	0.4	0.2
Silage	4.7	4.5
Straw	0.6	0.5
Other feeds	0.2	0.4

Hill herds: as for upland herds except silage 5.5 t/head to allow for longer winter period

Table 7.23 Feed budgets for growing beef cattle

Grazing
Target liveweight (t/ha) at 250 kg N/ha

May	2.2
June	2.0
July	1.7
August	1.6
September	1.4
October	1.4
Average	1.7

Increase by 4 kg for each extra kg of N

Silage and concentrates (t/head)

	Silage (25% DM, 10.5 ME)	Concentrates
Overwintered store cattle and finishing suckled calves	3	0.3
18-month beef	5	0.9
Silage beef (15–16 months)	6	0.8
Cereal beef (11–12 months)	*	1.6

* 0.2 t straw/head to maintain rumen function.

of Ruminant Livestock, Supplement No. 1. Commonwealth Agricultural Bureaux, Farnham Royal, Bucks, pp. 1–45.

Forbes, J.M. (1983) *The Voluntary Food Intake of Farm Animals*. Butterworths, London, pp. 1–206.

Fuller, R. (1988) *Suckled Calf Production*. Chalcombe Publications, Marlow Bottom, Bucks, pp. 1–85.

Gibb, M.J. & Treacher, T.T. (1978) The effect of herbage allowance on herbage intake and performance of ewes and their twin lambs grazing perennial ryegrass. *Journal of Agricultural Science, Cambridge*, **90**, 139–47.

Hodgson, J. (1975) The influence of grazing pressure and stocking rate on herbage intake and performance. In *Pasture Utilisation by the Grazing Animal* (ed. by J. Hodgson & D.K. Jackson), Occasional Symposium No 8, British Grassland Society, pp. 93–103.

Lonsdale, C.R. (1989) *Straights: Raw Materials for Animal Feed Compounders and Farmers*. Chalcombe Publications, Marlow Bottom, Bucks, pp. 1–87.

Ministry of Agriculture, Fisheries and Food (1975) *Energy Allowances and Feeding Systems for Ruminants*. Technical Bulletin 33. HMSO, London, pp. 1–79.

Ministry of Agriculture, Fisheries and Food (1984) *Energy Allowances and Feeding Systems for Ruminants*. Technical Bulletin 433. HMSO, London, pp. 1–85.

Ministry of Agriculture, Fisheries and Food (1986a) *Nutrient Allowances for Cattle and Sheep*. P2087. HMSO, London, pp. 1–6.

Ministry of Agriculture, Fisheries and Food (1986b) *Feed Composition*. Chalcombe Publications, Marlow Bottom, Bucks, pp. 1–69.

Orskov, E.R. (1987) *The Feeding of Ruminants: Principles and Practice*. Chalcombe Publications, Marlow Bottom, Bucks, pp. 1–90.

Osbourn, D.F. (1967) The intake of conserved forages. *Fodder Conservation* (ed. by R.J. Wilkins), Occasional Symposium No. 3, British Grassland Society, pp. 20–8.

Van Soest, P.J. (1982) *Nutritional Ecology of the Ruminant*. O & B Books, Corvallis, Oregon, USA, pp. 1–374.

Wahed, R.A. and Owen, E. (1986) The effect of amount offered on selection and intake of barley straw by goats. *Animal Production*, **42**, 473.

Wilkinson, J.M. (1985) *Beef Production from Silage and Other Conserved Forages*. Longman, London, pp. 1–140.

Wilkinson, J.M. (1988) *Silage UK*, 6th edn. Chalcombe Publications, Marlow Bottom, Bucks, pp. 1–185.

Chapter 8: Alternative Forages

by P.S. JARVIS

Introduction

The main forage crops in the UK and many other countries for cattle are conserved grass in the form of hay or silage, otherwise straw. Economic and nutritional considerations have led to a quest for alternative forages.

Feeding dairy cows, dairy heifers, suckler cows and beef animals is a mixture of science and art. Any ration needs to be balanced for energy, protein, minerals, vitamins and water, to meet the required production objectives. Energy sources will include starches, sugars and digestible fibre, whilst protein will be of rumen degradable and digestible undegradable protein and will contain a wide range of amino acids. The ration must be palatable, digestible, appetizing and free from dirt, stones, harmful bacteria and moulds. Some feeds are enhancers of dry matter intake (DMI), whilst others substitute for existing ingredients in the ration. Thus brewers grains, sodium hydroxide-treated straw, maize, etc. are enhancers of DMI whereas, for example, barley and wheat substitute for each other.

Table 8.1 Winter ration criteria for Friesian/Holstein dairy cows

	Milk yield (kg/day)			
	35	25	18	Dry
Minimum DM (%)	38	33	26	22
Energy density	12.0	11.4	10.8	9.5
Minimum MADF fibre (%)	15	18	22	25
Approximate DMI	20.9	17.1	14.7	9.3

Note: protein guidelines are 400 g DCP for maintenance and 60–65 g DCP/kg milk, with sufficient undegradable as well as degradable protein in the ration.
For Jersey cows with milk yields of 25, 18, 13 and 9 kg respectively, the protein requirements are 350 g DCP for maintenance and 70–75 g DCP/kg of milk.

The UK Ministry of Agriculture, Fisheries and Food and the Agricultural and Food Research Council have published standards for energy, protein and the major minerals for maintenance and production for lactating and fattening animals. Knowledge is incomplete, and the art of feeding stock relates to adjusting feeds, introducing different ingredients and measuring and observing the results.

The figures shown in Table 8.1 act as a starting point in the compilation of dairy cow rations, particularly as feeds can vary in analysis. Alternative forages will need to fit the criteria laid down for each animal's production. However some forages, such as maize and lucerne, are DMI enhancers and so they can be perfectly satisfactory at lower energy densities in winter rations.

Dairy heifers, calving at two years old, need to grow at 0.7–0.8 kg/head daily to attain a satisfactory calving weight, and beef animals in the final stages of fattening require growth rates in excess of 1 kg/head daily.

Total farm profitability determines whether or not alternative forages feature in a farming system. Factors to be considered include soil type, labour availability, working and fixed capital requirements, value for money, yield variability, rotational considerations and feeding facilities. The majority feature in winter rations, but kale and stubble turnips are often grazed in the summer and early autumn, while lucerne and red clover are versatile protein sources in the summer. They can be grazed (with caution because of bloat) or conserved as silage. Red clover is usually in a grass ley mixture, but lucerne is generally grown as a pure stand.

A brief description will be given for some of the crops available together with their use and integration in cattle rations.

Forage maize (corn)

The typical analysis of forage maize silage per kg dry matter (DM) is:

DM = 28 per cent, metabolizable energy (ME) = 10.8 MJ, digestible crude protein (DCP) = 70 g, neutral detergent fibre (NDF) = 360 g, modified acid detergent fibre (MADF) = 215 g
Minerals: Ca = 3.9 g, P = 1.8 g, Na = 0.2 g, Mg = 2.4 g
Yield on National Institute of Agricultural Botany (NIAB) plots = 12.0 t DM/ha

Maize silage is best stored in long, narrow clamps to limit the amount of heating and hence spoilage when the clamp is opened. Most maize is grown in the southern counties of Britain but as more early-maturing varieties are being bred, the frontiers are being pushed further north.

The true value of maize (corn) is often underestimated by conventional equations. Maize silage costs less to produce than grass silage, and is complementary to it. In a dull, wet summer, the ME can be under 10 but is still as good as most grass silages made in similar weather. Generally, it is a high-energy, low-protein conserved forage that has limited fibre and is low in minerals, particularly calcium, phosphorus, sodium, copper, zinc, iodine and manganese. The greater the proportion of maize in the ration, the more deficiencies need to be corrected.

A typical ration for a dairy cow yielding 25 kg milk might include 32 kg grass silage, 14 kg maize silage, 1 kg soya bean meal, 5.5 kg maize gluten and 0.15 kg high phosphorus minerals. Research work, particularly by Phipps (pers. comm.) has shown that by including at least 25 per cent of the silage as maize increases forage DMI, lowers the cost and increases milk production and hence the weight of fat and protein. The response is greater with 63 per cent digestibility ('D' value) silage compared with 68 D grass silage. With a ration based on 40 : 60 grass : maize silage and 6 kg concentrates, DMI and milk yield were increased by 2.8 and 2.9 kg respectively compared with grass silage and 6 kg concentrates. Maize silage combines well with lucerne silage, but needs an addition of 1–2 kg straw to provide fibre.

Maize silage can be used as the sole source of forage for dairy cows. An example ration for a cow producing 25 kg milk would be 27 kg maize silage, 3.5 kg caustic treated straw, 2 kg molasses, 2 kg sugar beet pulp, 3 kg maize gluten, 1 kg fishmeal, 2 kg soya bean meal and 0.3 kg mineral/vitamin supplement. As the DM of maize silage increases, so does the DMI.

Maize silage can be introduced to young cattle at under three months old, but additional protein, vitamins and minerals are necessary. Typically, a 300 kg heifer growing at 0.65 kg/day requires 5.1 kg DM of maize silage, 0.2 kg 50 per cent vegetable protein and one per cent non-protein nitrogen (urea) added to maize silage; 1 kg of a 34 per cent protein/mineral/vitamin supplement would also be suitable.

Bull beef animals have higher intakes of maize than grass silage. A beast weighing 300 kg needs 6 kg DM of maize silage plus 1.5 kg of a 34 per cent protein/mineral/vitamin concentrate supplement to gain 1 kg/day. This quantity of supplement is kept constant over a range of weights so that the crude protein of the complete ration declines as the animal matures.

Maize fits well into a grass silage system and can be self-fed or forage-box fed. It can be fed as a green crop prior to harvest, and used as a buffer feed in spring for cows at pasture.

Fodder beet

The typical analysis of fodder beet per kg DM is:

DM = 18.3 per cent, ME = 11.9 MJ, DCP = 34 g, NDF = 127 g, MADF = 83 g
Minerals: Ca = 3.9 g, P = 1.8 g, Na = 2.4 g, Mg = 1.4 g
Yield on NIAB plots = 14.2 t DM/ha (excluding the value of fodder beet tops (leaves), which can add up to 30 per cent to the DM)

Ensiled tops are higher in protein minerals (especially phosphorus) and fibre and can complement the diet, but are difficult to harvest and utilize efficiently. Fresh tops can contain harmful oxalic acid and lead to calcium problems but the problem is reduced with wilting. Thus they can cause scouring and milk fever in freshly calved cows.

Fodder beet is used primarily as a low-cost concentrate replacer for dairy cows, at a maximum of 4–4.5 kg DM (22–25 kg fresh weight). As a high-energy source, it will need to be balanced by additional degradable and undegradable protein. In limited cases, it can be used as part of the maintenance ration but additional protein, fibre (as hay or straw) and minerals will be required.

For a dairy cow yielding 25 kg milk, with 40 kg grass silage producing more than maintenance, 15 kg of fodder beet, 4 kg maize gluten and 2.25 kg of a proprietary 20 per cent protein, high-energy concentrate complete the ration. A mix of other dry concentrates such as barley and soya bean meal can replace maize gluten.

Harvested fodder beet can be fed from a hopper or behind an electric fence provided that sufficient feed space is available to avoid uneven intakes between cows in the herd. It is more commonly fed as part of a complete diet in a forage wagon, but the beet must be free from dirt and preferably finely chopped or shredded to integrate in the ration.

Strip-grazing beet in the field produces a multitude of problems: poisoning from tops (even when topped this can be via secondary growth in the spring), waste of feed and food troubles (see Chapter 28).

When used as a concentrate replacer, fodder beet enhances the butterfat and protein percentages in the milk, but observations suggest that it depletes the compositional quality when used as part of the maintenance ration.

A combination of fodder beet and soya bean meal can add to DMI and hence milk yield and quality, particularly replacing a 10.8 ME grass silage. The grass silage uptake has been shown to decrease from 9.6 to 7.0 kg DM/cow per day. When fodder beet was added to a poorer silage and with no soya bean meal, compositional quality was not improved. As well as lowering the ration cost, fodder beet partially acts as a concentrate replacer.

Fodder beet should be finely chopped or shredded in the rations for dairy heifers over one year old and are changing their teeth. For these animals average grass silage up to 2 kg DM (11 kg fresh weight) of fodder beet can be fed in place of sugar beet pulp to ensure good growth rates and conception. Using a straw-based ration, a 300 kg heifer growing at 0.8 kg/day could receive 3 kg straw, 14 kg fodder beet, 1.2 kg barley and 1 kg soya bean meal. If ammonia or urea-treated straw is used, 11 kg fodder beet and 1 kg barley could produce the desired results. Alternatively, 2 kg DM from both fodder beet and brewers' grains with *ad libitum* straw should produce a palatable and productive ration. Amounts will, of course, be increased as the animals grow.

Gleadthorpe Experimental Husbandry Farm (1984, 1985) developed a fodder beet system that explored its low cost when compared with concentrates for Friesian × Hereford heifers and steers. Crushed beet was introduced when the animals weighed 200 kg. Both fishmeal and soya bean meal have been used as the protein sources with minerals and straw also added if necessary.

In many cases, fodder beet requires much additional capital for sowing, harvesting, storing, cleaning and chopping the beet, but it can be grown in most areas of the UK and other temperate areas. In a wet autumn on heavy soils, harvesting can be difficult, but it is a relatively cheap source of energy. Mangels, which have a DM of 10–15 per cent, are in the main similar to fodder beet for feeding but crop yield is less.

Swedes

The typical analysis of swedes per kg DM is:

DM = 10.5 per cent, ME = 13.1 MJ, DCP = 64 g, NDF = 140 g, MADF = 114 g
Minerals: Ca = 3.5 g, P = 2.6 g, Na = 1.5 g, Mg = 1.1 g
Yield on NIAB plots = 7 t DM/ha

The crop is generally grown in the cooler west and north of Britain. Fungal problems such as powdery mildew and club-root can limit crop yields.

Swedes have a low protein and high energy content, but a relatively low yield of DM. They are used primarily for beef and sheep as well as for human consumption.

Swedes could be utilized by dairy cows on a similar DM basis to fodder beet, but are more costly to produce. Despite their low DM (10.5 per cent) they are likely to be DMI enhancers. Similarly, they can be fed to dairy heifers by incorporation in straw-based rations. The low DM of swedes could assist consumption, but chopping or slicing is advantageous. Swedes may be grazed *in situ*, especially by sheep.

Stubble turnips (leaves and roots)

The typical analysis of stubble turnips per kg DM is:

DM = 8.0 per cent, ME = 11.6 MJ, DCP = 130 g
Figures for fibre levels and minerals are not available
Yield on NIAB plots = 3.8 DM/ha (relates to the tops and that portion of the root that is above ground)

These quick-growing turnips are a very useful catch crop being sown in the spring as a prelude to a grass reseed in the autumn or after winter barley in July as a break crop.

Stubble turnips are grazed by dairy cows *in situ* behind an electric fence in midsummer and autumn, particularly where grass production is limited. In the summer, stubble turnips and *ad libitum* ammonia-treated straw complement grass, while in the early autumn the same combination can substitute for a limited amount of silage on free-draining soils. Stubble turnips can also be fed to sheep and suckler cows, but are little used for dairy heifers and beef animals because they are unlikely to be constrained by an electric fence. The cost per unit of energy is similar to grazed grass. Fungal problems such as powdery mildew and alternaria leaf spot can limit crop yields.

Kale

The typical analysis for kale per kg DM is:

DM = 13.6 per cent, ME = 12.6 MJ, DCP = 119 g, NDF = 208 g, MADF = 161 g
Minerals: Ca = 12.1 g, P = 3.5 g, Na = 1.2 g, Mg = 1.4 g (varieties differ in analysis)
Yield on NIAB plots = 8.6 t DM/ha

Kale can be grown in most areas of the UK but yields can be adversely affected by dry weather.

Protein and minerals are contained in the leaves and carbohydrates and fibre occur in the stem. Thus, the proportion of leaf to stem influences the feed value of kale.

Kale is a low DM, high-protein feed that is high in calcium, but low in phosphorus, copper, manganese and iodine. Goitrogens can interfere with iodine use in the dairy cow (see p. 221). Excessive amounts of kale can lead to haemolytic anaemia (see p. 613).

In the past, kale was strip-grazed in the autumn and up to midwinter and, together with hay, provided the maintenance portion of the dairy cows' ration. The practice has been largely curtailed as herds moved towards autumn calving, and a continuity of feed during the winter season became necessary. In addition, foot troubles were very common and udders needed additional washing. Currently, kale is grazed *in situ* in the summer and early autumn in a similar fashion to stubble turnips with ammonia-treated straw. It tends to be fed to mid- and late-lactation cows and should not exceed 30 per cent of the ration. In practice, 3–4 kg DM/head per day are consumed together with 1–2 kg of ammonia-treated straw. Kale can be cut and carted to all classes of stock, and may be strip-grazed by sheep in winter.

Forage rape

The typical analysis of forage rape per kg DM is:

DM = 14 per cent, ME = 9.5 MJ, DCP = 144 g (no fibre figures are available)
Minerals: Ca = 9.3 g, P = 4.2 g, Na = 2.3 g, Mg = 2.1 g
Yield on NIAB plots = 5.4 t DM/ha

Rape can be grown in most areas of the UK. Forage rape can be used as a catch crop like stubble turnips and kale but is lower yielding than the latter and higher yielding than the former. The principles of feeding and the reservations on use of forage rape are similar to kale. Forage rape can cause taints in milk and should be introduced into the ration slowly. It can be grazed *in situ* from July to December, or be zero-grazed.

Lucerne

The typical analysis of lucerne silage per kg DM is:

DM = 29 per cent, ME = 9.5 MJ, DCP = 134 g, NDF = 464 g, MADF = 357 g
Minerals: figures are not available, but it is claimed to be high in minerals, except sodium, and to have good buffering capacity in the rumen
Yield on NIAB plots = 14.7 t DM/ha

Lucerne is a perennial crop, lasting four years, grown on alkaline soils in dry areas.

Lucerne silage, like most legumes, has high intake characteristics due to the composition of the cell walls. In practice, the energy value to the animal is at least 1 MJ higher than the feed analysis, and DMI can be enhanced by 20–30 per cent. It is claimed that the protein is of a better quality than in grass silage. Lucerne silage is conserved in a clamp, but additives are necessary for good preservation because lucerne has low carbohydrate levels. Leaf loss should be avoided. Lucerne can also be used to make good quality big bale silage for dairy cows, and hay for racehorses.

Self-feeding layers of lucerne silage in a grass silage clamp should be avoided for dairy cows because it tends to go mushy. In winter rations for dairy cows, 4–5 kg DM of both lucerne and maize silage with 0.5–2 kg straw can form the basis of a highly productive winter ration (see section on maize, p. 99). It could also be fed with fodder beet. Lucerne silage is rarely fed to beef cattle or dairy heifers because only limited quantities are available, but could form a balanced ration with maize silage, fodder beet and straw to produce the required liveweight gain.

Lucerne is not normally grazed as dairy cows can suffer from bloat (see p. 637), except at the end of the growing season, i.e. October and after the first severe winter frost.

Red clover

The typical analysis for red clover silage per kg DM is:

DM = 22 per cent, ME = 8.8 MJ, DCP = 135 g
Figures are not available for the fibre levels and mineral content, but like lucerne, red clover has high intake characteristics and the ME is likely to be close to 10 MJ/kg DM
Yield on NIAB plots = 13.5 t DM for first harvest year, and 11.1 t/ha for the second harvest year

Unlike lucerne, red clover tends to be grown in the wetter areas of the UK, but like lucerne it can decrease nitrogen use and reduce the production costs of conserved fodder.

Red clover is not often grown as a pure stand by dairy farmers but as part of a three to four year ley with Italian, hybrid and early perennial ryegrasses for conservation. Typically, red clover is 20 per cent of the mixture as seed weight, but the number is large as clover has smaller seeds than the ryegrasses. Winter rations based on silage from the above mixture should encourage higher forage intakes and lessen the need for concentrate-type foods. However, red clover silage when compared with grass silage fed to dairy cows produced higher milk yields, higher percentages of protein and lactose, but a lower percentage of butterfat for early- and midlactation cows, but the lactation milk yield was not significantly higher. The grass/red clover sward has been grazed with no adverse effects from bloat. Sheep and young stock have also grazed the ley in the autumn with benefit. Lambs fed on pure red clover swards, again used cautiously, have shown liveweight gains increased by 30 per cent. Red clover silage has been given to young stock and beef animals have shown an increased growth rate of 14 per cent compared with grass silage (Thomas *et al.*, 1982).

Peas

The typical analysis for pea silage per kg DM is:

DM = 25.9 per cent, ME = 8.8 MJ, DCP = 146 g, NDF = 517 g, MADF = 384 g
Minerals: Ca = 12.7 g, P = 4.4 g, Na = 0.4 g, Mg = 2.0 g
Yield (estimated) = 7 t DM/ha

Pea silage can be a byproduct from the production of vining peas and may be more like straw. Peas can be grown on their own, but need some physical support and are usually sown in conjunction with spring barley on the basis of 40:60 peas:barley by seed weight. Newman & Luffman (1984) have produced the arable silage mixture (barley was cut at the cheesy stage) with a DM of 43.2 per cent, ME of 10.2 MJ and DCP of 147 g. They observed that the silage yield at 10 t DM/ha was very palatable. Depending on the stage of lactation, when fed to 200 dairy cows in Somerset, it produced rises in DMI between 10 and 20 per cent over grass silage. (Dry matter intake of grass silage tends to be in the range of 7–10 kg depending on the quality and quantity of the silage.) The arable silage mixture can also be fed to dairy heifers and beef animals. Peas are not an easy crop to establish and whole crop cereal silage may be preferred.

Sainfoin

A typical analysis for sainfoin silage per kg DM is:

DM = 24 per cent, ME = 8.4 MJ, DCP = 124 g
Figures for fibre and minerals are not available
Yield (estimated) = 7.5 t DM/ha

Sainfoin is a perennial legume that is not easy to establish. It has low-yielding, low-intake characteristics. The protein is more rumen undegradable than in grass silage, and so it can provide 50 per cent more absorbed protein than lucerne. Its main advantage is that animals do not suffer from bloat when it is fed, due to the presence of tannins (see p. 637).

Rye

The typical analysis for grazed rye per kg DM is:

DM = 23 per cent, ME = 9.5 MJ, DCP = 88 g
Figures are not yet available for fibre and mineral content
Yield (estimated) = 7.7 t DM/ha

Rye is grown on its own or in a mixture with Italian ryegrass to produce an early bite in the spring on light land with a low pH. It is usually strip-grazed by dairy cows once daily and its feed value often decreases rapidly. Zero-grazing is possible. Any surplus can be conserved as big bale silage and used for any class of stock. In some areas it is followed by forage maize and could be drilled after an early maturing variety of maize in the autumn. Many dairy farmers prefer buffer

Table 8.2 Analysis of byproducts fed to dairy cattle

Food	DM (%)	ME (MJ)	DCP (g)	NDF (g)	MADF (g)	Ca (g)	P (g)	Na (g)	Mg (g)
Brewers' grains	22.0	11.7	189	572	219	3.3	4.1	0.1	1.5
Cabbage	10.6	13.7	181	586	140	7.2	4.5	1.2	1.5
Carrots	13.0	12.8	62	–*	–	5.9	3.4	0.8	1.8
Parsnips	15.0	13.3	67	–	–	–	–	–	–
Potatoes	20.4	13.3	80	73	39	0.4	2.0	0.2	1.0
Pressed sugar beet pulp	25.4	12.3	60	557	259	9.0	1.1	0.6	2.0
Apples	13.6	12.2	–	111	101	0.5	0.9	0.1	0.3
Apple pomace	23.0	8.7	–	503	375	1.7	1.4	0.2	0.6

*–, no reliable information available.

feeding of silage in late spring or other combinations of feed to growing small areas of rye.

Triticale

Feed analysis figures are not available for triticale, which is a hybrid of wheat and rye. Triticale can perform a similar function to rye, and is said to have lower DM yields than rye in the earlier part of the season, but its digestibility stays at a higher level than rye as the crop matures. Feeding value is likely to be similar to whole crop silage. If cut in mid June, it can have a DM of 25 per cent and an ME of 9.6 MJ. Both sugar and fibre levels are higher than grass.

Whole-crop silage: whole wheat

A typical analysis for whole-wheat silage (Newman, pers. comm.) per kg DM is:

DM = 50 per cent, ME = 10.7 MJ, crude protein = 18 per cent, NDF = 400 g, pH = 8
Yield (estimated range) = 7–10 t DM/ha

In the past, whole-crop cereal silage has not performed well. The Agricultural and Food Research Council's Institute for Grassland and Environmental Research has recently shown that, when preserved with sufficient added urea, resulting in no fermentation occurring, whole-crop wheat has a potentially high intake. The alkalinity of the product positively assists rumen function, increases DMI and hence milk quality for dairy cows and growth rates for beef animals. (Wilkinson and Stark, 1990).

Whole-crop wheat silage can be fed with molasses to supplement grass or maize silage in the winter or for buffer feeding in the spring, or without supplement to dry stock.

Wet byproducts used in dairy cow rations

The products shown in Table 8.2 can be incorporated in winter rations for dairy cows and other stock. They are likely to be fed with straw and other ingredients for other cattle, and to supplement grass silage and act as a concentrate replacer for dairy cows.

Vegetable waste, e.g. Brussels sprouts, cabbages and cauliflowers from vegetable processing plants, could have a similar feed value to kale. Potato waste, pressed sugar beet, peas and beans are occasionally available. Good storage facilities and the avoidance of waste are necessary for the above products. They will all need to fit in with the ration criteria for the appropriate class of stock.

References

Gleadthorpe Experimental Husbandry Form (1984) In *Gleadthorpe Experimental Husbandry Form Annual Review*, pp. 15–17.

Gleadthorpe Experimental Husbandry Form (1985) in *Gleadthorpe Experimental Husbandry Form Annual Review*, pp. 38–40.

Newman, G. & Luffman, B.J. (1984) Lucerne, red clover and forage peas: management, utilization and incorporation into feed systems. In *Occasional Symposium of the British Grassland Society* (ed. by D.S. Thompson), pp. 147–51.

Thomas, C., Aston, K., Daley, S.R. & Hughes, P.M. (1982) A comparison of red clover with grass silage for milk production. *British Society of Animal Production Winter Meeting, Harrogate.*

Thomas, C., Aston, K. & Daley, S.R. (1985) Milk production from silage, 3. A comparison of red clover and grass silage. *Animal Production* **41**, 23–31.

Wilkinson, J.M. & Stark, B.A. (1990) *White crop cereals — making and feeding cereal silage.* Chelcombe Publications pp. 1–86.

PART 2
DISEASE

Chapter 9: Diagnosis and Differential Diagnosis in the Cow

by P.J.N. PINSENT

The clinical attitude

Veterinary clinicians must develop certain special attributes in relation to their environment. They must be inquisitive, questioning, curious and observant. They must notice everything around them, and, if possible, explain it. They must always be critical in the true sense of the word. They spend their lives diagnosing disease and must understand quite clearly that, as health is normality, then disease is simply *deviation from normality*. From this, it follows that veterinary surgeons will never be able to detect and recognize disease, i.e. deviation from the normal, until they know the normal. They must learn the normal in all domestic species in many different circumstances. For normality is relative, not absolute. It is relative to breed, age, nutrition, the stage of lactation or pregnancy, management, and many other factors.

Thus normality is relative to environment. The veterinarian, therefore, must consider the environment as critically as he does the patient. Is it suitable? Does it predispose to, or even cause, the abnormality present in the patient? Does it cause stress? Remember that the environment can only be appreciated if one considers the animal's viewpoint: for example, if it is thought that the ventilation in a calf house is suspect, it may well be advisable to get your head down among the calves!

If it is accepted that disease is often related to environment, nutrition, or management, then it follows that in an adverse environment other animals in the group may also be affected. In such circumstances, it is always well worthwhile looking carefully at the rest of the group, if necessary, animal by animal. It may well be that others are showing the same signs albeit to a lesser extent. Such an observation may be very helpful not only in diagnosis, but also from the viewpoints of treatment and prevention.

The veterinarians of today must concern themselves with the health of the herd as well as the individual and it is almost negligent to omit from the examination of the individual cow, a look, however brief, at the other stock in the group.

The other side of the coin is that, in unusual environmental conditions, when you are not certain whether the cow's response is normal or not, it is often very helpful to look at the rest of the group. If they are all showing the same response, then either they are all abnormal, which is unlikely, or they represent normality, in which case, the patient is also normal.

It should be remembered that the owner and his staff are an important part of the patient's environment, and can play a large part in the disease process and progress. They, equally with, or perhaps even more than, other environmental factors, merit critical assessment. Are they competent? Are they humane? Are they interested? Are they truthful? Have they contributed to the disease process? They merit critical study, for the staff are inextricably involved with their animals and the one cannot be considered without the other.

The important diagnostic principles that should always be followed are shown below.

1 Be systematic.
2 Adopt a routine that is found suitable and stick to it.
3 Take nothing on trust.
4 Apply continual critical assessment to oneself and monitor one's own attitudes and techniques.
5 Consider all the time:
   (a) Is there a problem?
   (b) If so, then define it.
   (c) Having defined it, what is best done about it?

The clinician's approach to the clinical case

There is nothing magical about clinical work. It depends upon care, patience, thoroughness, method and logical routine; a routine of examination that covers all the likely eventualities. Once having evolved such a procedure, there should be no short cuts without good reason, and, however cursory some sections of the examination, for various reasons, sometimes have to be, nothing should be omitted without due consideration.

The clinical examination

THE OWNER'S MESSAGE

The owner's message (usually termed the owner's complaint) should include name and full address, and may reach the clinician by direct word of mouth, by telephone, or frequently nowadays, by radio telephone direct to his car. The owner's complaint will also include the type of animal and the main presenting syndrome, e.g. a scouring cow, a downer cow, a convulsing cow, or a bloated cow.

There are a limited number of main presenting syndromes, and the clinician should learn differential lists for each of them, to include only the major differential conditions, not the rarities. It should be remembered when considering the differential lists that the common things occur commonly; that is why they are common!

The clinician should know the main presenting syndrome and its differential list, and during the journey to the farm should consider the following points.

1 The time of year. Many diseases are seasonal, e.g. the coughing calf indoors in November probably has a viral or bacterial based pneumonia, but the coughing calf at grass in August probably has husk.
2 The part of the country. Each type of country has its own disease problems, e.g. in the hills one meets malignant catarrhal fever, bracken poisoning, and piroplasmosis, while in intensive lowland dairying areas one meets coliform mastitis, milk fever and hypomagnesaemia.
3 The individual farm. The clinician will often know that a specific farm has a particular disease problem, e.g. a parasitic problem among the young stock, because they are overcrowded and underfed.
4 The type of management. For example, heavily stocked cubicle yards with straw bedding often lead to coliform mastitis.

Such patterns of disease become second nature to veterinary surgeons, and always hold good for the part of the country in which they work, although revision might be necessary in a practice 400 miles away.

The clinician will, therefore, arrive at the farm with a diagnosis already half formed. It will be adaptable, not dogmatic, a *working hypothesis*, to be confirmed or refuted; however, it is quite remarkable how often this hypothesis stands up to the test of full clinical examination, and, more importantly, refutes the presence of any other disease process.

Thus, if the clinician knows that the cow to be visited is showing convulsive signs at pasture, that it is early May, that it is an intensive dairy area in Britain and that the farm fertilizes heavily for an early bite, the chances that the disease condition is anything other than hypomagnesaemia are too remote to be significant. Nevertheless, a clinical examination, however brief, is always necessary.

HISTORY

History is all important and the foundation of diagnosis.
1 Immediate history is the story of the present illness.
2 Past history is anything in the animal's earlier life that may be relevant, e.g. calving and service dates, something similar at the same point in a previous lactation, and so on.
3 Herd or group history is important when adverse nutritional or management factors may be relevant to the present illness.

History taking is an art — it does not come naturally, but must be learnt and practised. After a few pleasant introductory words, questioning can begin while walking to the animal, which may be approached, but should not, if at all possible, be disturbed. First, look. Check the owner's statements mentally by reference to the animal and the surroundings. Do not hurry the owner at first: let him or her talk, then ask your own questions, checking each statement and following a routine that suits you. You are not wasting time for you are, meanwhile, carrying out the next two parts of the clinical routine.

Do not ask leading questions in the hope of saving time, or in the hope of confirming one's half formed diagnosis, for they often produce inaccurate or misleading answers. Human nature being what it is, owners may either agree with you because they think they ought to, or disagree because they are contra-suggestive.

Study the owner or stockworkers. Are they reliable? Are they telling the truth? Are they covering up errors in management? Are they guessing? Every clinician must be interested in the human animal; after all, it is the owner whom you serve, advise, encourage, or console. In a way, the owner is as much your patient as the cow. Admittedly, owners seldom deliberately falsify their story, but it is wise to beware the guilty one, the bombastic one, the one who knows it all, or the one involved in the sale or purchase of the affected animal.

DESCRIPTION

A formal description is more relevant to the examination of a horse, but it is often very useful for the clinician to classify the animal under observation mentally while the history is unfolding, e.g. a young Friesian cow, recently calved, and heavily in milk. It is always dangerous to be uncertain as to the exact type of animal under examination as it may lead to loss of face in discussion of the case, and occasionally, even to serious error.

PRELIMINARY INSPECTION

Like the description, this inspection, *note* inspection not examination, takes practically no time, and is carried out during history taking.

At this stage, do not touch, do not disturb. Stand well back. Put the picture in its frame. One is looking for the deviations from normality that constitute disease, so:

1 one must know the normal;

2 if the animal is frightened, pushed about or even handled, abnormalities may appear due to annoyance and fear. The minutiae that might have given a diagnostic lead will be masked. Condition, vigour, demeanour, respiratory pattern, appetite, rumination, faecal passage and type, and response to environment, should all be noted.

PRELIMINARY EXAMINATION

The animal may now be touched but it is essential to proceed quietly, with as little fuss as possible. This stage of the examination includes the rate and character of the pulse, the temperature, and a check on skin, eye, membranes, udder, and ruminal movement. Although pulse character and rate are very important, it is frequently quite impossible to examine the pulse properly in a modern dairy cow that has been separated from the others, driven into a crush, and clamped by the neck. It is usually not possible to do more than check the heart and heart rate with a stethoscope.

The clinician may well have arrived at a diagnosis at this stage, but if not is probably aware of the system of the body involved. In this case, he may only need to confirm his views, by examination of that system and by checking out the other systems quickly, even mentally.

Nevertheless, the position may still be far from clear, and the clinician will then have to embark upon a systematic examination. The procedure so far described will have taken no more than a few minutes, but if a full systematic examination becomes necessary, the case becomes much more time consuming.

SYSTEMATIC EXAMINATION

This includes all the manual and instrumental techniques necessary as part of such an examination, even including surgical intervention in some cases. The clinician, according to training and inclination, may interpret the word systematic as meaning (i) thorough, starting at the nose and finishing at the tail or (ii) system by system, in which case a mental list of the systems or sections that should be examined can be ticked off mentally when satisfied.

There is merit in adopting the second routine. It enables one to examine first the system or disease section that seems most likely to be affected from the preliminary evidence. Should the provisional diagnosis be confirmed, then a great deal of time will be saved, for it will only be necessary to check the remaining systems briefly, even, in some cases, mentally, to make sure that there is no other disease or lesion present. If there is no provisional diagnosis in mind, then it is reasonable to begin the systematic examination with the digestive system. In cows, this is the most likely cause of illness in obscure cases. Subsequently, the less important systems and sections can be examined as necessary.

A logical list of systems and disease groups for examination is as follows.

1 Digestive system.
2 Respiratory system.
3 Circulatory system.
4 Urinary system.
5 Genital system.
6 Locomotory system.
7 Nervous system.
8 Skin.
9 Sense organs.
10 Lymphatic system.
11 Liver.
12 Udder.
13 Parasite problems.
14 Metabolic disease.
15 Allergies.

The last five headings on this list are, of course, not systems: nevertheless, they are very important disease sites (liver and udder) or disease groups that are logically considered as entities on the clinician's list.

LABORATORY AND SPECIAL EXAMINATIONS

These are very important today, although increasing costs and the decline of dairying have unfortunately decreed that most laboratory work, apart from statutory Ministry investigations, or that done in the practice, is limited to the diagnosis of herd problems, rather than individual cow disease.

It is important that the clinician should never become slave to the laboratory. The laboratory investigation is intended to confirm or refute the provisional diagnosis (working hypothesis) already in your mind.

Clinical examination comes first. Laboratory results can be inaccurate, irrelevant, and confusing as well as expensive, but if used logically and critically, they can be of great help.

Laboratory investigations include: haematology, biochemistry, bacteriology, parasitology, serology, biopsy (histology) of tissues or fluids, and finally, necropsy.

Even after full examination, one may not have a complete diagnosis. However, there should be sufficient evidence to make a provisional diagnosis, which will allow a logical course of treatment and, where relevant, prevention. The clinician must be prepared to think, form a working programme even on insufficient evidence, have enough confidence to convince the owner, and enough adaptability to modify the programme tactfully if, and when, new evidence appears.

Owners, of course, are only partly interested in diagnosis. *Prognosis* is much more important to them. Will the cow get better? Will she be fully productive again? Is she worth treating? And today, unfortunately, another factor enters the equation. Will it be inconvenient to treat the cow; will she need nursing or extra care? If so, she is likely to be slaughtered, provided that she has antibiotic clearance and is likely to pass meat inspection.

The main presenting syndromes

It is not intended to discuss here the detailed techniques of the clinical examination of the various body systems. Every clinician has learnt these techniques as part of basic training, and there is excellent coverage in many text books, e.g. Boddie's *Diagnostic Methods in Veterinary Medicine* (1970). Instead, this chapter sets out to consider the differential diagnosis of some, although by no means all, of the main presenting syndromes that occur from day-to-day in the dairy cow.

Drooling at the mouth (kiddling, slobbering)

This is due to factors causing excess salivation, or factors preventing normal swallowing, or combinations of both.

Bacterial or viral lesions in mouth

Although foot-and-mouth disease has not occurred in Great Britain and some other countries for a number of years, it must never be forgotten (see Chapter 37(c)). The consequences of failure to recognize this disease are quite terrifying. Any salivating bovine animal, whether lame or not, whether pyrexic or not, must be treated as a possible case of foot-and-mouth disease until the clinician is satisfied that it is not. Other pyrexic diseases with oral lesions may give cause for concern, particularly bovine virus diarrhoea (BVD)/mucosal disease (see p. 660), infectious bovine rhinotracheitis, infectious bovine rhinotracheitis (IBR) (see p. 256) and occasional cases of malignant catarrhal fever, but, fortunately, the mouth lesions and signs caused by these three diseases are usually relatively superficial and mild.

Actinobacillosis causes mechanical difficulty in tongue movement. The lesion is obvious, but painless even when ulcerated (see p. 627).

Calf diphtheria is limited to the young animal, causes pain as well as difficulty in mastication or suckling, and produces inflammatory swelling with necrosis of the mucous membrane of the cheek (see p. 214).

Foreign bodies

These are rare in the mouths of cattle, but the lids of cans occasionally become wedged between the lower molars and the cheek. Rarely, a stick becomes impacted between the rows of lower molars, or a molar itself loosens (see p. 626).

Interference with swallowing

This may be due to paralysis of the fifth or seventh cranial nerves which, in turn, may be due to listeriosis, meningeal abscesses, or, particularly in the case of the 7th nerve, to trauma to the side of the head or face.

Fifth nerve paralysis makes the cow unable to close her mouth completely. The lips are in apposition but the teeth are not, a fact which is easily checked by flicking the lower jaw upwards, when the clicking together of upper and lower molars may be heard. Fifth nerve paralysis may often lead to accumulation of partly masticated food or cud in the pharynx, producing marked discomfort and gagging.

Seventh nerve paralysis causes unilateral or bilateral paralysis of the lips and cheek, and if of central origin, as in listeriosis (see p. 703), also causes flaccidity of the eyelids, with resultant keratitis and drooping of the ear on the affected side. This condition also leads to dropping of the cud bolus out of the mouth on the affected side, and thus, ultimately, to loss of condition.

Oesophageal choke, particularly in the high oesphageal position, causes anxiety, even distress, with arching of the neck and profuse salivation. Choke may also cause varying degrees of ruminal tympany (see p. 631).

Dilatation and diverticulum of the oesophagus, particularly in the low cervical position, may produce similar, though milder, signs, as accumulation of food in the diverticulum may eventually lead to blocking of the oesophageal lumen, with resultant accumulation of food and saliva above the lesion.

Actinobacillosis of the oesophageal groove may lead not only to low-grade ruminal tympany but also to reflux of ruminal and reticular fluid into the mouth, so that in shippen-housed (i.e. tied) cows, a pool of such fluid may be found in the manager in the morning (see p. 627).

Excess salivation of CNS origin

This may be seen in lead poisoning, for the toxin affects the salivary nucleus. Blindness and aimless wandering in the cow, abdominal pain and convulsions with bellowing in the calf, should help the diagnosis.

In the 'licking mania' ketotic complication of milk fever or in 'nervous acetonaemia' (see p. 590) excess salivation is due to the compulsive chewing so characteristic of the disease.

Rhododendron poisoning

This may cause profuse salivation, and even vomiting, as well as diarrhoea (see p. 615).

Organophosphorus compounds

These may also cause salivation and diarrhoea (see p. 618).

Acute photosensitization syndromes

These may well cause profuse salivation, as well as lacrimation, jaundice and, later, the onset of necrosis of the non-pigmented skin areas (see p. 686).

Acute dyspnoea

This condition, as in very severe pneumonia, may cause obvious salivation as a result of mouth breathing.

Acute anaphylactic shock

This often causes profuse drooling of saliva as well as tachypnoea, subnormal temperature, cold extremities, oedema, and a very rapid heart (see p. 758).

Vomiting (see p. 630)

Vomiting is very rare in the cow and, to all intents and purposes, only occurs in *laurel* and *rhododendron poisoning* (see p. 615). Very occasionally a peptic ulcer of the abomasum will cause problems (see p. 649). Regurgitation of rumen fluid or content (false vomiting) may occur in cases of acute bloat (see p. 637), or where there are lesions in the oesophageal groove, e.g. actinobacillosis or a foreign body ('wire') (see p. 643).

Occasionally, cases of oesophageal dilatation and diverticulation may accumulate material above the obstruction until it overflows into and out of the mouth.

Acute abdominal pain (colic)

It is interesting that acute colic pain of the type seen in the horse is relatively rare in cattle, and several of the syndromes that cause the most acute pain are not, in fact, obstructive gut lesions, as one would expect, and may not even involve the alimentary tract at all.

Acute gut obstruction

This may be due to the following causes.
1 Abomasal torsion (see p. 648).
2 Torsion of caecum, colon, or ileum or common mesentery (see p. 653).
3 Strangulated mesenteric hernia.
4 Strangulated scrotal hernia.
5 Gut tie: the entrapment of gut in peritoneal tears at the edge of the internal inguinal ring due to castration by traction in the slightly older animal.
6 Intussusception (see p. 654).
7 Obstruction of ileum by the stalk of a lipoma.

Abomasal or large gut torsion produces a degree, sometimes very considerable, of right-sided abdominal distension, not normally seen in small gut obstructions. In gut tie, there may be considerable distension in the inguinal region, whilst scrotal hernia obviously produces distension of the scrotum on the affected side. It is, however, very easy for the clinician to overlook scrotal or inguinal swelling unless aware of the possibility. These acute obstructive conditions cause the most acute colicky abdominal pain in the very early stages, but such pain is often very transient and by the time the case is presented to the veterinary surgeon, temperature is falling, pulse rate is rising, body surfaces are becoming cold and even clammy, and a dull toxaemic and shocked appearance develops as circulatory obstruction, necrosis, and gangrene of the obstructed gut supervenes. Intussusception is sometimes an exception in that many cases of bovine intussusception, particularly if large gut is involved, show little more than depression and dullness even in the early stages. Rectal examination is a useful diagnostic procedure.

Acute enteritis (see p. 656)

Acute enteritis, particularly salmonellosis (see Chapter 13), is similar to acute cereal over-eating, e.g. barley poisoning, in that some cases show spectacularly acute abdominal pain, often with some degree of tympany, which remains noticeable for a considerable time, often several hours, before the characteristic profuse diarrhoea begins. Laparotomies have been performed on a number of occasions at this stage of the disease in the belief that the condition was one of acute gut obstruction. Once diarrhoea appears, temperature falls often to normal or below, while signs of dehydration, electrolyte imbalance and shock appear.

Acute fermentative colic

This condition, involving the caecum and colon and producing right flank tympany, may occur on rich pasture, particularly in wet weather, and may be difficult to differentiate from acute obstructive conditions. Fortunately, these conditions generally respond to analgesics and antispasmodics before serious diagnostic errors occur.

The passage of a calculus down the ureter

This may produce the most spectacular colicky pain, which fortunately is usually relatively transient. Diagnosis is obviously extremely difficult (see p. 560).

Photosensitization involving teats

Acute photosensitization (see p. 326) in cattle, e.g. Ayrshires with sparingly pigmented teats and udders, can produce an inflammatory exudative lesion of teats and skin of the udder that is so painful that the cow behaves exactly as if suffering from an acute abdominal catastrophe. Diagnostic error will only be avoided if the clinician remembers the invariable rule that whatever may seem to be affecting a cow, the udder and teats must always be examined.

Acute abdominal distension

This is one of the important and relatively common presenting syndromes in the cow. All causes of abdominal distension in the cow are covered by the memory rhyme (the seven F's), which runs as follows: fat, fetus, fluid, flatus, faeces, food or foreign body. Severe abdominal distension may originate at several sites.

RUMINAL

Dietary ruminal impaction

This occurs in housed fattening cattle on store diet, hay or straw, with limited water. The massive ruminal impaction, absence of ruminal movement, raised temperature and pulse rate, painful frequent abdominal grunt, and hard scanty faeces, produce a syndrome requiring differentiation from *acute traumatic reticuloperitonitis* ('wire') (see p. 643) in its very early stages, although the impactive mass in the 'wired' rumen is never so great.

A similar condition, although much less severe, may occur in dairy cows tied in shippens during the winter should the water bowl cease to function, a mishap that frequently escapes the attendant's notice, and is always worth checking. Modern systems of building and management have markedly decreased the incidence of these two conditions.

Impaction of the rumen with grain (see p. 634) occurs in cows that have broken into a food store and eaten greedily, but even when the attendant is unaware of this, or will not admit it, the nature of the case generally becomes apparent in two to three days when profuse diarrhoea, staggering, recumbency, subnormal temperature, rapid pulse rate, and other evidence of toxic effects occur in severe cases. In cases seen soon after ingestion of large quantities of grain, palpation of the left sublumbar fossa may produce the same sensation as handling a sack of grain. If, as is generally the case in Britain, the grain is barley, the interim period of impaction, with arched back, grunt, depression and moderate tympany is usually transient, and within a few hours the profuse diarrhoea so characteristic of barley poisoning appears.

Vagus indigestion (see p. 641)

This condition is usually a complication of 'wire' that has produced adhesions, involving the medial wall of the reticulum and the cranial sac of the rumen, interfering with the function of the vagus nerve receptors in their walls. The atonic rumen, gradually filling with water and saliva, eventually produces a massive left-sided fluid distension in a cow steadily losing body condition.

Acute ruminal tympany (see p. 637)

Acute ruminal tympany presents relatively little diagnostic difficulty. The condition includes clover and kale bloat, and oesophageal obstruction (choke). The history, environmental circumstances, season of the year, and the gagging, retching, and salivating associated with most cases of choke are generally reasonably conclusive, although in very acute cases, of course, it pays to relieve the tympany via the left sublumbar fossa before worrying too much about the aetiology.

It is worth remembering that a thirsty cow, housed overnight in old-fashioned accommodation and released to drink its fill of very cold water, may easily become, transiently, quite alarmingly tympanitic, due presumably to the chilling effect of the frosty water on the rumen musculature.

The acute ruminal tympany of a cow that, for one reason or another, e.g. milk fever, has collapsed into lateral recumbency, should not require mention. It is, however, surprising that it is still quite commonplace to find that such a cow has not been supported in sternal recumbency, as the condition demands.

PERITONEAL

Acute diffuse peritonitis (see p. 655)

This condition occurs when the special ability of the bovine peritoneum to withstand and localize peritoneal infection fails for various reasons, allowing a virulent diffuse exudative process to spread across the peritoneal cavity. Usually, the condition stems from the breakdown of the defensive mechanisms isolating 'wire' in reticular diaphragmatic adhesions, but the leakage or rupture of a superficial liver abscess may produce the same result.

The peritoneal cavity fills with thin evil smelling pus of *Actinomyces (Corynebacterium) pyogenes*: there are widespread adhesions, temperature falls, pulse rate rises, scanty diarrhoea develops, body condition falls away, the cow is toxic and painful. The fluid wave is very obvious and confirmation by paracentesis is easy. The condition most likely to cause confusion is the massive milky ascites that may follow extensive liver damage and obstruction to the portal circulation. Inspection and examination of peritoneal fluid provides straightforward differentiation.

Peritoneal tympany

Peritoneal tympany, a gas-filled abdominal cavity, may occur following perforation of an abomasal ulcer at a point free of attached omentum, causing acute pain over much of the anterior abdomen, particularly on the right side. Grunting, tooth grinding, falling temperature and rising pulse rate are followed by progressive peritoneal tympany due to leakage of gas from the abomasal lumen into the abdominal cavity.

ABOMASAL

Dilatation and/or torsion of abomasum (see p. 648)

Dilatation and/or torsion of the abomasum on the right produces right-sided distension, very marked in cases

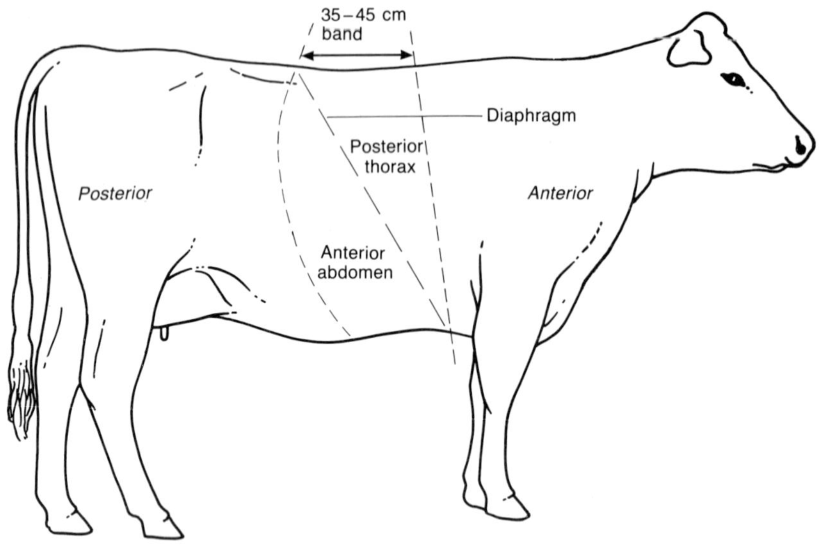

Fig. 9.1 Lateral view of cow showing anterior abdominal/posterior thoracic area.

of torsion, which also causes acute and even colicky pain.

Acute left abomasal displacement (see p. 645)

This condition produces significant abdominal distension of the left flank, but such cases are exceptional.

All abomasal cases are amenable to diagnosis by normal auscultation methods.

INTESTINAL

Acute tympanitic fermentative intestinal colic

This condition, which usually resolves without too much difficulty, can produce massive right-sided distension.

Torsion of caecum and colon on the common mesentery (see p. 653)

This serious and usually fatal complication of fermentation and atony also produces massive right-sided distension. Differentiation depends upon demeanour, rectal examination, pulse rate, and upon progress of the case following initial medication.

UTERINE

Hydrops amnion and allantois (see p. 479)

These conditions produce very marked abdominal distension. Diagnosis is helped by rectal examination. Uterine rupture producing extra-uterine pregnancy in the last third of pregnancy is marked by the formation of much fibrinous exudate in an abdomen filled with free uterine fluid and containing fetus and membranes. Such an abdomen is distended and shows a fluid wave which, on rectal examination, appears to be unassociated with the uterus. There is abdominal pain, rapid pulse, and often severe illness. Diagnosis depends upon an accurate history and the ballottement of a fetus in the lower abdomen, even though rectal examination reveals a partially involuted uterus.

Anterior abdominal/posterior thoracic pain

The organs and structures enclosed within a 35–45 cm band encircling the cow immediately behind the withers provide a group of diseases of great importance to the bovine clinician. Viewed from a lateral position, the diaphragm divides this area into the posterior thorax anteriorly and dorsally, and the anterior abdomen ventrally and posteriorly (Fig. 9.1).

The band described encircles lungs, mediastinum, heart, pleural cavity, and great vessels in front of the diaphragm, and rumen, reticulum, omasum, abomasum, liver, gall-bladder, spleen, and the anterior part of the peritoneal cavity posteriorly with much of the greater and lesser omental sheets. Differential diagnosis is often difficult and is not helped by the fact that both thoracic and abdominal lesions occur within this imaginary belt.

The classical and traditional condition affecting this area is traumatic reticulo-peritonitis ('wire') (see p. 643) and it is very convenient to use this condition, less common nowadays, but well known and recognized, as a yard-stick with which to compare the numerous other conditions of the posterior thorax and anterior abdomen.

The possibility of overlooking a penetrating foreign body, a serious mistake for both patient and clinician, is always at the back of one's mind when examining a bovine abdomen. It is always a considerable relief if one can eliminate the possibility of a foreign body and its complications, and such a process is, of course, very important to the surgeon when considering the site of a possible exploratory laparotomy. Nevertheless, neither the confirmation nor the refutation of a provisional diagnosis of traumatic reticulitis is easy without exploratory laparotomy. Thus, the clinical syndrome presents such wide variations in both the extent and intensity of signs that it is probably true to say that the only constant clinical sign is the presence of some degree of pain in the anterior abdomen. The range of differential diagnosis is therefore wide, and includes several groups of clinical conditions each capable of confusion by virtue of exhibiting one or more of the signs associated with reticulitis.

The acute clinical syndrome not infrequently encountered at the onset of the condition includes complete inappetence, and ruminal and reticular atony, resulting in ruminal impaction and slight tympany, with absence of ruminal movement and cudding. Constipation may also be a feature. Temperature may be 40–40.5°C (104–105°F) with a pulse rate of 80–90/minute. There is a marked drop in milk yield. The painful focus in the anterior abdomen results in general rigidity with arched back and protruding neck, disinclination to lie down, and spontaneous grunting accentuated by movement, defaecation, and micturition, and very marked on pinching the withers or applying upward pressure to the xiphisternal region.

This acute syndrome is by no means constant, even at the onset of reticulitis, and when present usually abates in 24–36 hours as the intensity of pain lessens, and varying degrees of ruminal and reticular motility return. Temperature tends to fall into the 39–39.5°C (102–103°F) range, pulse rate may be in the normal range or slightly raised, appetite, although poor, is not completely absent, ruminal impaction and tympany largely disappear, and faeces regain normal consistency. The painful rigid stance relaxes and although the back remains somewhat stiff and arched, pain may require elicitation by the clinician rather than being obviously spontaneous. Rumination, however, nearly always remains absent, or irregular and occasional.

In some cases, the only clinical signs are slightly depressed appetite and rumination, subnormal milk yield, and indications of pain so slight that they amount to no more than unwillingness to depress the back, so that even mild and painless diseases such as acetonaemia have to be considered in differential diagnosis.

The acute and subacute syndromes described above are, of course, essentially those of localized peritonitis, and pictures similar in broad outline will result from other causes of localized peritonitis, although the veterinarian may be able to differentiate the focus of pain.

1 Penetration of the involuted uterus or the vaginal fornix by a catheter or damage to the anterior vagina at service may produce a picture similar save for considerably less interference with alimentary motility, and for pain response on pressure over the posterior abdomen or on rectal examination. Such injuries frequently evoke straining, indicating the need for vaginal examination.

2 Postoperative peritonitis may well provide a syndrome similar to that of moderately acute traumatic reticulitis, but the fact of recent operation and the possibility of peritonitis resulting therefrom will be obvious to the clinician, particularly after procedures such as trocharization for the relief of bloat.

3 Perforation of an abomasal ulcer (see p. 649) may present a picture broadly similar to that of acute traumatic reticulitis if seen in the early stages before diffuse peritonitis, collapse and death occur. There is likely, however, to be acute pain over a much wider area of the anterior abdomen, particularly on the right side, than is the case in reticulitis. Any temperature rise is likely to be transient only, but the pulse rate will be considerably in excess of that expected in reticulitis and may exceed 100/minute. There will be grinding of the teeth and loud groaning as well as grunting of a similar type to that seen in acute reticulitis. The cow will not eat, is greatly depressed, and remains largely recumbent. In a proportion of cases, though by no means all, the abdomen becomes distended with gas, presumably by leakage through the perforation, and a state of true peritoneal tympany develops. This syndrome must also be considered in the differential diagnosis of acute abdominal distension.

4 A peritonitis syndrome varying from a very acute picture associated with shock to a subacute picture sometimes associated with straining is occasionally met with as the result of penetration of the rectum by a foreign body, usually a broom or pitchfork handle, introduced through the anus by an attendant with sadistic tendencies. Such a lesion is always detectable by rectal examination.

5 The more acute lesions of tubercular peritonitis (see p. 670), as seen in the breakdown forms of the disease, occasionally produce an abdominal syndrome similar to

that of traumatic reticulitis. Unless there are obvious coincidental signs of tuberculosis, diagnosis is made only on opening the abdomen with the intention of performing rumenotomy when the blood-streaked, caseating and even exudative lesions of the acute disease may be only too obvious. This syndrome is now rare in civilized countries but might occur should the disease again break out.

Having considered the differentiation of traumatic reticulitis from other causes of peritonitis, one must now be prepared to differentiate moderately severe forms of the disease from conditions which, although not involving peritonitis, cause pain in the anterior abdomen or posterior thorax. This question of pain in the anterior abdomen or posterior thorax is, of course, very important in the diagnosis of reticulitis, for one must remember that the reticulum, diaphragm, liver, abomasum, omasum, heart, pleurae, oesophagus and the posterior lung areas all lie approximately along the vertical line between the point at which one pinches the withers and the point at which one applies the bar.

Bacterial endocarditis (see p. 561)

Classically described and reviewed by Rees Evans (1957), bacterial endocarditis obviously requires differentiation from other cardiac diseases, but it is not generally realized that, in its earlier stages, before signs of venous congestion and circulatory stasis supervene, endocarditis can easily be confused with traumatic reticulitis. Pain, often intermittent in nature, and causing rigidity of stance with abduction of the left, or both, elbows, and discomfort when pressure is applied to the withers, xiphisternum, and left ventral aspect of the chest, is probably due to infarction of the lungs or myocardium, but is not unlike that due to a foreign body penetrating the reticulum. Once venous congestion is clinically obvious, the fact that the heart is diseased becomes apparent, and from this point the clinician must eliminate other cardiac diseases, particularly traumatic pericarditis.

Previous to the development of venous congestion, accelerated respirations with dyspnoea and coughing on exercise, the peculiar 'shifting' lameness of endocarditis, the tendency towards a markedly high pulse rate even when temperature is responding to antibiotics, and the presence, in some cases, of recognizable abnormality of heart sounds, may all help in differentiating endocarditis from reticulitis. The author is cautious on the subject of heart sounds, for although he has frequently been assured by skilled cardiologists that a murmur will always be audible in this disease, he has frequently failed to detect one in cases with a right-sided lesion. It is noticeable that endocarditis cases tend to retain a relatively bright demeanour, and reasonable appetite until the late stages of the disease. The white cell picture is of limited value as many cases present total and differential counts similar to those produced by a penetrating foreign body, although there is a tendency for both total white cell count and neutrophil percentage to be higher than in that disease.

Certain cases of pneumonia and pleurisy
(see Chapter 43)

These conditions, particularly the latter, exhibit signs of posterior thoracic pain that may simulate reticulitis and careful auscultation of the chest is necessary in an attempt to confirm the presence of abnormal thoracic sounds. Pleurisy is very painful in the early dry stages, but becomes painless as effusion develops. Respirations are rapid and shallow, but as effusion builds up, they become deep and swinging.

Impaction of the abomasum (see p. 650)

Impaction of the abomasum, involving primarily the pyloric outlet, with large quantities of fibrous foodstuffs, sand or gravel may occur very occasionally. There is a slow diminution in appetite and milk yield, and progressive ruminal impaction comprising solid food material with, occasionally, a little gas. Rumination ceases and constipation occurs. Temperature is never more than slightly raised, but pulse rate may eventually exceed 100/minute. At first, there is slight anterior abdominal pain only, but as the disease progresses, pinching of the withers and pressure over the xiphisternum are resented markedly. Pain may, in contradistinction to the case in reticulitis, be evoked by pressure over the anterior part of the right flank. The white cell picture may be in the normal range or similar to that of 'wire'. Although the patient becomes much weaker and more depressed than is the case in reticulitis, it is doubtful whether differentiation will be made before exploratory laparotomy reveals the distended doughy abomasum.

The author believes that true abomasal impaction is very rare, and that most of the cases described as abomasal impaction in the past have shown distension of the fundic portion of the abomasum with material like dry rumen contents, and an accumulation of fluid within the rumen, which suggest very strongly that they are, in fact, cases of 'vagus indigestion'.

Painful conditions of the liver

These obviously present a problem in differentiation within the group of diseases causing pain in the anterior abdomen or posterior thorax. The liver is a very difficult organ from the clinician's viewpoint. It is anatomically inaccessible, and, in spite of the considerable volume of work carried out in recent years, there are still no entirely satisfactory tests of liver function in the bovine species.

The cow has large reserves of liver tissue, and very considerable damage may occur without the production of a clear-cut syndrome. Liver biopsy is of limited value in that the portion of liver obtained may be quite unrepresentative of the whole, and the author prefers to make an incision behind the last rib, in the right sublumbar fossa, sufficiently large to allow a manual examination of the liver, and even, using a small torch, limited visual examination. A biopsy specimen can, if required, be obtained through such an incision with the minimum of risk.

Pyelonephritis (see p. 560)

In its more severe forms pyelonephritis produces pain that, although not sited in the anterior abdomen, can easily lead to confusion with traumatic reticulitis particularly as the white cell count is also usually raised. It may be said that, in spite of the raised temperature and pulse rate, the arched back, and the grunt not infrequently present, urine examination leaves the diagnosis beyond doubt. Nevertheless, failure to observe the urine may easily lead to error.

Impaction of the omasum

Another confusing condition, which is practically impossible to diagnose in life, is impaction of the omasum. The disease, which is fortunately very rare, produces slow weight loss, inappetence, low-grade anterior abdominal pain, and general dullness. Ulceration and necrosis of the abomasal leaves are found at post-mortem examination.

Diaphragmatic hernia (see p. 655)

In cattle diapragmatic hernia produces signs much more suggestive of anterior abdominal pain, particularly reticulitis, than of any thoracic involvement. It is, in fact, probable that many cases arise due to weakening of the diaphragmatic muscle by previous foreign body ('wire') damage. The hernial ring is usually small, involving parts of the reticulum, and sometimes the omasum. The resulting low-grade pain may actually be due to areas of peritonitis caused by the original 'wire'. The interference with reticulum and omasum, due to the constriction of the hernial ring and the development of adhesions, sometimes leads to 'vagus indigestion'.

Uterine torsion

It is worth remembering that the occasional cow which develops uterine torsion very early in parturition may show subacute or chronic abdominal pain with progressive inappetence and constipation. Such a case may show little or no further signs of developing labour.

Cases of acute traumatic reticulitis (see p. 643) *with ruminal impaction requiring differentiation from other conditions presenting this feature*

These conditions are discussed in the section on ruminal impaction and include dietary ruminal impaction in yarded cows on fibrous feeds, e.g. hay or straw, with limited access to water. A less spectacular ruminal impaction may occur in dairy cows tied in shippens during the winter should the water bowl cease to function or in groups when the water supply is reduced or ceases, e.g. freezing, bursts in piping, etc.

Impaction of the rumen with grain shows varying degrees of ruminal distension and discomfort for varying periods before diarrhoea supervenes.

Subacute and chronic ruminal tympany (see p. 637) do occur in traumatic reticulitis, particularly in the early stages, and often superimposed on a degree of ruminal impaction. A number of other conditions also result in slight ruminal tympany, which forms a differential group in its own right (see chronic bloat, p. 118).

Cases of traumatic reticulitis (see p. 643) *requiring differentiation from other causes of anterior abdominal pain and conditions causing stiffness and rigidity of stance*

Tetanus (see p. 567) is not infrequently misdiagnosed as reticulitis in the first instance. Not only is there subacute tympany, but the arched back, stiff unbending stance, and marked constipation of tetanus can be quite confusing.

Bilateral solar ulcer (see p. 357), *laminitis* (see p. 360) *and other hind foot lesions* (see Chapter 28). Similarly, but with less justification, cases of bilateral solar ulcer, laminitis, and other painful bilateral hind foot lesions may cause similar confusion.

Injury to lower cervical vertebrae. Occasionally, cows suffer injury to the lower cervical vertebrae, resulting in pain, stiffness and reluctance to bend the lower neck or back, and such cases have sometimes been diagnosed as traumatic reticulitis.

Complications of, and sequelae to, traumatic reticulitis (see p. 643) *causing confusion in diagnosis of anterior abdominal/posterior thoracic pain*

1 Cases are encountered where a piece of wire loose in the reticulum, by reason of its shape, repeatedly pricks the reticular wall and is then dislodged, producing minor episodes of pain and localized peritonitis that rapidly resolve. By the time operation has been decided upon, the animal is substantially normal and surgery is withheld, only for the syndrome to be repeated after varying intervals of time. It is possible that such 'pricks' should be included with transient phases of abomasal displacement as the reason for many of the 'non-specific inappetence' cases so well known to every bovine clinician.

2 A difficult problem is the case where traumatic reticulitis is strongly suspected and rumenotomy carried out, only to find that in spite of the presence of definite reticular adhesions, no foreign body can be found. There are three possibilities. Firstly, the adhesions may be longstanding and bear no relation to the present illness, i.e. the diagnosis is incorrect. This possibility can be checked by applying digital pressure to the adhesions — if pain is provoked, they are probably pertinent to the present ill health. Secondly, the foreign body may have become dislodged and passed down the gut, or even regurgitated, in which case prognosis is good. Thirdly, the foreign body may have passed completely through the reticular wall and be buried in adhesions and reactionary tissue beyond. Here the prognosis is obviously grave.

One can only advise a wait-and-see policy, but such cases do present difficulties in the management of clients who expect the production of a foreign body and, in its absence, are frequently inclined to doubt the diagnosis and regard the operation as an error on the part of the clinician.

3 An occasional, but nevertheless difficult, case is the cow from whose reticulum a foreign body has previously been removed and which now, weeks or months later, is showing a clinical syndrome suggestive of 'wire'. Has there, in fact, been a penetration by a further foreign body; or are the signs due to further infection or abscess formation in the old adhesions? In cases that do not respond promptly to antibiotic therapy, it is always wise to re-operate for even if no further foreign body is involved, an abscess may be found that can be drained into the reticulum.

4 A further group of conditions occur where a foreign body penetrating the reticulum has since penetrated a further organ. Signs, in these cases, are usually related largely to this secondary occurrence and the signs, all-important prognostically, of the primary foreign body aetiology tend to be masked. The classical example of this type of condition is traumatic pericarditis, producing a syndrome very well recognized, but presenting considerable difficulty at times in differentiation from endocarditis.

Penetration of the thoracic cavity to produce suppurative pneumonia or pleurisy also occurs, tending to produce a subacute thoracic syndrome with progressive loss of condition. It is of considerable importance prognostically to know whether such a condition is due to a penetrating foreign body or not and it is often extremely difficult, in the presence of pain in the posterior thorax, to decide whether pain exists in the anterior abdomen as well. The white cell picture will not help, and exploratory laparotomy may be necessary as a diagnostic aid.

Similarly, foreign body penetration of the liver may occur causing a large area of suppuration, which may produce a clinical picture similar to the acute liver-fluke syndrome previously mentioned, but with reticulo-ruminal interference as well. Extensive liver lesions of this type occasionally interfere sufficiently with the bile ducts to cause jaundice.

5 Occasionally, traumatic reticulitis leads to acute diffuse peritonitis, the abdomen filling with pus and producing abdominal distension, toxaemia, depression, weakness and diarrhoea, leading to death (see abdominal distension, p. 113).

6 Vagus indigestion is also a complication of traumatic reticulitis (see abdominal distension, p. 113).

Chronic bloat (chronic and subacute ruminal tympany) (see p. 637)

All conditions producing low-grade ruminal tympany must fall into one or other of two main groups: (i) those affecting normal rumino-reticular tone and motility, and (ii) those causing partial obstruction to the escape of gas from the rumen, motility and tone remaining normal.

CONDITIONS AFFECTING NORMAL RUMINO-RETICULAR TONE AND MOTILITY

Chronic inflammatory lesions of the mucous membrane and wall of the reticulum and the oesophageal groove

Actinobacillosis of these sites is the most important condition of this group. The smooth painless fibrous plaque of this disease interferes both with eructation and rumination, producing a mild tympany most obvious after feeding. If the oesophageal groove is badly affected, there is often a prolonged retching gurgling noise as the cow makes laboured attempts to bring up the first bolus of a new period of rumination. There may be drooling from the mouth.

Therapeutic response is normally rapid enough to be considered diagnostic.

Occasionally, inflammatory thickening and *A. pyogenes* abscessation of the area resulting from foreign body lacerations and partial penetrations may occur, also affecting eructation and rumination.

Inflammatory changes (peritonitis)

Inflammatory changes involving the serous lining of rumen, reticulum, or even abomasum are more important, leading to poor motility and even atony of the rumen–reticulum. The classic syndrome in this group, as already mentioned, is *traumatic reticulo-peritonitis ('wire)*. Even in longstanding cases, where some degree of rumen movement has returned, there may well be chronic ruminal tympany often superimposed on low-grade ruminal impaction.

A peptic abomasal ulcer sufficiently advanced to involve the peritoneal lining may well form omental adhesions, and may even perforate among these adhesions, so that there is no leakage into the peritoneal cavity itself. Such a cow, instead of dying within 24–36 hours of acute diffuse peritonitis, toxaemia and shock with massive peritoneal tympany, as described under abdominal distension, will pass into a state of intermittent low-grade pain, abnormal or negligible rumino-reticular movement with slight and intermittent ruminal tympany. There will be lethargy, weight loss and intermittent diarrhoea.

Acidosis (see p. 634)

This shows its classical features in barley poisoning, but many recently calved high-yielding cows on a high-energy diet develop milk acidosis after each feed. The slight ruminal tympany, plus near-diarrhoeic faeces in a lethargic cow with suboptimal appetite and milk yield is familiar in intensive dairy herds.

Vagus indigestion (see p. 640)

Occasional cases of vagus indigesion (see complications of traumatic reticulitis, p. 118 and abdominal distension, p. 113) show an accumulation of ruminal gas forming a marked, but chronic, tympany that may even mask the fluid present.

Tetanus (see p. 567)

Tetanus frequently produces a moderate tympany (see rigidity of stance and gait, p. 117).

Cold water

Under ruminal distension, the effect of cold water on the ruminal musculature is mentioned. In some herds, in which all the cows water at troughs in the yard, the whole herd may show a degree of post-drinking tympany.

Botulism (see p. 556)

With its generalized muscle weakness, botulism shows subacute tympany as a minor part of a fatal progressive disease.

CONDITIONS CAUSING PARTIAL OBSTRUCTION TO THE ESCAPE OF GAS FROM THE RETICULO-RUMEN

Motility and tone being normal, these conditions will cause low-grade tympany.

Oesophageal wall lesions (see p. 630)

Usually traumatic in origin, these include *oesophgeal stricture*, *oesophageal wall abscesses*, *oesphageal dilatation* and *oesophageal papillomata*, which are usually sited at the cardia.

Lesions causing external pressure on the oesophagus (see p. 631)

These lesions will also produce chronic tympany. They include *thymic lymphosarcoma* in young cattle and *enlarged posterior mediastinal lymph nodes* in the adult. Such enlargement is an important cause of chronic tympany and is usually due to one of three infective organisms: *A. pyogenes*, *Actinobacillus ligneresi* and, in earlier years, *Mycobacterium bovis*.

Diaphragmatic hernia (see p. 655)

This condition also not infrequently leads to chronic tympany.

DIAGNOSIS OF CHRONIC AND SUBACUTE RUMINAL TYMPANY

Diagnosis depends firstly upon a careful clinical examination to decide whether the tympany is related to a specific alimentary condition, or whether it is due to loss of gastric tone as a result of a more general disease. If the condition is primarily alimentary, and one believes there is no oesophageal obstruction, then auscultation should be carried out to check that the left flank tympany is ruminal and not abomasal (i.e. left displacement). Auscultation should leave one in no doubt, although it is not always easy to distinguish between a gas-filled abomasum, early vagus indigestion and reticular actinobacillosis.

The liver

The liver is practically impossible to examine clinically by normal methods. It is unfortunately true that unless one adheres to a strict routine, it is only too easy to examine a cow without even thinking about the liver. The liver has many functions and failure, therefore, may produce a variety of signs.

Signs include lethargy, slow weight loss, anaemia, low-grade or acute abdominal pain, massive abdominal haemorrhage, ascites, abdominal distension, chronic venous congestion, ataxia, ventral oedema, photosensitization, endocarditis, encephalopathy, dyspnoea with pulmonary thrombosis, massive nasal haemorrhage and, occasionally, jaundice. All these conditions may originate in hepatic disease. Also, one must consider the diverse problems of the high-yielding cow calving down with a very fat liver predisposing to metritis, coliform mastitis, ketosis, low solids, milk fever and even infertility.

The liver, it seems, is not only the site of specific disease conditions in its own right, but also may be a background factor predisposing to disease in other organs and systems. In the face of this diversity of signs, all one can suggest is that the clinician should always consider the possibility of liver disease when examining a cow. He/she is then unlikely to miss liver pathology when it occurs.

Laboratory tests, e.g. haematology, serum proteins, serum enzymes (aspartate aminotransferase (AST), serum alkaline phosphatase SAP, and particularly gamma-glutamyl transferase) may be helpful, though by no means conclusive. Paracentesis may occasionally help in the presence of ascites, while liver biopsy is at least theoretically useful. Unfortunately, these techniques are expensive and the farmer of today is very unwilling to authorize them in any but the most valuable of individual cows.

So consideration of the liver must be as rigid a rule as checking the udder, and a mental list of the syndromes involved in hepatic disease can be a great help.

Abscessation

This is usually due to *Ac. pyogenes* or *Fusobacterium necrophorum en route* from the rumen, and probably only clinically significant when extensive. Obviously, cereal over-eating and other conditions likely to damage the rumen wall will predispose to liver abscesses.

Complications of hepatic abscessation may be very serious.

1 Rupture into the abdominal cavity leading to an acute diffuse peritonitis.

2 Rupture into a major vessel, leading to major haemorrhage, shock and sudden death.

3 Vena cava thrombosis, usually where the vena cava passes through the diaphragm. It may produce hepatic portal obstruction leading to abdominal distension and ascites; but it may produce pulmonary thromboembolism leading to pulmonary abscessation. There will be a painful cough, and dyspnoea, with rupture of abscesses into blood vessels producing severe and often recurrent haemorrhage via the nose and mouth.

Hepatic necrosis

Hepatic necrosis due to *Fusobacterium* invasion causes pyrexia, inappetence, lethargy, rapid pulse, weight loss, ataxia and occasionally signs of anterior abdominal pain. The presence of jaundice is variable, but is diagnostically helpful when it occurs.

Cholecystitis

This condition is rare and difficult to diagnose. Such cases show ataxia, anterior abdominal discomfort and jaundice, with lowered appetite and milk yield. Temperature may be raised.

It is interesting that jaundice is much more likely to occur in obstructive hepatic conditions than in parenchymatous change.

Cirrhosis

Cirrhosis in cattle, for all practical purposes, means liver fluke infestation. This condition must never be forgotten. It occurs in adults as well as young stock, in herds as well as individuals, and although wasting, submaxillary oedema, and anaemia may well be present, the disease may merely cause chronic unthriftiness and suboptimal yield during the winter months, thus needing differentiation from a nutritional energy deficit. In fact, both problems may occur in the same herd particularly between parturition and peak yield.

It is worth remembering that in severe fluke infestation, constipation is more likely than diarrhoea, and that during the migratory stage of the young flukes, a low-grade abdominal pain syndrome may occur that requires differentiation from 'wire'.

Liver fluke infestation (see p. 238) has far reaching effects. It may lead to infertility, presumably due to weight loss, to low milk solids, and to salmonellosis, or to endocarditis due to bacteria passing to the liver and then into the circulation.

Cirrhosis also results from ragwort poisoning, causing weight loss, ataxia, encephalopathy, occasional jaundice and terminal tenesmus in the affected animal. The encephalopathy produces blindness, head pressing and dragging of the hind fetlocks reminiscent of lead poisoning in the adult cow. Ragwort poisoning during the grazing period may well trigger photosensitization.

Other syndromes involved in liver disease

Tuberculosis (see p. 609) and *neoplasia* of the liver are relatively rare. Neoplasis includes lymphosarcoma and adenocarcinoma, and is, to all intents and purposes, impossible to diagnose in life, while fatty livers may follow bacterial or chemical toxicity, but are much more common as the result of overfeeding.

The fatty liver syndrome (see p. 598), resulting from excessive weight gain prepartum, has gained prominence in recent years, but is probably less common today. The syndrome may be involved in many diseases in early lactation.

Constipation

Quite apart from the acute gut obstruction syndromes, constipation may occur in diverse circumstances in cattle.

1 Unsuitable fibrous diet, e.g. straw, may produce ruminal impaction.
2 Insufficient water intake may produce ruminal impaction.
3 External pressure on the gut, e.g. fat necrosis (see p. 655), lymphosarcoma (see p. 530), adhesions.
4 Pain:
(a) postoperative pain;
(b) injured back — faeces dry out in rectum;
(c) injured anus and rectum — painful bladder.
5 Weakness or paresis: milk fever, broken back. Constipation is, of course, a very useful differential sign of milk fever.
6 Some poisons, e.g. lead (see p. 617) and ragwort.
7 Pyrexia.
8 Anaemia. e.g. fluke (see p. 238), piroplasmosis (see p. 726). In both these diseases, constipation becomes very marked in long-standing cases.
9 Ketosis: mild constipation is a frequent clinical sign (see p. 590).
10 Hypocalcaemia (see p. 577).

Constipation is, of course, rare in dairy cattle.

Diarrhoea

Varying degrees of diarrhoea are normal today in intensive dairy herds feeding concentrates and silage.

Not all conditions causing diarrhoea originate primarily in the digestive tract, but from the viewpoint of differential diagnosis, it is best to consider all conditions causing diarrhoea together.

Acute diarrhoea

1 Most toxaemic conditions produce diarrhoea, e.g. diffuse peritonitis, acute mastitis (staphylococcal, coliform, or *A. pyogenes*), acute septic metritis, traumatic pericarditis. These conditions all involve damage by bacterial toxins, and the diarrhoeic faeces tend to be relatively scanty, but dark and sticky.
2 Several acute septicaemic diseases are associated with acute enteritis and diarrhoea, e.g. anthrax (see p. 551), transit fever (see p. 253) and other forms of acute pasteurellosis (see p. 563), and, of course, salmonellosis (see Chapter 13).
3 Some virus diseases, e.g. malignant catarrhal fever, or the BVD/mucosal disease complex (see p. 660).
4 Several plant poisons, e.g. solanin from green potatoes, water dropwort (see p. 616) and rhododendron (see p. 615).
5 Several chemical poisons, e.g. arsenic (see p. 613) and certain organophosphorus compounds.

Chronic diarrhoea

1 Johne's disease (see p. 664): the classical form of chronic diarrhoea with loss of weight, particularly from the hindquarters, ventral and submaxillary oedema and anaemia.

2 Tuberculosis of the intestine (see p. 609), very rare today, is always secondary to pulmonary lesions, and is similar, clinically, to Johne's disease.

3 Ulceration of the abomasum (see p. 649) produces scanty and intermittent diarrhoea in a cow losing weight, becoming anaemic, and showing signs of low-grade anterior abdominal pain. Erosion of such an ulcer into a blood vessel in the abomasal wall produces more profuse, tarry, faeces and may cause death.

4 Amyloidosis is very rare indeed (see p. 759).

5 Lymphosarcoma of large gut is also very rare in cattle.

Herd diarrhoea

1 Winter scours, or winter dysentery, has long been recognized as an acute, pyrexic, and occasionally slightly dysenteric condition, which races through a housed dairy herd in winter conditions, and then dies out with minimal long-term damage. There has been discussion as to the aetiological organism, various viruses and *Campylobacter* spp. having been incriminated (see p. 659).

2 Various nutritional diarrhoeas.

(a) Spring grass.

(b) Frosted roots or kale.

(c) Fodder beet poisoning, which causes a hypocalcaemia-like syndrome and diarrhoea.

(d) Acidosis (see p. 654), whether due to excessive root feeding, or more commonly due to excessive cereal overload. The classical acidosis syndrome is that of barley poisoning with its acute abdominal pain and low-grade tympany, followed by profuse diarrhoea (see p. 615).

3 Mineral deficiencies, e.g. copper (see p. 263) and cobalt (see p. 261) deficiency, producing chronic diarrhoea with weight loss and anaemia.

4 Parasitic diarrhoea, e.g. parasitic gastroenteritis (see p. 231) and coccidiosis (see p. 243), largely affecting young stock.

5 Toxicity, e.g. antibiotic contamination of the feed.

There is no easy way to diagnose the diarrhoeic animal. It is necessary to consider all environmental factors, including nutrition, stage of lactation, season of year, housing or pasture; whether the condition is an individual animal or herd problem, and whether it is acute or chronic in nature.

Other signs besides diarrhoea may indicate whether the faecal changes are due to a primary gut problem, or are secondary to a systemic disease.

Finally, one must utilize whatever laboratory tests for bacteria, parasites, viruses, or minerals are available under the circumstances. Even so, there will be one-off conditions, rarely met with in one's practice area, which will, from time to time, elude the diagnostic net!

Tenesmus (straining)

This condition occasionally occurs in cattle. *Coccidiosis* (see p. 243) in calves is an excellent example due to painful inflammatory changes in the hind gut. The *BVD/mucosal disease* (see p. 660) complex in young stock may have the same effect. Straining is also seen in the late stages of *ragwort poisoning* (see p. 618), in occasional cases of *terminal intussusception* (see p. 654), and sometimes in *urolithiasis in the male* (see p. 226).

It may also follow *sadistic human behaviour*, when sticks or broom handles have been forced into the rectum, frequently penetrating the wall of the hind gut some 30–45 cm (12–18 inches) proximal to the anus.

Occasionally, there will be sufficient straining to pass hard dry faeces in the cow with milk fever of some hours duration, to produce transient doubt in the attendant's mind as to the possibility of there being a further calf *in utero*. Obviously, the most frequent causes of straining in the cow are obstetrical, e.g. parturition, dystokia or vaginal injury.

Rectal examination may make things much worse if tenesmus is marked, but a look at the mucous membrane just within the anus with a pencil torch may be very helpful. In coccidiosis and the BVD complex, particularly, the acutely inflamed nature of the hind gut often spreads right to the anus itself.

The unthrifty or emaciated cow

Starvation

Even in developed countries today, starvation can still be seen in the poorer and more backward areas as a primary condition, much more frequently appears as a relative energy deficit in high-yielding cows near peak yield. In the period from parturition to peak yield, it is frequently associated with ketosis.

Ketosis (see p. 590)

Ketosis is nothing more nor less than energy deficit and may if untreated produce very severe weight loss.

Liver fluke infestation (see p. 238)

Liver fluke infestation, reaching its most dangerous in terms of liver damage in the late autumn and winter months when autumn-calved cows are at peak yield and possibly in energy deficit, accentuates the whole picture of energy deficit and ketosis.

Chronic hypomagnesaemia (see p. 583)

In cold windy weather in late winter, heavily pregnant cattle develop a state of chronic hypomagnesaemia as a result of low food intake and cold, becoming thinner and poorer until some additional stress triggers off the acute convulsive phase.

These four conditions, interconnected to varying degrees, account for much of the unthriftiness found in dairy herds. A further condition which may also be involved is copper deficiency.

Copper deficiency (see p. 263)

Copper deficiency, either in its own right, or resulting from molybdenum excess. In the latter case, there will be diarrhoea, but many herds exist in a low-grade copper deficiency, particularly at the beginning of the grazing season, when the rapid grass growth dilutes the copper uptake, with weight loss and infertility the only signs.

Other conditions leading to weight loss

On an individual animal basis, Johne's disease, which does not always cause diarrhoea in the early stages, and, historically, tubercular emaciation are important causes of weight loss, as are abomasal disorders such as left displacement and ulceration. Chronic liver disorders, e.g. ragwort toxicity or multiple abscessation may also result in poor thriving to the point of emaciation before clear-cut aetiological pointers appear.

A number of other conditions lead to weight loss and suboptimal yield, but reasonable and sensible clinical examination should produce a definitive diagnosis without real problems. These conditions include the following.

1 Lameness (laminitis, solar ulcer and white line lesions) (see p. 360), often ignored by farmers who completely fail to realize the serious nature of the long-term effects.
2 Chronic pyelonephritis (see p. 560), which should be obvious provided the clinician remembers to examine the urine.
3 Actinobacillosis of the tongue or oesophageal groove area, already discussed on p. 110–111.
4 Paralysis of the fifth or seventh cranial nerve.
5 The long-term toxic and depressing effects of mastitis, metritis, or postoperative peritonitis with adhesions and peritoneal abscessation.

The 'downer' cow (see pp. 368, 594)

A 'downer' cow used to be defined as a cow that remained recumbent after treatment for milk fever due to a continuing *hypophosphataemia*. But, by general usage, the term has come to mean any cow recumbent at, or near, parturition, and thus there is a large differential list.

Preparturient

1 Liver fluke (see p. 238) and/or starvation. These cows may have cirrhotic livers. They are thin, weak and lethargic, but not ketotic.
2 The fat cow syndrome (see p. 598). Occasionally, grossly fat preparturient cows with pathologically fatty livers may become recumbent.

Parturient

1 Prolonged dystokia may lead to exhaustion.
2 Rupture of cervix or uterus leads to recumbency through shock and is quickly fatal.
3 Traction injuries.
 (a) Sacroiliac disarticulation (see p. 377).
 (b) Obturator paralysis (see p. 366).
 (c) Torn adductor muscles (see pp. 369, 380).
 (d) Fractured pelvis (see p. 374).
 (e) Fractured femur (see p. 373).
 (f) Peroneal paralysis, which is much more likely to occur after milk fever than after parturition, because it is secondary to muscle atony in recumbency (see p. 367).

Parturient and Postparturient

Complications of milk fever (see p. 577)
1 Fractures and muscle injuries (see p. 370).
2 Ruptured gastrocnemius (see p. 380).
3 Peroneal paralysis (see p. 367).
4 Sciatic nerve paralysis (sensory and motor) (see p. 367).
5 Pressure ischaemia of hindleg or legs, which may lead to ischaemic muscle degeneration, particularly the semimembranosus and semitendinosis muscles. Serum

AST and creatine phospho-kinase levels rise markedly (see p. 368).
6 Ketosis and licking mania (see p. 590).
7 Failure of serum phosphate to rise with calcium (see p. 588).
8 The cows seems bright and well, but stays down. Never attempt to make a cow with milk fever get up before it is entirely ready to do so.

Notice that the following conditions are all important in the differential diagnosis of the 'downer' cow (see pp. 368, 594).
1 Acute staphylococcal (see p. 296) or coliform (see p. 297) mastitis.
2 Acute septic metritis (see p. 428).
3 Hypomagnesaemia (see p. 583).
4 Cereal over-eating: acidosis (see p. 634).
5 Fodder beet poisoning (see p. 615).
6 Botulism: a condition increasing in frequency and associated with the feeding of big bale silage. Diagnosis is aided by a normal temperature, slow pulse rate, and slowly progressive generalized muscular weakness affecting both voluntary and involuntary muscle (see p. 551).
7 Internal haemorrhage, with fast pounding heart, white membranes, rapid respirations and often a subnormal temperature. Diagnosis of the 'downer' cow is never easy, unless there is an obvious major fracture.

It is important that every 'downer' cow should be given full doses of calcium and phosphorus, and possibly also magnesium. It may be very logical to argue that a particular cow cannot possibly be a case of hypocalcaemia, but it is easy to be wrong. It is much safer to treat, just in case. With reasonable care no harm can be done.

Once satisfied that metabolic possibilities have been covered, a careful examination of the available parts of the skeleton should be carried out, but may not be very fruitful. It is not easy to assess injuries to the legs of 'downer' cow deep in sludge or slurry!

It is vital that the udder and the uterus should be properly checked, and, as far as the udder is concerned, *every* quarter must be examined however difficult access may be.

The cow ill during or after calving

There is no excuse in cases of periparturient illness for the taking of any form of short cut. The clinician must be satisfied that the cow has not developed any form of milk fever, and even when satisfied, it may be wise to give calcium/magnesium/phosphorus mixture subcutaneously as a precautionary measure.

The uterus must be examined to make sure that it is not infected, and not damaged, and, above all else, that there are no more calves within. Even after removing the third calf, the uterus should be checked for the fourth!

It is essential that the udder is properly examined. A parturient dairy cow may be very ill and dangerously toxaemic before the udder shows more than a small crepitating area just above the teat, and that may be all that is noticeable in some cases.

Pyrexia of unknown origin (PUO)

Obviously, many conditions may cause a marked rise of temperature in a cow, but a lethargic cow with a temperature of 40.5–41°C (105–106°F) is more likely to be a case of incipient mastitis than anything else, and should always be treated as such in the absence of other signs.

The next possibility is an active pulmonary hyperaemia as an early stage of pneumonia, while an acute septicaemic condition, such as salmonellosis may show pyrexia and little else for some 8–12 hours before diarrhoea supervenes. During this period, the total white cell count may be as low as 1500–2000 mm^3, with a neutrophil percentage of less than 10 per cent.

One should remember that *anthrax* (see p. 551) is also an acute septicaemic condition, and there have been many cases of early anthrax where lethargy and a temperature of 41–42°C (106–108°F) are the only signs present. In young stock, severe diarrhoea, often blood-stained, with injected membranes, may supervene within a few hours to be followed by ataxia, collapse and death. In the adult cow, it is not infrequent for the hyperpyrexic early anthrax picture to be followed by collapse, subnormal temperature, clammy skin, cyanotic mucous membranes, restlessness and anxiety, followed quickly by coma and death. The clinician must beware of a stage in this process when the cold recumbent cow is easily mistaken for a severe milk fever case. Realization will come when it is seen that injection sites are trickling dark blood, while spreading haematomata appear where a vaginal examination has been performed, the teats have been handled, or the stockworker has gripped the cow's nose.

Sudden death

This is a dangerously misleading heading. Very many cows that the owner regards as cases of sudden death, are in fact cows found dead, which is quite a different matter. A cow found dead may well have taken 12 hours or more to die, depending on the diligence of the stockworker and when the cow was last seen.

If one can assume that sudden death means that a cow has collapsed and died, if not immediately then within the hour, then the differential diagnosis is fairly clear-cut.

Acute infections

1 Anthrax: every case of sudden death is anthrax until proved otherwise (see p. 551).
2 Blackleg (see p. 558): usually young stock but may occur in young adults. The lesion is usually obvious at post mortem. The causal organism is *Clostridium chauveoi* and bruising of muscle groups predisposes to the problem (see p. 557).
3 Wound gas gangrene infections: other clostridial organisms involved in wound infections, usually obvious at post mortem (see p. 559).

Occasional cases of acute coliform (see p. 297) infections, salmonellosis (see Chapter 13), and pasteurellosis (see p. 253), may produce a very rapid, sudden and unexpected death.

Acute pasture conditions

1 Bloat: classical signs and environment, with a reasonably clear post-mortem picture, provided that the carcass is examined within an hour or so of death (see p. 637).
2 Hypomagnesaemia: classical convulsive syndrome on spring grass. The carcass is often covered with debris, sweat and mud, with signs of convulsive movement in the grass for a considerable distance around (see p. 583).
3 Fog fever: occurs in late summer or early autumn. As it is a herd problem there are usually other animals with signs. The lungs show a fairly characteristic post-mortem picture (see p. 624).

Electrocution and lightning strike (see p. 762)

There may be no signs whatsoever on the carcass, particularly in electrocution cases. The behaviour of neighbouring cows, if there is any witness, may help in electrocution, while it goes without saying that if a cow is to be struck by lightning, there must be a thunderstorm.

Accident or catastrophe

Road traffic accidents do occur but strangulation and asphyxiation as a result of faulty yokes and feed trough fittings are probably more common.

Catastrophes also include such events as a wire in the reticular wall being forced in one movement into the heart. The perforated abomasal ulcer leading to shock, peritoneal tympany and toxaemia is also included in this grouping.

Acute haemorrhage

This may result from the following.
1 Wire penetration into a great vessel.
2 Mammary vein rupture following injury.
3 Teat vessel haemorrhage following injury.
4 The rupture of a coronary vessel.
5 The erosion of an abomasal vessel into an artery in the abomasal wall.
6 Damage to uterine or vaginal vessels after forced traction in dystokia cases.
7 The erosion of a hepatic abscess into a major vessel.
8 A thromboembolic pulmonary lesion originating from liver (see p. 675).
9 A superficial haemangioma, often sited dorsally in the lumbar sacral area.
10 Occasional acute cases of the pyrexia, pruritis and haemorrhage syndrome (see p. 686) bleed from the gut, and all other tissues. They also show raised temperature, severe general pruritis, and aggressive behaviour before collapse and death.

It should be noted that all these haemorrhagic syndromes, with the exception of rupture of a coronary vessel, may not necessarily produce immediate death, but may instead produce a cold, staggery and severely anaemic animal with rapid pulse rate, rapid respirations, loudly beating heart and subnormal temperature. Early anthrax, peracute salmonellosis, acute babesiasis, and acute bracken poisoning may produce the same collapsed and anaemic syndrome.

Acute anaphylactic reactions (see p. 758)

There may be much saliva around the mouth with oedema of the larynx, pharynx, eyelids, skin of face and head, etc. On the other hand, the only lesions may be pulmonary.

Poisons (see Chapter 41)

Theoretically, a number of poisons may cause sudden death in the cow but, practically, sudden death by poisoning will be due to one of the following.
1 Yew (see p. 621).
2 Water dropwort (see p. 616).
3 Bracken: acutely haemorrhagic (see p. 619).
4 Strychnine: rarely found today.

5 Arsenic: rarely found today (see p. 613).
6 Lead: may cause sudden death in calves, but not usually in cows (see p. 617).

Jugular stasis (cording)

Care must be taken in the interpretation of jugular stasis. There is often confusion between jugular stasis and jugular pulsation, and it must be emphasized that jugular pulsation may occur in perfectly normal cows, especially if the head is held low as while grazing.

Jugular stasis may occur in conditions involving space-occupying lesions in the anterior mediatinum, e.g. thymic lymphosarcomata in young stock, mediastinal lymphosarcomata in the adult, or large mediastinal abscesses.

Nevertheless, the more common causes of jugular stasis (distension) stem from the heart itself.

Traumatic pericarditis (see p. 566)

Previously the most common form of cardiac disease in the cow, this condition has now become relatively rare in Great Britain.

Chronic vegetative endocarditis (see p. 561)

This condition has become much more frequent. It is probable that 30 years ago, many cases of endocarditis were missed completely for the clinician was so used to 'wire' and pericarditis that all cases of congestive heart failure were diagnosed as pericarditis and sent to the knacker's yard after the most superficial examination.

There are a number of important clinicial differences. The pericarditis case is much more toxaemic and therefore more depressed. Transition from relative health to acute illness is much more sudden, although there may, of course, have been low-grade reticulitis signs at some previous stage. Pain is more marked and very readily elicited by wither pinching. Cardiac sounds start with slight friction sounds synchronous with the heart beat, which is usually more than 100/minute. Within a day or so, the tinkling splashing sounds indicative of gas/fluid production within the pericardium can be heard, and in a further day or so the sac is grossly distended with pus, and splashing and tinkling have ceased. The heart sounds are now muffled and may, in fact, be louder on the right side because the pressure of the distended pericardium against the left thoracic wall tends to extend the whole structure across to the right.

Gross jugular and mammary engorgement and dependent oedema will now be present at jaw, neck, brisket and lower abdomen. Pulse rate may well reach 140/minute.

Endocarditis, on the other hand, runs a more gradual course. For some time, the picture may be one of low-grade anterior abdominal pain, plus a temperature rise to 40–41°C (104–106°F). Pain is felt over a much wider area of the chest. The pulse rate is not generally very greatly raised at first. The cow is often relatively bright and may even eat a little, but exercise tolerance is very poor. Heart sounds, at first, are often no more than loud, and even later in the disease it is not always possible for ordinary mortals to hear the cardiac murmur that is stated to be invariably present in this disease. The reason for this seems to be that, in most cases, the lesion is right sided.

At first, therefore, and for several days at least, vegetative endocarditis falls within the anterior abdominal/posterior thoracic pain grouping, and is easily mistaken for 'wire'. There may even be a wire, for although most cases derive the valvular infection from the rumen via the liver, from the udder, uterus, pharynx or feet, occasional cases are met in which the primary pyogenic focus is a penetrating reticular foreign body. It is interesting that, in most cases of vegetative endocarditis, the white cell count and the temperature fall during antibiotic treatment, but the pulse rate is unaffected.

Eventually, jugular congestion, shifting lameness, dependent oedema, pulmonary signs, and even haematuria, may all appear.

In right-sided cases, pulmonary thromboembolism may cause marked thoracic pain, whilst ascites and engorged mammary and jugular veins are very noticeable. In left-sided cases, pulmonary congestion causes dyspnoea and coughing with less pain, but haematuria due to renal infarction is more likely.

Myocardial abscesses

Myocardial abscesses of considerable size may sometimes occur producing a clinical picture similar to that of endocarditis, but with lower temperature rises, and a slower course.

Other causes of jugular stasis

Fatty degeneration of the heart, and *tubercular pericarditis*, are usually masked by more obvious systemic signs of the respective diseases.

'Redwater' (blood or blood pigments in urine)

With very few exceptions, disease of the urinary tract in cattle produces significant urinary haemorrhage, and the differential diagnosis obviously includes the numerous haemolytic conditions producing urinary haemoglobin.

Obviously, therefore, when presented with a 'redwater' case, the first stage in diagnosis is to decide whether the case is one of haematuria or haemoglobinuria. Microscopical examination or centrifuging the urine will supply the answer, but usually the simple expedient of standing some urine in a container for a few minutes, while clinical examination is proceeding, will give a satisfactory answer. The clinician must remember that many cows with redwater are not presented as such, for stockworkers rarely notice, or even see, a cow urinate except by chance. If asked whether the urine is normal, the invariable answer is that it must be or it would have been noticed. This is wishful thinking, upon which no reliance can be placed.

Once differentiation between blood and blood pigment has been made, diagnosis becomes much easier.

Haematuria

1 Chronic cystic haematuria (enzootic haematuria (see p. 620) or chronic bracken poisoning (see p. 619)).
2 Pyelonephritis (see p. 560).
3 Calculi (see p. 226).
4 Neoplasia other than is involved in (1).

These four conditions show primary lesions within the urinary tract.

Enzootic haematuria (see p. 620) has a regional incidence dependent upon the prevalence of bracken. It tends to occur in older cows brought up on the farm, and the blood in the urine, slight at first and slowly increasing, contains very little pus or exudative material.

Pyelonephritis (see p. 630) is much more likely to be encountered in dairy herds, but is, for some reason, a rare disease today in Britain compared with its incidence in the 1950s and 1960s.

There are systemic signs varying from very acute to very mild, but diagnosis is greatly assisted by the presence of pus, debris and renal casts, as well as blood, in the urine. Rectal examination may help and the presence of pain is another differential point, for enzootic haematuria is painless and afebrile. Bacteriology on the urine of pyelonephritis may, in fairly early cases, produce a culture of *Corynebacterium renale* which is the primary causal organism. Remember that the pain, the temperature, and the arched back invite confusion with 'wire' unless the clinician keeps pyelonephritis in mind in such cases, particularly in the first third of lactation, and insists on inspecting a urine sample.

Urolithiasis (see p. 226) occurs largely in the young male, and other signs such as straining, the absence of significant amounts of urine and, eventually, 'water belly' overshadow the presence of blood spots in the urine.

Neoplasia of the urinary tract, other than that due to chronic bracken poisoning, is very rare.

A number of conditions occur in which haematuria is but one of a number of fairly obvious systemic signs, so that the urinary blood, when present, is not important in diagnosis.

1 Vegetative endocarditis (see p. 561).
2 Septicaemic conditions, e.g. anthrax (see p. 551) and acute pasteurellosis (see p. 563).
3 Acute bracken poisoning: a disease with markedly raised temperatures and generalized haemorrhages, which behaves like an acute septicaemia and probably is one.

It is worth remembering that very high doses of sulphonamides may theoretically produce crystalluria and haematuria, but sulphapyridine, the sulphonamide that most frequently produced these signs, is no longer used.

Haemoglobinuria

Piroplasmosis is an acute, pyrexic, and acutely haemolytic tick-borne disease of certain areas of Britain and other countries caused by *Babesia divergens*. The clinical signs include profuse diarrhoea, followed by stubborn constipation in a non-premune cow, progressive anaemia, with very rapid pulse rate, loudly pounding heart, and deep port wine coloured urine (see p. 726).

Bacillary haemoglobinuria is a peracute and rapidly fatal pyrexic disease due to *Clostridium haemolyticum* (now renamed *Cl. oedematiens* Type II). It affects young stock in certain rough hill areas, but is of relatively little importance overall (see p. 553).

Postparturient haemoglobinuria is seen during the weeks following parturition in cows in certain parts of eastern Scotland and occasionally in England. It is non-febrile, but progressive and frequently fatal due to very severe anaemia, and is possibly associated with root and straw feeding, and abnormalities in phosphorus metabolism. It is too rare today to be of real significance (see p. 589).

Kale and rape poisoning are too well known to merit detailed consideration. Large quantities are required and wilted kale is much less likely to cause problems. It is worth remembering that rape in excess may also produce abdominal pain, nervous signs and/or dyspnoea (see p. 613).

Leptospira icterohaemorrhagiae produces haemoglobinuria in the calf, but this is most unlikely to occur in the adult(see p. 569).

Very cold water, thirstily drunk, may cause haemoglobinuria in the calf, but not in the adult.

Copper toxicity, rare in cattle, may apparently produce haemoglobinuria (see p. 613).

Cows breathing badly (hyperpnoea and dyspnoea)

The clinician must not assume that rapid respirations in cattle necessarily indicate the presence of pneumonia. Cattle 'blow' for many reasons.

Physiological

Cattle breathe more rapidly when full after feeding, after exercise, in hot and humid weather, and when they are nervous or frightened. A herd coming in for milking on a hot summer afternoon after a mile walk from lush grazing may all appear dyspnoeic! When asked to comment on a cow's respiratory pattern, it is always worth comparing it with that of neighbouring cows.

Pathological

Respiratory rates.
1 Increase markedly in many diseases due to pyrexia.
2 Increase and become jerky in acutely painful conditions, e.g. septic feet, acute laminitis (see p. 256).
3 Increase in acute toxaemic conditions, e.g. summer mastitis, coliform mastitis, acute septic metritis.
4 Increase in metabolic disease, e.g. hypomagnesaemia (see p. 583) or acidosis (see p. 634).
5 Increase markedly with a much shallower thoracic excursion in conditions that prevent full pulmonary expansion, e.g. ruminal tympany, ruminal impaction and pleural effusion.
6 Increase in conditions in which the upper respiratory tract is blocked at least in part, e.g. malignant catarrhal fever, IBR (see p. 256) and pharyngitis.
7 Increase and become shallow in conditions that interfere with the function of the respiratory muscles, e.g. tetanus (see p. 567).
8 Increase very markedly in severe anaemic conditions, e.g. piroplasmosis and haemorrhage.
9 Increase and become laboured in conditions that, for various reasons, decrease the amount of active lung tissue, for example:
(a) active pulmonary congestion prior to pneumonia;
(b) chronic venous congestion, e.g. vegetative endocarditis;
(c) acute anaphylactic conditions (see p. 758);
(d) 'fog fever' (acute pulmonary oedema and emphysema) (see p. 674); and
(e) pneumonia (see p. 202).

Acute nervous and convulsive syndromes

Nervous symptoms occur relatively frequently in cattle of all ages, and vary from mild signs of ataxia and head pressing on the one hand to hyperaesthesia, circling, muscular tremors, aggression, collapse and convulsions, on the other.

Acute hypomagnesaemia (see p. 583)

This condition occurs in dairy cattle on heavily fertilized high-protein pasture at turnout in spring, and again in the autumn. It also occurs in winter and early spring in beef cattle on exposed pasture. Hyperaesthesia, with muscular tremors of face, eyelids, ears and muscles of the head and neck, is followed by strabismus, generalized muscular tremors and collapse in generalized clonic convulsions.

Transit tetany

This occurs during transport, largely in preparturient cattle under stressful conditions. Signs are similar to those of hypomagnaesemia, but blood may be low both in magnesium and calcium.

Spongiform encephalopathy (see p. 708)

This is a 'new' condition recently observed in Britain that shows more slowly developing hyperaesthesia with ataxia and behavioural changes prior to collapse. These changes include apprehension occasionally amounting to panic, obsessive licking of nose and lips, semaphoring of ears, refusal to pass through doorways, kicking off the milking clusters in the parlour, reflex kicking at other times, and muscular tremors of neck and shoulders.

Hepatic encephalopathy (see p. 695)

Hepatic encephalopathy, occuring as a complication of certain forms of liver disease, e.g. ragwort (see p. 618) or other forms of plant poisoning, is due to the effect upon the brain of ammonia released from the damaged liver. Signs are ataxia, dullness, slow circling, head pressing and collapse. Occasional periods of excitement are seen.

Tubercular meningitis (see p. 215)

Now almost forgotten, tubercular meningitis was seen in half-grown cattle as a sequel to congenital tuberculosis affecting first the liver and then the brain. Ataxia, stumbling, bellowing, and an incoordinate aggression with head pressing followed by collapse were frequently seen in this condition. In the days of horned cattle, fracture of one or both horns often occurred as a result of head pressing. Blindness in one or both eyes might also occur.

Lead poisoning (see p. 617)

In the adult lead poisoning produces blindness and aimless wandering, often complicated by trauma due to collisions with walls, trees, etc. Bellowing frequently occurs.

Rape poisoning (see p. 613)

Rape poisoning may produce excitement, aggression, blindness and bellowing, a nervous syndrome which may be complicated by dyspnoea, haemoglobinuria and constipation.

Listeriosis (listerellosis) (see p. 703)

Listeriosis occasionally occurs in silage-fed cattle producing an initial pyrexia followed by hyperaesthesia, a tendency to aggression, circling, head pressing, facial paralysis with drooping of one or both upper eyelids, and keratitis. One or both ears may also be involved, and occasionally the fifth cranial nerve as well as the seventh is affected so that chewing and swallowing are impaired, and food becomes impacted in the pharynx and mouth.

Ketosis (acetonaemia) (see p. 590)

Ketosis is normally a sign of energy deficit in high-yielding dairy cattle between two and six weeks after calving. The condition may well be subclinical, doing no more than reducing yield. At its worst, it produces inappetence for concentrates, lethargy and constipation, with a normal or subnormal temperature and pulse rate.

Occasionally, a nervous form occurs producing ataxia and excitement, with marked head signs, the patient licking itself and anything within reach in an obsessive fashion, holding the bars of the shippen or parlour in its teeth, and chewing to such an extent that tongue and lips may bleed forming a bloodstained froth. Ketone bodies are present at high levels in blood, milk and urine.

Occasionally, this licking frenzy may occur as a complication of milk fever. It is known as 'licking mania' and believed to be ketotic in origin.

Acute inflammatory, exudative and/or haemorrhagic lesions in the brain

Acute inflammatory, exudative, and/or haemorrhagic lesions within the brain may cause marked excitement bordering on mania before collapse occurs. This picture may occur in *anthrax* (see p. 551), in which case diagnosis will be helped by generalized haemorrhage and oedema; and is also sometimes seen in *malignant catarrhal fever* companied by marked nasal and ocular discharge, with heat and pain over the sinuses of the head. Horns, if present, feel hot and in cattle with white horns become very reddened and may, in fact, become loose. There is usually profuse diarrhoea.

CONVULSIVE SYNDROMES THAT ARE RELATIVELY FREQUENT AMONG CALVES

Lead poisoning (see p. 617)

This is still common causing abdominal pain, blindness, salivation and convulsions with marked bellowing and leading rapidly to death.

Magnesium tetany

In beef calves fed dam's milk alone without supplement magnesium tetany appears at 12–16 weeks of age producing star gazing, stilted gait, muscular tremors and hyperaesthesia leading to convulsions and death. Abdominal pain, blindness and bellowing are not features of magnesium tetany.

Gammexane (gamma BHC) poisoning (see p. 614)

This condition due to feeding milk in buckets contaminated with gammexane, after mixing insecticides, and causes very severe clonic convulsions and death.

Linseed poisoning (see p. 613)

The acute dyspnoeic picture with gasping and muscular spasm that follows the feeding of warm wet linseed to calves may look much like a convulsive picture unless one is aware of the signs of prussic acid poisoning.

Muscular dystrophy (see pp. 222, 266)

Calves dying of heart failure due to the cardiac form of muscular dystrophy will normally be housed calves fed only on dam's milk. Vitamin E intake may therefore be low, and at two to three months of age any sudden excitement, such as the arrival of the dam at feeding time, may trigger off a cardiac failure episode with cyanosis and anoxia which, nevertheless, may superficially resemble a convulsive syndrome.

Cerebrocortical necrosis (see p. 701)

Cerebrocortical necrosis (CCN) occurring in housed or yarded calves may produce star gazing, hyperaesthesia and ataxia but, occasionally, leads to a severe convulsive picture.

References

Boddie, G.F. (1970) *Diagnostic Methods in Veterinary Medicine*, 6th edn. Oliver and Boyd, Edinburgh.

Rees Evans, E.T. (1957) Bacterial endocarditis of cattle. *Veterinary Record,* **69**, 1190–202.

THE CALF

Chapter 10: Outline of Clinical Genetics

by G.B. YOUNG

Genetics in hereditary diseases corresponds to the microbiology of infections. Before Pasteur's contribution to bacteriology, infections were crudely controlled by isolation, but his work greatly improved preventive measures. Similarly, genetics greatly improves the precision in controlling hereditary diseases.

Many genetic problems are complex and exhibit a spectrum from being entirely genetic to entirely environmental. The genetic component may be divided into major gene and polygenic effects. Polygenes each have a small effect and produce continuous variation. Most disease due to major genes is, however, also influenced by minor genes and many diseases currently considered polygenic may in reality be affected by relatively few major genes.

Observations and experimentation indicate that, like the well-studied *Drosophila*, cattle carry a genetic load of deleterious major genes producing gross abnormality and of deleterious polygenes producing subfertility, increased disease susceptibility and poor physique. With current knowledge many polygenic constitutional defects can only be studied biometrically, but the final aim is to recognize individually every gene and its location on specific chromosomes. Recombinant DNA technology now makes this theoretically feasible.

Deleterious major genes

Every body system is subject to abnormal inheritance. Indeed, if, as the embryo unfolds, a defect occurs early, several subsequent systems may be involved producing a syndrome. Environmental disturbances, or other genes sometimes inherited differently but affecting the same developmental pathway can produce identical diseases or syndromes.

Genetic diseases affect all ages from conception to senility. Congenital malformations, observed at birth, may be genetic or due to maternal effects such as infections, nutritional deficiencies or drugs. Genes control the synthesis of proteins and, when defective, generally result in an enzyme reduction or deficiency — the one gene/one enzyme hypothesis.

Molecular genetics has developed the concept of control genes, influencing structural genes, but most genetic diseases are still thought of in terms of structural or chromosomal mutations.

Genetic epidemiology

All cattle breeds possess several genetic diseases, some common to many breeds, others specific to individual breeds. Several hundred have been described and many more are known.

Most persist at a low frequency. Some appear almost sporadically in many different herds over the years. Others are concentrated in a few herds in sudden outbreaks. Occasionally, a defect increases until individual or collective action reduces its frequency. If breeders relax its frequency increases again, producing a cyclical pattern.

Economic loss

Calf loss may reach 20 per cent within a herd for several years, as in Galloway tibial hemimelia. Maternal mortality may be high as in prolonged gestations in many breeds. Difficult parturitions reduce yield and late abortions result in long dry periods. In later developing defects, e.g. hip dysplasia, only cull value is obtained. The bull has to be replaced, the breeding programme is disrupted and pedigree sales drop. Counterselection substantially reduces economic selection.

Few breeders escape genetic disease at some time. Economic data is not available on either the direct loss due to major deleterious genes or the greater indirect loss from counterselection. Genes capable of producing defects are, however, abundant and most cattle probably carry several. Only fear of inbreeding and continual selection against defects prevents more frequent outbreaks.

Modes of inheritance

Inheritance is duplicate: each individual has two genes (units of inheritance) for a particular character or function at each locus on the chromosomes. A parent passes one on a random basis to an offspring, the other coming from the second parent. Chemically, genes are nucleic acids (DNA) and the fine structure of the gene has been elucidated, but for most clinical purposes the gene may still be regarded as the unit of inheritance.

Dominant genes

In regular dominance every carrier is affected. The disease is generally inherited from one parent and half its offspring are affected. A new dominant gene producing a severe effect tends to be lethal and produces single isolated effects. Surviving dominants produce relatively minor defects, e.g. notched ears in Ayrshires.

Irregular rather than regular dominants are more common in cattle. An individual may carry the gene but not manifest it due to intangible environmental effects or modifying genes (incomplete penetrance). Half of its offspring also carry the abnormal gene but a proportion similarly do not manifest it, producing irregular segregation ratios.

Hereditary ataxia in Aberdeen Angus illustrates this inheritance. Transmitting bulls mated to non-carrier cows leave around 25–40 per cent of calves affected instead of the expected 50 per cent, so penetrance is from 50 to 80 per cent.

Some late-developing defects, such as arthritic conditions in bulls, could, in theory, be due to dominants. The bull would not exhibit the disease until old, and bred from, and because of culling, the relationship and ratios between bull and offspring might not be easily noticeable.

Semidominant genes

These are quite common in cattle. A single gene produces a defect but a double dose increases its severity. In the single dose, the abnormal gene converts a Kerry into the small, more desirable, Dexter, but a double dose produces monsters. Matings of Dexters produce on average 25 per cent, Kerry types, 50 per cent Dexter types and 25 per cent bulldog monsters (see p. 145).

Many dwarves exhibit this inheritance. Often, as in snorter dwarves in Herefords, the carrier conformation is only slightly different from normal and slightly better (heterozygote advantage). Selection for carriers then spreads the disease. At the limits, one-quarter of the calves are defective.

Recessive genes

A single dose does not show in a carrier because of the normal dominant gene. The defect only appears with a double dose. Neither parent is affected yet the defect has come from both parents.

In carrier matings one in four of the offspring are normal (RR), two are carriers (Rr), and one will be affected (rr). This is true on average but not for individual or small groups of matings. Moreover, pure recessives giving exact ratios are rare, even with the traditional genetic model of *Drosophila*.

The abnormal gene is usually considered neutral in carriers but in some cases, probably more than is currently understood, it may be detected biochemically. Carrier recognition is a major field of genetics and should always be sought in major recessive outbreaks in cattle.

Recessive defects may also have reduced penetrance. Since the frequency of recessive homozygotes is generally low, if further reduced by incomplete penetrance, inheritance is best described simply as irregular, and calculating the penetrance of a recessive is generally unprofitable.

Recessive defects often appear following line breeding. A breeder obtaining good daughters from one bull is often tempted to use related bulls on these. These related males may carry the same recessive gene derived from a common ancestor. Some second matings are thus between carriers and defects appear. The pedigrees of affected animals often reveal common ancestors within a few generations.

Sex-limited and sex-linked genes

Many cattle diseases are limited to one sex, for example, testicular hypoplasia. The other sex, however, plays an equal role in inheritance and the defective genes are in the non-sex autosomes. This inheritance must be distinguished from sex-linked recessive inheritance where the abnormal gene is carried on the X chromosome and a carrier cow transmits the disease to half her bull calves, and leaves half her heifer calves as carriers; a cow with a double dose of the harmful gene would show the disease. Since sex-linked recessives are not transmitted by unaffected bulls, they are rare in cattle.

Multiple alleles

Each locus on the chromosome may have not just two but several genes present. Various combinations of these genes may produce a gradation of severity of a condition. For example, a series of multiple alleles reducing melanism successively dilutes coat colour from normal agouti to albinism. Multiple alleles may contribute to the variation in clinical expression of many diseases. They are also a common form of inheritance in many disease-related biochemical variants.

Irregular inheritance

Many, indeed most, genetic diseases of cattle are inherited irregularly. They do not provide simple genetic ratios and are characterized by sporadic incidence and occasional concentration within families. Arthrogryposis in Charolais, characterized by calves with twisted limbs (see p. 147), cleft palates and a twisted spine, illustrates the problem. More than half of all artificial insemination (AI) bulls produce a few defective calves but a few (about 5 per cent) leave around five per cent of affected calves.

Cryptorchids provide another example of non-Mendelian inheritance. Cryptorchidism is frequently sporadic. Most extensively used sires leave some cryptorchids. Many cryptorchids leave mainly normal offspring and most cryptorchids have normal parents. Occasionally, however, affected or normal bulls sire a higher proportion of affected offspring than average. Their incidence also increases markedly on inbreeding. Cryptorchidism thus has a genetic component and probably both male and female contribute to its occurrence.

Such defects result from unknown environmental factors and genetic susceptibility, either recessives or dominants, exhibiting a very sensitive threshold of manifestation.

Genetic polymorphism

This is a discontinuous variation which persists in a population apparently more or less at random. Cattle blood groups are an obvious example. Their relative proportions are not maintained by a balance between mutation increasing the defect and selection removing genes in affected animals. Most, however, will probably be ultimately shown to affect fitness. Many may be relics of resistance mechanisms to much earlier plagues.

Chromosomal abnormalities

Structural chromosomal mutations, such as duplications, deficiencies, inversions, translocations and alterations in chromosomal number, are not uncommon in cattle. Large chromosomal breakages produce complete sterility and small breakages subfertility. Both are inherited like irregular dominants. Bulls with low conception rates due to minor chromosomal abnormalities pass the defect directly to their sons.

Many chromosomal defects, often difficult to detect, are probably present in early embryos, and account for a considerable proportion of early embryonic mortality and some reduction in conception rate. The uterus, however, acts as a clearing house for such defects and few progress to birth.

Epidemiology and control

Breeds are generally organized hierarchically. A few top herds supply bulls to less influential breeders who in turn supply commercial producers. If a harmful gene spreads in the top strata these bulls spread carriers through the breed. Similarly, if the defect is eliminated from the top herds then sires free from the defective gene slowly reduce the defect in the other herds. The origin and increase of a harmful mutant in the top herds is probably due to mutation and genetic drift.

Control is the sum of the control efforts of individual breeders. Affected herds select against the gene, and breeders soon learn from which herds to reduce their purchases. The distribution of non-carrier bulls reduces the incidence.

The desirability of control will vary with the severity and frequency of the defect. A defect causing dystokia justifies considerable counterselection, but a minor defect like colobomata very little. Strong selection against a defect may also relax selection for important economic characters.

Controlling dominants

A regular dominant spreads directly down through a breed but such direct transmission is rare in cattle except for minor defects such as some forms of polydactyly. If required culling all affected animals eliminates the defective gene.

Dominants exhibiting incomplete penetrance, however, commonly spread directly. The lower the penetrance, the greater the likelihood of this occurring. If penetrance is high a few offspring will pinpoint a carrier parent and transmitters can be culled. If penetrance is low, control is more difficult, since many offspring are required to detect carriers.

Controlling recessives

At breed level, epidemiology and control depend on the gene frequency. This is simply the proportion of genes of a particular type in the population. Since each animal has two of these genes, the proportion of carriers is approximately twice the gene frequency, and the incidence of affected individuals is the square of the gene frequency. Thus, if the incidence of a recessive defect is 1 per cent, the gene frequency is 10 per cent and the proportion of carriers about 20 per cent. Even a low incidence of defects thus implies large numbers of carriers.

Moreover, this gene frequency will be the average for the whole breed and much higher frequencies will occur in farms that have used carrier males recently. Thus the outbreaks and frequencies will be patchy with some farms heavily affected and others with few or no defects. This often renders measurement of the incidence of a defect in a breed difficult. A useful guide is that a defect attracts notice when around 1 per cent of calves are affected in the breed so that about 18–20 per cent of animals are carriers.

Reduction in frequency can be rapid if the initial frequency is high but is slower as the frequency decreases or if the initial frequency is low. Thus breeders can rapidly reduce a recessive defect at high levels but eliminating it completely is very difficult.

The main difficulty in selecting against a recessive is the large number of carriers that cannot be recognized on visual inspection. However, if all bulls and cows producing defects are culled, experience shows the incidence of the defect soon drops to acceptable levels.

Controlling an irregularly inherited defect

In a disease like arthrogryposis all bulls leaving defects cannot be culled but only bulls transmitting most frequently. Similarly, in defects like cryptorchidism control is based on not using affected animals or close relatives and this is effective in maintaining a low frequency.

Irregular defects like cryptorchidism would only increase if affected animals were continuously used. Why they persist at a low level despite generations of natural and artificial selection is unknown although carrier advantage may be suspected.

Genes exhibiting good and bad effects

Some pleiotropic genes or closely linked gene complexes produce both desirable and undesirable effects and selection for the good effects may spread the gene. For example, some genes producing desirable coat colours also cause infertility. Selection for the coat colour may thus spread infertility or maintain it at a low level, as in white heifer disease.

A gene may be beneficial when single but harmful in a double dose as in selection for the desirable conformation in American beef breeds resulting in unconscious selection for carriers.

Inheritance involving advantageous and disadvantageous effects may be much more common in cattle than suspected.

Assessing controls

Excessive controls, such as compulsory recording of all abnormalities are sometimes advocated. Controls are essential, particularly where a defect has become a problem, but they should be kept in proportion. They should be kept to the minimum level necessary, so that selection for efficient production can proceed as rapidly as possible.

Investigating genetic diseases

Inheritance may be suspected when other factors are excluded, the defect runs in families and previous reports implicate genetics. Since environmental defects may simulate genetic conditions and similar clinical defects have different genetic causes inheritance in the affected herd should be investigated.

Inheritance exists when one bull has sired all the defects and another contemporary bull has left none when mated to similar females in a similar environment. However, such controls are often not available and a properly designed experiment may be necessary.

If line breeding is being practised a new defect is probably genetic. If recessive, both sexes are affected equally and the incidence within a herd seldom rises above 15–20 per cent. The disease may disappear as unaffected males are brought in. Since environmental changes are often made simultaneously confusion may arise.

Simple recessive defects resemble each other fairly closely — one dropsical calf tends to be similar to another. Where considerable variation in clinical appearance or age of onset is present a simple recessive is unlikely.

In cattle, and especially in a small herd, establishing the exact inheritance may be difficult. Often all that can be said is that the disease runs in families and comes from either one parent only or, alternatively, the genetic factors are present in both parents.

Breed differences are also suggestive of genetic disease but not conclusive because of possible confounding between breed and environment. This is particularly true where infections or mineral deficiencies are involved.

Pedigree analysis

A few generations intensively studied are better than long pedigrees. A list of normal and affected animals born during and immediately prior to the outbreak, their sex, sire, dam and maternal grandsire is generally adequate. This list will indicate if simple genetic ratios exist.

With recessives one out of four offspring of carriers are affected, but in practice the common ratio obtained is one in eight. This occurs when two carrier males are used successively. The first carrier leaves on average half of his daughters carriers (as well as half his sons). In mating the second carrier bull to the carrier daughters, one out of the four offspring are defective. About one in two × one in four or one in eight of the second bull's offspring are defective.

Care has to be taken with pedigrees since as many as 10 per cent may be inaccurate. Few pedigree investigations fail to produce anomalous cases.

Differentiating genetic and infectious diseases

Genetic and infectious diseases may, on occasion, be confused. Their epidemiology can be similar, with deleterious genes or infectious agents radiating out from heavily diseased foci. Moreover, many infectious diseases through close contact are familial and genetic resistance may be present, enhancing the familial aspects. Pathology may even be similar, since an invading organism can affect the same developmental pathway as a deleterious gene. The crucial distinctions are the isolation of an infectious agent and experimental transmission of the disease or the establishment of fairly clear-cut genetic ratios, preferably the former.

Genetic counselling

A breeder should be advised to change the bull immediately, thus eliminating the appearance of the defect and reducing the carrier incidence in offspring. Continuous use of non-carrier bulls gradually reduces the number of carriers.

If a carrier male has had only restricted use all his daughters should be culled. However, where the herd has many carrier females, culling should be gradual to avoid decimating the herd. Known carriers and low-producing females should be culled first. Where the abnormal gene occurs in a particularly good strain its frequency should be reduced rather slowly so as to preserve the strain intact, i.e. some defects should be suffered to maintain production qualities.

In a serious outbreak a breeder might test a male on about 20 of its daughters or half sisters, or on 10 known carrier females. Generally, however, test mating is expensive and best avoided.

Control of defects inherited as irregular dominants or in a non-Mendelian fashion, follows the same principles. The bull should be changed and transmitting females culled.

When a defect rises in frequency, the breed society should seek veterinary advice. After ensuring that the disease is recognizable, both clinically and pathologically, its mode of inheritance and methods of control are then explained to breeders so they can counterselect most effectively. Prenatal diagnosis and selective abortion, although feasible, should only have limited application in valuable animals in cattle practice.

Genetic defects and artificial insemination

Artificial insemination centres seldom suffer outbreaks of genetic disease because they avoid inbreeding, particularly in the larger units, and rapidly withdraw bulls transmitting defects. Although most bulls carry several defective genes, few leave many defects in their progeny since their cow population is unlikely to have a high gene frequency for the same defect. While a carrier bull leaves half his daughters carriers, each time a non-carrier is used on the succeeding daughter's generations, the carrier incidence is halved.

Automatically eliminating bulls leaving three or so affected offspring is rather rigid. Selection against bulls leaving calves causing maternal mortality, late developing defects, or leaving three affected calves in their first 100 offspring should be more intense than against bulls producing unimportant defects, or producing a few abnormalities among several thousand normal calves. Again, a few defects among several thousand normal calves is tolerable from a bull transmitting efficient production.

When an undesirable gene is increasing an AI centre should buy bulls from sources thought to be free. Even with limited numbers of offspring and a low gene frequency carrier bulls should soon be detected. For a serious condition, bulls might be progeny tested on known carrier females.

Testing all bulls on their daughters would test for any deleterious gene. Since most bulls probably carry several such genes, the bulls available would be limited. Where older bulls are being used, the test might be of some value, although low production in the inbred daughters would be a disadvantage.

Generally, AI, because of its scientific basis and monitoring procedures, is an agent for reducing rather than increasing defects.

Genetic defects and egg transplanting

Routine egg transfer permits intense selection among females and potentially concentrates even further the genetic base. It thus enhances the risk of spreading genetic defects. Provided proper surveillance is instituted and donors transmitting defects rapidly withdrawn, like AI, it should however decrease rather than increase genetic disease.

Polygenic deleterious genes

There is very marked individual variation in fertility, in susceptibility to infections and metabolic diseases and in conformation and physique. The genetic part of continuous variation is considered to be due to many additive genes, each with a small effect. They produce a bell-shaped distribution whose mean can be shifted by selection.

Multifactorial inheritance, particularly from field data, is measured by a heritability estimate — the ratio of genetic influences to all influences (genetic and environmental). Heritability estimates tend to vary widely according to the method of calculation and the particular field data chosen and are commonly averaged to obtain a generalized more reliable estimate. Individual estimates have to be treated with great caution, especially when used to predict rates of progress under selection. Strictly speaking they apply only to the population from which they are obtained and their predictive value is limited to a few generations at most.

Sterility and infertility genes

Infertility genetics is little understood. Although there is substantial automatic natural selection present for fertility, the marked decline in fertility with inbreeding and its restoration on crossbreeding demonstrates the existence of many infertility and subfertility genes.

Difficulties and inaccuracies in statistically measuring fertility, and the different indices used, have produced very different estimates of its heritability. Most studies suggest the heritability of pregnancy rate in cattle is low, almost zero. Some based on sire/son comparisons, however, suggest figures as high as 40 per cent.

Intense selection for yield is thought by some workers to lower fertility. It can be argued that a few per cent decrease in pregnancy rate might be overestimated in comparison with high yield. Lengthening calving intervals, however, markedly reduce profitability and selection for fertility should remain a high priority with some culling of sons of bulls with low pregnancy rate.

Semen volumes and sperm numbers, concentration, motility and morphology show marked age, breed, weight and individual variation. Semen characteristics are considered to be moderately heritable (15–20 per cent) and should respond to selection to improve semen quality but progress would be slow. The correlation between sperm characteristics and fertility is, however, not entirely clear and some semen standards may be unnecessarily high. Specific sperm defects, e.g. knobbed sperm, are often due to single genes and should be strongly selected against. Testicular size and conformation are also influenced considerably by genes. The difference in libido between beef and dairy bulls is sufficient to indicate the strong genetic influence in libido.

At the herd level most infertility problems are transient and non-genetic. Similarly, repeat breeding in individual cows is usually of environmental or management origins. Oestrus expression, however, probably has a considerable genetic component associated with hormonal differences.

Calving difficulties

Genetic selection for yield and growth rate increases body size and larger cows inevitably have increased calving problems. Friesians, for example, have more difficulties than Jerseys or Ayrshires. At the extreme limit in pure, large, continental breeds cows can only produce a few calves before becoming sterile. Counter-selection is impossible as long as growth rate is given priority and the only remedy is Caesarean section.

Susceptibility and resistance genes

Susceptibility and resistance genes are widespread and genetic variation in disease resistance has always been demonstrated when adequately sought. Animals relatively resistant to one disease are often susceptible to another. Resistance is sometimes polygenic but, with increasing research, it has often been found to be dependent on relatively few genes.

In natural epidemics an invading organism frequently spreads rapidly causing heavy mortality. Some genetically resistant animals almost invariably survive and subsequently multiply. After initial oscillations, host and parasite settle down to coexist. Initially acute diseases tend to become chronic as genetic immunity develops.

Before control, selection for resistance genes must have been intense. This effect is still obvious in tropical countries, for example, where Zebus are markedly more resistant to local disease than exotic breeds. In grading up by crossbreeding a proportion of Zebu genes has to be retained and indeed in high-disease areas improvement of indigenous cattle may be preferable. For many large countries resistance genes dictate a stratified breeding programme from pure exotics to pure indigenous cattle. In tropical countries genotype–environment interactions are of prime significance.

In European cattle the most obvious example of genetic resistance is in mastitis. There are marked breed differences. Heritability estimates vary enormously but are probably around 10–15 per cent. Daughters of infected dams are more susceptible and some bulls transmit substantially more mastitis than others. In one extensive survey most mastitis cases were daughters of relatively few AI sires.

Selection to raise the frequency of mastitis-resistance genes, even with AI, although feasible, would be difficult. Many daughters, perhaps 250, would be required to classify the bull. Currently sires' daughters are classified mainly on first lactation yield when mastitis is infrequent and the effect of AI on mastitis incidence is probably neutral. It is dangerous to assume that selection for high heifer yield automatically implies selection for health, as many diseases occur in later lactations.

Calf scours and pneumonia also have a genetic component, associated with colostral antibody. This varies genetically, as does the vitality of the calf, influencing its suckling ability.

The greatest progress in artificially selecting for disease resistance depends on detecting biochemically resistant and susceptible animals. Considerable progress is being made on this front centring around immune response genes. These control the ability of the animal to produce antibody against certain specific antigens. The *Ir* genes are on the part of the chromosome that contains the genes controlling the acceptance of tissue grafts, the histocompatibility genes. These latter can be detected serologically and both *Ir* genes and histocompatability genes form a multiple allelic series.

As knowledge of this gene complex increases and the genetic basis of immunity is understood in finer detail, positive selection for resistance to disease may become more feasible. Artificial insemination, egg transplanting and, ultimately, gene transfer are the obvious instruments.

Selection for disease resistance is likely to be profitable, however, only where vaccines are not available, although in some cases genetically more resistant animals respond more effectively to vaccines. Both approaches may in some circumstances be complementary.

Metabolic disease genetics

Individual variation in susceptibility to metabolic disease is well demonstrated by milk fever. It has a heritability estimate of around 20–25 per cent and a repeatability of about 20 per cent indicating how susceptible cows can be. There are also breed variations, Channel Island breeds being particularly liable. Breed variation in hypomagnesaemia and acetonaemia also exists.

The anaemia common in high-yielding cows provides one of the best experimental examples of the strength of biochemical individuality. In one unpublished twin study, despite marked prolonged nutritional and weight differences, haemoglobin, red blood cells, packed cell volumes and mean haemoglobin concentrations were all so highly determined by individuality that pair members closely resembled each other in blood pattern, despite the nutritional differences within and between pairs. Individual differences overshadowed the nutritional effect.

Such individual differences indicate the need for caution in interpreting disease status from blood analysis in individuals. Because of individual variation normality is difficult to define. A single animal with a low haemoglobin may not be anaemic but merely exhibiting a normally determined low value. Blood tests are generally most valuable at the herd level in preventive medicine.

Selection for increasing yields is putting dairy cows under increasing stress and metabolic diseases are steadily increasing in developed countries. Both milk fever and acetonaemia are basically diseases of high yielders and almost unknown in less-developed countries.

Disease genetics and cattle improvement schemes

These are essentially interwoven. Improvement schemes carry risks as well as rewards. Those based on AI and egg transplants steadily to improve rates of progress involve the risk of inbreeding depression.

Inbreeding depression

Since relatively few males are required to avoid inbreeding, in theory it presents little problem in improvement schemes.

As technology reduces bull numbers and AI sires are followed by their sons more care will be necessary. Using a few score bulls for several million cows should not cause serious inbreeding provided sons are not chosen repeatedly from only the very best sires, causing an undue concentration on very few sires. However, after many decades, such a system could cause a serious accumulation of inbreeding effects. Remedies would include importations, using stored semen or splitting the breed into small units and exchanging bulls. Similarly, with egg transplanting overconcentration on a few mothers has to be avoided.

In practice, however, more inbreeding may be occurring than is generally suspected and with inadequate recording the risks may be being underestimated.

Intense single-character selection

Single-character intense selection in all species reduces fertility and frequently produces other undesirable correlated responses. The balanced homeostasis of the animal is upset. At the extreme it often uncovers major defects, e.g. pygmies in downward selection for weight.

Intense selection for yield in dairy cattle increases mastitis, udder oedema and metabolic diseases. The genetic, early, high-peak yields in dairy cows, much higher than in any other species, induces stress. High yielders also suffer increased digestive disorders, foot problems and calving difficulties. High yielders, although more profitable, thus require expensive health care, particularly to maintain mammary function.

The genetic reduction in fertility associated with high yield is probably sufficiently serious to reassess current selection programmes in dairy cattle. Increased efficiency of production, rather than yield alone, should be the objective.

Balanced selection

In future, greater emphasis is likely to be placed on balanced selection. Factors like growth rate and mature size, body conformation and composition, food intake and efficiency and perinatal mortality and disease resistance are likely to be built into selection indices. Selection will probably also occur under controlled conditions as well as using field data. The aim will be better balanced and healthier animals and hence more profitable dairy cattle.

Positive selection for health

Selection and longevity in dairy cows

The very short lifespan of dairy cows (and bulls) is probably due to poor management and particularly inadequate fertility control. Genetic selection for health and longevity could, however, contribute substantially to better health. In livestock, positive eugenics is possible.

Longevity has a considerable genetic component independent of yield. The heritability of survival to the sixth lactation may be around 20 per cent. Theoretically, selection for longevity at the end of the first lactation is possible but would require too many daughters and measurements to be economically feasible. As biochemical individuality is explored in greater depth it may become possible.

Bull mothers

A simple approach to improving health, and longevity is to place a much greater emphasis on older bull mothers, cows that have successfully over five or six generations resisted mastitis, metabolic disease and infertility. This approach is now being implemented.

Crossbreeding

Crossbreeding schemes, even those where the primary objective is blending different maternal and paternal characters, greatly improve health and vigour.

The simplest explanation of hybrid vigour is that the load of recessive deleterious genes, which can be exposed on inbreeding, are covered up by normal alleles on crossbreeding. Crossbreeding is extensively used in beef production, particularly where hardiness is vital, as in exposed hill areas.

Systematic crossbreeding schemes are being used in some Scandinavian, eastern European and tropical countries but generally have been little developed in western Europe.

The best schemes of cattle improvement, maximizing both health and efficiency, are probably based on combining crossbreeding and selection and using selection indices. Dairy cattle improvement is only in its infancy and with increasing research and development such schemes are likely to develop in the West.

Health recording schemes

Another approach to genetically improving health is a greater emphasis on health recording schemes. Currently, the most effective of these are devoted to improving fertility control, particularly regular calving and improved heat detection and, to a lesser extent, early detection of metabolic breakdown. With improved design, however, they are likely to detect bulls transmitting undesirable qualities such as mastitis susceptibility and poor heat expression.

Conclusion

In cattle improvement the future is likely to see a greater emphasis on selection for survival and efficiency as well as production, and genetics will become a core subject in cattle preventive medicine. With gene transfer enabling resistance genes to be built in to cattle, a new pasteurian age is developing and the prospects seem limitless.

Further reading

Brock D.J.H. and Mayo O. (editors) (1972) *The Biochemical Genetics of Man*. London and New York. Academic Press. pp. 1–725.

Emery A.E.H. (1983) *Elements of Medical Genetics*. Edinburgh, London, Melbourne, New York. Churchill Livingstone. pp. 1–283.

Hamori D. (1983) *Constitutional Disorders and Hereditary Diseases in Domestic Animals*. Amsterdam, Oxford, New York. Elsevier Scientific Publishing Company. pp. 1–728.

Lerner I.M. (1954) *Genetic Homeostasis*. New York, Wiley. pp. 1–134.

Nicholas F.W. (1987) *Veterinary Genetics*. Oxford, UK, Oxford University Press. pp. 1–580.

Pirchner F. (1983) *Population Genetics in Animal Breeding*. Second Edition. New York and London. Plenum Press. pp. 1–414.

Chapter 11: Congenital Conditions

by A.H. ANDREWS

Introduction

Most farmers will, at times, have calves that show defects of a varying degree at birth. Such defects, although congenital, may be due to genetic or environmental factors or their interaction. The overall level of incidence of congenital defects ranges considerably in surveys from 0.2 to 3.0 per cent. It should be remembered that genetic defects are not always apparent at birth. The incidence of all specific defects is very small, but detailed investigation of any system will often show slight deviations from the norm. Genetic causes can be inherited on a dominant, recessive or additive basis and often they are influenced by the environment. In many cases all that can be said about a particular condition is that it is familial. Factors connected with the environment are many-fold. Other problems are the result of bacterial or viral infections, nutritional deficiencies, chemical poisoning and physical insults. If the condition occurs in the early stages following fertilization (i.e. up to day 14 after fertilization), death of the embryo occurs and it is resorbed. During the embryo and organogenesis stage (15–44 days after fertilization) the effect is variable. In many cases there is death of the embryo with resorption or abortion, whereas in others the embryo remains viable and there is congenital absence, deficiency or disturbance in function. Once the fetus stage is reached (day 45 to birth) then again death can occur resulting, if early, in resorption, otherwise mummification or abortion and, if later, in stillbirth. In other cases the fetus survives and may be normal or suffer growth retardation, reduction in size or organic function, or the animal may become weak.

It is often difficult to diagnose the problem and to decide whether a congenital condition is inherited or not, and if it is, whether control of the condition is necessary. Often it is hard to ascertain the frequency of a problem, as farmers are reluctant to admit its presence and also how frequently it is occurring. In many cases with large herds and limited labour, abortions or deformities are often missed. When the condition is present in the offspring of bulls used in artificial insemination the frequency may again be hard to determine because of the disinclination of farmers to report the problem. An indication as to whether or not a problem is of genetic origin may be obtained from the type of defect apparent and the knowledge already available about the condition. Other evidence may be a sudden outbreak of a defect following the use of a new sire and which only affects calves of his parentage. In some cases there is evidence of a gradually increasing number of similar abnormalities that occurs over a number of years. Following an investigation, it may be shown that a defect is confined to a particular family within a herd or to the progeny of certain dams.

In most cases the history will show a much lower incidence of any inherited defect in crossbred animals than in pedigree ones. Some genetic problems are noted as being very common in certain breeds or families within the breed and this aids a tentative diagnosis of the condition, e.g. hip dysplasia in Herefords (see p. 382). The history should be indicative of a relationship between the condition and mating systems rather than the time of year, disease incidents, etc. The re-use of the same bull in repeat sire–dam matings may also indicate the inherited nature of the condition and its mode of inheritance, as also can sire–daughter or sire–half-sister matings, but these involve a considerable period of time before any mode of inheritance can be suggested or confirmed.

Some of the more common conditions are described under generalized headings of the systems involved.

Cardiovascular system

Ectopia cordis

This is an uncommon congenital abnormality where the heart is present outside the thoracic cavity. The cause is unknown. The heart is usually positioned in the region of the lower neck and can be seen pulsating when some distance from the calf. Some cases are displaced into the abdominal cavity.

Ventricular septal defects

These are the most common form of congenital heart lesion in calves. They vary in their size, which determines the severity of the signs and their location, but they are often high on the septum. In some cases the animal survives for many years with nothing untoward being suspected. The defects can be single or combined with abnormalities of the blood vessels. The defect allows blood to pass from the left ventricle to the right one.

The signs mainly depend on the size of the defect. If it is small the animal may grow normally, have a normal exercise tolerance and a normal life expectancy. Such cases are usually only detected when the animal is examined for some other reason. Occasionally, calves will suddenly drop dead with no premonitory signs at a few weeks to several months of age. In severe cases there will be some stunting in growth, decreased exercise tolerance and a varying degree of listlessness. Other calves will remain recumbent at birth and die soon afterwards. In the uncomplicated case there is no cyanosis, but on auscultation all animals have a systolic murmur that is very obvious and can be heard on both sides over a wide area of the chest. At necropsy there is an interventricular defect and this is often just ventral to the aorta. In some cases there may be an enlarged liver.

Multiple cardiac lesions

There are many of these but all tend to be uncommon. In most cases the animal is born dead, weak or stunted. Often other congenital defects are also exhibited. Tetralogy of Fallot is probably the most common and involves a ventricular septal defect with pulmonary stenosis, a dextroposed aorta and a secondary ventricular hypertrophy. Eisenmenger's syndrome is relatively similar to tetralogy of Fallot with a ventricular septal defect, a dextroposed aorta but there is no pulmonary stenosis. Other multiple cardiac lesions include a double aortic arch and a double outlet to the right ventricle.

The affected animals usually die. Those that survive show a very poor growth rate, severe dyspnoea when exercised, and lassitude. Cyanosis is present in many cases, particularly after exercise, although in Eisenmenger's syndrome, cyanosis may not develop until late. Auscultation of the heart will reveal a murmur.

Patent foramen ovale

This normally takes about seven to ten days to close completely in the normal calf. Patency is relatively common. In many cases there is little blood transport, but if it does occur it is usually from left to right and so there is normally no cyanosis. Hypertrophy of the right ventricle may sometimes arise. There are usually no signs unless other defects are present. Cyanosis is absent unless there is subsequent right ventricular hypertrophy.

Patent ductus arteriosus

Although patent during intra-uterine life, the ductus arteriosus closes within a day of birth and at least by five days old. The condition is relatively common and the cause is unknown. Blood passes from the aorta to the pulmonary artery. Signs are often limited other than poor exercise tolerance and lassitude. There is no cyanosis, but there is a continuous murmur often known as a machinery murmur as it increases and decreases with each cardiac cycle. The condition can be corrected surgically.

Aortic stenosis

This is very uncommon and is just below or at the aortic semilunar valves' attachments. Some animals show few signs, others show dyspnoea. There is a systolic murmur. Death can occur suddenly with respiratory distress.

Persistence of the right-sided aortic arch

This is rare, but when it occurs the oesophagus is encircled by blood vessels, causing constriction. There is usually regurgitation of milk after feeding and this normally starts at birth or soon afterwards.

Persistent truncus arteriosus

This condition occurs very rarely.

Abnormal origin of the carotid arteries

This may affect one or both arteries, which may derive from the pulmonary artery instead of the aorta. This results in weakness of the myocardium in the ventricle of the affected side due to anoxia, and leads to congestive heart failure.

Aortic coarctation

This is a constriction at the site of entry of the ductus arteriosus and results in a systolic murmur and poor pulse.

Cardiomyopathy

A condition often with polydipsia, hyperpnoea and dyspnoea for one to seven days before death has been described in Australian Poll Hereford calves with a tight curly hair coat. At post-mortem examination there is vascular congestion of the liver, spleen and lung with diffuse streaking of the entire myocardium. It appears to be a genetic condition, possibly associated with a simple autosomal recessive mode of inheritance.

Blood disorders

Factor XI deficiency

The main congenital coagulation deficiency reported in cattle involves factor XI (plasma thromboplastin antecedent). It has been reported in North America and recently in Britain. It has been shown to be present in some Holstein Friesian breed lines and is transmitted as an autosomal recessive trait. Factor XI protein is concerned at an early stage of the contact or intrinsic activation pathway of blood coagulation. This pathway converges with the extrinsic one due to tissue damage, resulting in the activation of factor X. Following activation the factor converts prothrombin to thrombin, which in turn changes soluble fibrinogen to an insoluble fibrin clot. Bleeding problems can vary from minor to profuse with haematuria and post-injection haemorrhage.

Skeletal defects

Achondroplastic calves (bulldog calves, chondrodystrophia fetalis)

Although it has been associated with the Dexter breed, it can also occur in the Friesian, Hereford, Jersey and Guernsey. It is basically a defect of interstitial growth. The condition is mainly a recessive gene except that it is dominant in the Jersey. When Dexters are mated together 25 per cent of the offspring are bulldogs, 50 per cent are Dexters and 25 per cent are Kerry-type Dexters with long legs. Most calves are aborted at about seven months' gestation. The calves usually have very short limbs, flattened skulls with a foreshortened face and short nose. There are often abdominal hernias and anasarca. In many animals there is hydrocephalus due to the deformed cranium.

Osteopetrosis (metaphyseal dysplasia)

This has been recorded in black and red Aberdeen Angus and Hereford calves. It is thought to be due to an autosomal recessive gene. The calf may be born prematurely. At birth it is small and of low weight, with brachygnathia inferior (shortened mandible), protrusion of the tongue, impaction of the molar teeth, misshapen coronoid and condyloid processes, open fontanelle, thickened cranial bones, shortening of the long bones and a lack of bone marrow. Radiographs show the homogeneous bone shaft.

Atlanto-occipital fusion

This is rare and is due to a failure of the first cervical vertebra to separate from the occipit and thereby form a joint. It need not necessarily be apparent at birth. The main signs are ataxia with inability to coordinate limb movements. There are then abnormal flexures of the cervical region and recumbency.

Mandible and face abnormalities

The terms 'overshot' and 'undershot' are often used for these conditions, but they have variable definitions. Abnormal length of the upper and lower jaws is better termed superior or inferior prognathia and shortening of the upper or lower jaw is superior or inferior brachygnathia respectively. Most newborn calves show a degree of inferior prognathia, but this condition resolves. However, persistent inferior prognathia is more common than inferior brachygnathia (parrot mouth). The conditions are thought to be inherited. Problems can arise from impaction or non-apposition of the molar teeth. Extreme hypoplasia or agnathia are rare. Lateral deviation of the face with normal development of the mandible (campylognathia) is occasionally seen.

Vertebral column defects

Various abnormalities have been reported including lordosis (ventral deviation), kyphosis (dorsal deviation) and scoliosis (lateral deviation). Occasionally, there is partial or total agenesis of the posterior part of the spinal column; screwtails are reported in Red Polls and wrytails in Jerseys. Ankylosis of the intervertebral joints has been recorded.

Defects of the limbs and claws

Occasionally, duplication of all or part of the limb occurs and in other animals the whole or various bones of the limb are absent. One problem recently described is tibial hemimelia in Galloway cattle. Polydactyly or extra digits have occasionally been seen. A quite frequent abnormality is the partial or complete fusion of the digits (syndactyly). The condition is reported in the Holstein, Aberdeen Angus, Hereford and Chianina. It occurs more commonly in the front than the hind legs and the right limbs are more often affected. It can be inherited as a simple autosomal recessive trait. Duplication of the whole limb (polymelia) is very rare. It can be attached to the thigh of the normal limb by soft tissue and a pseudoarthrosis may develop between the femoral head and the pelvis.

Osteoarthritis

Although it can be nutritional in origin, it can also be inherited in Jersey and Holstein Friesian cattle. There are two main conditions, namely degenerative arthropathy, which mainly involves the hips, and degenerative osteoarthritis, which primarily affects the stifle joints. The latter condition develops in older cattle over a period of one or two years. The stifle shows crepitation and the limb is not raised much off the ground when walking. The articular cartilages show degeneration.

Achronchia

This condition involves the limbs having very long, thin distal extremities like a spider and the bones are brittle. It has been recorded in the Simmental breed. Often there is spinal curvature and inferior brachygnathia, which often affects other body systems.

Displaced cheek teeth

The lower mandible tends to be shorter and narrower than normal with abnormal eruption or impaction of the cheek teeth.

Lymphatic system

Inherited lymphatic obstruction

This has been reported in Ayrshire calves and is caused by the autosomal recessive condition. The lymph nodes tend to be small and the lymphatic vessels are large and tortuous. The condition results in oedema, which varies from slight to severe. The calves may be born dead. The oedema may be so gross as to cause dystokia. Oedema can be of the head, neck, ears, tail and legs. In slight cases there is oedema of the legs and these animals may survive. Accessory lobes may be present at the base of the ears.

Alimentary tract defects

Cleft Palate (palatoschiasis)

This can occur as an individual condition but is normally associated with other conditions, particularly arthrogryposis.

Harelip

This has been recorded in cattle but its mode of inheritance is not known. Occasionally, ingestion of lupin (*Lupinus sericeus*) can result in the condition.

Smooth tongue (epitheliogenesis imperfecta linguae bovis)

This is seen in the Holstein Friesian and Brown Swiss. It is the result of an autosomal recessive gene and leads to the filiform lingual papillae being small. The animals tend to be in poor condition with a poor coat and increased salivation.

Atresia ilei

This condition has occasionally been reported and there is disruption of patency. The signs are of a distended abdomen and this may lead to dystokia. Some cases are due to a recessive gene.

Atresia coli

This has been recorded in Aberdeen Angus and other breeds. The calves only survive a few days.

Atresia ani

This may be inherited and is seen in several breeds including the Friesian. The animal is usually born bright, but will usually die within a week unless surgical relief is provided.

Muscular system defects

Congenital flexure of the pastern joints

This is common and present in most breeds. In the Jersey it is considered to be caused by an autosomal recessive gene. The calves show knuckling over on one or both front pasterns, and occasionally the hind limbs are also affected. The condition is usually reversible and most calves recover within about six weeks. In some cases it may be necessary to splint the limbs. Manganese deficiency in the dam can also lead to the condition as can locoweed or poison vetch (*Astragalus* and *Oxytronis* spp.).

Arthrogryposis ('curled calf disease') (see pp. 380, 720)

By definition this is a permanent joint contraction. The condition is normally bilaterally symmetrical and the forelimbs are affected more than the hind limbs. The muscles show marked atrophy, they are pale in colour and there is replacement of many muscle fibres with fat. Cleft palate is often also present. The condition is common in the Charolais breed where it is a recessive gene. The gene is probably more prevalent than it should be because carrier dams appear to have advantages in improved longevity and fertility. Infection of the fetal calf by akabane virus can result in the condition, as can lupin (*Lupinus sericeus*) ingestion.

Muscular hypertrophy (double muscling, muscular hyperplasia, culard)

This is a characteristic with some production potential in that some muscles have increased numbers of muscle fibres. The condition is seen in the South Devon, Limousin, Charolais and Belgian Blue and the degree of skeletal muscle involvement varies. It occurs most commonly in the hind limbs with a rounding of the hindquarters. The muscles affected have deep grooves along the intermuscular septa and this may be seen in the muscles of the shoulder, back, rump and hindquarters. Many of the animals tend to stand in a stretched position. The calves tend to be less viable at birth and because of the increased muscle size dystokia is common. In the Belgian Blue dystokia results partly from a narrowing of the dam's pelvis.

Multiple tendon contracture

This has been recorded in Shorthorn cattle and results in dystokia due to the calf's limbs being fixed in extension or flexion. There is a lack of mobility of the limbs and often positioning is abnormal. The problem involves the tendons and there is limb muscle atrophy. The calves are born dead or are destroyed because they are unable to stand. The condition is thought to be inherited by a single recessive gene.

Joint hypermobility

The cause of the condition is unknown but in Jersey calves it is a single autosomal recessive gene. The joints are very mobile and can be bent into very abnormal positions with overextension and flexion of all or most of the upper fore and hind limb joints.

Achondroplastic deviation

Most cases appear to be inherited as a single recessive characteristic and involve the Aberdeen Angus and Hereford breeds but cases have been reported in the Holstein and Shorthorn. The calves have short legs, a wide, short head and the mandible protrudes far in front of the dental pad. The eyes bulge and the tongue protrudes. Breathing is stertorous with the forehead protruding and the maxilla distorted.

Nervous system defects (see p. 698)

Hydrocephalus

This is uncommon in calves and can be inherited or congenital (see p. 697). It is often associated with other deformities, e.g. congenital achondroplasia. The condition is seen in the Holstein and Hereford and is inherited. Infection of the fetus with akabane virus can produce the problem and it is thought vitamin A deficiency can contribute to the condition. It can result from obstruction to the drainage of cerebrospinal fluid from the ventricles or cranial malformation. In both conditions the animals are born dead or die in a few days. There are usually ocular defects.

Cerebellar hypoplasia

This is also known as Hereford disease, but is seen in the Holstein and Shorthorn and appears to be genetic. During pregnancy, infection with mucosal disease virus can produce the condition (see p. 599). The cerebellum tends to be small, tough and leathery or even absent. Most calves are obviously affected at birth; there is swaying of the neck, with inability to stand and blindness occurring in severely affected animals. Less badly affected calves have exaggerated and incoordinated limb movements. The animals are conscious and able to drink. Some will survive for several months.

Inherited cerebellar ataxia

This condition is described as being due to a single autosomal recessive gene. It is seen in the Holstein, Jersey and Shorthorn and the signs are similar to cerebellar hypoplasia, although they are not apparent at birth. The gross lesions are minimal and consist of a wet glistening appearance to the cerebellar white matter, which appears on histology to be reticulate.

Cerebellar abiotrophy (premature ageing)

This condition is seen in Hereford and Simmental calves and appears when four to eight months old. There is the sudden onset of ataxia, which then progresses slowly. The animals are not blind. Calves remain strong but become recumbent or decline slowly into a spastic ataxia. Histologically, there is ageing or degeneration of the cerebellar neurones.

Congenital spasms

The condition has only been reported in the Jersey and there is a continual tremor of the head, neck and limbs. The animal cannot walk and it may die in a few weeks.

Familial ataxia and convulsions

These have been reported in Aberdeen Angus calves and appear to be an incomplete dominance. The signs are seen within a few hours of birth but can occur when two or three months old with the sudden onset of tetanic spasms, which last for three to twelve hours. In mild cases there is a stiff, exaggerated movement but in the severe form there may be convulsions with recumbency, opisthotonus and paddling of the forelimbs. Following the initial signs there is a residual ataxia with a goose-stepping action, which lasts weeks or months. Necropsy shows lesions of degeneration of the cerebellar cortex Purkinje cells. Diagnosis depends on age, signs and their remission.

Progressive ataxia

This has been recorded in the Charolais in Britain and subsequently in France. The signs do not develop until the animal is about a year old and they are seen as a progressive ataxia. The animal has increasing difficulty in rising until it may become permanently recumbent. Histologically, there is a myelin degeneration of the white matter of the cerebellum and internal capsule.

Idiopathic epilepsy

This condition occurs when the calves are a few months old and mainly involves the Brown Swiss. It is inherited as a dominant characteristic. The convulsions are epileptiform and are seen when the calf is stimulated. They disappear once the animal is one to two years old.

Lysosomal storage diseases

There is a generalized glycogen storage problem in beef Shorthorns with muscle weakness, incoordination of gait and eventual recumbency. In the Friesian there is a GM_1 gangliosidosis where there is an accumulation of ganglioside (GM_1) in the nervous tissue due to reduced activity of the enzyme β-galactosidase. At about three months old the animal begins to grow more slowly, is blind and has a staring coat.

Mannosidosis

The condition has been recorded in Aberdeen Angus and Murray Grey cattle in New Zealand, Australia and recently in Britain (see p. 696). It is inherited as an autosomal recessive trait and is a deficiency of a specific lysosomal hydrolase enzyme, α-mannosidase, and this causes the accumulation of mannose and glucosamine in secondary lysosomes. The signs develop from one to fifteen months old and most animals die by one year. There is, at first, slight hind leg ataxia, then a fine lateral head tremor, slow vertical head nodding, aggression and loss of condition. Diagnosis is based on reduced tissue and plasma levels of α-mannosidase. Histologically, accumulations of mannose and glucosamine are seen in the nerve cells, fixed macrophages and epithelial cells of the viscera. Tissue and plasma levels of α-mannosidase are about half the normal in heterozygous animals and can thus be detected.

Spastic paresis (see pp. 387, 685, 700)

There is an extension of the stifle and tarsal joints of one or both hind limbs. The condition is seen in the Friesian, but other breeds can be affected. Signs are not usually present until the animal is several weeks or months old, when they start to progress. Contraction of the Achilles tendon, gastrocnemius and superficial flexor tendons overstraighten the hock joint, so that the os calcis is moved cranially towards the tibia. Usually, one leg is more affected than the other and this limb may appear shorter. In the later stages of the severe cases, the leg may swing backwards and forwards like a pendulum. The condition is considered to be inherited but, where only small numbers of an AI bull's offspring are affected and the animal is of high genetic merit, it has been suggested that it should still be used as a sire. Surgery can relieve the condition but the animals should not be used for breeding. Recently, analysis of cerebrospinal fluid concentrations of homovanillic acid, the main metabolite of dopamine, has shown levels to be lower in spastic paresis calves than normal contemporaries. The possibility of a disorder in dopamine metabolism has therefore been suggested as a possible cause of the condition.

Neonatal spasticity

This condition involves a single recessive characteristic in the Jersey and Hereford. The animal is born normal but within the first week it develops convulsions of the head, neck and limbs, preceded by neck deviation and bulging eyes.

Periodic spasticity

This has been recorded in the Guernsey and Holstein breeds. It appears to be a single recessive character with incomplete penetrance and is often not noticed until the animals are adult. Early signs involve the hind end, with difficulty in rising, the hind limbs are stretched backwards and the back depressed. The back muscle may fasciculate and the condition progresses from a few seconds duration to last up to 30 minutes. The animal cannot walk during the attack.

Inherited congenital myoclonus

The condition does not involve oedema of the central nervous system and is therefore described as inherited congenital myoclonus (see p. 695). It is inherited as an autosomal recessive gene and is seen in America, New Zealand and Australia to affect Hereford and polled Hereford-cross calves. It has also been reported in Britain in the Hereford, Jersey and South Devon. Animals are usually produced after a shorter than normal gestation period. They are bright and alert but recumbent, often in lateral recumbency and some are unable to move their head. There is extension and crossing of the hind limbs with hypersensitivity to noise and touch. Often when animals are encouraged to stand there are myoclonic spasms with the body becoming rigid. At necropsy there is usually damage to the hip joints, probably secondary to myoclonic contractions. There is no oedema of the central nervous system. The main differential diagnosis is maple syrup urine disease. No treatment is possible and the same mating pattern should not be used again.

Maple syrup urine disease

This condition is like a branched-chain ketoacid decarboxylase deficiency and is possibly inherited as an autosomal recessive gene. It is very uncommon but may be seen in polled Hereford calves (see p. 695). There are higher than normal concentrations of branched-chain amino acids in plasma and/or serum, urine, cerebrospinal fluid and formalin-fixed cerebral tissue. It has been suggested that the condition is analogous to branched-chain ketoacid decarboxylase deficiency or maple syrup urine disease. There is dullness, opisthotonus and recumbency and a poor response to touch or auditory stimuli. At post mortem there is severe stratus spongiosus. The main differential diagnosis is inherited congenital myoclonus.

Congenital pastern paralysis

The defect is lethal due to prolonged recumbency and in Red Danish cattle at birth can take the form of opisthotonus, muscle tremor with spastic extension of the limbs and exaggerated tendon reflexes. There is neuronal degeneration in many parts of the brain and spinal cord. In the Norwegian Red Poll a similar condition is seen but only involving opisthotonus and muscle tremors.

Perosomus elumbis

This occurs very occasionally in ruminants. There is aplasia or hypoplasia of the spinal cord caudal to the thoracic area. This results in rigidity of the hind limbs, there is muscle atrophy and no joint movement. Most cases are born dead.

Ocular defects (see p. 713)

Reports of ocular defects in cattle are few. Anophthalmia and microphthalmia occur infrequently. Entropion is also very rare. Dermoids can occur on the eyelids, conjunctiva and cornea, but they are commonest on the third eyelid.

Exophthalmus with strabismus

This has been recorded in the Hereford and is combined with strabismus in Shorthorns and their crosses in Britain and Jerseys in America. The signs, particularly in the Shorthorn, are usually delayed until a year old, although occasionally young calves are affected. The condition is progressive and defective vision is observed first, followed by protrusion and deviation of both eyeballs medially with difficulty in focusing. The condition is considered to be inherited as a recessive gene, but some occur in cases of cerebellar hypoplasia or mucosal disease.

Colobomata

These problems appear to have a high prevalence in the Charolais. There is an absence of part of one or more of the structures of the eye. The condition occurs during early gestation, when the eye is developing. Although always bilateral, it may not be symmetrical and it is usually found associated with the optic disc and the tapetum nigrum below the disc. The retina is involved and in some animals the choroid and sclera are also affected. The condition is present at birth and does not progress. The mode of inheritance has been debated, but a dominant gene with incomplete penetrance, autosomal recessive or polygenic inheritance have all been suggested. Signs are not usually apparent although an ophthalmoscopic examination will reveal the lesion. The very severely affected animal can be blind, and a few others are considered to be hyperexcitable due to the defective vision.

Congenital cataract

Lens opacity is present from birth. The condition has been recorded in the Friesian, Hereford, Jersey and Shorthorn. Some cases in the Holstein and Jersey are considered to be due to an autosomal recessive gene. A form of nuclear cataract in Friesian and Friesian-cross calves appears to be more common in calves born in the summer months and is considered to be of environmental origin. The condition is bilateral and not progressive. In most animals the degree of involvement of each eye is similar. In severe cases blindness is apparent. It is not always possible to examine the fundus of the eye, but in most affected calves there is no abnormality of the retina or optic disc (see p. 718).

Persistent hyaloid vessels

These are quite common and are the vestige of the earlier development of the eye. They have no practical significance.

Skin defects

Symmetrical alopecia

This is apparently inherited as a single autosomal recessive characteristic in Holstein cattle. It involves animals born with a normal hair coat but which is then lost in a symmetrical pattern over the body. It occurs between six weeks and six months of age and affects both pigmented and non-pigmented areas.

Congenital hypotrichosis

Several forms are recorded that vary both in inheritance and degree. There may be partial or complete loss of hair and the condition is present at birth. In some instances the animals will grow satisfactorily provided there is sufficient shelter.

Epitheliogenesis imperfecta

This condition can occur in either sex and reports include Holstein, Ayrshire and Jersey calves. Most animals die within a few days of birth. It is considered to be caused by an autosomal recessive gene. There are normally areas of varying size devoid of skin or mucous membrane. The defects are often distal to the tarsal and carpal joints. Lesions may also occur on the muzzle, tongue, hard palate, cheeks and nostrils.

Keratogenesis imperfecta (baldy calves)

The condition appears a few months after birth and is lethal. It has been observed in the Friesian and is due to an autosomal recessive gene. The skin tends to develop alopecia, there is a loss of body condition and the horns do not grow. The skin then becomes scaly, thickened and folded, particularly on the neck and shoulders. There is alopecia and raw areas may develop, particularly on the knees, hocks, elbows, axillae and flanks. The joints tend to be stiff and there is overgrowth of the hooves.

Inherited parakeratosis (lethal trait A46)

This is possibly an autosomal recessive condition. It is seen in Friesian cattle and is thought to be due to an increased zinc requirement. The signs are usually seen about four to eight months after birth with alopecia and parakeratosis of the limbs, muzzle and under the jaw. The animal becomes stunted and, if untreated, it dies in about four months. At necropsy there is thickened skin with thick crusts over the skin lesions. The spleen shows hypoplasia. Diagnosis depends on low serum zinc levels (normal 12–27 μmol/l; 80–120 mg/100 ml) and history of parakeratosis. Therapy must continue for the rest of the animal's life and as a calf about 0.5 g zinc oxide or 1 g zinc sulphate daily is required. The dose should be increased as the animal grows older.

Interdigital hyperplasia

This condition is particularly seen in the Hereford and it is considered to have a genetic predisposition. The condition tends to be present in the older animal and can be surgically removed, but has a tendency to recur.

Albinism

Varying types occur. In partial albinism the coat colour is normal for the breed or a dilute colour, but the iris is blue and white centrally, with a brown border. Incomplete albinism is characterized by a white or mainly white coat and the iris may be blue, grey or white. The condition is inherited by an autosomal dominant gene. In complete albinism the coat is pure white and the iris white or pink. The condition is inherited as a simple autosomal recessive trait.

Familial acantholysis

This has been recorded in Aberdeen Angus calves. There is a loss of skin at the carpal and metacarpal joints and coronet, where there is horn separation. The defect is one of defective collagen in the basal and prickle layers.

Congenital ichthyosis

This is also known as fish scale disease in that there is alopecia and the presence of a horny epidermis.

Body cavity defects

Umbilical herniae (navel ruptures)

These are found with a low frequency in several breeds, but especially the Friesian and Holstein. It would appear in some cases to be due to the environment, following infection, to a dominant gene with incomplete penetrance, or autosomal recessive genes. In one study of the progeny of Holstein bulls, more cases occurred in the female than the male offspring. In the male many umbilical herniae are missed unless a conscious effort is made to look for the defect. This is due to the hernia occurring just anterior to the prepucial orifice. If the hernia is small it may not need to be treated. Larger hernias may need surgical repair by suturing across the hole or surgical webbing may need to be introduced. Many cases are inherited and the animal should be recorded as often the hernia is hard to detect in the adult. Do not breed from affected cattle.

Inguinal herniae

These occur far less commonly than umbilical herniae. Little is known about aetiology.

Scrotal herniae

Like inguinal herniae, these are rarely seen but can occur in the Sussex breed. Little is known about the aetiology, but there is a familial trait.

Schistosoma reflexus

This is a group of conditions in which there is a longitudinal fissure in the body wall. The cause is unknown, but it may be due to the failure of the somatopleure of the blastodermic vesicle to close. At birth the vertebral column is angulated with the head and tail showing approximation dorsally. The abdominal and thoracic organs lie free in the dam's uterine cavity.

Diaphragm defects

These occur occasionally and, depending on size and position, they may or may not involve abdominal organ herniation.

Reproductive system defects

Testicular hypoplasia (see p. 492)

This occurs sporadically in all breeds of bull. The problem can be bilateral or unilateral as well as being partial or complete. The left side is more commonly affected. Work on gonadal hypoplasia in Swedish Highland cattle showed an inherited origin and this is probably also the case in British breeds.

Cryptorchidism

There is incomplete descent of the testicles into the scrotum and this may be unilateral or bilateral, although the former is more common. Bilateral cryptorchidism usually produces a sterile animal. The condition occurs in most breeds including the Friesian and Hereford. Although studies of aetiology are few, it is considered to have an inherited basis.

Wolffian duct aplasia

This is normally seen in the area of the epididymal head.

Ovarian aplasia

This occurs occasionally with or without other reproductive abnormalities.

Ovarian hypoplasia

As with testicular hypoplasia, this has mainly been recorded in the Swedish Highland breed where it is inherited.

Müllerian duct aplasia

Various forms can occur and all are uncommon, but the main form is uterus unicorni.

Duplication of the reproductive tracts

This can occur as a deficient union or exaggerated union of the Müllerian ducts. They can result in a partial or complete duplication of the cervix or uterine body or vaginal septa.

White heifer disease

The condition used to be common in the white Shorthorn with up to 10 per cent of them being affected. It is now rare, but can be found in other breeds. There are varying degrees of involvement. In all cases there is partial or complete persistence of the hymen. This may be the only abnormality, but in other animals there are abnormalities cranial to the hymen. These defects may include the absence of the cranial vaginal cervix, uterine body or horns. The ovaries are functional and in most cases there is a distension of the normal organs due to the accumulation of the products of secretion.

Prolonged gestation

This has been recorded in most dairy breeds and in some cases it has an inherited origin. There are two main forms of the condition.

1 Prolonged gestation with fetal giantism. In these animals the fetus continues to grow *in utero* before parturition 21 to 100 days late. The cow usually calves with no udder development or ligament relaxation and usually first stage labour is minimal, necessitating a Caesarean section. The calves tend to be heavy, have well-erupted teeth and a good coat growth. The adrenals of the calves are hypoplastic and following delivery most are weak and die in hypoglycaemic crisis. The condition is the result of an autosomal recessive gene.

2 Prolonged gestation with adrenohypophyseal hypoplasia. This is due to a recessive gene and it is mainly recorded in the Channel Island breeds. The gestation length is increased by weeks or months and parturition occurs about seven to fourteen days after the calf's death. There is again no udder development and few signs of parturition. The calf in this case is small and ceases to grow after the seventh month of gestation, so it can often be delivered by manual traction. It may show disproportionate dwarfism, craniofacial defects that may cause hydrocephalus, alopecia and abdominal distension. There is no or only partial development of the adenohypophysis.

It should be remembered that the gestation period of some of the larger beef breeds such as the Charolais, Simmental and Limousin is longer than for the Friesian or most British beef breeds.

Hermaphroditism

Both true and pseudohermaphrodites occur. In the true form there are gonads of both sexes, although they may be combined into an ovo-testis. In the pseudohermaphrodite, cattle are genetically female with female gonads but they have partial masculinization of the external genitalia. The animals usually exhibit normal oestrous behaviour and on investigation have normal ovaries. However, the vulvar orifice is usually small and displaced ventrally.

Freemartinism

This is seen in twins where a female is developing with a male and this affects about 11 out of 12 such twins. The calf contains both normal 60,XX chromosomes and a few 60,XY (male) chromosomes. Occasionally, a female calf will be born singly with this abnormality and this is due to the death of the other twin. Freemartins are usually sterile.

The external genitalia resemble a female, but the vulva is smaller than normal. Later a tuft of hair develops at the vulva and in many cases a well-developed clitoris is found. Internally, there is a varying amount of agenesis or hypoplasia of the Müllerian system and stimulation of the Wolffian system. The ovaries tend to be hypoplastic and the vagina is usually non-patent, which allows diagnosis of the condition in the calf by the passage of a probe. However, occasionally the vagina is tubular and terminates at the normal position of the cervix, which is absent. The uterus tends to be two thick cords and there are two thin ducts that extend from the gonads to the intrapelvic urethra. There are often seminal vesicles present.

Urinary system defects

Pervious urachus

The defect occurs occasionally in calves. However, it may go undetected for weeks or even months, particularly in the male. Urine is discharged in a dribble from the urachus. All urine may be passed via the urachus although in some cases passage is also via the urethra. The condition may lead to cystitis and, as the umbilicus does not heal, there is often omphalophlebitis, septicaemia and polyarthritis. Surgical correction of the condition is possible and can be successful.

Other defects

Congenital porphyria

This is very rare. It is mainly seen in the Friesian and Holstein. It is caused by a simple recessive gene and occurs more frequently in the female than the male. There is increased porphyria in the blood and urine leading to the accumulation of the product in the tissues. The teeth tend to be pink or brown in colour and this can be seen in the newborn. The urine is red or purple and animals will develop cutaneous photosensitization and anaemia. There are high levels of uroporphyrins and coproporphyrins in the blood.

Familial polycythaemia

The condition is seen in the Jersey and is inherited as a simple autosomal recessive trait. There are early deaths. Those alive have poor growth, congestion of the mucosae and dyspnoea. There is a reduced erythrocyte count, packed cell volume and haemoglobin concentration.

Congenital goitre

This is an inherited condition but animals can be kept alive although mortality is high. Goitre also occurs when iodine deficiency affects the gestating dam (see p. 221).

Anomalous twins

There is faulty division in monozygotic twinning and this results in various abnormalities. There are varying degrees of conjunction, but double-headed monsters are most often seen. Others have a single head and the posterior part of the body is divided. In some cases the separation of the vertebral column may be almost complete, resulting in Siamese twins. Occasionally, small amorphous monsters called amorphous globosus or acardiac twins occur. They are related to double monsters and identical twins. They are found attached to the fetal membranes of the other calves and comprise an outer skin enclosing adipose tissue.

Chromosomal translocations

There are always 60 chromosomes present in the normal bovine. Translocation is the fusion of two morphologically distinct chromosomes. The most common is 1/29 translocation where there is fusion between number 1 and 29 pairs; it is also referred to as the Robertsonian translocation. It has been recorded in the Swedish Red and White breed, Charolais, Red Poll, British White and other breeds. The condition appears to be of importance in that there is reduced fertility in such animals due to early embryonic death.

Chapter 12: Calf Diarrhoea

by G.A. HALL, P.W. JONES AND J.H. MORGAN

Introduction

Diarrhoea in the neonatal calf is a serious welfare problem and a cause of economic loss due to mortality, treatment costs and poor growth. Calf diarrhoea is an example of a complex or multifactorial disease, resulting as it does from an interaction between the calf, its environment and nutrition and infectious agents (Fig. 12.1). Successful control of an outbreak will depend on recognition of the important factors in that outbreak and correction of the problems. Identification of the infectious agents involved is important because it permits a logical approach to disease control. Appropriate advice on nutrition, colostrum feeding, vaccination, hygiene and the use of antibiotics can only be given if it is clear which infectious agents are present and what their contribution to the disease process might be.

Causative mechanisms in diarrhoea

The digestive tract may be regarded as a high fluid flow system in which 80 per cent of the fluid contained within it is secreted into it and 20 per cent is ingested. Secreted fluid originates from salivary glands, gastric mucosa, pancreas, liver and small and large intestinal mucosa. Of the water that enters the digestive tract, 95 per cent is absorbed. Diarrhoea may be defined as an increase in faecal water loss due to increased faecal water content or to increased volume of faeces excreted or to a combination of both. The occurrence of diarrhoea indicates an imbalance between absorption and secretion of water and electrolytes. Only a slight imbalance in the equilibrium between secretion and absorption, in favour of secretion, may lead to severe diarrhoea because very large volumes of fluid are fluxing in both directions. There are several possible causes of imbalance.

Altered ion transport

Diarrhoea due to altered ion transport is caused by reduced absorption of sodium ions by villous enterocytes (Fig. 12.2), by increased secretion of chloride ions by

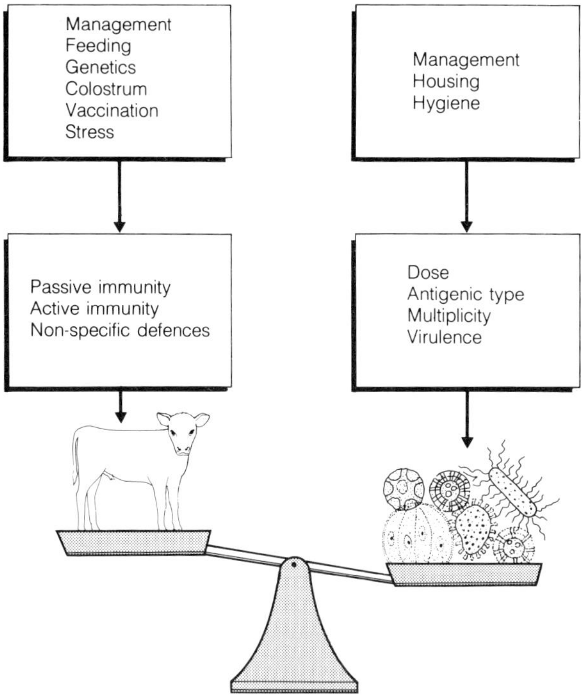

Fig. 12.1 Interactions between management, the calf and enteric agents. Reproduced from Morgan (1990).

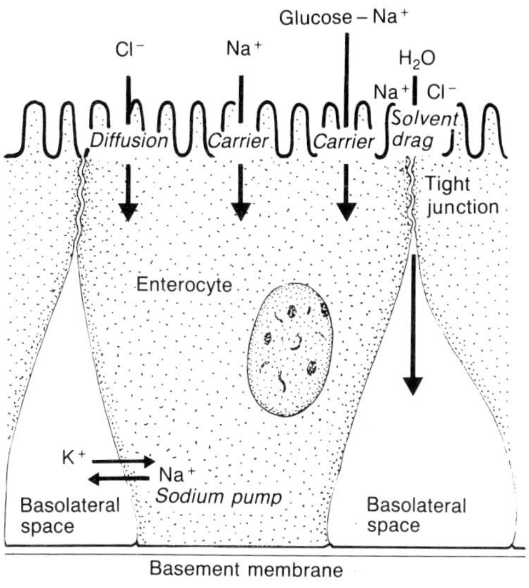

Fig. 12.2 Line drawing illustrating some mechanisms of movement of sodium and chloride ions and water from the intestinal lumen into basolateral spaces. The sodium pump expels sodium ions from the villous enterocyte into the basolateral space. Sodium ions diffuse along the electrochemical gradient created by the sodium pump, through the enterocyte luminal surface membrane, where passage is assisted by glucose-dependent and glucose-independent carrier systems. Chloride ions and water follow the movement of sodium ions.

crypt cells (Fig. 12.3) or by both mechanisms acting together. These changes are stimulated in calf diarrhoea by bacterial enterotoxins produced by enterotoxigenic *Escherichia coli* (Fig. 12.4). These bacteria, held on the gut surface by fimbrial adhesins, release enterotoxins. The subunit A of the heat-labile toxin activates adenylate cyclase located on the basolateral membrane which, in turn, raises the production of intracellular cyclic adenosine monophosphate (cyclic-AMP). Increased production of cyclic-AMP reduces sodium ion absorption by villous cells (Fig. 12.5) and consequently water absorption is reduced. At the same time secretion of chloride ions, and therefore water, is stimulated in crypt cells (Fig. 12.6). The heat-stable enterotoxin activates guanylate cyclase, stimulating intracellular synthesis of cyclic guanosine monophosphate (cyclic-GMP), which probably stimulates secretion and reduces absorption, although the precise mechanisms are not known (Fig. 12.5).

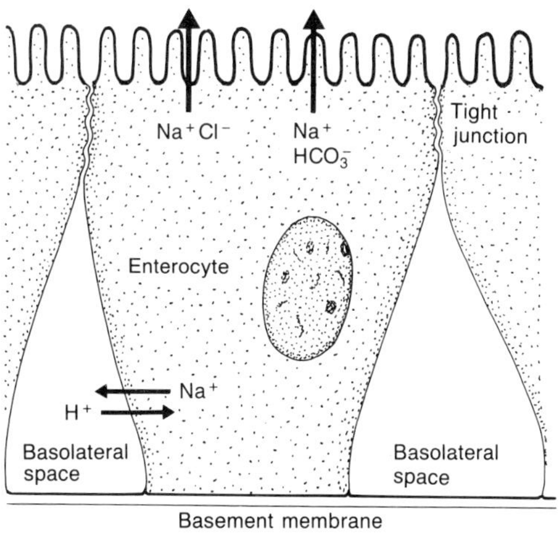

Fig. 12.3 Line drawing, illustrating some mechanisms of sodium secretion by crypt enterocytes. Sodium ions are secreted through the luminal surface and chloride and bicarbonate ions and water transported within the sodium ions.

Passive malabsorption

Diarrhoea may be the consequence of water malabsorption (Fig. 12.7). If malabsorption occurs then normal secretory processes and fluid loss due to tissue hydrostatic pressure will continue and will cause diarrhoea. Water malabsorption will follow a direct reduction of active uptake of sodium ions from the intestinal lumen. Malabsorption also occurs when morphological

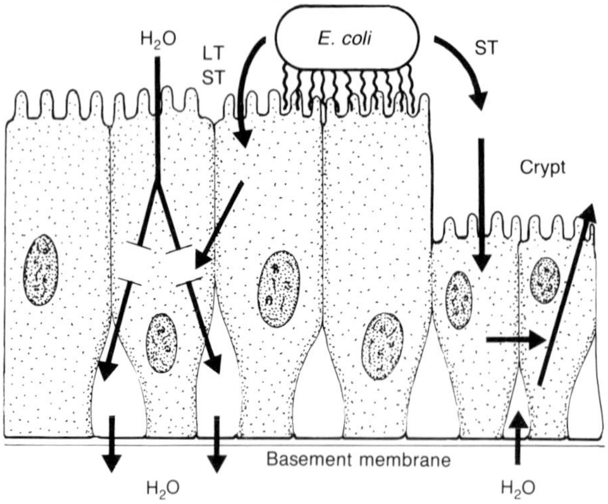

Fig. 12.4 Line drawing to illustrate the mechanisms by which enterotoxigenic *E. coli* cause diarrhoea. Bacteria are attached to the enterocyte surface by fimbriae and secrete heat-labile enterotoxin (LT) or heat-stable toxin (ST), which act on metabolic pathways in villous enterocytes to block water absorption and on metabolic pathways in crypt enterocytes to stimulate water secretion.

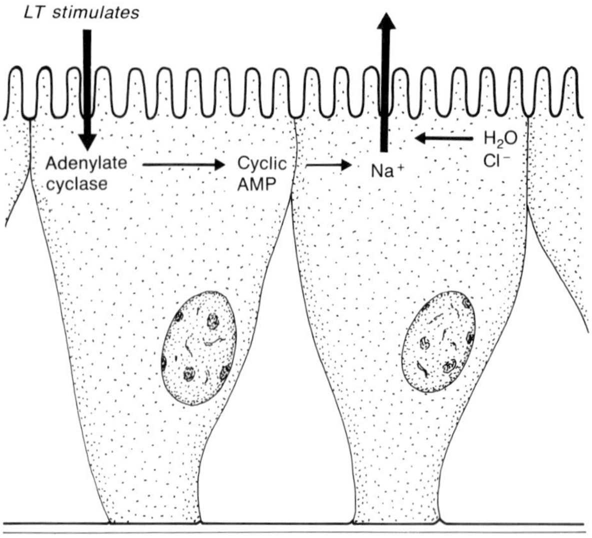

Fig. 12.6 Line drawing illustrating the effects of heat-labile enterotoxin (LT) on the secretion of sodium ions by crypt enterocytes. LT increases production of intracellular cyclic-AMP and this stimulates secretion of sodium ions, which carry with them chloride ions and water.

changes reduce the absorbing surface area. The best example of such morphological change is villus stunting produced by viral enteritis. The mature villous enterocytes can be regarded as the functional compartment of the small intestine, with absorption as one of the principal functions. A substantial reduction in the number of villous enterocytes causes a corresponding loss of function. Furthermore, crypt hyperplasia occurs in viral infections and immature secretory cells migrate onto the villus, increasing secretory capacity. In addition to loss of absorptive capacity there is also loss of digestive capacity, therefore maldigestion occurs, which can lead to an osmotically induced diarrhoea.

Intestinal motility

Increased intestinal motility may contribute to the development of diarrhoea, resulting in decreased transit

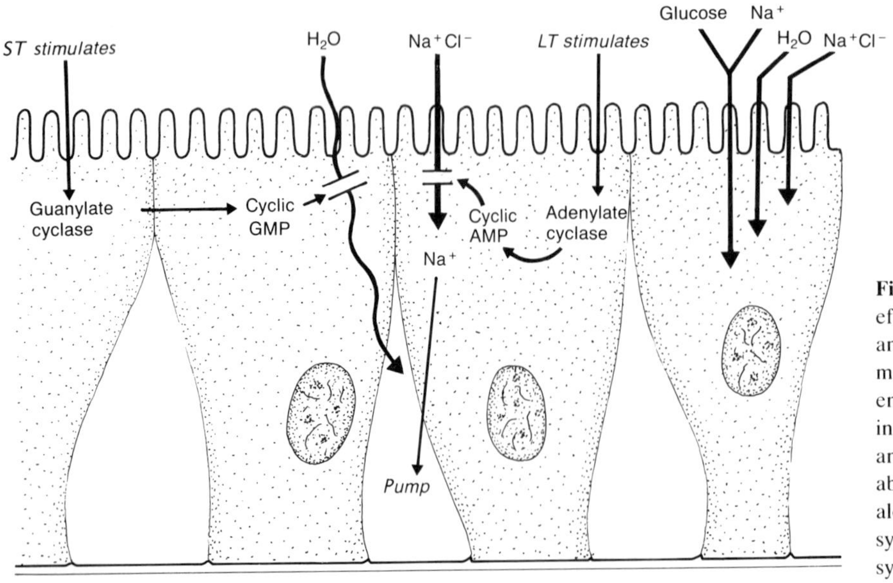

Fig. 12.5 Line drawing illustrating the effects of heat-stable enterotoxin (ST) and heat-labile enterotoxin (LT) on movement of water through villous enterocytes into basolateral spaces. ST inhibits water absorption via cyclic-GMP and LT, acting via cyclic-AMP, blocks absorption of sodium ions and water along the glucose-independent carrier system. The glucose-dependent carrier system is not affected by either toxin.

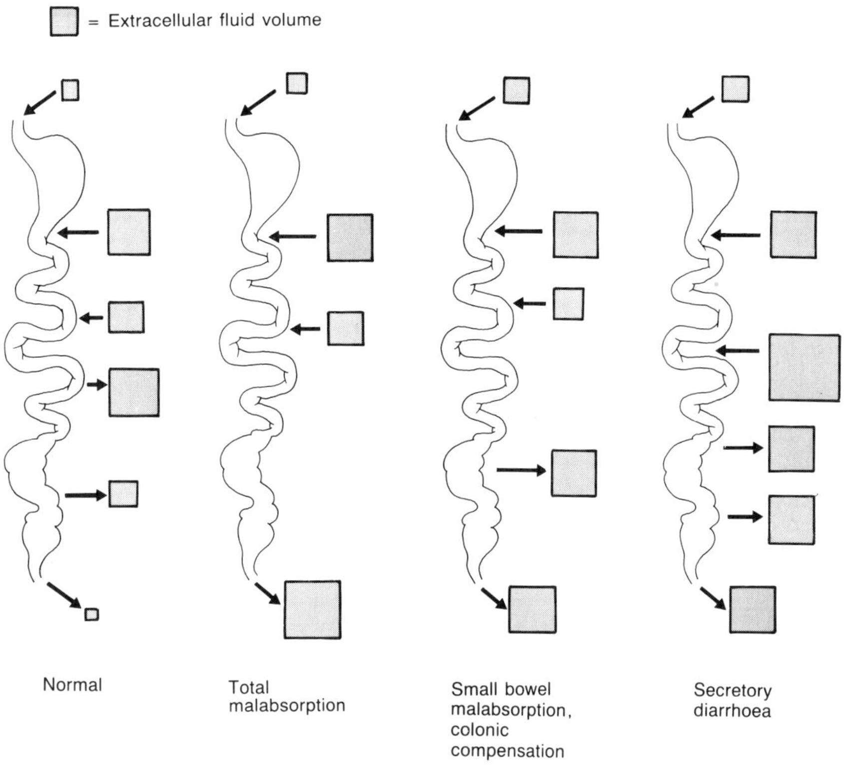

Fig. 12.7 Fluid fluxes in normal growing pigs (40 kg) and pigs with diarrhoea. Volumes of fluid entering and leaving the intestines are drawn in proportional size to the extracellular fluid volume shown at the top. Most water is absorbed by the distal small intestine and colon in pigs of this age and colonic compensation is likely to be much less in neonatal pigs. Reproduced from Argenzio R.A., Pathophysiology of neonatal diarrhoea. *Agri-Practice* (1984) **5**, 25–32, by kind permission of the author and publishers.

time and insufficient time for normal absorption. The role of motility is now considered to be less important than was thought previously.

Osmotic effects

Lactose, the major sugar in cows milk, is split into glucose and galactose by the enzyme β-galactosidase (lactase), which is located on microvilli of jejunal enterocytes. These monosaccharides are rapidly absorbed and therefore they have little osmotic effect. Viral enteropathogens destroy mature enterocytes, thus creating a transient deficiency in β-galactosidase. Consequently, lactose passes undigested to the colon together with an osmotic equivalent of water. It may be inferred from studies of pigs, goats and horses that the consequences of increased lactose in the colon depends on the balance between input of lactose and the fermentative capacity of the colonic microbial flora. If the calf possesses a well-developed colon and colonic microbial flora and the amount of lactose entering is not excessive because of restricted dietary intake and/or slight intestinal damage, then the lactose will be fermented to short-chain fatty acids. These will be absorbed through the colonic mucosa, a process that facilitates the absorption of sodium ions and water by the colonic mucosa. These processes are 'anti-diarrhoeal' (Fig. 12.8). In a young animal, with a poorly developed colon and colonic microflora, there may be little fermentation of lactose that remains in the lumen, holding water and contributing to the diarrhoea (Fig. 12.8). In an animal with a well-developed colonic microflora, dumping of large amounts of lactose into the colon as a result of *ad libitum* feeding and severe intestinal damage, results in hyperfermentation and the production of lactic acid rather than short-chain fatty acids. Lactate is poorly absorbed and draws water into the colon by osmosis, exacerbating the diarrhoea. These mechanisms explain why withholding milk from calves with rotavirus scour reduce the severity of the diarrhoea (Fig. 12.8).

Tissue hydrostatic pressure and increased permeability

Tissue hydrostatic pressure results in a continual seepage of water from the mucosa into the lumen and this can contribute to the pathogenesis of diarrhoea if malabsorption is present. Seepage may be increased by inflammation of the mucosa, which allows greater leakage of fluid between enterocytes. In very severe inflammatory conditions, for example acute salmonellosis, the epithelium may be so extensively damaged as

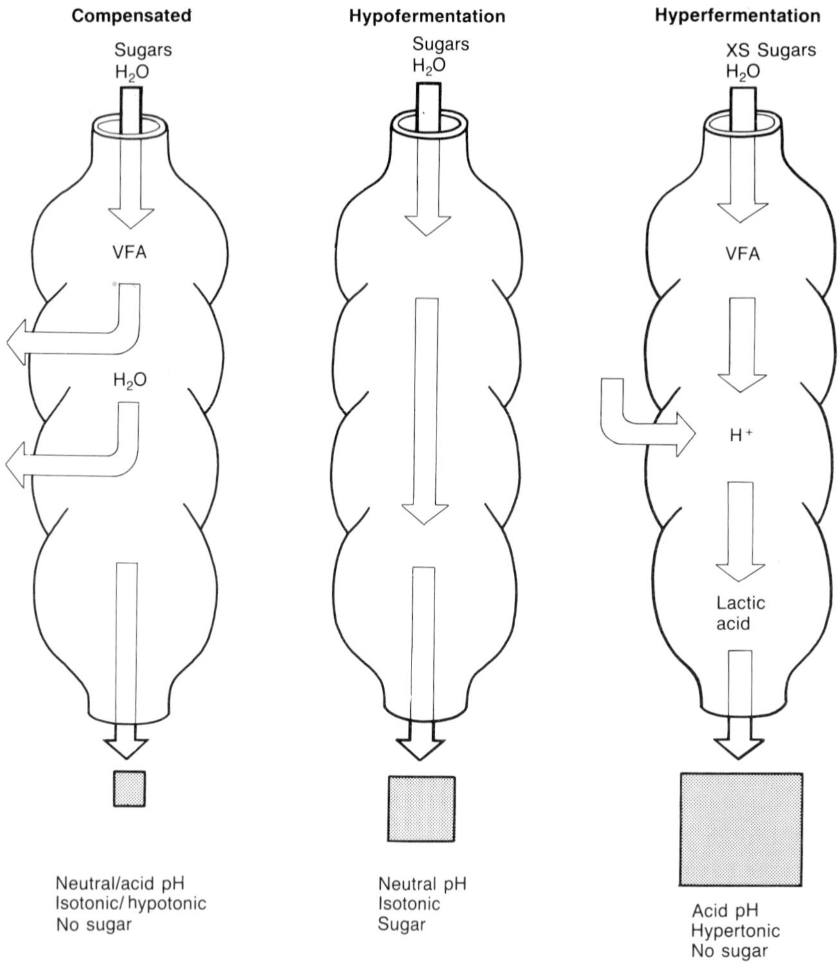

Fig. 12.8 Three alternative consequences of a small intestinal maldigestion and malabsorption, as seen in rotavirus infection. In the 'compensated' situation, the colonic flora is well developed and microbial fermentation of the moderate amounts of malabsorbed carbohydrate yields volatile fatty acids (VFA). These are rapidly absorbed, stimulating water absorption and promoting colonic compensation so that diarrhoea does not occur. If the colon and colonic flora are poorly developed there is hypofermentation and consequently no compensation, and diarrhoea occurs. If the colonic flora is well developed and is overloaded with sugar, hyperfermentation occurs and lactic acid is produced that promotes osmotic diarrhoea. Reproduced from Argenzio, R.A., Pathophysiology of neonatal diarrhoea. *Agri-Practice* (1984) 5, 25–32, by kind permission of the author and publishers.

to allow erythrocytes to leak from capillaries, through the epithelium into the lumen; clearly other blood constituents will be lost also.

Types of diarrhoea

Having examined the various pathophysiological processes that can give rise to diarrhoea, two general types of diarrhoea can be recognized.

Secretory diarrhoea

A diarrhoea resulting from net movement of fluid into the gut lumen despite fasting. Faeces are characteristically isotonic with plasma, watery and alkaline, and the volumes produced are usually large. The faeces are alkaline because sodium and bicarbonate ions are secreted by the ileum. In compensation, the colon may be exchanging potassium ions for sodium ions. Acute secretory diarrhoea is always caused by a bacterial infection.

Osmotic diarrhoea

A diarrhoea where the faeces may have high osmolality due to unabsorbed molecules with osmotic activity, usually of dietary origin. Faeces may contain undigested lactose and faecal pH will vary, depending on the amount of lactose fermented to short-chain fatty acids or lactic acid. Osmotic diarrhoea may also be thought of as a diarrhoea caused by malabsorption and maldigestion. Faecal volume is smaller than in secretory diarrhoea and the diarrhoea is reduced or abolished by fasting.

Role of the large intestine

Most diarrhoea in the calf originates in the small intestine and as a result small intestinal function has received most study. It is evident that the large intestine, particularly the colon, is a very important site of water absorption and consequently may contribute to the development of diarrhoea if its functional capacity is overwhelmed or impaired by the fermentative mechanisms described above. Similarly, its function may be impaired by infection with *Cryptosporidium*, coronavirus or enterohaemorrhagic *E. coli*. Ingesta entering the colon from the small intestine may be damaging. Marked damage to the colonic epithelium has been reported in recent studies where bile salts were infused into the colon of the pig. Rapid transit of small intestinal contents into the colon could, theoretically, cause damage by this mechanism.

Effects of diarrhoea and their clinical signs

The systemic effects of diarrhoea, which eventually culminate in death, are precipitated by a single event, the loss of extracellular fluid. Endogenous secretion into the gastrointestinal tract in 24 hours may equal the extracellular fluid volume. Loss of 15 per cent of the extracellular fluid volume leads to clinical signs and loss of 30 per cent results in death.

Diarrhoea causes changes in plasma constituents that are similar regardless of the cause of the diarrhoea (Fig. 12.9). When neonatal colostrum-fed calves were experimentally inoculated with coronavirus, the water and electrolyte losses were severe (Lewis & Philips, 1978). Faecal water loss increased 28-fold, faecal volume increased 22-fold and faecal water content increased from 73 to 94 per cent. Renal water loss was reduced to 30 per cent of normal and there were severe losses of sodium and chloride ions and considerable losses of bicarbonate and potassium ions. There was loss of body weight, 12.7 per cent between onset of diarrhoea and death. Plasma volume decreased by 40 per cent leading to a 39 per cent increase in haematocrit and a 33 per cent increase in plasma protein concentration. The increase in plasma protein concentration was lower, possibly because of protein loss by catabolism or by leakage into the intestinal lumen. Both these values vary widely between individuals and are of little value in assessing severity of fluid loss.

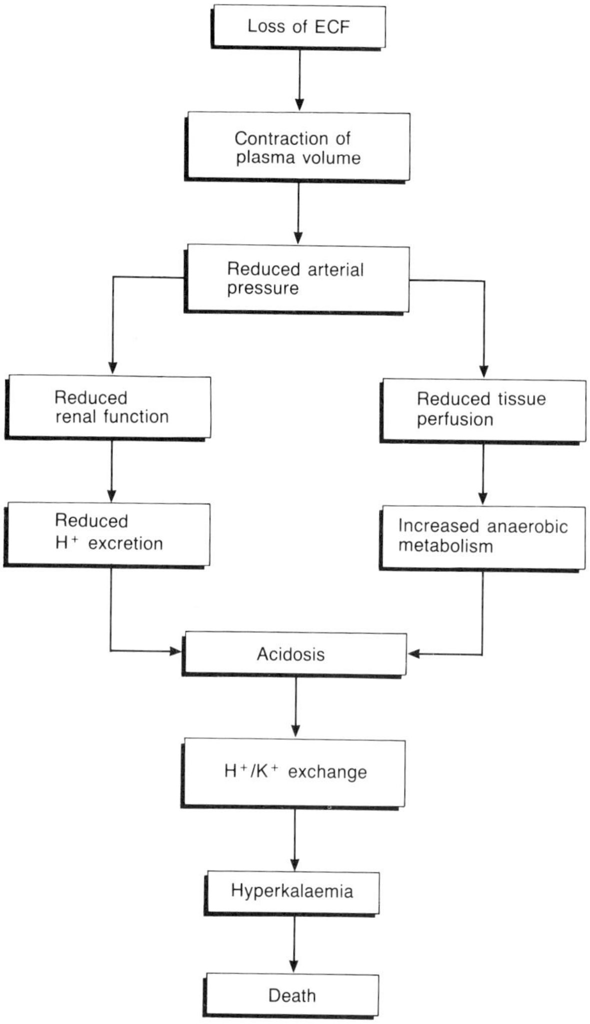

Fig. 12.9 The systemic consequences of diarrhoea. Reduction of extracellular fluid volume leads to acidosis, an exchange of extracellular H^+ for intracellular K^+ leading to hyperkalaemia causing cardiac failure. Reproduced from Argenzio, R.A., Pathophysiology of neonatal diarrhoea. *Agri-Practice* (1984) **5**, 25–32, by kind permission of the author and publishers.

Contraction of plasma volume gives rise to the clinical signs of sunken eyes and 'tenting' of skin folds; it leads to a fall in arterial blood pressure, which stimulates peripheral vasoconstriction. Peripheral vasoconstriction, in its turn, leads to poor tissue perfusion with blood, localized ischaemia and lower metabolic activity so that the temperature of peripheral tissues falls, approaching ambient temperature prior to death; the extremities, the ears and mouth, feel cold. Rectal temperature increases until near to death when it falls rapidly to below normal.

Acidosis is an important consequence of diarrhoea and a number of factors contribute to its development. A major factor is loss of bicarbonate ions in faeces and, additionally, there may be absorption of acids produced by microbial fermentation of lactose in the large intestine. Loss of extracellular fluid (dehydration) causes decreased perfusion of the kidney with blood causing reduced renal function, which leads to decreased excretion of hydrogen ions by the kidney. Finally, lactic acidosis may develop because of increased production of lactate following peripheral hypoxia, and decreased utilization of lactate due to decreased delivery of lactate to the liver. The ability of the liver to use lactate for gluconeogenesis may be impaired because of increased intracellular concentration of hydrogen ions. Indeed, the liver may become a lactate producer rather than a lactate utilizer. The calf attempts to reduce acidosis by panting to increase exhalation of carbon dioxide. Intracellular acidosis occurs in parallel with the fall in the blood pH. Intracellular production of hydrogen ions increases and hydrogen ions move into cells. This movement of hydrogen ions into cells forces potassium and sodium ions to be lost and hyperkalaemia develops. However, potassium is also lost in the faeces, so that the plasma concentration may, theoretically, be increased, normal or decreased depending on the rate of loss from plasma into faeces, and from cells into plasma. In general it is increased. The loss of potassium ions from cells into the interstitial fluid causes levels of intracellular potassium to fall and levels in interstitial fluid and plasma to rise and, consequently, adjacent to cells, the ratio of extracellular potassium : intracellular potassium is reduced. This redistribution of potassium causes a reduction in the resting potential of cell membranes, which has serious and eventually lethal effects on cardiac muscle function. As the concentration of potassium ions in plasma rises, heart rate falls and there is a decreased amplitude, or loss of the P wave. The activity in plasma of the myocardial enzymes lactate dehydrogenase isoenzyme 1, creatinine phosphokinase 1 and aldolase is raised indicating cardiac damage. Thus death from acute severe diarrhoea in the calf appears to be due to potassium cardiotoxicosis.

Metabolic and hormonal changes

Hypoglycaemia frequently occurs in acute severe diarrhoea of calves especially young calves near death. Anorexia, decreased absorption of nutrients, minimal glycogen reserves, inhibited gluconeogenesis, increased glycolysis due to reduced tissue perfusion and anoxia and insulin-like effect of bacterial endotoxins on liver may contribute to the hypoglycaemia. Signs of hypoglycaemia are weakness, lethargy, convulsions and coma. Hypoglycaemia stimulates corticoid secretion; plasma concentration of corticosterone and hydrocortisone are elevated in calves with diarrhoea and are higher in calves that die. Theoretically, corticosteroids help counter hypoglycaemia by stimulating gluconeogenesis but their effects may be blocked. Plasma aldosterone concentrations are increased in calves with diarrhoea probably due to acidosis, hypovolaemia, hyperkalaemia and hyponatraemia. The actions of aldosterone are helpful in that sodium and water retention is increased as is excretion of potassium and hydrogen ions. There is, however, decreased renal function, which limits the helpful actions of aldosterone.

Infectious agents

The elucidation of the infectious causes of calf diarrhoea has been a major area of progress over the last 20 years. For many years, salmonellas were the only known cause, but in 1967 it became clear that a small number of strains of *E. coli* caused a watery diarrhoea and subsequently these came to be known as enterotoxigenic *E. coli* (ETEC). Rotavirus was the first viral enteropathogen to be recognized, followed by coronavirus and more recently calici-like virus, astrovirus and Breda virus. *Cryptosporidium* was found to cause diarrhoea in calves approximately 10 years ago and *Campylobacter* spp. became regarded as putative pathogens at the same time; subsequent studies, which will be reviewed later, indicated that campylobacters do not cause diarrhoea in calves, although they are an important enteropathogen in man. Most recently, *E. coli* have been identified that cause diarrhoea without producing enterotoxins; these include strains that infect the large intestine and cause mild dysentery, the enterohaemorrhagic *E. coli* (EHEC), and strains comparable to human enteropathogenic *E. coli* (EPEC).

Deciding whether a particular putative infectious agent is an important cause of calf diarrhoea is a laborious process starting with the detection of the agent in faeces from a calf with diarrhoea. A pure inoculum must be prepared from faeces that may contain many bacteria and viruses. The pathogenicity of the inoculum is confirmed by experimental inoculation of a susceptible host, reproducing the disease and re-isolating the pathogen from the experimentally infected animal. An accurate and rapid diagnostic test must be devised so that the prevalence of the agent in association with field disease can be surveyed.

Bovine rotavirus

The agent

Rotavirus is a new genus within the family Reoviridae. The virus contains double-stranded RNA in 11 segments. Particles have a wheel-like appearance; a wide hub formed by the core, spokes formed by 20 outer capsomers and an often ill-defined outer rim (Fig. 12.10). Incomplete particles lacking the outer capsid layer are frequently seen in faeces. Almost all bovine rotaviruses share a common antigen and have been

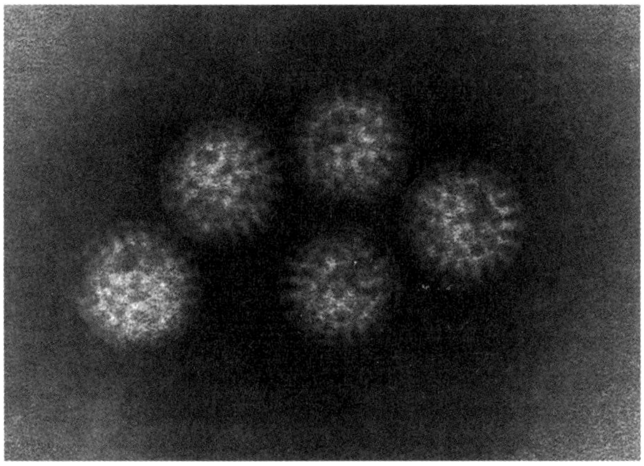

Fig. 12.10 Transmission electron micrograph of a cluster of five bovine rotavirus particles. Visible are the wide hub, spokes formed by the capsomers and the outer rim. (Courtesy of Dr J.C. Bridger, Institute for Animal Health, Compton.)

classified as group A rotaviruses. There is antigenic variation within group A rotaviruses, which can be detected by cross-neutralization tests. This variation has been used to divide the group A rotaviruses into serotypes. There are strains that lack the group A antigen that have been isolated from pigs, chickens and humans and these are sometimes referred to as atypical rotaviruses or non-group A rotaviruses.

Epidemiology

Bovine rotavirus is universally present in all cattle herds. Calves become infected by the faecal–oral route when colostrum feeding has stopped and levels of colostral antibody are falling in the small intestine. The incubation period varies from 15 hours to five days and is followed by virus excretion, which commences in the second week of life. Many infections are subclinical but a proportion result in diarrhoea, thus accounting for the peak incidence of 'white scour' at about 10 days of age. Initially, calves are dull and are often reluctant to eat; they may appear to have abdominal distension. Diarrhoea develops, which may be watery at first, but it rapidly becomes pale yellow or white and pasty and may contain mucus; dehydration commonly develops. Excretion of copious amounts of yoghurt-like faeces is typical of rotavirus infections that are uncomplicated by other enteropathogens and the faeces are thought to have this appearance because they represent the passage of partially digested or undigested milk. The severity and duration of disease are variable, clinical signs usually last four to eight days and under field conditions infections may be fatal. Occurrence of pyrexia is variable, but when it occurs it is usually mild.

Pathogenesis

Rotaviruses infect mature enterocytes, located on the surface of villi. Particles are detected in the cytoplasm, usually in dilated cisternae of the endoplasmic reticulum. Masses of granular or finely fibrillar virus precursor (viroplasm) containing virus cores are present outside the cisternae. Particles released from viroplasm pass into the cisternae; some bud through the membrane of the endoplasmic reticulum and acquire an envelope. Viral multiplication within the cells initiates degenerative changes, the cell exfoliates and the rapid loss of large numbers of cells leads to fusion and stunting of villi. The columnar epithelium is replaced by enterocytes that are cuboidal or squamous and the epithelium contains increased numbers of immature cells from the crypts (Fig. 12.11). In very severe cases the villi may be obliterated leading to a totally flat epithelium. The pathogenic process may commence in the upper jejunum and progress along the small intestine to the ileum, producing a wave of damage as described by Mebus *et al.* (1971), although observations by others suggest that this is not so. There is variation in pathogenicity between strains; whilst some strains may only damage a limited length of upper jejunum, others may damage the entire length of the small intestine. Some poorly virulent strains are able to infect enterocytes, replicate within them and cause enterocyte loss, but not at a sufficiently rapid rate to outpace repair mechanisms and cause lesions and diarrhoea. The existence of strains of low virulence has implications for accurate diagnosis of rotavirus diarrhoea because it may be assumed that such strains could be excreted by calves with diarrhoea caused by other enteropathogens. To be confident in a diagnosis of rotavirus diarrhoea, it is necessary to identify rotavirus in the faeces of significantly more diarrhoeic calves than in age-matched, clinically normal calves on the same farm. On the basis of present knowledge, groups of four affected and four normal calves are adequate.

The changes in intestinal structure affect its function. Loss of mature enterocytes with their lactase and their replacement with immature enterocytes containing less lactase results in a reduced capacity of the mucosa to digest lactose, especially in the jejunum. Because the surface area of the small intestine is reduced, there is reduced ability to absorb the glucose and galactose that is produced from the digestion of lactose. Thus lactose accumulates in the large intestine, where by virtue of

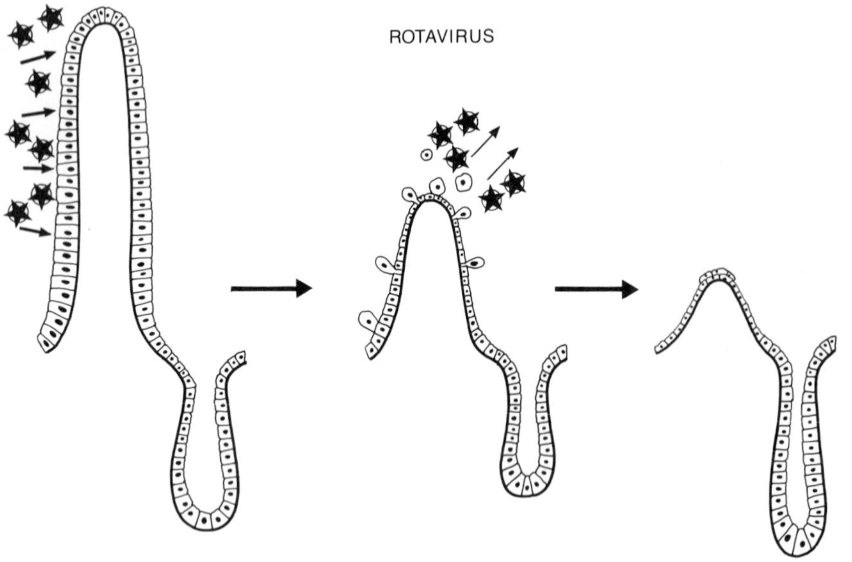

Fig. 12.11 Line drawing illustrating the development of the small intestinal lesion in rotavirus infection. Mature enterocytes are infected and virus replication causes enterocyte death and sloughing. Villi stunt and the surviving enterocytes are cuboidal or squamous. Mitosis increases in the crypts, which elongate. ✱ represents a virus particle.

its hypertonicity it prevents absorption of water from faeces and contributes to the development of water loss and dehydration. Bacterial fermentation of the lactose may increase the osmotic effects. As a result of enterocyte loss, the population of enterocytes on the villi changes from mature cells with digestive and absorptive function to predominantly immature cells with secretory function. The number of cells in the crypts (secretory cells) also increases. Thus the functional balance may change from absorption to secretion.

Prevention

Virtually all calves that have sucked colostrum will have serum antibody to rotavirus, which can be detected by a number of tests. These antibodies, however, do not protect against infection and disease because for protective purposes neutralizing antibody is required in the gut lumen. This is because the entire disease process occurs on the mucosal surface and if antibodies are to interfere with the pathogenic process they must be present in the gut contents that bathe the mucosal surface; luminal antibodies neutralize virus and prevent initial infection and spread of infection from enterocyte to enterocyte. There is recent evidence, however, suggesting that serum antibodies, which originated from the colostrum of hyperimmune cows, can be transferred to the gut where they are protective. Following natural infection, calves are immune to disease; this is thought to be the result of an active mucosal immunity provided by IgA and cell-mediated mechanisms. Repeated episodes of re-infection without signs occur throughout life, maintaining herd immunity and the virus in the population and environment.

Colostrum contains antibodies to rotavirus that help protect the calf against infection and disease. The concentration of antibody in colostrum and early milk declines rapidly, reaching levels that are thought to be non-protective three to four days after parturition (Fig. 12.12). Under farm conditions, where rotavirus is always present, it is clear that infection is delayed rather than prevented by feeding colostrum immediately after birth; rotavirus excretion frequently occurs in the second week of life and this is clearly a period when calves are susceptible to infection and disease. For calves reared artificially, some protection might be obtained during this period by feeding stored surplus colostrum, which will contain some antirotaviral antibody.

The first vaccine, marketed in the USA, was a live attenuated vaccine for oral administration to calves at birth. It aimed to stimulate active immunity in the calf. Although, in some trials, it protected calves against experimental challenge, its efficacy in the field appeared limited. The reasons for lack of efficacy are unknown but possibly they include inactivation of vaccine virus by neutralizing colostral antibody, low antigenicity of the vaccine strain or lack of cross-protection between the vaccine strain and field strains. More recently, active vaccination of the calf has been succeeded by providing enhanced passive protection to calves by vaccinating dams with inactivated vaccines. Because rotavirus is endemic in herds, cows have antibodies to

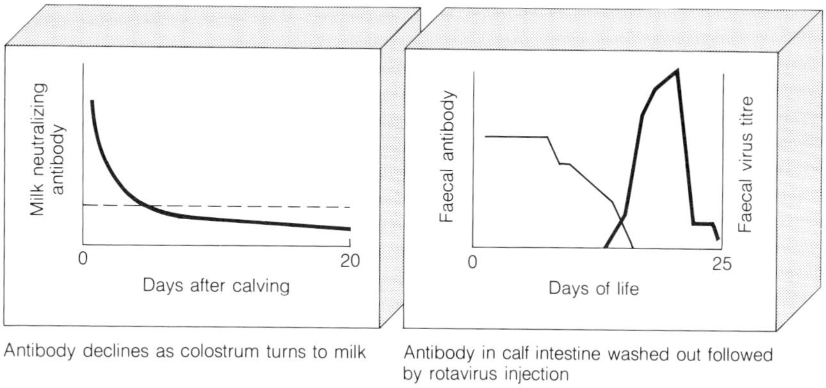

Fig. 12.12 Graphical illustration of changes that occur in neutralizing antibody to rotavirus in cows milk after calving and faecal antibody to rotavirus and faecal virus in the early days of a calf's life. Reproduced from Morgan (1990).

rotavirus in their serum and parenteral administration of a single dose of inactivated virus boosts these pre-existing serum antibodies. Consequently, the concentration of antibody in colostrum and milk is increased and antibody is present in milk for longer than in unvaccinated animals. This approach has been tested by several groups and appears to have been effective in all but one, in which calves sucking hyperimmunized heifers developed diarrhoea after challenge at seven days of age. In a second study, continual feeding of colostrum from vaccinated dams prevented disease following experimental challenge and in a third, hyperimmune colostrum fed as 1 per cent of a milk replacer diet prevented infection and disease following experimental challenge. Under farm conditions, feeding calves a diet that contained 10 per cent colostrum from vaccinated dams delayed the onset of diarrhoea and reduced its incidence, duration and severity during a natural outbreak of scour in which rotavirus, *E. coli* (K99) and *Cryptosporidium* were involved. Feeding colostrum from non-vaccinated cows gave less protection but more protection than when no colostrum was fed.

Thus, dam vaccination can be useful. The protective effect will vary with the level of antibody in colostrum and milk and the amount consumed. This system is suitable for suckled calves and for artificially reared calves if hyperimmune colostrum is saved and added to milk replacer diets; it is no use to the farmer who buys in his calves from market because he has no access to colostrum. Dam vaccination may delay rather than prevent diarrhoea. Strains of rotavirus exist that cause disease in calves aged four months and it is possible that calves exposed to such strains would become infected and scour when passive protection was removed. There is evidence, however, that disease which occurs as passive protection wanes is less severe than that seen in the totally susceptible calf. Consequently, feeding normal or immune colostrum even if it did not give total protection might reduce disease severity. If active immunity can develop in the presence of passive antibody in the gut, then prolonged feeding of hyperimmune colostrum will prevent disease, not just delay it, because when feeding passive antibody is stopped, natural exposure to virus will have occurred and a natural immunity will be present. The evidence for the development of active immunity in the presence of passive antibody is variable. In one study, bovine colostrum was fed to gnotobiotic piglets that were inoculated with porcine rotavirus. They did not develop diarrhoea but they did produce antibodies to porcine strains and were immune to further challenge. On the other hand, the failure of the avirulent vaccine in calves was attributed partially to blocking by colostral antibody.

A fourth potential limitation of the dam vaccine, indeed of all vaccines, is the extent to which one strain will protect against the wide range of strains that occur in the field. In theory, we might expect this to be limited in rotaviruses since *in vitro* cross-neutralization tests show marked lack of neutralization between some strains. In practice, however, this does not seem to be a problem. Experience with a commercially available dam vaccine has shown that whilst neutralizing antibody to the homologous strain is increased, neutralizing antibody to heterologous strains is also raised, although to a lesser extent. The vaccine virus also increases neutralizing activity to porcine and simian rotaviruses. Much will depend on the rotaviruses that the cow has experienced prior to vaccination.

The ideal immunoprophylactic system would be to provide initial passive protection by hyperimmune colostrum with active vaccination of the calf whilst it is passively protected so that active immunity will be stimulated as passive protection wanes. The first part of this system is available.

Diagnosis

Diagnosis of rotavirus disease is based on the detection of virus or virus antigen in the faeces. Examination of faeces in the electron microscope has been the standard technique used in laboratories and the virus is usually easier to detect if it has been purified and concentrated. The value of this diagnostic method is limited by the requirement for an electron microscope and an expert operator and as a result research laboratories have devised alternative methods. Fluorescein-labelled antibodies have been used to detect virus antigen in faecal smears and in cell cultures inoculated with faecal preparations. The sensitivity of the cell culture method has been enhanced by increasing the chance of cell infection by centrifuging the inoculum onto the cells or by adding trypsin to the cells in culture. Immunoelectrophoresis, radioimmunoassay and complement fixation tests of faeces have also been developed, but all require sophisticated laboratory equipment. Enzyme-linked immunosorbent assays (ELISA) have been developed for rotavirus and a plate ELISA is used by many diagnostic laboratories. Some diagnostic laboratories use the polyacrylamide gel electrophoresis method, which has proved to be equally satisfactory. The diagnostic kits available to practice laboratories in the UK are a dot ELISA, a latex method and a plate ELISA system. The plate ELISA system requires a minimum of equipment and also tests for bovine coronavirus and $K99^+$ *Escherichia coli*; a modification to the system has permitted the detection of *Cryptosporidium*.

The identification of rotavirus particles or antigen in the faeces of calves with diarrhoea does not automatically lead to a diagnosis of rotavirus disease in the outbreak. Rotavirus antigen was detected in 50 per cent of faeces from healthy calves aged one to two weeks in a study in which an ELISA test was used. Thus, in order to reach a sound diagnosis, and using that test to identify excretors, it was necessary to show that significantly more than 50 per cent of diarrhoeic calves were excreting rotavirus. This was achieved by examining faeces from four calves with diarrhoea and four matching normal calves on the farm. The number of calf faeces that will need to be examined in an investigation of an outbreak will depend on the ability of the diagnostic test in use to detect excretion by normal calves.

Management

The management of an outbreak of rotavirus diarrhoea, once it has been diagnosed, should be based on the twin concepts of reducing exposure to infection and enhancing resistance to infection. Good hygiene is unlikely to be completely successful in controlling spread of infection because rotavirus is endemic and highly infections, but it will help to reduce the build-up of infection throughout the calving period and thus reduce the infectious challenge to which calves are exposed; several studies have recorded beneficial results from good hygiene. To assist good hygiene, calving accommodation and calf pens should be designed for ease of cleaning and with adequate drainage. An 'all-in, all-out' policy should be adopted where possible, especially in units rearing purchased calves. Pens should be cleaned between batches, steamed, disinfected and allowed to dry. Disinfectants that have been reported to be affective against rotavirus are 0.25 per cent formaldehyde, 2 per cent phenol, 1 per cent sodium hypochlorite, 0.25 per cent propiolactone, quaternary ammonium compounds and iodophores. Mixing calves of different ages should be avoided and stress should be limited by staggering management interferences such as castration, dehorning and change of accommodation.

Increasing resistance to infection can be achieved by promoting general calf health and by stimulating specific immunity. Early colostrum intake is vital for general calf health and, thereafter, milk or good quality milk substitute should be fed regularly and at the correct temperature. Extended feeding of stored colostrum to prolong the period when passive antibody is present in the gut lumen is helpful in restricting infection with rotavirus. Vaccination of cows in late pregnancy is a method of enhancing the levels of anti-rotavirus antibody in the colostrum and milk and has been shown to be very effective in suckler systems and in systems feeding milk substitute, if hyperimmune colostrum is collected and added to the milk substitute.

The use of antibiotics in rotavirus diarrhoea is not indicated, unless enteropathogenic bacteria are thought to be a contributory cause. Sick calves should be isolated to reduce build-up of infection in the calf pens and facilitate the provision of rehydration therapy. Once isolated, it is beneficial to replace milk with oral electrolyte solution so as to reduce the development of osmotic diarrhoea and commence the process of rehydration.

Bovine coronavirus

The agent

Bovine coronavirus (BCV) is a member of a group of viruses with a characteristic morphology seen in the

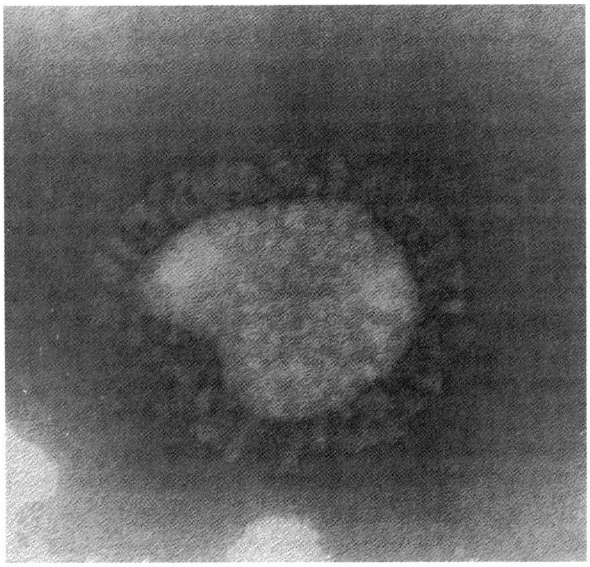

Fig. 12.13 Transmission electron micrograph of a single particle of bovine coronavirus. The particle has an irregular shape and is covered by a corona of peplomers. (Courtesy of Dr J.C. Bridger, Institute for Animal Health, Compton.)

electron microscope (Fig. 12.13). The virions, which contain single-stranded polyadenylated RNA are pleomorphic spherical particles 70–220 nm in diameter with a corona of widely spaced club-shaped surface projections (peplomers), which are 20 nm long. Bovine coronavirus has two types of peplomer of different length. There is only one serotype of bovine coronavirus.

Signs

Calves usually become infected with coronavirus when they are between one and three weeks old, although disease may occur in calves up to three months of age. Transmission of infection is by the faecal–oral route, but the recent demonstration of infection in the upper respiratory tract allows the possibility of faecal–respiratory and respiratory–respiratory transmission. Calves develop diarrhoea in a manner virtually identical to rotavirus; studies of experimental inoculations suggest that the incubation period is 20–30 hours. Generally, coronavirus diarrhoea is more watery and of greater severity than rotavirus diarrhoea, leading more rapidly to dehydration and acidosis. The severe diarrhoea also leads to substantial losses of sodium, potassium, chloride and bicarbonate ions. Fluid yellow faeces are passed at first and these turn to a yellow liquid containing milk clots and mucus. Depression, fever and anorexia occur and clinical signs of disease usually last four to five days.

Pathogenesis

Bovine coronavirus infects mature enterocytes located on the surface of villi and epithelial cells of the upper respiratory tract. The small intestine is severely damaged due to sloughing of infected cells, especially the ileum, and cells on the surface and in the crypts of the large intestine are also killed. Infection of the upper respiratory tracts does not appear to cause lesions. Virus particles are assembled in the cytoplasm by a budding process through the rough endoplasmic reticulum. They are subsequently transported through and accumulate in the Golgi complex and released from the cell by lysis. The range of lesions seen in the small intestine are identical to those produced by rotavirus and repair can occur rapidly because small intestinal crypt cells are largely unaffected. Virus damage to colonic crypt cells results in atrophy of the mucosal ridges and dilated crypts containing dead exfoliated cells. The mechanisms by which the intestinal damage caused by bovine coronavirus results in diarrhoea are thought to be the same as described for rotavirus. The presence of severe lesions in the ileum, caecum and colon, areas of the small and large intestine that absorb water may account for the more watery nature of the diarrhoea seen in BCV infections. It is not clear whether or not strains of BCV vary in virulence, as is seen in bovine rotaviruses.

Prevention

It is probable that immune responses to BCV will be similar to those seen in rotavirus infection; calves that have recovered from coronavirus diarrhoea are protected against reinfection. Colostrum may be protective, as it is against rotaviruses, but there is no vaccine available in the UK to boost the levels of anticoronavirus antibody in colostrum and early milk.

Diagnosis

Bovine coronavirus is universally present on all cattle farms, as indicated by the presence of antibodies in all adults. Diagnosis of coronavirus disease, like that of rotavirus disease, is based on the detection of virus or virus antigen in intestinal tissue or faeces. Examination of faeces in the electron microscope, including immune electron microscopy, has been the standard technique used in laboratories, but the value of these diagnostic methods is limited by the requirement for an electron microscope and an expert operator. Cell culture of bovine coronavirus from faeces is possible in a number of cell lines but this is a technique reserved for use in research laboratories. Fluorescein-labelled antibodies may be used to detect virus antigen in faecal smears and in cryostat sections of tissues collected at necropsy. Care should be taken if diagnosis is to be based on examination of tissues because virus-infected enterocytes may be sloughed due to autolysis if the tissue is not collected under terminal anaesthesia or within a few minutes of death. Also, if tissues are collected late in the disease process, infected cells may not be present, even though the villi are stunted and diarrhoea is still present. Assays using ELISA have been developed for detection of bovine coronavirus and are used by diagnostic laboratories. The existence of bovine coronavirus excretion by clinically normal calves is recorded, although it is not seen as commonly as is rotavirus; this may be due to the insensitivity of diagnostic tests or subclinical infections may be uncommon.

Management

An outbreak of BCV diarrhoea should be managed in the same way as an outbreak of rotavirus diarrhoea; that is, aim to reduce exposure to infection and enhance resistance to infection. Good hygiene is unlikely to be completely successful in controlling spread of infection because bovine coronavirus is endemic, but it will help to reduce the build-up of infection throughout the calving period; management methods that encourage good hygiene have been described.

Increasing resistance to infection can be achieved by promoting general calf health, as described previously. The immunoprophylactic approach of vaccination of cows in late pregnancy to enhance the levels of anti-coronavirus antibody in the colostrum and milk cannot be adopted in the UK because there is no vaccine available. The use of antibiotics in BCV diarrhoea is not indicated, unless enteropathogenic bacteria are thought to be a contributory cause. Sick calves should be moved to isolation facilities to help prevent a build-up of infection and to facilitate the provision of rehydration therapy. Once isolated, it is beneficial to replace milk with oral electrolyte solution so as to reduce the development of osmotic diarrhoea and commence the process of rehydration. Diarrhoea induced by BCV is often more watery than that caused by rotavirus, possibly because the colon is less able to absorb water because it is damaged by the infection. The watery diarrhoea is likely to lead to severe dehydration and rehydration therapy is more likely to be required in calves with BCV diarrhoea.

Calici-like virus (Newbury agent)

Particles of calf calici-like virus measure approximately 33 nm in diameter and have an indefinite feathery outline with dark hollows on the surface. Some particles have a 10-spiked sphere morphology. The virus was first detected in faeces of calves with diarrhoea and the pathogenic process has been studied in gnotobiotic calves. As far as is known, the disease is confined to the unweaned calf, although a gnotobiotic calf aged 60 days was susceptible to infection and disease. In gnotobiotic calves, clinical signs of enteric disease are identical to those seen in rotavirus infections and the lesions are comparable to those produced by rotavirus and BCV.

Two antigenically distinct isolates of Newbury agent have been identified and infection with either virus did not protect against clinical illness following infection with the other virus three weeks later. There are no specific diagnostic tests for the calf calici-like viruses, other than electron microscopic examination of faeces concentrated and purified by ultracentrifugation. They might be suspected as the aetiological agent in cases that appeared clinically similar to rotavirus, but are negative for rotavirus and other enteropathogens. Calves with diarrhoea caused by a calici-like virus may be managed as though they were infected with rotavirus.

Astrovirus

Astrovirus is a descriptive name for viruses with a star-like pattern on their surface in the electron microscope. They have a diameter of 28–30 nm and contain single-stranded RNA. Astroviruses have also been detected in faeces of lambs with diarrhoea where the virus infected enterocytes causing mild villus stunting in the mid small intestine. Astroviruses have been detected in calf faeces in association with diarrhoea but experimental infection of gnotobiotic calves with astrovirus did not cause diarrhoea. Nevertheless, antibodies to astrovirus are widespread in cattle sera, having been found in 11 out of 22 herds in the UK and in 30 per cent of cattle sera examined in the USA. Recently, astroviruses were shown to infect and damage the specialized epithelium of the dome villi (Fig. 12.14) in the Peyer's patches of calves. These calves did not develop diarrhoea, but severe diarrhoea occurred in mixed infections of astrovirus and rotavirus or astrovirus and Breda agent. It is probable that astroviruses are not pathogenic on their own, but may increase the severity of the disease produced by other enteropathogenic viruses. There are no routine tests to detect

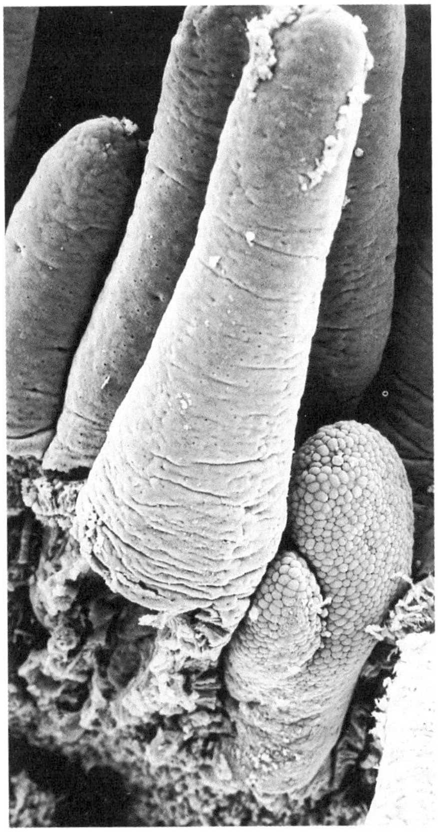

Fig. 12.14 Scanning electron micrograph of calf small intestine illustrating absorptive villi and a dome villus covered by a characteristic epithelium, which is thought to be specialized for antigen uptake and which has been shown to be susceptible to infection and damage by bovine astroviruses.

astroviruses in faeces, but in the research laboratory they can be identified by electron microscopic examination of faeces concentrated by centrifugation.

Breda virus

This virus was first described as causing calf diarrhoea in the USA in 1982. Particles were described as either spherical or kidney shaped, with peplomers. Thus the virus resembles coronavirus superficially, but is antigenically distinct and has been classified into a new family of enveloped RNA viruses, the Toroviridae. Three isolates have been placed into two serotypes. Experimental calves inoculated orally with Breda virus developed a profuse, watery, bright-yellow diarrhoea and they became anorexic, depressed and dehydrated.

Virus replication, as detected by immunofluorescence, occurred in the jejunum and especially in the ileum and colon, where both crypt and villous enterocytes were infected. Lesions were similar to those produced by coronavirus. Jejunal and ileal villi were stunted and there were crypt abscesses in the small intestine and particularly in the colon. There were areas of necrosis of the surface epithelium of the colon.

There are no tests available commercially which detect Breda virus in faeces. Electron microscopy of faeces and thin sections through ultracentrifuge pellets may be used in the research laboratory and, because all isolates of Breda virus possess common antigens, antibodies to these can be used in an immunofluorescent test of intestinal sections and in an ELISA test. Examination by ELISA of over 200 faeces from UK calves with diarrhoea failed to detect Breda virus. However, in a separate study, antibodies to Breda virus were detected in 55 per cent of cattle sera.

Escherichia coli

Three groups of *E. coli* have been identified that appear to cause diarrhoea in calves. Strains that elaborate a heat-labile enterotoxin or a heat-stable enterotoxin are called the enterotoxigenic *E. coli* (ETEC). A second collection of strains exists that colonize the small intestinal mucosa and cause diarrhoea, but do not elaborate enterotoxins. Characteristically, these strains attach closely to the luminal surface of enterocytes, often in cup-shaped depressions or on cytoplasmic protrusions, described as 'pedestals'. This attachment of bacteria to the enterocyte surface usually results in the microvilli being effaced and the lesion has been named the 'attaching and effacing' (AE) lesion (Fig. 12.15). Comparable strains cause diarrhoea in children and are called enteropathogenic *E. coli* (EPEC). It is appropriate to use this term for equivalent calf strains, but care is required because the term enteropathogenic *E. coli* has been used in the veterinary literature for many years to describe strains associated with diarrhoea, regardless of their pathogenic mechanism.

A third group of strains colonizes the surface of the large intestine and causes a mild dysentery. These strains also cause AE lesions but because they cause blood to be lost into the lumen of the large intestine, they are called enterohaemorrhagic *E. coli* (EHEC); once again comparable strains cause a similar disease in children. Some EPEC and EHEC, but not all, produce a toxin that kills Vero cells *in vitro* and is called Verocytotoxin (VT) or Shiga-like toxin (SLT). This toxin does not cause AE lesions, but is probably involved in the pathogenic process. *Escherichia coli* that produce VT are referred to as VT^{+} *E. coli* or VTEC. VTEC have been isolated from calves with diarrhoea,

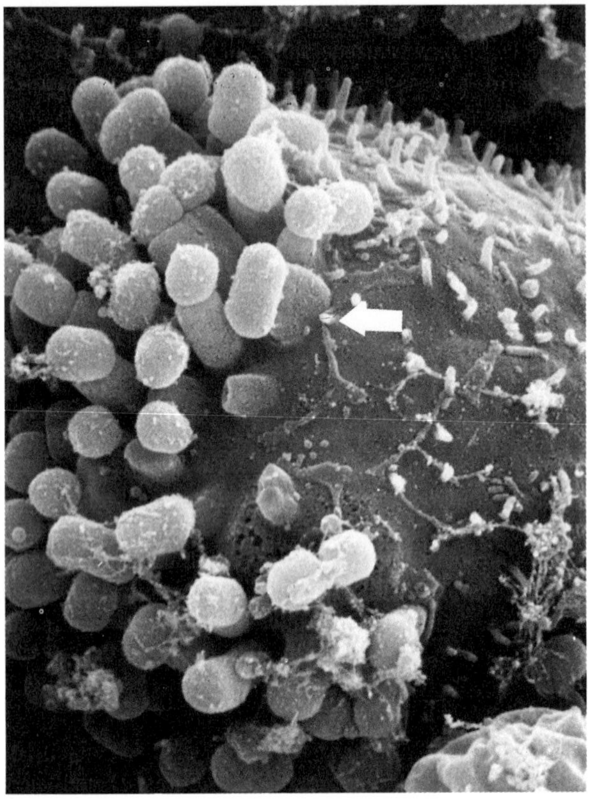

Fig. 12.15 Scanning electron micrograph of an enterocyte in the colonic mucosa of a gnotobiotic calf inoculated experimentally with an enterohaemorrhagic *E. coli* (strain S102–9). Bacteria are attached closely to the surface of the enterocyte, often on 'pedestals' (arrow) and the microvilli have been effaced.

but they may also be present in the faeces of healthy calves. In an epidemiological study, they were found to be as common in the faeces of healthy calves as in the faeces of calves with diarrhoea. Therefore, designation of an *E. coli* as a VTEC may not necessarily define it as an isolate capable of causing diarrhoea and demonstration of a VTEC in the faeces of a calf or calves with diarrhoea does not constitute a diagnosis of the cause of the diarrhoea.

ENTEROTOXIGENIC *E. COLI*

Enterotoxigenic *E. coli* most commonly cause diarrhoea in calves under three days old. In experimentally infected newborn calves the incubation period is 12–18 hours. Calves are depressed and anorexic and rapidly dehydrate and die. In calves ETEC diarrhoea can be diagnosed clinically because it causes disease in very young calves and because it produces a very profuse and much more watery diarrhoea than any other of the calf enteropathogens.

Enterotoxigenic *E. coli* possess two virulence attributes (determinants) that distinguish them from nonpathogenic strains: ability to adhere to the mucosal surface of enterocytes and, as mentioned previously, ability to produce enterotoxins (see Fig. 12.4).

Adhesion is mediated by filamentous protein structures called fimbriae, sometimes called pili or adhesins, which bind to specific receptors on the enterocyte cell membrane. Adhesion mediated by fimbriae does not bring the bacterium in close contact with the enterocyte luminal surface as is the case with EPEC and EHEC. The microvilli are unaltered and 'cups' and 'pedestals' are not seen. The presence of receptors is affected by age, and susceptibility to infection is greatest in the newborn calf when expression of receptors is greatest. These fimbriae are antigenic and so many of them are known by their antigenic name (e.g. K99, F41). Their adhesive ability allows ETEC to overcome the peristalsis of the small intestine by sticking to the mucosal surface. The adhesion antigens commonly found in ETEC of calves are K99 and F41; they often occur together but may be present independently. $K99^{+}$ strains are also capable of inducing diarrhoea in pigs, foals, lambs, goats and possibly other ruminants. Adhesion of the bacterium to the enterocyte surface confers another advantage to the bacterium because enterotoxins are released close to their receptor sites. The ability of ETEC to produce fimbriae and enterotoxins is determined by genes that are usually carried on a single plasmid and thus occur together. It is adequate, therefore, to diagnose ETEC infection by detecting either the enterotoxin or the adhesin.

Detection of adhesins forms the basis of the diagnostic tests for ETEC because they are easier to detect than enterotoxins. Special culture media may be required to encourage ETEC to express adhesins because, in general, K99 and F41 are poorly produced by bacteria *in vitro* although they are readily produced by bacteria growing in the gut. Once expressed they can be detected using specific antisera in agglutination, haemagglutination or ELISA tests.

It is helpful to understand the mechanisms of absorption and secretion in the small intestine before considering how the enterotoxins produced by ETEC cause diarrhoea. Absorption occurs through the activity of the mature villus enterocyte. Sodium ions are transported out of enterocytes through the basolateral cell membranes into the basolateral spaces by an energy-dependent mechanism, the sodium pump. This creates a concentration gradient extending from the lumen into the enterocyte. Sodium ions, followed by chloride ions diffuse along the concentration gradient from the lumen through the microvillous surface, assisted by a brush border carrier system. The osmolality in the basolateral spaces increases and water passes from the lumen along the osmotic gradient (see Fig. 12.2). There are several carrier systems that assist the entry of sodium ions; one system does not utilize the products of digestion, another utilizes glucose, which is specifically absorbed through the luminal surface of enterocytes and each molecule of glucose carries with it a molecule of sodium. Chloride ions and water follow and this flow of water traps additional sodium and chloride ions by solvent drag (Fig. 12.2). Carrier systems for amino acids and citrate also transport sodium ions and water through the intestinal mucosa. These carrier systems, particularly the glucose carrier system, are particularly important in rehydration therapy. Secretion occurs from crypt cells; sodium passes into the intestinal lumen taking chloride and bicarbonate ions and water with it (Fig. 12.3). Cyclic-AMP stimulates this secretory activity.

The heat-stable enterotoxin (ST) is the enterotoxin usually produced by ETEC strains from calves. Two forms of ST occur (ST_A and ST_B) but only ST_A occurs in calves. Both forms stimulate guanylate cyclase activity within enterocytes, causing increased levels of intracellular cyclic-GMP, which inhibits absorption by villous enterocytes but has no effect on secretion.

The heat-labile enterotoxin (LT), rarely produced by calf ETEC strains, is made up of two subunits. Subunit A stimulates adenylate cyclase activity within enterocytes. Subunit B assists entry of subunit A into enterocytes. Adenylate cyclase raises the levels of cyclic-AMP in mature villous enterocytes and crypt cells. In mature villous enterocytes, cyclic-AMP inhibits the independent pathway for the absorption of sodium ions and therefore of chloride and water (see Fig. 12.5). In crypt cells, it stimulates sodium secretion, which takes with it chloride and water (see Fig. 12.6).

Although the main mechanism for the pathogenesis of diarrhoea is attributed to enterotoxins, which do not cause visible damage to the gut, experimental infections of gnotobiotic and conventional calves, both colostrum fed and colostrum deprived, have revealed a pathology associated with ETEC infections that probably contributes to the development of diarrhoea. Villi become stunted and fused together and the enterocytes change shape from columnar to cuboidal. These cells are probably immature enterocytes and these changes indicate an increased rate of enterocyte loss.

Immunoprophylaxis against ETEC-induced diarrhoea is based on the use of immune colostrum. Dam vaccination is used to stimulate high levels of antibody in the colostrum and this approach is particularly successful because calves are susceptible to this disease for only the first few days of life when colostrum is fed. Vaccines containing the K99 fimbriae, or dead bacteria with the K99 antigen expressed on the surface, are used because adhesion is an important component of the pathogenic process.

It is possible to recognize clinically an outbreak of calf diarrhoea caused by ETEC. An outbreak characterized by the rapid onset of severe, very watery diarrhoea, which quickly causes dehydration and collapse and is frequently fatal and occurs in calves that are less than 48 hours old, is likely to be caused by ETEC. Faecal bacteriology will confirm the diagnosis. ETEC diarrhoea is not common in the UK, but outbreaks have been associated with poor housing and management at calving.

The immediate response must be rapid isolation and treatment of sick calves by rehydration with an electrolyte solution; several are available commercially and those that combat acidosis are to be preferred. Rehydration may be given by intravenous infusion if the calf is unable to feed and intravenous infusions may be changed to oral administration as the calf recovers strength. Less severely dehydrated calves may be treated only by oral rehydration. The biochemistry of oral rehydration will be discussed later. Antibiotics, especially if given orally, will be useful in this disease that is caused by bacteria. However, fluid therapy is the first priority because calves may die of dehydration before any beneficial effects are obtained from antibiotic therapy. Following immediate management of an outbreak with fluid therapy and antibiotics, it may be appropriate to introduce dam vaccination. It should be possible to eliminate the infection from the herd with the use of antibiotics, dam vaccination and good hygiene. ETEC with the K99 antigen are absent from most farms and disease prevention should concentrate on exclusion of the infection by good herd security.

ENTEROPATHOGENIC *E. COLI*, ENTEROHAEMORRHAGIC *E. COLI* AND VEROCYTOTOXIN-PRODUCING *E. COLI*

There are no specific clinical signs of diarrhoea caused by EPEC and VTEC although a yellow watery diarrhoea has been reported. The mean age of calves with diarrhoea caused by EHEC was 15 days. Calves maintained a normal appetite and did not develop pyrexia, but a mild diarrhoea containing blood was seen. In prolonged cases there was dullness, signs of abdominal pain, dehydration and weight loss.

Although the EPEC, EHEC and VTEC are capable of causing diarrhoea in calves and have been associated with outbreaks of disease, it is difficult to diagnose their specific involvement. Presence of frank blood in the faeces is suggestive of EHEC, especially if salmonellas and *Cryptosporidium* are not isolated from faeces. The presence of these enteropathogens will be suggested by the failure to find other agents and possibly by the finding of *E. coli* in association with the mucosa of the small or large intestine. An *in vitro* test has been developed for research use that detects *E. coli* capable of causing AE lesions; if this test is adopted by diagnostic laboratories, diagnosis will be improved. Affected calves should be rehydrated and receive antibiotic therapy.

Campylobacter spp.

The related campylobacters, *Campylobacter jejuni* and *C. coli*, have been recognized recently as important enteric pathogens of man. They are the most common cause of diarrhoea in developed countries and they are one of the three most common causes of diarrhoea in developing countries; *E. coli* and rotavirus are the other two enteropathogens of major importance. Recognition of the importance of campylobacters followed marked improvements in culture techniques that improved isolation and identification from faeces. They have been isolated from healthy and diseased domestic animals and poultry for many years and, not unexpectedly, the most common sources of infection in human outbreaks are fresh poultry, minced meat and unpasteurized milk.

The recognition of animal products as the source of human infection has prompted a re-assessment of the importance of *C. jejuni* and *C. coli* in causing enteric disease of farm animals. Since the 1930s, campylobacters have been thought of as the cause of an enteric disease of housed adult cattle in the winter; syndromes referred to as 'winter dysentery', 'winter scours', 'vibrionic enteritis'. The above association has, however, been questioned and more recently a coronavirus has been implicated as the cause of winter dysentery (see p. 659). The association of campylobacters with calf diarrhoea has been examined in experimental infections and in case-control studies of field outbreaks. The results have shown that *C. jejuni* is present on all farms and most case-control studies have failed to demonstrate an association between excretion of this organism and calf diarrhoea. In the majority of experimental studies, inoculation of calves with *C. jejuni*, even using high doses, resulted in colonization without diarrhoea. *Campylobacter jejuni* may be detected in up to 80 per cent of weaned calves, indicating that isolation of this organism from calves with diarrhoea does not constitute a diagnosis. *Campylobacter coli* is less commonly isolated from cattle and experimental inoculations and case-control studies indicate clearly that it is non-pathogenic. *Campylobacter fetus* subsp. *fetus* and *C. hyointestinalis* are also commonly isolated from cattle of all ages, but most evidence suggests that they are not a cause of intestinal disease.

Cryptosporidium

Cryptosporidium is an enteric coccidia recognized commonly in calves. The organisms are spherical or ovoid parasites that adhere to the microvilli of enterocytes, particularly in the ileum, but also in the large intestine. Cryptosporidia exhibit three important differences from other enteric coccidia: excreted oocysts are directly infective to new hosts, cryptosporid are not host specific so that infection can spread between mammalian species, including man, and finally they are unaffected by existing anticoccidial drugs.

The life cycle commences with the ingestion of oocysts containing sporozoites, which become trophozoites. In the asexual phase of the life cycle the trophozoites mature to schizonts containing eight merozoites, which are liberated and infect new enterocytes to form a second generation of merozoites. In the sexual phase, macrogametes fuse with microgametes and give rise to zygotes, which form oocysts. Sporozoites form within oocysts in the intestinal lumen, or whilst they are still attached to the surface of enterocytes so that oocysts excreted in the faeces are directly infective to new hosts without an obligatory period of maturation outside the host body. Consequently, infection can spread rapidly within a group of calves and the pattern of spread is similar to that seen with rotavirus and not similar to that seen in *Eimeria* spp.

Cryptosporidiosis is seen in neonatal calves, usually when they are aged one to two weeks (peak 11 days old), at about the same time as they develop rotavirus diarrhoea. Most calves appear to become infected, but not all develop diarrhoea. Subclinical infections are not thought to be the result of passive protection by colostral antibodies because experiments have shown that antibodies that are fed are not protective; subclinical infections remain unexplained. Experimental infections indicate an incubation period of two to five days and close association between occurrence of diarrhoea and excretion of oocysts. Depression and anorexia accompany the profuse watery green diarrhoea, which contains mucus and occasionally blood. Diarrhoea may be intermittent and lasts two to 14 days (usually about seven) and causes dehydration. Morbidity is usually high and mortality low, although some outbreaks have been associated with high mortality. Dehydration and acidosis do not appear to be the cause of death as is the case with acute viral or bacterial enteritis.

Infected mucosae (Fig. 12.16) are congested and villi are stunted in the ileum. Enterocytes in the small and large intestines become cuboidal or squamous and crypts may become dilated and filled with exfoliated cells and neutrophils. The lamina may become infiltrated with mononuclear inflammatory cells, neutrophils and eosinophils. Cryptosporidia appear to cause diarrhoea by destroying mature enterocytes, but by an unknown mechanism. The population of mature enterocytes is reduced in size and numbers of immature cells are increased. Mucosal lactase activity is markedly depressed and there is reduced ability to digest and absorb food. Intestinal secretion may be enhanced due to the increased numbers of secretory cells in the mucosa.

The self-limiting nature of natural and experimental infections and the widespread detection of antibodies indicates that immune responses occur that are protective. No further information is available on immunity.

Cryptosporidiosis can be diagnosed by detection of oocysts in faecal smears. Several staining methods are available, of which the Giemsa stain, the modified acid fast method and auramine are the most widely used. Alternatively, mucosal smears of ileum may be stained with Giemsa or histological sections of ileum stained by haematoxylin and eosin. The histological method is of little value if autolysis is advanced because the enterocytes will have sloughed from the mucosal surface. The most reliable method is to make and stain smears of oocysts concentrated from faeces using flotation techniques.

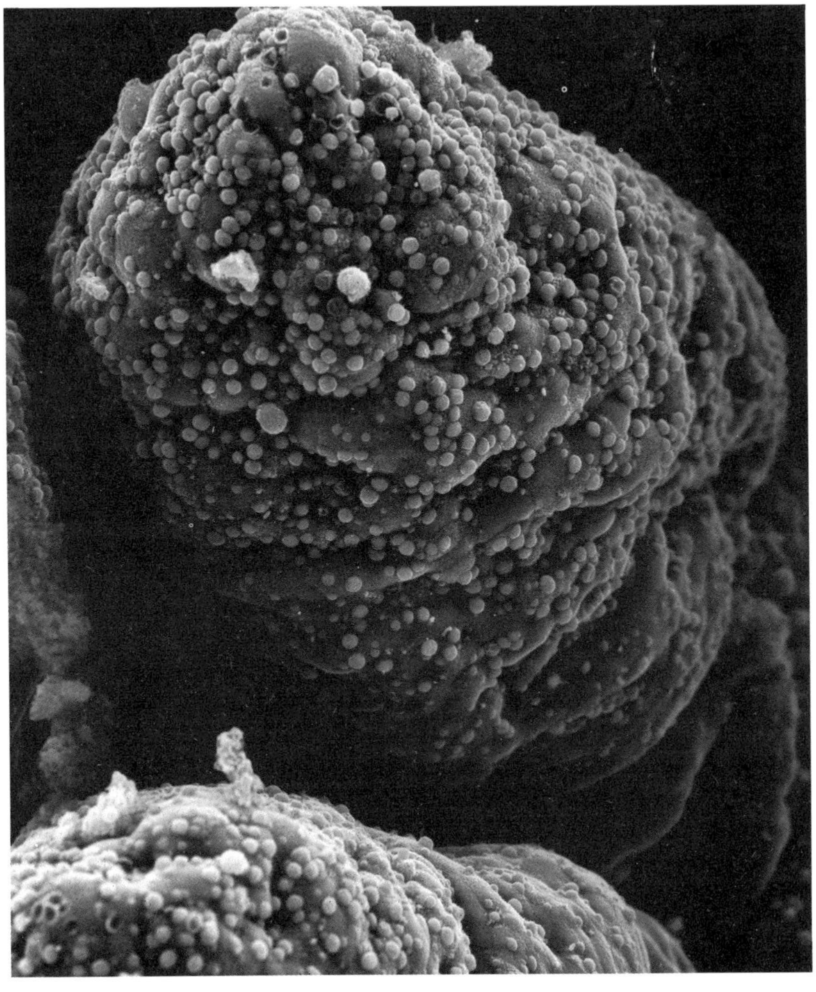

Fig. 12.16 Scanning electron micrograph of the ileal mucosa of a calf naturally infected with *Cryptosporidium*. The surface of the villi is heavily infected and partially exfoliated enterocytes are present at the tip of the villus.

Management of an outbreak presents problems, because although a large number of chemotherapeutic agents have been tested for efficacy against *Cryptosporidium*, none has been found to be effective. A mixture containing 100 g sulphaquinoxaline, 1 g vitamin B_2, 3 g vitamin B_{12} and 10 g vitamin K_3, dissolved in 2.5 l of water was found to be helpful. Mortality was reduced from 40 per cent to 4.7 per cent when calves were fed 100 ml twice daily for 10 days. Most workers recommend high levels of hygiene as the best approach to control, but oocysts are extremely resistant to a variety of disinfectants, including iodophor, cresylic acid, sodium hypochlorite, benzylkonium chloride, sodium hydroxide and aldehyde-based disinfectants. Ammonia and formalin are effective disinfectants and the organism is susceptible to freezing and thawing and to temperatures over 50°C. Steam cleaning is strongly recommended.

Investigating an outbreak of calf diarrhoea

The investigation should start with a farm visit, to examine the calves clinically and establish a picture of calf husbandry and of the outbreak. Enterotoxigenic *E. coli* diarrhoea can be suspected on the basis of age of affected calves and faecal consistency. Some practitioners can smell salmonellosis! Faeces, not rectal swabs, should be collected as soon as possible after the onset of diarrhoea and before treatment commences and should be examined for rotavirus, coronavirus, *Cryptosporidium* and *Salmonella* spp. Samples from very young calves with watery diarrhoea should be tested for $K99^+$ *E. coli*. Faeces should be collected from affected calves and age-matched healthy calves on the farm; a minimum of four calves in each category. Faecal collection should continue if the outbreak persists, to monitor for changes in enteropathogens being excreted. Where a problem persists, or no diagnosis has been reached, samples may be sent to a research laboratory for examination by electron microscopy or for the detection of EPEC, EHEC and VTEC. A post-mortem examination of a calf submitted alive to a laboratory may help to elucidate the significance of results of faecal examination and indicate the presence of other agents not detected by faecal examination. Laboratories are frequently asked to assist in the diagnosis of the aetiology of calf diarrhoea outbreaks on the basis of samples submitted from one or two calves only. Clearly this is pointless, because diagnosis of disease caused by an endemic agent is based on the detection of the agent in a higher percentage of the faeces of calves with diarrhoea than in healthy calves on the same farm. Where data are not available from healthy calves on the same farm, results from other studies may be considered. Rotavirus and *Cryptosporidium* have rarely been found in more than 50 per cent of randomly selected healthy calves and coronavirus is usually detected in less than 25 per cent. Figures above these values may be taken as a tentative diagnosis.

Salmonellas, which may be suspected clinically, are often only detected qualitatively. Merely isolating these bacteria is relatively meaningless; quantitative bacteriological techniques should be used to demonstrate excretion of large numbers of bacteria from calves with diarrhoea. It is only worth looking for K99 adhesins where the outbreak is suggestive of ETEC, i.e. if calves under one week of age are affected and there is severe watery diarrhoea.

Epidemiology

On a farm basis, the infectious agents that have been associated with neonatal calf diarrhoea can be divided into three groups: those infections that are usually absent but may be introduced and cause an outbreak of disease (ETEC, *Salmonella* spp.); the ubiquitous agents (rotavirus, coronavirus, astrovirus and *Cryptosporidium*) that are invariably present on every farm; and those agents for which inadequate epidemiological data are available (calici-like virus, Breda virus and VTEC). Although there is evidence to support the view that all the above infectious agents are able to cause diarrhoea in calves, it is clear that their presence in the intestinal tract does not inevitably lead to disease and they are not all equally important in the aetiology of calf diarrhoea.

The prevalence of these agents in calves with diarrhoea in southern Britain, as determined from 45 outbreaks of calf diarrhoea is shown in Fig. 12.17 (Reynolds *et al.*, 1986); another survey examined outbreaks in northern England and southern Scotland (Snodgrass *et al*, 1986). Rotavirus was associated most frequently

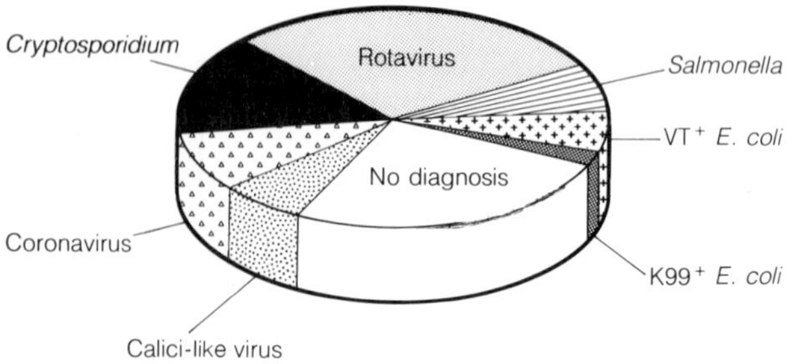

Fig. 12.17 Prevalence of pathogenic agents in calf diarrhoea.

with calf diarrhoea and was most common on dairy farms and single-suckler beef units (Fig. 12.18). *Cryptosporidium* was associated with calf diarrhoea slightly less often than rotavirus and was more common in beef suckler units than dairy farms. In southern England, salmonellas occurred in 25 per cent of outbreaks and were most often a problem for rearers of calves bought-in from markets. Enteropathogens were not detected in 31 per cent of faeces of calves with diarrhoea. Rotavirus and *Cryptosporidium* were excreted by up to 50 per cent of normal calves, and on the basis of this evidence an outbreak of rotavirus-induced or *Cryptosporidium*-induced diarrhoea should only be diagnosed if more than 50 per cent of calves with diarrhoea are excreting either enteropathogen. Coronavirus was detected rarely in clinically normal calves and it was invariably associated with disease, usually in outbreaks with high mortality. Convenient tests are not available to detect calici-like viruses in faeces; they are detected for research purposes by examination of purified faeces in an electron microscope. As a result, little epidemiological data on these viruses are available. However, calici-like viruses were detected in 26 per cent of outbreaks studied in the survey in southern Britain. They have been classified as ubiquitous on the basis of this evidence. Results of two surveys show that diarrhoea caused by ETEC was uncommon in the UK at that time; this may still be the situation. Intermittent excretion of ETEC may occur throughout life, often unassociated with diarrhoea, making interpretation of diagnostic findings difficult and emphasizing the need for quantitative bacteriology.

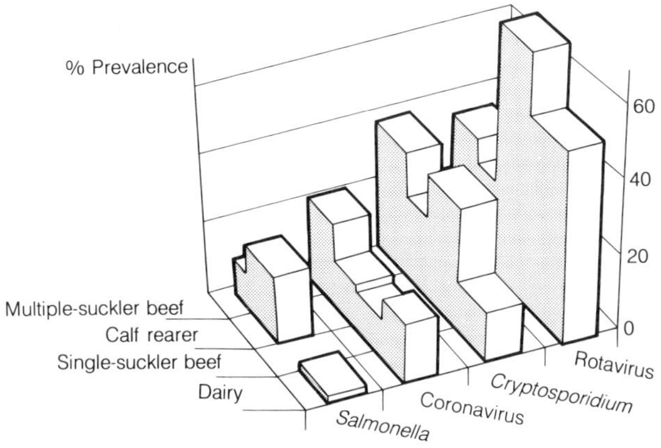

Fig. 12.18 Correlation of farm type with prevalence of pathogens in calf diarrhoea. Reproduced from Morgan (1990).

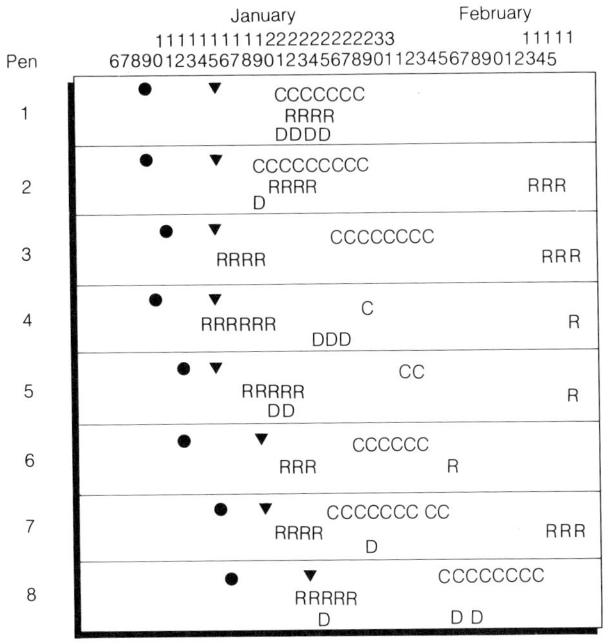

Fig. 12.19 The spread of rotavirus and *Cryptosporidium* between calves in adjacent pens. (●) Day of birth, (▼) day of move to rearing pens. C, *Cryptosporidium* excretion; R, rotavirus excretion; D, day of diarrhoea. Reproduced from Morgan (1990).

Mixed infections

With the recognition of enteropathogenic agents and the development of diagnostic tests, it has been possible to look at outbreaks of diarrhoea and at individual animals to assess the importance of mixed infections. Results of surveys of faeces of calves with diarrhoea indicate that although single infections may result in diarrhoea, the likelihood of diarrhoea occurring increases with the number of enteropathogens present. When 21 moribund calves with diarrhoea were examined in detail by necropsy, two or more enteropathogens were detected in 19 calves (Hall *et al.*, 1988). The most common combination of enteropathogens revealed by these studies has been rotavirus and *Cryptosporidium* and the way in which these infections can overlap in rearing pens is illustrated in Figs. 12.19 and 12.20. Studies of distribution of infection of the gut mucosa with these two agents and the severity of the lesions have shown that either agent, as a single infection, might not cause sufficient intestinal damage to cause diarrhoea, but together they could. A study of the intestinal pathology of normal calves that were excreting rotavirus showed that there were severe lesions in the anterior small intestine and mild lesions in the mid small intestine, but the lower small intestine and large intestine were normal (Reynolds *et al.*, 1985). *Cryptosporidium*, however, infects and damages the lower small intestine and the large intestine, so that in a

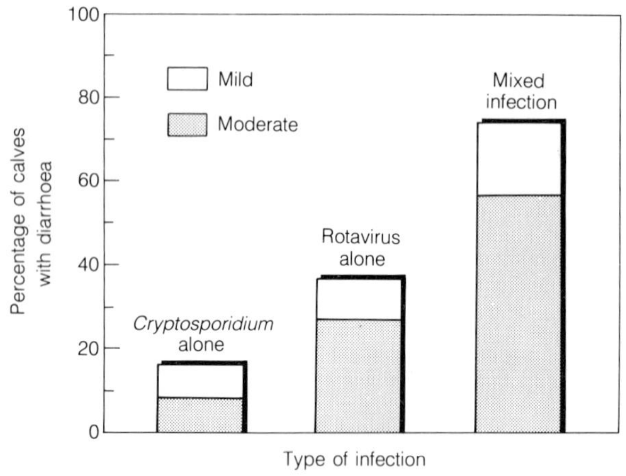

Fig. 12.20 Occurrence of diarrhoea in farm calves infected with either rotavirus or *Cryptosporidium* and in mixed infections.

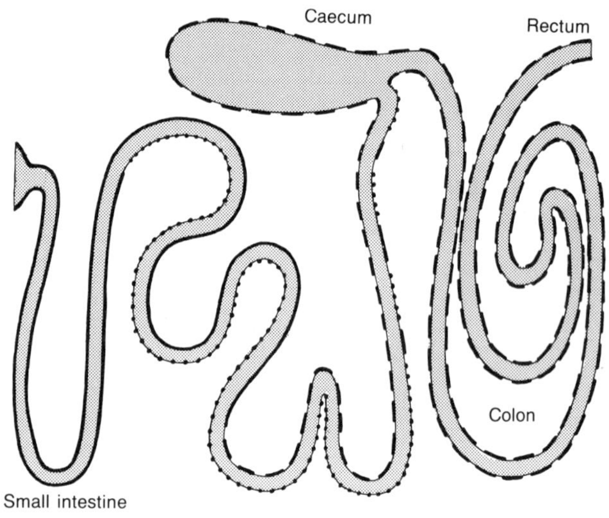

Fig. 12.21 Line drawing illustrating the small and large intestines of the calf and indication of those parts susceptible to infection by rotavirus (-----) and those susceptible to infection by *Cryptosporidium* spp. (–––). Reproduced from Hall (1989).

combined infection the cumulative damage would be sufficient to cause diarrhoea (Fig. 12.21). Similarly, if simultaneous infection with coronavirus and either rotavirus or calici-like virus occurred there would be cumulative damage because the former infects and damages the lower small intestine and large intestine, whilst the latter infects and damages the upper small intestine. The concept that mixed infections involving rotavirus, *Cryptosporidium*, coronavirus and calici-like virus cause cumulative damage in the small and large intestines is based on information presently available concerning the predilection sites of these pathogens. There is, however, evidence that different strains of rotavirus and coronavirus may have different predilection sites within the small intestine and this could affect the development of cumulative damage.

Many of the recognized enteropathogens infect and damage the small intestine and coronavirus, Breda virus, EHEC and *Cryptosporidium* also damage the large intestine. However, assuming that diarrhoea is more likely to occur when both the small and large intestines are damaged, there is a need to study the infectious agents that damage the large intestine. Diarrhoea was often associated with infections and lesions throughout the small and large intestines in a study of the pathology of 21 calves with diarrhoea in southern Britain (Hall *et al.*, 1988); coronavirus and bacteria adherent to the mucosal surface were associated with the lesions in the large intestine. The results indicate that these bacteria, some of which were EHEC, were contributing to the development of diarrhoea. Evidence from field studies also suggests that mixed infections are important in the development of diarrhoea. In a longitudinal study of calves, from birth to weaning, only 15 per cent of calves that excreted *Cryptosporidium* sp. and 37 per cent of calves that excreted rotavirus experienced diarrhoea, but in calves in which the two infections occurred together, 75 per cent developed diarrhoea (Fig. 12.20).

Rotavirus and ETEC were the infectious agents first identified as able to cause diarrhoea in calves and, as a result, combined inoculations with these agents were studied by several groups. The interaction between these two agents was studied despite the fact that ETEC cause diarrhoea in calves that are less than 48 hours old, whereas the mean age of calves with rotavirus diarrhoea is 10 days. The conclusions reached from these studies were that combined infections were more severe, although it was unclear whether this was due to additive effects or synergism. Also, it appeared that infection with rotavirus increased colonization of the small intestine by ETEC and might render a calf susceptible to ETEC at an age when it would normally be resistant to infection and disease by virtue of its age.

Management of diarrhoea

A knowledge of the chronology of fluid, electrolyte, hydrogen ion, hormonal and energy substrate changes resulting from diarrhoea is a necessary prelude to the development of the best supportive therapy. The first priority is to treat fluid depletion, i.e. restore extracellular fluid volume so as to counter shock and acidosis. It is then appropriate to consider the use of drugs.

Rehydration

Intravenous fluid therapy will be required in severely dehydrated, moribund animals; an isotonic polyelectrolyte solution containing Na^+, K^+, Cl^- and acetate is ideal. Initially, the concentration of potassium in the fluid should be at physiological levels, because hyperkalaemia probably exists, but as dehydration is countered, the concentration of potassium may be increased to counter depletion.

Oral fluids are very satisfactory in the less severely affected animals. They are usually isotonic with plasma and contain sufficient K^+ and HCO_3^- to replace faecal losses and Na^+ and glucose in equimolar amounts. Preparations are available commercially that are formulated to utilize the pathways of absorption of glucose, amino acids and citrate, which carry water with them. These formulations counter acidosis by inclusion of bicarbonate and citrate, which is metabolized to give bicarbonate ions. Energy is supplied as glucose and citrate. Commercially prepared oral rehydration solutions are sophisticated formulations and should always be used where possible, but in the absence of a commercial formulation, a suitable recipe is shown below.

Add to a litre of water
- 3.5 g NaCl
- 2.5 g $NaHCO_3$
- 1.5 g KCl
- 20.0 g glucose

The method of oral administration may be important in calves. Electrolyte solution passes directly into the abomasum and intestine when it is drunk naturally, but electrolyte given by stomach tube is deposited in the rumen and may remain there and absorption may be delayed. However, if the calf will not drink, use of a stomach tube is indicated. As a rule of thumb, if a calf is in lateral recumbency, use intravenous therapy, if it can lift its head but cannot drink, use the stomach tube and if it can drink, encourage it to take electrolyte solution by mouth.

The efficacy of oral rehydration varies with the type of diarrhoea. In secretory diarrhoea, the sodium–glucose absorption system is unaffected by bacterial enterotoxins and glucose/electrolyte solutions are very effective in rehydrating the animal. Nevertheless, the diarrhoea continues and this should be stressed to the client (Fig. 12.22). The small intestine may be so severely damaged in very severe viral infections that oral electrolyte solutions are ineffective. In less severe viral infections, for example many rotavirus infections of calves, sufficient functional surface may remain for oral electrolytes to be effective. As a general guide, if faeces are acidic or contain sugar oral electrolyte solutions may be ineffective.

Nutrition

There is conflicting opinion on the ideal level of nutrition in diarrhoeic calves. On the one hand, it has been pointed out that the energy requirements of a newborn calf are approximately 2500 kcal/day, equivalent to 600 g of glucose. The glucose content of 10 l of oral glucose/electrolyte solution containing 80 mM glucose is 144 g, which does not supply sufficient energy. Therefore, feeding glucose/electrolyte solution puts the calf into a negative energy balance, causing a general weakening due to catabolic processes. The advantages of fasting are that the problem of undigested carbohydrates reaching the colon, with the effects previously discussed, is avoided. These effects are most likely to occur in virus-induced diarrhoea where maldigestion and malabsorption occur; overfeeding is undesirable in these cases and restricted feeding may be indicated. A rational approach is to feed electrolyte solution alone for two days and subsequently add increasing amounts of milk to the electrolyte. Mixing electrolyte solution and milk does not appear to interfere with clotting of milk in the abomasum. With suckled calves, separate the calf and the cow, feed electrolyte and then allow the calf to suck the cow.

Drugs

Theoretically, a number of drugs might be helpful in the control of diarrhoea. Cholinergic antagonists and adrenergic agonists should block secretion by blocking the entry of calcium ions into secretory crypt cells. The phenothiazines are theoretically useful together with inhibitors of prostaglandins. In practice, however, the drugs available have been found to have undesirable side-effects and although many antisecretory drugs have been investigated, none have been found suitable for clinical use and none are available for the treatment of calf diarrhoea.

In severe dehydration, rehydration must be the first priority. If indicated, antibiotics may be used to control bacterial infections once the possibility of death from dehydration has been eliminated. There are two situations where the use of antibiotics is indicated; infections with *Salmonella* spp. or with pathogenic *E. coli* (ETEC, EHEC and VTEC). Broad-spectrum antibiotics and antimicrobials have been used widely as a primary form of treatment of calves with neonatal

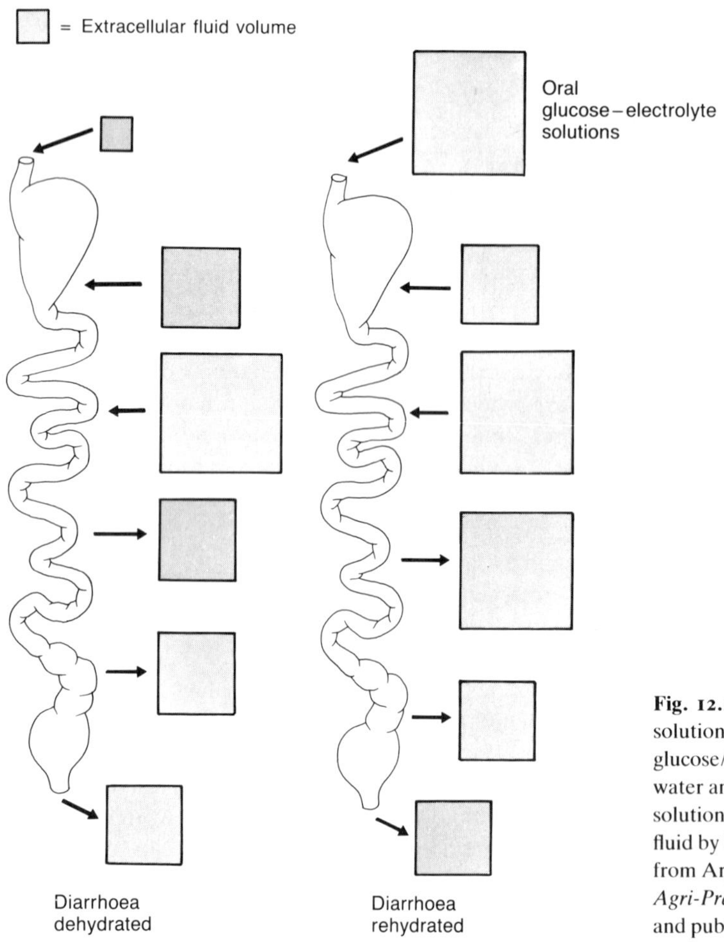

Fig. 12.22 Effect of orally administered glucose/electrolyte solution of fluid fluxes in secretory diarrhoea in the pig. Where glucose/electrolyte solution is not given, there is a net loss of water and dehydration develops. Where glucose/electrolyte solution is given, the diarrhoea continues but there is a net gain of fluid by intestinal absorption and rehydration occurs. Reproduced from Argenzio R.A., Pathophysiology of neonatal diarrhoea. *Agri-Practice* (1984) **5**, 25–32, by kind permission of the author and publishers.

diarrhoea, without sound reasons in many cases. Most therapeutic trials for treatment of diarrhoeal calves with antibiotics have been uncontrolled or used small numbers of animals and have not, therefore, been convincing. Recently, however, the value of antibiotic therapy in undifferentiated calf scour was studied in a large number of calves on six farms (Grimshaw, 1987). Calves were examined each day and a decision made on clinical condition and necessity for treatment. Antibiotics reduced mortality from 26 per cent to less than 10 per cent. The identification of a possible role for adherent bacteria in the colon of the calf, in the pathogenesis of diarrhoea, has strengthened the case for the use of antibiotics in undifferentiated calf diarrhoea.

The disadvantages of using antibiotics are that some directly damage the intestinal mucosa and may contribute to the development of diarrhoea. Antibiotics add significantly to production costs, they contribute to the problem of resistance factors in the enterobacteria, they may result in residues in meat and antibiotic use may result in the carrier state in *Salmonella* infections.

Environment

The impact of environment on the pathogenesis of calf diarrhoea may be discussed under the following headings: microbial environment, immunological environment, nutritional environment, genetic environment and physical environment.

Microbial environment

The enteropathogens that have been discussed are all excreted in faeces in very large numbers by clinically sick calves. It is clear, therefore, that once an outbreak is established the major source of infection is faecal contamination of the environment by clinically affected calves. Other animal sources, or reservoirs of infection have been described; rotavirus and coronavirus are excreted by calves and cows with subclinical infections and similar situations could be expected for the other enteropathogens, which have been investigated less well. Studies of dairy systems (Greene, 1983; McNulty & Logan, 1983) have shown the value of cleansing, disinfection and use of the 'all in all out' system in the control of diagnosed and undiagnosed calf diarrhoea. Calving accommodation and calf pens should be designed for ease of cleaning, steaming and disinfection and with adequate drainage. Pens should be well ventilated, but draught free. Pens and utensils should be kept clean, and pens kept dry with adequate straw. Cleansing and disinfection in the middle of a rotavirus outbreak was shown substantially to reduce the percentage of subsequent calves that were infected; once infection became re-established most calves became infected and diseased. In another study, calf mortality from septicaemia and enteritis was 3.8 and 3.9 per cent in successive years and, after improved management, was reduced to 1.2 per cent in the following year; the reduction in mortality was attributed to improved management. The important improvements were thought to be single penning of newborn calves, careful cleansing and disinfection of pens and use of oral electrolyte solutions. In a second study (Greene, 1983) involving 34 dairy farms and 8000 calves, the same author concluded that introduction of good hygiene and early colostrum feeding reduced morbidity in the next calving season from 36 per cent to 11.3 per cent and mortality from 5.4 per cent to 1.2 per cent. It was concluded that adding antibiotic therapy to the use of oral electrolytes did not improve treatment results. However, studies of this type, which use historical controls, have been severely criticized.

A controlled study of 16 dairy herds reported diarrhoea in 62 per cent of calves, which was reduced to 23 per cent in herds where management was improved (Moerman *et al.*, 1982). Six management practices were identified that increased the incidence of diarrhoea.

1 If the number of calving boxes was less than 10 per cent of the number of annual births.
2 If calves were housed in one room rather than two or more.
3 If there was direct contact between, or a short distance between, the calving boxes and the calf-rearing house.
4 If there was a delay of more than one hour before first colostrum intake.
5 If the number of calves born in the previous four weeks was greater than 10–15.
6 If there was worsening of general hygiene.

The same principles apply in beef systems (Radostits & Acres, 1980). Firstly, it is important to remove the source of infection from the calf's environment, or minimize it. Measures that can be adopted include the following.

1 Avoid confining the herd, especially at calving. Avoid using calving corrals or paddocks in which mud and faeces soon predominate and where animal density is high.
2 Regularly change the pastures that the herd grazes.
3 Do not calve cows and heifers on the pasture on which they have been held during winter; move them to clean areas just before calving.
4 Do not calve on the same area year after year. Avoid calving in barns and sheds where infection builds up rapidly, and ventilation and sunlight are restricted, encouraging survival of infection.
5 Choose a calving ground that is sheltered and well drained. Avoid creating local areas within calving grounds where animals congregate and infection builds up, i.e. restricted feeding or watering areas.
6 Calving areas should be cleaned up and left vacant during summer.
7 Isolate calves, as far as is possible, from the contaminated environment by removing calves from areas contaminated by diarrhoeic calves. Reduce crowding of calves by dividing the calving herd into small subgroups and dispersing newborn calves with their mothers soon after birth.

Immunological environment

Neonatal calves are more resistant to enteric infections when suckled than when fed artificial feeds, regardless of whether there is absorption of colostral immunoglobulins or not. This suggests that components of colostrum and milk that are not absorbed have an intestinal role in protecting the neonate. The other quite distinct protective function provided by the immune components of mammary secretions is their absorption to provide passive circulating antibody, which prevents invasion of micro-organisms.

SPECIFIC PROTECTIVE SYSTEMS IN COLOSTRUM AND MILK (see p. 803)

Immunoglobulins are concentrated from the cow's serum into colostrum from five weeks prepartum. The classes of immunoglobulins that are present in colostrum and milk are IgA, IgG_1, IgG_2 and IgM. IgA and IgG_2 each comprises 5 per cent of colostral immunoglobulins and IgM comprises approximately 7 per cent. The majority of colostral immunoglobulins (80–90 per cent) are IgG_1 and the concentration of IgG_1 in colostrum is three to twelve times that of maternal serum, because of selective secretion by the acinar epithelial cells of the mammary gland.

Colostral proteins are absorbed very rapidly and efficiently by the small intestine of the newborn calf.

The small intestinal villi are covered by highly vacuolated enterocytes, which are specialized in the uptake of macromolecules by pinocytosis. The ability to absorb macromolecules may persist for up to 24 hours after birth and its disappearance is known as 'closure of the gut'. Although the gut may remain 'open' for up to 24 hours, closure occurs rapidly after ingestion of the first feed. If the first feed is colostrum, all is well, but if the first feed is milk, the gut will 'close' and colostrum fed subsequently will not be absorbed. Thus, IgG_1 is absorbed into the blood of the calf in large amounts during the first 24 hours of life. All macromolecules presented are absorbed but IgG_1 is predominant and therefore it is absorbed in greatest amounts. IgA in milk provides a passive intestinal humoral immunity in other species. In ruminants the predominance of IgG_1 in milk suggests that it has a similar function.

The immune components of mammary secretions have two functions. Firstly, colostral antibodies absorbed into the circulation of the neonate provides passive circulating antibody, which prevents invasion of micro-organisms (e.g. septicaemic *E. coli*). Secondly, colostral antibodies that are not absorbed due to gut closure, and milk antibodies, act within the gut lumen, providing passive local immunity. Milk antibody has been shown to protect calves from ETEC, probably by anti-adhesive activity. Absorbed colostral antibody may also influence enteric infections because IgA is absorbed along with IgG_1 and some is resecreted onto mucosal surfaces.

Studies of the concentration of immunoglobulins in the blood of diseased calves showed that calves with the lowest levels of immunoglobulin had highest mortality; colisepticaemia was the major killer, either rapidly or via abscesses in the umbilicus, liver and joints. Calves with low levels of immunoglobulins may also show a greater incidence of diarrhoea.

The principal stimulus of antibody production by the mammary gland, against enteropathogens, results from gut infection. It may result, however, from presentation of infectious agents to the mammary lymphoid tissue, rather than to the gut. When newborn calves were infected with either *E. coli* or salmonellas and allowed to continue sucking their mothers, antibodies appeared in the milk that were attributed to infection of the mammary gland during suckling, resulting in the production of specific antibodies. Also, specific antibodies to enteropathogens may be secreted into milk even though the dam has not experienced the enteropathogen. This occurs if pathogenic and non-pathogenic (commensal) bacteria have common antigens that stimulate cross-reacting antibodies.

Colostral antibodies, if they are to be absorbed effectively or if they are to have a protective function in the gut lumen, must resist rapid degradation. The mechanisms that protect colostrum from degradation in the gastrointestinal tract are the low activity of pancreatic protease in the neonatal calf, the presence of a trypsin inhibitor in colostrum, the high buffering capacity of colostrum, the reduced secretion of acid in the abomasum in the first three days of life and the resistance of IgG_1 to proteolysis by chymotrypsin. The enterocytes of the newborn calf are specialized for non-selective macromolecule absorption by pinocytosis and vesicle transport. This process results in rapid and effective uptake of antibodies (IgG_1) because these are the major macromolecules in colostrum.

There are, in addition to protective immunoglobulins, non-specific protective systems in colostrum and milk (Reiter, 1978). Lactoferrin, an iron-binding protein present in colostrum and milk, inhibits bacterial growth, possibly by reducing availability of iron to bacteria. There are appreciable amounts in bovine colostrum but little in bovine milk. Citrate, also present in colostrum, competes for iron, making it available for bacteria. Therefore, normal colostrum is not bacteriostatic for *E. coli*, but once the citrate is removed colostrum is bacteriostatic. Conditions in the calf small intestine apparently favour the action of lactoferrin because citrate is rapidly absorbed from the calf small intestine and bicarbonate, which assists binding of iron and lactoferrin, is secreted into the small intestine. The antibacterial action of lactoferrin is enhanced by specific antibodies in colostrum. The lactoperoxidase/thiocyanate/hydrogen peroxidase system is inhibitory or lethal to bacteria via the production of an oxidation product. Lactoperoxidase is synthesized by the mammary gland, thiocyanate ions are present in milk and are secreted into the calf stomach and cow's milk contains glucose and glucose oxidase, which provide hydrogen peroxide; hydrogen peroxide is also produced by lactobacilli, which are the predominant bacteria in the flora of the stomach and small intestines of newborn calves. Thus, all the components of this protective system are present in the calf *in vivo*.

The absorption of colostral immunoglobulins is influenced by several factors and 20–50 per cent of calves attain inadequate serum IgG levels. The time of the first colostrum meal is an important determinant of serum immunoglobulin concentration; late feeding leads to lower levels. Also, first-milk colostrum has the highest concentration of immunoglobulins, therefore preparturient leaking or milking leads to poorer quality postparturient colostrum. Colostrum is secreted prepartum and once removed is not replaced. The amount of immunoglobulin absorbed varies with its concentration in the colostrum and this is more important than the quantity of colostrum consumed.

Maternal nutrition may affect colostrum production. Poor nutrition does not, apparently, influence the concentration of immunoglobulin in colostrum but decreases the amount of colostrum produced, therefore sucking calves achieve lower levels of serum immunoglobulin; heifers produce less colostrum than cows. A second feed of colostrum increases the absorption of immunoglobulin from the first feed, presumably because the second feed displaces colostrum from the upper gastrointestinal tract into the jejunum.

The presence of the dam improves the efficiency of absorption of immunoglobulins by the calf by up to 80 per cent. Lower serum levels are obtained if the calf and dam are separated at birth and colostrum is fed by bucket. The dam licks and cleans the newborn calf in the order: thorax, back, abdomen, head, neck and perineum. The placenta is then eaten. Suckling does not occur unless the licking process occurs. An easy parturition leads to early licking. Beef cows mother better than dairy cows; they lick longer and stand better to be sucked. The speed at which calves stand is important because they then start to seek the teats. If cows have calved standing then sucking is likely to start earlier. Field-born calves have higher levels of serum immunoglobulins than box-born calves. The cow is likely to be the primary object of teat-seeking attention but in a box the walls may confuse the calf. Low pendulous udders delay successful sucking.

Farmers should be encouraged to ensure that all calves receive a minimum of 2 l of colostrum soon after birth, within 6 to 9 hours, if possible. Practical recommendations to enhance colostrum uptake include the following.

1 Do not separate dam and calf until 24 hours postpartum.

2 Provide bedding to allow the calf to stand easily.

3 Encourage early feeding, which is very beneficial. The calf may need assistance to ensure this.

4 Keep a supply of frozen colostrum for use after prepartum leakage.

5 Encourage outdoor calving in warm weather; it is more likely to lead to higher levels of serum immunoglobulins.

Methods of measuring the concentration of immunoglobulins in calf serum include the following.

1 Single radial immunodiffusion: convenient, accurate and capable of measuring IgG_1, IgG_2 and IgA.

2 Zinc sulphate turbidity test: depends on the selective precipitation of immunoglobulin by zinc sulphate; there is good correlation between zinc sulphate turbidity and total immunoglobulin content of serum.

3 Sodium sulphite precipitation method.

4 Refractometry: measures total protein.

The immunoglobulin content of colostrum can be assessed simply and accurately with a hydrometer (Fleenor & Stott, 1980) and one designed specifically for the purpose is available in the UK.

Nutritional environment

Skim milk powders, which have been severely heat treated, and some non-milk proteins (e.g. soya) do not coagulate well in the abomasum. This may result in gastric stasis and reduced secretion of gastric acid and enzymes, which causes increased escape of undigested protein into the duodenum and reduced secretion of pancreatic enzymes. These events result in diarrhoea. Soya initiates immune-mediated intestinal damage in some calves and heated soya may contain substances that are directly damaging to the intestinal mucosa. Some feeding methods may upset the balance between the calf and the infectious agents to which it is exposed, thus precipitating diarrhoea. These include feeding cold milk, bucket feeding, high-fat diets and skim milk. Alternatively, feeding methods that are said to alleviate diarrhoea include use of acidified milk and fermented colostrum, even though it is less well absorbed than fresh colostrum.

Changes in the pasture being grazed by the dam may result in changes in milk composition causing diarrhoea in suckled calves. High-nitrogen fertilizers are said to inhibit milk coagulation. Cows deficient in calcium may also produce milk that does not coagulate. This results in gastric stasis and abomasal distension due to accumulation of secretions and diarrhoea occurs.

Genetic environment

Little is known of genetic effects but it has been reported that Ayrshire and Jersey calves are more susceptible to enteric disease than Friesians and that some breeds absorb colostrum better than others.

Physical environment

Hypogammaglobinaemia is more common in single-suckled beef herds where the stocking density is high, presumably due to poor mothering and supervision. Calf mortality is less if the person who looks after the calves is the farmer, or a member of his family.

Single penning helps reduce the spread of infection, as do solid walls between pens. Aspects of the physical environment that contribute to the development of diarrhoea by stressing calves are inclement weather, particularly snow and rain, cold wet bedding and crowding.

References

Fleenor, W.A. & Stott, G.H. (1980) Hydrometer test for estimation of immunoglobulin concentration in bovine colostrum. *Journal of Dairy Science*, **63**, 973–7.

Greene, H.J. (1983) Minimise calf diarrhoea by good husbandry: treat sick calves by fluid therapy. *Annales de Recherches Veterinaires*, **14**, 548–55.

Grimshaw, W.T.R. (1987) Efficacy of sublactam–ampicillin in the treatment of neonatal calf diarrhoea. *Veterinary Record*, **121**, 162–6.

Hall, G.A., Reynolds, D.J., Parsons, K.R., Bland, A.P. & Morgan, J.H. (1988) Pathology of calves with diarrhoea in southern Britain. *Research in Veterinary Science*, **45**, 240–50.

Hall, G.A. (1989) Mechanisms of mucosal injury: animal study. In: *Viruses and the Gut, Proceedings of the Ninth BSG: SK&F International Workshop*, 27–29.

Lewis, L.D. & Philips, R.W. (1978) Pathophysiologic changes due to coronavirus-induced diarrhoea in the calf. *Journal of the American Veterinary Medical Association*, **173**, 636–42.

McNulty, M.S. & Logan, E.F. (1983) Longtudinal survey of rotavirus infection in calves. *Veterinary Record*, **113**, 333–5.

Mebus, C.A., Stair, E.L., Underdahl, N.R. & Twiehaus, M.J. (1971) Pathology of neonatal calf diarrhoea induced by a reo-like virus. *Veterinary Pathology*, **8**, 490–505.

Moerman, A., de Leeuw, P.W., van Zijderveld, F.G., Baanvinger, T. & Tiessink, J.W.A. (1982) Prevalence and significance of viral enteritis in Dutch dairy cattle. In *Proceedings XIIth World Congress on Diseases of Cattle, Amsterdam*. Vol. 1, pp. 228–36.

Morgan, J.H. (1990) Epidemiology, diagnosis and control of indifferentiated calf diarrhoea. *In Practice*, **12**, 17–20.

Radostits, O.M. & Acres, S.D. (1980) The prevention of epidemics of acute undifferentiated diarrhoea of beef calves in western Canada. *Canadian Veterinary Journal*, **21**, 243–9.

Reiter, B. (1978) Review of the progress of dairy science: antimicrobial systems in milk. *Journal of Dairy Research*, **45**, 131–47.

Reynolds, D.J., Hall, G.A., Debney, T.G. & Parsons, K.R. (1985) Pathology of natural rotavirus infection in clinically normal calves. *Research in Veterinary Science*, **38**, 264–9.

Reynolds, D.J., Morgan, J.H., Chanter, N., Jones, P.W., Bridger, J.C., Debney, T.G. & Bunch, K.J. (1986) Microbiology of calf diarrhoea in southern Britain. *Veterinary Record*, **119**, 34–9.

Snodgrass, D.R., Terzdo, H.R., Sherwood, D., Campbell, I., Menzies, J.D. & Synge, B. (1986) Aetiology of diarrhoea in young calves. *Veterinary Record*, **119**, 31–4.

Further reading

Acres, S.D. (1985) Enterotoxigenic *Escherichia coli* infections in newborn calves: a review. *Journal of Dairy Science*, **68**, 229–56.

Angus, K. (1987) Update: Cryptosporidiosis in domestic animals and humans. *In Practice*, **9**, 47–9.

Argenzio, R.A. (1984) Palthophysiology of neonatal diarrhoea. *Agri-Practice*, **5**, 25–32.

Michell, A.R., Bywater, R.J., Clarke, K.W., Hall, L.W. & Waterman, A.E. (eds) (1989) *Veterinary Fluid Therapy*. Blackwell Scientific Publications, Oxford.

Pearson, G.R. & Logan, E.F. (1986) Pathological and immunological aspects of neonatal enteritis of calves. *Veterinary Annual*, **26**, 68–75.

Roy, J.H.B. (1990) The Calf. In: *The Management of health*. Volume 1, 5th edn. Butterworths, London.

Saif, L.J. & Smith, K.L. (1985) Enteric viral infections of calves and passive immunity. *Journal of Dairy Science*, **68**, 206–28.

Snodgrass, D. (1986) Prevention of calf diarrhoea by vaccination. *In Practice*, **8**, 239–40.

Chapter 13: Salmonellosis

by P.W. JONES

Introduction

Salmonellosis is a collective description of a group of diseases caused by bacteria of the genus *Salmonella* with signs that vary from severe enteric fever to mild food poisoning. The genus *Salmonella* belongs to the family Enterobacteriaceae, a large group of facultatively anaerobic Gram-negative rods, which also contains *Escherichia coli*.

The genus is subdivided into serotypes, which are grouped into five subgenera on the basis of their biochemical reactions. Subgenus I contains the 'typical' salmonellas isolated mainly from warm-blooded animals, whilst subgenera II to V are usually, but not exclusively, isolated from cold-blooded animals and the environment. Subgenus III contains serotypes previously included in the genus *Arizona* and subgenus V includes atypical strains, often formerly included in subgenus I. The serotypes (or serovars) within a subgenus cannot, with rare exceptions, be distinguished biochemically and differentiation is on the basis of the possession of somatic (O) antigens and diphasic flagellar (H) antigens in the Kauffmann–White scheme. The antigenic formula consists of three parts delimiting the O antigens and the H antigens, which may occur in two phases. O antigens have arabic numbers (at present 1–67) and H antigens have letters in phase 1 and letters and numerals in phase 2 since the same antigens may occasionally occur as phase 1 or phase 2 in different serotypes. Thus the common cattle pathogen *Salmonella dublin* has the antigenic formula 1,9,12:gp:– denoting that it is distinguished by the presence of O antigens 1, 9 and 12 and H antigens g and p. It does not have a second phase. The other common cattle pathogen *S. typhimurium*, which is diphasic, has the formula 1,4,5,12:i:1,2. When initiated the scheme comprised 44 serotypes and varieties organized in five O-groups (A–E) but it has since expanded to include over 2000 serotypes organized in 48 O-groups.

The antigenic formulae of serotypes commonly involved in disease in cattle is shown in Table 13.1.

The names given to the serotypes do not follow the usual rules of nomenclature. The first serotypes to be identified, such as *S. typhi*, *S. choleraesuis*, *S. abortusovis*, *S. typhimurium*, were given names that indicated the disease with which they were associated or their common animal host, and these names, which have become accepted by clinical microbiologists, continue to be used. Types isolated subsequently bear the name of the town or region in which they were first isolated, such as *S. dublin*, *S. liverpool*, *S. crossness*, *S. bareilly*, or are designated solely by their antigenic formulae. As an aid to epidemiological studies many of the commonest serotypes have been further subdivided into phagetypes, biotypes or plasmid-types. All of the serotypes are, however, very closely related on the basis of pathogenicity, serology, biochemical reactions and DNA hybridizations and the proper status of the serotypes within the genus should probably be a single species divided into a number of subspecies.

All serotypes of *Salmonella* are pathogenic for man, animals or both. Some serotypes such as *S. typhi*, *S. paratyphi A* and *S. sendai* appear to be strictly 'host-adapted' and cause disease only in man. Similarly, *S. abortusovis* and *S. pullorum* cause disease in sheep

Table 13.1 The antigenic formulae (Kauffmann–White scheme) of *Salmonella* serotypes commonly isolated from cattle in the UK

Serotype	Antigens		
	Somatic	Flagella	
		Phase 1	Phase 2
S. saintpaul	*1*,4,[5],12	e,h	1,2
S. derby	*1*,4,[5],12	f,g	–
S. agona	*1*,4,12	f,g,s	–
S. typhimurium	*1*,4,[5],12	i	1,2
S. agama	4,12	i	1,6
S. bredeney	*1*,4,12,*27*	l,v	1,7
S. heidelberg	*1*,4,[5],12	r	1,2
S. indiana	*1*,4,12	z	1,7
S. stanleyville	*1*,4,[5],12,*27*	z_4,z_{23}	[1,2]
S. montevideo	6,7,*14*	g,m,[p],s	[1,2,7]
S. virchow	6,7	r	1,2
S. infantis	6,7,*14*	r	1,5
S. mbandaka	6,7,*14*	z_{10}	e,n,z_{15}
S. newport	6,8	e,h	1,2
S. enteritidis	*1*,9,12	g,m	[1,7]
S. dublin	*1*,9,12,[Vi]	g,p	–
S. panama	*1*,9,12	l,v	1,5
S. anatum	3,10	e,h	1,6
S. give	3,10	l,v	1,7
S. havana	*1*,13,23	f,g,[s]	–

–, flagella antigens occur in first phase only.
[ ], not always present.
1,*14*,*27*, phage-determined, not always present.

and poultry respectively, while a second group of 'host-restricted' types, which includes *S. dublin* and *S. choleraesuis*, cause disease primarily in one animal species, in this case cattle and pigs respectively, but are opportunist pathogens of others. A third, and by far the largest group of 'ubiquitous' types, typified by *S. typhimurium*, cause disease in a wide variety of animals including cattle and humans.

Salmonellosis as a disease of humans, cattle, sheep, pigs and poultry is manifested clinically by one of three major syndromes: a peracute systemic infection, an acute enteritis or a chronic enteritis. In humans, this ranges from the generalized typhoid infection, through the less severe paratyphoid infections to a mild gastro-enteritis. The majority of serotypes produce a mild to severe gastroenteritis that only rarely becomes generalized and severe infections are most often encountered in very young, old or immunologically-compromised patients. It is generally accepted that *Salmonella* gastroenteritis is a zoonotic disease, mainly contracted by consuming large numbers of salmonellas in food of animal origin or foods contaminated with animal products in which the salmonellas have proliferated. There is, however, convincing evidence not only that infection can be a sequel to the consumption of small doses but that direct person-to-person contact is involved in many outbreaks.

The cycle of infection between man and farm animals is often called the '*Salmonella* cycle'. Whilst it is accepted that infections in the human population are usually associated with the consumption of animal products such as eggs, milk and meats it is not always realized that it is possible for the farm animal population to become infected by direct contact with man or the waste products of man such as sewage and sewage-polluted waters. It is further complicated by the possibility of the spread of disease by wild animals such as rats, birds and insects and by the recycling of animal products and wastes from one animal species to another. Thus an understanding of salmonellosis, and the eventual solution of the current disease problems may only arise from an interrelated study of the disease in many animals and the manner in which the bacteria responsible contaminate the environment and pass from one animal to another.

The '*Salmonella* cycle' is shown in diagrammatic form in Fig. 13.1. It must, however, be emphasized that some of the links in the cycle are tentative and that the main source of infection for humans is animal products and the principal sources of infection for domestic animals are other animals of the same species and contaminated feed.

The disease in farm animals differs from the disease in humans, where the majority of cases represent comparatively minor discomfiture, by having a high morbidity and mortality even when treated. Until recently salmonellosis in animals in the UK was characterized by the large proportion of infections caused by the 'host-adapted' and 'host-restricted' serotypes: *S. choleraesuis* in pigs, *S. abortusovis* in sheep, *S. pullorum* and *S. gallinarum* in poultry, and *S. dublin* in cattle. Recently, apart from the latter, these serotypes have virtually disappeared in the UK although they remain important in other parts of the world. Salmonellas may be carried by animals in the absence of clinical signs and this is probably the normal situation in pigs and poultry although *S. enteritidis* (phagetype 4) has recently become associated with clinical disease in the latter.

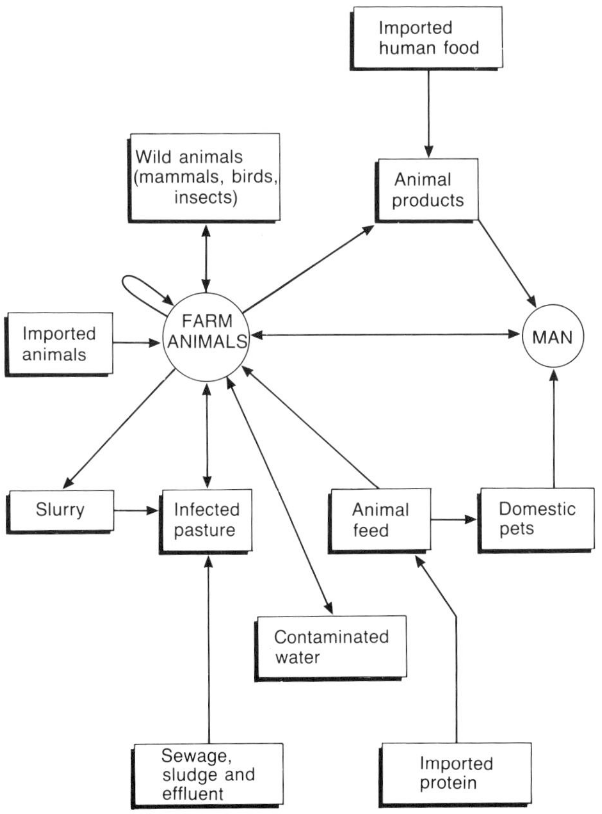

Fig. 13.1 The '*Salmonella* cycle'.

Salmonellosis in cattle

In cattle the disease, which has been recognized for almost two centuries, has a world-wide distribution and has been associated primarily with *S. dublin* and *S. typhimurium*. Other serotypes infect cattle more sporadically and these 'exotic' serotypes have become more common in the UK during the past 25 years, although during the last 10 years approximately 100 serotypes other than *S. dublin* and *S. typhimurium* have only accounted for about 10 per cent of incidents. The number of outbreaks caused by the 'exotic' serotypes has declined in the last few years. There was a dramatic rise in the incidence of salmonellosis in cattle between 1960 and 1969 due to an increase in isolations of *S. dublin*. This was followed by an equally dramatic decline in both *S. dublin* and total incidents and a slight rise in *S. typhimurium*. Over the last 10 years the incidence has remained about the same and at present *S. dublin* and *S. typhimurium* are isolated at about the same frequency with the former being more common in adults and the latter more common in calves. A feature of *Salmonella* infections in all species, however, is a continual fluctuation in the proportions of the serotypes involved. It is common for a serotype to be introduced to the country and to establish in one or more species, possibly as the predominant serotype, and then to decline without any apparent reason or without the intervention of public health or veterinary authorities. The recent predominance of *S. hadar* in poultry and the human population is a good example and it may possibly be predicted that the present epidemic of *S. enteritidis* phagetype 4, which has replaced *S. typhimurium* as the predominant serotype in poultry and the human population, will follow the same course. It is always possible, therefore, for the relative importance of *S. typhimurium* and *S. dublin* to change and the relative importance of these two serotypes in cattle should not be judged on the basis of isolations over only a few years.

Another feature of salmonellosis in calves during the last three decades has been the development of strains resistant to one or more antibiotics. This has occurred almost exclusively in a relatively small number of phagetypes of *S. typhimurium* and has been the subject of considerable debate on the use of antibiotics prophylactically, therapeutically and as growth promoters in calves. The problem was first recognized in the 1960s when the number of antibiotic-resistant strains isolated from cattle rose from less than 3 per cent at the beginning of the decade to more than 60 per cent by 1965 and most of the isolates belonged to one phagetype (type 29). This phagetype disappeared at the end of the decade and the proportion of antibiotic-resistant isolates declined but by the end of the next decade the proportion had again risen to approximately 60 per cent. This was due to the emergence of two closely related types (193 and 204) and was associated with the development of chloramphenicol resistance. Although these two phagetypes also subsequently declined they have been replaced during the last decade by the closely related phagetype 204c. This phagetype, which has become endemic, particularly amongst market-purchased calves and in the calf-rearing trade, represented less than 15 per cent of isolations in 1981 and 1982 but by 1985 accounted for about 80 per cent of isolations. As in previous outbreaks 204c has also declined in the last few years but it is resistant to a wide range of antibiotics, which both complicates treatment of the disease in calves and presents dangers to the human population. Fortunately, although it has been responsible for several dramatic outbreaks in humans, it is not at present as prominent in humans as in cattle and its importance has been overshadowed by the recent epidemic of *S. enteritidis* phagetype 4.

Strains of *S. dublin* isolated in the UK, unlike *S. typhimurium*, have remained comparatively sensitive to antibiotics. In contrast, strains isolated in Holland, Belgium, Germany and the USA are usually resistant to a number of antibiotics. A recent study has shown that in Dutch and German strains resistance is chromosomally mediated, although it was probably determined previously by the carriage of plasmids. Strains from the USA, which were unusual in being sensitive to chloramphenicol, differed from Dutch strains in possessing R-plasmids in addition to the 48 MDa 'virulence associated plasmid' (see below). The reason for the difference between British isolates and those from North America and Europe has not been explained satisfactorily but is usually attributed to the selection pressure of antibiotics in animal feed. Presumably the same pressure is exerted in the UK as elsewhere and is equally applied on *S. dublin* as on *S. typhimurium*. Multiple-antibiotic-resistant strains of *S. dublin* resistant to chloramphenicol began to be reported in the UK from 1979 and the chloramphenicol resistance was transmissible, although located on R-plasmids distinct from those carrying the same resistance genes in *S. typhimurium*. Perhaps the emergence of multiply-resistant *S. dublin* strains in the UK is at an early stage, although the serotype seems to be less endowed with plasmids than *S. typhimurium* and perhaps has difficulty in their accumulation and replication.

Epidemiology

Salmonellosis occurs in calves in all months of the year but there is a peak of disease associated with all serotypes between October and December with a low incidence in June and July. This is associated with calving patterns rather than a true seasonal increase and reflects the distribution of calvings in dairy herds. Similarly, since the source of calves sold through markets to fattening units is bull calves from dairy herds and surplus cross-bred heifer calves from dairy and beef units, there is also a seasonal incidence in fattening units since most outbreaks in calves occur within a few weeks of purchase from markets.

The importance of salmonellosis as a disease of calves was recently demonstrated by a survey carried out by researchers at the Institute for Animal Health, Compton and described in detail later in this chapter. In this survey samples of faeces from diarrhoeic calves on 45 farms in the south of England were examined for the presence of a variety of putative enteropathogens including salmonellas, rotavirus, calicilike viruses, coronavirus, K99$^+$ *E. coli*, cryptosporidia and campylobacters. Salmonellas were isolated from 12 per cent of diarrhoeic calves in 24 per cent of diarrhoea outbreaks. In 37 of the outbreaks, samples were taken from normal calves of similar age to the calves with diarrhoea and a comparison between isolation rates from healthy and diarrhoeic calves was prepared. Salmonellas were isolated from 12 per cent of diarrhoeic calves compared with only 3 per cent of normal calves thus showing a clear association of the organism with disease ($P < 0.001$). Salmonellas were associated with an outbreak of severe dysentery on six farms while single cases of typical salmonellosis occurred in three outbreaks and salmonellas were detected with other agents as part of a diarrhoea problem in two outbreaks where dysentery and pyrexia were not recorded. This highlighted the problem of arriving at a diagnosis in an outbreak of enteritis when several organisms may be involved as part of a disease syndrome. Since salmonellas may be carried by apparently healthy animals isolation of the organism, unless it is present in large numbers ($>10^5$ g of faeces), is not proof of the cause of disease. There was a correlation between the type of farm and the isolation of salmonellas from diarrhoeic calves. Diarrhoea was more likely to be associated with salmonellas in units (calf-rearer, multiple-suckler) where large numbers of calves were purchased from markets although a large number of isolations were also made from calves on dairy farms.

Cattle are probably infected with salmonellas by the oral route although respiratory and conjunctival infection may also occur. The dose required to initiate infection is thought to be high. The experimental infectious dose for calves has been variously estimated as between 10^5 and 10^{11} organisms although doses in excess of 10^8 are normally required, while the dose for adult cattle is approximately 10^{11} orally and greater than 10^8 intravenously. However, it is probable that animals are infected naturally by much smaller doses since factors such as concurrent parasitism (particularly fascioliasis), ketosis, metritis, mastitis, cystitis, pneumonia, viral infection, dietary changes, pregnancy, food and water deprivation and other stress factors such as freezing, wet weather or worming are known to lead to increased susceptibility. Natural infections have been described where animals are thought to have been infected with very small doses particularly in feed. In one such outbreak dairy cows were infected from a component of feed containing less than three *S. mbandaka*/g and the infection spread to their calves.

The primary host defence to salmonellas is probably the stomach or the rumen. In monogastric animals, gastric acidity is responsible for eliminating a large proportion of invading organisms. In ruminants, salmonellas are eliminated rapidly from the rumen where the concentration of fatty acids and low pH are sufficient to inhibit their growth. When this concentration is altered by, for example, starvation and refeeding, salmonellas are able to grow. Similar reactions probably occur in the caeca of calves. Other barriers to infection include peristalsis, intestinal mucus, lysozyme, lactoferrin and the normal bacterial flora of the intestine; absence of a fully developed intestinal flora may, in part, account for the comparative lack of resistance of young animals to salmonellosis. In calves, colostrum, whether normal or immune, is particularly important and animals that have not received colostrum or have received insufficient amounts are particularly susceptible. It is also possible that resistance to salmonellosis in cattle may be under genetic control. Several researchers have commented on the variations in susceptibility to salmonellosis amongst breeds of cattle; for example, Friesians are thought to be less susceptible than Channel Island calves. In mice initial growth of salmonellas is controlled by two alleles; *Ity*, which is involved with the ability of macrophages to kill salmonellas and *Lps*, which confers resistance to the effects of endotoxin. A third allele, *Xid* (X-linked immune deficiency), controls the ability of mice to produce antibodies. It has recently been suggested that a single, dominant, autosomal gene may also be involved in the resistance of chickens to salmonellosis and, although the analysis of such genes in cattle will be more difficult, it is likely that similar mechanisms will be identified in future.

The source of most outbreaks is probably animal-to-animal contact, although there are distinct differences in the epidemiology of the disease in adults and calves, and between serotypes. Infected cattle may excrete up to 10^8 salmonellas/g of faeces and contamination of the environment in the proximity of other cattle by excreting animals will obviously be a potent source of infection. In an outbreak of *S. saintpaul* infection in two large dairy herds infection rapidly spread from cows to their calves, presumably by contact with the contaminated environment of calving barns, and all calves that eventually became infected were excreting salmonellas within 72 hours of birth. Dairy calves may thus become infected by contact with their dam, other calves or the contaminated environment and the collection of calves for intensive rearing, which involves transport to markets and dealers' premises, produces an ideal environment for dissemination. There is good evidence that *S. typhimurium* has become established in the environment of the calf trade in the UK. When *S. typhimurium* gains a foothold in calves subjected to this treatment it spreads so rapidly that entire herds in rearing premises may become infected. It is not surprising that *S. typhimurium*, and particularly multiple-drug-resistant types, such as phagetype 204c, have become endemic in market-purchased calves in the UK and in Europe.

There have been several recent reports that demonstrate the importance of salmonellas in market-purchased calves and in rearing units. One of these was a survey of almost 600 market-purchased calves supplied to 11 rearing units. Frequent swabbing of the calves indicated that less than 1 per cent were infected when they arrived at the rearing units but within the next six weeks over half the calves became infected and, surprisingly, this was not reduced by feeding antibiotics prophylactically or by penning the calves separately. In fact, salmonellas were isolated more frequently from calves kept in individual pens than from calves penned in groups. The calf units examined in this survey were cleaned and disinfected between batches of calves and yet salmonellas could still be isolated from the environment after cleaning in over half of the units. In a similar study of a calf unit in Berkshire, which bought calves from local markets, 250 calves were examined over a two-year period and 51 were shown to be infected with one of four different phagetypes of *S. typhimurium*. Phagetype 204c that was multiply-antibiotic-resistant was isolated at the beginning of the survey. This was eventually removed by destocking and a rigid hygienic programme. The calf units were steam-cleaned, after which *S. typhimurium* 204c was still isolated from environmental samples. Following further steam-cleaning and washing with disinfectant the organism was no longer detectable in the environment but was detectable from the next batch of calves introduced to the units. Although it is not certain that this was the result of environmental contamination the organism was not isolated from the calves on arrival. Subsequent batches of calves (20 or 30 per batch) were examined on arrival and three further serotypes, *S. typhimurium*, *S. agama* and *S. binza* were isolated (Table 13.2). Salmonellas were subsequently isolated from 20 per cent of calves that developed diarrhoea on the farm.

Both of these surveys amply demonstrate that infection in a limited number of calves can spread rapidly in young, susceptible animals subjected to the stress of the marketing and rearing systems and once established it may be difficult to remove the organism from an infected environment. It may also be possible that salmonellas which cannot be recovered on normal bacteriological media may, although non-recoverable, remain viable and infective for animals.

The manner in which animals in previously uninfected dairy herds become infected is more problematical, and the source of infection may vary from serotype to serotype. Most outbreaks are probably associated with the introduction of infected stock or contaminated feed but polluted water supplies, the spreading of contaminated animal manures and human sewage sludge on pasture, and contamination of pasture or feed by scavenging birds may also be involved. Outbreaks have also been described where the probable source of infection was direct human contact. Insects may also be involved in mechanical transmission since in the author's experience it is difficult to contain salmonellosis outbreaks when animals are kept in units that are not insect-proofed and similar difficulties have been described in rearing *Salmonella*-free pigs unless fattening units were rendered fly-proof.

Table 13.2 Isolation of salmonellas from batches of calves on arrival at a rearing farm in Berkshire

Batches of calves examined	27
Salmonella-positive batches	10 (37%)
Number of calves examined	650
Salmonella-positive calves	13 (2%)
Serotypes isolated	
S. typhimurium	9 calves
S. agama	3 calves
S. binza	1 calf
Of the 10 positive batches	
8 contained only 1 *S. typhimurium*-infected calf	
1 contained³ *S. agama*-infected calves	
1 contained 1 calf infected with *S. typhimurium* and 1 calf infected with *S. binza*	

The epidemiology of *S. dublin* in dairy herds differs from that of other serotypes. *Salmonella dublin* has a precise geographical distribution. The organism has remained established in adult cattle in Wales and in southwest and northwest England. It is thought that this distribution may, in part, be due to an association between *S. dublin* and *Fasciola hepatica* although this may be fortuitous and merely indicate that both are influenced by similar climates and survive better in wet conditions. *Salmonella dublin* probably persists on farms in these areas because recovered animals remain infected and excrete the bacteria in their faeces either continuously or intermittently. Elsewhere in the UK, the disease is predominantly one of calves in calf-rearing units rather than adults and it is introduced to the units with the introduction of infected animals.

Animals which excrete salmonellas continuously ('active carriers'), usually in concentrations of up to 10^5/g of faeces, can be detected by bacteriological examination, which will also detect 'passive carriers' — animals that ingest salmonellas in their feed and pass them in their faeces without actual infection of the intestine or the mesenteric lymph nodes. When removed from an infected environment these latter stop excreting. Active excretion is usually a sequel to clinical enteritis or septicaemia and infected animals may excrete for many years and perhaps for life. It may also develop in animals that have not shown clinical signs, although this probably occurs only in cases of concurrent fascioliasis. In such cattle, *S. dublin* is characteristically present in the gall-bladder and alimentary contents without necessarily colonizing the rest of the animal. However, although active excretors are an obvious source of infection for other cattle, and although the source of calf infection is assumed to be adult cattle, field studies have shown that the majority of calves infected with *S. dublin* are home-bred on farms where there is no clinical evidence of adult salmonellosis. This is characteristic of the disease and has led to a search for other sources of infection. Many of the infections occur in closed herds; other sources of infection such as feed are not appropriate to a 'host-restricted' serotype such as *S. dublin* and although contaminated streams may be implicated this gap in the epidemiology is usually explained by the existence of 'latent carriers'. These are animals that have salmonellas somewhere in their tissues or alimentary tract but only rarely excrete the organisms in their faeces. It has been suggested that infection with *S. dublin* is mainly latent, but is activated by stress, particularly at parturition, and the birth of congenitally infected calves to latent carriers or to cows that excrete *S. dublin* only intermittently would explain the occurrence of disease in calves on farms where searches for active carriers are unsuccessful. It is possible to detect greater numbers of excretors by bacteriological examination of faeces taken at calving and surveys have revealed animals which, although found to be infected with *S. dublin* at necropsy, were not detected as carriers by previous faecal sampling. It has not proved possible, however, to create such animals experimentally and serological tests for their detection have been singularly unsuccessful. Serum agglutination tests (SAT) may detect a proportion of actively infected animals but they do not detect latent carriers and antiglobulin, haemagglutination and complement fixation tests are equally unsuccessful, although they may be useful in detecting active carriers and infected herds. Delayed hypersensitivity skin tests can distinguish vaccinated from unvaccinated calves and are a reliable means of detecting systemically infected animals but they may, unfortunately, also detect recovered animals. It is possible that many unexplained outbreaks may be the result of human contact or extended survival of the organism in the environment, although most evidence, particularly from field studies, would favour the latent carrier hypothesis. The problem may be solved in future by the application of some of the newer techniques in molecular biology, and particularly the polymerase chain reaction (PCR), which are capable of detecting very small numbers of organisms.

In contrast to *S. dublin*, infection with other serotypes does not appear to result in active or latent carriers. Adult cattle usually excrete for a maximum of a few weeks following infection and excretion that is detected for longer periods probably reflects recontamination from the environment although the establishment of some 'exotic' serotypes such as *S. saintpaul* for up to a year have been reported. Similarly, *S. saintpaul* has been shown to be retained in the tissues of calves for up to eight weeks after excretion had apparently ceased.

Pathogenesis

Most research on the pathogenesis of salmonellosis (Fig. 13.2) has been carried out in mice and the results extrapolated to other species. However, in calves it would appear that salmonellas probably adhere to and penetrate epithelial cells of the Peyer's patches of the small intestine and caecum. Evidence is also accumulating that this may involve M cells and may account for the host specificity of some serotypes by providing a specialized epithelium cell to which they may adhere. The mechanism of penetration is unclear but may involve translocation by macrophages, endocytosis or entry through tight junctions that have degenerated. Penetrating organisms pass through the epithelium to the lamina propria where they induce an inflammatory reaction and are engulfed by neutrophils and macrophages. In mice the epithelium is subsequently repaired and salmonellas surviving in the intestine are rapidly cleared such that within 24 hours of infection it is difficult to isolate invading organisms from the intestine. In calves, salmonellas appear to continue to proliferate

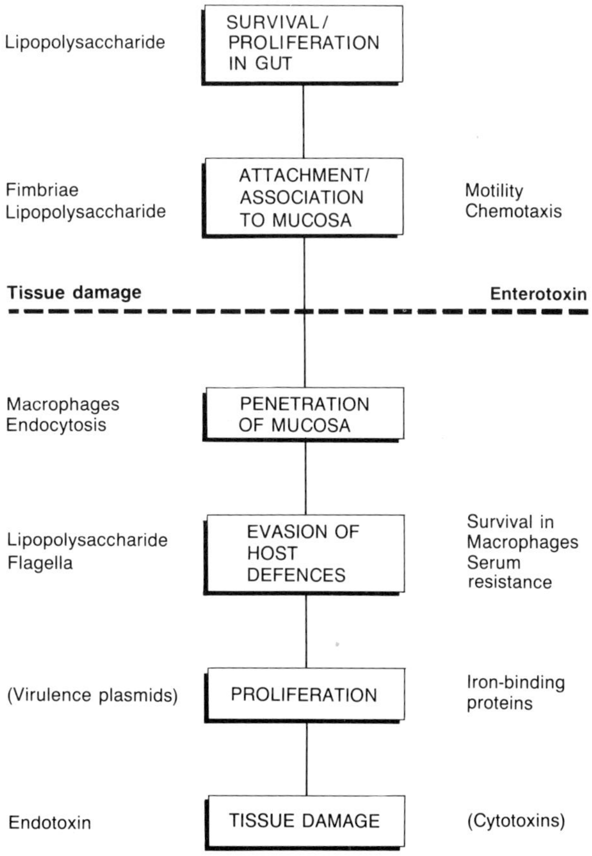

Fig. 13.2 A tentative pathogenesis of salmonellosis.

either within the intestinal mucosa or within the lumen and as many as 10^8 salmonellas/g can often be isolated from the faeces within 24–48 hours of infection. There is still considerable debate about the mechanisms that may allow salmonellas to evade intracellular killing in phagocytic cells or indeed as to whether the principal site of replication is within cells or extracellularly. Regardless of this controversy, it is clear that the sequel to initial invasion is enteritis, which may or may not be accompanied by systemic spread and septicaemia. In the latter, bacteria, which are not contained within the lymph nodes draining the gut, spread via the efferent lymphatics. Bacteraemia ensues and the salmonellas are removed by the reticuloendothelial tissues, principally of the liver and spleen. Release of endotoxin results in haemorrhages, leucopenia, leucocytosis, hypotension, hypoglycaemia and shock, although some of the tissue-damaging effects of salmonellas may also be due to the release of cytotoxins distinct from endotoxin.

The signs of enteritis are described later. In calves, the most severe damage occurs in the ileum where the villi are shortened and denuded of enterocytes, which detach and are extruded. As the disease progresses other parts of the alimentary tract become involved and the associated lymph nodes are enlarged, oedematous and congested. The role of enterotoxins in this process is open to debate since damage does not occur in the absence of invasion. Since the elucidation of the role of enterotoxins in diarrhoea caused by shigellas, vibrios and *E. coli*, many researchers have attempted to demonstrate the role of a similar toxin in salmonellosis. Many of the tests used to demonstrate enterotoxins in other groups of organisms such as ligated ileal loops, skin permeability assays and various cell culture assays may also be shown to be positive when applied to salmonellas. However, although putative enterotoxins have been purified and shown to be widespread amongst salmonellas, many groups of workers have been unable to reproduce the results of others and a definitive role for enterotoxins in the disease process has not been demonstrated. Fluid accumulation in enteric salmonellosis is thought to result from the activation of the adenylate cyclase system, which could be dependent upon the release of prostaglandins induced either by enterotoxins or as part of the inflammatory response brought about by bacterial invasion. Confirmation awaits the construction of isogenic, enterotoxin-positive and -negative strains that can be used to demonstrate the role of putative toxins *in vivo*.

A description of all the properties of salmonellas involved with their pathogenicity and virulence is beyond the scope of the discussion presented here but a tentative summary is given in fig. 13.2. One aspect that probably merits further description is the recent discovery of plasmids, which may be involved in the ability of many of the most important serotypes to cause severe disease. The existence of large molecular weight plasmids in many serotypes of *Salmonella* has been described for more than 20 years. Originally, because their role was unknown they were described as 'cryptic plasmids' but more recently it has been shown that the large plasmid harboured by many of the important serotypes, including *S. typhimurium*, *S. dublin* and *S. enteritidis*, is characteristic of the serotype and they have become known as 'serotype-specific plasmids' or 'virulence plasmids'. Naturally-occurring, plasmid-free strains and strains cured of the plasmid are avirulent in mice in which the normal disease is septicaemia. In calves infected experimentally, plasmid-containing strains cause enteritis and a generalized systemic infection while plasmid-free strains induce enteritis in the absence of the generalized reaction. It thus appears that plasmid genes are involved in the ability of salmonellas to proliferate within the host and that in cattle both plasmid and chromosomal genes are essential for the expression of the full disease. In this context it is interesting that some of the phagetypes of *S. typhimurium* regularly isolated from disease outbreaks in calves do not contain 'virulence plasmids' and this may explain the variation in the degree of severity of the disease observed in the field. Genetic analysis has revealed a region essential for virulence, which is conserved in all serotypes that harbour 'virulence plasmids' and several genes involved in the control of virulence have been identified.

Signs

ADULTS

The disease in adult cattle is usually sporadic, although *S. dublin* has become endemic in some areas of the country and on some farms, and acute and subacute forms are recognized. In the characteristically severe form of the disease produced by *S. dublin* in adult cattle the onset is usually sudden. Fever, dullness, anorexia and abruptly depressed milk yield at first associated with firm faeces, which may contain blood, is rapidly followed by severe diarrhoea. The faeces often become watery and contain large numbers of salmonellas (up to 10^8/g). The fever usually persists for several days, then animals rapidly become cold and recumbent and death, which may be preceded by abortion, occurs in approximately 75 per cent of untreated animals between four to seven days from the onset of clinical signs. In some animals the disease is more protracted and cattle may become emaciated and dehydrated and show signs of abdominal pain. A milder disease characterized by diarrhoea and abortion, or abortion in the absence of other clinical signs, from which animals usually recover, also occurs. A similar disease is produced by other serotypes including *S. typhimurium*, although in these cases abortion is a less frequent event. Survivors of *S. dublin* infections often remain as carriers, possibly for life, while infection with other serotypes seldom results in the carrier state although excretion of types such as *S. saintpaul* for up to two years after infection has been reported.

CALVES

In calves, disease usually occurs between two to six weeks after birth. Characteristically, calves become dull and anorexic and develop a fever. Diarrhoea follows, which in young calves involves the excretion of faeces with the colour and consistency of putty. This may be bloodstained and may contain fibrin and mucus. Eventually, the faeces become dark brown and watery with an offensive odour. More rarely the faeces are heavily bloodstained, become stringy due to the presence of undigested milk and pseudomembrane formation and may contain shreds of necrotic intestinal linings. In older calves the faeces is usually watery, dark brown and offensive. The calves become very weak and dehydrated and death usually occurs after five to seven days of illness in untreated individuals. The disease is very variable; in some calves, especially those two to three days old, bacteraemia and septicaemia occur and the animals collapse and die without diarrhoea. In other animals the disease may be so mild as to pass unnoticed or may be associated with diarrhoea in the absence of systemic disease. Diarrhoea may be prolonged in some calves, which may eventually die as a result of dehydration, electrolyte loss and acid–base imbalance. In both calves and adults systemic infection may lead to complications such as pneumonia, meningitis, osteitis and polyarthritis and gangrene may occur when the disease has been prolonged. Mortality from acute salmonellosis may be as high as 60 per cent and all calves may become infected. Recovered calves do not normally appear to become carriers of either *S. dublin*, *S. typhimurium* or the exotic serotypes and consequently infected calves do not grow into infected adults. However, the disease is often slow to resolve and salmonellas have been isolated from calves up to six months after their initial infection.

The disease produced by different serotypes in calves is usually similar, although the peak incidence of disease and mortality with *S. dublin* is at four weeks of age compared with three weeks for *S. typhimurium*. Calves from dams infected with *S. dublin* may be infected from birth and these are particularly likely to succumb to septicaemia rather than enteritis.

Diagnosis of salmonellosis

It will be apparent from the description above that diagnosis of salmonellosis presents several difficulties. The clinical signs and findings at post-mortem examination are not unique to salmonellosis and although a tentative diagnosis may be made this should be confirmed in diseased animals or at necropsy by isolation of the organism. Diseased animals showing signs of enteritis usually excrete large numbers of organisms in their faeces and counts, rather than enrichment cultures, should be used (see below). For this reason faecal samples rather than swabs should be taken and these should obviously be obtained before administration of antibiotics. It may also be possible to isolate the organism from oral secretions and by blood culture, although these are less reliable than faeces cultures and must be taken with care to avoid contamination. Animals that have died of salmonellosis usually have large numbers of salmonellas distributed throughout their tissues and samples of spleen, liver, hepatic and bronchial lymph nodes will yield counts in excess of 10^6 organisms/g. Similar concentrations will also be present in the wall and contents of the gut and associated lymph nodes. Samples should be taken from the gut and internal organs in order to distinguish animals that have died of enteritis without septicaemia. Samples of fetal fluids, vaginal mucus and cotyledons should be taken from animals that have aborted. Counts will again give a more reliable result since the cotyledons from animals that have aborted due to *S. dublin* infection will usually contain between 10^8 and 10^{10} organisms/g.

Identification of carriers by bacteriological examination is more difficult and an attempt must be made to distinguish 'active carriers' from 'passive' excretors and 'latent carriers'. Faeces samples are more reliable than swabs and should distinguish 'active' or 'persistent' excretors whose faeces usually contain in excess of 10^5 salmonellas/g. Animals should not be assumed to be excretors on the basis of one isolation, nor should they be considered to be free of infection unless at least three negative faecal samples have been obtained.

Even in this latter case 'latent carriers' and animals that will eventually clear the infection, and yet are still harbouring salmonellas, will be missed. There may be an advantage in taking samples from adults at calving although care must still be observed to distinguish 'passive carriers'. Traditionally, samples of gall-bladder or bile have been taken to identify carriers at slaughter. Unfortunately, these may not always contain salmonellas unless animals are infested concurrently with *Fasciola hepatica* and a variety of tissues including alimentary contents and superficial lymph nodes need to be examined. It has been possible, in the author's experience, to isolate salmonellas from the walls of the omasum, abomasum and rumen or from lymph nodes such as the bronchial node, prescapular node and retropharyngeal node when all other tissues have been negative. Similarly, the author has only very rarely isolated salmonellas from the tonsil although this has been the preferred site of other investigators.

Identification of infected herds may be achieved by faecal samples but this may present similar difficulties to identifying individual infected animals, particularly in the case of *S. dublin*. A simple, less expensive and probably more reliable method is to take samples of slurry where this is available. Milk filters were very useful in this respect but the recent change to the use of in-line metal filters has removed this method as a realistic option.

A variety of enrichment techniques and isolation media are available for the cultivation of salmonellas. They rely on promoting the selective growth of salmonellas whilst inhibiting the growth of contaminants and identification on the basis of colony morphology and biochemical reactions. The choice of media depends upon the environment from which the organism must be isolated and often depends upon the subjective choice of bacteriologists who specialize in *Salmonella* isolation. The topic is too large to discuss in detail here although the author has found that a range of liquid enrichment media and the use of at least two types of solid isolation media are necessary to guarantee the isolation of the majority of serotypes. Once isolated, the identification of salmonellas to genus level is carried out on the basis of biochemical reactions for which a variety of rapid kits are now available. Further identification is carried out by slide and tube agglutination tests, which define the serotypes according to the Kauffmann–White scheme (see p. 182). Since a large number of differential sera are required this is usually the province of dedicated laboratories. Important serotypes such as *S. typhimurium* and *S. enteritidis* may be further subdivided by phage-typing, plasmid analysis or a variety of molecular techniques such as DNA or RNA fingerprinting. Although used for research purposes a phage-typing scheme for *S. dublin* is not available in the UK and this serotype is subdivided into biotypes. Unfortunately, although seven distinct, stable biotypes have been identified the majority (approximately 75 per cent) of strains isolated in the UK belong to the same biotype and the scheme is of little use in epidemiological investigations.

A number of serological techniques are also used in an attempt to identify *Salmonella*-infected animals (see p. 187). Unfortunately, no single test has proved useful in distinguishing all infected animals, some of which do not mount an antibody response, and all suffer from an inability to distinguish infected animals from others which, although previously infected, no longer harbour the organism. Various techniques such as enzyme-linked immunosorbent assay (ELISA) or nucleic acid probes that will detect small amounts of antigen have been developed but they have yet to be evaluated.

Control measures and vaccination

Attempts to control salmonellosis in cattle have involved the use of strict hygiene measures, antibiotics, and vaccination, either singly or in combination. Most of the control measures are obvious from the discussion presented above and the role of antibiotics and vaccination is described below.

To prevent the introduction of salmonellosis to herds it is necessary to provide animals with uncontaminated feed and water, to control ingress of rodents and birds and limit human contact. When adult stock have to be 'bought-in' these should be quarantined and examined bacteriologically. Exacerbating factors such as ketosis and liver-fluke infestation should be controlled and particular care should be taken in maintaining the health and hygiene of animals at calving. This should include the use of individual calving boxes and thorough cleaning between animals. Calves should be encouraged to absorb sufficient colostrum. To prevent acquisition of infection in calf-rearing units only good quality calves from herds of known health history should be purchased. They should be singly penned in solid-sided pens and strict hygiene should be observed during feeding and cleaning. Units should be run on an all-in, all-out basis and calf-houses should be thoroughly cleaned (preferably by steam-cleaning, disinfection or fumigation) between batches. In the event of a disease outbreak affected animals should be quarantined and restrictions should be placed on the movement of susceptible stock. Human contact with infected animals should be restricted and strict hygiene should be observed when moving between groups.

During the course of an extensive outbreak of salmonellosis due to *S. saintpaul* in two large dairy herds, investigated by the author, many methods to control infections and reduce mortality were attempted. These included the use of an autogenous vaccine, which had no effect on mortality but reduced the duration of faecal excretion, and treatment with oxytetracycline and ampicillin, which reduced mortality and the number of persistent excretors. Other measures included restriction of movement of stock and personnel, the use of impermeable clothing and disinfectant sprays, removal of predisposing factors such as dietary imbalance, reduction of stocking densities, segregation of susceptible animals, prompt antibiotic treatment of sick animals and removal of 'persistent excretors'. These measures were designed to reduce the level of environmental contamination. This is primarily due to contamination with the faeces of diarrhoeic animals and 'persistent excretors' from which calves may be infected either at birth, particularly when communal calving facilities are used, or when housed in the same buildings as adults. Once infected, calves may excrete such large numbers of organisms (up to 10^8/g of faeces) that less than 0.1 g of faeces may contain a lethal dose for other calves. Thus any measure that reduces environmental contamination may help to break the cycle of infection. Methods that appeared successful in this particular outbreak were prompt antibiotic treatment of sick calves, removal of adult carriers, reduction in stocking densities and segregation of susceptible animals.

Salmonellosis may be spread from farm to farm and amongst cattle on infected premises by the disposal or use of animal wastes on pastures as a fertilizer. The number of organisms contained in such materials is usually low and the risk can be reduced to an acceptable level if sensible restrictions are observed. The following code of practice based on work carried out at the Institute for Animal Health and designed further to reduce the number of salmonellas should be followed.

1 When possible slurry should be spread on arable land or land used for conservation. Salmonellas do not survive for long enough on grass to be a danger in hay, nor do they survive efficient silage making.

2 Composted waste may safely be spread on pasture to be grazed by animals but slurry should be stored for at least one month prior to spreading.

3 Pasture treated with stored slurry should not be grazed for at least one month after spreading. If the slurry cannot be stored, this interval between spreading and grazing should be extended. In addition, since young animals may be more susceptible to salmonellosis they should not be allowed to graze pasture dressed with slurry for at least six months after spreading.

4 The principal danger to cattle occurs when fresh unstored slurry, particularly pig slurry or poultry manure, must be applied to pasture. This danger can be reduced by using low application rates and by leaving pasture as long as possible before grazing.

5 Consideration should be given to mechanical separation of slurry. This produces a solid fraction that readily composts and a liquid fraction in which salmonellas die off rapidly.

6 Slurry should not be spread by equipment, such as a rain-gun, which involves the production of spray.

These recommendations were designed to reduce the risk of infections from animal wastes but they may be applied, with minor modifications, to the disposal of human sewage sludge on agricultural land. However, water authorities disposing of sewage sludge produce their own codes of practice that should be followed.

Prevention of salmonellosis by vaccination has been attempted since the late nineteenth century. There has been considerable scientific debate on the relative importance of humoral and cell-mediated immunity but it is now generally agreed that solid immunity probably depends on both humoral and cellular responses. Although the humoral response is not totally protective it plays an important role in the suppression of infection in its early stages although a cellular response is probably required for complete elimination of the organism. In consequence, both live and killed vaccines have been used for the prevention of salmonellosis in cattle and attempts have been made to protect calves actively and passively by transfer of maternal antibody in colostrum.

In the UK only inactivated vaccines are available. The inactivated vaccine, which is licensed for use in both adults and calves, is a formalin-killed preparation of *S. dublin* and *S. typhimurium* that also contains *E. coli*. This vaccine has been the subject of recent field and experimental tests and has been shown to be effective when used to induce antibodies in adults, which could be transferred to calves in colostrum.

However, most investigators have believed that cell-mediated immunity is necessary to provide solid protection and the majority of recent attempts at vaccination have utilized living, attenuated cells. These have either been naturally occurring avirulent strains, laboratory-derived or mutated strains, or more recently, genetically engineered strains. These have included rough strains and the part-rough *S. dublin* mutant (strain

51) derived by H. Williams Smith which, although virulent in mice, was of reduced virulence for calves. This strain, which proved successful in protecting calves experimentally against both *S. dublin* and *S. typhimurium*, was made available in the UK as a commercial vaccine. The vaccine, which performed well in field trials, was usually given to calves parenterally one week after birth. Vaccinated calves were said to develop immunity within a few days of administration and probably remained protected for a minimum of three weeks. It was, however, reported that the vaccine did not protect against a heavy challenge unless the vaccine dose was increased to a level at which it was potentially virulent. It may also have been more virulent in stressed animals, may have aggravated pre-existing enteric and respiratory disease and may, rarely, induced anaphylactoid reactions. This vaccine is no longer available.

Another group of rough vaccine strains, with a block in the enzyme uridine-diphosphate-galactose-4-epimerase, have been tested experimentally in cattle. Rough mutants although avirulent are poorly immunogenic. Galactose-4-epimeraseless (Gal E) mutants, however, although rough *in vitro* due to an inability to produce smooth-type lipopolysaccharide, are smooth and immunogenic *in vivo* when galactose is supplied exogenously. Even though they are smooth *in vivo* they are avirulent because of a restriction in their ability to colonize the tissues of their host due to galactose-induced bacteriolysis. In other words, they remain viable in the host long enough to induce an immune response but since they are capable of accumulating galactose, but not able to break down the excess, they eventually lyse. Unfortunately, although Gal E mutants were successful in protecting calves against experimental challenge, their potential as commercial vaccines has not been exploited because of doubts about their safety.

Recent research on live vaccines has concentrated on the use of genetic constructs. Amongst the first of these, originally produced in the USA, were strains deficient in the use of certain aromatic compounds generally known as *Aro* deletants or *Aro*− strains. These strains were modified by transposon mutagenesis and are deficient in an enzyme of the aromatic synthetic pathway; they are unable to synthesize chorismate from which *p*-aminobenzoic acid, a precursor of folate, and dihydroxybenzoate, a precursor of the iron-binding protein enterochelin, are produced. In the absence of *p*-aminobenzoic acid and dihydroxybenzoate, which are not found in mammalian tissues, they will not grow. *Aro*− strains of *S. dublin* and *S. typhimurium* have been produced and tested experimentally in calves. They induce good protection when administered orally or parenterally, are able to cross-protect against challenge with heterologous serotypes and are safe. They do not establish in the host, do not cause side-effects and are genetically stable. Their only disadvantages are that not all constructs are equally protective and that they may not be able to protect calves less than three weeks of age. More recently, constructs deficient in more than one enzyme or constructs with auxotrophic mutations have also been produced. These strains, which because they have two or more independent mutations are even safer than strains with a single mutation, have also been shown to be effective vaccines for calves and may even be able to protect animals within the first month of life. As yet none of these strains are available commercially for use in the UK.

Another vaccine strain that depends upon limited replication in vaccinated animals has been used in Germany. This is an avirulent, non-reverting, streptomycin-dependent strain of *S. dublin* that is normally administered orally. It is claimed that this strain protects against both *S. dublin* and *S. typhimurium* and when used with a killed vaccine in older calves and adults has eradicated salmonellosis from large areas of eastern Germany.

Since calves may become infected within the first few days after birth and the peak of mortality occurs between three to four weeks of age, passive protection by vaccination of adult animals would appear to be the ideal way of protecting calves. Unfortunately, attempts at passive protection have met with conflicting results. Recently, however, an experimental vaccination regimen based on dam vaccination and prolonged colostrum feeding has been described. Cows were vaccinated with formalin-inactivated *S. typhimurium* approximately seven weeks and two weeks preparturition. Calves were given the opportunity to suck from their dam for 48 hours following parturition and were then fed cold, stored colostrum from their own dam for a further eight days. These calves were resistant to a normally lethal challenge of *S. typhimurium* or *S. dublin* given five days after birth and excreted salmonellas in their faeces for only a short period after infection. Mortality was also reduced in calves that sucked from a vaccinated dam and were then fed on normal colostrum and in calves born to unvaccinated cows and later fed on 'immune' colostrum. The degree of protection was correlated with the amount of passive antibody measurable in the faeces of calves by ELISA. The presence of maternal antibody may interfere with active vaccination of calves using either inactivated or live vaccines. However, schemes based on dam vaccination have recently proved successful in field trials in Germany and Israel and these results suggest that vaccination of pregnant cattle may be a useful method of controlling outbreaks of salmonellosis in dairy herds. It may also be used to confer resistance upon young calves at the time when they are sold in markets and thus limit the amount of infection in calf-rearing units.

Vaccines may have an important role to play in the prophylaxis of bovine salmonellosis but until improved vaccines become available they will not be a substitute for good husbandry and hygiene.

It is not intended to discuss treatment of animals infected with salmonellosis in detail here since this is based on the use of antibiotics and fluid replacement therapy as described earlier for *E. coli* (see p. 175). Although antibiotics are not used in the treatment of gastroenteritis in humans their use is justified for bovine salmonellosis, which is a systemic disease with a high mortality in the absence of treatment. The disease in cattle is similar to systemic infections such as typhoid and paratyphoid in humans where antibiotics are used routinely.

The concern with the use of antibiotics is that they have the potential of predisposing to colonization with salmonellas, increasing levels and duration of excretion by carriers and of selecting for antibiotic-resistant strains. The effect of antibiotics on an animal and its resident micro-organisms will depend upon the dose level, duration of administration, and antimicrobial spectrum of the antibiotic. The effects of antibiotics to which salmonellas are sensitive at therapeutic doses must be distinguished from the effects of the same antibiotic at subtherapeutic concentrations and the effects at either concentration of antibiotics to which salmonellas are insensitive. Similarly, since the antibiotic may have an effect upon the salmonellas or the normal flora or both, the age of the animal host is important since age is often the principal factor in determining the composition of the normal flora. An antibiotic to which salmonellas are sensitive, used at the correct therapeutic dose, may be predicted to reduce excretion. The same antibiotic at a subtherapeutic dose may lead to increased multiplication of salmonellas due to a suppressive effect on the activity of growth-suppressing normal flora. Similarly, the use of an antibiotic to which salmonellas are resistant, but the normal flora sensitive, may be expected to result in increased multiplication and excretion.

Antibiotic therapy in uncomplicated *Salmonella* gastroenteritis in humans has not been recommended for more than 40 years. Therapy apparently does not shorten or otherwise alter the clinical course of infection and has frequently been shown to prolong post-convalescent excretion. Antibiotics have also been shown to prolong excretion in laboratory mice and streptomycin has even been used to render mice more susceptible to experimental infection. However, antibiotics have been used extensively to treat salmonellosis in cattle without undue complications. It should be clear from the remarks above that the antibiotic sensitivity of the organism should be determined and the information used to choose the preferred antibiotic. The use of antibiotics for prophylaxis is more controversial and most authorities have reported that medication with antibiotics has no part to play in the prevention of salmonellosis. The use of antibiotics in the treatment of an outbreak of *S. saintpaul* infection has been described above. In the same outbreak antibiotics were successfully used prophylactically and have also been used to effect a bacteriological cure in adult carriers and calves.

Chapter 14: Digestive Disorders of Calves

by R.W. BLOWEY

Introduction

The young calf is particularly susceptible to digestive disorders, with the major presenting clinical sign of scouring (diarrhoea) being a significant cause of economic loss due to ill-thrift and death. Immediately after birth the calf is exposed to a wide range of infectious agents, to which it must develop an immunity. Many calves are hand-reared and consequently within a few days their diet may change from whole milk to milk substitute. Later they must learn to eat solid food, to be weaned at six to eight weeks old. Such rapid changes of feed and feeding systems, in combination with a changing immune status, render the calf susceptible to a wide variety of infectious diseases and nutritional disorders. Infectious conditions are described elsewhere in this book (see Chapters 12, 13). This chapter discusses the common nutritional disorders.

Abomasal milk clot failure and milk scour

Abomasal volume in the newborn calf is 1.5 l. It has a neutral pH, thus allowing the first feed of colostrum to pass through unclotted, so that immunoglobulin molecules can be absorbed whole through the intestinal epithelium. Initially, renin coagulates milk (optimally at pH 6.5), with clot formation within minutes of ingestion. The clot contracts, expressing the whey proteins (albumin and globulin), minerals and lactose in liquid whey, which begins its passage into the duodenum 5–10 minutes later. After two to three days the number of parietal cells in the abomasal epithelium increases and they begin to secrete hydrochloric acid. Abomasal pH falls. This converts pepsinogen secreted by chief cells into the active form of pepsin. Both pepsin and renin are capable of clotting milk and both can digest the milk protein casein, but pepsin is most effective at pH 5.2 and, additionally, can digest a wider range of proteins. The pepsin digestion system is not fully developed until approximately seven to ten days old and until that stage calves should, ideally, receive either whole milk or substitute consisting of whole milk. Similarly, the very young calf has an immature intestinal digestion. Pancreatic proteases can cope with whey proteins, pancreatic lipases with fat and intestinal lactase degrades the milk sugar lactose into glucose and galactose. The ability to digest starch does not develop until the calf is at least seven days old and full activity of maltase, sucrase and amylase systems, allowing the calf to digest non-milk carbohydrate, is not complete until three weeks old.

Figure 14.1 is a 'flow' diagram of digestion in the young calf. Complete digestion of the abomasal milk clot (or 'curd') by lipases and proteases may take 6–8 hours and hence calves fed twice daily are only without nutrients for a short period. Calves left with their dams may suckle seven to ten times each day and any remaining curd forms a nucleus for the next milk clot.

If abomasal milk clot formation is poor, then whole milk spills over into the duodenum, where casein cannot be digested. In addition to altering the osmotic

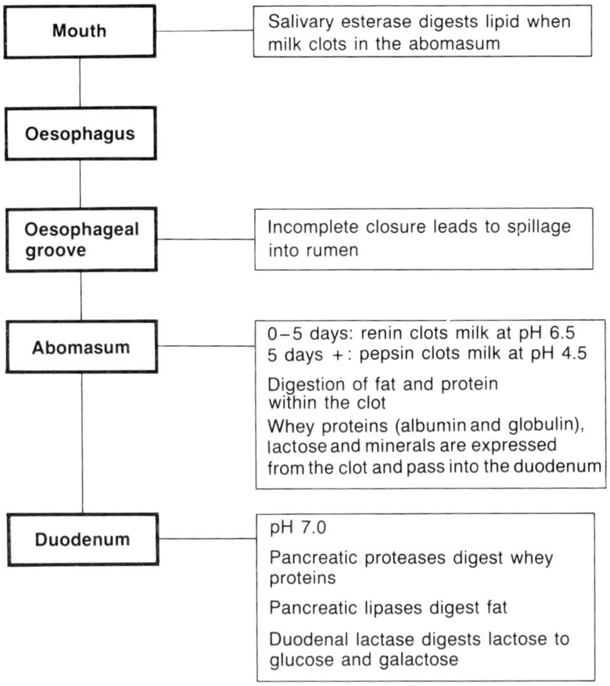
Mouth
Salivary esterase digests lipid when milk clots in the abomasum
Oesophagus
Oesophageal groove
Incomplete closure leads to spillage into rumen
Abomasum
0–5 days: renin clots milk at pH 6.5
5 days +: pepsin clots milk at pH 4.5
Digestion of fat and protein within the clot
Whey proteins (albumin and globulin), lactose and minerals are expressed from the clot and pass into the duodenum
Duodenum
pH 7.0
Pancreatic proteases digest whey proteins
Pancreatic lipases digest fat
Duodenal lactase digests lactose to glucose and galactose

Fig. 14.1 Flow diagram of digestion in the young calf.

balance, this provides an excellent medium for bacterial fermentation in the lower intestine and scouring results. Similarly, if excessive quantities of milk are provided (greater than 1.5 l for the young calf), or if a hungry calf is allowed to gorge itself, then abomasal digestive processes become overloaded and whole milk spills into the duodenum. This can also be a problem with suckler calves, especially if the dam is a 'milky' Friesian or Holstein crossbred animal. Although the calf may suckle every few hours, overloading and dietary scouring can still occur. This is particularly common if cows are put with the calves only twice daily.

On bucket-rearing systems a variety of management factors can lead to poor abomasal milk clot formation. These include:

1 nervous or stressed calves, for example feeding immediately after arrival from market, dehorning or some other stressful procedure;

2 irregular feeding times;

3 milk substitute fed at the wrong temperature or incorrect strength (see p. 196); and

4 inflammation of the abomasum (see p. 199).

Many enzyme systems are induced, that is, enzyme activity develops following exposure to substrate. Calves should therefore be reared on a single type of milk substitute and, preferably, from a single batch purchased to cover the whole rearing period. A sudden change in the ingredients of the milk substitute could lead to incomplete digestion of protein, fat or carbohydrates, which later undergo putrefactive fermentation in the lower intestine, resulting in malabsorption, a fetid diarrhoea and weight loss. Such calves are more susceptible to colonization by pathogenic *Escherichia coli* and salmonellae.

Irregular feeding and its influence on abomasal pH can also have an effect on the susceptibility of a calf to infection. Most ingested enteric infections are killed at an abomasal pH below 4.5. The very young calf, which for the first few days of life has an abomasal pH of 6.5, is particularly susceptible to infection therefore. However, this is counteracted by surface-active antibodies contained in whole milk and colostrum. In the older calf, the acidity of the empty abomasum, i.e. after complete digestion of the curd 6–8 hours after the previous feed, may fall to as low as pH 2.0. Following a feed of milk, pH rapidly rises towards neutrality (e.g. pH 6.5), the extent and persistence of this rise depending on the volume and nature of the liquid milk ingested. With warm whole milk, abomasal pH falls to below 4.2 within 3 hours of a meal and bacterial killing once again becomes effective. Figure 14.2 indicates the periods required for other feeds.

Clearly, calves that develop a poor abomasal milk clot, or that have other abomasal disorders (e.g. abomasal dilation, p. 199), resulting in increased pH values, will be more susceptible to infection. In addition, improperly digested fats passed in the faeces produces steatorrhoea, with subsequent hair loss over the legs and perineal region (Plate 14.1). Affected calves will be unthrifty and in poor condition, due to poor absorption of nutrients.

Treatment with oral electrolytes for two to three days and dietary correction is normally effective.

Problems with milk substitutes

A full review of liquid feeds and feeding systems is beyond the scope of this book. Those interested should consult more authoritative texts such as Webster (1984). Because of the immaturity of the pepsin–HCl system, calves should receive colostrum and whole milk for the first three to four days of life. Most conventional milk substitutes are based on skim milk powder (SMP), to which is added lipids and fats from a variety of sources, all highly emulsified to ensure even suspension throughout the milk when it is reconstituted. These SMP substitutes should clot in the abomasum. Addition

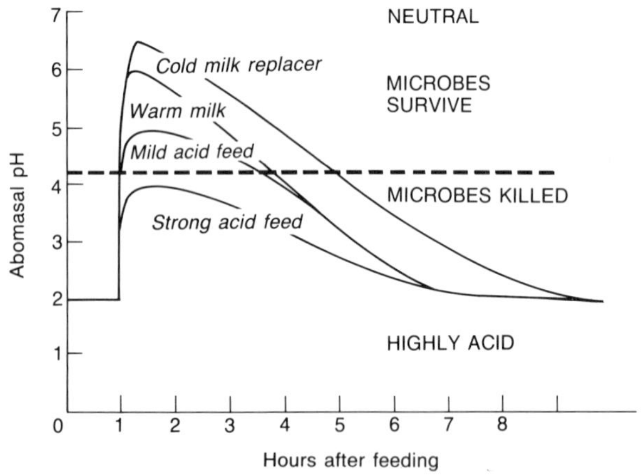

Fig. 14.2 The effect of type of milk and milk substitute on abomasal pH (taken from Webster, 1984).

of weak organic acids (e.g. citric or fumaric) reduces pH to 5.7 and thus improves keeping quality. Fully acidified milk powders, with a pH of approximately 4.2, have an even better keeping quality. As casein would clot at this low pH it cannot be used and strong acid powders primarily consist of whey proteins (albumin and globulin) with added fat. Without casein they do not clot in the abomasum, but this does not seem to produce any increase in digestive problems. Such 'zero' replacers (so-called because they contain no skim milk powder) are commonly used in *ad libitum* calf feeding systems.

If skim milk powder is overheated during manufacture, casein is denatured, abomasal milk clot formation is poor, undigested casein passes into the small intestine and scouring may result from putrefactive bacterial fermentation. Most proprietary milk substitutes are carefully monitored and the majority of problems associated with their feeding are managemental in origin. The first golden rule must be *to read the manufacturer's instructions*. To achieve even dispersal of the product, and especially of the fat, many manufacturers recommend that milk is mixed at a higher temperature (45–50 °C) and then cooled to just above blood heat (42 °C) before feeding. A thermometer is needed to do this. The temperature cannot be judged manually. On a hot day milk will feel cool and consequently may be fed too hot. On a cold day the temperature may be overestimated and the milk substitute consequently fed too cold. Milk substitute mixed below the optimum temperature produces an inferior product. Added protein and minerals sediment to the bottom of the bucket and are wasted. In addition, poorly dispersed fats remain as a layer on the surface of the milk, forming a ring around the calf's muzzle after feeding, which produces secondary alopecia (Plate 14.2). If a long row of calves is fed from a single container, the milk for the last calf can be appreciably cooler. Again fat will rise to the surface and alopecia may develop on the muzzle. A fall of only 6 °C in the temperature of the milk fed will *double* the time taken to form the abomasal clot. Undigested milk may then leak from the abomasum, thus reducing its nutritive value and possibly inducing diarrhoea. Conversely, however, if milk is fed too hot calves simply will not drink it, but no adverse effects have been observed. It is interesting to compare this with our own liking for hot drinks.

Milk fed at the wrong strength can cause problems. Powder is normally added at 125 g/l for twice daily feeding and 150 g/l on once daily systems. Abomasal milk clot will be optimal at these concentrations. If too dilute, clot formation is poor. Milk should not, therefore, be fed 'half strength' for scouring calves, as this may retard clot formation. Although some proprietary electrolyte preparations state that they can be used with whole milk and improve clotting time, there is some evidence that the clot thus formed is less stable. In general, therefore, it is best to avoid diluting milk substitutes and if electrolytes are to be given, they should be fed separately. Similarly, calves should not be allowed to drink large volumes of water immediately after milk, as this will have the effect of diluting the milk.

Probably the biggest problem with milk substitutes comes from careless mixing. Stirring with the hand is simply not adequate: a whisk, whether manual or mechanical, is essential. Carelessly mixed powders leave lumps and a sediment of protein in the bottom of the bucket and poorly dispersed fat rises to the top. Trials have shown that up to 60 per cent of the oils in a replacer may be wasted in this way, producing poor growth, stunted calves and possibly scouring due to inadequate abomasal clot formation.

Oesophageal groove dysfunction

From as early as two weeks of age the young calf begins picking at hay, grass or other solid foods. Bacteria ingested with this food, initially *E. coli* and lactobacilli, initiate ruminal fermentation. With increasing age, the rumen becomes progressively more anaerobic and an adult ruminal flora eliminates the early organisms. The inability of *E. coli* and salmonellae to survive for significant periods in the rumen is one reason for encouraging early ruminal development. However, at this age rumen fermentation alone would be unable to provide adequate nutrients for the rapidly growing calf and milk needs to continue 'monogastric' digestion in the abomasum. Milk entering the rumen is both wasteful and dangerous and its passage directly into the abomasum is achieved via the oesophageal groove. In the anterior wall of the dorsal sac of the rumen there is a muscular channel that runs from the distal end of the oesophagus into the rumino-omasal orifice, as shown in Fig. 14.3. A reflex action from suckling results in muscular closure of this groove, to form an enclosed pipe, and milk is then transferred directly into the abomasum. As the calf gets older, the thought of being fed and the sight, sounds and stimuli associated with the arrival of its milk will be sufficient to evoke closure. It is most important that closure occurs prior to feeding and hence the establishment of a standardized feeding regimen is vital. The calf needs to know that it is about to be fed, that a pleasurable event is forthcoming. Feeding times should be consistent each day. Milk should be provided at the correct and consistent temperature, in the same amount at each feed and of a similar taste and consistency. Stressed calves, for example, those that have just arrived from market, may not achieve groove closure and should therefore be given electrolyte solutions for their first feed. Similarly, calves should not be moved, handled, dehorned, etc. immediately before feeding. Slow drinkers present a problem. While the milk is warm, oesophageal groove closure may be adequate. However, if the bucket is left in front of the calf it may drink later, with possible milk spillage into the rumen. Some calves fail to learn to drink adequately and must be finger or teat suckled until weaning, although this is preferable to reluctant drinking with inadequate groove closure. Bucket height and teat position are important. The bottom of the bucket must be at least 30 cm above the floor of the pen, which means that it must be raised as straw bedding accumulates. Unfortunately, it is all too common to see calves on their knees trying to drink from a bucket some way below pen level. Teats for milk substitute should be positioned such that the calf has sufficient space to stand back to suckle and at a height that allows its nose to be tilted upwards and the oesophagus at least horizontal.

Milk spilt into the rumen undergoes rapid fermentation. This may produce an acute and sometimes fatal bloat and colic, within 15–30 minutes of feeding. In more chronic cases, ruminal development is retarded and abnormal products of digestion pass into the intestine, producing scour. Chronic pain restricts food intake and therefore growth and development. The Charolais calf in Plate 14.3 has a typically distended left flank caused by ruminal bloat. The superficial haemorrhage resulted from trocarization with a needle. A pasty scour is evident on the tail.

Treatment of oesophageal groove closure is, in effect, treatment of chronic bloat and is discussed in the next section.

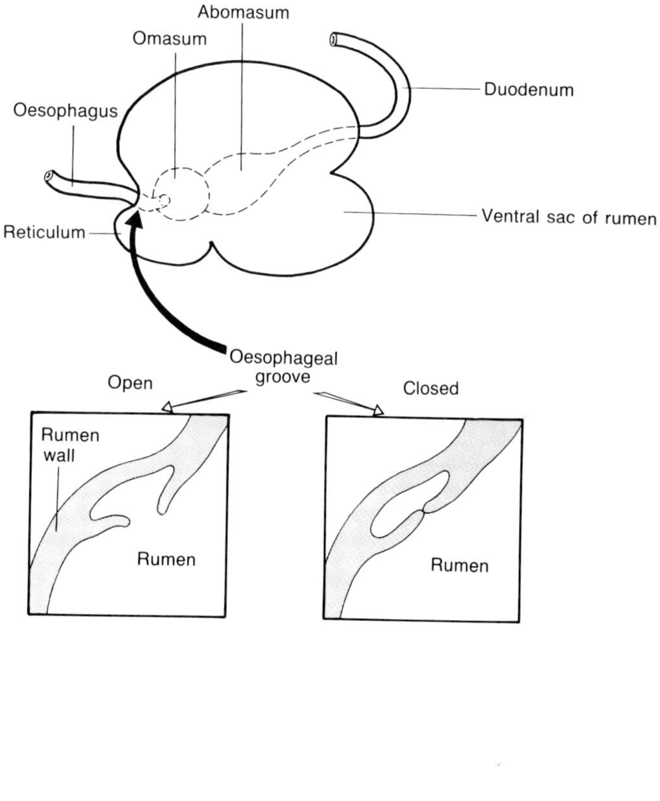

Fig. 14.3 The oesophageal groove (Blowey, 1988).

Ruminal bloat (see p. 637)

The development of normal rumen function is a complex process and any interference can produce bloat. Organisms ingested with feed from approximately two weeks onwards eventually establish an anaerobic fermentation. It is the ingestion and subsequent fermentation of solid feed that stimulates the rapid expansion in *size* of the rumen, although full development is not complete until 12 weeks old, when the rumen comprises approximately 80 per cent of the total volume of the four stomachs. During this period, development of the rumen *papillae* is affected by the type of food offered. Inadequate long fibre and fermentation of a high-concentrate diet leads to low ruminal pH and acidosis. This can restrict development of papillae to such an extent that inflammation and ulceration of the ruminal wall permits bacterial 'leakage' and subsequent hepatic abscessation. The addition of 10–15 per cent chopped straw to concentrates, especially high-starch products, will improve rumen fermentation, thereby increasing the overall digestibility of the ration and promoting increased dry matter intake, since high acidity depresses the activity of cellulolytic bacteria. Calves that do not have hay on offer should therefore be bedded freshly each day, with ample palatable straw. Long fibre encourages rumination and subsequent saliva production, which in turn both neutralizes and dilutes ruminal acidity. Silage or other forages may be used, but it seems critical that the fibre length is 5.0 cm or above. It has been suggested that concentrate intakes in heifer calves being reared for dairy replacements should be restricted, as this will encourage greater consumption of forage and the development of a larger rumen, capable of sustaining greater intakes later in life.

Irregularities at any stage of rumen development can lead to bloat, but the two most common causes are oesophageal groove failure, with subsequent fermentation of milk in the rumen, and acidosis caused by high level feeding of improperly formulated concentrates. The bloat is a gassy bloat, caused by ruminal atony. The rate of ruminal contractions and subsequent eructation and gas release varies with the physical presentation of the diet, as shown in Table 14.1, and with dietary constituents. High-forage diets produce greater ruminal activity than high concentrate.

Table 14.1 Effect of the physical form of diet on ruminating behaviour of calves 6–9 weeks old (from Webster 1984, adapted from Hodgson, 1971)

	Grass pellets	Long or chopped grass
Eating (min/24 h)	132	276
Ruminating (min/24 h)	138	459
Eating (min/kg DM)	85	320
Ruminating (min/kg DM)	70	535
Dry matter intake (g/24 h)	1553	862

Signs

Typically, bloat is seen 15–30 minutes after a feed of milk or concentrate. Mild cases may deflate spontaneously over 3–4 hours, as ruminal contractions recommence. More protracted cases may remain bloated until the next feed, because bloat depresses feed intake and is therefore, to an extent, a self-perpetuating phenomenon. Death frequently occurs with acute cases. Affected calves are uncomfortable, with bouts of colic, often leading to kicking at their abdomen. Many develop a chronic scour (see colour plate 14.3), leading to general poor growth and unthriftiness.

Treatment

The syndrome may develop in both preweaned and postweaned calves and treatment is similar, the method used depending on the severity of the condition. Acute bloat must be deflated, either using a large bore needle through the rumen wall or, preferably, by stomach tube. Oral antibiotic will depress gas production. Penicillin may be the drug of choice, since lactobacilli proliferate in both acidosis and milk fermentation. Withdrawal of food and feeding electrolyte solutions for three to four days, removes the fermenting substrate. Calves should then be returned to liquid milk for a week and eventually reintroduced to solid food. Even then, a proportion of cases recur and in many instances this treatment is, for a variety of reasons, impractical. In such cases the construction of a permanent ruminal fistula in the triangle between the most caudal point of the last rib and the lumbar transverse processes is indicated. Under local anaesthesia, the rumen wall is sutured to the skin. Although rumen contents may spill onto the flank, this does not appear to upset the calf and in many animals the improvement in growth and general condition following surgery is dramatic. A proportion of fistulae seal spontaneously after six to twelve months. Others require surgical correction, although this is not normally performed for beef animals.

On farms where bloat is a common problem, feeding and management systems should be examined, especially in relation to the encouragement of early ruminal development. Highly nutritious concentrates should be offered from two to three weeks old onwards, preferably in small amounts each day, to ensure freshness and palatability. Water should be freely available, especially on once daily milk feeding. Inadequate access to water restricts concentrate intake and occasionally a long drink by a thirsty calf with a dry rumen leads to rapid fermentation of concentrates and subsequent bloat. In this respect the placing of buckets is important. Water should always be freely available, but the calf must be 'programmed' to regard it as a drink, namely without stimulating the oesophageal groove closure reflex. However, milk is a food and as soon as the calf has finished, replace the milk bucket with another containing concentrate. The calf immediately puts its head in and starts to eat, thus encouraging concentrate intake and, at the same time, discouraging excessive water drinking. Even so, occasional calves will still drink to excess, looking bloated and uncomfortable when they do so. In such cases, water is best withheld until 2–3 hours after the feed of milk, accepting the risk of bloat following rapid fermentation of dry ingested concentrates.

Rumen impaction and 'pot-bellied' calves

This condition is almost the reverse of bloat, in that it is associated with overconsumption of dry, fibrous and relatively indigestible foods, sometimes compounded by inadequate access to water. It may be a group problem, or the result of inadequate trough space, when the smaller members of the group get pushed out and have to exist on forage alone.

Postweaning feeding is a critical stage of the calf's development. The rumen is not fully mature, being more acid (i.e. lower pH) than the adult and unable to synthesize sufficient microbial protein, relative to energy, to meet the calf's high requirements for growth. Preweaning, milk has passed directly into the abomasum and this source of undegradable protein must be replaced by high-quality undegradable foods, e.g. fishmeal or linseed meal, after weaning. The higher the growth rate required, the higher will be the requirement for additional undegradable protein. As feed conversion is much more efficient at a younger age (Table 14.2), it is still cost-effective to feed expensive, nutritious diets to freshly weaned calves.

If the diet largely consists of poor-quality forages, the calf's growth will be stunted, and the rumen will be distended with slowly fermenting foods. Affected calves have a 'pot-bellied' appearance, i.e. the lower abdomen is distended, often on the right as well as the left flank. Ruminal contractions may be slow and the rumen feels 'doughy' on palpation. In an extreme case, where poorly grown calves left without food for many hours were allowed unlimited access to palatable straw, the author has seen severe illness and even death due to ruminal impaction. However, this is rare. Abomasal impaction is described on p. 651.

Table 14.2 The effect of age on feed conversion (taken from Blowey, 1988)

Body weight (kg)	Feed conversion ratio
50	2 : 1
100	3 : 1
300	5.5 : 1
500	8.5 : 1

Abomasal ulceration and dilatation

Abomasal ulceration is common in artificially reared calves, the majority of cases being asymptomatic and seen only at post mortem (for example in veal calves). Surprisingly, perhaps, the incidence is higher in those veal calves that have had access to forage. Many clinical cases are seen at two to three weeks old, when they first start eating solid food, or in animals that have developed pica, often as a result of chronic illness. These points suggest that ulcers result from large, inadequately digested particles of hay or straw, passing from the rumen to the abomasum. There is undoubtedly an increase in ulceration in calves with trichobezoars (hair balls), but whether the hair balls lead to ulceration, or whether chronic ulceration stimulates the calf to lick and eat hair (in the same way as chronic ruminitis) is uncertain. Ulceration occurs in association with abomasal dilation (see p. 200) and may also result from ruminal acidosis and starch overload, allowing undigested starch to spill over into the abomasum. Fungal hyphae are visible microscopically in a proportion of ulcers and may be involved in the pathogenesis.

Signs

The majority of ulcers in calves are subclinical. Some may haemorrhage, producing melaena and anaemia, which is occasionally fatal. Others produce a localized peritonitis of the abomasal serosa, whilst perforating ulcers lead to acute peritonitis and death. The three-week-old Friesian calf in Plate 14.4 was recumbent, in considerable pain, with a subnormal temperature

(37.5 °C) and sunken eyes. Regurgitated rumen contents are visible at the mouth. Death followed within 2 hours, despite abomasal drainage, lavage and parenteral metoclopramide. On post mortem (Plate 14.5) two large ulcers, one perforated with a white diphtheritic lining, were present, typically on the greater curvature of the abomasum.

Treatment

The treatment of abomasal ulcers is largely symptomatic. Valuable calves with extensive haemorrhage may be given a blood transfusion, but bleeding ulcers are less common in calves than in adult cattle. Kaolin has been used, but probably antacids such as magnesium oxides or magnesium silicate give a better response. Metoclopramide at 0.5–1.0 mg/kg body weight has been used to alleviate abomasal atony (Biggs *et al.*, 1989). Drainage and lavage may be indicated in concurrent abomasal dilation and ulceration. Antibiotics are indicated when peritonitis is suspected.

Abomasal dilatation

Also known as abomasal bloat, this condition of unknown aetiology produces a shock syndrome in calves, typically at two to three weeks old, namely when they first start eating solid good. Many cases are fatal. Affected calves are very dull, with sunken eyes and subnormal temperature, and are often reluctant or unable to stand. Enteritis may occur, but it is not a consistent feature. The enlarged abomasum, distended by excess fluid and occasionally with gas to produce tympany, can be ballotted on the lower right flank. The accumulated fluid has a much higher pH (range 5–7) than a normal calf with an empty abomasum (pH 2–3), thus allowing the bacterial count to increase to 10^5–10^9 ml, with coliforms predominating. A normal calf has an abomasal pH range 2–4 and a bacterial count of 50 000/ml, with mainly staphylococci and *Bacillus* species and very low numbers of *E. coli*. This has led to the proposal that abomasal dilation is an enterotoxaemia, similar to 'watery mouth' in young lambs (Price, 1989).

Abomasal drainage may be achieved by deep insertion of a stomach tube. With the calf in lateral recumbency on a straw bale and its head hanging down, the excess fluid is discharged under gravity. The abomasum can then be flushed two to three times with electrolyte solutions and, if treated symptomatically for shock and acidosis and fed electrolytes for 24–48 hours, recovery rates are acceptable. Metoclopramide at 0.5–1.0 mg/kg body weight has been reported useful to overcome abomasal atony (Biggs *et al.*, 1989), but the current author has met with very limited success.

In those cases that reach post mortem, a degree of abomasal ulceration, sometimes with fungal hyphae, is often present.

Acute abomasal bloat may also occur in milk substitute-fed calves within 20–30 minutes or less after feeding. Affected animals are seen in severe distress, kicking at the distended abdomen or rolling on the floor. Some cases are fatal, others respond to relaxant therapy, for example pethidine or mepramizole. On post mortem the milk has often failed to clot, but no other lesions are seen and the cause remains unknown. It has been suggested that it is more common with infrequent and irregular feeding times.

Postweaning nutritional scour

A pale grey or browny-yellow scour is not uncommon in calves after weaning. In some calves growth is not significantly affected, while others become thin, severely stunted and may even die. Pyrexia is either mild or absent. Microscopic and cultural examination of faeces fails to reveal significant pathogens. Symptomatic treatment with antiprotozoals (e.g. amprolium), antibiotics or kaolin/chlorodyne preparations may help, but often recovery is simply a feature of increasing age.

The aetiology is unknown and it is probable that no single factor is involved. Suggested causes include poor ruminal development preweaning (see p. 198), use of inappropriate concentrates postweaning (for example, adult dairy rations containing high levels of allergenic vegetable protein and/or inadequate undegradable protein), feeding finely ground high-starch cereals, leading to chronic ruminitis and acidosis, or sudden feed changes, e.g. from a coarse mix ration to pelleted food. Calves can often achieve higher intakes of pelleted feeds and may gorge themselves. Infectious conditions such as late exposure to rotavirus or coronavirus, or primary BVD infection may also be involved.

Reducing concentrate to 0.75 kg/day of a high-quality product fed twice daily and increasing access to palatable, but reasonably coarse, hay may be beneficial but in the majority of cases improvement is gradual with increasing age. Severely affected calves should be returned to a milk diet.

Colic (see p. 651)

Colic is commonly seen in young calves. It occurs in association with many of the syndromes described earlier in this chapter, namely oesophageal groove dysfunction, acidosis, ruminal bloat, ruminal impaction, abomasal ulceration and abomasal dilatation. True intestinal spasmodic colic occurs and may precede enteritis and subsequent diarrhoea. Colic may also be a sign of a more serious abdominal disorder, for example torsion of the root of the mesentery, intussusception, acute peritonitis, cystitis with urethral obstruction or atresia ani/coli. The latter condition is seen within 24–48 hours of birth.

Treatment of colic therefore depends on the diagnosis and is discussed in the relevant section.

References

Biggs, A.M., Dainton, J.T. & Tucker, M.E. (1989) Metoclopramide for preventing watery mouth. *Veterinary Record*, **124**, 312.

Blowey, R.W. (1988) *A Veterinary Book for Dairy Farmers*, 2nd edn. Farming Press, Ipswich, pp. 1–456.

Blowey, R.W. & Weaver, A.D. (1991) *A Colour Atlas of Diseases of Cattle*. Wolfe Publications Ltd, London.

Orskov, R. (1987) *The Feeding of Ruminants*. Chalcombe Publications Ltd, Marlow, Bucks, pp. 1–90.

Price, T.P. (1989) A treatment of calf enterotoxaemia. In *Proceedings of British Cattle Veterinary Association 1988–1989*, pp. 185–93.

Webster, J. (1984) *Calf Husbandry Health and Welfare*. Granada Technical Book, pp. 1–202.

Chapter 15: Calf Respiratory Disease

by A.H. ANDREWS

Introduction

Bovine respiratory disease (BRD) in calves in the developed world occurs under two main management systems. The first involves young, housed calves, usually dairy bred and either reared for beef or as dairy replacements. These are weaned from their dams within a few days of birth and then fed milk substitute or milk until weaned, usually between five and eight weeks of age. Under such conditions these calves can succumb to one of two different respiratory syndromes. Often one will lead into the other. The first is a problem of slow, insidious onset known as chronic or cuffing pneumonia, whereas the second is more sudden and acute in occurrence and is given a variety of names, the most common being calf pneumonia, acute pneumonia or enzootic pneumonia.

The second problem is in a management system involving weaned suckled calves, usually six months to two years old and mainly reared outside. This disease occurs following transport and housing and results in a condition best described as transit fever or shipping fever (see Chapter 18). All the syndromes are best defined by the circumstances in which they occur because their aetiology is complex and mainly multifactorial in nature. This involves the susceptibility of the animal, the environment in which it is kept, the management of the animal as well as the various disease agents to which it is subjected. In many BRD problems the causal agents will be similar in each of the syndromes and it is only the management conditions that will be different.

Enzootic and cuffing pneumonias

The aetiology of pneumonia in young calves is extremely complex in both the acute and the chronic form. It is fair to suggest that the disease is multifactorial. It is usually seen in calves reared indoors, particularly when they are reared for beef production and so have moved farms at an early age. Most cases occur between two and five months and usually following weaning from a milk-substitute diet. The causes of the problem are partly infectious agents, the environment, management and the animals themselves.

Epidemiology

Chronic. It is very difficult to determine the incidence of chronic or cuffing pneumonia as most affected calves are not treated and they do not die. In addition, by the time and animals reach slaughter weight or are culled the residual damage is minimal. However, in a survey of dairy-bred animals reared on a farm it was found that 11 per cent had significant pneumonic lesions and it was estimated that this resulted in a 7.2 per cent reduction in liveweight gain (Thomas *et al.*, 1978).

Acute. Very few studies have been undertaken into the incidence of this condition. However, Thomas (1978) obtained health records for 12 beef farms in 11 British counties. The records covered 11 050 animals between 1970 and 1977. Mortality of bought-in calves is variable according to the rearing system used. However, a figure of 5.5 per cent is usual and it can be suggested that about half these deaths are due to enzootic pneumonia. This was seen in the Thomas study, which showed a death rate of 2.7 per cent from pneumonia out of a total mortality of 5.9 per cent. The overall number of animals treated for pneumonia was 32.6 per cent although the levels on individual farms varied from 3.1 to 52 per cent. It should also be remembered that some calves require more than one treatment for pneumonia. Again, there are few records for this but a level of retreatment of 10 per cent of all susceptible animals is probably not unrealistic. The recorded level was 8.9 per cent being treated on more than one occasion over a five-year period (Thomas, 1978) in a group of 2040 animals of which 22 per cent became ill initially. Another problem is that besides mortality, calves may become chronically affected and fail to thrive. Culling probably doubles the mortality due to disease and a level of 3.6 per cent was found in the study by Thomas. The reduction in liveweight gain in animals treated for pneumonia but which were not culled or died, compared with those untreated, was found to be 2.6 per cent (Thomas *et al.*, 1978).

Aetiology

A large number of different infectious agents have been isolated and suggested to be involved in the aetiology of both chronic and acute calf pneumonia. Often the enzootic form is called 'viral pneumonia'. However, it is generally considered this term is a misnomer as it presupposes the aetiology and in most cases, even when viral agents are present, they only form part of the disease complex. It is usually considered that the most important agents involved in the chronic or cuffing form are mycoplasmal. They include *Mycoplasma dispar* and *Ureaplasma* spp. When it comes to the acute form there is a very long list of pathogens. Many have been seen in the disease but may not necessarily have produced the problem experimentally (see Table 15.1). However, certain agents do seem to be more commonly involved. Thus the three main mycoplasmal agents are *M. bovis*, *M. dispar* and *Ureaplasma* spp. In the case of viruses, those most commonly implicated are bovine

Table 15.1 Infectious causes of enzootic pneumonia. The cause is often multifactorial, probably often mycoplasmal infection followed by viral and bacterial causes

Viruses	Mycoplasma	Bacteria
Respiratory syncytial virus (BRSV)*	*Mycoplasma bovirhinis*	*Pasteurella haemolytica**
Parainfluenza virus II	*M. dispar**	*P. multocida**
Parainfluenza virus III (PI3)*	*M. mycoides* subsp. *mycoides*	*Actinomyces* (*Corynebacterium*) *pyogenes**
Reovirus types 1,2,3 (Reo)	(little importance in Europe)	*Streptococcus pneumoniae*
Bovine viral diarrhoea virus (BVDV)*	*M. alkalescens*	*Staphylococcus aureus*
Adenovirus types 1,2,3,4	*M. arginini*	*Strep. bovis*
Enterovirus	*M. bovis**	*Staph. epidermidis*
Rhinovirus type 1 (RV)	*M. bovigenitalium*	*Strep. mitis*
Infectious bovine rhinotracheitis	*Acholeplasma laidlawii*	*Strep. faecalis*
(IBR)*	*A. modicum*	*Aerococcus wiridans*
	A. axanthum	*Acinetobacter* sp.
	Ureaplasma spp.*	*Micrococcus luteus*
	Leach's group 7 mycoplasmas	*Staphylococcus* spp.
		Neisseria spp.
		*Chlamydia**
		Actinobacillus lignieresii
		Klebsiella spp.
		Corynebacterium bovis
		C. xerosis
		Streptococcus spp.
		Aerococcus sp.
		Haemophilus sp.
		*Haemophilus somnus**
		Aeromonas sp.
		Bacillus sp.
		Alcaligenes faecalis
		Micrococcus roseus
		Micrococcus spp.
		Escherichia coli
		*Fusobacterium necrophorum**

*Thought to be the most important causes.

respiratory syncytial virus (BRSV), parainfluenza III (PI3) virus, infectious bovine rhinotracheitis (IBR) and bovine viral diarrhoea (BVDV) virus.

The bacterial pathogens involved are a very long list and one or more tends to be isolated from most cases of disease. It is often postulated that these may be secondary invaders after primary damage by mycoplasma or viruses. The most commonly isolated organisms are *Pasteurella haemolytica*, *P. multocida* and *Haemophilus* spp., especially *Haemophilus somnus*. In addition, cases that involve toxaemia often include *Actinomyces* (formerly *Corynebacterium*) *pyogenes* and *Fusobacterium necrophorum*. The involvement of bacteria in this complex condition of enzootic pneumonia is also enforced by the fact that in most naturally occurring outbreaks of disease there is some clinical response following the use of antibiotics.

The environment

Various factors in the environment tend to be considered to be important. There is a popular belief that the disease is often associated with low environmental temperatures and a high humidity (see p. 786). Often a respiratory problem is associated with a sudden drop in temperature 24 to 72 hours previously. It is thought that the cold may allow infection to flare up partly by affecting the respiratory defence mechanisms and it also allows disease spread by encouraging calves to huddle together. It appears that the alveolar macrophages, ciliated and mucus-secreting cells are susceptible to the environment and cold stress inhibits clearance from the lungs. In the cold, animals reduce heat loss by slowing down their respiratory rate and by a partial reduction in the pulmonary ventilation rate (Webster, 1981b). This causes a reduced pulmonary oxygen tension and it has been shown that hypoxia reduces the clearance rate of some organisms in mice (Green & Kass, 1965), and there is a reduction in mucociliary rate and alveolar phagocytic activity (Thomson & Gilka, 1974). The probable role of hypoxia in respiratory infection is indicated by the fact that most lung consolidation occurs in the ventral parts of the apical and cardiac lobes and these tend to be the areas of lowest oxygen tension and the slowest rate of clearance of pathogens (Veit *et al.*, 1978).

At times, outbreaks of disease occur with a high temperature and a low humidity. Thus rearing at a temperature of 21 °C (70 °F) and 47 per cent relative humidity (RH) predisposed Friesian and Jersey calves to respiratory disease compared with those kept at a temperature of 14 °C (60 °F) and 36 per cent RH (Roy *et al.*, 1971). It does seem that a high relative humidity may be beneficial at a high environmental temperature as it increases the sedimentation rate of airborne particles and thereby reduces the bacterial count of the environment. These factors have formed the basis for the establishment of the sweat box system for pigs (Gordon, 1963) and this is why water drips are often used in buildings for veal production.

Although it is generally recognized that respiratory disease commonly occurs at certain times of the year, and under certain weather conditions, it is only recently that attempts have been made to determine why. In housed dairy-bred calves on one farm two peak levels of enzootic pneumonia occurred; the first was between October and December and the second from February to May (Thomas, 1978). A study of a veal-calf unit over a 14-month period showed extensive outbreaks of disease in October, April and early June (Miller *et al.*, 1980).

The relationship between season and respiratory disease is probably partly due to management influences, particularly the housing of animals in close proximity, thereby assisting in the build-up and transfer of infection. However, the correlation between weather and disease is harder to prove, and in a disease outbreak involving veal calves no relationship was found (Miller *et al.*, 1980). A sudden drop in environmental temperature is often followed one to three days later by an outbreak of respiratory disease in housed, dairy-bred calves or housed single-suckler calves (Wiseman, 1978). Pneumonia in Irish calves housed in naturally ventilated buildings also tended to be precipitated by change in weather, such as frost, rain and wind or damp, humid conditions (Bryson *et al.*, 1978).

Body temperature regulation in cattle is well developed, so they can tolerate both heat and cold (Webster, 1981a). However, draughts in buildings can result in chilling, which increases the metabolic rate and perhaps reduces resistance to infection (Webster, 1981b), but high relative humidity on its own does not chill cattle (Webster, 1979). Webster (1981b) therefore postulated that the main effect of weather was compounded by the building itself. Thus a badly constructed building with poor ventilation would reduce ventilation rate, and the water-carrying capacity of the air would be detrimentally affected by bad ventilation and possibly poor drainage. Such conditions could lead to the relative humidity remaining at more than 90 per cent for several days, and this in turn would increase the survival and spread of pathogenic organisms. Some support for this view has been obtained by work showing an increased survival of small airborne bacteria at high relative humidities (Jones & Webster, 1981). There is thus an increase in the number of infective particles that are not removed in the nasal passages and these are deposited further down the respiratory tract, possibly causing disease.

Management

The time of weaning appears to be important in that more lung lesions are found in calves weaned at five weeks than those on an *ad libitum* substitute diet until 14 weeks old (Roy *et al.*, 1971). The reason for this is not clear but it might be due to the lower levels of energy intake, or lower availability of a micronutrient (Roy *et al.*, 1971) or perhaps inhaled dust or fungal spores, which are more prevalent when dry feed is eaten, exacerbate the problem (Lacey, 1968), or due to weaning being less stressful or the calf more resistant to respiratory disease at an older age.

There is a relationship between colostral antibody levels and respiratory disease (Thomas & Swann, 1973). This apparent resistance to disease might be due to the ingestion of increased levels of specific antibody or due to an indirect effect resulting from a reduced amount of enteric disease, or possibly the gradual reduction in passive immunity allowing a more orderly exposure of the calf to respiratory pathogens. When colostral antibodies are low there is a relatively fast loss of antibody, which may then allow the invasion of many pathogens (Williams *et al.*, 1975).

The purchase of a large number of calves from different sources for dairy and beef production and keeping them in the same housing allows the easy spread of potential respiratory pathogens to other animals in close proximity. It is considered by many authors (Wiseman, 1978) that it is the collection of a large number of young calves of a similar age and putting them into the same air space that is the main reason for the problem of pneumonia in intensively reared calf systems. It is not always accepted that the number of calves in a single air space is more important than the air space or floor area per calf. Other factors involved in increasing disease levels are the inadequate cleaning and disinfection of the building between batches, as well as not allowing the accommodation sufficient rest between calf intakes. In some cases younger animals are mixed with an older group, thereby allowing transmission of micro-organisms from the old, apparently clinically normal animals. Economic considerations may also influence the picture if there is a reluctance to employ preventive measures such as vaccination, etc. Several management procedures such as castration, disbudding and weaning all appear to have an effect on the level of disease. The importance of microbial agents is indirectly indicated by the importance of adequate uptake of colostrum (Phillips, 1975; Thomas, 1979).

The calf

There appear to be some breed differences in susceptibility to respiratory disease and Friesian and Jersey calves are more likely to be infected than Ayrshire or Hereford × Friesians (Roy, 1980). It has been postulated that this may be due to an increased skin thickness in some breeds, which provides better insulation.

Signs

Chronic. The condition is one of gradual onset. There is generally no illness and so the calf is bright, eats well, but it may have a slight mucoid or mucopurulent oculonasal discharge. The temperature is normal or slightly raised at 38.5–39.5 °C (101–103 °F); the respiratory rate may be at any level from normal to 100 per minute with a normal pulse. There is a dry, explosive cough that is usually produced singly. On auscultation there are noises of whistling, wheezing or squeaking and these are more commonly heard at expiration, although often they occur at both inspiration and expiration. The sounds are most common in the anterior and ventral parts of the chest.

Acute. Although one calf may be seen to be ill to begin with, several animals will usually become sick within the next 24–48 hours. There is normally a reduction in feed intake of the group and widespread coughing will be apparent. The affected animals appear dull and the head tends to be carried lower than normal. There is inappetance, pyrexia (40–40 °C, 104–107 °F) and a dull coat. Other signs including a mucoid or mucopurulent oculo-nasal discharge, tachypnoea (respirations are usually over 40 per minute), dyspnoea and hyperpnoea are normally present. In all but very severely ill calves there tends to be an increase in the amount of coughing; the cough itself may be of a harsh, dry, hacking type, but in others it will be moist. Pinching the upper trachea often elicits a cough. On auscultation of the thorax there are usually loud, harsh sounds or whistling, wheezing or squeaking. These sounds may be present at inspiration or expiration, but more commonly they are heard at the latter and in some cases there are fluid sounds such as bubbling or gurgling, which will be audible in the cranio-ventral parts of the lungs. In some bacterial infections, where there is marked consolidation, few sounds are present.

Necropsy

Chronic. Lesions tend to be confined to the ventral parts of the lung lobes and involve, in decreasing severity, the apical, cardiac and cranial parts of the caudal lobes. The area involved may be 5–40 per cent of the lung tissue and it tends to be red or purple in colour and to be indurated. Histologically, there are accumulations of lymphocytes in the peribronchiolar tissue and it is this that produces a cuff; macroscopically it is seen as a mottling of the lesion's cut surface. When accumulation is great, then the lymphocytes can cause a narrowing of the bronchiolar lumen and cause the surrounding alveoli to be compressed. Resolution of the lesions occurs over several months provided that they are uncomplicated. The bronchial and mediastinal lymph nodes are usually enlarged and there is often a fibrinous pneumonia.

Acute. Within the clinical entity of acute pneumonia there are three types of pathological entity that can be recognized involving the lungs (Pirie, 1979).

1 Type 1. There is localized consolidation particularly of the cranial lobes and the tissue is dark red, friable and there is no gross evidence of necrosis. Interstitial emphysema may be present. Histologically, there is an absence of peribronchiolar cuffing, but there is necrosis of the bronchiolar epithelium. The changes are often suggestive of a viral infection, but in many cases the presence of a virus cannot be proven because of the absence of inclusion bodies or positive immunofluorescence. PI3 infection can be suspected when there is alveolar and bronchiolar epithelium proliferation and eosinophilic intracytoplasmic inclusion bodies are present. RSV infection can result in alveolar epithelium hyperplasia and large multinucleate syncytial cells. Bronchial collapse occurs with adenovirus infection due to bronchiolar necrosis; there are basophilic and eosinophilic intranuclear inclusion bodies in epithelial and other cells. Intranuclear inclusion bodies, particularly in the epithelial cells of the trachea and bronchi, are seen in IBR.

2 Type 2. There is often marked consolidation of the cranial lobes with red or red/grey hepatization with widespread tissue necrosis and in many cases suppuration and this may involve up to 70–80 per cent of the lung. This type of lesion is often characteristic of bacterial infection. Extensive consolidation and suppuration are particularly seen in *A. pyogenes* and *F. necrophorus* infections.

3 Type 3. This is characteristic of calves that suddenly develop respiratory distress. The syndrome is often called atypical interstitial pneumonia. At post-mortem examination there is interstitial emphysema, pulmonary oedema and congestion, with alveolar epithelial hyperplasia and hyaline membrane formation.

Besides the lungs, there is usually gross enlargement and congestion of the mediastinal and bronchial lymph nodes. In some cases there is fibrinous pleurisy and the heart may be enlarged with epicardial and endocardial haemorrhages. Sero-sanguinous fluid may be present in the thorax and pericardial sac (Thomas, 1979).

Diagnosis

Chronic. Several animals are affected and are usually indoors. The problem is gradual in onset and although the animals show respiratory signs they are bright and eat well. The respiratory signs include single, dry coughing.

Acute. Again this affects a group of calves. Respiratory signs are present and the animals are usually obviously ill. Nasal swabs can be taken for bacterial, viral or mycoplasmal identification and the last two groups require placement in transport medium. Fluorescent antibody tests are available for most of the more important viral causes. Even when a potential pathogen is recovered it does not always mean that it is the same agent as is causing trouble in the lungs. Paired serum samples can be taken two weeks apart. This may indicate the cause but is only of value if control measures can then be implemented for the future.

Differential diagnosis

Chronic. This needs to be differentiated from acute pneumonia but in the latter case the animal is ill. Inhalation pneumonia is likely only to involve a single animal, which again is ill, and there is usually a related history. Tuberculosis may cause problems but usually there is a herd history and the dam may be showing signs. Muscular dystrophy (see p. 222) can produce respiratory signs but usually such animals have a fast pulse rate and raised serum creatine kinase aspartate and aminotrans-ferase levels. Congenital heart defects (see p. 144) will usually only involve one animal and there is a heart murmur, possibly with signs of cyanosis. Salmonellosis can result in signs but the calf is noticeably ill with diarrhoea.

Acute. Chronic pneumonia is a major differential diagnosis but the animals are not really ill in such cases. Uncomplicated IBR infection (see p. 256) could cause difficulties but there are mainly upper respiratory signs and a noticeable conjunctivitis. Salmonellosis (Chapter 13) will usually present with enteric signs. Although mucosal disease (see p. 660) can give rise to respiratory signs, there is usually also diarrhoea and, in some, mouth ulceration. Inhalation pneumonia mainly involves a single animal and there is an appropriate history. Tuberculosis will be detected by a history of disease in the herd. Congenital heart defects (see p. 144) involve a single animal and there is usually a heart murmur. Calf diphtheria (see p. 214) results in stertor and is again a single animal problem. Malignant catarrhal fever affects single animals and there is lymph node enlargement, corneal opacity and often nervous signs present.

Treatment

Chronic. Therapy is usually not necessary unless the calf is showing severe coughing. Several antibiotics are of use, including tylosin at 4–10 mg/kg (2–5 mg/lb) body weight, oxytetracycline at 10 mg/kg (5 mg/lb) body weight, spiramycin at a dose of 20 mg/kg (10 mg/lb) body weight or spectinomycin at 20–30 mg/kg (10–15 mg/lb) body weight. The macrolide antibiotics (tylosin, erythromycin, spiramycin) are all concentrated in the lungs and have good efficacy against mycoplasmal infections.

Acute.

1 Antimicrobials. If more than 30 per cent of the animals are affected and need treatment it is probable that many others are incubating the condition, so that it is often a good policy to persuade the farmer to treat all the cattle in the group. As with most disease, the earlier treatment is started, the less the mortality and the fewer the animals that have to be culled because of chronic disease. The drugs commonly used are given in Table 15.2. The therapeutic agent administered should have a broad spectrum of activity and ideally it should be bactericidal. The choice will most probably have to be based on previous successful usage on that farm or elsewhere. It is best not to use long-acting preparations because if there is no response to treatment it will make the initiation of subsequent therapy very difficult. If an animal dies then culture of swabs from the lung, bronchial and mediastinal lymph nodes and the subsequent antibiotic sensitivity of the isolates may be of use. The ideal is to culture swabs from material in carcasses that have not been treated. The culture of nasal or pharyngeal swabs from live infected calves is of dubious value as it cannot be certain that the organism cultured will be the same as the one causing disease in the lungs.

Therapy should be continued for three to five days, depending on the drug used and the response to treatment. In acute cases the choice of antimicrobial agent is normally dictated by those that can be given intravenously. Intratracheal administration of antibiotics has been advocated by some practitioners and in such cases those in aqueous solution are preferable to those in organic solvent. No antibiotic is at present licensed in Britain for this route of administration. Those compounds most commonly used have included erythromycin, trimethoprim and sulphadoxine.

2 Corticosteroids. Some of the compounds available are shown in Table 15.3. The drugs commonly in use today include betamethasone, dexamethasone, prednisolone, flumethasone and triamcinolone. These compounds only provide symptomatic relief and do not cure the condition. Many people consider them to be overused (Pirie, 1979), but often an animal will show little or no improvement on antibiotic therapy alone, only to recover rapidly once corticosteroids are added to the treatment regimen. Their action is to suppress all stages of inflammation regardless as to whether the cause is physical, chemical or immunological in origin. Thus in the acute stage, corticosteroids reduce vasodilation, oedema formation and leucocyte infiltration (Eyre, 1978). The drugs also have a 'euphoric' effect on the dull animal and this may allow the calf to eat and otherwise speed its recovery (Pirie, 1979).

The main problem with corticosteroids is the unselective suppression of inflammation that therefore includes those parts of the inflammatory and immune response, such as macrophage infiltration, which are concerned with the control and removal of infectious organisms. In such an environment an organism can multiply and spread within the animal. This may be the agent that caused the pneumonia or an opportunist organism that enters the body. The reduction in the immune response can also increase the ability of the same organisms to reinfect the animal following recovery. It is therefore essential that antibiotic therapy is administered concurrently with corticosteroid therapy and in most circumstances it is probable that a bactericidal drug is indicated rather than a bacteriostatic drug. Adequate therapeutic doses of the antibiotic should be given and maintained for sufficient time. Another problem with the prolonged use of cortico-

Table 15.2 Some of the antimicrobial compounds used in calf pneumonia therapy

Antimicrobial compounds	Bactericidal (C) or bacteriostatic (S)	Route of administration	Dosage (mg/kg)	Dosage (mg/lb)
Amoxycillin	C	i.v., s.c., i.m., oral	7	3.5
Ampicillin	C	i.v., s.c., i.m., oral	2–7	1–3.5
Ceftiofur	C	i.m.	1.1	0.5
Chloramphenicol	S	i.v., s.c., i.m., oral	4–10	2–5
Danofloxacin	C	i.m.	1.25	0.6
Erythromycin	S	i.m.	2.5–5	1.25–2.5
Oxytetracycline	S	i.v., s.c., i.m., oral	10	5
Penicillin plus streptomycin	C	s.c., i.m.	10–20 10–15	5–10 5–7.5
Spectinomycin	C	i.v., i.m., oral	12.5–30	6.25–15
Spiramycin	S	i.m., oral	20	10
Sulphadimidine	S	i.v., s.c., oral		
initial			200	100
maintenance			100	50
Sulphamethoxypyridazine	S	i.v., s.c., i.m.	22	11
Sulphapyrazole	S	i.v., s.c., i.m.	30–100	15–50
Tilmicosin	S	s.c.	10	5
Trimethoprim and sulphadiazine	C	i.m., oral	15–22.5	7.5–12
Trimethoprim and sulphadoxine	C	i.v., i.m.	15	7.5
Tylosin	S	i.m., oral	4–10	2–5

Table 15.3 Corticosteroids used in respiratory disease in calves

Drug	Dose per animal (mg)
Betamethasone	2–10
Cortisone	up to 500
Dexamethasone	2–5
Flumethasone	0.5
Hydrocortisone	up to 300
Prednisolone	up to 20
Triamcinolone	up to 5

steroids is that there is a risk of inducing permanent adrenal insufficiency, but this has produced little worry in cattle.

3 Non-steroidal anti-inflammatory drugs (NSAIDs). These drugs are salicylate-like compounds and although many are not registered for use in cattle, they do help reduce inflammatory reactions by blocking the synthesis of prostaglandins and inhibiting kinin formation (see p. 860). They also antagonize the actions of some of the chemical mediators in the lungs such as 5-hydroxytryptamine (5-HT) and histamine, which are mainly released from mast cells in response to antibody–antigen reactions (Pirie, 1979). Besides an anti-inflammatory action, NSAIDs have two properties that corticosteroids do not possess, namely they are antipyretic and analgesic. Until the availability of flunixin these compounds were little used in Britain although they are frequently prescribed in Holland where corticosteroids are not allowed to be used for respiratory diseases in calves. The main drugs available are shown in Table 15.4. The drugs most commonly available in Britain are flunixin meglumine, meclofenamic acid and phenylbutazone.

4 Antihistamines. These drugs have been used in the past but most clinicians have found them to be of little use in calf pneumonia. This is probably because the

Table 15.4 Non-steroidal anti-inflammatory drugs

	Route of administration	Dose*
Acetyl salicylic acid	Oral	1.0–4.0 g/animal
Flunixin meglumine	Injection	2.2 mg/kg (1.0 mg/lb)
Ibuprofen	Oral	10 mg/kg (5 mg/lb)
Indomethacin		
Mefenamic acid		
Meclofenamic acid	Oral	2.2 mg/kg (1.1 mg/lb)
Naproxen	Oral	10 mg/kg (5 mg/lb)
Phenylbutazone	Oral/injection	4.4 mg/kg (2.2 mg/lb)
Sodium meclophenamate		

* Doses are only guidelines. Note that most of the drugs are not registered for use in cattle.

main chemical mediator of cattle is not histamine but 5-HT. The histamine that is released occurs very quickly following the antibody–antigen reaction so that antihistamines can only be of use in the early stages of the inflammatory response (Pirie, 1979).

5 Sympathomimetics. These drugs (see Table 15.5) are all adrenaline-like and their actions to a varying degree are similar to it. Adrenaline causes an increased heart rate followed by slower, more powerful contractions mediated by the aortic and carotid reflexes. The resulting increased blood pressure causes passive dilatation of the blood vessels of the brain, lungs and heart. The blood supply to the skin, kidneys and alimentary tract is reduced. There is a decrease in the permeability of the capillaries and so a reduction in oedema formation occurs. Bronchial relaxation takes place allowing easier lung aeration.

Although both adrenaline and isoprenaline are of some use in relieving respiratory signs, they are little used because of their stimulatory effects on the heart. This is because adrenaline acts on many types of receptors that are designated α and β, those of the heart and lung being β_1 and β_2 receptors, respectively. Recent work has produced compounds that will act on only one type of receptor and not on the others. Thus salbutamol acts specifically on the bronchial receptors and is a specific bronchodilator.

6 Xanthine derivatives. Those commonly in use are etamiphylline camsylate and diprophylline, but others are available and are given in Table 15.6. Their actions are relatively similar to those of adrenaline. There is stimulation of the central nervous system where caffeine is the most powerful, myocardial stimulation where aminophylline and diprophylline are strongest, bronchodilation and diuresis. Their main uses in respiratory disease are bronchodilation and, to a secondary extent, fluid removal. The mild action of these drugs compared with substances such as adrenaline means that they are all relatively safe.

7 Expectorants. One drug used at present as a spas-

Table 15.5 Sympathomimetics used in the treatment of respiratory disease

	Route of administration	Dose
Adrenaline 1 in 1000	s.c., i.m.	0.2–0.4 ml/50 kg (100 lb)
	i.v.	0.1–0.2 ml/50 kg (100 lb)
Amphetamine*	s.c., i.m.	0.2–0.6 mg/kg (0.1–0.3 mg/lb)
Clenbuterol**	i.v., i.m. oral	0.8 μg/kg (0.4 μg/lb)
Isoprenaline**		
Methylamphetamine*	s.c., i.m.	0.1–0.3 mg/kg (0.05–0.15 mg/lb)
Salbutamol**		

* Amphetamines are indirect-acting sympathomimetic compounds and because of their abuse in humans they can no longer be prescribed in Britain and other countries by veterinary surgeons.

** These drugs are not registered in some countries for use in cattle respiratory conditions.

Table 15.6 Xanthine derivatives that can be used in respiratory disease

	Route of administration	Dose
Aminophylline	oral	0.15–0.3 g/calf
	s.c.	0.3–1.5 g/calf
Diprophylline	i.v., i.m.	0.12–0.5 g/calf
Etamiphylline camsylate	i.m., s.c., oral	0.7–1.05 g/calf
Theobromine	oral	1.0–2.0 g/calf

molytic is bromhexine hydrochloride, which can be given orally or by intramuscular injection at a dose of about 0.5 mg/kg body weight for five to seven days. Its action is mainly to reduce the viscosity of mucus and thereby help in its expulsion, resulting in improved respiratory function. Other expectorants are often used in chronic cases of coughing. These include a mixture of strychnine hydroxide, arsenic trioxide and ferric ammonium citrate green at a dose of about 5 ml orally twice daily, or diphenhydramine hydrochloride, ammonium chloride, sodium citrate and menthol at 5–10 ml orally two or three times daily. There is limited benefit from the antihistaminic action of diphenhydramine hydrochloride in cases of calf pneumonia.

8 Antisera. Several antisera are available that have been produced either in cattle or horses against *P. multocida*, the septicaemic and pneumonic strains of *P. haemolytica* and, in some cases, diplococci. Little experimental work is available to demonstrate their efficacy or lack of it and so their use is speculative (Thomas, 1979). As has already been indicated there are numerous organisms involved in the aetiology of calf pneumonia and it would be only right to expect benefit in some cases where the organisms in the antisera are a major factor in the disease process.

9 Supportive therapy. During the disease phase many animals become partially or completely anorexic and it has been suggested that multivitamin injections, particularly of the vitamin B group may be of use in overcoming any temporary deficiencies that might occur as the result of the low storage of vitamins (Thomas, 1979). As vitamin A is of use in epithelial repair it may be advantageous to inject this compound to ensure speedy respiratory mucosal regeneration.

10 Nursing. As with many other diseases, although nursing is important, it is often neglected. Affected animals should be removed from the in-contact group partly to reduce spread of infection and also to allow access to feed and water away from competition. Food supplied should be highly palatable and non-dusty to encourage uptake. The environment of the convalescent calf should include plenty of bedding, and draughts must be avoided. The provision of oxygen by means of a mask and reducing valve has been used in animals at indoor agricultural and fatstock shows.

11 Vaccination. It is possible to obtain rapid confirmation as to the aetiology of outbreaks of calf pneumonia. If the cause is viral it is possible to use live vaccines and to vaccinate in the face of an outbreak. This can be very effective provided it is undertaken in the early stages of disease among the group. It appears to produce non-specific interferon followed by good specific immunity to the virus vaccinated against. To be effective a live vaccine needs to be used and it must be administered intranasally.

Prevention

As the disease is multifactorial, preventive measures include attention to management as well as possible vaccination. Thus ensuring there are no more than 30 calves in any one air space as well as making sure that different age groups are not mixed is helpful. If disease tends to follow particular patterns it is best to alter the time of undertaking stressful procedures such as weaning, castration and disbudding. Often ensuring castration and disbudding are undertaken more than two weeks before weaning can be helpful. Increasing the duration of feeding milk substitute can also be useful, as well as ensuring weaning is not undertaken at a time when this is likely to result in pneumonia. Gradual weaning is often helpful, particularly when cattle are fed in groups on a milk dispensing machine that will provide feed throughout the 24 hours.

When calves are home-reared, it should be ensured that they receive adequate amounts of colostrum. All calves should be given adequate good quality feed. If calves are bought-in they should be examined at entry and any which show purulent ocular or nasal discharge rejected. Calves should not receive dusty or overmilled feed. As disease occurs on the same farms year after year, the time when disease starts should be noted and checked to see if it can be associated with any changes in management, etc. Calves bought as batches should be kept together and not mixed with other batches. An all-in all-out policy for rearing calves is best advocated. Ideally, calves should be reared before and after weaning in the same building for at least a month and preferably longer.

There are various vaccines available and, as might be expected with a disease of such complex aetiology, the results experienced by different farmers and veterinary surgeons are extremely variable (see p. 809). In some cases this may be due to the type of vaccine used. It is thought that the age incidence of enzootic pneumonia may well coincide with the decline in colostral immunity. Thus peak onset of pneumonia in housed calves is often at two to four months old when concentrations of serum IgG_1, IgG_2 and IgA are at their lowest (Corbeil *et al.*, 1984). It must also be remembered that several of the pathogens involved in the disease complex are immunosuppressive. These organisms include *M. dispar*, ureaplasmas and *M. bovis* as well as BRSV. In consequence, vaccination of calves where the organisms are already present in the animals is likely to reduce the immune response.

Dead vaccines are used to provide immunity against *P. multocida* and septicaemic and pneumonic strains of *P. haemolytica*. It is probable that a new, more efficacious *P. haemolytica* vaccine will become available following successful experimental work (Gilmour *et al.*, 1979). A killed polyvalent vaccine is available for bovine parainfluenza III virus, bovine adenovirus III, bovine reovirus I, bovine viral diarrhoea and infectious bovine rhinotracheitis virus. This is given by intramuscular injection and on farms where disease occurs before six weeks old the first two doses are given two or four weeks apart with a third dose at 10 to 12 weeks old. Few trials have been conducted into efficacy, but those available do suggest it is of limited value (Phillips *et al.*, 1973; Morzaria *et al.*, 1978). Subsequently, modified live intranasal vaccines have been available. A study of the live vaccine in the absence of disease showed virus could be isolated from most animals (10/11) and there was seroconversion in 7/11 (Lucas *et al.*, 1982). Although good immunity was conferred to animals by modified live vaccination, it was shown that some cattle became carriers after exposure to field strains of IBR (Nettleton & Sharp, 1980).

A dead vaccine has been produced against *M. bovis*, but it has had only limited success experimentally. There are several live vaccines used in Europe including ones against respiratory syncytial virus and parainfluenza III virus. A vaccine for PI3 has been licensed and it is possible others will eventually be available in Britain and elsewhere.

From experience, the vaccines themselves do appear to have variable results on individual farms. This is probably due to the type of vaccine used, i.e. live or dead, other underlying pathogens, the level of infective dose and whether or not the particular pathogens present in the vaccine are responsible for disease on that farm. There is a particular problem for farmers who continually buy-in batches of calves as the pathogens introduced with each group are likely to be different. Thus it is very difficult to create a suitable vaccination policy to prevent pneumonia, unless several vaccines are used to cover most of the major pathogens. Such a policy is obviously costly and at times very wasteful as it will result in immunization for diseases that are not present. This has led to the suggestion that in such units it is best to make a diagnosis as to the likely cause of enzootic pneumonia in the first animal(s) to be affected. If the agent is primary viral then the calves can be vaccinated in the face of an outbreak.

References

Bryson, D.G., McFerran, J.B., Ball, H.J. & Neill, S.D. (1978) Observations on outbreaks of respiratory disease in housed calves. I: Epidemiology, clinical and microbiological findings. *Veterinary Record*, **103**, 485–9.

Corbeil, L.B., Watt, B., Corbeil, R.R., Betzen, T.G., Brownson, R.K. & Morrill, J.L. (1984) Immunoglobulin concentrations in serum and nasal secretions of calves at the onset of pneumonia. *American Journal of Veterinary Research*, **45**, 773–8.

Eyre, P. (1978) Pharmacological considerations of current methods of therapy. In *Respiratory Diseases in Cattle. Current Topics in Veterinary Medicine Volume 3* (ed. by W.B. Martin), pp. 409–16. Martinus Nijhoff, The Hague.

Gilmour, N.J.L., Martin, W.B., Sharp, J.M., Thompson, D.A. & Wells, P.W. (1979) The development of vaccines against pneumonic pasteurellosis in sheep. *Veterinary Record*, **104**, 15.

Gordon, W.A.M. (1963) Environmental studies in pig housing. IV. The bacterial content of air in piggeries and its influence on disease incidence. *British Veterinary Journal*, **119**, 263–73.

Green, G.M. & Kass, E.H. (1965) The influence of bacterial species on pulmonary resistance to infection in mice subjected to hypoxia, cold stress and ethanol intoxication. *British Journal of Experimental Pathology*, **46**, 360–6.

Jones, C.R. & Webster, A.J.F. (1981) Weather-induced changes in airborne bacteria within a calf house. *Veterinary Record*, **109**, 493–4.

Lacey, J.C. (1968) The microflora of fodders associated with bovine respiratory disease. Journal of General Microbiology, **51**, 173–7.

Lucas, M.H., Roberts, D.H., Sands, J.J. & Westcott, D.V.E. (1982) The use of infectious bovine rhinotracheitis vaccine in a commercial veal unit: antibody response and spread of virus. *British Veterinary Journal*, **138**, 23–8.

Miller, W.M., Harkness, J.W., Richards, M.S. & Pritchard, D.G. (1980) Epidemiological studies of calf respiratory disease in a large commercial veal unit. *Research in Veterinary Science*, **28**, 267–74.

Morzaria, S.P., Maund, B.A., Richards, M.S. & Harkness, J.W. (1978) Results of a small field trial with a multicomponent inactivated respiratory viral vaccine. In *Respiratory Diseases of Cattle. Current Topics in Veterinary Medicine, Volume 3* (ed. by W.B. Martin), pp. 497–508. Martinus Nijhoff, The Hague.

Nettleton, P.F. & Sharp, J.M. (1980) Infectious bovine rhinotracheitis virus excretion after vaccination. *Veterinary Record*, **107**, 379.

Phillips, J.I.H. (1975) Bovine respiratory disease. In *Veterinary Annual*, 15th issue (ed. by C.S.G. Grunsell & F.W.G. Hill), pp. 13–15. Wright, Bristol.

Phillips, J.I.H., Clegg, F.G., Halliday, C.J., Cross, M.H., Hardy, R. & Maund, B.A. (1973) An examination of two bovine respiratory disease vaccines. *Veterinary Record*, **92**, 420–4.

Pirie, H.M. (1979) *Respiratory Diseases of Animals*, pp. 68–70. Notes for a Postgraduate Course, Glasgow Veterinary School.

Roy, J.H.B. (1980) *The Calf*, 4th edn. Butterworth, London.

Roy, J.H.B., Stobo, J.F., Gaston, H.J.G., Anderton, P., Shotton, J.M. & Ostler, D.C. (1971) The effect of environmental temperature on the performance and health of the preruminant and ruminant calf. *British Journal of Nutrition*, **26**, 363–81.

Thomas, L.H. (1978) Disease incidence and epidemics — the situation in the UK. In *Respiratory Diseases of Cattle. Current Topics in Veterinary Medicine, Volume 3* (ed. by W.B. Martin), pp. 57–65. Martinus Nijhoff, The Hague.

Thomas, L.H. (1979) *Respiratory Disease in Housed Calves*, pp. 1–22. Booklet 2181. MAFF Publications, Middlesex.

Thomas, L.H. & Swann, R.C. (1973) Influence of colostrum on the incidence of calf pneumonia. *Veterinary Record*, **92**, 454–5.

Thomas, L.H., Wood, R.D.P. & Longland, J.M. (1978) The influence of disease on the performance of beef cattle. *British Veterinary Journal*, **134**, 152–61.

Thomson, R.G. & Gilka, F. (1974) A brief review of pulmonary clearance of bacterial aerosols emphasizing aspects of particular relevance to veterinary medicine. Canadian Veterinary Journal, **15**, 99–107.

Veit, H.P., Farrell, R.T. & Troutt, H.F. (1978) Pulmonary clearance of *Serratia marcescens* in calves. *American Journal of Veterinary Research*, **39**, 1646–50.

Webster, A.J.F. (1979) Housing and husbandry of the veal calf. In *Veterinary Annual*, 19th issue (ed. by C.S.G. Grunsell & F.W.G. Hill), pp. 49–53. Scientechnica, Bristol.

Webster, A.J.F. (1981a) Optimal housing criteria for ruminants. In: *Environmental Aspects of Housing for Animal Production*. Proceedings of 31st Easter School, University of Nottingham School of Agriculture (ed. by J.A. Clark), pp. 217–32. Butterworths, Sevenoaks.

Webster, A.J.F. (1981b) Weather and infectious disease in cattle. *Veterinary Record*, **108**, 183–7.

Williams, M.R., Spooner, R.P.L. & Thomas, L.H. (1975) Quantitative studies on bovine immunoglobulins. *Veterinary Record*, **96**, 81–4.

Wiseman, A. (1978) Influence of environment on respiratory disease. In *Respiratory Diseases of Cattle. Current Topics in Veterinary Medicine, Volume 3* (ed. by W.B. Martin), pp. 149–57. Martinus Nijhoff, The Hague.

Chapter 16: Other Calf Problems

by A.H. ANDREWS

Joint or navel ill (see p. 384)

Joint or navel ill is a common problem in the calf. At birth there is a sudden change from the fetal circulation to that of the newborn calf. The blood vessels in the umbilical cord rapidly lose most of the blood within them but still remain patent, thereby allowing the introduction of infection. Infection can be caused by a single organism or a mixture. A wide variety can be involved including *Streptococcus* spp., *Escherichia coli*, *Erysipelothrix insidiosa*, *Pasteurella multocida*, *Actinomyces (Corynebacterium) pyogenes* and *Fusobacterium necrophorum*. The problem normally arises from calving taking place in conditions with poor hygiene. Often the calf will not have had sufficient intake of colostrum and usually the navel will not have been treated.

Infection enters the umbilicus and may result in a local reaction at the point of entry into the body, between the muscle layers or in the peritoneum. In other cases entry is via the urachus and can lead to local infection. Otherwise the bacteria may pass via the umbilical vein to the liver and then in the blood to the body. When infection is present in the blood it may cause a septicaemia or eventually result in chronic illness due to localization in organs such as the heart, brain, eye and most often the joints.

Signs

The signs vary and can be restricted to local inflammation of the navel or the abdominal wall muscles. In such cases the navel is swollen, soft and usually painful. The umbilical blood vessels are swollen at their base. Localized peritonitis may be difficult to detect. Where there is septicaemia, the calf rapidly becomes ill with depression, pyrexia (40.5 °C, 105 °F) and accelerated respiratory and pulse rates. The mucous membranes become reddened and there are often petechial haemorrhages. There may be a varying degree of dehydration, followed later by acidosis, recumbency and death.

In cases of bacteraemia that localize, the signs are often missed for several weeks or even months. In some animals there is inappetance, dullness and an intermittent slightly raised temperature (39–40 °C, 103–104 °F). Other signs depend on the organs affected. When there is local infection of the urachus the animal will become unthrifty and slightly slow to move. There may be a slightly raised tail with micturition. In animals with localization in the heart valves, endocarditis results with a heart murmur. If the eye is involved there is panophthalmitis with hypopyon. In the case of meningitis there is likely to be nystagmus, hyperaesthesia and tonic–clonic convulsions. The most common form is joint ill and one or more joints may be involved. In many cases there is bilateral involvement with pain and swelling, commonly of the carpal joints. Aspiration of the affected joints usually reveals thick pus. The animal tends to become lame and to have an altered stance.

Necropsy

Post-mortem examination may reveal the presence of infection in the umbilical vessels, which are swollen and contain blood. There may be localized peritonitis. In the septicaemic form petechial and ecchymotic haemorrhages are evident on the subserosa and submucosa of various organs. In the more chronic form various organs will show inflammation and abscessation.

Diagnosis

Diagnosis is aided by the presence of a swollen navel as well as by the signs. There may be a neutrophilia and blood culture may be helpful. The main difficulty is in differentiating the condition from other forms of enteritis, septicaemia and locomotor problems such as muscular dystrophy (see p. 222).

Treatment and control

Treatment of the septicaemia will usually involve the use of antimicrobials, which in the main should be given intravenously. Appropriate antibiotics include amoxycillin, ampicillin, oxytetracycline, sulphonamides or potentiated sulphonamides. Chloramphenicol can be of use. In less severe cases other treatments such as penicillin and streptomycin may be given by the parenteral routes. The duration of therapy should be at least five days. If the animals are dehydrated, parenteral or oral electrolyte solutions will be required. In the more localized forms involving the navel or urachus, the infected material should be removed. There are problems in the treatment of localized chronic infection such as joint ill. In some cases the use of potentiated sulphonamides or lincomycin by injection has given good results. Surgical opening of the joints with removal of pus and affected tissue and joint flushing can be useful.

Control is dependent on whether the calves are on their farm of origin or have been bought-in. If the former, then all navels should be dipped immediately after birth in an appropriate disinfectant. Tincture of iodine or iodine teat washes are useful for this purpose. Generally they allow the navel to be sterilized and help to cause desiccation. Antibiotic aerosols are used but it is often difficult to ensure the whole navel is completely covered. In purchased animals the navels should be examined, and calves with enlarged navels rejected. The joints of the animals should also be inspected. The navels should be dipped in an appropriate disinfectant solution on arrival at the farm.

Oral and laryngeal necrobacillosis

This is also known as calf diphtheria and there are two forms, oral which is most common, and laryngeal. The condition is caused by *Fusobacterium necrophorum*.

Oral form

This is quite common and is usually sporadic in occurrence although there may be outbreaks where hygiene is poor. In such cases it is probably spread by dirty milk pails, machine teats or feeding containers. Individual cases sometimes occur where fibrous and coarse food is offered. Although mainly seen in housed calves, it can also occur at pasture. Affected calves are usually up to three months old and often have intercurrent disease, nutritional deficiency or their teeth are erupting. The incubation period is about four days.

Signs

The major sign is a swelling of the cheek, particularly in the region of the first cheek teeth. The calf is often bright and active with a normal temperature. Opening the mouth reveals a necrotic swelling in the cheek, in which may be impacted food material, and there may be a foul smell. The animal may salivate a little. In a few cases there is also involvement of the tongue, which may become swollen and protrude from the mouth. Neglected cases may extend to the nasal cavity, pharynx, lungs, abomasum and coronets of the legs.

Necropsy

On post mortem oral lesions are usually well circumscribed with an area of oedema and a necrotic centre. If the necrotic area is lost, an ulcer is seen.

Diagnosis

The main differential diagnoses are foreign bodies in the mouth, papular stomatitis, mouth and jaw injuries and mucosal disease. All are quite easy to eliminate by thorough oral examination.

Laryngeal form

This form is less common and is sporadic in occurrence. It has been seen in animals up to and over a year old.

Signs

These cattle tend to be dull with inappetance or anorexia. Often there is pyrexia (40.5 °C, 105 °F) and there may be stertor. Usually respirations are dyspnoeic to a varying degree. There is a cough that is moist and painful. Palpation of the larynx is resented and can elicit the cough. The mouth may be foul smelling. Many of these animals do not respond well to treatment and the diphtheritic area may become detached resulting in sudden asphyxiation or lung infection.

Necropsy

The lesion in the larynx is normally well embedded into the laryngeal cartilage. When lung lesions occur there are necrotic areas present surrounded by a catarrhal pneumonia.

Diagnosis

The main differential diagnoses are laryngeal oedema, laryngitis and vocal cord paralysis. These may be hard to eliminate unless an endoscopic examination is undertaken or an exploratory laryngotomy is performed.

Treatment

In either case the animal should be isolated from the others. It should have its own feed and water buckets. In the oral form, parenteral or oral therapy is usually successful. Suitable antibacterial agents include oxytetracycline, potentiated sulphonamides, streptomycin, sulphonamides orally or parenterally or penicillin parenterally. Therapy for three to five days is usually sufficient. When the animal is inappetant it should be encouraged to eat. In the laryngeal form, therapy needs to be continued for longer and should be parenteral. If breathing is very laboured then it may be necessary to undertake a tracheotomy and insert a tracheal tube. In some cases success is only achieved by surgical removal of the necrotic area and then using an intratracheal tube until the laryngeal oedema has reduced.

Control

If more than a single case occurs, hygiene should be improved. The calves should be fed with their own buckets and quality feed should be used. The milk and water buckets should be cleaned and disinfected after each feed and the feed bucket disinfected at least twice a week. Occasionally, it is necessary to give oral antibiotics as a prophylactic measure. Suitable agents include chlortetracycline and oxytetracycline.

Meningitis

This is an inflammation of the meninges. The condition is uncommon and most often occurs following a pre-existing disease such as septicaemia. The organisms that can be involved are usually bacteria and include *Listeria monocytogenes*, *Escherichia coli*, *Pasteurella multocida* and *Haemophilus somnus*. A secondary meningitis can follow infection with *Mycobacterium bovis*. Although most cases are haematogenous in origin, a few result from spread of local infection or can follow disbudding, skull injuries, otitis media or frontal sinusitis. In most instances meningitis is the result of central infection causing local swelling and inflammation around the nerve trunks. Spinal meningitis will often lead to hyperaesthesia of the body, muscular tremors in the limbs and neck and an arched back.

Signs

The condition usually starts with a sudden onset of pyrexia and in many cases toxaemia. There is hyperaesthesia to any cutaneous sensation and muscular tremors of the neck and head with opisthotonus and paddling movements of the limbs. There may be ocular lesions with hypopyon and ophthalmitis. The animal may appear blind and the pupillary reflex may be sluggish. Ophthalmoscopic examination may show the retinal irises to be engorged with oedema of the optic disc.

Necropsy

On post-mortem examination the meninges are thickened and opaque, especially ventrally, and there is engorgement of the meningeal vessels with haemorrhaging. The cerebrospinal fluid (CSF) is often cloudy.

Diagnosis

This is difficult in the live animal but the nervous signs are an indication and there is a leucocytosis. Confirmation can only be obtained by examination of the CSF, showing it to be cloudy with a high white cell count and possibly bacteria present. The differential diagnosis includes coccidiosis (see p. 243), septicaemia, vitamin

A deficiency (see p. 220), hypomagnesaemia (see p. 219) and poisoning with various substances (see Chapter 41).

Treatment and control

Treatment involves the use of a broad-spectrum antimicrobial that will penetrate the blood–brain barrier. The potentiated sulphonamides or chloramphenicol are probably most useful and the latter may be preferable because high levels diffuse into the CSF. Prevention is difficult but should involve the rapid treatment of all septicaemias, otitis or local injuries. Disbudding should always be undertaken with care.

Otitis

Otitis media and externa both occur. The condition has recently been more frequently diagnosed in calf-rearing units in America and Britain. The cause is unknown but most outbreaks have been preceded by enzootic pneumonia and it is thus possible that an ascending infection occurs along the Eustachian tube. In some outbreaks up to 30 per cent of calves have been involved. In individual cases of otitis media there may be extension from an otitis externa or from navel infection via the haematogenous route. The organisms involved vary but vitamin A deficiencies have been reported in some outbreaks. The external ear is such that there are streptococci and staphylococci present. When there is middle ear infection these two species may be present, or *P. haemolytica*, *Haemophilus* spp. or *Neisseria catarrhalis*.

Signs

In otitis externa the animal is well and has a normal temperature but the ear tends to be droopy with a foul-smelling purulent discharge. In middle ear infection, unless bilateral, the head is rotated and there is a degree of incoordination. The animal is often dull and there is inappetance. Radiography may show rarefaction of the tympanic bulla.

Diagnosis

This condition is differentiated from brain or spinal abscesses or injury by the rotation of the head.

Treatment and control

Treatment of the external form is relatively simple and involves the local application of antibiotics, in practice often from intramammary tubes. Suitable antibiotics include cloxacillin, chlortetracycline and penicillin and streptomycin. Otitis media is much less satisfactory to treat and involves puncturing the tympanic mucosa, irrigation with antiseptic solutions and local and parenteral antibiotics. Prevention is difficult as the cause is often unclear but it should involve adequate treatment of all cases of calf pneumonia.

Bovine papular stomatitis (BPS)

This is caused by a virus of the genus parapoxvirus. The condition is very common throughout the world. Lesions can occur in any age of animal and both sexes. However, most lesions are seen in young cattle. The virus causes pseudo-cowpox in cows (see p. 322). The organism has a high morbidity and is found in the saliva and nasal secretions. Spread is by contact. The disease is usually of little importance except in the differential diagnosis of other oral lesions, although occasionally it can be of financial significance. The condition found is variable but can be seen in calves of seven days old. It can be transferred to others, particularly following a bite, cut or scratch. Most lesions are local but may take many weeks to heal. Occasionally, systemic signs occur.

Signs

The lesions vary in severity. The mild form is the most common with the animal remaining healthy, eating well with no evidence of pyrexia, diarrhoea or respiratory distress. The lesions tend to be ring-like and pathognomonic. The periphery of the lesion is a thin red zone, within which is a white, slightly raised area of hyperplasia, with a yellow or brown centre due to tissue necrosis. Lesions heal from the middle outwards. Most involve the rhinarium and mouth and are often found near erupting teeth. Occasionally, a second type of lesion is a brownish-purple colour and usually the size of the ring lesions. It heals from the middle outwards producing a horseshoe shape lasting from four days to about two weeks. However, areas of lesions may last several months overall.

The severe form is less common and often associated with other intercurrent disease, e.g. parasitism. Lesions are slightly raised, diffuse and roughened, and are yellow or grey in colour. They are seen in any part of the mouth and can involve marked sloughing of the mucosae. As the more diffuse lesions heal an underlying circular form often remains. In some cases saliva is held in the mouth making the lips wet.

Necropsy

Death from BPS is rare. Most lesions are in the mouth or rhinarium but may occasionally be seen in the oesophagus, rumen, reticulum and abomasum. Typically, there are no vesicles and on histology there is a ballooning degeneration of the stratum spinosum cells, which may contain eosinophilic intracytoplasmic inclusion bodies.

Diagnosis

Diagnosis is dependent on examining the lesions, the animal remaining healthy, viral isolation, histopathology and use of an electron microscope. Immunity can be measured by the serum neutralization test but levels are usually low. The main conditions to be differentiated are foot-and-mouth disease, mucosal disease, malignant catarrhal fever, rinderpest, vesicular stomatitis and mycotic stomatitis.

Treatment

Treatment is not justified but in severe cases concurrent infections can be treated. Antibiotic therapy is recommended to resolve secondary infections. Prevention is not practical at present but the condition is less severe in healthy herds so good nutrition and freedom from parasites are important.

Calcium, phosphorus and vitamin D deficiency (see p. 391)

These conditions are all closely related and it is best to consider them together. All three compounds can lead to primary and secondary deficiency, but conditions relating to their lack are very rare in calves. The diseases of the skeleton that do occur are usually associated with faulty mineral supply rather than vitamin D problems.

Calcium is well absorbed in the calf's small intestine. Therefore, primary deficiency is extremely unlikely, as is secondary deficiency, which could possibly occur if very high levels of cereals were fed without additives or high phosphorus levels were used. The daily calcium requirement of calves is 10–30 g ($\frac{1}{3}$–1 oz) depending on size and growth rate.

Phosphorus is very efficiently absorbed from milk, but less so from dry feeds. Primary deficiencies may resemble rickets. Secondary problems resulting from low vitamin D levels, high calcium or high vitamin A are rare. Phosphorus deficiency is widespread due to the types of soil present in an area. Leaching by rain or constant removal by cropping can lead to phosphorus-deficient soil. Excessive calcium, iron or aluminium can also result in the problem. The optimum calcium : phosphorus ratio is 2 : 1.

Vitamin D is usually provided by good quality hay and exposure to sunlight. Present feeding systems include supplementation of milk substitutes and so do not normally predispose to the problem, although lush green feeds contain much carotene and other substances that have anti-vitamin D properties. The optimal daily intake is 7–12 iu/kg body weight (3.5–6 iu/lb).

Signs

The signs are usually only seen in the best-growing calves. There is some degree of lameness, particularly of the forelimbs, which are bent forwards or laterally. The limb joints and costochondral junctions are swollen. In some calves the back will be arched and in severe cases the tail is elevated. There may be a marked tendency to lie down.

Necropsy

On death the animal is in poor condition. The ribs are easily cut and the limb bones are soft with thin, compact bone and they are easily fractured. The joints tend to be enlarged with thickened epiphyseal cartilage.

Diagnosis

Diagnosis is usually on clinical signs. The alkaline phosphatase level will be raised. The levels of serum calcium and phosphorus will depend on the cause of the condition but phosphorus will be low if it is due either to vitamin D or phosphorus deficiency. Radiographic examination shows the bones to lack density and the ends have a diffuse appearance. The epiphyses tend to be widened and irregular. The ash content of the bone is reduced from 60 per cent to 45 per cent and the ash : organic matter ratio will be reduced from the normal 3 : 2. The main problems to be differentiated are copper deficiency (but the plasma and/or liver copper concentrations will be low), arthritis and epiphysitis.

Treatment and prevention

Treatment varies according to the cause. In minor Ca : P imbalances sufficient vitamin D is all that is necessary. Where the skeletal deformities are pronounced, treatment will have only limited effect. Otherwise in calcium deficiency check there is no excess phosphorus present. Calcium should be provided but not to excess as this may cause other deficiencies. If phosphorus is deficient, dicalcium phosphorus or disodium phosphate should be used. The ratio of calcium : phosphorus of 2 : 1 should be provided by the diet. A vitamin D injection of 3000–5000 iu/kg body weight will provide adequate levels for one to three months. Response to treatment is usually slow. Prevention requires ensuring adequate levels of minerals and vitamin D in the diet. Bone meal and dicalcium phosphate are ideal sources of both calcium and phosphorus but they are expensive. Ground limestone is a useful cheap method of ensuring adequate calcium in the diet, but its overuse can result in other mineral deficiencies.

Copper deficiency

This is either primary due to a lack of copper in the diet or secondary when the dietary level is adequate but there is a failure in digestion, absorption or metabolism of the copper. In calves, deficiency can be seen at a few weeks old although it is much more common when three or four months old. This is because copper is stored in the liver and there is preferential absorption from the dam. Milk contains little copper although levels are high in colostrum. In the milk-fed animal absorption in the small intestine is high (up to 80 per cent) but this falls as the animal becomes a ruminant (2–10 per cent). Milk substitutes tend to be supplemented with copper and so most cases arise in calves sucking their dams or at grass. Problems often occur in the spring or summer when the mineral content tends to be lower.

Primary deficiency depends on the soil type and is common on sandy soil, particularly where there is much rain and leaching, and on peat. Secondary deficiencies are probably more numerous than primary. They can be due to high molybdenum levels and this effect is increased by the presence of sulphur, which may be in the form of protein. High levels of iron, zinc, lead, cadmium and calcium carbonate also reduce copper absorption.

Copper is concerned with the formation of cytochrome oxidase, which regulates oxidation processes and electron transfer in tissues. It is also part of the enzyme lysyl oxidase, which is used for elastin or collagen synthesis and deficiency results in skeletal defects and blood vessel fragility. Copper is also present in caeruloplasmin, which releases iron from stores into plasma for erythropoiesis and deficiency results in anaemia.

Signs

The signs of *primary deficiency* are that the calves have a reduced growth rate; sometimes there is a scour but not usually as pronounced as in secondary deficiency. There may be a stilted gait with some ataxia developing after exercise, but recovery occurs after rest. Ribs and limb bones may develop spontaneous fractures, the shaft thickness may be reduced and there is osteoporosis. Thickened epiphyses, particularly in the fetlock region, may be noted, and stiffness of the joints.

Secondary deficiency is usually seen in calves sucking the dam or grazing. There is again a stiff gait and unthriftiness. Molybdenosis is characterized by severe scours. Some calves become very lame with epiphyses that are painful to palpate and usually the distal ends of the metapodial bones are enlarged. On radiography there is a thickened irregular epiphyseal plate, and the metaphyses are thickened. In some animals depigmentation of the hair occurs.

Necropsy

On post mortem there is usually emaciation with anaemia seen as thin, watery blood and pale tissues. Where copper levels are low there are deposits of haemosiderin in the liver, kidney and spleen. The limb bones may show evidence of rarefaction and fracture. A thickening of the epiphyseal plates, particularly of the metapodial bones, may be present. In the small intestine there may be villous atrophy. Histologically, the bones show osteoporosis.

Diagnosis

In practice the majority of cases are diagnosed because of the area where the animals have lived, and most calves will be sucking a cow or at pasture. The signs give an indication of the condition and it usually affects several animals. Examination can involve looking for anaemia with a reduced erythrocyte count ($2–4 \times 10^{12}$/l; normal, $5–10 \times 10^{12}$/l) and low blood haemoglobin (5–8 g/100 ml; normal, 8–15 g/100 ml). Plasma copper levels are low (normal, >15 μmol/l; deficient, <0.9 μmol/l) as are liver levels (normal, 100–200 p.p.m. drymatter (DM); deficient, <50 p.p.m. DM). Cytochrome oxidase (normal, >7.0 μmol/g wet liver) and caeruloplasmin levels are low. Copper can also be estimated in the diet, pasture and soil. Often response to copper therapy gives an indication.

Treatment

When therapy is undertaken it is important to confirm the presence of copper deficiency, as overdosing is toxic. Oral administration of 1.5 g copper sulphate is very useful, but requires constant handling of the calves. Parenteral administration of copper can overcome the problem. Copper sulphate has been used at a dose level of 200 mg/calf. A methionine copper complex can be administered as a deep intramuscular injection at a dose of 40 mg/calf, as can diethylamine copper oxyquinoline sulphonate at a rate of 0.24 mg/kg body weight by subcutaneous injection and copper edetate as a subcutaneous injection of 50 mg. Experiments in sheep have shown high doses of copper methionine subcutaneously to be safer than calcium copper edetate and diethylamine copper oxyquinoline (Mahmoud & Ford, 1981) but it was considered that this might have been the result of the rapidity of absorption depending on the route of injection. A comparison of the efficacy of copper preparations in cattle showed copper edetate to be best with copper diethylamine oxyquinoline sulphonate 19 per cent worse, aqueous copper methionate 36–48 per cent worse, and cupric sulphate producing the second-best result. The injections also cause a local reaction with copper diethylamine oxyquinoline sulphonate giving least damage, copper edetate producing an intermediate reaction and copper methionate causing most swelling (Suttle, 1981a).

Prevention

Prevention is to ensure that the level of copper in the diet of dams and calves is at least 10 mg/kg body weight. When deficiency has been determined it may be necessary routinely to inject or drench the cattle. However, no such programme should be undertaken unless a sample of the animals has been checked to ensure blood copper levels are low. The timing of the first injection (in severely affected herds) is at about six weeks old, but subsequent injections need to be based on further blood sampling. Copper sulphate can be used as a drench at a level of 1.5 g weekly. Cupric oxide needles have been used to alleviate hypocupraemia in heifers (Suttle, 1981b). A form of soluble glass has been used to release copper slowly from an intraruminal bolus. The use of pasture dressing annually with 5.6 kg/ha (5 lb/acre) copper sulphate is effective. As there is a possibility of poisoning, animals should not graze the pasture until after heavy rain or three weeks after application. The copper supplementation of water has been advocated (Farmer *et al.*, 1982). Salt licks containing 0.5 per cent copper sulphate are safe in use but are not permitted in all countries.

Hypomagnesaemic tetany of calves (see p. 583)

The condition occurs most commonly in calves on high-milk or milk-substitute intakes that are receiving little other feed. It results from a hypomagnesaemia that may be associated with hypocalcaemia. The young calf has a serum magnesium level similar to the dam and receives extra magnesium in its colostrum. However, milk is deficient in this element and if it constitutes most of the feed then there will be a gradual fall in circulating magnesium levels. This is partly allayed by the absorption of magnesium from bones. The calf is also able to absorb magnesium very efficiently from the small and large intestine in early life but this capacity reduces so that by three months old it becomes poor. The problem is often seen in veal or suckler calves after two months of age. Occasionally, hypomagnesaemia is seen in the young calf about two weeks old and this is due to poor absorption, which can occur with diarrhoea, the feeding of liquid paraffin or the use of fibrous feed, which increases salivation and thereby causes the body to lose magnesium. A calf requires 1–5 g daily, according to size and growth rate.

Signs

In the early stages there is hyperexcitability to stimuli with increased ear movements, interspersed with the ears being held back. There tends to be opisthotonus, ataxia and head shaking. The animal may have trouble drinking from a bucket on the ground. The temperature is normal and the pulse rate rapid. Later on there are muscular fasciculations with jaw champing, frothing at the mouth and a spastic gait. Convulsions may occur starting with the calf stamping its feet, pricking its ears, retracting its eyelids and the head being held up. The animal may fall and show tonic–clonic movements of the legs with uncontrolled passage of urine and faeces, a fast pulse over 200/minute with heart sounds audible away from the chest and respirations ceasing. The temperature is often raised to 40.5 °C (105 °F) due to muscular exertion. If the convulsions are severe the pulse is often imperceptible, cyanosis develops and the animal dies within about 30 minutes. In some cases there are periods of relative normality between bouts of convulsions.

Necropsy

On post-mortem examination there is usually extensive haemorrhage and congestion of the organs including the aorta, mesentery, pericardium, gall-bladder and intercostal walls.

Diagnosis

Diagnosis depends on the history of the feeding regimen used or presence of diarrhoea as well as the signs present and serum magnesium levels (normal, 0.9–1.4 mmol/l, 2.2–3.4 mg/100 ml). Clinical signs may occur at 0.12–0.33 mmol/l (0.3–0.8 mg/100 ml). In animals that die the Ca : Mg ratio in the caudal vertebra or rib bone is increased from a normal of 70 : 1 often to over 90 : 1. The aspartate aminotransferase and creatine kinase levels also tend to be raised because of the increased muscular activity. The main differential diagnoses involve conditions resulting in clonic convulsions. These include tetanus (but the course is usually longer) (see p. 567), arsenic, lead or mercury poisoning (but in all these there is colic and diarrhoea and with lead there is blindness). Strychnine poisoning can occur and results in a stiff gait. Hypovitaminosis A may well result in night blindness. Encephalitis (which may be viral or bacterial in origin) or meningitis may be difficult to determine. *Clostridium perfringens* (*welchii*) type D produces apparent blindness and a raised blood glucose level (normal, 2.5 mmol/l, 45 mg/100 ml).

Treatment and prevention

Treatment should include the use of magnesium sulphate (50 ml of 25 per cent solution) subcutaneously and possibly calcium borogluconate intravenously. Magnesium given intravenously can lead to medullary depression and cardiac embarrassment. If necessary the animal should be sedated with acepromazine or xylazine. When the problem is the result of diarrhoea then this should be rectified. The condition in the older calf is prolonged and there will be greatly reduced magnesium levels in bone, etc. Thus these animals will need to be supplemented with 2–4 g magnesium oxide or 4–8 g magnesium carbonate daily.

Prevention involves the provision of roughage, usually as good quality hay, from ten days of age. This is difficult in suckler calves but can be overcome by feeding the cows with magnesium oxide (calcined magnesite) at a level of 60 g daily. Magnesium can also be given to calves in the form of magnesium bullets or in molassed creep feed.

Vitamin A deficiency

The condition results from a deficiency of the fat-soluble vitamin A or its dietary precursor carotene. Secondary deficiency can arise where there is sufficient vitamin A/carotene in the diet but it does not reach a normal tissue level due to a failure in digestion, absorption or metabolism. In calves the condition may result in skeletal changes, which can affect the brain or spinal cord. The condition can be congenital or postnatal and is often partly due to the nutritional status of the dam. Usually, a diet of green food will provide sufficient of the precursor carotene and hence vitamin A. Thus problems do not occur at pasture until there are periods of prolonged drought, which can cause deficiency in the calves of affected dams or beef calves about six months old.

The condition is more common in housed animals fed diets likely to be deficient in vitamin A such as straw, cereals or sugar beet pulp. The dam's nutrition is important in that carotene in green food does not pass across the placental barrier until it is converted to vitamin A. It can then be taken up by the fetus and stored in the liver, as also can the vitamin A in water-soluble injections or fish oils. Colostrum is a major source of vitamin A for the calf and the introduction of extra carotene or vitamin A to the dam's diet precalving can be useful. The vitamin A requirement for a pregnant cow is about 80 iu/kg body weight daily and that for a calf is about 40 iu/kg.

Calves that are fast-growing, stressed or in a high environmental temperature require more vitamin A. Many factors that influence the vitamin A and carotene contents of feeds can lead to secondary deficiencies. Vitamins C and E help to prevent vitamin A loss, and the uptake of the vitamin is inversely proportional to the phosphate present in the diet. The vitamin is not very stable and so pelleting of the rations, storage at high temperatures and rancidity all decrease the content of the diet. Wood preservatives such as chlorinated naphthalenes inhibit carotene conversion to vitamin A and prolonged oral use of liquid paraffin or other mineral oils can produce a deficiency. Vitamin A is used to produce visual purple for the retina, normal epithelium and bone, and for normal CSF absorption.

Signs (see p. 719)

Congenital. Calves are born blind due to impingement of bone on the optic nerve. Other signs are due to increased CSF resulting in syncope with the calves showing tonic–clonic convulsions, ventral flexion of the head and neck, retraction of the eyeballs and tetanic closure of the eyelids. The calves are not blind. They may die during convulsions. In some outbreaks the affected calves develop severe diarrhoea and occasionally otitis media.

Postnatal. One of the most common lesions is the presence of large amounts of brown, bran-like scales in the coat and this is particularly seen in fast-growing animals. A reduction in growth rate may occur but is usually also the result of other deficiencies combining with that of vitamin A. Classical xenophthalmia with thickening and whitening of the cornea is unusual. When it does occur, it may be accompanied by serous ocular discharge. Nervous signs usually start with ataxia and weakness of the hind limbs and then the forelimbs. Increase in CSF pressure results in nerve compression and can lead to fainting with animals showing tonic–clonic convulsions for up to half a minute. The signs are similar to those for congenitally affected animals. Night blindness is more likely to be seen in yearling cattle.

Necropsy

Following death it may be possible to see the constrictions of the optic nerve, or the cranial cavity or vertebral cord may be reduced in size leading to injury to the spinal nerve roots. Histologically, there is squamous metaplasia of the interlobular ducts of the parotid salivary gland that is pathognomonic. The epithelium of the prepuce, reticulum and rumen shows hyperkeratosis. The liver may show focal necrotic areas.

Diagnosis

Diagnosis depends on post-mortem findings, plus a history of a lack of green feed and the signs. The deficiency can be confirmed by determining plasma vitamin A levels (normal, 25 µg/100 ml; deficient, $<$10 µg/100 ml) and CSF pressure (normal, $<$100 mm H_2O).

The condition needs to be differentiated from hypomagnesaemia where the animal is not blind, lead poisoning where there is abdominal pain, tetanus where there is no blindness and *Clostridium perfringens* (*welchii*) type D where there are high blood glucose levels. Bacterial and viral encephalitis and meningitis (see p. 215) usually result in pyrexia.

Treatment and prevention

Treatment involves the parenteral administration of aqueous vitamin A at a rate of 400 iu/kg body weight. The animals often respond quickly to treatment even where convulsions are occurring. Subsequently, an adequate level of vitamin A should be present in the diet (40 iu/kg). Often in practice daily allowances are doubled. Green feed or early-cut hay, good quality silage or dried grass should be given. However, very high daily levels of vitamin A supplementation in the diet can lead to exostoses on the digits and loss of epiphyseal cartilage. This produces lameness, ataxia and poor hoof development. Where it is difficult to supplement the diet, injections of vitamin A can be used every two weeks at a rate of 5000 iu/kg.

Iodine deficiency

This can be the result of a primary lack of iodine. Secondary deficiency is recorded following high intakes of brassicas, high calcium ingestion, heavy bacterial contamination of feed or water, a low level intake of linseed meal or other plants containing cyanogenetic glycosides. Iodine deficiency occurs in most parts of the world where there is a high rainfall and there is little exposure to oceanic iodine. Soils with a high calcium content are likely to be deficient. The condition is mainly seen in the newborn calf of a deficient dam. Iodine forms part of the hormone thyroxine, and a deficiency will result in the pituitary increasing the production of thyrotrophic hormone. This in turn leads to goitre. Calves born alive are prone to die if chilled, etc.

Signs

Many of the affected calves are aborted or stillborn and usually there is evidence of thyroid enlargement (goitre). If the animal is born alive it will be weak and disinclined to suck. Occasionally, the gland will be felt to pulsate. Very rarely areas of alopecia are apparent.

Necropsy

The thyroid glands are enlarged and heavier than usual (normal fresh weight 6.5 g). Histologically, there is thyroid hyperplasia.

Diagnosis

Diagnosis depends on the area or a diet containing goitrogenic plants. There is thyroid enlargement in the calves and several heifers or cows abort or produce stillborn or weak calves. Plasma protein iodine levels are low (normal, 2.4–4.0 µg/100 ml). The thyroid weight is increased and the iodine content of the gland is low (normal, 15.6–39.0 mmol/kg DM; deficient, 9.5 mmol/kg DM). Differential diagnosis is mainly to eliminate other causes of abortion (see Chapter 34).

Treatment and prevention

Treatment is to ensure that the calf sucks and is kept in a warm, draught-free environment. Thyroid extract can be used at a dose of 1–2 mg/kg body weight (0.5–1 mg/lb). Intravenous sodium iodide can be used at a dose of 5–7 g for the young calf, but it is not without risk; potassium iodide can be used orally at about 3 g per calf. Iodism (iodine poisoning) can sometimes develop.

Prevention involves allowing the dams adequate iodine in the diet. A recommended level is 0.8 mg/kg DM for pregnant and lactating cows. The level for calves should be 0.12 mg/kg DM.

Iron deficiency

Iron deficiency is not common in cattle and the primary condition is mainly seen in veal calves without access to roughage. The secondary condition usually follows heavy infestation with sucking lice such as *Haematopinus eurysternus* and *Linognathus vituli* or after haemorrhage. The primary condition can occur in veal calves or others fed predominantly raw milk or unsupplemented milk substitute. The calf has only sufficient iron for about three weeks after birth and milk is a poor source of iron. In the case of veal calves there is an attempt to maintain iron levels low to keep the meat white. Over half the iron in the body is in the form of haemoglobin with small amounts present in myoglobin and in enzymes used for oxygen utilization. The normal blood haemoglobin values for adult cattle are 8.0–15.0 g/100 ml. However, the value in a calf at birth is 12.9 g/100 ml, dropping to 10.4 g/100 ml on a diet of milk and solid feed (Holman, 1956). The calf's daily iron requirement is 50 g and as only about 2–4 g are received from the cow's milk there is a need to supplement with hay, straw and cereals. The only source of iron for veal calves on slats without roughage is the milk substitute and this needs to be supplemented. Levels less than 19 mg soluble iron/kg DM of feed are likely to result in problems.

Signs

The main sign is a reduction in appetite followed by reduced weight gain. The mucous membranes tend to become pale, but death is extremely rare.

Necropsy

Necropsy findings are of pale muscles with the blood thin and watery and clotting slowly. The liver tends to be enlarged and there is moderate anaemia. Diagnosis depends on the history of the diet and signs. It can be confirmed by haematological examination demonstrating a reduced erythrocyte count and low haemoglobin value. The serum iron level is low (normally 30 mol/l, 167 μg/100 ml when born, reducing to 12μmol/l, 67 μg/100 ml at three weeks). The main differential diagnoses are those of copper and cobalt deficiency but signs additional to the anaemia will be present.

Treatment and prevention

Treatment usually involves the injection of 1 g of iron weekly to each calf as iron dextran or 0.5–1.0 g iron as ferric polygalactofuranose. Vitamin B_{12} is also often used at levels of 5–10 μg/kg body weight. Prevention is by supplying milk substitute containing an iron concentration of 25–30 mg/kg DM. This will ensure that the animal has a normal appetite and growth and it will help to produce pale meat suitable for veal (Bremner *et al.*, 1976). This is because the level is sufficient to give an acceptable blood haemoglobin without there being enough to produce much myoglobin. Most milk substitutes for calf rearing contain considerably more iron.

Selenium/vitamin E deficiency (see p. 266)

Vitamin E and/or selenium can be deficient and result in muscular dystrophy, also known as white muscle or fish flesh disease. It can be seen at any age after birth. Selenium deficiency is mainly dependent on the area where crops are produced. Soils derived from granite or pumice are deficient. Alkaline soils encourage selenium absorption by plants. The condition appears to be becoming increasingly important, probably due to the increased cost of bought-in feeds causing farmers to use more home-produced crops for their animals. The accepted level of selenium in feeds is 0.1 mg/kg DM. Selenium is mainly used by the body in the production of the enzyme glutathione peroxidase.

Vitamin E deficiency is much more dependent on the type of crop grown and its storage, etc. Vitamin E levels tend to be high in green pasture, silage, dried grass or kale. Adequate levels of the vitamin are also present in cereal grains, well-cured fresh hay, maize silage and brewers' grains, but deficiencies can occur on poor quality hay, straw or root crops unless there is a suitable supplement provided. Vitamin E tends to deplete with storage. Calf diets high in unsaturated fatty acids, as can occur where cod liver oil, fishmeal, soya bean meal or linseed oil are fed, may become deficient due to their oxidation, resulting in rancidity and the destruction of vitamin E. Storage of grains when wet or with propionic acid can also reduce the vitamin E level. Normal levels for growing cattle are considered to be 150 mg of α-tocopherol, and for the calf, milk substitutes should contain antioxidants and 300 iu/kg DM α-tocopherol.

The condition affects muscles, particularly cardiac, skeletal and diaphragmatic. Deficiency can occur in suckler calves sucking mothers with low selenium or vitamin E levels or in artificially reared calves on deficient diets. The condition results from unsaturated fatty acids entering the muscle cells where they accumulate. They are oxidized to lipid peroxides, which result in degeneration and calcification. It is believed vitamin E helps prevent lipid peroxide formation within the muscle cells whereas selenium compounds with many unsaturated points are known as polyunsaturated fatty acids and these are particularly common in vegetable oils, which therefore predispose to peroxide formation.

Signs

The signs vary in degree and in the sudden death syndrome the calf appears perfectly healthy but while drinking or normally within 30 minutes of feeding the animal will suddenly collapse. Death is usually within a minute of collapse. Mortality is 100 per cent.

Acute muscular dystrophy is again sudden in origin. The animal becomes dull and lies in lateral recumbency. There is respiratory distress, a heart rate often elevated to 150–200 beats/minute and irregular. The rectal temperature is normal, the calf is fully conscious and has normal eye reflexes. Most calves die within 6–18 hours and the mortality approaches 100 per cent.

The most common form seen is subacute muscular dystrophy and the morbidity is variable between about 10 and 40 per cent of calves. The signs depend on the muscles affected. The animal may stand stiffly; it is reluctant to move and when it does it may have a stiff gait. The calf is often weak and will not stand for long. However, it is fully conscious with normal appetite, normal temperature and usually normal respiratory rate, but the heart rate may be raised. In many cases the gait is abnormal and it moves by rotation of the hocks. In some cases the affected muscles are swollen and firm on palpation. It has been shown that there is increased susceptibility to infectious diseases such as calf pneumonia due to delayed lymphocytic response.

Necropsy

On necropsy of calves with the sudden death syndrome there are often no macroscopic lesions. Other cases may show congestion of the liver and lungs. The heart shows a slight pallor of the myocardium. Histologically, lesions not otherwise apparent can be detected with a haematoxylin basic fuchsin–picric acid method and these are considered to be peracute myocardial degeneration. In acute muscular dystrophy there are localized streaks in the diaphragm and skeletal muscles. In the latter they tend to be bilaterally symmetrical white or grey areas in the muscles. In the heart there may be cardiac hypertrophy and myocardial degeneration with pulmonary congestion and oedema. Histologically, there is no inflammation but changes vary and include hyaline degeneration and coagulative necrosis. In subacute muscular dystrophy there is usually no cardiac involvement but the skeletal muscles show bilateral grey or white areas.

Diagnosis

Diagnosis depends on the area and diet provided as well as the signs. Decreased glutathione peroxidase levels occur (usually 20 μmol/min) and the normal level of selenium in the blood is 0.63 μmol/l. There are raised plasma creatine phosphokinase and aspartate transaminase levels. The blood tocopherol level can be useful (normal, 770 μg/100 ml). Otherwise liver and kidney levels of selenium can be examined (normal, 3 and 30 μmol/kg DM). Response to treatment can be determined as a means of diagnosis.

Treatment

Therapy can involve the use of vitamin E and/or selenium depending on the cause of deficiency. The dose of D_2-α-tocopherol is about 6 iu/kg body weight. Selenium can be injected as 0.1–0.15 mg/kg sodium selenite. Long-acting selenium injections are obtainable. The combined injections have become available and produce acceptable results. Selenium can also be given in the form of reticular bullets or in soluble glass. The diet should provide sufficient vitamin E and selenium. Cows with calves at foot or in late pregnancy can be given a combined vitamin E/selenium injection to supplement their calves.

Prevention

For prevention growing calves should be given a supplement at the rate 0.1 p.p.m. selenium of the total ration and 150 mg/head of α-tocopherol daily. Cows should receive a supplement of vitamin E during the last two months of pregnancy. Injections of selenium and vitamin E can be used; selenium bullets or soluble glass intraruminal boluses are also of value. Pastures can be top-dressed with fertilizer containing sodium selenite 75–150 g/ha (1–2 oz/acre) or foliage dusting or spraying can be undertaken at 17.5 g/ha ($\frac{1}{4}$ oz/acre). Analysis of pasture should be undertaken to determine that toxic levels of selenium are not produced; this can occur at levels of 0.5 mg/kg. Selenium can be added to the drinking water.

Zinc deficiency

This can be either primary due to a lack of zinc, or secondary due to impaired uptake. It is usually seen in calves from six to ten weeks old, particularly in the period after weaning, and most commonly they are housed. Usually, calves do not show signs on diets containing 40 p.p.m. zinc, but it is probable that calcium and highly fibrous diets reduce zinc availability and perhaps low copper levels reduce uptake. A congenital condition occurs in Freisan calves resulting in an increased 3 in requirement (see p. 151).

Signs

Signs usually occur about two weeks after the deficient diet is introduced. The main signs are of poor growth with possible stunting. There is alopecia and parakeratosis often affecting the limbs, muzzle, vulva, anus and tail head. There are fewer lesions on the main part of the body. In some cases any wounds or abrasions will take longer to heal. Most animals do not die but skin biopsies show increased thickness of all skin components and the stratum corneum contains nucleated epidermal cells.

Diagnosis

Diagnosis is partly on the lesions and a biopsy shows parakeratosis. Normal plasma zinc levels are 9–18 μmol/l (80–120 μg/100 ml). Serum alkaline phosphatase, albumin and amylase levels fall whereas serum globulin levels rise. The calves usually start to respond to therapy in about a week.

Treatment and prevention

Treatment involves oral medication with zinc sulphate at a level of 2 g weekly, or 1 g weekly by injection is useful. Any calcium oversupplementation should be corrected and fibrous roughage should be reduced. A diet containing 50 p.p.m. zinc should prevent the condition. Weekly oral medication with 0.5 g zinc sulphate can be helpful. Long-term control can be obtained with zinc-containing fertilizer.

Furazolidone poisoning

Furazolidone is a common form of prophylactic medication in calves, which can result in problems of toxicity. There are two syndromes, one of which (the acute) involves overdosing at levels of 20–30 mg/kg body weight and the classic condition results from long-term feeding of low levels, often 2 mg/kg. Both are usually the result of poor mixing, which allows some animals in a group to receive more than the others. Mortality in both cases in high and the chronic form may be seen several days after furazolidone feeding ceases.

Signs

In the acute form there are nervous signs with hyperexcitability, including muscle tremors, arched back and possibly circling, convulsions and death normally within a few days. When the chronic condition occurs there tend to be necrotic lesions and haemorrhages in the mouth and lower gut. This results in melaena or dysentery.

Necropsy

After death few lesions are seen in the acute condition but when chronic there are haemorrhages and necrosis in the alimentary tract. Haemorrhages are present on the peritoneal and pleural surfaces and there is decreased myelopoiesis in the bone marrow.

Diagnosis

Diagnosis depends on the signs and feeding the compound and can be confused with bracken poisoning (see p. 619) or anthrax.

Treatment and prevention

Little therapy can be given in either case but in the acute form furazolidone feeding should be stopped at once. Noise should be kept to a minimum and excitement should be avoided. Sedatives such as acepromazine, xylazine or magnesium sulphate can be helpful. In the chronic form little can be done, except perhaps to give blood transfusions. Prevention involves the correct dosage of furazolidone being offered to calves and it should be thoroughly mixed. If given with milk substitute from a bulk container the milk must be constantly agitated. Furazolidone in the micronized form or combined with diethyl sulphoxide or other nitrofurans will reduce the risk. Therapy with furazolidone, whether medicinal or prophylactic, should not be repeated.

Iodism

The overuse of sodium or potassium iodide in therapy for conditions such as actinobacillosis, iodine deficiency or ringworm can lead to iodism. The signs depend partly on the form of administration. If intravenous the animal can show considerable discomfort with dyspnoea, staggering and tachycardia. When given subcutaneously there is swelling following injection for about two days and local discomfort for about two hours after administration. In the oral form the coat becomes stary, with a scaly skin and often a fine, white dandruff. There is excessive lacrimation and nasal discharge with, in some cases, a degree of inappetance. If problems arise in treatment from the intravenous route then the iodine should be given subcutaneously or orally. When signs occur following oral administration, treatment should be discontinued.

Cerebrocortical Necrosis (CCN, polioencephalomalacia)

Aetiology

It is a deficiency of thiamine caused by endogenous thiaminase. Thiaminase has been found to be produced by *Clostridium sporongenes* and certain *Bacillus* spp. which can be found in cases of CCN. However, this does not mean they are the only factors.

Occurrence

It is a sporadic condition which can occasionally occur as outbreaks. Most animals affected are fast-growing, well-nourished animals between 6 and 18 months old. It can occur following deprivation of food pasture to good grazing.

Similar syndromes can be produced experimentally by feeding large amounts of bracken or horsetail which contain high levels of thiaminase. Amprolium is also a specific thiamine antagonist and has also been used experimentally. Molasses toxicity results in a similar problem due to a fall in the proprionate levels. Thiamine is naturally synthesized in the rumen. It forms an essential component of several enzymes used in glucolysis in the brain. Deficiency in thiamine results in increased blood pyruvate levels and a decrease in the lactate: pyruvate ratio as well as a depression of the erythrocyte transketolase level. This causes an interference with normal carbohydrate metabolism and the cerebral cortex in particular requires the oxidative metabolism of glucose.

It is possible that thiamine deficiency might have a direct metabolic effect on the neurones, particularly in the calf which is very dependent on the pentose pathway of metabolism in which the transketolase enzyme limits the rate of activity. Thiamine pyrophosphate is a coenzyme for several carbohydrate metabolic reactions and it is associated with transketolase in the pentose pathway of glucose oxidation. There tend to be marked cerebral oedema and cerebral necrosis and the signs are mainly the result of an increase in intracranial pressure.

The morbidity is usually low but occasionally up to 25 per cent. However, mortality can be 25 to 50 per cent if not treated early, with higher levels in young cattle (six to nine months) than older ones.

Signs

In acute cases there is a sudden onset of nervous signs including blindness, muscle tremors, particularly of the head and neck, head pressing, jaw champing and frothy salivation. Animals tend to be hard to handle and in the early stages signs may be intermittent. Although the animal appears blind, and the menace reflex is absent, the palpebral and pupillary reflexes are present. The convulsive signs soon become continuous with the animal becoming recumbent. The signs are then of opisthotonus, nystagmus, optic disc oedema, often strabismus and clonic tonic convulsions which become worse when the animal is stimulated. The temperature is normal, the ruminal movements are normal but the heart rate is variable. Calves often die in one to two days although older animals show signs for a longer period. Recovery following therapy may well take two to four days or longer.

The signs of the subacute form last for a few hours to several days and include blindness, head pressing and standing. The condition will resolve in some cases. However, in an outbreak of CCN some of the animals show anorexia, partial impairment of eyesight and a mild depression. Almost all of the animals recover within 24 hours of therapy.

Although recovery may occur, some animals may still remain blind. The longer the time between onset of signs and therapy, the less favourable the prognosis. When cattle remain dull and anorexic after three days' treatment they are unlikely to recover and should be a slaughtered.

Necropsy

Most of the animals do not show any gross changes in the body other than the brain. There is usually increased intracranial pressure with a yellowing and compression of the dorsal cortical gyri. The cerebellum tends to be compressed into the foramen magnum and recovered animals show decortication of the motor area and occipital lobes. Histologically there is bilateral necrosis of the dorsal occipital and parietal cerebral cortex and also, occasionally, the thalamus, basal ganglia, laterial geniculate bodies and mesencephalic nuclei. Cerebellar lesions also occur.

Diagnosis

Diagnosis can be made from the following:

1 History — age of animals, a change in feeding and the condition of the animal.

2 Signs — blindness, normal palpebral and pupillary reflexes; normal ruminal movements, normal temperature but otherwise many nervous signs.

3 Blood pyruvate and lactate levels are increased.

4 Urine pyruvate levels increased.

5 Erythrocyte transketolase activity reduced.

6 Pyruvate kinase levels are much increased.

7 Thiamine levels in erythrocytes, blood and plasma may be in the normal range.

8 Blood creatine phosphokinase (CPK) levels may occur.

9 Thiaminase levels increased in rumen liquor and in faeces.

10 Haematology virtually normal although total and differential counts may show a mild stress reaction.

11 Increased cerebrospinal fluid pressure, 200–350 mm saline (normal 120–160 mm saline).

12 Histology — bilateral necrosis in cerebral cortex (bisect brain longitudinally, put one half in buffered formalin, the other is deep-frozen).

13 Green fluorescence of brain then exposed to long-wave ultraviolet light.

Differential diagnoses are shown in Table 16.2.

Table 16.1 Differences in thiamine levels within certain tissues of the body in animals with or without cerebrocortical necrosis. (After Edwin *et al.*, 1979.)

	CCN (±SEM)	Not CCN (±SEM)
Liver dry (ug/g)	2.5 ± 0.43	11.1 ± 2.11
Heart dry (ug/g)	2.5 ± 0.56	13.2 ± 2.12
Brain dry (ug/g)	1.8 ± 0.37	7.7 ± 1.52
Erythrocyte transketolase (% TPP effect)	172	15

Table 16.2 Differential diagnoses.

Disease	Differential diagnoses
Listeriosis	Unilateral facial paralysis, pyrexia
Lead poisoning	Abdominal pain, diarrhoea, no pupillary reflex, no ruminal movements
Coenuriasis	Slow onset, circling
Molasses poisoning	Similar to cerebrocortical necrosis but history of feeding large quantities and also glucose levels full whereas thiamine levels remain normal
Amprolium poisoning	Similar to cerebrocortical necrosis but history of feeding it
Bracken or horsetail poisoning	Similar to cerebrocortical necrosis but highly unlikely to cause such a manifestation other than experimentally
Haemophilus somnus	Infection, but usually pyrexia and neutrophilia

Treatment

Thiamine hydrochloride should be administered intravenously at a dose of 10 mg/kg (5 mg/lb) BW, the dosage should be repeated every three hours or so for five treatments. A response will occur in 24 hours if animals are caught in the early stages, otherwise recovery is slowly progressive over several days. Multivitamin injections are often used but although they are suitable for follow-up therapy, in the initial stages insufficient thiamine will be administered unless very large doses are given.

Nursing is important and the cattle should be presented with wholesome food including at least 50 per cent good quality roughage. Rumen liquor from cattle on predominantly roughage diets may be helpful. The use of dried brewers' grains can help the conditions as they contain high levels of thiamine and others of the B vitamin group. Levels of 0.5–1.0 kg/300 kg BW (1–2 lb/6 cwt) have been suggested.

Control

The precipitating factors for CCN are still not known, which makes it difficult to recommend preventive measures. As the condition is the result of endogenous thiamine activity, provision of extra thiamine is of limited value. Most natural feeds contain thiamine at a level of 2 ppm and this, plus the vitamin synthesized in the rumen, is normally sufficient. Provision of adequate amounts of roughage should prevent the condition and a level of 1.5 kg roughage per 100 kg BW is suggested.

Urolithiasis

Urinary calculi are either organic or inorganic. The organic type are less common and form casts or urinary deposits. The inorganic ones tend to be crystalline and are more common. The condition is usually seen in calves that are housed, with milk substitute as their main source of feed or in weaned growing animals fed high levels of concentrates. Some pastures are problem areas, which can be due to high plant oestrogen, oxalate or silica levels. Most calculi in housed animals contain calcium or magnesium ammonium phosphate although struvite and oxalate deposits occur at times. At pasture, carbonates of calcium, magnesium and phosphorus are most common. Vitamin A deficiency has been suggested as a precipitating factor both indoors and when cattle are grazing. The urinary pH has an influence and phosphate and carbonate calculi form more readily in an alkaline than an acid urine. Binding of the calculi occurs with mucoprotein in the urine and this is seen more frequently when oestrogens from plants or growth promoters are present, or the ration is pelleted.

Urolithiasis can occur in all animals fed a predisposing diet regardless of sex; however, the condition is mainly seen in the male because signs are not normally observed unless some form of urethral blockage occurs. More cases are found in castrated than entire animals. Calculi can lodge anywhere in the urethra but occur most commonly at the sigmoid flexure of the penis with the region of the ischial arch being the second most common site.

Signs

Most of the signs are associated with partial or complete blockage of the urethra. This is seen as frequent attempts to urinate, which may be accompanied by the passage of small amounts of urine, often blood-tinged, or the attempts are unproductive. Calculi may be present on the prepucial orifice hairs. There is usually evidence of mild to severe colic with kicking at the belly, paddling movements and tail swishing. In most untreated cases with complete urethral obstruction, there will be perforation of the urethra or bladder rupture. When either takes place there is usually a period of relief from abdominal pain. When bladder rupture has occurred the urine enters the abdomen, which becomes distended and there is a fluid thrill present on percussion. In those with urethral perforation, urine tends to dribble under the skin, causing ventral abdominal distension, which will start to progress anteriorly. In most cases there is some toxaemia and possibly uraemia and this is seen as inappetance, with increasing dullness of the animal, which will ultimately become comatosed and die.

Necropsy

At necropsy there is usually some degree of cystitis, often with urinary deposits present in the bladder. When the bladder ruptures there is much fluid in the abdomen and in those cases of urethral perforation there will be erosion in the area of the calculus and urine, possibly with cellulitis, present subcutaneously. The position of the calculus can be ascertained by the passage of a catheter.

Diagnosis

The diagnosis depends on the history, particularly of the area and feeding as well as the sex of the animal and signs. If there is bladder rupture then the fluid can be aspirated from the abdominal cavity. It is often difficult to determine that urine is present without its odour and appearance. Urinary crystals may be present on prepucial hairs and these should be analysed. The main differential diagnoses are ascites, intussusception and constipation.

Treatment

Treatment of the condition is primarily by surgery. If the animal is nearing slaughter and there is no bladder rupture or urethral perforation then casualty slaughter is best. Otherwise, treatment is usually only successful in the early stages and all treated animals and others in the group must be carefully examined for several days subsequently. It may be possible to perform a urethrotomy and remove the calculi. Provided the stones are distal to the ischial arch then the provision of a urethrotomy in the perineal region may overcome the problem and, if it proves impossible to remove the calculi, the opening can be made permanent. Medical treatment can include hyoscine butylbromide injected intravenously or intramuscularly at a dose of 20–40 mg/animal, or 5–10 ml of protein-free pancreatic extract possibly repeated once or twice. Acetylpromazine can give useful results acting as a smooth muscle relaxant. Withdrawal of concentrates may assist the condition and the provision of salt water following relief of the blockage is useful.

Prevention

Prevention is partly dependent on feed alteration, and precipitation of phosphate can be avoided by having a correct ratio of calcium to phosphorus, which should be at least 1.2 : 1, but levels up to 2.5 : 1 have been suggested. The concentration of magnesium in the diet should be kept at 10 W and this means that the maximum amount of magnesium oxide that should be added to the diet is 200 g/t ($\frac{1}{2}$ lb/ton) of feed. In the concentrates, up to 3 per cent salt has been recommended and it is thought to have an ionic effect rather than just causing diuresis. Such diets should only be used where there is always free access to water. The addition to feed of urinary acidifiers such as ammonium sulphate or phosphoric acid can be helpful. In animals at pasture the use of salt in the water can reduce the concentration of silicic acid in the urine, thereby preventing silica calculi formation. Adequate water supplies must always be available at pasture and areas likely to produce urolithiasis are best grazed by female cattle.

References

Bremner, J., Brockway, J.M., Donnelly, H.T. & Webster, A.J.F. (1976) Anaemia and veal calf production. *Veterinary Record*, **99**, 203–5.

Edwin, E.E., Markson, L.M., Shreeve, J., Jackman, R. & Carroll, P.J., (1979) *Veterinary Record*, **104**, 4–8.

Farmer, P.E., Adams, T.E. & Humphrics W.R. (1982) Copper supplementation of drinking water for cattle grazing molybdenum-rich pastures. *Veterinary Record*, **120**, 253–72.

Holman H.H. (1956) Changes associated with age in the blood picture of calves and heifers. *British Veterinary Journal*, **112**, 91–104.

Mahmoud, D.H & Ford, B.J.H. (1981) Injection of sheep with inorganic injections of copper. *Veterinary Record*, **108**, 114–17.

Suttle, N.F. (1981a) Comparison between parenterally administered copper complexes of their ability to alleviate hypocupraemia in sheep and cattle. *Veterinary Record*, **109**, 304–7.

Suttle, N.F. (1981b) Effectiveness of orally administered cupric oxide needles in alleviating hypocupraemia in sheep and cattle. *Veterinary Record*, **108**, 417–20.

GROWING CATTLE

Chapter 17: Endoparasites and Ectoparasites

by S.M. TAYLOR AND A.H. ANDREWS

Endoparasites

Although cattle of all ages may become infected with many species of parasites, clinical disease caused by parasitism is mainly observed in groups of animals under 18 months of age, especially when two preconditions coincide:

1 the availability of large numbers of the infective stages of the parasite (a variable that is usually dependent on the relationship between the bionomics of the parasite and suitable maturation conditions);

2 the presence of susceptible cattle grazing on the contaminated area.

When these two conditions are fulfilled, the resultant simultaneous maturation of large numbers of parasites in a specific host organ produces severe tissue disruption and the consequent signs associated with the parasite involved. The gastrointestinal tract, lungs and liver are the organs most commonly affected. It is prudent, therefore, when considering the diagnosis and treatment of parasitic disease to inquire whether the two preconditions have existed, and to involve their separation as part of the therapeutic and prophylactic advice given.

Parasitic gastroenteritis

The term itself is currently specifically associated with the presence of large numbers of nematodes in the abomasum and intestines rather than any other endoparasites. The nematodes in the abomasum are generally considered to be the primary pathogens, with those in the intestines playing a lesser but synergistic role.

Temperate areas

The predominant worms in the abomasum are those of the genus *Ostertagia* with *O. ostertagi* the most important and numerous. In the small intestine *Cooperia oncophora* and *Nematodirus helvetianus* are commonest.

There are two common forms of ostertagiasis, type I and type II, and since they are the result of different manifestations of the bionomics of *O. ostertagi* will be described separately.

TYPE I OSTERTAGIASIS

This form of the disease is characterized by a profuse watery diarrhoea in calves at grass. The faeces, because of the grass diet, is usually green. There is rapid loss of weight in severe cases, coupled with a slight hypoalbuminaemia due to protein loss and in chronic cases this can eventually result in submandibular oedema. It is most common in late summer and autumn in northern temperate areas.

Aetiology and epidemiology

The direct cause is the ingestion over a relatively short period of large numbers of the infective larvae of *O. ostertagi*. The presence of such large numbers of larvae is a result of several epidemiological interactions, a working knowledge of which is necessary if the best advice on treatment and prophylaxis is to be offered.

The annual pattern of fluctuations of infective larval numbers on calf grazing was described by Michel (1969), and can be seen in Fig. 17.1, which shows that the number of infective larvae in northern temperate areas is lowest in May and June but rises to a peak in late August and September. Summarized, the pattern arises from the following sequence of events. Calves put out to graze in April or May, on grazing that has been used for cattle (and especially calves) during the preceding year, ingest some of the infective larvae remaining on the pasture from the contamination produced in the previous summer. These infective larvae develop into adults in approximately three weeks and egg laying commences. The rate of hatching of these eggs is influenced by temperature and availability of moisture, and providing the latter is present increases as the temperature rises, reaching a peak in midsummer. The larvae thus hatched in May, June and July migrate or are washed out of faecal pats on to surrounding herbage to await ingestion by the eventual host. Their numbers are maximal in late July, August or early September, the precise timing depending on the climate in the area involved during the year in question. In normal climatic years in the British Isles the maximum number of infective larvae is found in southern England in late July, and in the west of Scotland and Northern Ireland in mid to late August. Wet summers produce an earlier peak but numbers of

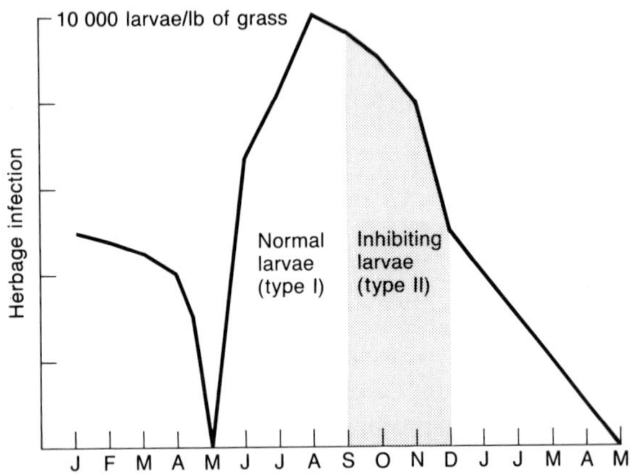

Fig. 17.1 Normal annual pattern of worm larvae on pasture in northern temperate countries.

infective larvae decrease more quickly than normal due to more rapid depletion of the numbers in faecal pats and to dilution due to the more abundant grass growth under these conditions. Conversely, in dry summers the build-up is delayed; release of larvae from faecal pats does not take place under the autumn rainfall and the larval contamination is maximal thereafter.

Parasitic gastroenteritis normally occurs when calves or non-immune older cattle are grazed on pastures on which a large number of infective larvae are present. Typical cases occur in dairy herds where autumn-borne replacement calves are put out to graze for the first time in April or May. The pastures used are frequently close to the farmhouse to enable both ease of inspection and rehousing should weather conditions deteriorate. For these reasons the same fields frequently have the same use each year. The calves remain on the fields until midsummer, excreting eggs that initiate the midsummer larval increase. At that point, when grass in such paddocks requires resting the farmer has aftergrass available after conservation for silage or hay. The calves are transferred to the aftergrass with or without anthelmintic treatment. Shortly afterwards, by which time the grass in the original fields has recovered slightly, spring-borne calves are put out on to it. If no prophylactic measures are taken, the inevitable result of severe type I ostertagiasis ensues a few weeks later in the latter calves, caused by ingestion of massive numbers of infective larvae by fully susceptible cattle over a relatively short period of time.

Pathogenesis

Ingested infective larvae of *O. ostertagi* develop in the gastric glands in the abomasal mucosa, emerging 18–21 days later as adults. Whilst in the mucosa their presence produces distension of the parasitized acini, which in turn causes several pathological and biochemical lesions. Firstly, the hydrochloric acid-producing parietal cells in the acini are destroyed and replaced by rapidly dividing undifferentiated cells that do not produce acid. If the infection is severe and lesions extensive a thickened hyperplastic gastric mucosa results, little acid is produced and the pH of the abomasum rises from pH 2 to pH 7, and the intercellular junctions are disrupted. The change in pH has several major consequences. Above pH 4.5 pepsin ceases to be active in protein digestion; at pH 6 and above pepsinogen is not converted to pepsin and remains unaltered in excess and is reabsorbed into the bloodstream via the ruptured intercellular connections, raising the blood pepsinogen concentration. At the same time blood proteins such as albumin can leak outwards into the lumen. As a result of the rise in pH the abomasal contents become less bacteriostatic and bacterial overgrowth of the damaged wall results.

Signs

When all the above events occur the intestinal metabolism is also affected and the classical signs of acute diarrhoea, inappetance and weight loss commence.

TYPE II OSTERTAGIASIS

This form of the disease is usually found in yearlings in the late winter or spring following their first season of grazing. Affected cattle can be housed or outwintered.

Aetiology and epidemiology

As with type I disease the direct cause is the simultaneous maturation of large numbers of *O. ostertagi*. The circumstances surrounding the event require some additional explanation, since the normal time of the disease is not when infective larvae on the pasture are most abundant.

Infective larvae present on pasture after September and ingested from that time until the following spring undergo a change in their normal parasitic development, which results in a period of delayed development at the early fourth larval stage while within the abomasal wall. The behavioural change has been shown to be more common in some strains of *O. ostertagi* than others and to be brought about by either cold or desiccation in their preparasitic exposure (Armour *et al.*, 1969). In the late autumn, calves that have not had adequate prophylactic treatment may harbour many thousands of such larvae but relatively few normally developing larvae or adult worms. Type II ostertagiasis results when these inhibited larvae resume their development in the last winter or spring, the emerging larvae producing the same lesions as those causing type I disease.

ATYPICAL FORMS OF PARASITIC GASTROENTERITIS

Parasitic gastroenteritis in beef herds

This is not usually a problem in spring-calving herds, since most of the infective larvae are consumed by the adult cows, which normally have enough immunity to prevent a high percentage of worms establishing and producing eggs. The calves that might transmit the infection are too young to consume much grass in the early part of the season. As a result the peak of infective larval numbers does not develop until September or October when most calves are weaned, treated and housed. Conversely, in autumn-calving herds in which calves are weaned in the following spring and grazed in the same manner as dairy replacements, the same epidemiological picture can result, i.e. type I ostertagiasis will occur in the absence of preventative measures.

Early-season type I ostertagiasis

In areas where climatic conditions allow autumn-born calves to be put out in March or early April, the number of infective larvae remaining on pasture can be sufficiently high to cause normal type I disease from 4 to 6 weeks after going to grass.

Nematodiriasis in calves

Parasitic gastroenteritis due to large infections of the nematode *Nematodirus battus* have recently been observed. Normally recognized as a parasite of sheep, it has recently been observed to be able to be transmitted by cattle, both on farms where annual alternation of sheep and cattle has taken place and even where cattle only are kept, and has caused severe outbreaks of diarrhoea in calves.

Parasitic gastroenteritis in adult cattle

Although uncommon, since most cattle acquire immunity by the age of 18 months, occasional individual cases can occur. Bulls that are grazed on calf paddocks and cows, which due to debilitating intercurrent diseases such as fascioliasis may have some of their normal immune reactions depressed, can both suffer from type II ostertagiasis.

Diagnosis

Affected animals are invariably presented with diarrhoea, which may be present to a greater or lesser degree in all members of the group. Younger animals are frequently the most severely affected. There will be a history that indicates grazing on potentially infected pasture during the preceding four to eight weeks in the case of type I ostertagiasis or during the previous late summer and autumn for type II ostertagiasis.

Specific diagnosis (see Table 17.1) can be assisted by the following tests.

Table 17.1 Differentiation between type I and type II ostertagiasis

	Type I	Type II
Seasonal incidence	Predominantly July–November; occasionally April–May	February–May
History	Usually in calves at grass for the first time, heavily stocked (8–10/ha). Occasionally in beef yearlings during the second year's grazing, and in individual cows and bulls transferred from hill herds to more intensive systems	*Always* in calves that grazed on heavily stocked pasture during the previous autumn, usually in younger members of group. Can also occur in bulls grazing calf paddocks. Occurs usually when housed or within 3 weeks of being put to grass
Clinical signs	Profuse green diarrhoea; will only usually recur once approx. 10 days after treatment. Rapid loss of body weight. Morbidity high, mortality low	Intermittent profuse diarrhoea. Recurs every two weeks until supply of inhibited fourth stages is exhausted. Morbidity low, mortality high
Laboratory findings*	Not usually anaemic PCV > 0.3 RbC > 7×10^6/mm^3 Hb > 10 g/100 ml Serum pepsinogen 2–5 iu	Mild anaemia PCV 0.22–0.26 RbC 5.6 ± 10^6/mm^3 Hb 8.4 ± 0.5 g/100 ml Serum pepsinogen 2–8 iu
Post mortem	pH abomasal contents >5.0 >50 000 adult *O. ostertagi* Severe abomasal reaction	pH abomasal contents >5.0 >50 000 adult *O. ostertagi* plus large numbers of immature fourth stages Severe abomasal reaction

* PCV, packed cell volume; RBC, red blood cell; Hb, haemoglobin.

1 Faecal egg counts. Despite the dilution of faeces caused by diarrhoea, the nematode egg counts will be in excess of 1000 eggs/g. Counts may be higher in less severely affected calves that have not yet become severely diarrhoeic. In older animals and in some individuals in type II cases the faecal egg counts may be low enough to be misleading, and if suspected the results of other tests should be borne in mind.
2 Plasma pepsinogen. In healthy calves the normal level of plasma pepsinogen is less than 1 international unit (iu) of tyrosine. In affected calves the level will normally be greater than 3 iu, and in very severely diseased individuals up to 4.5 iu. It should be pointed out that in adult cattle the normal pepsinogen level can be 1.5–2 iu, almost that found in calves in the prepatent period of type II ostertagiasis. Plasma pepsinogen levels in adults therefore should be carefully evaluated.
3 Plasma gastrin. The plasma concentration of the hormone gastrin has been shown to rise at the time of patency in experimental infections and to peak at levels between 500–1000 pg/ml. Although still under investigation it may be used as a substitute for plasma pepsinogen in the future.
4 Post-mortem findings. In both type I and type II ostertagiasis the abomasum (providing the animal has remained untreated) will contain large numbers of adult *O. ostertagi*. The number can vary from 50 000 to 1 000 000 in extreme cases. In type II disease pepsin digest of the abomasal mucosa or incubation in lukewarm normal saline will reveal large numbers of inhibited fourth stage worms. The pH of the abomasal contents will be raised to pH 4.5.

Treatment

Type I disease can be treated with almost any of the anthelmintics currently available such as levamisole, benzimidazoles or ivermectin. Type II disease requires the use of some of the modern longer acting benzimidazoles or pro-benzimidazoles or, especially, ivermectin, all of which are more effective in removing both adult and inhibited fourth stage parasites. Levamisole is much less effective for type II disease as it has a poor efficiency against inhibited worms due to its rapid excretion (see p. 80).

Prevention

As for most parasitic diseases, prevention is more cost-effective than treatment. Since there are no vaccines yet available for gastrointestinal nematodes, numerous schemes that combine grazing management and anthelmintic therapy have been developed. The methods fall into three types: (i) evasive; (ii) suppressive; and (iii) dilution.

Evasive strategies. The basis of this category (also called the 'Weybridge' system) was first enunciated by Michel (1968) at the laboratory of the same name. Using the knowledge of the epidemiology of parasitic gastro-enteritis that had then become available, Michel pointed out that if susceptible cattle were removed from infected to uninfected grazing just before the summer increase in infective larval numbers, serious parasitism could be avoided. When combined with anthelmintic treatment at the time of movement the system reduces the level of nematode worm egg contamination on the clean grazing. In essence, therefore, the system involves taking no prophylactic action until early July. At that time, pasture which has not been used for cattle grazing that year is available after grass has been taken for silage making or some other form of conservation.

The calves are given anthelmintic treatment before being moved to it. The timing of the treatment can vary with the pharmacokinetics of the anthelmintic used and its effect on nematode eggs if contamination of the aftergrass is to be avoided. For instance, the longer acting benzimidazole anthelmintics (oxfendazole, albendazole, fenbendazole) are ovicidal within a few hours after treatment and their slow rate of excretion means that cattle are protected from infection with susceptible parasites for approximately 30 hours after treatment. They can therefore be put back safely onto the contaminated grazing for 24 hours after treatment before transfer to the aftergrass. The same technique can be applied with ivermectin, which although not ovicidal has an even longer half-life and will inhibit further infections for at least one week. On the other hand, levamisole has a rapid excretion rate and is also not ovicidal. If reduction of contamination as well as nematode removal is intended, cattle treated with levamisole require to be yarded after treatment at least overnight if not for 24 hours. After this first treatment in early to mid-July, and depending on the availability of grass and its previous grazing history the calves may require no further treatment until housed in late autumn, although in practice many are treated four to six weeks after the first movement. Although highly effective and the most economical method of prophylaxis when carried out carefully, it should be pointed out that although excellent for control of gastrointestinal nematodes it is not completely effective in the prevention of lungworm infection caused by *Dictyocaulus viviparus*.

Suppressive strategies. These have been introduced gradually since the mid 1970s and are also based on knowledge of the epidemiology of the infections. Unlike the evasive systems, which allow natural infection and pasture contamination to take place in spring and early summer, the basis of these methods is to suppress egg production during that period (Fig. 17.2). If pasture contamination is prevented or reduced, the summer increase of infective larvae is of such proportions as to cause a negligible risk of severe parasitism. Suppression is carried out by two different methods: (i) repeated anthelmintic treatments with standard preparations, the interval between which is determined by the pharmacokinetic properties of the chemical used; or (ii) the use of a device, usually an intraruminal bolus, which has a continuous slow release of the active anthelmintic for periods from 60 to 120 days. Such boluses are usually administered by balling-gun at or just before susceptible calves are put out to grass in the spring, although recent experiments have shown that they can also be effective when given in midsummer to prevent infection in calves grazing previously contaminated fields. The length of prophylactic activity varies between different climatic areas and nematode species, e.g. in southeastern areas of the UK suppression for eight weeks after being put to pasture in spring may be sufficient, but in wetter western areas it may require to be prolonged for a further 5 weeks and if lungworm infections are present on the farm for up to 15 weeks.

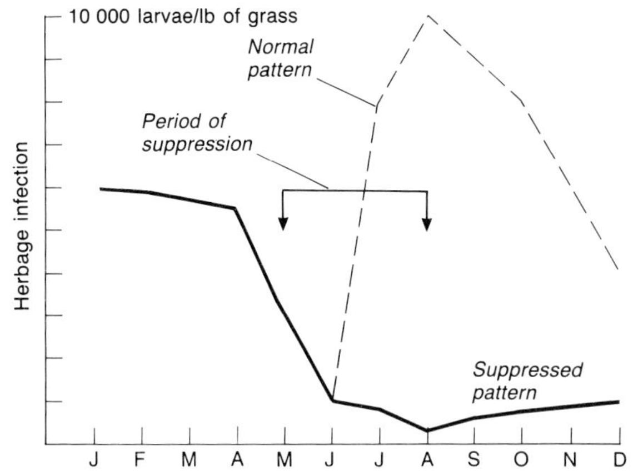

Fig. 17.2 Rationale for anthelmintic suppression.

Dilution strategies. Originally described in New Zealand as the Ruakura method (McMeekin, 1954) and further amended by Leaver (1970), the methods consist of the grazing of paddocks in relays by groups of calves followed by groups of older cattle. The basis of the technique is that the greater consumption of infective larvae by the immune or partially immune adults will delay and reduce the build-up of infective larvae on the paddocks. Initially, no anthelmintic treatments were given, but in modern practice the method is frequently combined with either of the evasive or suppressive techniques.

The advantages and disadvantages of each of the

three preventive methods are summarized in Table 17.2.

Parasitic bronchitis

Dictyocaulus viviparus is almost the sole cause of severe pulmonary helminth infections in cattle. Occasionally, other parasites are found but rarely in numbers sufficiently large to cause disease. In general, calves at grass from midsummer to autumn are those most frequently clinically affected, but heavy infections in animals of any age previously uninfected will produce signs. It is most prevalent in dairy-type calves, but is also common in weaned beef calves. The range of signs can vary from occasional coughing to severe respiratory distress, and is a reflection of the number of infective larvae ingested during a relatively short period.

Aetiology and epidemiology

The immediate cause of clinical symptoms is the ingestion two to four weeks previously of large numbers of infective larvae of *D. viviparus* by non-immune cattle. Experimentally, severe infections can be induced by a single administration of larvae at a rate of between 25 and 50 larvae/kg body weight. Typically, an affected calf weighing 300 kg will have ingested between 7500 and 15 000 L3 (3rd stage larvae). This is a much smaller infection than is required to cause parasitic gastroenteritis by *O. ostertagi*, and is an indication of lesser margin for error involved in ensuring adequate prophylaxis.

Table 17.2 Advantages and disadvantages of the prophylactic methods for gastrointestinal parasites

Method	Advantages	Disadvantages
Evasive	Low labour cost Low anthelmintic cost Not likely to lead to anthelmintic resistance in nematodes	Does not protect against lungworm Reduces the flexibility of pasture usage in the late summer
Suppressive	If carried out for long enough will reduce the chances of lungworm infection More likely to lead to anthelmintic resistance in target nematodes	Higher labour or anthelmintic costs especially in the case of slow-release boluses Allows more flexible use of grazing
Dilution	Lower anthelmintic costs	Requires excellent fencing and high labour costs and is generally used only in well organized dairy farms Is not effective for prevention of lungworm infection

The epidemiology is more complex and infections are also much less predictable than are those of gastrointestinal nematodes, principally because at present not all details of larval survival and transmission are known. Infections are more prevalent in wetter areas especially those in the west of the British Isles. One of the major differences between *D. viviparus* and gastrointestinal nematodes that has an influence on the unpredictability of infections is that the female worm produces eggs containing fully developed larvae, which are passed in the faeces. These become infective within a much shorter time than the eggs of *Ostertagia* species and hence in optimal conditions can produce a rapid increase in their numbers. In addition to rapidity of maturation to infectivity, larvae are also dispersed from faecal pats by some of the following means: (i) ascending the common faecal fungus *Pilobolus* and being propelled into the air on discharge of the sporangium, to be carried by wind to adjacent areas; (ii) although unverified, there is evidence that earthworms or coprophagous beetles may act as transport hosts; (iii) also unverified, it has been reported that the European hare (*Lepus europaeus*) can be infected, although experiments have shown that the smaller blue hare (*L. timidus*) common in Ireland is refractory to infection. In addition to these means of dispersal it has been shown that infective larvae can remain viable in soil as well as on pasture over the winter, and that small numbers of adult worms and hypobiotic larvae can survive and overwinter in infected animals despite their hosts having some immunity to further infection, only to mature and propagate larvae during the following spring.

Pathogenesis

After ingestion, infective larvae penetrate the intestinal mucosa, moult to the L4 stage of their life cycle and migrate via bloodstream and lymphatic channels to the lungs. This takes place approximately one week after being consumed, and up to this point no clinical effects are observed in the host. After that period, larvae break out of blood vessels into alveoli and small bronchioles, after which they moult to become young adults, and as they increase in size they ascend the bronchiolar tree towards the large bronchioles and bronchi. Larvae are first found in faeces from the 25th day after infection.

Signs

Clinical signs appear during the second week after infection and their severity depends on the number of developing worms. The signs range from occasional to repeated coughing, with a noticeably increased respiration rate in the worst affected. By the third week, severely affected cattle do little else except stand in a characteristic head extended position with rapid shallow breathing and frequent coughing.

Although most calves if not severely affected will recover after treatment, a small percentage will suffer a relapse of clinical signs in the absence of fresh infection. The precise aetiology of this is uncertain but autopsy reveals an oedematous rubbery lung with alveolar epithelialization observed microscopically.

Necropsy

The pathological progression during maturation progresses from alveolitis and bronchiolitis to bronchitis and severe emphysema, sometimes with superimposition of a secondary bacterial pneumonia. If left untreated after patency even moderate infections can progress in severity due to aspiration of eggs and hatched larvae back into previously unaffected alveoli and smaller bronchioles, resulting in bronchitis and pneumonia.

Diagnosis

Affected cattle are invariably presented with varying degrees of respiratory abnormality, and since similar signs can occur as a result of infection by a variety of pathogens, careful differential diagnosis is advisable. The grazing history and time of the year in northern temperate areas invariably involve cattle grazing established pasture previously used by other cattle plus the appearance of clinical signs between July and October. Since the caudal lobes of the lung are more frequently affected, adventitious lung sounds are usually more apparent from these areas, in contrast to those from viral pneumonias, which usually affect the cranial and medial lobes. Confirmation of the diagnosis by identification of larvae in faeces or sputum samples can only take place after patency, which takes place approximately 25 days after infection, although it should be noted that in adults that are suffering from a re-infection the infection usually does not reach patency.

Treatment

In order to kill the worms and larvae present in the lung tissues, anthelmintic treatment is essential. The most effective are ivermectin, levamisole and some of the more recently developed benzimidazoles or probenzimidazoles, such as oxfendazole, fenbendazole, albendazole and netobimin. Severely affected animals may also require antibiotic therapy to control secondary bacterial pneumonia and if anorexia has been present rehydration with electrolytes may also be helpful. In most outbreaks a range of severity is observed and it is frequently advisable to house the worst affected cattle, especially if climatic conditions would be stressful even to healthy calves. In addition, because treatment of severe cases can exacerbate signs farmers should be warned of the possibility. In outbreaks involving adult dairy cows care should be taken that the anthelmintic used does not prevent sale of milk products for a prolonged period until a withholding time long enough to allow excretion of the drug has passed. The drug with the shortest withholding period is levamisole, and experience has shown that in such cases cows can be treated with it in small batches each day, the most severely affected first, in an effort to reduce the sale of milk as little as possible (see p. 823).

Prevention

There are two major methods available, the first relying on inducing immunity and the second on suppression of infections.

Vaccination (see p. 810). Immunity can be stimulated by the use of a live vaccine, which takes the form of two doses of 1000 infective larvae irradiated by gamma-irradiation. Calves should be two months old before vaccination and the doses separated by four weeks and preferably both doses given before going to grass in the spring or before the time of earliest challenge in outdoor calves. Although the vaccine induces excellent protection against clinical disease it does not completely prevent all worms from natural infections completing their life cycle, so that the parasite can be maintained at a very low level on pasture grazed by vaccinated cattle. If the farmer neglects to vaccinate, parasite numbers can quickly increase sufficiently, if weather conditions are favourable, to affect non-immune cattle within their first grazing season.

Suppression. On farms where calves have suffered lung damage due to viral pneumonia, vaccination may be inadvisable because of the possibility of exacerbation of the existing lesions. Under these circumstances it has been found that regular anthelmintic treatments throughout the grazing season can suppress infection sufficiently to minimize the danger of clinical disease and at the same time allow some immunity to be induced by the natural ingestion of infective larvae from pasture, which are subsequently killed before completion of their life cycle. The method has also been successfully applied to normal healthy calves, but it requires to be carried out and monitored carefully, since there are potential problems in its use. Firstly, the length of time during which anthelmintic suppression is required may vary between areas with different climatic patterns and farming practices. In general in the British Isles it is necessary to provide anthelmintic cover until mid-August. The methods of application require that the anthelmintic must be extremely effective against all stages of the parasitic life cycle of the nematode. Those anthelmintics used fairly successfully have been injections of ivermectin at three, eight and thirteen weeks after going to grass on 1 May, and an intermittent-release intraruminal bolus designed to administer a therapeutic dose of oxfendazole approximately every three weeks for 130 days. The level of immunity stimulated depends on the number of larvae ingested from pasture, and since this can be highly variable some cattle in a group may have inadequate resistance to future infection should they be exposed to it. As a result, careful monitoring is necessary after cessation of anthelmintic treatment and some thought required to plan cattle husbandry during the subsequent year.

Stephanurosis (kidney worm)

Aetiology and epidemiology

This is mainly an infestation of pigs but it can infect calves and is due to *Stephanurus dentatus*. The adult is up to 45 mm in length.

The condition is found in the tropical and subtropical countries of Africa, East and West Indies, Brazil, Hawaii, Philippines, Australia and southern Europe where pigs are kept but in calves adult worms do not develop. The larvae cause damage to the liver parenchyma during migration and produce thrombosis of the abdominal blood vessels, which may be fatal. Aberrant larvae can encapsulate anywhere in the host but the majority are found in all parts of the kidney. The eggs produced in the pig form hatch to produce first stage larvae. These develop to third stage infective larvae if there is warmth and moisture. The larvae are often ingested by earthworms and these act as a vector for infection. The infective larvae are otherwise susceptible to cold or drying. Transmission is either by ingestion, which may include earthworms or by skin penetration. In the host they pass to the liver where they remain for a considerable time before going to other parts of the body.

Signs

They are mostly of anaemia, ill thrift and ascites. Many infestations are without signs.

Necropsy

Necrotic lesions with thrombosis in the mesenteric blood vessels and hypertrophy of the mesenteric lymph nodes are likely to be found. In a few cases there may be haemorrhages and abscesses in the lungs and kidneys.

Diagnosis

This will depend on the presence of calves grazing areas with infected pigs. An immunodiffusion test can be used. There is a marked eosinophilia.

Treatment and control

Fenbendazole at high doses may be effective. Calves should not graze pastures recently used by pigs.

Fascioliosis

Fascioliasis in cattle is a chronic wasting disease caused by the presence in the liver and bile ducts respectively of immature and adult trematodes of the genus *Fasciola*. The disease is found in vast areas of the world, with the smaller *F. hepatica* (3.5 × 1 cm) in temperate countries and the larger *F. gigantica* (7.5 × 1 cm) in tropical regions the commonest species. Calves and yearlings are most commonly affected but any age of animal may be susceptible. Although it may take place at any time of the year, infection is most prevalent during autumn in temperate areas with the resultant effects of disease becoming apparent in winter and spring.

Aetiology and epidemiology

F. hepatica. Multiplication of the parasite is partially climatically regulated, since its life cycle involves an intermediate host that requires adequate moisture and a suitable ambient temperature. The intermediate hosts are various species of snail of the genus *Lymnaea*, which are found on wet mud surfaces. In the British Isles, *L. truncatula* is the species involved. It prefers a neutral or slightly alkaline habitat, but can survive in fairly acid conditions such as peaty hills, although under such conditions individual snails remain small and the population low. At its maximum it can have a shell length of 1·cm. The snail population fluctuates, being least in winter and greatest in June and July, especially in years when late spring rainfall has been above average, when large numbers accumulate and are therefore available for transmission of *F. hepatica*.

Briefly summarized the life cycle of *F. hepatica* is as follows. The adult parasite in the bile ducts is a hermaphrodite and can be self- or cross-fertilized. Large numbers of eggs are produced by each parasite, which pass from the ducts to the gall-bladder and are subsequently passed into the intestine on contraction of that organ. Eggs are then passed in the faeces, but will not hatch unless moist and until an ambient temperature of 10 °C is reached. Hatching at temperatures between 22 and 26 °C takes nine days, but under normal temperatures in the months of May and June in the British Isles, it can take four weeks. On hatching, the released miracidium must locate and penetrate the foot of *L. truncatula* within three hours. Once in the snail, the parasite undergoes multiplication through stages of sporocyst and rediae and reaches the cercarial stage after a minimum of two months, although in colder temperatures it may take up to 16 weeks or should winter intervene complete development may cease until the following spring. Under natural conditions within the British Isles, cercariae from summer infections are released from snails between late August and October, and in some areas from overwintered infections in April or May. On release from the snail, which must take place in conditions of wetness, the cercariae swim to the nearest plant, encyst on its leaves and become the infective stage, termed metacercariae, several hundred of which can arise from one miracidium. Metacercariae on herbage can survive for several months and can therefore maintain the infection from one year to the next.

Cattle become infected by ingestion of grass on which metacercariae are encysted. The metacercariae excyst in the small intestine, the wall of which they penetrate to reach the peritoneal cavity where they move to the liver and invade its capsule. At this point the flukes are very small (about 1 mm) but as they burrow through the liver parenchyma they gradually increase in size and in primary infections in cattle will reach the bile ducts after six to eight weeks, when they mature and become egg-laying adults 10–12 weeks after ingestion. In response to the presence of fluke in the liver parenchyma, the liver of cattle produces a more intense fibrous reaction than that of sheep, and the resultant cirrhosis is much more severe and is longer lasting. The liver cells of cattle do not regenerate as do those of sheep, and the result of even moderate infection in cattle is a more fibrous liver parenchyma than in most other species.

Within the bile ducts, the adult flukes suck blood and the spines on their cuticle cause multiple small haemorrhagic lesions. In cattle, the resultant fibrous reaction within the bile ducts is also more severe than in sheep and the bile ducts walls thicken and become gradually calcified thereafter (Fig. 17.3). The result of the fibrous reaction during a primary infection in both bile ducts and parenchyma of cattle shortens the life span of adult flukes in the ducts to a maximum of 1.5 years and reduces the chances of flukes from subsequent infections being able to complete their life cycle. Cattle therefore become largely resistant to further infections, most of which do not become patent and the few flukes that do so may take much longer than normal to reach patency and survive in bile ducts for a relatively short time.

F. gigantica. Although similar in many respects to *F. hepatica* it is not found in western Europe, but is widespread within tropical and subtropical climatic regions. The intermediate hosts are also snails of the genus *Lymnaea* but the species are more aquatic than those transmitting *F. hepatica*, and thrive in swamps, drainage channels and artificially flooded areas. As a result the epidemiology is closely tied to the periods of maximum rainfall, the snails being infected and development in the snail completed within these periods. Cercariae are shed towards the end of the wet season and encyst on herbage and even on the water surface at the start of the dry season.

The parasitic life cycle is similar to that of *F. hepatica* but each phase takes slightly longer with the result that patency of primary infections take three or four weeks longer than *F. hepatica*, eggs being found in faeces from 13 to 16 weeks after ingestion of metacercariae.

Signs

There is a progressive loss of weight with anaemia and occasionally oedema.

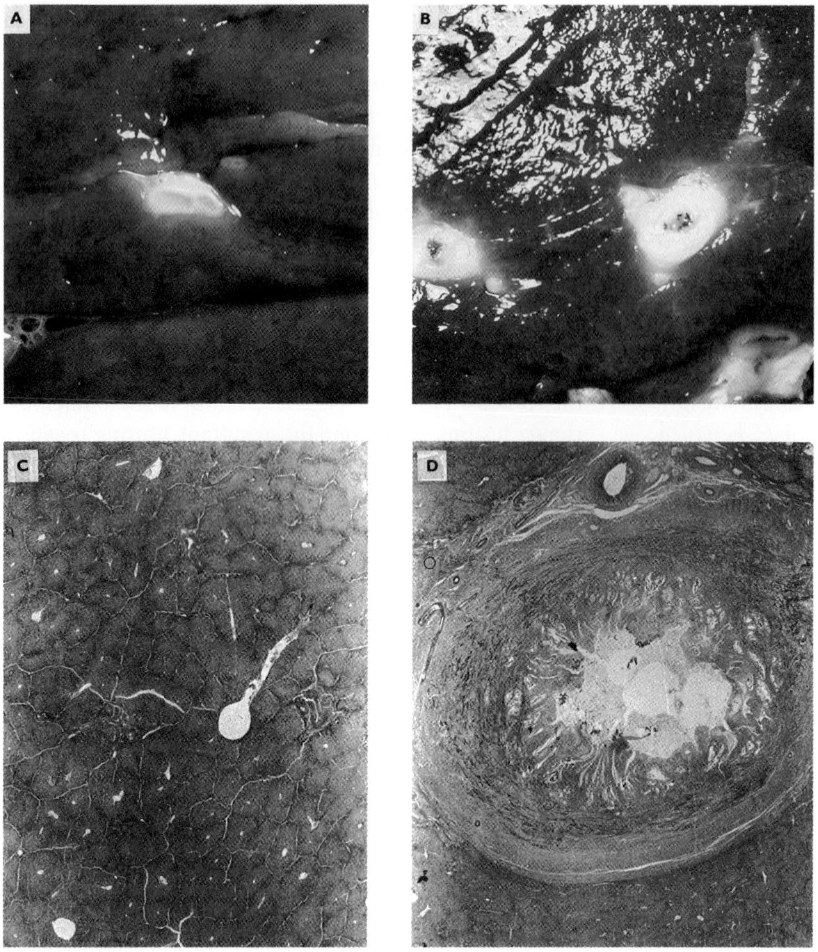

Fig. 17.3 (A) Normal and (B) liver-fluke infected bovine liver. (C,D) Microscopic sections of the same stained to show fibrous tissue.

Diagnosis

The disease is characterized by a gradual loss of condition that is exacerbated if the quantity and quality of feeding is suboptimal. A chronic anaemia develops and the packed cell volume (PCV) drops to approximately 20%. Erythrocytes are hypochromic but normocytic, and while the leucocyte count may be slightly raised, the percentage of eosinophils in a differential count is greatly increased and may consist of up to 20 per cent of the total white cell count. In cows the total milk yield and the non-fat solids proportions may be reduced.

Diagnosis can be confirmed by the presence of fluke eggs in faeces samples, but detection is not always as simple as in sheep, especially in adults since even in patent infections excretion of eggs is intermittent. Examination of plasma shows a hypoalbuminaemia, and during the migration phase the plasma glutamate dehydrogenase (GLDH) is raised. Once the epithelium of the bile duct walls becomes diseased, the plasma concentration of gamma-glutamyl transpeptidase (GT) rises and this is a useful diagnostic indicator.

Treatment

Affected cattle are treated by administration of a fasciolicide. Of those currently used for cattle the commonest are oxyclozanide, rafoxanide, nitroxynil, albendazole, netobimin and triclabendazole. All will remove more than 90 per cent of adult flukes from the bile ducts, but they have variable efficiencies against the immature stages migrating through the liver. The most effective is triclabendazole, which will remove developing flukes from a few days after ingestion. Rafoxanide and nitroxynil are effective against six-week-old flukes at normal dose rates and at increased dose levels affect those four weeks old. Albendazole, netobimin and oxyclozanide at normal dose rates remove only adult flukes from the bile ducts, but are suitable for lactating dairy cows, since oxyclozanide requires no milk withdrawal and albendazole and netobimin a three-day interval (see p. 823).

Prevention

There are four methods available that are used individually in suitable circumstances or can be combined in an attempt to give a more rapid reduction in the prevalence of the parasite.

1 Prophylactic use of anthelmintics to reduce both the number of flukes in cattle and the number of eggs excreted. This is by far the commonest practice and involves treatment of cattle once or twice annually. In the British Isles such treatments take place in the autumn and late spring.

2 If the areas of snail habitat are delineated and small and they can be drained. This is usually not cost-effective for fluke control alone if the sites are extensive.

3 Small snail habitats can be fenced off during the time of greatest infection.

4 Snail habitats can be treated with molluscicide. There can be environmental objections since many which were formerly in use were toxic to many species in addition to snails. The most satisfactory is *N*-tritylmorpholine, which although not available in the UK is used in many tropical countries.

Paramphistomosis (stomach fluke disease, intestinal amphistomiasis)

Aetiology and epidemiology

The cause of acute paramphistomiasis in Africa is *Paramphistomum microbothrium*. Other *Paramphistomum* spp. and *Cotylophoron* spp. are found in ruminants in Africa and tropical and subtropical regions. In Asia, *Calicophoron* spp. are found and one species occurs in Africa. *Carmyerius* spp. is seen in Africa, India, Pakistan and the Middle East.

It has been recorded in a severe form in Australia, India and the USA. The life cycle is indirect and similar to that of *Fasciola*. It involves aquatic snails that are adapted to a variety of locations. Disease only occurs where there is a massive concentration of the infected planorbid snails. The metacercariae are ingested and the immature flukes develop in the duodenum where they may be seen in the mucosa. The flukes are 3–4 mm long and 1–2 mm wide. They also develop in the abomasum but are less common. They then migrate through the abomasum to the rumen and reticulum where again few are found. The prepatent period is very variable, being between one and a half to four months. Most outbreaks occur in the late summer, autumn or early winter when pastures are being contaminated with cercariae. Although all ages of cattle are susceptible, infestation is most commonly seen in yearlings. Fewer infestations occur in the adult, suggesting some degree of immunity.

Signs

Acute This is due to a massive infestation in calves. There is a persistent fetid diarrhoea without blood or mucus. There is anorexia, weakness, marked loss of condition, and then recumbency. In some cases there is submaxillary oedema and a pallor of the mucosa. Death occurs in about one to two weeks after signs develop.

Chronic In heavy infestations of adult flukes there is a chronic loss of weight, a dry coat and anaemia.

Necropsy

In the acute case there is severe inflammation of the duodenum and abomasum as the parasite penetrates deeply into the mucosa and sometimes the muscularis layer, and there is haemorrhage. There is muscular atrophy, subcutaneous oedema and fluid accumulation in the body cavities. Large numbers of small, immature, flesh-coloured flukes are present in the lumen. In less acute cases the duodenum is thickened and congested. There is fluid in the abdominal cavity.

Diagnosis

Most disease occurs with immature flukes and so it is not easy to detect in the live animal but it can be missed at post mortem. Often other parasitic infestations are present, which again causes paramphistomiasis to be overlooked. However, the history and area where the cattle are grazing can give some indications. There is a reduction in the red and white blood cells and a hypoalbuminaemia. Differential diagnoses include copper and cobalt deficiencies, liver fluke, parasitic gastroenteritis, Johne's disease in the adult and poisoning.

Treatment

Few of the modern trematocides have been tested against paramphistomiasis but there is no reason to believe that they may not be helpful. Brotianide at

55 mg/kg is effective against adult flukes but less so against the immature stages. Diamphenithide should be effective in the early stages, and niclosamide at 90 mg/kg has some efficacy against the immature parasite.

Control

Drainage of low-lying areas and destruction of the soil will considerably reduce infestation. The most susceptible animals, i.e. calves and immature cattle, should be kept away from likely snail habitats. Routine treatment against *Paramphistomum* before they mature and can infect snails is of use.

Schistosomosis (bilharziosis)

Aetiology and epidemiology

There are several parasites in the genus *Schistosoma*. *Schistosoma bovis* is found in African, Asian and southern European cattle. *Schistosoma mattheei* occurs in cattle in Central and southern Africa and can infect man. *Schistosoma indicum* is found in India and Pakistan as is also *S. spindale*, which can also occur in South East Asia and Indonesia. *Schistosoma japonicum* occurs in the Far East. *Schistosoma nasale* is again found in India and Pakistan and is unusual in that the adult occurs in the mucosal veins of the nose. Several minor species occur involving *S. curassoni*.

Various species of the parasite are widespread and the adults live in veins. Unlike most flukes, *Schistosoma* spp. are not hermaphroditic and the longer male carries the long slender female, which is up to 25 mm long, in a gyroectoplasmic canal. Infection can be via the skin or gut. After penetrating the skin the schistosomulae (young flukes) pass via the lymphatic system to the right side of the heart. They then go via the lungs into the circulation and then to the liver. They mature in the portal veins before migrating to their final area, usually the mesenteric veins, but they are also found in the urinary bladder veins in the case of *S. mattheei* and in the nasal mucosal veins in *S. nasale*. When infection is oral the gut is penetrated and the immature stages pass to the liver via the blood.

Once mature, eggs are produced that can hatch within minutes if conditions are right. The free-swimming microdiae penetrate snail hosts producing sporocysts, daughter sporocyst and cercariae but there are no redia. The cercariae must infect the final host within one or two days or they die off as there is no metacercarial stage. There are various genera of snails involved depending on the species of *Schistosoma* (Table 17.3). All the snails like mud except for *Oncomelonia* spp., which are aquatic.

Table 17.3 Intermediate snail hosts of *Schistosoma* spp.

Species	Intermediate snail host genus
S. bovis	*Bulinus* and *Physopsis*
S. indicum	*Indoplanorbis*
S. japonicum	*Oncomelania*
S. mattheei	*Bulinus*
S. nasale	*Lymnaea* and *Indoplanorbis*

In many areas of Africa most of the cattle are infected but there are very few signs. Young cattle are more likely to be ill.

Signs

The main signs are of diarrhoea, which may contain blood and mucus, and is intermittent. There is a loss of condition and reduced resistance to other diseases. Death occasionally occurs. Infestation with *S. nasale* causes a mucopurulent nasal discharge with dyspnoea. Chronic cases develop nasal granuloma.

Necropsy

In severe infestation there are small grey–white granules in the gastrointestinal tract with petechial haemorrhages and ecchymosis. The ileocaecal body may be enlarged and haemorrhagic. Granulomas may also be scattered through the liver parenchyma as well as the lungs and bladder. In *S. nasale* infestation there may be nasal granulomas.

Diagnosis

The signs and grazing history help but it is difficult to diagnose unless faeces are taken or nasal discharge if *S. nasale* is present. The eggs are large and characteristically spiral. As the eggs hatch quickly they need to be fixed in 10 per cent formalin.

Differential diagnosis involves coccidiosis, trypanosomiasis, poisoning and Johne's disease.

Treatment

Trichlorophan, an organophosphorus compound, can be used parenterally, or niridazole or thioxanthane derivatives such as becanthane or hycanthane may be used. Treatment must be performed carefully otherwise a large number of dead schistosomes will produce emboli and lead to hepatic infarction or portal occlusion.

Control

Immunity to the disease occurs but varies with the *Schistosoma* spp. Control involves keeping cattle away from areas frequented by the intermediate host. Molluscicides can be of some benefit.

Coccidiosis

Bovine coccidiosis almost invariably affects groups of cattle less than one year old, although it does occasionally occur in older animals. It is manifested by enteritis, diarrhoea and in severe cases dysentery. Not all members of the group are equally affected and light infections are self-limiting; severe infections can be fatal if untreated. The disease is caused by the ingestion over a short period of large numbers of oocysts of *Eimeria* species by non-immune cattle, the larger the infective dose producing the most severe signs. *Eimeria* are species specific, and although there are 13 species that have been isolated from cattle, *E. zuernii* and *E. bovis* are much the commonest and most pathogenic. They are found everywhere in the world where cattle are farmed.

Aetiology and epidemiology

The presence of large enough accumulations of oocysts to cause disease is the result of farming practices that allow groups of cattle, which frequently have been stressed by transport and by mixing with others, to ingest food or water contaminated by faeces. It can happen either indoors on straw bedding, which is both damp and contaminated with faeces, or outdoors around drinking or feeding troughs. It can take place at any time of the year so long as conditions prevail that produce adequate moisture and temperature for oocysts to survive and become infective, but frequently occurs three or four weeks after groups of purchased calves are mixed. In North America it has also been associated with the sudden stress of extreme temperature reductions in midwinter.

After ingestion, the oocyst is disrupted, releasing eight sporozoites each of which penetrates an intestinal epithelial cell and develops into a trophozoite. Multiple fission within the trophozoite produces a schizont, which after a few days ruptures the cell to release a large number of merozoites, which in turn invade other epithelial cells. There are up to four generations of schizogony depending on the species involved. The location of the cells invaded is important for the pathogenicity of the species, e.g. *E. zuernii* and *E. bovis* both invade cells in the lower ileum and later schizogony and gametogony (the term used to describe the sexual stages) take place in the epithelial cells of the caecum and colon. The gametocytes are formed deep in the epithelium and their rupture causes severe disruption of the lining of the caecum with resultant haemorrhage into the lumen. After gametogony, oocysts are formed that subsequently are passed in faeces. They are not immediately infective but require to undergo sporulation, in which the sporocyts and sporozoites are formed ready for further infection. The last process requires adequate moisture and warmth and takes 24–72 hours. The total life cycle from ingestion to patency occupies 15–17 days for *E. zuernii* and 15–20 days for *E. bovis*. Oocyst production during infection with a single species lasts for five to twelve days but may be prolonged in multiple species infections. The oocysts are very resistant to external conditions and will survive for up to two years in suitable environments with adequate moisture. They can resist moderate frosts down to $-8\,°C$ for two months, but are susceptible to drought, high temperatures and the chemical action of ammonia.

Signs

The presenting signs of diarrhoea or dysentery accompanied sometimes with severe straining in a group of calves leads to suspicion of coccidiosis.

Diagnosis

Examination of faeces samples for the presence of large numbers of oocysts can confirm the diagnosis. Care should be taken in interpretation of oocyst counts since small numbers are present in the faeces of many normal calves, and in severely affected diarrhoeic calves the main oocyst production phase may have passed or their numbers be misjudged due to the dilution factor of liquid faeces. Occasionally, calves may exhibit nervous signs the reasons for which are as yet obscure, and viral diseases that have cerebral affects should be considered.

Treatment

Two considerations need to be borne in mind. Firstly, severely affected calves will require individual treatment with an anticoccidial and, if deemed advisable, fluid therapy with electrolytes and injections of antibiotics to control secondary bacterial injections. Anticoccidial treatments include injections of sulpha drugs or the oral administration of sulphadimidine at 140 mg/kg body weight daily for three days, or amprolium at 10 mg/kg for four or five days. It should be remembered that overdose with amprolium, which is a thiamine antagonist, has been associated with producing cerebrocortical necrosis (CCN) so care should be taken to give the correct dose.

Secondly, prophylactic treatment for other calves in the group should be assessed, depending on the numbers involved. Monensin included in the diet at 16.5 p.p.m. of the diet, either continuously to suppress all infection or for two cycles of medication for a week separated by a week when it is removed, can protect from the infection and allow sufficient immunity to be stimulated. Sulphadimidine can also be used prophylactically at 35 mg/kg, but it should be borne in mind that as light infections are self-limiting such treatments may not be cost-effective.

Other measures should be taken to reduce the chances of infection, i.e. removal of food contaminated with faeces, better siting of feeding and water troughs so that faecal deposition on food and in water is made less likely. If the problem is a recurring event with each batch of calves, thought should be given to a short period of anticoccidial treatment after two weeks of exposure to possible infection so that incipient infections are disrupted but sufficient stimulation of immunity has been allowed to take place. A potent anticoccidial of a novel chemical type, toltrazuril, has been used experimentally in this manner with great success and may constitute a significant future advance in the prophylaxis of the disease.

Sarcosporidiosis (sarcocystosis)

Aetiology

The cause is *Sarcocystis*, a coccidial protozoan that has a predator–prey life cycle. The indirect hosts are dogs, cats and man and each may contain several species of sarcocyst, each one specific for a different intermediate host. *Sarcocystis hirsuta* is present in the ox and cat species, *S. cruzi* in the ox and dog and *S. hominis* in the ox and man. In the final host the *Sarcocystis* spp. undergo an enteric cycle with oocysts in the cells producing sporocysts in the faeces. On entry to some intermediate hosts those infected via the dog undergo schizogamy in blood vessel endothelial cells before passing to the muscle. Those of the cat are not pathogenic and are found in the oesophagus, and throughout the tissues of the intermediate host produce microscopic cysts. If cattle are grazing and ingesting a few oocysts this probably results in a strong immunity. Signs develop about 26 days after infection.

Signs

Usually, no signs occur but, following ingestion of massive doses, calves may develop anorexia, fever, emaciation and anaemia. Adults can suffer pyrexia, emaciation and abortion.

Necropsy

There are usually petechial and ecchymotic haemorrhages throughout the body, especially in the heart, brain, liver, lungs, kidneys and muscle. Some animals show emaciation, lymphadenopathy, anaemia and ascites. Death is usually due to necrotizing endocarditis. Histologically, schizonts can be found in the endothelium throughout the body and haemorrhages, lymphatic infiltration and oedema occur in the tissues and organs.

Diagnosis

This is usually based on post-mortem findings.

Treatment

There is no satisfactory treatment but amprolium has been used to reduce the severity of infection.

Control

This is difficult but involves keeping carnivores away from cattle. Infection in dogs and cats can be avoided by cooking the meat.

Taenia saginata

Taenia saginata is a cyclophyllidean tapeworm, for which man is the final host. It is transmitted to man by the ingestion of the intermediate larval stage in undercooked beef. Although the larval stage can be found in any age of cattle, viable cysts are found mainly in cattle up to two years of age. The presence of the parasite in the muscles of cattle does not cause clinical signs unless the animal is very heavily infected and the myocardium is involved, but because it is a zoonotic infection its presence can cause significant losses to the beef industry, especially in developing countries. In countries where sanitation standards are high it is a decreasing problem that on average is found in 0.5 per cent of bovine carcasses, with occasional heavy infections occurring under unusual circumstances. In those areas of Africa, Asia and parts of Latin America where human sanitation methods are rudimentary or non-existent and local customs favour ingestion of raw or undercooked beef, the prevalence may be up to 20 per cent.

Epidemiology

The adult tapeworm inhabits the intestines of man. Its scolex has no hooks, and apparently moves up or down the intestine depending on whether the host has eaten recently or not. When the host's stomach is empty the scolex moves back up the intestine towards the duodenum, and these movements produce hunger pains and vague intestinal discomfort. Fully grown the tapeworm may reach a length of 8 m. Mature egg-filled (about 25 000) proglottids are shed from its posterior end and are passed in faeces or wriggle out of the host's anus nocturnally. Anal pruritis and occasional diarrhoea are usually the only signs apart from the aesthetic and hygienic conditions involved.

The eggs are resistant to external conditions. They are inactivated within two weeks if desiccated, but are known to survive for 16 days in raw sewage, 71 days in liquid manure, 159 days on pasture and 200 days in sewage sludge. No normal method of handling sewage can inactivate them other than total incineration or extensive heat treatment. Extended periods of sludge digestion with or without heat may affect viability but technical proof is lacking. Chemical disinfectants other than some containing copper at very high pH (11.5) are not ovicidal.

Two-thirds of outbreaks in developed countries have been shown to be associated with the spreading of sewage sludge on agricultural land. The remainder have been presumed to be caused by spread of seagulls feeding at sewage plants and passing viable eggs through them on to grazing land, or by accidental flooding of pasture by contaminated effluent streams from sewage plants. Migrant labour from less developed countries and infected stockmen have been implicated in some isolated local multiple infections.

Once ingested, the egg hatches and the liberated oncosphere travels via the bloodstream to striated muscular tissue, including the myocardium. It develops in the muscle and reaches infectivity three months after ingestion, when it is recognizable as a whitish fluid-filled cyst with a diameter of approximately 1 cm, known as a cysticercus. It becomes enclosed in a thin fibrous capsule. Cellular immune reaction around it gradually increases and the capsule becomes thickened, eventually leading to the death of a high proportion of the cysticerci within 18 months and resistance to further infection, although some may survive for several years. After death the contents of the cysts become caseous and finally calcified. The masseter, tongue and heart muscles were generally considered preferential sites and are still examined carefully during meat inspection at abattoirs, in preference to damaging more expensive cuts of meat by the multiple incisions that would otherwise be necessary.

Control

There are no drugs suitable for ante-mortem treatment. Carcasses that are found to be infected are normally treated in one of two ways.

1 If lightly infected they are frozen to a temperature of −10 °C for a minimum of 10 days, after which any previously viable cysticerci will have been killed.

2 Heavily infected carcasses are usually condemned as unfit for human consumption and rendered after heat treatment into animal feedstuffs. The thermal death-point of cysticerci is 57 °C and meat for human consumption should be raised to at least that temperature if the possibility of infection is to be avoided.

***Echinococcus granulosus* and hydatid cysts**

There are two species of the taeniid tapeworm *E. granulosus*. The first is *E. granulosus granulosus*: the adult is found world-wide in the intestine of dogs and many wild Canidae but *not* the red fox. The intermediate form, the hydatid cyst, is found in domestic and wild ruminants, man and pigs, but *not* horses and donkeys. The second is *E. granulosus equinus*, which is almost exclusively found in Europe: adults parasitize the dog and the red fox, and horses and donkeys are the exclusive intermediate hosts.

Cattle therefore are affected by hydatid cysts of *E. granulosus granulosus*. The majority of hydatid cysts cause little apparent disease as they are situated in the liver or lung, their presence only becoming disclosed at abattoirs. Occasionally, they develop in sites where their gradually increasing size causes pressure on vital organs, the resultant disease being dependent on the organ and system affected.

Aetiology and epidemiology

The adult worms parasitize the small intestine of the dog. They are small worms, consisting of four segments and length 0.6 mm. Large numbers may be present in infected animals, each releasing one gravid segment daily containing many eggs, which are resistant to normal external climatic conditions and remain infective for up to two years. After ingestion by cattle or other hosts the oncosphere penetrates the wall of the intestine and is carried via the bloodstream to the liver or other organs where they lodge and start to grow to become hydatid cysts. Growth is relatively slow and may take at least one year to reach a diameter of 20 cm. In restricted sites the cyst assumes the shape of the space available, and daughter cysts may be formed and spread to other organs. If growth takes place in the omentum or mesentery cysts can become very large. There is usually little cellular reaction around cysts in cattle. Since most cattle in developed countries are slaughtered in abattoirs there is little chance of further spread unless casualties are fed to farm dogs or packs of hounds. In underdeveloped countries or where carcasses are not disposed of, wild Canidae ingesting the offal become infected, the brood capsules from within the hydatid cyst evaginating, the scolex attaching to the intestinal wall and reaching adulthood and patency some six weeks later. Infection in dogs is usually symptomless.

Treatment and control

Affected cattle are not treated specifically for hydatidosis, principally because of the difficulty of diagnosis, but also because anthelmintics are only now becoming available for treatment of infected human beings. Activity against larval forms has been claimed for praziquantel and albendazole although most cysts are excised.

Prevention is directed to ensuring that dogs do not become infected, either by regular treatment, the most effective anthelmintic being praziquantel, or by preventing the ingestion of infected offal.

Toxoplasmosis

Toxoplasmosis is a protozoan zoonosis that can infect any species of vertebrate. It is mainly recognized as being most pathogenic for sheep, however, it occasionally causes human illness, and it can cause significant disease in cattle.

Aetiology and epidemiology

The parasite involved is *Toxoplasma gondii*. It has a two-host life cycle with both sexual and asexual stages. The definitive hosts are cats, both domestic and wild, which become infected by eating raw infected meat from the intermediate host, which can be any other species of vertebrate but is frequently a rodent. Once ingested the infective cysts are digested, each releasing large numbers of bradyzoites. They penetrate intestinal epithelial cells and undergo a coccidia-like series of schizogonies and finally gametogony in the small intestine to produce oocysts in faeces within one and a half weeks after ingestion of cysts. The cat then excretes oocysts for approximately two weeks. Oocysts remain viable for 17 months on pasture and if they contaminate animal feed any animal consuming it becomes infected.

Within the intermediate host, development is asexual. The oocyst wall is disrupted releasing eight sporozoites, which reach the lymph and blood vessels after penetrating the intestinal epithelium. The tachyzoites, as they are now called, are spread throughout the body to muscles, heart, lungs, liver, uterus and central nervous system, where they penetrate cells and multiply asexually. It is during this phase that the intermediate host becomes ill. After each multiplication, the infected cells rupture releasing 8–16 tachyzoites for further spread. After some days of such divisions the host develops some resistance to the organism and the spread of tachyzoites ceases, but is replaced by the formation of slow-growing cysts, each of which eventually contains large numbers of bradyzoites. Normally these remain until ingested, but should the host's immunity be reduced by other disease the invasive process can recommence. The tissue cysts are susceptible to freezing and cooking to 70 °C for 30 s and therefore consumption of adequately cooked infected meat is harmless.

The organism is ubiquitous. Blewett (1983) reviewed the serological surveys that have been carried out in domestic animals and came to the estimate that antibody was present in 6.5 per cent of horses, 12.5 per cent of cattle, 23.5 per cent of pigs, 30 per cent of sheep and 40 per cent of cats. He also postulated that different animals vary in susceptibility to infection and in the rate of loss of antibody, and concluded that cattle return to a seronegative status much more rapidly than do sheep, which are as a result a more reliable indicator of the actual prevalence of the infection.

Diagnosis

At autopsy or in abattoirs the most common findings are multiple necrotic granulomatous foci in internal organs. Histopathological examination is necessary for confirmation. *In vivo* cattle are presented with vague pyrexic disorders sometimes affecting the central nervous system. If pregnant cows are affected, stillborn or weak calves that die within a few days of birth may result. Such calves frequently manifest nervous signs such as tremors of the head or neck, teeth grinding or convulsions.

Serological diagnosis can be made using a variety of tests such as indirect immunofluorescence or enzyme-linked immunosorbent assay (ELISA), or the Sabin–Feldman dye test. Because of ease of carrying out the test, an ELISA using both anti-IgM and anti-IgG for detection of both acute and chronic infection is currently being developed.

Treatment and control

Treatment of acutely infected animals can be attempted by the use of pyrimethamine and sulpha compounds such as sulphadiazine or sulphadimidine. Results in animals have been disappointing compared with those in mice and humans. These drugs affect tachyzoites but not bradyzoites so that total elimination of the parasite is not possible. Recent experiments with the ionophore monensin have shown prophylactic activity in sheep, but there are no reports of its use in cattle (Buxton *et al.*, 1987). Other preventative measures include prevention of cat faecal contamination of animal food and adequate destruction of infected carcasses.

Bunostomiosis

Bunostomiosis in cattle is caused by the hookworm *Bunostomum phlebotomum*. It mainly affects cattle up to one year old and causes a range of signs from unrest and mild abdominal pain to diarrhoea and eventually anaemia depending on the stage of the infection and the number of worms present. It is more prevalent in subtropical and tropical regions than in temperate; this distribution has become especially marked during the last decade as the worm, which does not occur in large numbers, seems especially sensitive to some of the modern anthelmintics and may now be absent from those areas where frequent suppressive anthelmintic treatments have been applied.

Aetiology and epidemiology

Bunostomum phlebotomum parasitizes the small intestine of cattle. Adults can reach 3.0 cm in length and are characterized by a large buccal capsule with lateral cutting teeth and a tooth-like structure in its base, which is the duct of an oesophageal gland. The worms suck blood, which can induce anaemia and in large numbers cause diarrhoea.

The eggs from adult females pass out with faeces. Depending on climatic conditions, a parasitic infective larvae, which is susceptible to desiccation, will develop under optimal conditions of adequate moisture and warmth within one week. The infective larvae can infect susceptible cattle in either of two ways.

1 By penetration of the skin after which it enters the bloodstream and passes to the lung, emerging into the alveoli and after further moulting up the bronchial tree to the pharynx, where it is then swallowed and passes to the intestine to mature.

2 By direct ingestion after which it burrows into the intestinal wall during development to emerge as an adult.

The prepatent period is eight weeks. The worm flourishes in conditions of adequate moisture and warmth and thus is generally a subtropical problem, but disease has been recorded in countries as far north as Scotland, where it has been seen in cattle maintained indoors on damp straw bedding.

Signs

Heavy percutaneous larval infections cause restlessness, stamping and itching. Once in the intestine adults suck blood and cause haemorrhagic anaemia and hypoalbuminaemia, and small numbers (about 2000) in comparison to other gastrointestinal nematodes, other than *Haemonchus placei*, will cause very severe disease and death.

Diagnosis

It is difficult to diagnose when prepatent and mild anaemia is the main sign. When patent it should be differentiated from other parasites that cause haemorrhagic anaemia, e.g. *H. placei* and *F. hepatica*, and those deficiencies such as cobalt or copper that adversely affect erythropoiesis.

Treatment and control

The parasite is sensitive to modern anthelmintics and can be controlled by their suppressive or strategic use. Other measures in housed cattle should be the provision of dry bedding and its replacement when soiled. Once infected and treated, cattle normally develop a strong immunity to the parasite.

Haemonchosis

Haemonchiasis is manifested by haemorrhagic anaemia and diarrhoea, and is caused by the presence in the abomasum of *Haemonchus placei* (synonym *H. similis*). As with bunostomiasis it is mainly pathogenic in immature cattle, since infection in the first three years of life usually produces a strong immunity to re-infection. It also has a similar distribution, being commonest in subtropical and tropical countries but present in most temperate countries and able to cause disease during any unusually warm periods of weather.

Aetiology and epidemiology

Adults of *H. placei* suck blood from the surface of the abomasum. They are fairly large in comparison to other abomasal nematodes and measure 3 cm in length when fully grown. In the female the ovaries and intestine are spirally intertwined to give the worm its 'barber-pole' appearance and nickname. The male has large barbed spicules, and both sexes a small lancet in the buccal capsule.

Female *H. placei* are very prolific egg producers and can lay up to 10 000 eggs daily. The eggs are passed in faeces and undergo a typical trichostrongyline development to infective larvae. The time taken to reach this stage varies considerably between temperate and subtropical climatic areas. In the former, it may take several weeks in contrast to four days under suitable conditions. The conditions for development of *Haemonchus* spp. have been studied in some detail, and it has been concluded that they require a temperature in excess of 18 °C and rainfall of 5.3 cm/month for maximum translation, but can develop provided the mean minimum temperature is not less than 10 °C. As a result of the combination of fecundity and rapid infective development in favourable conditions, pasture can become quickly contaminated with huge numbers of infective larvae. In the subtropics acute infections can therefore be found in susceptible young cattle, whereas in temperate areas infections are more likely to be chronic. Under adverse conditions in the tropics, e.g. dry seasons, infective larvae can undergo hypobiosis in a similar manner to *Ostertagia* spp., and resume development shortly before the rainy season commences.

Once ingested, larvae undergo two moults before becoming adult in 26–28 days, when infections become patent. After the first moult, the L4 larvae and subsequent adults suck blood, leaving haemorrhagic spots on the abomasal epithelium, and the resultant blood loss is the major pathogenic sequelae. However, in large infections, the pH of the abomasal contents may be increased in the same way as in ostertagiasis, with the resultant digestive disturbance, raised plasma pepsinogen, possible bacterial overgrowth and diarrhoea. Once patent, peak egg production from females is normally reached between six and seven weeks after infection and may continue for a further six to eight weeks. Cattle, unlike sheep, develop resistance to the worm and unless immunologically compromised by intercurrent illness or malnutrition the population decreases rapidly thereafter and the animal remains fairly resistant for the remainder of its life.

Signs

There are two types of clinical picture. The first occurs in severe primary infections and presents severely anaemic, weak and sometimes diarrhoeic young cattle. The second is found in chronic lesser infections and typically causes weakness, lethargy, weight loss, a less acute anaemia, hypoproteinaemia, submandibular oedema and anasarca.

Diagnosis

Diagnosis can be confirmed if the infection is patent by the examination of faeces samples, which may reveal very high faecal egg counts. The plasma pepsinogen level may be raised. The grazing and past parasitic history may be helpful in differentiating from other causes of anaemia or diarrhoea such as fascioliasis, bunostomiasis, copper or cobalt deficiencies, babesiosis, coccidiosis, bacillary haemoglobinuria and malnutrition.

Treatment and control

Anthelmintic treatment is the primary consideration and *H. placei* is susceptible to levamisole, ivermectin and modern benzimidazoles as well as the flukicides rafoxanide, clorsulon and nitroxynil. This should be coupled with movement to uninfected pasture. Prevention can be achieved using similar methods as those described for ostertagiasis.

Hypodermatosis (warbles)

Hypodermatosis is the term used to describe infection with and the lesions caused by the larvae of two species of the fly genus *Hypoderma*, *H. bovis* and *H. lineatum*. The disease is characterized by damage to dorsal flesh, hides, oesophagus, central nervous system and occasionally death due to anaphylaxis (see p. 678).

Aetiology and epidemiology

The adult flies are distributed in the northern hemisphere, excluding the most northerly arctic regions. There are two species *H. bovis* and *H. lineatum*. *Hypoderma bovis* favours the northern parts of their habitat areas and *H. lineatum* the southern and warmer areas, but both species can occur simultaneously. The adult flies have a yellow abdomen characterized by a broad stripe of black hairs. They are active in warm weather, generally in Europe between the months of June and August. Their presence upsets cattle, which run to avoid them and in doing so injure themselves on fences or other obstacles. The females of *H. bovis* deposit eggs singly on hairs, frequently above the hocks on the hind legs; the eggs of *H. lineatum* are laid in rows, from whence its name was derived, usually on the lower part of the body and in places where both adult and eggs are difficult for cattle to dislodge. The eggs adhere strongly to the hairs. They hatch in four to six days and the first stage larvae crawl down to the skin, which they penetrate, and proceed to migrate through soft tissues towards their overwintering sites. This movement takes several weeks, and by late autumn *H. bovis* has reached the epidural fat within the vertebral column and *H. lineatum* the submucosa of the oesophagus. The larvae remain in these sites during the winter, moulting to their second stage of development. At the end of the winter they resume migration both reaching the subdermal tissue along the back in the spring. They make a hole in the overlying skin through which they respire while developing to the third stage, which reaches a length of 2–3 cm and is characterized by rows of small spines on the posterior margin of most of its segments and posterior spiracles on a terminal tuberosity. The creamy-white larvae emerge from the back of the animal in April and May and fall to the ground to continue development by pupation, eventually emerging as adults five weeks later. They have a short lifespan as adults, mating, laying eggs and dying within two weeks of emergence.

Pathogenesis

The larvae are most pathogenic during two phases of their development. The first is during the late autumn and winter when they are in the epidural fat or oesophageal wall respectively. If present in large numbers, or if treated and killed *in situ*, the anaphylactic reactions may cause damage to the spinal cord that can result in either spinal paralysis or difficulty in swallowing and eructation, which can lead to bloat. The second is during their pre-emergence development, where they damage the subdermal tissue and skin of the back and cause subsequent downgrading of hides and trimming of carcasses, and cause irritation and loss of growth in the live animal.

Signs

In the late autumn and winter, occasionally there can be damage to the spinal cord resulting in paralysis, difficulty in standing or bloat. In the spring, there are swellings under the skin 55–75 cm either side of the midline containing pus, a breathing hole and a third stage larva.

Diagnosis

If disease results during their winter development, the symptoms have to be differentiated from other causes of spinal or oesophageal paralysis. There is an ELISA test available that detects antibody to migrating larvae and, although originally designed to aid eradication programmes, it may be helpful in diagnosis. When larvae are in their pre-emergence sites on the back their presence is unmistakeable since no other condition causes similar lesions, especially if a heavy infection is present.

Treatment

The larvae are susceptible during their migration to systemic organophosphorus insecticides and the anthelmintic ivermectin. Care should be taken not to treat cattle when larvae are in their overwintering sites, as death *in situ* and subsequent lysis may result in anaphylaxis. For that reason statutory eradication policies have compulsory treatments applied before mid-November, coupled where necessary with inspection and further treatments in the following spring.

The organophosphorus treatments are normally applied dermally as pour-on preparations. A large number are available, the most popular currently being phosmet and crufomate. Mass treatment has resulted in eradication from many islands although it has proved more difficult on large land areas. Ivermectin, although highly effective, is not normally used in mass eradication campaigns since its primary use is as an anthelmintic. Although prophylaxis against adult flies is not actively undertaken, slow-release devices such as ear tags impregnated with organophosphorus compounds or synthetic pyrethroids do reduce the possibility of oviposition by adults.

Ectoparasites

Lice (pediculosis)

Lice are ubiquitous parasites of cattle. In large numbers they cause skin irritation and have been associated with anaemia and may act as vectors of pathogenic organisms (see p. 682).

Aetiology and epidemiology

Lice are host-specific parasites and are classified into two types: (i) sucking lice and (ii) biting lice. Five species infest cattle, four sucking and one biting. The former are *Haematopinus eurysternus* and *H. quadripertusus*, 'short-nosed' sucking lice; *Lignognathus vituli* 'long-nosed'; and *Solenopotes capillatus* 'small blue' sucking lice. The biting species is *Damalinia bovis*. As might be construed the sucking lice have mouthparts adapted for piercing skin and sucking blood; the biting lice ingest skin and hair detritus, blood and scabs. Each species has a preferential area on animals but if large numbers are present can be found anywhere on the body surface. Normally, *H. eurysternus* and *D. bovis* are found on the poll, neck and head and the latter also along the mid-dorsal region of the body. *Lignognathus vituli* and *S. capillatus* also favour the head, neck and frequently the ventral surface of the neck, dewlap and axillae. *Haematopinus quadripertusus* is restricted to subtropical areas and is usually found in the area of the tail and posterior lumbar regions.

The life cycle of lice is direct. Adults live for approximately one month during which time they lay a few hundred eggs, which are tightly attached to hair by a glue-like substance produced by the louse. The eggs hatch within a few days and the first nymph, which resembles a small softer adult, emerges. It undergoes three moults to second and third stage nymphs and finally adults, each nymphal stage taking one week. The entire life cycle from egg to adult occupies approximately three weeks.

There are seasonal variations, especially marked in temperate areas, in the number of lice found on cattle. In these areas numbers on susceptible cattle increase during autumn and early winter, peaking in late winter and early spring. There are two reasons for this: (i) cattle are frequently housed in autumn and lice are easily transferred from infested to non-infested animals, and (ii) climatic conditions favour louse activity; strong sunlight and high skin temperatures have been shown to inhibit lice and the converse occurs in winter. Within groups of infested cattle there are always those that carry heavier burdens than others, and it is generally accepted that very large louse populations are indicative of stress or intercurrent illness, poorly fed cattle parasitized by nematodes and trematodes being frequently and characteristically louse infested.

The pathogenic effects of louse infestation have been the subject of much research. It is now considered that light or moderate infections have little effect on cattle. Heavy infestations lead to skin irritation, scratching and rubbing, with resultant damage to hides. Some reports have indicated that large sucking lice burdens may also cause anaemia and weight loss, although it has also been noted that these effects can be prevented by adequate high quality nutrition. Lice may also act as vectors for blood-borne organisms, and have been implicated in the transmission of *Eperythrozoon wenyoni*.

Signs and diagnosis

Louse infestations are usually evident by the presence of eggs adherent to hairs, on the edge of bald areas and on parting of hair careful examination of preferential niches with a magnifying lens will reveal adults and nymphs.

Treatment and control

Lice are fairly easily killed by the application of organophosphorus, amitraz or synthetic pyrethroid preparations, either as sprays, pour-ons or dusting powders. The residual activity of synthetic pyrethroids is generally of longer duration. This aspect is important because for complete removal of all lice the activity must not only kill adults but nymphs emerging from eggs. The anthelmintic ivermectin because of its long half-life is also extremely effective, removing all sucking and more than 98 per cent of biting lice. For preventative purposes, housed cattle can be treated at housing, sometimes complemented by removal by electric clippers of a 15 cm band of hair from the poll to the root of the tail.

Mange

Mange is the descriptive term used for infection of animals by mites, the smallest arthropods of the order Acarina. They are obligate parasites transmitted from infected to non-infected animals by direct contact. There are four species that parasitize cattle and two others which are facultative parasities of them and other animals (see p. 602).

Aetiology and epidemiology

Although of the same order, the mites have different morphologies and habitats, and some are classified as 'burrowing' and others as 'non-burrowing'. For these reasons they are described separately.

Non-burrowing mites. One species, *Chorioptes bovis*, is specific to cattle. *Psoroptes ovis*, although primarily a parasite of sheep, can become permanently adapted to cattle. Non-specific mites are those species of harvest mites present on pasture, the larvae of which can infest many different species of animals: the mite species are *Neotrombicula* and *Eutrombicula*.

1 *Chorioptes bovis*. The most common mite found on cattle. It reaches a length of 0.75 mm, and is recognizable by its cup-shaped suckers on short unjointed pedicels. It is seen most frequently during autumn and winter in housed cattle, frequently on the hind legs but also on the neck, the head and root of the tail. It is a surface feeder, and produces mild hair loss, lesions increasing in size only slowly. The lesions are obviously itchy as affected cattle will rub affected areas on walls, doors, etc., incurring damage to the skin and subsequent quality of the hide after death.

2 *Psoroptes ovis*. This mite is normally found on sheep and is the cause of sheep scab, which is notifiable and government regulated in many countries. The mite is a similar size to *C. bovis* but is characterized by long jointed pedicels with funnel-shaped suckers on the legs. Although similar to *P. ovis* from sheep, which is transferrable experimentally both to cattle and rabbits the rarity of cases of mites transferring from sheep to cattle and vice versa in nature has led to the conclusion that some adaptation to specific hosts takes place, and that infection of sheep by cattle strains does not occur.

The mite, although a surface feeder, is much more irritant than *C. bovis* since its mouthparts are adapted for piercing skin, causing the formation of serious vesicles, which can coalesce and eventually become scabs. The life cycle is typical for both *P. ovis* and *C. bovis*. Female mites lay approximately 90 eggs. The hatching of eggs and subsequent development from larva to nymph to adult occupies approximately 10 days. Adult mites can live for a maximum of six weeks.

Affected cattle become restless because of the skin irritation. The areas commonly affected are the abdomen, tail root and perineum, and they can become further damaged by scratching. In extreme cases animals may cease to feed adequately and lose weight.

3 *Forage mites*. The adults and nymphs of the family Trombiculidae are free-living on pasture. Eggs are laid on soil, and larvae crawl on to vegetation and to animals that lie on or brush through the foliage. The larvae are skin-piercers, causing vesicles. Animals become hypersensitive to their secretions and the subsequent rubbing and scratching increases the damage to skins.

Burrowing mites

1 *Sarcoptes scabiei*. Mites of this species are host specific although they are morphologically identical to those infesting other animal species. The adults are slightly larger than half the size of *P. ovis* and *C. bovis*. They are characterized by a rounded shape and the presence of triangular scales on the posterior of the dorsum. Adult females burrow tunnels in the epidermis. They lay eggs in tunnels, hatching taking place within a week. The hatched larvae crawl to the surface and create further epidermal tunnels in which they moult through the stage of nymphs to become adults. Males and females mate either in tunnels or on the skin surface and the cycle resumes, the entire length of which occupies three weeks.

Sarcoptes scabiei infections cause extreme irritation. On cattle the preferred sites are the neck and the lumbar area adjacent to the tail, resulting in the colloquial description of 'neck and tail mange', but it can be found in other areas. Early small lesions exhibit hair thinning and slightly thickened scaly skin, but soon the irritation and resultant rubbing combined with expansion of infected areas results in total loss of hair and thickened, crusted and excoriated skin. Affected animals may become so preoccupied with the irritation that they reduce their food intake leading to loss of weight or milk production, and secondary bacterial infections may ensue on the most severely rubbed lesions.

2 *Demodex bovis*. This mite is considered to be a normal commensal found on bovine skin; as for all members of the family Demodicidae it becomes pathogenic only when the efficiency of the immune controls of its host is reduced. The mites are characteristically cigar shaped, 0.2 mm long, with four pairs of short legs close to the anterior end. Their preferred niches are in hair follicles and sebaceous glands and because of this deep location are not transmitted unless prolonged contact occurs. For this reason it is presumed that the young become infected shortly after birth during feeding from their mother, and as a result lesions are

usually seen in cattle on the muzzle, head, neck and back. The lesions take the form of small 0.75 cm diameter nodules and are follicles or glands filled with mites and caseous pus. In some countries a high proportiön of hides may be affected, but in the UK the average prevalence is 17 per cent (Urquhart *et al.*, 1987). The lesions do not normally seriously affect cattle and treatment is not usually necessary.

Diagnosis

All of the mites are too small to be easily seen with the naked eye, and microscopic examination of skin scrapings is necessary, as it is for differentiation of most skin conditions. Mites are normally most easily found in scrapings taken from the edge of lesions. The scrapings are boiled in sodium or potassium hydroxide and centrifuged prior to examination of the sediment by microscope.

Treatment and control

Mites are affected by amitraz, some organophosphorus compounds, synthetic pyrethroids and the anthelmintic ivermectin. For topical applications the problem is to ensure that the chemical can come into contact with the parasite and it may be necessary to remove scabs before application. The organophosphorus compounds used frequently are phosmet, propetamphos and diazinon, and the synthetic pyrethroids flumethrin, deltamethrin and cypermethrin. Organophosphorus compounds and ivermectin should not be used on dairy cows giving milk for human consumption unless withdrawal periods are observed.

References

Armour, J., Jennings, F.W. & Urquhart, G.M. (1969) Inhibition of *Ostertagia ostertagi* at the early fourth larval stage. II. The influence of environment on host or parasite. *Research in Veterinary Science*, **10**, 238–44.

Blewett, D.A. (1983) The epidemiology of ovine toxoplasmosis. I. The interpretation of data for the prevalence of antibody in sheep and other host species. *British Veterinary Journal*, **139**, 537–45.

Buxton, D., Donald, K.M. & Finlaysan, J. (1987) Monensin and the control of experimental ovine toxoplasmosis: A systemic effect. *Veterinary Record*, **120**, 618–19.

Leaver, J.D. (1970) A comparison of grazing systems for dairy herd replacements. *Journal of Agricultural Science, Cambridge*, **75**, 265–72.

McMeekin, C.P. (1954) Good rearing of dairy stock. Bulletin Department of Agriculture New Zealand No. 228.

Michel, J.F. (1968) The control of stomach worm infections in young cattle. *Journal of British Grassland Society*, **23**, 165–73.

Michel, J.F. (1969) The epidemiology and control of some nematode infections. *Advances in Parasitology*, **7**, 211–82.

Urquhart, G.M., Armour, J., Duncan, J.L., Dunn, A.N. & Jennings, F.W. (1987) *Veterinary Parasitology*. Longman Scientific, Harlow, pp. 1–286.

Chapter 18: Respiratory Disease

by A.H. ANDREWS

Shipping fever (transit fever, pasteurellosis)

Epidemiology

The condition is an important respiratory problem in groups of weaned suckled calves that have been sold, often via a market, hence the terms transit fever or shipping fever. They are usually over six months old and under two years. During part of the sale transactions they will probably have been mixed and grouped with other batches of animals of similar age during transport, at the market or following arrival at the finishing farm. Most cases occur within the first month of their entry to the fattening unit and most cases are seen at least 10 days after arrival (Andrews *et al.*, 1981). The disease is characterized by an illness of sudden onset with dullness, pyrexia and anorexia. It is an acute exudative bronchopneumonia with toxaemia as well as much fibrin present in the exudate and often accompanied by fibrinous pleurisy (Blood & Radostits, 1989). The condition is common in North America, Europe and Britain. It is particularly prevalent in the American cattle feedlot industry and is the largest cause of mortality in that system. In a Colorado survey 75 per cent of all clinical disease in yearling cattle and 64 per cent of all post-mortem diagnoses were due to respiratory disease (Jensen *et al.*, 1976). The morbidity and mortality rates vary considerably but a level of up to 35 per cent and a mortality of 5–10 per cent of those affected or 0.75–1 per cent of the susceptible population is often quoted (Blood & Radostits, 1989).

Aetiology

The aetiology of the condition is still open to disagreement. It is considered to be stress or management induced with the participation of infectious agents. The infection has been thought to be primarily viral, mainly due either to parainfluenza III (PI3) virus or infectious bovine rhinotracheitis (IBR) virus, followed by secondary infection with either *Pasteurella multocida* or *Pasteurella haemolytica* (Pirie, 1979). *Pasteurella haemolytica* biotype A serotype 1 is considered to be the most common isolate although biotype T strains have also been found. *Pasteurella haemolytica* biotype A produces a heat-labile cytotoxin that is ruminant specific destroying leucocytes (Sherwen & Wilkie, 1982). *Pasteurella multocida* infection is only isolated occasionally. Recently, it has been proved experimentally that *P. haemolytica* biotype A1 can produce the disease as a primary agent in non-immune calves (Shoo, 1989). Disease does depend on administering the organisms into the lungs either intratracheally (Friend *et al.*, 1977; Gibbs *et al.*, 1983) or intrathoracically (Houghton & Gourlay, 1984; Panciera & Corstvet, 1984). However, the exact mechanism by which the organisms enter the lung and result in lesions is not yet known. Other evidence of *P. haemolytica* involvement is that calves previously exposed naturally to the infection are much more resistant to experimental and natural pneumonic pasteurellosis (Confer *et al.*, 1984).

Although *P. haemolytica* can be isolated from the nasal passages it is only in small numbers when calves are healthy and unstressed. The organisms can be present in low numbers in the tracheal air but are not considered to be normal inhabitants of the lungs (Grey & Thomson, 1971). However, as the calves are transported, move to market and then enter the feedlot, the number of *P. haemolytica* biotype A1 increases in the nasal tract, the tracheal air and then the lungs, where bronchopneumonia can result (Frank & Smith, 1983). Thus management factors are important. The effects of stress are extremely difficult to quantify and have not been successfully undertaken experimentally to produce transit fever. However, transportation of yearling cattle does result in a rise in plasma fibrinogen levels, which is indicative of stress (Phillips, 1984). Increased fibrinogen levels also occur following confinement in unfamiliar surroundings and deprivation of food and water. In addition, it seems that cattle suddenly introduced to a diet consisting of large amounts of cereal are more prone to respiratory problems (Wilson *et al.*, 1985).

The environment tends to be important in that disease seems to be related to the season of the year (Andrews, 1978), fluctuations in daily ambient temperature and increased concentration of airborne particles 2.0–3.3 μm in diameter (MacVean *et al.*, 1986). Calves kept at a constant temperature of 16 °C (60 °F) showed minimum levels of nasopharyngeal bacteria at a relative humidity between 65 and 75 per cent. However, bacterial counts tend to rise at humidities on either side of this range (Jones & Webster, 1981).

The interrelationship of different micro-organisms and transit fever still needs further elucidation. However, cattle entering feedlots with low serological titres to IBR, bovine respiratory syncytial virus (RSV) and *Mycoplasma dispar* were at greater risk of being treated for BRD (Rosendal & Martin, 1986). It has also been shown that IBR, PI3, bovine virus diarrhoea (BVD) and RSV are all associated with acute respiratory disease (Martin & Bohaz, 1986).

In many outbreaks of transit fever it is likely that the stress of movement plus mixing with other calves, the introduction to housing and a new diet are sufficient to initiate disease. The main organism involved is usually a *Pasteurella* species, especially *P. haemolytica* biotype A1. Spread of infection is optimized by crowded conditions in transport and markets. It is also probable that as animals go down with disease and pass on the infection, the organism increases in virulence. This can be seen in some outbreaks in which disease can be traced from individual animals to other members of the same group and then to other groups (Andrews, 1976).

Signs

The peracute form is unusual but results in sudden death with no premonitory signs.

In the acute form the animals are dull and inactive with excessive oculo-nasal discharges, which may be mucupurulent. There is usually anorexia although the cattle still drink, and a marked fever (40–41 °C, 104–106 °F). There is rapid (40+/minute), shallow breathing and a soft, productive cough, which tends to increase with exercise. On auscultation there are bronchial sounds over the anterior and ventral parts of the lungs, which become louder as the condition continues. In some cases squeaks and high-pitched sounds are heard, together with a pleuritic rub. Later signs can include dyspnoea with marked abdominal breathing and an expiratory grunt. Diarrhoea occurs in a few animals. There is usually a favourable response to therapy.

Necropsy

Death is usually the result of anoxia and toxaemia although occasionally in young cattle there is septicaemia. Usually, over one-third of the lung shows marked consolidation and the ventral parts of the apical and cardiac lobes are most involved. Initially, there is lung congestion and then hepatitis with exudate and, in some animals, emphysema. Bronchitis and bronchiolitis are usually catarrhal, often with serofibrinous pleurisy and a fibrinous pericarditis. There is usually much pleural effusion.

Diagnosis

This depends on the history of age, recent movement, weaning or housing. The signs also help with severe respiratory signs involving the anteroventral parts of the lungs and pyrexia. Post-mortem findings of lung consolidation and pleurisy are present, and impression smears show bipolar staining organisms with methylene blue. *Pasteurella haemolytica* or *P. multocida* may be isolated from nasal swabs in live animals or lungs at post mortem and their antibiotic sensitivity determined. Serology for antibody rise can be undertaken, as also can haematology but often the findings are variable.

Differential diagnosis

Differential diagnosis includes enzootic pneumonia (see p. 202) but this usually occurs in younger calves with a different history. Infectious bovine rhinotracheitis (see p. 256) usually shows mainly upper respiratory signs and a conjunctivitis. Fog fever (see p. 236) is mainly apparent in older cattle at grass after a pasture move in the autumn. Parasitic bronchitis (see p. 236) is present in cattle following grazing. Acute bronchopneumonia would be almost identical except for bacteriological isolation. Contagious bovine pleuropneumonia is severe in all age groups of cattle and the affected animals suffer severe pain and toxaemia with a high mortality.

Treatment

Therapy for shipping fever is given in Table 18.1. Treatment should begin early. Most cattle will usually show some improvement within one to three days of initiating treatment. Complete recovery may take four to seven days. Where severe outbreaks occur it may occasionally be necessary to use mass medication by water as most ill cattle still drink well.

Prevention and control

Although the disease of transit fever is sporadic, many of the conditions that predispose to the problem can be defined. This should mean that methods of prevention should be relatively easy to institute. Ideally, the calves would be weaned at least two weeks prior to leaving the farm of birth (Andrews, 1976). They would be introduced to the type of feed to be provided on the rearing farm. In addition, they would be batched in groups that would go direct from the farm of birth to the rearing farm. In reality this does not happen as the farmer producing the calves hopes that by selling them at market he will obtain a better price than by selling direct. In addition, the first farmer will be little concerned about the subsequent disease status of his calves once they have left his farm for sale. This makes the possibility of vaccination prior to movement difficult.

As cattle go through markets, disease prevention tends not to be practised because many of the factors enhancing the likelihood of a disease outbreak are outside the control of the purchasing beef rearers.

Table 18.1 Therapy for shipping fever

Drug	Method of administration	Dose (mg/kg)	Dose (mg/lb)	Duration
Amoxycillin trihydrate	s.c., i.m.	7	3	Daily for 3–5 days
Ampicillin trihydrate	s.c., i.m.	5–10	2.5–5	Daily for 3 days
Ceftiofur	i.m.	1.1	0.5	Daily for 3–5 days
Chloramphenicol	i.m.	10	5	3–4 times daily for 3 days
Danofloxacin	i.m.	1.25	0.6	Daily for 3–5 days
Erythromycin	i.v., i.m.	5	2.5	Daily for 3 days
Oxytetracycline	i.v., s.c., i.m.	10	5	Daily for 3 days
Oxytetracycline (long-acting)	i.m.	20	10	Usually once
Penicillin/dihydrostreptomycin	i.m.	(20–30 000 iu/kg)	(10–15 000 iu/lb)	Daily for 3 days
		20	10	
Penicillin (long-acting)				
benzathine	i.m.	5	2.5	Usually once
procaine	i.m.	6	3	Daily for 3–5 days
Spectinomycin	i.v., i.m.	10–20	5–10	Daily for 3–4 days
Spiramycin	i.m.	20	10	Daily for 2–3 days
Sulphadimidine	i.v., s.c., oral	150	75	Daily for 3 days
Tilmicosin	s.c.	10	5	Usually once
Trimethoprim and sulphadiazine	i.m.	4	2	Daily for 3–5 days
		20	10	
Trimethoprim and sulphadoxine	i.v., i.m.	3	1.5	Daily for 3–5 days
		12.5	6	
Tylosin	i.m.	4–10	2–5	Daily for 3–5 days
mass medication		10	5	Daily for 5–7 days
Oxytetracycline	oral	100	50	Daily for 5–7 days
Sulphadimidine	oral	5	2.5	Daily for 5 days
Trimethoprim and sulphadiazine	oral	25	12.5	

All animals should be provided with good quality feed and adequate ventilation. Corticosteroids, e.g. betamethasone, dexamethasone, are often found to help in reducing the level of exudation. Flunixin meglumine may be useful in reducing inflammation, and *Pasteurella* antisera may also be helpful.

Thus they cannot control the time before moving, the transport of the animals from the farm of origin, their mixing with other cattle or the conditions present at market. Likewise they will probably have little direct say as to how the animals are transported or their mixing with other groups before their entry to the rearing farm. It is only once the cattle reach the rearers that control measures can be undertaken. Obviously, they can ensure that the animals are kept in as satisfactory an environment as possible and are only lightly stocked. This is best done by having the animals outside but this is resisted by most farmers because of the inconvenience and extra labour required. The new ration for the cattle can also be introduced slowly.

The problem is worse in North America where calves often travel vast distances. Here various preconditioning programmes are undertaken. It is advised that calves should be fed prior to weaning and kept in the same place once the dams are removed. Following weaning, regular checking of the calves several times a day should be practised. When animals are travelling they should be given adequate periods of rest and offered feed and water. They should also be well bedded during transit. Some farmers inject multivitamin preparations before moving and vaccines can be used, including those against *Pasteurella* and PI3 virus.

In many countries antibiotics are used following the move. These have given variable results mainly due to predicting when injections should be undertaken. This is because most problems occur about seven to ten days after entry to the feedlot or farm. When used, it is probably best to give long-acting preparations and initiate therapy when the first animals show disease. Use of antibiotic medication in the feed or water is a common practice in North America and while it appears to reduce mortality it has no effect on morbidity.

Vaccination

If it is considered that *P. haemolytica* and at times *P. multocida* form an important part of the disease syndrome of transit fever then it might be possible to obtain some protection by vaccination. Various vaccines are present in Europe but currently only two are available in Britain.

In North America various *Pasteurella* bacterins and viral vaccines have been used to assist with the control of transit fever. Their efficacy appears to be low and literature reviews suggest that at present there is little evidence to show the efficacy of such vaccines under feedlot conditions (Myers, 1984).

Recently in North America several new vaccines have become available. One of these is a *P. haemolytica* vaccine/bacterial extract. This has been shown to be effective to controlled challenge provided two doses of vaccine have been administered prior to challenge (Sherwen & Wilkie, 1988). Response in a field trial has however only shown a slight decrease in morbidity of disease, with slight improvement in relapse rates and response to treatment (Bateman, 1988; Jim *et al.*, 1988).

Infectious bovine rhinotracheitis

Aetiology

Infectious bovine rhinotracheitis (IBR) is a highly infectious and contagious disease of cattle. It is caused by a virus known as bovid herpes virus 1 (BHV 1). It is generally considered that there are several strains of the virus, although often the differences between the strains are not easily shown in the laboratory. The disease is seen in North America, Europe and Africa. It is considered that the outbreak of severe respiratory disease that occurred in Great Britain in the mid-1970s was due to a new strain being imported.

While the disease is primarily one of cattle, it can also infect deer, goats and pigs. The main sources of infection between animals are nasal discharge (or eye discharge), when it is affecting the respiratory system, and vaginal or preputial discharges, semen, or the fluids and tissues of the fetus when the infection involves the reproductive tract.

Epidemiology

In most cases of respiratory infection disease is spread by aerosol. The genital form of the disease is contracted venereally . As respiratory infection is spread via the air, it can spread by direct contact between the animals or where the cattle are in the same air space, i.e. there is air contact. This can only be avoided by ensuring the walls extend from floor to ceiling and there is no contact with other animals either at the front of the pens or with other groups on either side. However, generally there is a need for close sustained contact between groups. This is why disease is often slow to spread within and between groups. It often takes two to five weeks to spread in a group. However, unexplained outbreaks of IBR do occur on isolated farms.

Latent infection. There is a problem with BHV 1 in that it is able to become a latent infection. Thus once an animal is infected with a strain of the virus or vaccinated with a live viral vaccine, the virus may remain in the animal for the rest of its life without it showing any signs of illness. The site of latency is arguable but the virus can be found in the trigeminal nerve of clinically normal cattle. However, if the animal is stressed at all, such as when moved or calving, or becomes ill, the virus may be shed. Shedding can also occur in bulls when mating. This shedding may be, but is often not, accompanied by any signs of disease. Corticosteroid injections may promote virus shedding. The level of this latent infection is variable but can be up to 10 per cent of clinically normal animals. In addition, while most of these cattle will show antibody levels to the BHV 1 virus, some do not. Thus all cattle in herds where disease occurs have the capacity to spread disease even when there are no clinical signs of disease present in the herd. The only way of knowing whether or not disease is present is to look at the results of blood tests. If a blood test shows an antibody titre (positive response) to BHV 1 in cattle other than calves it means that the animal(s) have been exposed to infection and could possibly be carriers. If a blood test from an animal is negative it generally means that the animal is unlikely to have been exposed to infection, but it does not completely rule out the possibility that the animal is a latent carrier of disease. Thus tests on individual animals are of limited significance; however, on a herd basis repeated negative tests indicate that it is highly unlikely infection is present. When tests show several animals with antibody levels in the herd then infection is present. The calf that receives colostrum from its infected mother will also show a positive antibody level to the test although not necessarily being infected. The antibody provided from the colostrum will usually remain for one to six months, depending on the amount received from the mother.

Incubation period. The incubation period for the disease is very variable. Experimentally, it usually takes three to seven days. However, in most beef units disease occurs about 10–20 days after introduction of infected or susceptible animals. Longer incubation periods do occur. This is quite likely when it is considered that latent carriers may not be shedding virus at a particular time.

Signs

Respiratory disease. This disease is the most common form. It is usually seen in cattle over six months old but can occur at a younger age. The signs vary considerably but typically they tend to be worst in animals from about six months to two years old.

1 Mild disease. This is just a conjunctivitis, i.e. slight reddening to the lining of the eye and eyelids with some discharge, usually watery and clear (see p. 716). This often occurs when the disease strain is mild or degree of infection is low, or the animal is resistant.

2 Subacute disease. This is commonly seen in adult cattle and often is of only short duration. There is a marked rise in temperature lasting only a day or two (40 °C, 104 °F). Often there is a marked drop in milk yield. Again the lining of the eyes is reddened with discharge and this also involves reddening of the lining of the nose with nasal discharge. The animals will salivate and there may be a short, expressive cough. Breathing is rapid and shallow. The animals recover in 10 to 14 days.

3 Acute disease. The signs are as in the subacute form but the temperature tends to be higher (40–41 °C, 104–106 °F). These signs are particularly present in growing cattle between six months and two years old. The respiratory signs are more likely to include a cough and there is some respiratory distress. The discharge from eyes and nose tends to become profuse, yellow, thick and purulent. The lining of the nose may show grey areas, which consist of dead tissue that smell and are shed. The signs tend to last a lot longer before recovery occurs.

4 Peracute disease. The animals develop very high temperatures (42 °C, 108 °F) with eye and nasal discharge, respiratory distress, cough and then death in about 24 hours.

Some cattle may die owing to complications and this is particularly so in the six month to two year age group. Here mortality may reach 10 per cent or more. However, it is usually only about 1 per cent. Some cattle keep a stertor (snoring breathing) for many months. Some become 'puffers' with bouts of respiratory signs including distress when breathing, loss of appetite and cough. These usually have a secondary bronchopneumonia and die in weeks or months after losing condition. Often they become recumbent before death.

Characteristically, there is a sudden outbreak of disease involving the respiratory tract. This will initially involve the group of cattle to which infection has been introduced. It will then tend to spread round all the other groups and ages of cattle. This can often take a few weeks or many months, dependent on the strain of virus, the level of infection and the degree of exposure to infection of each group. Characteristically, an outbreak in a group reaches a peak at about two or three weeks after its start and is over between the fourth and sixth week.

Reproductive form. In most cases the reproductive and respiratory forms are not seen together.

1 Infectious pustular vulvovaginitis. This is an infection of the vulva and vagina often lasting several weeks. It results in the discharge of pus from the vulva, usually in small quantities. There is reddening of the lining and pustule presence. In some cases infection causes irritation in the vagina resulting in frequent urination and possibly increased straining.

2 Infectious bovine penoposthitis. Bulls show a small amount of purulent discharge from the prepuce. The surface of the penis and prepuce may be reddened with haemorrhages and small necrotic areas.

3 Endometritis. Infection of the uterus, with discharge, poor conception rates and short returns to oestrus, can occur if semen is infected.

4 Abortion. This is becoming increasingly common and occurs some weeks or months after the animal is infected. Abortion is usually at six to eight months of pregnancy and often the placenta is retained following abortion. In some cases of infection calves are born weak at the normal time.

Generalized/alimentary form. This is seen in young newborn calves and is recorded mainly in America. It occurs when calves receive little or no immunity in the colostrum and are then subjected to infection. The animals show a severe temperature reaction, they do not eat and they salivate. The lining of the nose is red. The eyes may show a conjunctivitis. In addition, the lining of the mouth and the soft palate (at the back of the throat) are reddened with mucus present. The opening to the trachea, i.e. the pharynx, is also reddened with much discharge present. There is usually severe respiratory distress with a bronchopneumonia. Some calves show severe diarrhoea and dehydration.

Central nervous system/encephalitic form. This is seen in calves under six months old and involves brain signs. The animals show incoordination with bouts of excitement and depression. In other cases there are convulsions, bellowing and blindness with salivation. This nervous form is rare.

Other infections. Reports of infections of the udder and intestinal tract have been made. However, these are rarely the only systems affected.

Necropsy

Respiratory form. In uncomplicated cases, lesions are restricted to the upper respiratory tract terminating at the upper bronchi. Inflammation of the muzzle and the nasal cavities varies from some congestion and petechiation with mucoid exudate, to a fibrinopurulent exudate with necrosis of the nasal mucous membranes. The submandibular and retropharyngeal lymph nodes tend to be swollen and oedematous. There is a laryngotracheobronchitis, which varies from a mild congestion of the mucous membranes with a mucoid discharge to large areas being covered by a necrotic layer of exudate (Pirie, 1979). In some cases there is pulmonary emphysema and secondary exudative bronchopneumonia, which may be purulent or necrotizing. Histologically, the mucous membranes show acute catarrhal inflammation and in some cases the epithelium and larynx tend to be infiltrated with neutrophils, lymphocytes, plasma cells and macrophages. In naturally occurring infections, inclusion bodies appear to be absent.

Abortion. Aborted fetuses often show marked autolysis and focal necrotic hepatitis.

Alimentary form. Epithelial necrosis of the turbinates, oesophagus, rumen and abomasum. Inclusion bodies are often evident in the surviving epithelium.

Nervous form. A non-suppurative encephalitis occurs particularly affecting the cerebral cortex and internal capsule.

Diagnosis

This will depend on the type but in the alimentary form it will depend on a history of IBR in the herd with virus present in the faeces or nasal swabs and possible necrotic areas on the turbinates. The nervous form is difficult to differentiate except that there is probably an IBR outbreak in the herd. At post-mortem examination the turbinates may show necrotic lesions.

In the respiratory form the history is that a new animal or group has entered the herd. In most cases several animals will be affected and besides varying degrees of respiratory signs there will usually be a conjunctivitis with copious, initially serous, ocular discharge. There may be necrosis of the nasal mucosa but this is absent in the mouth. The virus can be isolated in upper nasal or ocular swabs and is detected by fluorescent antibody staining. Otherwise paired blood samples will show a rise in titre to the enzyme-linked immunosorbent assay (ELISA) test. Other tests used include the serum neutralization test, indirect haemagglutination test, complement fixation test and virus neutralization test.

Treatment

There is a considerable divergence of opinion as to whether or not to use antibiotic treatment. If the disease appears to be uncomplicated, and this is unusual, then there would appear to be little point in therapy. If, however, as in most cases, there is secondary lung involvement, then therapy is justified. At the start of an outbreak all cases should be isolated as soon as possible because although it may not stop spread of the disease, the first animals are often clinically the worst affected. If antimicrobial agents are to be used, all ill calves should be treated for three to five days with any one of a number of drugs, including penicillin and streptomycin, oxytetracycline, ampicillin, trimethoprim and sulphadiazine, sulphadimidine, sulphamethoxypyridazine and sulphapyrazole. The animal should be given good, wholesome feed and it should be encouraged to eat and drink. Some farmers have vaccinated their calves with live vaccine after the start of an outbreak, with good results, but to be successful infection must not have become established. It should be remembered that for effective protection, vaccines should be introduced before the onset of infection. Several compounds have been found that are active against herpes viruses. However, many are toxic, but one drug, acyclovir, has been shown to be safe and may in the future be tried in animals.

Control

Management. It is best to keep a closed herd. However, in America, and also Britain, infection has been found in closed herds. Any new animal entering a known uninfected herd should be blood tested prior to entry. If the test is negative the animal should be isolated for a month and then retested. The use of corticosteroids may allow detection of virus in swabs of carrier animals. If the tests are all negative the animal can be allowed to enter the herd. The risks then of the introduction of infection are small. If the animal suffers a respiratory problem while in isolation the second test should not be until two or three weeks after the end of the episode. Some farmers may need to go to these lengths to keep their pedigree herds free from disease, because many European countries will not accept exports unless they are shown to have a negative titre for IBR. The same conditions at present govern the entry of bulls to some artificial insemination (AI) centres.

Vaccination. An inactivated multicomponent vaccine has been available for a long time. The vaccine could be given as doses two to four weeks apart with a third injection at 10–12 weeks old. Its efficacy has at times been questioned. Subsequently, live IBR vaccines have become available. They are given by intranasal inoculation and should be administered 24–48 hours after entry to the farm. Ideally, calves should be vaccinated 10 days prior to any movement. Beef calves can be vaccinated about two weeks or so before they are weaned. One vaccine is temperature sensitive and so only replicates in the upper parts of the respiratory tract. However, the vaccine can still produce circulating antibody levels in some cattle, which will preclude their export or their sale to AI centres. Another vaccine does replicate in organs other than the lungs and produces a good systemic immunity. The vaccines provide effective immunity but they do allow the replication and re-excretion of the IBR virus, which can thus spread infection to non-vaccinated animals.

References

Andrews, A.H. (1976) Factors affecting the incidence of pneumonia in growing bulls. *Veterinary Record*, **98**, 52–5.

Andrews, A.H. (1978) Some factors influencing respiratory disease in growing bulls and the effect of treatment on liveweight. In *Respiratory Diseases in Cattle*. Seminar in CEC Programme of Coordination of Research in Beef Production, Edinburgh, 8–10 November 1977 (ed. by W.B. Martin), pp. 169–80. Martinus Nijhoff, The Hague.

Andrews, A.H., Cook. G.L., Pritchard, D.G., Morzaria, S.P. & Gilmour, N.J.L. (1981) Observations on a respiratory disease outbreak in weaned suckled calves. *Veterinary Record*, **108**, 139–42.

Bateman, K.G. (1988) Efficacy of *Pasteurella haemolytica* vaccine/bacterial extract in the prevention of bovine respiratory disease in recently shipped feedlot calves. *Canadian Veterinary Journal*, **29**, 838–9.

Blood, D.C. & Radostits, O.M. (1989) Pneumonic pasteurellosis of cattle (shipping fever pneumonia). In *Veterinary Medicine*, 7th edn, pp. 663–73. Baillière Tindall, London.

Confer, A.W., Panciera, R.J. & Fulton, R.W. (1984) Effect of prior exposure to *Pasteurella haemolytica* antiserum on experimental pneumonic pasteurellosis. *American Journal of Veterinary Research*, **45**, 2622–4.

Frank, G.H. & Smith, P.C. (1983) Prevalence of *Pasteurella haemolytica* in transported calves. *American Journal of Veterinary Research*, **44**, 981–5.

Friend, S.C., Thomson, R.G. & Wilkie, B.N. (1977) Pulmonary lesions induced by *Pasteurella haemolytica* in cattle. *Canadian Journal of Comparative Medicine*, **41**, 219–23.

Gibbs, H.A., Allan, E.M., Selman, I.E. & Wiseman, A. (1983) Experimental bovine pneumonic pasteurellosis. *Veterinary Record*, **113**, 144.

Grey, C.L. & Thomson, R.G. (1971) *Pasteurella haemolytica* in the tracheal air of calves. *Canadian Journal of Comparative Medicine*, **35**, 121–8.

Houghton, S.B. & Gourlay, R.N. (1984) Bacteria associated with calf pneumonia and their effect on gnotobiotic calves. *Research in Veterinary Science*, **37**, 194–8.

Jensen, R., Pierson, R.E., Braddy, R.M., Saari, D.A., Lauerman, L.H., England, J.J., Keyvan, F.A.R., Collier, I.J.R., Horton, D.P., McChesney, A.E., Benitez, A. & Christie, R.M. (1976) Shipping fever pneumonia in yearling feedlot cattle. *Journal of the American Veterinary Medical Association*, **169**, 500–6.

Jim, K., Guichon, T. & Shaw, G. (1988) Protecting feedlot calves from pneumonic pasteurellosis. *Veterinary Medicine*, **83**, 1084–7.

Jones, C.R. & Webster, A.J.F. (1981) Weather induced changes in airborne bacteria within a calf house. *Veterinary Record*, **109**, 493–4.

MacVean, D., Franzen, D.K., Keefe, T.J. & Bennett, B.W. (1986) Airborne particle concentration and meteorological conditions associated with pneumonia incidence in feedlot calves. *American Journal of Veterinary Research*, **47**, 2676–82.

Martin, S.W. & Bohaz, J.G. (1986) The association between serological titres in infectious bovine rhinotracheitis virus, bovine viral diarrhoea virus, parainfluenza III virus, respiratory syncytial virus and treatment for respiratory disease in Ontario feedlot cattle. *Canadian Journal of Veterinary Research*, **50**, 351–8.

Myers, L.C. (1984) Questions on the efficacy of cattle vaccines. *Journal of the American Veterinary Association*, **184**, 5–7.

Panciera, R.J. & Corstvet, R.E. (1984) Bovine pneumonic pasteurellosis: model for *Pasteurella haemolytica* and *Pasteurella multocida*-induced pneumonia in cattle. *American Journal of Veterinary Research*, **45**, 2532–7.

Phillips, W.A. (1984) The effect of assembling and transit stresses on plasma fibrinogen concentration of beef calves. *Canadian Journal of Comparative Medicine*, **48**, 35–41.

Pirie, H.M. (1979) *Respiratory Diseases of Animals*, pp. 68–70, 71–4. Notes for a Postgraduate Course, Glasgow Veterinary School.

Rosendal, S. & Martin, S.W. (1986) The association between serological evidence of *Mycoplasma* infection and respiratory disease in feedlot cattle. *Canadian Journal of Veterinary Research*, **50**, 179–83.

Sherwen, P.E. & Wilkie, B.W. (1982) Cytotoxin of *Pasteurella haemolytica* acting on bovine leucocytes. *Infection and Immunity*, **35**, 91–4.

Sherwen, P.E. & Wilkie, B.W. (1988) Vaccination of calves with leukotoxic culture supernatant from *Pasteurella haemolytica*. *Canadian Journal of Veterinary Research*, **52**, 30–6.

Shoo, M.K. (1989) Experimental bovine pneumonic pasteurellosis: A review. *Veterinary Record*, **124**, 141–4.

Wilson, S.H., Church, T.L. & Acres, S.D. (1985) The influence of feedlot management on an outbreak of bovine respiratory disease. *Canadian Veterinary Journal*, **26**, 335–41.

Chapter 19: Trace Element Disorders

by N.F. SUTTLE

Introduction

The full impact that trace element disorders can have on the health of cattle was seen when Europeans attempted to carry their methods of animal production to the New World and to the Antipodes. The geologically young soils bordering Australia, and forming the Florida peninsula and the interior of New Zealand's North Island were a graveyard for many an animal until the therapeutic effect of newly discovered essential trace elements became known. Crop and pasture growth was also limited by some of the deficiencies but these were the more easily diagnosed because they produced characteristic foliar abnormalities. The animal's needs were more difficult to delineate because they lacked clinical definition and persisted where the more modest needs of the plant had been met. Since those pioneering days, trace element disorders have been described in many areas of the world and they continue to appear when new methods of production are introduced. The following descriptions of specific disorders concentrate on the more commonly encountered deficiencies of cobalt (Co), copper (Cu) and selenium (Se).

Four terms will occur frequently in each section and require definition.

1 Depletion. The reduction of body stores of the element.

2 Deficiency. The presence of subnormal concentrations of the element in the bloodstream or other body compartments.

3 Disorder. The malfunction of trace element-dependent body processes (subclinical disease).

4 Disease. The presence of visible clinical abnormalities.

The definitions become particularly important when attempts are made to describe the trace element status of cattle biochemically, with a view to distinguishing between the four states or confirming disease when clinical signs are non-specific.

Cobalt disorders

Clinical signs

All ruminants require a dietary supply of Co for the synthesis of the essential vitamin B_{12} by rumen micro-organisms. Cattle are less susceptible to a lack of Co than sheep but when they succumb, they develop essentially the same clinical abnormalities in the same order: anorexia, loss of body condition, muscular wasting and finally an anaemia that is both normochromic and normocytic. In the early stages of the disease, the hair coat can become rough and discoloured and may be repeatedly licked. Appetite may become depraved (pica). Eventually, the skin becomes thin and fragile and the mucous membranes pallid. The clinical picture is thus one of a 'pining' or 'wasting' disease, indistinguishable from many other causes of ill-thrift. Cobalt-deficient cattle may be more susceptible to parasite and microbial infections than normal cattle (MacPherson *et al.*, 1987a).

There is a neurological disease that affects cattle in Australia when they graze *Phalaris tuberosa* pastures called 'Phalaris staggers'; it can be prevented by Co dosage but not by administration of vitamin B_{12} and is, therefore, not a classical deficiency syndrome. The response to Co may arise through the neutralization of fungal neurotoxins by the element (Lee & Kuchel, 1953).

Aetiology

The only known functions of Co arise from its place at the centre of the corrin ring of two cobalamin (Cbl) molecules, methyl- (Me) and adenosyl- (Ado) Cbl, which have contrasting functions in the body. MeCbl acts as a coenzyme to methionine synthetase and is linked to folate metabolism, using methyltetrahydrofolate as the methyl group recipient. Deficiencies of this coenzyme can theoretically impair methionine synthesis and the bioavailability of folate and cause formiminoglutamic acid (FIGLU) to appear in urine. AdoCbl enables propionate to be used for gluconeogenesis via succinate and the tricarboxylic acid (TCA) cycle, acting as coenzyme to methylmalonyl-CoA isomerase: insufficiency causes methylmalonic acid (MMA) to accumulate.

The anorexia and anaemia that are successive debilitating consequences of deficiency may reflect the dysfunction of first AdoCbl, then MeCbl. Loss of appetite has been linked to increased blood propionate concentrations but the accumulation of other abnormal metabolites, e.g. MMA and the disturbance of rumen fermentation (McDonald & Suttle, 1986; Rice *et al.*, 1989) may also affect appetite. Loss of appetite probably compounds the effects of a diminishing supply of glucose precursors. The anaemia of Co deficiency may reflect the role of MeCbl in DNA synthesis and red cell maturation (Chanarin *et al.*, 1981).

The basic cause of Co deficiency disorders is a simple nutritional deficit that can be traced to impoverished soils in which crops or pastures have grown. Interactions can occur in the soil that leave most of the Co in unavailable forms. Cobalt can be adsorbed onto iron and manganese oxides, particularly at high soil pH. If extraction with 0.43 M acetic acid yields <0.3 mg Co/kg air-dry soil, deficiencies may develop. The diet should contain >0.05 mg Co/kg dry matter (DM) (Winter *et al.*, 1977). Interactions in the animal have been postulated because Co can be incorporated into various analogues of B_{12} by the rumen microbes (Dryden & Hartman, 1971). There is thus competition for Co in the rumen between different forms of the vitamin. Cobalamins are selectively absorbed in association with intrinsic factor but other analogues may find their way into the bloodstream or tissues: whether they then compete with or supplement the action of cobalamins has yet to be elucidated. However, it seems likely that ruminants would have developed protective mechanisms, if they are needed, against analogues so copiously produced in the rumen.

Necropsy

At necropsy, cattle suffering from Co deficiency show the hallmarks of starvation. There is little body fat except in the liver, which is often pale and friable due to fatty infiltration. In severely affected individuals hypoplasia of the bone marrow will be found while the spleen contains haemosiderin.

Diagnosis

Coresponsive disorders are best diagnosed through responses in growth or health to Co or B_{12} supplementation in controlled trials (e.g. Duncan *et al.*, 1986). The biochemical confirmation of deficiency from the assay of plasma B_{12} in cattle is more difficult than in sheep for a number of reasons. Firstly, plasma B_{12} concentrations do not appear to show the same response to Co supplementation as they do in sheep. Oral doses of Co ten times higher on a body weight basis than those that increase plasma B_{12} in sheep (Field *et al.*, 1988) are ineffective in cattle (N.F. Suttle and J. Brebner, unpublished data). High plasma B_{12} concentrations (>500 pg/ml) are rarely found and values often fall to exceedingly low levels (<100 pg/ml, e.g. Reid & McQueen, 1985) before cattle fail to thrive, though there are exceptions (e.g. Duncan *et al.*, 1986). Secondly, the assay of B_{12} by the more favoured radioisotope binding method is susceptible to interference from non-specific binders (Wright *et al.*, 1982; Millar *et al.*, 1984) and possibly from analogues of B_{12} in the plasma (Halpin *et al.*, 1984). The transport proteins for B_{12} in plasma, the transcobalamins, show quantitative differences from man (Polak *et al.*, 1979) as well as seasonal anomalies (Millar *et al.*, 1984), which may influence B_{12} assay by certain methods. The results of assays of B_{12} in bovine plasma are therefore likely to vary substantially between laboratories and assays of the analogue component by difference, using specific and non-specific binders, may not always have been quantitative.

There is little information on liver B_{12} concentrations in cattle or their relationship with plasma B_{12}. Diagnostic thresholds for sheep have long been extrapolated to cattle; thus values <0.10 μg/g fresh liver have been taken to indicate moderate to severe deficiency and values >0.19 have been regarded as normal. Australian studies have confirmed the validity of the lower limit for grazing calves (Winter *et al.*, 1977).

The diagnosis of Co disorders from the presence of abnormal metabolites in the blood and urine is well established in sheep and non-ruminants but has only recently been extended to cattle. Quirk & Norton (1988) found that heifers grazing pastures low in Co (0.036 mg/kg DM) remained healthy and excreted no MMA or FIGLU in urine, despite low plasma B_{12} concentrations (96 pg/ml). After calving, milk yield was unaffected but low B_{12} concentrations in the milk (42–86 pg/ml) caused depletion of plasma B_{12} in their calves (59–74 pg/ml) and growth retardation, which was accompanied by increased urinary excretion of FIGLU. They concluded that MMA was less reliable than FIGLU as an index of dysfunction but their method for MMA was relatively insensitive (30 μmol/l). Assay of plasma MMA has been advanced as a measure of functional B_{12} status in sheep with concentrations >5 μmol/l taken to be abnormal (Rice *et al.*, 1987): as yet plasma MMA has not been tested for the confirmation of Co deficiency in cattle.

Treatment or prevention

Although there are clearly differences in B_{12} metabolism between cattle and sheep, there is no evidence that these affect the methods of treating and preventing disorders. The injection of B_{12} as cyano- or hydroxycobalamin, 2–6 mg/50 kg liveweight, provides protection for several weeks even though responses in plasma B_{12} soon dissipate. Heavy cobalt oxide pellets, given in pairs or singly with a 'grinder', improve the B_{12} status of growing and adult cattle for several months (Judson *et al.*, 1981; Quirk & Norton, 1988) as does the soluble glass bolus (Allen *et al.*, 1985). The effectiveness of infrequent oral doses of Co in anthelmintics, as is practised with sheep (Field *et al.*, 1988), has not been tested but weekly doses of 35–70 mg Co without anthelmintic are said to be effective (Underwood, 1966). Cobalt supplementation via the drinking water can be practised where there is a piped water supply (MacPherson, 1983).

Recent evidence that volatile fatty acid (VFA) production by rumen microbes is influenced by Co deficiency (McDonald & Suttle, 1986; Rice *et al.*, 1989) might suggest that there is an advantage for the oral route over the injection route, since only the former meets the needs of the microbes for B_{12}. Comparisons between methods have rarely been conducted but one at least showed no advantage in calf growth for oral Co versus injected B_{12} (Judson *et al.*, 1981).

Administration of Co on a group basis via licks containing 0.1 per cent Co or mineral mixes containing up to 0.4 per cent Co may provide an inexpensive means of prevention but could not be guaranteed to treat all individuals.

The best long-term strategy on certain soil types will be to apply Co salts, such as hydrated $CoSO_4$ at 2–3 kg/ha, every three to four years. Responses may, however, be short-lived on sandy soils and negligible on calcareous or recently limed soils.

There is virtually no risk of overdosing with cobalt but this should not be used as an excuse to overfeed Co to animals whose capacity to synthesize and absorb B_{12} is strictly limited.

Copper disorders (see Chapter 16)

Clinical signs

The sequence and severity of signs associated with a lack of dietary Cu in cattle depend upon the rate and stage of development at which it occurs. There are no definitive reports of teratogenic or neurological effects, comparable with swayback in sheep (cf. Richards & Edwards, 1986). In the growing calf, loss of hair colour, growth retardation and changes in metatarsal conformation are the earliest signs of abnormality followed by diarrhoea and finally anaemia (Mills et al., 1976; Suttle & Angus, 1976). Cardiac hypertrophy has been reported in experimentally depleted calves (Leigh, 1975) and this may be an early manifestation of the myocardial degeneration that can cause sudden death after prolonged deficiency in the field (Bennetts *et al.*, 1941). Addition of small amounts of the Cu antagonist, molybdenum (Mo), to the diet (2 mg/kg DM) accelerates rather than changes these clinical manifestations of disorder (Suttle & Angus, 1976). At much higher Mo concentrations (>10 mg/kg DM), animals may develop diarrhoea immediately upon exposure to the antagonist (Suttle, 1988).

Infertility has long been associated with Cu deficiency in cattle but there is little published evidence that deficiency leads to impaired reproduction unless Mo is involved (Phillippo *et al.*, 1982, 1987b). Molybdenum-induced deficiency is associated with delays in the onset of oestrus, impaired conception rate and anoestrus: these abnormalities have yet to be induced by other antagonists of Cu such as Fe (Phillippo *et al.*, 1987b). Copper-responsive infertility in cattle given Mo, therefore, is not necessarily Cu dependent and may result from the direct or indirect suppression of the release of luteinizing hormone (Phillippo *et al.*, 1987b).

Anaemia is a late sign of Cu deficiency in growing calves (Suttle & Angus, 1976) and may be associated with Heinz body formation in the periparturient cow (Black, 1981). The *in vitro* viability and/or function of neutrophils from Cu-deficient cattle is poorer than that of cells from normal cattle (Jones & Suttle, 1981; Boyne & Arthur, 1986) but there is no evidence yet for impaired resistance to infections *in vivo*.

Aetiology

Most Cu deficiencies in cattle are induced: they are induced in the rumen where the anaerobic degradation of sulphur(S)-rich, fibrous feeds leaves little of the ingested Cu in a soluble form. After weaning, less than 10 per cent of the total Cu input is absorbed during passage down the gastrointestinal tract and the percentage can be reduced to as little as 1.2 per cent by small increments in dietary Mo (Suttle, 1978). Again it is transformations in the rumen that are pivotal: extrapolating from sheep, it appears that the progressive substitution of S^{2-} for O^{2-} in molybdate creates thiomolybdates, which complex Cu and bind it to the solid phase (Price *et al.*, 1987). Surplus trithiomolybdate ($MoOS_3$) is absorbable and capable of changing the distribution of Cu in the blood (Mason *et al.*, 1986) and tissues (Wang *et al.*, 1987). Just how important the systemic effects of thiomolybdates are under normal grazing conditions has yet to be determined because the 'tell-tale' appearance of abnormal fractions such as TCA-insoluble copper has been restricted to experimental situations (Wang *et al.*, 1988).

Most cases of Cu-responsive growth retardation in cattle are associated with abnormally low ratios of Cu : Mo in the herbage (<3.0; Phillippo, 1983) and it has been suggested that they may reflect direct effects of Mo on the central control of appetite (Phillippo *et al.*, 1987a). It is, however, premature to discount the role of Cu (Suttle, 1988) and factors that influence Cu status should not be ignored. Copper absorption in cattle is as sensitive to Mo inhibition as it is in sheep (Suttle, 1978) and the equations derived for grazing sheep to predict Cu absorption (Suttle, 1983b) should give an approximate weighting for cattle. High S intakes from the diet (Suttle, 1983b) or drinking water (Smart *et al.*, 1986) also suppress Cu absorption. Poor Cu absorption, and hence deficiency problems, will therefore be more common on lush, immature, S-rich swards than on brown, mature swards. Copper is also absorbed better from hay than from fresh grass of similar S content (Suttle, 1983a). Ensiled grass is a good source of absorbable Cu while S concentrations are low (about 2 g/kg DM), but availability probably falls rapidly as concentrations rise to 3 g/kg DM if cattle share the characteristics of sheep (Suttle, 1983b). High iron (Fe) concentrations also lower Cu status in cattle (Bremner *et al.*, 1987; Phillippo *et al.*, 1987a) and there is debate over whether or not the antagonism requires the presence of moderate amounts of dietary S (Suttle, 1988).

The principal determinants of hypocuprosis in grazing cattle are probably soil Mo, soil pH (high values encourage Mo uptake), sward maturity, rainfall (or irrigation), fertilizer use and soil ingestion rather than the Cu content of the soil or herbage on all but the most impoverished, sandy soils.

Shortage of absorbable Cu leads to (i) rapid depletion of liver stores, (ii) a lowering of caeruloplasmin synthesis and a drop in plasma Cu, and (iii) a reduction in cuproenzyme activities in the erythrocyte and tissues. Although cytochrome oxidase and superoxide dismutase have been the most studied, others such as lysyl oxidase and dopamine hydroxylase will almost certainly follow the non-ruminant pattern in showing disorder (Prohaska, 1987). Effects on growth, cardiac function and bone development cannot be attributed to a particular enzyme deficiency with certainty. Even the depigmentation once attributed to diminished tyrosinase activity must be open to other explanations now that it is known to be produced by Co as well as Cu deficiency (Judson *et al.*, 1982). Connective tissue defects, including those in the ligamentum nuchae, are probably due to lysyl oxidase deficiency leading to defective cross-links in elastin. Digestive disturbances may result from disruption of mitochondrial respiration and villous atrophy (Fell *et al.*, 1975) but enhanced inflammatory reactions to gut parasites cannot be ruled out in grazing animals (Suttle *et al.*, 1989).

Necropsy

The pathology of bovine Cu deficiency is largely unhelpful because the histological changes underlying the clinical signs, like the signs themselves, are nonspecific. The earliest and most dramatic lesions are likely to be those affecting the epiphyseal growth plates in the costochondral junctions and metatarsal/metacarpal bones. These can become overgrown to the point that they spill over to leave islets of collagen distal to the plate in various states of irregular calcification and fibrotic replacement (Irwin *et al.*, 1974; Suttle & Angus, 1976). Gross degenerative changes are also seen in connective tissues such as the ligamentum nuchae (Mills *et al.*, 1976). In severe cases showing diarrhoea, villous atrophy in the duodenal and jejunal regions is likely to be seen (Fell *et al.*, 1975; Suttle & Angus, 1976) but is indistinguishable from that caused by gut parasites.

The anaemia of Cu deficiency in the bovine is similar to that of Fe deficiency, i.e. macrocytic and hypochromic (Bennetts *et al.*, 1941). Cardiac lesions including fibrosis of the myocardium have been reported in natural outbreaks only once, over 40 years ago, in Australia (Bennetts *et al.*, 1941). While cardiac hypertrophy was seen in some experimentally depleted calves, which took a like time to develop clinical signs (Leigh, 1975), it was not present in others that were depleted more rapidly (Suttle & Angus, 1976).

Attention has been switched recently from the lesions that underlie the expected and familiar clinical signs to those which, though less spectacular, occur earlier and may underlie the debilitating effects of the disorder. Fell and his associates (Fell *et al.*, 1985; Fell, 1987) have found basement membrane defects in the pancreatic acinar cell, the duodenal enterocyte and kidney tubule, pointing to perhaps a common early failure of proteoglycan organization.

It remains to be seen whether Mo can cause distinctive histological or ultrastructural changes at central sites such as the pineal body which may be crucial to the development of disorder (Phillippo *et al.*, 1987b) and whether or not these are Cu dependent.

Diagnosis

Since none of the clinical signs of Cu deficiency given above is specific, diagnosis must be supported by biochemical tests showing subnormal tissue Cu status. Because availability has such a major effect on Cu uptake, herbage or dietary Cu concentrations alone are almost worthless and should be accompanied by measures of Mo and S and predictions of available Cu (Suttle, 1983b). Even then, other factors such as initial Cu reserves, other dietary antagonists (Fe and ingested soil), breed differences in susceptibility and the rate of animal production may determine the outcome of events. In establishing Cu as a limiting factor to production in a new area, a response to a specific Cu treatment affords the best assessment though not necessarily showing Cu deficiency to be the primary cause (cf. p. 264).

The conventional criteria of Cu status, i.e. liver and blood Cu concentrations, are most dependable when herbage Mo concentrations are low (<5 mg/kg DM). Under these circumstances the ranges 10–20 mg Cu/kg DM for liver and 3–9 µmol Cu/l for plasma can be regarded as 'marginal' as individual values: as group means, they indicate that some individuals are likely to benefit from Cu supplementation and that cheap measures to improve Cu status would be prudent. At higher dietary Mo concentrations (35 mg/kg DM), changes in the distribution of Cu in the plasma and liver may complicate the assessment of Cu status (Wang *et al.*, 1988). With high Mo concentrations (>5 mg/kg DM) in pasture, 'teart'-like conditions may operate for critical periods, with animals responding to Cu while normocupraemic. It remains to be seen whether supplements that achieve normocupraemia invariably provide a sufficient defence against Mo-induced infertility and whether other parameters such as plasma Mo or plasma Fe concentrations have merit for diagnosing Mo-induced ill health (Phillippo *et al.*, 1987a, b).

Treatment or prevention

The treatment of Cu deficiency is achieved readily by single oral doses of Cu or parenteral injections of the element. In animals close to market weight the use of chelates of Cu with ethylene diamine, tetra-acetic acid (EDTA), glycine or methionine may result in unacceptable, 'cold' abscesses at the injection site, whether given subcutaneously or intramuscularly. Use of water-soluble complexes such as the hydroxyquinoline sulphonate and heptonate will avoid abscess formation but increase risks of acute toxicity (e.g. Suttle, 1981).

Prevention of deficiency and disorder can be achieved to varying degrees of precision and duration with oral and parenteral supplements. Copper oxide particles are more effective than serial injections, providing protection for several months (Judson *et al.*, 1985; Rogers & Poole, 1988). Soluble glass boluses are likely in time to give equally sustained protection and are particularly suited to the extensive grazing situation (Allen *et al.*, 1985; Judson *et al.*, 1985; Givens *et al.*, 1988). During periods of supplementary feeding or housing, the use of Cu salts as forage additives or cereal supplements commends itself. Where food supplements are not given, the free-access mineral is likely to afford protection to the majority of the individuals in herds that take to it. If Cu proves to be useful as an antidote to Mo rather than an essential nutrient in some situations by rendering toxic thiomolybdates or molybdate less available, a particular pattern of Cu provision (e.g. slow rumenal release or steady dietary supplementation) may have advantages over other forms of supplementation.

Selenium disorders (see p. 222)

Clinical signs

Selenium deficiency in cattle can impair development throughout life. The suckling calf can develop chronic skeletal and cardiac myopathy if the dam's diet is low in Se (Hidiroglou *et al.*, 1985) while the calf on pastures deficient in Se can suffer growth retardation before (Morris *et al.*, 1984) and after weaning (Gleed *et al.*, 1983). In spring, calves can develop acute myopathy with myoglobinuria when turned out to graze. Selenium supplementation has improved conception rate in cows (McClure *et al.*, 1986) and heifers (MacPherson *et al.*, 1987b). At parturition, cows of low Se status are more likely to retain the placenta than Se-supplemented cows (Trinder *et al.*, 1969) and they are the more susceptible to metritis and cystic ovaries (Harrison *et al.*, 1984). Selenium deficiency also affects the circulatory system: the growing calf can develop a Heinz-body anaemia (Morris *et al.*, 1984) and when calving coincides with turnout, the cow which is both Cu and Se deficient may be vulnerable to haemolysis and haemoglobinuria (Black, 1981).

Despite the variety of clinical signs caused by a lack of Se, it is rare for more than one sign to appear in a single herd. Problems of muscular dystrophy have not been reported in the many studies of retained placenta, which is probably the commonest Se-responsive condition in cattle. Similarly, growth retardation and muscular dystrophy have not been reported in the one outbreak of disorder. Selenium deficiency in cattle has been associated with impaired phagocyte function *in vitro* (Boyne & Arthur, 1979) prompting speculation that Se deficiency would lead to decreased resistance to disease but these suggestions have not been confirmed in experimental (Reffett *et al.*, 1988) or field studies. Improvements in calf survival in herds on diets of marginal Se concentration (0.03–0.05 kg Se/kg DM) have been reported but vitamin E as well as Se was given and the role of Se alone is unclear (Spears *et al.*, 1986).

Aetiology

The principal function of Se in animals relates to its intracellular presence in the antioxidant enzyme glutathione peroxidase (GSHPx), which uses various potentially dangerous peroxides as substrates. Recently, Se has been linked with iodine metabolism in ways that indicate a separate function independent of GSHPx (Arthur *et al.*, 1988). While the basic cause of Se disorders is obviously a shortage of the element in the diet, which in turn can be traced to soil formations also deficient in Se (Kubota *et al.*, 1967; Watkinson, 1983), other factors are probably involved in field outbreaks of Se-responsive disease. Calves fed experimental diets of exceedingly low Se content (0.01–0.02 mg/kg DM) indoors can be depleted of Se to the point that they have undetectable activities of GSHPx in their blood and yet do not develop myopathy (Arthur, 1988; Reffett *et al.*, 1988). In one study (Arthur, 1988) the failure to induce myopathy was the more surprising because the diet was also low in vitamin E, which shares the role of antioxidant defence with Se in the tissues.

The importance of dietary sources of oxidant stress was demonstrated by workers in Belfast (Rice & McMurray, 1982) who showed that the addition of polyunsaturated fatty acids (PUFA) to diets deficient in vitamin E and Se, simulating the composition of PUFA-rich spring grass, will precipitate myopathy. Other stresses may yet be required to induce myopathy because Arthur (1988) has shown that feeding of PUFA-rich grass indoors to calves deficient in Se and vitamin E did not precipitate the disorder, whereas grazing the same grass produced acute myopathy. He suggested that exercise or some other component of the environmental change at turnout contributed to the development of muscle damage. The excitable behaviour of the calf will of course result in increased activity of muscles involved in locomotion, circulation and respiration and exercise is known to induce oxidant stress and exacerbate the effects of vitamin E deficiency (Jackson, 1987). It is highly likely that the intense and sometimes prolonged muscular activity of the uterus at parturition makes it particular vulnerable to Se (and vitamin E) deficiency. Adverse weather conditions have been implicated in outbreaks of acute myopathy (Allen *et al.*, 1975). The cause of Se-responsive disorders is thus multifactorial.

Diagnosis

The differential diagnosis of Se-responsive disorders is complicated by the non-specific clinical signs of disease: most can be attributed to vitamin E deficiency while others, such as retained placenta and growth retardation, have many possible causes of both nutritional and non-nutritional origin. It follows from the extreme tolerance of low plasma and blood Se (or GSHPx) concentrations in the absence of exacerbative factors that measures of Se (or GSHPx) alone cannot confirm a disorder. Neither is there likely to be a simple relationship between dietary Se concentration and incidence of disease.

Very small differences in Se status may determine vulnerability. In the study of Hidiroglou *et al.* (1985) for example, myopathy occurred in calves in one year when blood GSHPx declined from 29 to 19 iu/g haemoglobin (Hb) and plasma Se from 11 to 6 ng/ml, but not in the next when the respective falls were 51 to 28 iu/g Hb and 16 to 13 ng/ml. Pasture Se was consistently low at 0.02–0.04 mg/kg DM. In a survey of the Se status of cattle in northeast Scotland (Arthur *et al.*, 1979), it was noted that while 85 per cent of herds had a blood Se status <0.05 µg/ml, a threshold below which a risk of clinical disease was suggested (Anderson *et al.*, 1979), only 10 per cent had a recent history of myopathy; the winter diets mostly contained <0.05 mg Se/kg DM.

The clinically significant thresholds for dietary and blood Se concentrations probably vary with the Se-responsive condition and the dietary supply of vitamin E. Incidence of retained placenta can be reduced in cows receiving diets of higher Se content (0.04–0.05 mg/kg DM (Trinder *et al.*, 1973) than those giving freedom from myopathy. Likewise, thresholds for blood GSHPx activities and Se concentrations probably need to be set higher than 0.05 mg/l for normal reproduction (Trinder *et al.*, 1973; McClure *et al.*, 1986).

In monitoring Se status, the assay of GSHPx has largely replaced that of whole blood Se because it is easier to assay yet highly correlated with blood Se concentration. Enzyme activities have been converted to blood Se equivalents (e.g. Anderson *et al.*, 1979) for comparative purposes. Interpretation of blood GSHPx activities is, however, complicated by many factors. Despite almost two-fold differences in the specific activities of GSHPx (activity/unit Se) between sheep and cattle (Anderson *et al.*, 1978), the same diagnostic threshold has been used for both (activity equivalent to 50 ng/ml; Anderson *et al.*, 1979). Provided that the specific activities are equally different for the substrates encountered *in vivo* and the two species have similar requirements in terms of intracellular enzyme activity, the lower specific activity in the bovine could mean that physiologically equivalent Se concentrations are 50 ng/ml for cattle and 25 ng/ml for sheep. The slow turnover of erythrocytes ensures that blood GSHPx activity reflects past rather than present Se supply. The data of Hidiroglou *et al.* (1985) indicate that it may take four months for blood GSHPx fully to reflect an improved Se supply and just as long to reflect a waning supply. Plasma Se responds immediately to such changes and is a useful adjunct to blood GSHPx in assessing Se status.

The measurement of GSHPx activity is subject to wider interlaboratory variation than most analyses in the clinical context: Rice *et al.* (1987) have identified some important variables. The use of an assay kit will help to standardize results but differences can still arise and each laboratory should determine and quote its own Se equivalence for GSHPx activity. Results are variously reported per ml blood, per g haemoglobin and per ml cells: while these will be highly correlated with each other within laboratories, the use of common conversion factors for comparative purposes may introduce errors.

The greatest limitation of blood GSHPx for monitoring disorder is that the target tissue in Se deficiency is muscle not blood. Furthermore, there are wide variations between muscles in their GSHPx content (Anderson *et al.*, 1978) and in the lipid composition of their membranes (Rice & Kennedy, 1988). Measurement of blood GSHPx alone is unlikely to reflect the risk of lipid peroxidation and hence myopathy in crucial muscles.

Treatment or prevention

The many different methods for administering Se orally and parenterally have been reviewed (Allen, 1983; MacPherson, 1983) and three were compared by MacPherson and Chalmers (1984). Long-term supplementation can be achieved by both routes: by administering heavy metal (iron oxide) (e.g. Hidiroglou *et al.*, 1985; McClure *et al.*, 1986) or soluble glass boluses (Judson *et al.*, 1985) orally and by injecting a relatively insoluble Se salt, barium selenate, in an oily base (MacPherson & Chalmers, 1984; MacPherson *et al.*, 1987b) parenterally, blood Se concentrations have been increased for at least five months. Supplementing the drinking water (MacPherson & Chalmers, 1984), the pasture (by fertilizer application; Watkinson, 1983), or the winter diet (Stowe *et al.*, 1988) with Se also provides long-term protection. Stowe *et al.* (1988) concluded that a supplement of 2 mg Se/day upon an estimated intake of 0.5 mg/day was not sufficient to raise plasma Se in the periparturient cow to 'acceptable levels' (>0.6 ng/ml): nevertheless retained placenta and metritis was only half as prevalent in treated as in untreated cows.

It is questionable whether most forms of long-term Se supplementation are the most cost-effective way of treating what are usually short-term problems. The Se-responsive diseases associated with parturition and turnout are acute conditions that can be effectively treated or prevented by single injections of Se as selenite or selenate (e.g. Trinder *et al.*, 1969; Eger *et al.*, 1985; McMurray & McEldowney, 1977). There is considerable variation in dosage practice. For example, for the prevention of retained placenta, Se doses have varied from 2.3 to 50 mg: the highest dose rate, equivalent to 0.1 mg/kg liveweight is the most commonly used.

Selenium has generally been given with vitamin E and it is impossible to assess retrospectively whether there was invariably a need for both nutrients. The limited studies in which only one nutrient was given to some animals show that the benefit of providing vitamin E with Se varies from farm to farm (Trinder *et al.*, 1973). The need for dual supplementation may also depend on the nature of the clinical problem. A combination of oral vitamin E with parenteral Se reduced the incidence of retained placenta in one instance in which the separate treatments were ineffective but Se alone reduced the prevalence of metritis and cystic ovaries (Harrison et al., 1984). In the treatment of acute myopathy at turnout, McMurray and McEldowney (1977) found that vitamin E (2.8 mg/kg liveweight) was less effective than Se (0.0625 mg/kg liveweight) and added nothing when given with Se. In this situation cattle of low vitamin E status were turned onto grass of naturally high vitamin E concentration. The variable responses to vitamin E given with Se will be due largely to the wide variations found in the vitamin E status of housed cattle.

References

Allen, W.M. (1983) Parenteral methods of trace element supplementation. British Society of Animal Production Occasional Publication No. 7, pp. 87–92.

Allen, W.M., Bradley, R., Berrett, S., Parr, W.H., Swannack, K., Barton, C.R.Q. & Macphee, A. (1975) Degenerative myopathy with myoglobinuria in yearling cattle. *British Veterinary Journal*, **131**, 292–308.

Allen, W.M., Drake, C.F. & Tripp, M. (1985) Use of controlled release systems for supplementation during trace element deficiency — the administration of boluses of controlled release glass to cattle and sheep. In *Proceedings of Fifth International Symposium on Trace Element Metabolism in Man and Animals* (ed. by C.F. Mills, I. Bremner & J.K. Chesters), pp. 719–22. Commonwealth Agricultural Bureaux.

Anderson, P.H., Berrett, S. & Patterson, D.S.P. (1978) Glutathione peroxidase activity in erythrocytes and muscle of cattle and sheep and its relationship to selenium. *Journal of Comparative Pathology*, **88**, 181–9.

Anderson, P.H., Berrett, S. & Patterson, D.S.P. (1979) The biological selenium status of livestock in Britain as indicated by sheep erythrocyte glutathione peroxidase activity. *Veterinary Record*, **104**, 235–8.

Arthur, J.R. (1988) Effects of selenium and vitamin E status on plasma creatine kinase activity in calves. *Journal of Nutrition*, **118**, 747–55.

Arthur, J.R., Price, J. & Mills, C.F. (1979) Observations on the selenium status of cattle in the north-east of Scotland. *Veterinary Record*, **104**, 340–1.

Arthur, J.R., Morrice, P.C. & Beckett, G.J. (1988) Thyroid hormone concentrations in selenium-deficient and selenium sufficient cattle. *Research in Veterinary Science*, **45**, 122–3.

Bennetts, H.W., Beck, A.B., Harley, R. & Evans, S.T. (1941) Falling disease of cattle in the south-west of Western Australia 2. Studies of copper deficiency in cattle. *Australian Veterinary Journal*, **17**, 85–93.

Black, H. (1981) Post-parturient haemoglobinuria in Northland. Proceedings of the Sheep and Beef Cattle Society of New Zealand Veterinary Association's 11th Seminar, Massey University, Palmerston North, pp. 11–14.

Boyne, R. & Arthur, J.R. (1979) Alterations in neutrophil function in selenium deficient cattle. *Journal of Comparative Pathology*, **89**, 151–8.

Boyne, R. & Arthur, J.R. (1986) Effects of molybdenum and iron-induced copper deficiency on the viability and function of neutrophils from cattle. *Research in Veterinary Science*, **41**, 417–19.

Bremner, I., Humphries, W.R., Phillippo, M., Walker, M.J. & Morrice, P.C. (1987) Iron-induced copper deficiency in calves: dose-response relationships and interactions with molybdenum and sulphur. *Animal Production*, **45**, 403–14.

Chanarin, I., Deacon, R., Perry, J. & Lumb, M. (1981) How vitamin B_{12} acts. *British Journal of Haematology*, **47**, 487–91.

Dryden, L.P. & Hartman, A.M. (1971) Variations in the amount and distribution of vitamin B_{12} and its analogues in the bovine rumen. *Journal of Dairy Science*, **54**, 235–45.

Duncan, I.F., Greentree, P.L. & Ellis, K.J. (1986) Cobalt deficiency in cattle. *Australian Veterinary Journal*, **3**, 127–8.

Eger, S., Drori, D., Kadoori, I., Miller, N. & Schindler, H. (1985) Effects of selenium and vitamin E on incidence of retained placenta. *Journal of Dairy Science*, **68**, 2119–22.

Fell, B.F. (1987) The pathology of copper deficiency in animals. In *Copper in Animals and Man* (ed. by J. McC Howell & J.M. Gawthorne), pp. 1–28. CRC Press Ltd, Boca Raton, Florida.

Fell, B.F., Dinsdale, D. & Mills, C.F. (1975) Changes in enterocyte mitochondria associated with deficiency of copper in cattle. *Research in Veterinary Science*, **18**, 274–81.

Fell, B.F., Farmer, L.J., Farquharson, C., Bremner, I. & Graca, D.S. (1985) Observations on the pancreas of cattle deficient in copper. *Journal of Comparative Pathology*, **95**, 573–90.

Field, A.C., Suttle, N.F., Brebner, J. & Gunn, G. (1988) An assessment of the efficacy and safety of selenium and cobalt included in an anthelmintic for sheep. *Veterinary Record*, **123**, 97–100.

Givens, D.I., Zervas, G., Simpson, V.R. & Telfer, S.B. (1988) Use of soluble glass rumen boluses to provide a supplement of copper for suckled calves. *Journal of Agricultural Science, Cambridge*, **110**, 119–204.

Gleed, P.T., Allen, W.M., Mallinson, C.B., Rowlands, G.J., Sansom, B.F., Vagg, M.J. & Caswell, R.D. (1983) Effects of selenium and copper supplementation on the growth of beef steers. *Veterinary Record*, **113**, 388–92.

Halpin, C.C., Harris, D.J., Caple, I.W. & Petterson, D.S. (1984) Contribution of cobalamin analogues to plasma B_{12} concentrations in cattle. *Research in Veterinary Science*, **37**, 249–51.

Harrison, J.H., Hancock, D.D. & Conrad, H.R. (1984) Vitamin E and selenium for reproduction in the dairy cow. *Journal of Dairy Science*, **67**, 123–32.

Hidiroglou, M., Proulx, J. & Jolette, J. (1985) Intraruminal selenium for control of nutritional muscular dystrophy in cattle. *Journal of Dairy Science*, **68**, 57–66.

Irwin, M.R., Poulos, P.W., Smith, B.P. & Fisher, G.L. (1974) Radiology and histopathology of lameness in young cattle with secondary copper deficiency. *Journal of Comparative Pathology*, **84**, 611–21.

Jackson, M. (1987) Muscle damage during exercise; possible role of free radicals and the protective effect of vitamin E. *Proceedings of the Nutrition Society*, **46**, 77–80.

Jones, D.G. & Suttle, N.F. (1981) Some effects of copper deficiency on leucocyte function in sheep and cattle. *Research in Veterinary Science*, **31**, 151–6.

Judson, G.J., McFarlane, J.D., Riley, M.J., Milne, M.L. & Horne, A.C. (1981) Treatment of cobalt deficiency in calves. In *Proceedings of the Fourth International Symposium on Trace Element Metabolism in Man and Animals* (ed. by J. McC Howell, J.M. Gawthorne & C.L. White), pp. 191–4. Australian Academy of Science.

Judson, G.J., McFarlane, J.D., Riley, M.J., Milne, M.L. & Horne, A.C. (1982) Vitamin B_{12} and copper supplementation in beef calves. *Australian Veterinary Journal*, **58**, 249–52.

Judson, G.J., Koh, T.-S., McFarlane, J.D., Turnbull, R.K. & Kempe, B.R. (1985) Copper and selenium supplements for cattle: evaluation of the selenium bullet, copper oxide and the soluble glass bullet. In *Proceedings of the Fifth International Symposium on Trace Element Metabolism in Man and Animals* (ed. by C.F. Mills, I. Bremner & J.K. Chesters), pp. 725–8. Commonwealth Agricultural Bureaux, Farnham Royal.

Kubota, J., Allaway, W.H. & Carter, D.L. (1967) Selenium in crops in the United States in relation to selenium-responsive diseases of cattle. *Journal of Agricultural and Food Chemistry*, **15**, 448–56.

Lee, H.J. & Kuchel, R.E. (1987) The aetiology of *Phalaris* staggers in sheep. I. Preliminary observations on the preventive role of cobalt. *Australian Journal of Agricultural Research*, **4**, 88–99.

Leigh, L.C. (1975) Changes in the ultrastructure of cardial muscle in steers deprived of copper. *Research in Veterinary Science*, **18**, 282–7.

Mason, J.M., Woods, M. & Poole, D.B.R. (1986) Accumulation of copper on albumin in bovine plasma *in vivo* after intravenous thiomolybdate administration. *Research in Veterinary Science*, **41**, 108–13.

McClure, T.J., Eamens, G.J. & Healy, P.J. (1986) Improved fertility in dairy cows after treatment with selenium pellets. *Australian Veterinary Journal*, **63**, 144–6.

McDonald, P. & Suttle, N.F. (1986) Abnormal fermentations in continuous culture of rumen microorganisms given cobalt-deficient or barley as food substrates. *British Journal of Nutrition*, **56**, 369–78.

McMurray, C.H. & McEldowney, P.K. (1977) A possible prophylaxis and model for nutritional degenerative myopathy in young cattle. *British Veterinary Journal*, **133**, 535–42.

MacPherson, A. (1983) Oral treatment of trace element deficiencies in ruminant livestock. British Society of Animal Production Occasional Publication No. 7, pp. 93–106.

MacPherson, A. & Chalmers, J.S. (1984) Methods of selenium supplementation of ruminants. Veterinary Record, **115**, 544–6.

MacPherson, A., Gray, D., Mitchell, D.B.B. & Taylor, C.N. (1987a) *Ostertagia* infection and neutrophil function in cobalt-deficient and cobalt-supplemented cattle. *British Veterinary Journal*, **143**, 348–53.

MacPherson, A., Kelly, E.F., Chalmers, J.S. & Roberts, D.J. (1987b) The effect of selenium deficiency on fertility in heifers. In *Proceedings of 21st Annual Conference on Trace Substrates in Environmental Health* (ed. by D.D. Hemphill), pp. 551–5. University of Missouri.

Millar, K.R., Albyt, A.T. & Bond, G.C. (1984) Measurement of vitamin B_{12} in the livers and sera of sheep and cattle and on investigation of factors influencing serum vitamin B_{12} levels in sheep. *New Zealand Veterinary Journal*, **32**, 65–70.

Mills, C.F., Wenham, G.B. & Dalgarno, A.C. (1976) Biochemical and pathological changes in tissues of Friesian cattle during the experimental induction of copper deficiency. *British Journal of Nutrition*, **35**, 304–31.

Morris, J.G., Chapman, H.L., Walker, D.F., Armstrong, J.B., Alexander, J.D., Miranda, R., Sanchez, A., Sanchez, B., Blair-West, J.R. & Denton, D.A. (1984) Selenium deficiency in cattle associated with Heinz body anaemia. *Science*, **223**, 291–3.

Phillippo, M. (1983) The role of dose–response trials in predicting trace element deficiency disorders. British Society of Animal Production Occasional Publication No. 7, pp. 51–60.

Phillippo, M., Humphries, W.R., Lawrence, C.B. & Price, J. (1982) Investigation of the effects of copper status and therapy on fertility in beef suckler herds. *Journal of Agricultural Science, Cambridge*, **99**, 359–64.

Phillippo, M., Humphries, W.R. & Garthwaite, P.H. (1987a) The effect of dietary molybdenum and iron on copper status and growth in cattle. *Journal of Agricultural Science, Cambridge*, **109**, 315–20.

Phillippo, M., Humphries, W.R., Atkinson, T., Henderson, G.D. & Garthwaite, P.H. (1987b). The effect of dietary molybdenum and iron on copper status, puberty, fertility and oestrous cycles in cattle. *Journal of Agricultural Science, Cambridge*, **109**, 321–36.

Polak, D.M., Elliot, J.M. & Haluska, M. (1979) Vitamin B_{12} binding proteins in bovine serum. *Journal of Dairy Science*, **62**, 697–701.

Price, J., Will, M.A., Paschaleris, G. & Chesters, J.K. (1987) Identification of thiomolybdates in digesta and plasma from sheep after administration of ^{99}Mo-labelled compounds into the rumen. *British Journal of Nutrition*, **58**, 127–38.

Prohaska, J.R. (1987) Functions of trace elements in brain metabolism. *Journal of Comparative Pathology*, **67**, 858–901.

Quirk, M.F. & Norton, B.W. (1988) Detection of cobalt deficiency in lactating heifers and their calves. *Journal of Agricultural Science, Cambridge*, **110**, 465–70.

Reffett, J.K., Spears, J.W. & Brown, T.T. (1988) Effect of dietary selenium on the primary and secondary immune response in calves challenged with infectious bovine rhinotracheitis virus. *Journal of Nutrition*, **118**, 229.

Reid, T.C. & McQueen, T.P. (1985) Cobalt supplementation for beef cattle. In *Proceedings of Fifth International Symposium on Trace Element Metabolism in Man and Animals* (ed. by C.F. Mills, I. Bremner & J.K. Chesters), pp. 739–41. Commonwealth Agricultural Bureaux, Furnham Royal.

Rice, D.A. & Kennedy, S. (1988) Vitamin E: functions and effects of deficiency. *British Veterinary Journal*, **144**, 482–96.

Rice, D.A. & McMurray, C.H. (1982) Recent information on Vitamin E and selenium problems in ruminants. Roche Symposium Basle, Hoffman La Roche, pp. 1–19.

Rice, D.A., McLoughlin, M., Blanchflower, W.J., Goodall, E.A. & McMurray, C.H. (1987) Methylmalonic acid as an indicator of vitamin B_{12} deficiency in grazing sheep. *Veterinary Record*, **121**, 472–3.

Rice, D.A., O'Harte, F.P.M., Blanchflower, W.J. & Kennedy, D.G. (1989) Methylmalonic acid in the rumen of cobalt-deficient sheep and its effects on plasma methylmalonic acid. Proceedings of Nutrition Society, **48**, 141A.

Richards, R.B. & Edwards, J.R. (1986) A progressive spinal myelinopathy in beef cattle. *Veterinary Pathology*, **23**, 35–41.

Rogers, P.A.M. & Poole, D.B.R. (1988) Copper oxide needles for cattle: a comparison with parenteral treatment. *Veterinary Record*, **123**, 147–51.

Smart, M.E., Cohen, R., Christensen, D.A. & Williams, C.M. (1986) The effects of sulphate removal from the drinking water on liver copper and zinc concentrations of beef cows and their calves. *Canadian Journal of Animal Science*, **66**, 669–80.

Spears, J.W., Harvey, R.W. & Segerson, E.C. (1986) Effects of marginal selenium deficiency and winter protein supplementation on growth, reproduction and selenium status of beef cattle. *Journal of Animal Science*, **63**, 586–94.

Stowe, H.D., Thomas, J.W., Johnson, T., Martenuik, J.V., Morrow, D.A & Ullrey, D.E. (1988) Responses of dairy cattle to long-term and short-term supplementation with oral selenium and vitamin E. *Journal of Dairy Science*, **71**, 1830–9.

Suttle, N.F. (1978). Determining the copper requirements of cattle by means of an intravenous repletion technique. In *Proceedings of the 3rd International Symposium on Trace Element Metabolism in Man and Animals* (ed. by M. Kirchgessner), pp. 473–80. Arbeitskreis fur Tierenahrungforschung, Weihenstephan.

Suttle, N.F. (1981) Comparison between parenterally administered copper complexes of their ability to alleviate hypocupraemia in sheep and cattle. *Veterinary Record*, **109**, 304–7.

Suttle, N.F. (1983a) Effect of molybdenum concentration in fresh herbage, hay and semi-purified diets on the copper metabolism of sheep. *Journal of Agricultural Science, Cambridge*, **100**, 651–6.

Suttle, N.F. (1983b) Assessment of the mineral and trace element status of feeds. In *Proceedings of the Second Symposium of the International Network of Feed Information Centres* (ed. by G.E. Robards & R.G. Packham), p. 211. Commonwealth Agricultural Bureaux, Farnham Royal.

Suttle, N.F. (1988) The role of comparative pathology in the studies of copper and cobalt deficiencies in ruminants. *Journal of Comparative Pathology*, **99**, 242–57.

Suttle, N.F. & Angus, K.W. (1976) Effects of experimental copper deficiency on the skeleton of the calf. *Journal of Comparative Pathology*, **88**, 137–48.

Suttle, N.F., Knox, D., Angus, K.W. & Coop, R. (1989) Does dietary molybdenum enhance the inflammatory reaction to and rejection of gut nematodes in sheep? Proceedings of the Nutrition Society, **48**, 71A.

Trinder, N., Woodhouse, C.D. & Renton, C.P. (1969) The effect of vitamin E and selenium on the incidence of retained placentae in dairy cows. *Veterinary Record*, **83**, 550–3.

Trinder, N., Hall, R.J. & Renton, C.P. (1973) The relationship between the intake of selenium and vitamin E on the incidence of retained placentae in dairy cows. *Veterinary Record*, **93**, 641–4.

Underwood, E.J. (1966) *The Mineral Nutrition of Livestock*, pp. 147–61. Commonwealth Agricultural Bureaux.

Wang, Z.Y., Poole, D.B.R. & Mason, J. (1987) The uptake and intracellular distribution of ^{35}S-trithiomolybdate in bovine liver *in vivo*. *Journal of Inorganic Biochemistry*, **31**, 85–93.

Wang, Z.Y., Poole, D.B.R. & Mason, J. (1988) The effects of supplementation of the diet of young steers with Mo and S on the intracellular distribution of copper in liver and on copper fractions in blood. *British Veterinary Journal*, **114**, 543–51.

Watkinson, J.H. (1983). Prevention of selenium deficiency in grazing animals by annual top dressing of pasture with sodium selenate. *New Zealand Veterinary Journal*, **31**, 78–85.

Winter, W.J., Siebert, B.D. & Kuchel, R.E. (1977) Cobalt and copper therapy of cattle grazing improved pasture in northern Cape York peninsula. *Australian Journal of Experimental Agriculture and Animal Husbandry*, **17**, 10–15.

Wright, C.L., Taylor, C.N. & Greer, J.C. (1982) Estimation of serum vitamin B_{12}. *Veterinary Record*, **111**, 242.

ADULT CATTLE
Mastitis and Teat Conditions

Chapter 20: Anatomy, Physiology and Immunology of the Udder

by K.G. HIBBITT, N. CRAVEN AND E.H. BATTEN

Anatomy of the udder

Introduction

The mammary gland is essentially a skin gland. It is believed to have evolved by modification of a sweat gland and retains two common features: development by ingrowth of ectoderm; and a bilayered epithelium of inner secretory cells and outer myoepithelial cells, which by contracting promote flow of milk from the peripheral alveoli into the major ducts. Assuming the new function of catering for the immune welfare and nutrition of the neonate, the mammary gland has evolved into a highly branched compound structure with enormous numbers of dilated alveoli. This pattern allows for both synthesis and storage of milk on a large scale. Yet neither function is possible until the cow becomes pregnant, when the rudimentary and inactive gland undergoes massive growth to definitive structure and only then begins to synthesize secretion.

Early development of the udder

The first trace of mammary development appears in bovine embryos of 1.5 cm length as two short lines in the ectoderm running from the umbilicus caudally into the groin. Each line is several cells thick, but intense proliferation of cells in the basal layer at focal points produces an ingrowth, the mammary hillock (Fig. 20.1a). This soon enlarges into an ovoid mammary bud (Fig. 20.1b) invested by a condensation of inductive mesenchymal cells. As the rudiment of the duct system each mammary bud determines the site where a gland will form. By the seventh week of gestation in fetuses 9 cm long, four primary mammary buds are usually present, two on each side, defining the future quarters of the udder. Extra buds occasionally form and develop into supernumerary teats. Active proliferation of mesenchymal cells around the mammary bud lifts the epidermis into a rudimentary teat by the 8-cm stage. Simultaneously, vigorous proliferation of cells near the inner end changes the mammary bud into a solid cellular column, which elongates vertically into the mesenchyme (Fig. 20.1c) as the rudiment of the duct system, the future single galactophore. Meanwhile, division among the epidermal cells below the original bud produces an epidermal cone at the base of the duct primordium.

By the 19-cm stage the growing duct primordium is longer than the teat and slightly swollen at the inner end. Here a cavity or lumen appears and soon spreads proximally towards the teat apex. On reaching the epidermal cone the split remains narrow as the lumen of the future teat canal. Later this will open on the

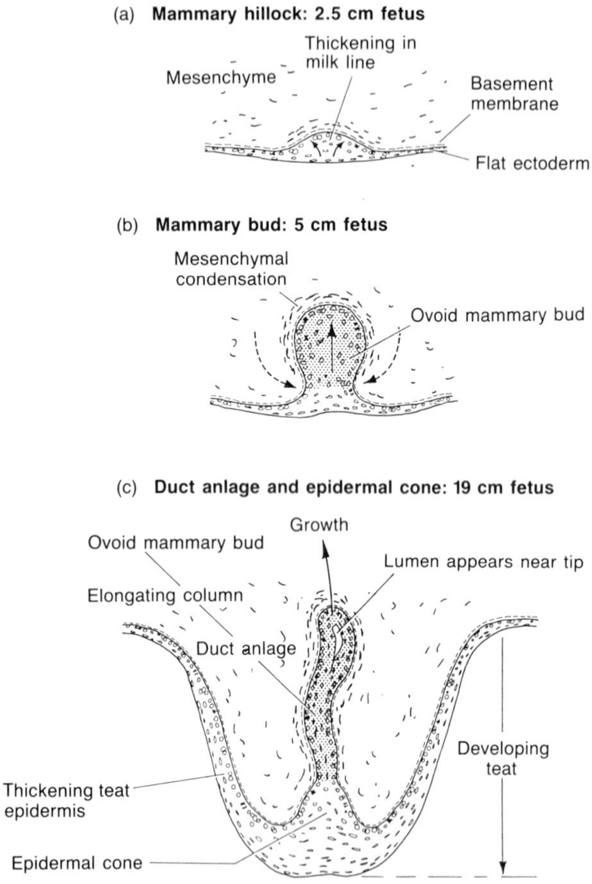

Fig. 20.1 (a) Transverse section of a mammary line at the level of a localized cellular proliferation, which forms a mammary hillock and determines where a gland will develop. (b) Later stage showing an ovoid mammary bud with cells more basophilic (stippled) than in the epidermis. A condensation of mesenchymal cells surrounds the bud. Curved broken arrows indicate growth of mesenchyme, which elevates a rudimentary teat. (c) Sustained proliferation (upper arrow) near the tip converts the mammary bud into a columnar vertical ingrowth, the precursor of the axial duct and storage sinuses. Meanwhile, division among the subjacent epidermal cells produces a cone, which later splits to form the lumen of the teat canal (From Turner, 1952).

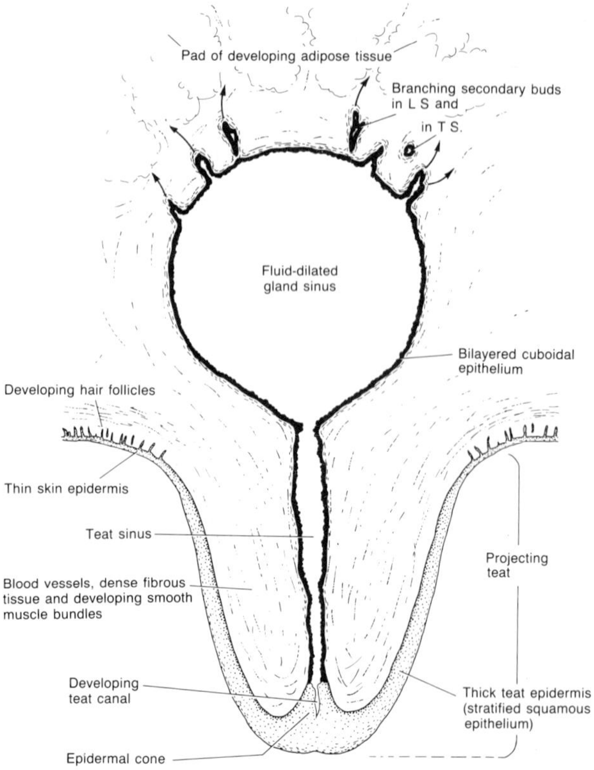

Fig. 20.2 Diagrammatic vertical section of the teat and mammary rudiment in a 35-cm fetus. Stratified epithelium is shown dotted. It appears distinctly thicker in the epidermal cone, where the teat canal lumen is forming, and over the surface of the teat rather than above it where hairy skin is differentiating. Derivatives of the original mammary bud are lined by double cuboidal epithelium (black) and comprise the narrow teat sinus leading from the fluid-distended gland sinus. Up to 10 short secondary buds project from the dome of the sinus and later will branch to form major ducts as they grow into the overlying cushion of fat. LS, longitudinal section; TS, transverse section (from Turner, 1952).

teat apex and both teat canal and superficial epidermis will be lined by a common, thick, stratified squamous, keratinizing epithelium.

By the 35-cm stage (Fig. 20.2) the growing duct rudiment has differentiated into three distinct regions.

1 An upper spheroid chamber distended with fluid represents the future gland sinus or milk reservoir.

2 A slightly longer mid-portion forms the more slender teat sinus.

3 A narrow teat canal within the epidermal cone, but still closed from the exterior by a plug of horny cells.

From the domed roof of the gland sinus several short solid epithelial cords, the secondary sprouts, project dorsally into the overlying pad of differentiating adipose tissue. When canalized these secondary sprouts represent the bases of the 10 or more major lactiferous ducts, which in the adult deliver milk into the gland sinus for storage. The teat sinus, gland sinus and duct bases are lined by a bilayered cuboidal epithelium. As also in the terminal alveoli, which differentiate later in pregnancy, the inner cells are potentially secretory, while the outer differentiate into myoepithelial elements. In contrast the lowest and narrowest part of the axial lumen, forming the teat canal, is lined by thick stratified squamous epithelium continuous with and identical to the glabrous epidermis of the teat. The latter is distinctly thicker, even in the fetus, than the epidermis above the teat where hair follicles differentiate from solid cellular ingrowths. The mesenchyme around and between the rudimentary epithelial ducts differentiates to provide blood vessels, lymphatics, small amounts of smooth muscle and an extensive fibroelastic stroma. Tracts of denser white fibrous and elastic tissue form the suspensory ligaments and dorsally numerous lobules form in the pad of adipose tissue.

Just before birth tertiary sprouts develop as short side branches from the secondary ducts, but thereafter the gland remains in an arrested state of development until puberty. Some extension to the ducts occurs during oestrous cycles, but full structural differentiation of the mammary gland is completed only during pregnancy under the influence of progesterone from the corpus luteum and other hormones. During the first half of pregnancy, intense cell proliferation at the blind ends elongates the ducts, which branch repeatedly establishing an extensive tree. At the peripheral tips of the large number of fine ducts thus formed narrow tubular prospective alveoli then differentiate. In the second half of pregnancy, protein secretion and lipid droplets slowly accumulate, dilating the alveoli into saccular chambers 120 μm across and filled with stored colostrum awaiting release in the first suckling after birth.

The adult bovine mammary gland

The cow's udder comprises four quarters, each an individual gland drained by a teat. The four secretory glands are structurally separate and function independently, without flow of milk between them. Receiving a large flow of blood and laden with stored milk, the lactating udder often weighs 50–60 kg. Support for this massive weight is provided by dense fibrous suspensory ligaments that insert into the pelvis and tendons of the abdominal wall. The ligaments spread laterally and ventrally over the udder, then coverge inwards to join paired median ligaments. These form a double vertical partition separating glands on the left from those on the right. Septa of interlobular connective tissue span between the lateral and medial ligaments and support the heavy lobules of parenchyma. As the medial ligaments contain relatively more elastin than the predominantly collagenous lateral ligaments the full udder drops in the midline and the teats become splayed outwards.

BLOOD SUPPLY

During the production of 20 kg of milk each day 9000 kg of blood circulate through the udder of the cow. Most of this rich supply arrives through the inguinal canal in the external pudendal arteries derived from the external iliac trunks. The udder also receives a subsidiary supply, cranially through the subcutaneous abdominal artery and caudally via the perineal artery. Numerous small veins leaving the parenchyma anastomose and converge around the base of the udder into a circular vessel that is drained by three trunks: the large subcutaneous abdominal vein, which passes cranially and penetrates the abdominal wall near the xiphoid cartilage; the external pudendal vein, which departs through the inguinal canal; and the perineal vein.

INNERVATION

The principal nerve supply derives from branches of the third and fourth lumbar nerves, which traverse the inguinal canal. Contributions from the first and second lumbar nerves supply the cranial, and from the perineal nerves the caudal regions respectively. These are mainly sensory nerves, but they carry from the caudal mesenteric plexus sympathetic fibres, which modulate blood flow by direct action on the arterioles. Whereas the skin and particularly the teats receive a rich sensory supply, nerves are sparser in the glandular parenchyma and chiefly, if not entirely, vasomotor: the secretory alveoli lack a nerve supply. After the skin is anaesthetized the deeper mammary tissue may be incised without apparent sensation.

MAMMARY GLAND: HISTOLOGICAL ORGANIZATION

Histologically classified, the lactating udder is a large, lobulated, compound exocrine gland with dilated alveoli storing milk. Each alveolus is a single or bifid sac, slightly longer than wide and distended to an internal diameter of 120–150 μm by milk (Fig. 20.3). The lining epithelium is bilayered. The inner secretory or alveolar cells vary from tall cuboidal (8 μm) in the partially empty gland to stretched squamous (3 μm) in full distension stated. Synthesis and release of milk constituents (fluid, casein, lactose and lipid) is continuous, until temporarily arrested by the distending pressure. The outer contractile myoepithelial cells are indistinct in routine sections, but staining for alkaline phosphatase reveals their spider shape, with branching processes embracing the curved contour of the alveolar wall (Fig. 20.4). Towards term and during lactation the large alveoli have a rich capillary supply and are packed closely together into polyhedral lobules about 2 mm across. The alveoli drain into intralobular ducts which,

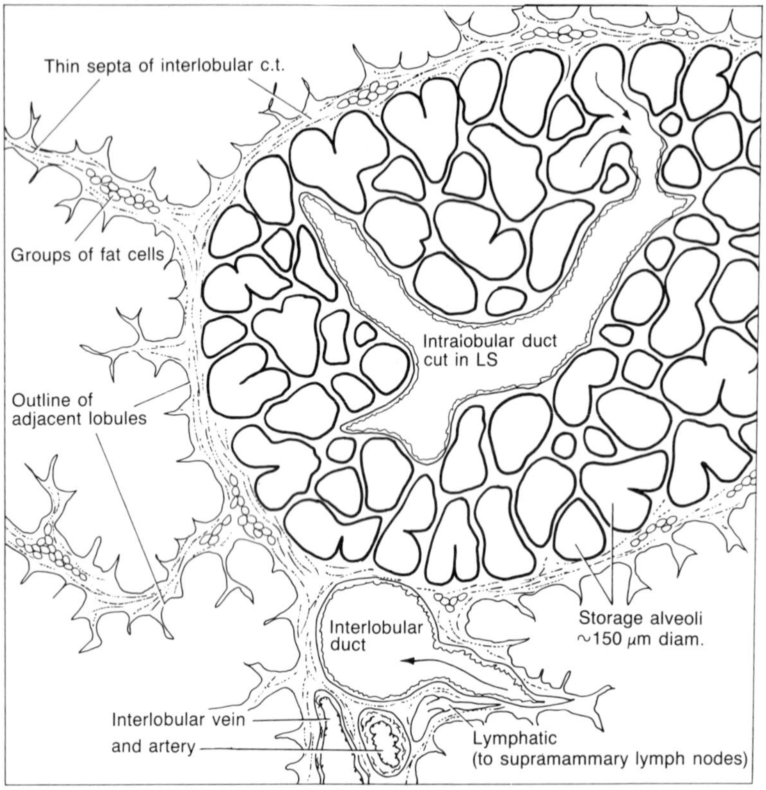

Fig. 20.3 Histological features of the lactating udder, showing large polyhedral lobules supported by thin septa of connective tissue carrying the distributing service vessels: interlobular ducts emerging (at lower right) from lobules, arteries supplying and veins draining the dense networks of perialveolar capillaries. Nearby collecting lymphatics carry a considerable flow of afferent lymph rich in lymphocytes, neutrophils and macrophages and during infections, e.g. mastitis, carrying antigens that induce immune responses in the supramammary lymph nodes.

In each lobule the alveoli tend to be similar in size, but are generally smaller, averaging 60 μm across, with a tall cobbled epithelium in lobules that released milk at the previous lactation. When fully distended with milk, as shown, alveoli approach 150 μm in diameter and have a thin stretched lining. Smaller profiles represent alveoli slices in oblique to tangential planes. Intralobular ducts drain milk from alveoli (curved arrows), but unless fortuitously sliced in longitudinal section are almost indistinguishable from the alveoli, being comparable in width and lined by identical secretory epithelium. c.t., connective tissue; LS, longitudinal section (diagram by E.H. Batten).

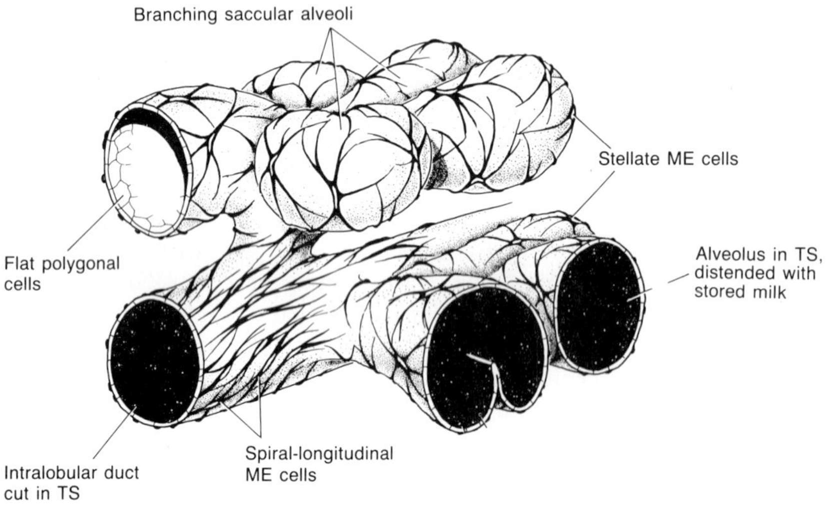

Fig. 20.4 Diagram showing several branching milk-distended alveoli of the lactating udder draining into a relatively wide intralobular duct. In the sectioned profiles fat droplets in the milk are shown white against a black background. Contraction of the network of stellate myoepithelial cells (cytoplasm black, nuclei white) expels milk from the alveoli into the intralobular ducts. In turn these become shortened and compressed by the contraction of the spirally aligned myoepithelial cells, which propel milk towards the larger interlobular ducts. ME, myoepithelial cells; TS, transverse section (after Linzell, 1961).

unlike those in salivary or lacrimal glands, are indistinct, since they resemble the alveoli in size, milk content and secretory lining. The heavy lobules are enclosed and bound together by thin septa of supportive connective tissue. This also carries distributing arteries and veins, lymphatics and the larger interlobular ducts, which converge and unite into major ducts opening into the gland cistern.

THE TEAT

Each teat has a single narrow teat canal, which dorsally opens into a wider teat cistern lined by bilayered epithelium. Normally, the teat canal is kept closed by sphincter action of the surrounding smooth muscle and elastic tissues. Thus in section the lumen is a narrow stellate crevice, with the lining of thick, keratinizing,

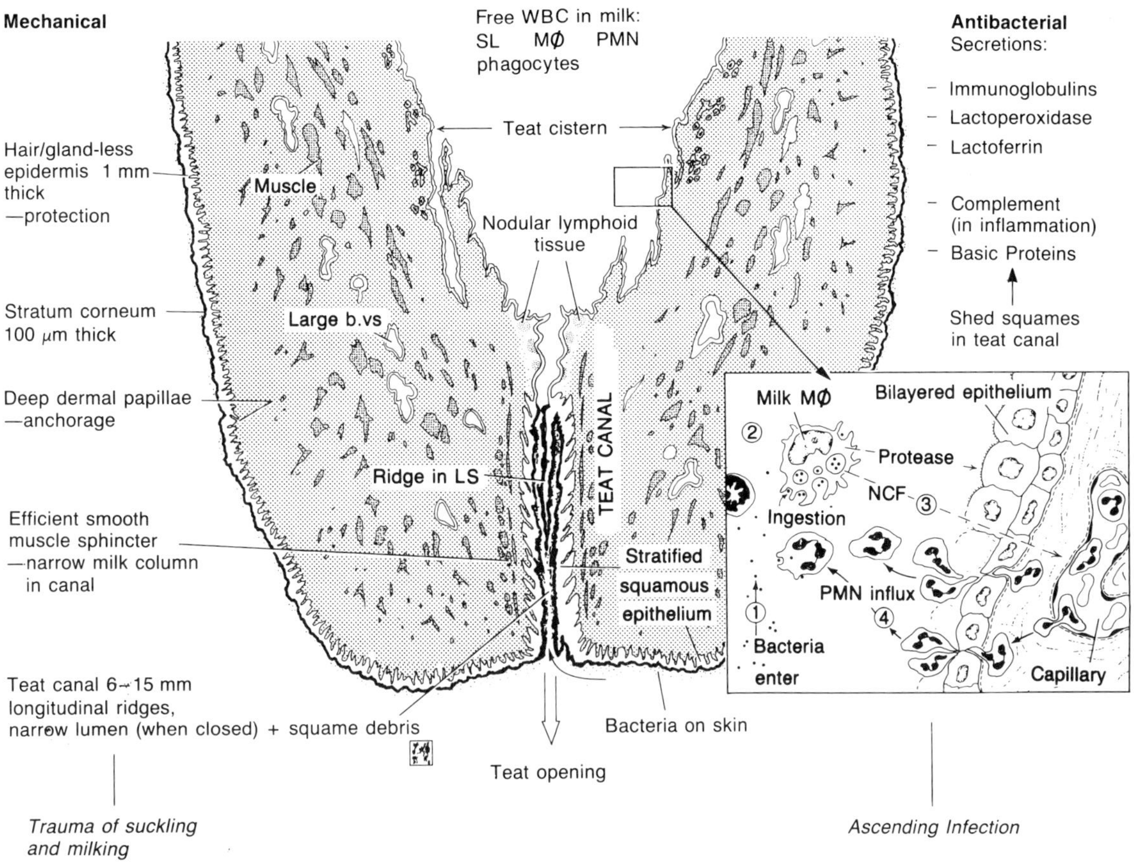

Fig. 20.5 Diagram of a vertical section of a cow's teat, showing on the left factors that protect against mechanical trauma during suckling or milking, and on the right defences against ascending infection by bacteria from the skin surface (curved arrow) entering the teat canal.
Milk normally contains shed epithelial cells, from both alveoli and ducts, squames from the teat canal, small lymphocytes (SL), macrophages (MØ) and neutrophils (PMN). As phagocytes the last two cell types often contain small droplets of fat ingested from the milk. Subepithelial plasma cells occur near the ring of nodular lymphoid tissue that surrounds the rosette or inner end of the teat canal, where the stratified, keratinizing lining gives way to a bilayered cuboidal epithelium of the teat cistern. Inset right summarizes the early response to mastitis-forming bacteria experimentally introduced into the teat canal. Bacteria (1) are ingested by milk macrophages (2), which release enzymes that damage and loosen the inner layer of the epithelium and neutrophil chemotactic factor (NCF), which induces (3) within 4 hours the emigration of large numbers of PMN from the subepithelial capillaries and venules. After insinuating through the cisternal epithelium the PMN (4) join with the macrophages in the ingestion and killing of bacteria. WBC, white blood cells; b.vs, blood vessels; LS, longitudinal section (diagram by E.H. Batten).

stratified squamous epithelium thrown into several longitudinal folds that almost meet centrally (Fig. 20.5). The teat is robustly constructed and well adapted to tolerate the shear stresses generated by a suckling calf or milking machine.

Structurally the teat wall comprises five distinct tissue layers: superficial epidermis, then dermis, intermediate layer, fibrous lamina propria and internally the epithelium of the teat canal. The teat is covered by thick, stratified squamous, keratinizing epidermis with neither hair follicles nor sweat and sebaceous glands. Whereas the thinner skin over the udder is relatively loosely attached and can freely be moved over the underlying glandular lobules, the teat skin is immobile and tightly anchored to the deeper fibromuscular core. This firm surface is well suited to withstand mechanical shear forces set up by suckling, hand or machine milking. In the lactating cow the teat epidermis is remarkable for three features.

1 In thickness about 1 mm, it is comparable with muzzle epidermis and some 12 times deeper than epidermis of hair skin (75 μm in frozen sections, which preserve the 30 layers of horny squames only 1 μm thick).

2 The protective stratum corneum is a compact layer, 100 μm deep and comprising as many overlapping layers of dead horny squames.

3 The underside is deeply papillated: epidermal

pegs interdigitate with narrow, deep intrusions of dermal connective tissue.

Over this interface the area of adhesive basement membrane is fivefold greater than in the flat underside of hairy epidermis. This interlocking pattern binds epidermis securely and inseparably into the dermis and dissipates shear stresses from the surface through the deeper tissues. The dermal fibrous mat continues into the dense fibromuscular layer, without the intervening loose superficial fascia typical of thin skin.

Beneath the epidermis the dermis carries a rich capillary network and numerous fine bundles of sensory fibres derived from lumbar nerves 2–4. Despite its thickness as a protection against wear, teat epidermis is highly sensitive, since the penetrating dermal papillae carry sensory nerves and endings to within 200 μm or less of the surface. This rich innervation receives tactile stimuli and relays to the central nervous system impulses that lead to the release of oxytocin from the pars nervosa into the blood. In turn, circulating oxytocin induces contraction of myoepithelial cells, promoting flow from the terminal alveoli and along the ducts during milk let-down. The deeper regions of the dermis contain dense collagenous tissue surrounding bundles of smooth muscle arranged mainly longitudinally.

The third or intermediate layer contributes much of the strength of the teat wall, as it contains numerous bundles of smooth muscle set in coarse fibroelastic tissue. These muscle bundles are aligned in longitudinal, circular and oblique planes. Major blood vessels are present, including distributing arteries, a complex plexus of anastomosing veins and numerous collecting lymphatics, which drain to the supramammary nodes.

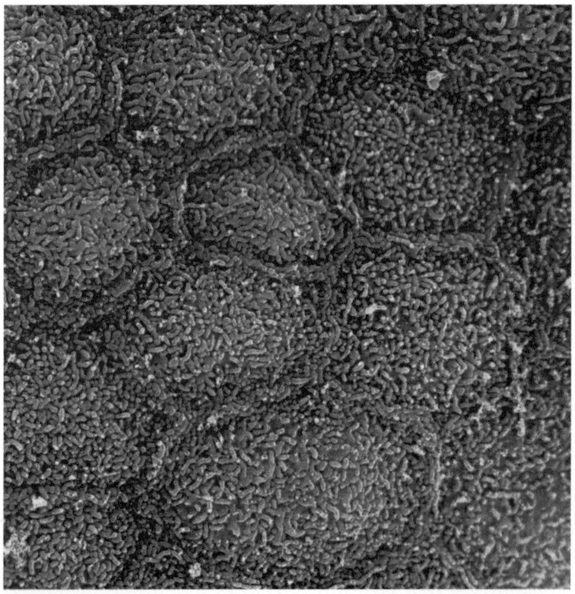

Fig. 20.6 Characteristic outline of teat epithelial cells covered with irregular microvilli (× 9000). From Collins *et al.* (1986).

The lamina propria resembles the dermis in its fibroelastic components, but carries more microvessels catering for the nutrition of the adjoining epithelium of the teat canal. During ascending infections with pathogenic bacteria, increased emigration from the local venules creates leucocytic infiltrations beneath regions where epithelial cells have been damaged, as explained in Fig. 20.5.

Both the teat cistern and the gland cistern dorsal to it are lined by a common bilayered cuboidal epithelium. Under scanning electron microscopy the superficial cells fit closely in hexagonal profiles densely covered with microvilli (Fig. 20.6). In the junctional region around the inner opening of the teat canal (earlier termed Furstenberg's rosette from the mucosal creases) the surface cells are more rounded and protruding, with sparser microvilli. In this region just beyond the barrier epithelium of the teat canal the lining may be a lymphoepithelium important in the uptake or penetration of invading antigens. Intraepithelial lymphocytes are profuse and both diffuse and nodular lymphoid tissue are present in the lamina propria. The accumulations of plasma cells and germinal centres (Fig. 20.7) often present there provide evidence of local humoral immune responses.

The physiology of lactation

Introduction

The secretion of milk by specialized mammary glands in the female for the nourishment of the newborn is the essential characteristic that distinguishes mammals from other animals. This feature is epitomized in the dairy cow which, as a result of intensive selection, has a disproportionately high output of energy in milk in relation to body size. Continuing improvements in milk yield and feed efficiency are the result of refinement of the genetic make-up of stock and improvements in management and nutritional practices. This focusing of effort on increasing milk production has prompted the facetious comment that the modern dairy cow should perhaps be regarded as an appendage of the udder rather than vice versa! Indeed, the readjustment of physiological processes that occurs in order to meet the extra metabolic demands of lactation involves not just differentiation and activation of mammary tissue but extends to changes throughout the body. Not the least

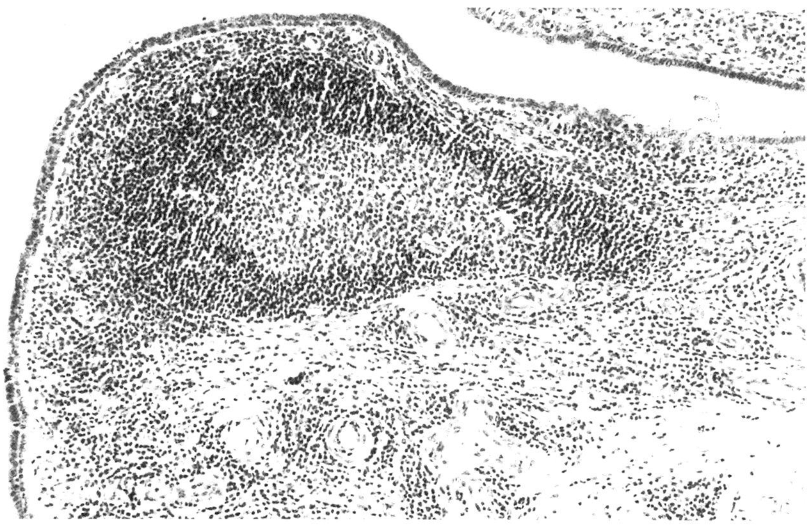

Fig. 20.7 A lymphoid nodule with germinal centre beneath the double cuboidal epithelium living Furstenberg's rosette (HE × 32). From Collins *et al.*, 1986.

of these is the hormonal regulation of nutrient utilization and partitioning between the mammary gland and other organs.

Milk is a complex secretion and its production is under complex control. By understanding the underlying physiology, the relevance of correct nutritional and husbandry practices in maintaining health and optimizing performance may be better appreciated.

Mammogenesis

Mammogenesis may be defined as the growth and differentiation of the mammary gland to the stage prior to active secretion. Since milk yield is ultimately dependent on the number of secretory cells and their activity, factors that influence the former during mammogenesis can have lasting implications for subsequent milk production.

From birth to puberty mammary growth is isometric, i.e. in balance with the growth rate of the whole body, but just prior to the onset of ovarian activity mammary growth becomes allometric (i.e. exceeds that of the body surface). Only during the first pregnancy does marked branching of the duct system and lobulo-alveolar development occur, with expanding parenchyma displacing adipose tissue within the mammary fat pad. Lobulo-alveolar proliferation accelerates as pregnancy advances with division of secretory cells continuing at least until the onset of lactation. Balanced mammary development exhibits a crucial dependence on hormonal stimulation. The hormones principally implicated include steroids (oestrogens, progesterone and adrenal corticoids) and protein hormones (prolactin, somatotrophin and placental lactogen). Thyroid hormones are possibly also involved. Many of these hormones interact synergistically to promote the different stages of mammogenesis. Oestrogens and somatotrophin are responsible for ductal development whereas progesterone and prolactin appear to regulate lobulo-alveolar proliferation. The additional presence of adrenal corticoids maximizes this growth. Placental lactogen may, in some species, also stimulate alveolar formation but in the cow relatively little enters the maternal circulation.

During the period of allometric growth just prior to puberty the administration of exogenous somatotrophin to heifers appears to promote an increase in mammary parenchyma. It is known that excess energy consumption during the period of allometric growth in heifers offered a high plane of nutrition results in lower mammary secretory tissue weight and is also associated with low milk production during subsequent lactation. It has been suggested that these effects of overfeeding during this critical phase of mammary development may in fact be caused by a decrease in endogenous levels of somatotrophin, as has been observed during high plane feeding. Thus the interplay between nutritional management and hormonal balance during mammogenesis may have important consequences for subsequent production.

Mammary development is partly reversed during advancing lactation when gradual involution occurs. These effects become more pronounced during the dry period. A period of non-lactation between successive lactations is an essential prerequisite for maximal milk production. Milk yields in the next lactation are definitely impaired if cows are dry for less than six weeks.

On the other hand there is little or no advantage to be gained in terms of an increase in subsequent lactation yield by extending the dry period to more than eight weeks.

Lactogenesis

The initiation of milk secretion (lactogenesis) in all mammals is closely coordinated with parturition. Parturition itself involves a complex interplay of endocrine controls with marked differences between species. There are two general concepts as to what constitutes the main lactogenic trigger, the positive stimulus of lactation-promoting hormones and the release from the inhibitory effects of progesterone. A peak in blood prolactin levels coincides with, but is not essential for, parturition. Suppression of prolactin release in cows inhibits the final stages of secretory cell differentiation and results in reduced milk yield. Thus elevation of prolactin (together with adequate amounts of adrenal corticoids) and the permissive effect of progesterone withdrawal, appear to provide the main lactogenic stimulus in the cow. An additional feature may be the removal near term of a locally produced inhibitory factor (possibly prostaglandin $F_{2\alpha}$).

Lactogenesis requires the preferential supply and uptake of nutrients by mammary tissue. Nutrient availability is enhanced by the disconnection of the fetal supply at parturition and increases in mammary blood flow and local selective nutrient uptake become evident.

Milk synthesis and secretion

The constituents of milk are synthesized mainly from small molecules absorbed from the blood, specific carrier systems probably assisting their entry into secretory cells. The blood supply provides not only precursors for milk synthesis but also adequate energy-yielding substrates to drive the synthetic processes.

Lactose (milk sugar) is a disaccharide composed of one molecule of glucose and one of galactose. In bovine milk its concentration, at about 4.8 per cent, is the most consistent of any constituent due largely to its influence in maintaining the osmolality of milk. Blood glucose is the main precursor of lactose but small amounts may also be formed from amino acids, glycerol and acetate. The final enzyme-catalysed step in lactose synthesis from glucose involves an enzyme, 'lactose synthetase', which is unique to mammary tissue. This is composed of two protein components and the availability of the second component, α-lactalbumin (a milk protein), determines the rate of synthesis of lactose, which occurs in the Golgi membranes of secretory cells.

Milk protein synthesis involves the assembly of different amino acids in a specific order along a chain. It takes place in the ribosomes of the rough endoplasmic reticulm (RER in fig. 20.8) of secretory cells, proteins destined for secretion being released into the lumina of the endoplasmic reticulum. Total amino acid nitrogen uptake by mammary tissue entirely accounts for the output of nitrogen in milk protein. However, the proportions of different amino acids absorbed by the glands are at variance with their appearance in milk protein, indicating that some are metabolized while others are synthesized by mammary tissue. The majority of milk proteins are synthesized locally and are unique to milk (e.g. caseins). However, certain blood proteins and similar proteins synthesized by plasma cells adjacent to secretory epithelia are also transferred into lacteal secretions — in large amounts in colostrum (*see below*).

The fat content of bovine milk varies widely between and within breeds and is influenced by diet and environmental factors. The majority of milk fat is in the form of triglycerides, which are assembled in or near the endoplasmic reticulum of secretory cells using fatty acids and glycerol synthesized in the cytosol. Approximately half of the fatty acids in milk are derived directly from the blood — chiefly those greater than 14 carbons in length. *De novo* synthesis of fatty acids utilizes volatile fatty acids arising from rumen fermentation, fatty acid synthesis from glucose being negligible in ruminants. Acetate and β-hydroxybutyrate are important precursors and contribute mainly to the synthesis of shorter-chain fatty acids. The glycerol required for milk triglycerides is partly derived from hydrolysis of blood lipids and partly by synthesis from glucose. Esterification of fatty acids with glycerol is followed by aggregation of triglycerides to form the characteristic fat droplets of secretory cells.

The mechanisms for cellular release of secretion differ for the various components of milk. Instead of combining into a large exocrine granule typical of zymogenic and serous cells, milk protein remains separate as multiple small granules. These are visible only ultrastructurally and present a large surface area, which facilitates rapid digestion. Non-immune protein, such as casein, is delivered from the rough endoplasmic reticulum to the Golgi complex, where through the agency of lactose synthetase, lactose is added. This causes the vesicles leaving the Golgi to swell osmotically. As they rise through the supranuclear cytoplasm the vesicles become tightly clustered around the sides of the lipid droplets, which lie free in the cytoplasm and may be up to 5 μm in diameter. Subsequently, membranes of the more superficial vesicles fuse with the apical plasmalemma and their content of protein, lactose, calcium and fluid is emptied into the alveolar lumen by conventional exocytosis. As the vesicles successively discharge, their inner walls remain over the surface of the protruding lipid as the milk fat droplet membrane. Ultimately undercut by the fusion of membranes between the lowest vesicles, the milk fat droplet is liberated into the lumen without damage to the cell and in a manner reminiscent of the shedding from an erythroblast of a pyknotic nucleus of comparable size.

The process of milk fat release is best termed microapocrine, since it does involve some loss of cell components — the membrane investing the lipid and beneath it usually a thin veil of cytoplasm, as illustrated in Fig. 20.8. About 5 per cent of droplets are signet-shaped, with a crescentic fragment of cytoplasm containing a few mitochondria or short profiles of rough ER. Immune proteins, such as various immunoglobulins arriving via the blood or derived from local plasma cells, are taken into the cell base by receptor-mediated endocytosis into coated vesicles, translocated through the cytoplasm and released at the apical membrane.

Mature milk is characterized by a high concentration of potassium and a relatively low sodium concentration similar to the situation within the secretory cells. Milk is 8 per cent water. The amount of water (and hence milk volume) is determined largely by the rate of lactose secretion since lactose is not reabsorbed across epithelial cell membranes and it exerts an important osmotic 'draw' within the milk duct system.

Milk ejection

In the interval between milkings, milk continues to be synthesized and secreted at a more or less constant rate into the alveolar lumina and thence to the large collecting ducts and sinuses. The resistance of the teat sphincter retains the milk in the sinuses but much of

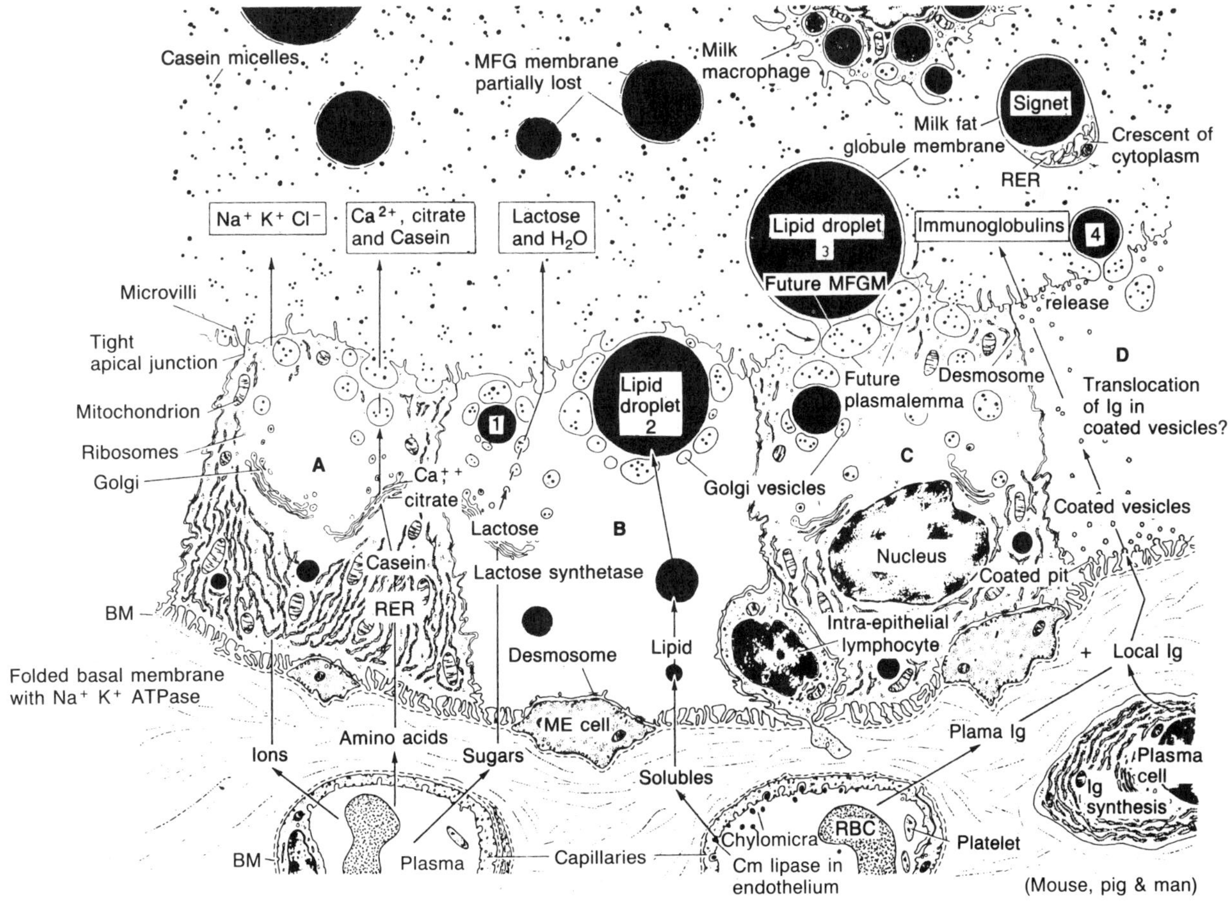

Fig. 20.8 Mammary alveolus secretory pathways. RBC, red blood cell; Ig, immunoglobulin; RER, rough endoplasmic reticulum; BM, basement membrane (diagram by E.H. Batten).

the milk remains within alveoli and will not flow out passively even when the teat sphincter is patent. Forcible expulsion is, therefore, required to remove this alveolar milk from the gland. Milk ejection is under neuroendocrine control.

The milk ejection reflex involves stimulation of nerve receptors in the skin of the teat. Mechanical stimulation triggers an impulse in afferent mammary nerves. This impulse is transmitted via the spinal cord and ultimately arrives in the posterior hypothalamus. Specialized neurones in this region synthesize oxytocin (a peptide hormone) and a carrier protein. In addition to receiving the afferent excitatory stimulus originating from the teat, the neurones also receive facilitatory and inhibitory impulses that arise in other parts of the brain. If the net result of these impulses is stimulatory, neurosecretory granules are released into blood capillaries from axons that terminate in the posterior pituitary. Thus following mechanical stimulation of the teats of cows, oxytocin increases rapidly in the blood, reaching a peak within 2 minutes.

In mammary tissue, contractile myoepithelial cells form a basketwork surrounding the alveoli. Oxytocin in mammary blood binds with high affinity to receptor sites on myoepithelial cells (Fig. 20.4), resulting in contraction of the cells and expulsion of the milk from the alveoli.

Although sucking and milking are the most potent and natural stimuli to elicit the milk ejection reflex, udder washing and even visual and auditory cues associated with milking routines can substitute, as the reflex becomes conditioned by experience. Stressful stimuli which involve the release of catecholamines and activity of the sympathetic nervous system can have negative influences on oxytocin release, mammary blood flow and oxytocin binding to myoepithelial cells, thereby inhibiting milk ejection. Myoepithelial cells also contract to an extent in response to direct mechanical stimuli, independently of oxytocin release. Palpation of the udder (or butting by calves) may trigger this local so-called 'tap reflex'.

Galactopoiesis

Frequent milk let-down and its removal from alveolar lumina assists in the maintenance of milk production (galactopoiesis) by preventing 'end product inhibition'. Nevertheless, the continued secretion of milk also depends on a continued hormonal drive, which induces and maintains the synthetic enzyme complement of secretory cells and also ensures an adequate supply of substrates. The chief hormones implicated in the maintenance of lactation are different from those responsible for lactogenesis.

The essential role of the pituitary gland in the maintenance of lactation in all mammals has long been recognized. The roles of the various pituitary hormones have been revealed by studies on hypophysectomized animals with hormonal supplementation or by the use of specific antagonists. In most species (i.e. rabbits, pigs, dogs, humans) prolactin has been identified as the key galactopoietic hormone and suppression of prolactin secretion by bromocriptine has a rapid effect in inhibiting milk secretion. In ruminants, however, suppression of prolactin secretion has only a partial (sheep) or no inhibitory effect (cows, goats) on lactation. In these species, somatotrophin (pituitary growth hormone) provides the main galactopoietic stimulus. The dose-dependent stimulation of milk yield in dairy cows that follows administration of somatotrophin has been known for many years. With the advent of recombinant DNA technology, commercial exploitation of this effect is now practicable and our knowledge of the role of somatotrophin has increased as a result of the considerable recent research on this topic.

The release of somatotrophin into circulation from the anterior pituitary is under the influence of various hypothalamic peptides that arrive in the hypophyseal portal blood supply; these include a specific somatotrophin releasing hormone and an inhibitory peptide, somatostatin. Thyroid hormone releasing hormone also enhances somatotrophin release and synergizes with the action of the specific releasing hormone. A direct effect of increased levels of somatotrophin is the induction in the liver and other organs of the synthesis of other peptides known as somatomedins or insulin-like growth factors (IGFs). IGFs in turn appear responsible for mediating many of the effects attributed to somatotrophin (Fig. 20.9).

It seems likely that somatotrophin does not exert its galactopoietic effect by direct stimulation of the udder. Rather it acts by partitioning available energy away from body tissues and towards milk production but the increased yield is not merely a passive response to an increased nutrient supply. There is also an increased synthetic activity per secretory cell. Administration of somatotrophin also elevates cardiac output and mammary blood flow. It is considered that this increase in blood flow is, at least in part, a consequence rather than a cause of the increased activity of mammary tissue.

The metabolic effects of administering supplementary somatotrophin to dairy cows are well documented. In early short-term studies, acute responses of hyper-

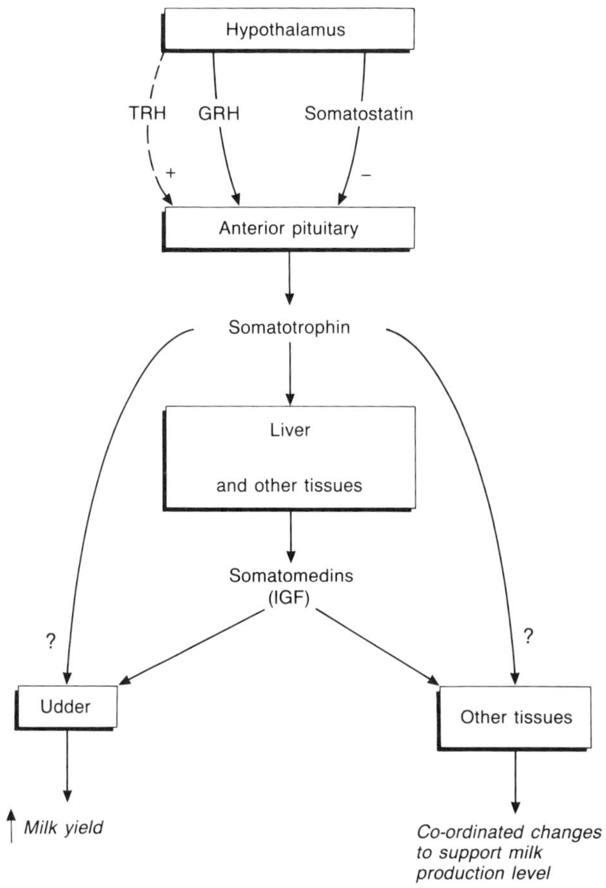

Fig. 20.9 Regulation of somatotrophin release and its effects on milk production. TRH, thyroid hormone releasing hormone; GRH, growth hormone releasing hormone.

glycaemia ('diabetogenesis') and elevation of circulating free fatty acids ('lipolysis') were reported. In contrast, there is now substantial evidence from studies where somatotrophin has been administered for long periods which indicates that the significant increases in milk yield are perfectly balanced by increased voluntary feed intakes and alterations in metabolism of body tissues such that steady-state concentrations of blood metabolites are maintained. These coordinated changes are consistent with the role of somatotrophin as a homeorhetic control, allowing a substantial shift in the partitioning of nutrients to the mammary gland.

The key role of somatotrophin in milk production is underscored by the evidence that cows selected for high genetic merit for yield show higher endogenous levels (basal and after stimulation) of somatotrophin than low yielders. Furthermore, somatotrophin levels decline with advancing lactation in line with milk production. Somatotrophin levels are also influenced by nutritional status independently of these genetic effects. Underfed cows have generally higher somatotrophin levels than those that are well fed, although this may be offset by a lower somatotrophin responsiveness of the underfed animals.

Other hormones with a suggested role in galactopoiesis include adrenal corticoids and thyroid hormones. In most species adrenal corticoids are essential for lactation but there is little evidence that plasma levels are a limiting factor. Thyroxine and tri-iodothyronine may have a stimulatory effect on milk yield via effects on metabolic rate.

Immediate increases in milk yield can be obtained by commencing three times a day milking, which indicates that the secretory capacity of mammary cells can be increased. Frequency of milking does not appear to affect endogenous somatotrophin levels. The mechanisms are not fully understood but may involve the removal of inhibitors.

Manipulation of lactation

The continuing steady increase in annual average milk yields of dairy cows is the result of judicious genetic selection and improvements in management, especially nutritional management. Experts expect these trends to continue for some years to come. However, a growing understanding of the physiological processes of lactation, together with advances in biotechnology, now make possible a variety of new ways to control and manipulate lactation.

Administration of somatotrophin to prepubertal heifers has been shown to increase mammary parenchyma but whether this translates into increased milk yields is not yet clear. Nevertheless, optimal nutritional management during this period is clearly of practical relevance in influencing mammogenesis and subsequent yield.

The hormonal manipulation of galactopoiesis has considerable commercial potential, both in a free market for milk products and for efficient quota management under a milk quota system. Biotechnology-derived somatotrophin in prolonged-release formulations are already available for commercial use in some countries (see p. 863). Endogenous somatotrophin production may also be enhanced by administering releasing factors or by immunization of animals against their natural inhibitory peptide, somatostatin. Research into such approaches is under way.

Developments in direct genetic transfers between mammalian cells make possible the insertion of extra somatotrophin genes which, if expressed, will enable cows to produce high endogenous levels of somatotrophin. The genes might be triggered by an external stimulus such as a dietary factor. Such transgenic 'super cows' could be propagated rapidly using modern reproductive techniques. Transgenic techniques might also be employed to modify the characteristics of the milk constituents produced.

There are also opportunities for optimizing milking procedures to exploit physiological controls of lactation more fully. Further automation of the milking process culminating in robotic milking may permit milking several times a day and, with some sophistication, optimal prestimulation, stripping and individual quarter milking.

Immunology of the udder and teat

Immunity in the mammary gland may be divided into two systems (see Chapter 27). Firstly, a non-specific system that offers a first line of defence when a pathogen invades, and frequently is able to resist the invasion of a number of potentially infectious agents. Secondly, if the nonspecific system fails, the tissues of the mammary gland can adapt and produce a specific defence against each infectious agent. Frequently this system, once developed, remembers the invading pathogen, which can be resisted by the specific defence system on a later occasion.

Non-specific immunity

Most infections of the mammary gland of the dairy cow enter through the teat canal so the teat provides a very important barrier to infection particularly since its exterior surface is frequently exposed to a most contaminated environment. The defences of the mammary gland may be considered under several headings.

The teat canal as a mechanical barrier

The length of the teat canal has no effect on the susceptibility of cows to mastitis but it has been reported in the literature that teat ducts from quarters susceptible to infection had a larger diameter than those from resistant quarters. Differences in teat duct patency might be expected to correlate positively with ease of milking but a relationship between milking characteristics and the incidence of intramammary infection is not universally accepted. Teat ducts with a temporary patency, such that a continuous unbroken column of milk is maintained for some time after milking, may offer a means of entry for micro-organisms and a way in which they may be transported upwards through the duct. In capillary columns of milk at 37 °C, micro-organisms are capable of rising rapidly in association with ascending milk fat globules. Any mechanism, therefore, that is likely to break the fat-rich milk column and prevent an upward passage of bacteria is likely to increase the mammary gland defences. Various suggestions have been made on how the teat duct closes, e.g. it may close in a spiral fashion 'wringing out' the last drops of milk, but as the streak canal has ridges arranged longitudinally a spiral wringing would not be effective. Teat canal keratin is a white wax-like material derived from the surface cells of the stratified squamous epithelium and which forms a network in the lumen of the canal, thereby trapping invading bacteria and disrupting the milk column. Another simple mechanical method of preventing organisms from penetrating the teat canal is the flushing action during milking. Organisms not adhering to the teat canal wall or the keratin mesh at the beginning of milking are soon flushed out. The higher infection rate of quarters at drying off has been attributed to the cessation of milking and the consequent failure to flush out pathogens. Later in the dry period, there is an increase in the antimicrobial properties of the canal, which may restrict bacterial multiplication.

Antimicrobial substances within the teat canal

Antimicrobial substances in the teat canal may contribute to the defence of the mammary gland. The antimicrobial role of esterified and non-esterified fatty acids, particularly myristic acid, palmitoleic acid and linoleic acid has been described. These fatty acids are present in the teat canal keratin and it was suggested that the unsaturated fatty acids were the most inhibitory.

Some proteins isolated from the teat canal also play an important role in the defence of the mammary gland. At physiological pH they carry a positive charge and bind electrostatically to the mastitis pathogens which, at the same pH, carry a negative charge. The inhibiting effect of the various concentrations of these proteins has been demonstrated *in vitro* on the growth of staphylococci and streptococci. This antimicrobial activity of these proteins was not seen when micro-organisms were incubated with whole keratin under *in vitro* conditions. The cationic protein under these conditions would have already bound to other negatively charged molecules in the keratin. In the living animal continuous synthesis of these cationic proteins would overcome such binding. Despite the antimicrobial environment within the teat canal, local colonization by Gram-positive cocci has been reported, but the growth is very feeble with a low percentage viability.

Antimicrobial substances in mammary secretions

Non-specific antimicrobial substances in mammary secretions also contribute to the defences of the mammary gland. Lactoferrin is an iron-chelating protein which, in the presence of bicarbonate, inhibits the growth of micro-organisms having a high iron requirement. The activity of this protein is inhibited by the presence of citrate. Lactoferrin is thought to exert its most protective effects in the mammary secretions during the dry period when its levels are high compared with those in full lactation. These higher concentrations of lactoferrin may also influence the defences of the dry gland through the modulation of leucocyte functions.

Another anti-bacterial system present in milk involves the enzyme lactoperoxidase. This enzyme, in the presence of thiocyanate and hydrogen peroxide, can produce a short-lived highly oxidative system that is bacteriostatic for Gram-positive and bacteriocidal for Gram-negative organisms. Thiocyanate is present in milk, particularly in animals fed on diets containing legumes or brassicas. Doubt has been expressed in the past over the source of hydrogen peroxide (H_2O_2). Phagocytosing neutrophils are likely to be one source of H_2O_2 and some can be produced by the metabolism of catalase-negative organisms such as streptococci. Another enzyme present in milk, xanthine oxidase, may also contribute by generating H_2O_2. Recent research has demonstrated that xanthine oxidase is present in the teat duct and secretory tissue of the bovine mammary gland. The action of xanthine oxidase on its substrate leads to a release of hydrogen peroxide, which is then available to the lactoperoxidase system.

In addition to the above, antimicrobial systems that operate locally within the teat canal are likely also to be operative in the milk itself and in deeper parts of the mammary gland. The role of lysozyme in bovine body fluids, including milk, is equivocal. Some authors doubt its existence and, if present, the concentration would be extremely low, but possibly increasing in mastitis. As yet no defensive role has been ascribed to lysozyme in bovine tissues.

Antimicrobial cationic proteins, as found in the teat canal, may also be present in milk during mild inflammation. These proteins possess similar properties to the cationic proteins in the milk cells and are thought to have left the cells by a process of reverse pinocytosis.

Earlier methods used by many workers attempting to demonstrate haemolytic complement were too insensitive, but more recently a sensitive microassay revealed that low levels of haemolytic complement are present in milk throughout lactation, albeit usually masked by the anticomplement activity of the milk. Complement levels are highest in colostrum, in inflamed glands and in late lactation. A high correlation between the levels of serum albumin and the third component of complement during an inflammatory response suggests that complement components are passively transferred into the milk but this relationship is not seen in normal milk. Although the defensive role of the classical complement pathway remains in doubt it has been established that complement-sensitive organisms, such as some strains of *Escherichia coli*, are killed by the alternative complement pathway. *In vitro* tests, however, do not support this since serum-sensitive strains of *E. coli* can be grown in milk drawn from the udder. It is possible, however, that *in vivo* a very mild inflammatory response is needed to elevate slightly the serum-derived complement in milk.

Specific immunity: lymphocytes

Lymphocytes are present in cows' milk at all stages of lactation and constitute 1–2 per cent of the milk cell population, which is low compared with that of human milk. Lymphocytes consist of T and B cells together with a population of lymphoid cells, which do not consistently carry markers of either T or B cells, the so-called null cells. The ratio of these cells (T : B : null) is similar to that in peripheral blood, but the percentage of B cells is slightly increased in dry gland secretions. Lymphocytes in mammary secretions are functionally competent, responding to mitogens and antigens. However, some responses of the T cells from mammary secretions to mitogens are lower than those of T cells from the systemic circulation. The precise reason for this difference in responsiveness is not clear, although it is known that mammary secretions contain soluble immunosuppressive factors that may be responsible. In addition, the T cell population in the mammary secretion may contain a greater proportion of suppressor cells which would inhibit responses.

Differences in the functional activity of T lymphocytes in blood and those in mammary secretions are evident as differing responses to specific antigens. Much of this work has been carried out using human mammary secretions and supports the view that lymphocytes in the mammary secretion form a distinct subpopulation. They belong to a mucosal immune system in which lymphocytes migrate from secretory surfaces of the body, e.g. the gut, to the mammary gland, but this is not the case in ruminants.

A similar migration occurs with B cells, but in the cow it has been suggested that following intestinal immunization there is a migration of antigen-stimulated IgG lymphoblasts and perhaps of antigen to the spleen and peripheral lymph nodes. This would be consistent with the appearance of serum-derived IgG antibodies in the colostrum and milk. When antigen is infused directly into the udder all classes of antibody, but particularly IgA and IgG_1, are produced locally from antibody-forming cells in the glandular stroma and in the regional supramammary lymph nodes.

Tissues in the terminal inner portion of the teat contain a high proportion of plasma cells, lymphocytes and macrophages, which may be involved in local immunity, and antibody-containing cells have been demonstrated in germinal centres in the distal Furstenberg's rosette of the teat cistern (Fig. 20.7). Of the plasma cells in this region 88 per cent synthesize IgG_1, 10 per cent IgM while only a few synthesize IgA. The distribution of these cells does not change in relation to the mammary secretory activity.

Although the homing of lymphocytes to the mammary gland appears to be well established in some species, not all migrate into the secretions; in the rat mammary gland some remain in the alveolar and ductal epithelium. These intraepithelial lymphocytes are likely to be the predominating cell types infiltrating bovine mammary tissues and remain in association with the epithelia after a *Staphylococcus aureus* infection. Information from other species may reveal the precise identity and function of these cells. In man a substantial proportion are T cells. Intraepithelial lymphocytes may form an important defence against infection at mucosal surfaces. Currently, there is a paucity of information on the role or even existence of NK and K cells in the bovine mammary gland; nevertheless, there is some evidence to suggest that lymphocyte activity in bovine mammary tissues may differ from that of other species.

Immunoglobulins in mammary secretions (see p. 336)

Milk contains most immunoglobulin classes in differing amounts that vary during lactation. IgG_1 is present in the largest concentrations and it passes from the blood to the milk by a process of selective transfer. During inflammation of the udder, IgG_2 and other proteins are transferred from the blood. Some immunoglobulins such as IgM and IgA are locally produced and they arise from cells of the lymphoblast–plasma cell series that are located close to glandular epithelium in various parts of the mammary gland. The distribution of immunoglobulin classes in blood, colostrum and milk is shown in Table 20.1.

Table 20.1 Immunoglobulin (mg/100 ml) in the blood and mammary secretions of the cow (from Lascelles, 1979)

	IgG_1	IgG_2	IgA	IgM
Blood serum	1400	1300	39	380
Colostral whey	4000–9000	250	470	540
Milk whey	40	6	11	9

It will be noted from Table 20.1 that colostrum has a markedly higher concentration of IgG_1 than serum. This concentration is associated with the presence of specific receptor sites for this immunoglobulin on the membranes of bovine mammary epithelial cells. There are suggestions in the literature that the levels of IgA in milk and colostrum have probably been underestimated because much of the IgA is associated with milk fat globule membranes, and some IgM may also be globule bound. The precise origin of IgG_2 and IgA in the mammary gland of the cow remains in doubt. A local synthesis of IgG_2 has been reported in the cow but this was not confirmed in the ewe. There appears to be less disagreement concerning the origin of IgM and IgA, which are thought to be largely derived from local synthesis in the mammary gland of the cow, but in the ewe the synthesis of these immunoglobulins appears to be confined to the period of mammary involution whereas in early and mid-lactation large amounts are transferred from the blood.

Inflammation of the mammary gland leads to a rapid increase in levels of immunoglobulin and other serum proteins, including complement, within the first few hours. In this situation IgM and IgG_1, together with serum-derived complement, control the growth of serum-sensitive coliform organisms. Phagocytosis by neutrophils is more efficient if they are coated with specific IgG_2 antibodies.

The precise role of IgA in the mammary gland of the cow remains in doubt. Some workers believe that it may block IgG- or IgM-mediated complement fixation, in which case it would have detrimental effects on the protection of the mammary gland in early infection. On the other hand, it may activate complement, but this may not be of great importance due to the low levels of complement in milk. There have been some reports that IgA antibodies assist the binding of bacteria to fat-globule membranes. This would hinder the mammary defence system by making the bacteria more difficult to phagocytose.

Phagocytic cell mobilization in the mammary gland and phagocytosis

The most effective system of udder defence against invading pathogens is the phagocytic activity of neutrophils. Normally, these cells are present in milk in very low numbers, the predominating leucocytes in the milk of healthy cows being macrophages and lymphocytes. Neutrophil numbers, however, rapidly increase in the very earliest stages of infection. The value of neutrophils in early infection was seen when unrestricted growth of bacteria occurred in the mammary gland of cows rendered neutropenic by the administration of anti-bovine leucocyte serum.

Neutrophil recruitment within the mammary gland is likely to be triggered by the presence of bacteria and bacterial products, which stimulate the formation of endogenous inflammatory mediators. These mediators lead to a margination of neutrophils in capillary vessels, cause a relaxation of endothelial cell junctions and allow a diapedesis of the neutrophils into the surrounding subepithelial connective tissues. The neutrophils in turn may release other inflammatory agents, further accelerating the process of neutrophil mobilization. The identity of the inflammatory mediators, which has been studied by a number of workers, includes prostaglandins produced by the cyclo-oxygenase pathway, leukotrienes produced by lipo-oxygenation and interleukins. Prostaglandins have been measured in bovine milk and shown to increase in concentration from 4 hours after the administration of intramammary endotoxin. Prostaglandins are synthesized in bovine mammary tissue and may also be generated by neutrophils.

Pathogens entering the mammary gland and causing mastitis are rarely invasive. Therefore, if an antimicrobial environment is to be produced in the mammary gland neutrophils must be present in the teat and lactiferous sinus regions, the ducts and in the alveolar lumen. Milk collects in the teat and lactiferous sinus regions and it is thought that neutrophils are attracted as far as the luminal surface of the two cell-thick epithelium by a concentration gradient of chemotactic factors originating from the lumen of the gland. Under these conditions, the neutrophils pass through the basement membrane and between the epithelial cells (Fig. 20.5). In severe staphylococcal infections the surface cells suffer toxic damage and in some cases this leads to large areas of epithelial erosion. Infections with *E. coli* frequently lead to more localized toxin-induced epithelial lesions and it is from these regions that the neutrophils migrate into the lumen.

A rapid neutrophil migration is essential for the efficient defence of the mammary gland following *E. coli* invasion, but particularly if the response occurs before the bacterial count in the milk exceeds 10^4/ml. Some cows, however, particularly if recently calved, fail to recruit neutrophils into their milk, and this lead to an unrestricted bacterial growth and severe damage within the mammary gland tissues. This situation may not be observed clinically since there may be a complete lack of inflammatory reaction. Nevertheless, these animals soon become severely ill and death may follow. Frequently, cows respond with a neutrophil recruitment but there is often a delay such that bacterial numbers may increase to a high level. Bacteria and neutrophils may then coexist in the mammary gland resulting in a protracted mastitis.

A rapid neutrophil response is also beneficial for controlling the growth of *Staphylococcus aureus* in mammary tissues, thereby preventing severe disease. A complete elimination of the organisms, however, rarely occurs and frequently a chronic subclinical disease remains in which small numbers of organisms are present in the milk, which has a permanently elevated cell count. These chronic infections may not be immediately obvious to the herdsman due to the very low grade inflammatory response in the tissues.

In any consideration of the immunology of the bovine mammary gland, availability of opsonins to permit the efficient phagocytosis of invading pathogens must be considered. The effector mechanisms of the phagocytes in the mammary gland may be activated by the Fc region of one or more classes of immune globulin and/or by fragments of the complement system bound to particles. Phagocytic cells have receptors for opsonins, where the opsonin is recognized and binds. This is linked with an effector unit that triggers the cell function. Different species of animals have different specificities for their receptors for different classes of immune globulin. Non-ruminant neutrophils have not been shown to bind to cytophilic antibody but cytophilic IgG_2 is active for ovine neutrophils and increases the bacteriocidal activity against *Staphylococcus aureus*. IgG_2 from immune bovine serum or milk whey will opsonize *E. coli*. Furthermore, the major opsonin for neutrophil phagocytosis of mammary gland pathogens using decomplemented non-immune bovine serum is IgM.

Further reading

Butler, J.E. (1974) Immunoglobulins of the mammary secretions. In *Lactation: a Comprehensive Treatise*, Vol. III (ed. by B.L. Larson & V.R. Smith), p. 217. Academic Press, New York.

Collins, R.A., Parsons, K.R. & Bland, A.P. (1986) Antibody containing cells and specialised epithelial cells in the bovine teat. *Research in Veterinary Science*, **41**, 50–5.

Cowie, A.T. (1977) Anatomy and physiology of the udder. In *Milking Machine* (ed. by C.C. Thiel & F.H. Dodd), pp. 156–78. National Institute for Research in Dairying, Reading.

Craven, N. & Williams, M.R. (1985) Defences of the bovine mammary gland against infection and prospects for their enhancement. *Veterinary Immunology and Immunopathology*, **10**, 71–127.

Hibbitt, K.G., Cole, C.B. & Reiter, B. (1969) Antimicrobial proteins isolated from the teat canal of the cow. *Journal of General Microbiology*, **56**, 365–71.

Larson, B.L. (ed.) (1985) *Lactation*. Iowa State University Press, Ames, Iowa.

Lascelles, A.K. (1979) The immune system of the ruminant mammary gland and its role in the control of mastitis. *Journal of Dairy Science*, **62**, 156–60.

Linzett, J.L. (1961) Recent advances in the physiology of the udder. In *Veterinary Annual* (ed. W.A. Pool). John wright and Sons, Bristol, 44–53.

Mepham, T.B. (ed.) (1983) *Biochemistry of Lactation*. Elsevier, Amsterdam, New York.

Peel, C.J. & Bauman, D.E. (1987) Somatotrophin and lactation. *Journal of Dairy Science*, **70**, 474–86.

Poutrel, B. (1982) Susceptibility to mastitis: a review of factors related to the cow. *Annales de Recherches Veterinaires*, **13**, 85–99.

Turner, C.W. (1952) The Mammary Gland. In *The anatomy of the udder of cattle and domestic animals*. Lucas Brothers Publishers, Columbia, 176–83, 203–7.

Weber, A.F., Kitchell, R.L. & Sautter, J.H. (1955) Mammary gland studies. 1. The identity and characterisation of the smallest lobule unit in the udder of the dairy cow. *American Journal of Veterinary Science*, **16**, 255–63.

Chapter 21: Mastitis

by A.J. BRAMLEY

Introduction

Mastitis is the most prevalent infectious disease of adult dairy cattle. Several species of bacteria, fungi, mycoplasmas and algae have been isolated from the natural disease or have been shown to reproduce it experimentally. The predominant species are listed in Table 21.1. Infrequently, aseptic mastitis occurs due to hormonal imbalances or local trauma. Furthermore, many clinical cases of mastitis that are due to infection are negative on bacteriological culture of the mammary gland secretion (Bulletin, 1987a).

The inflammation, characteristic of mastitis, may be undetectable without the use of diagnostic tests applied to the milk or secretion. This is termed subclinical mastitis. The subclinical stage may be prolonged or proceed rapidly to clinical mastitis in which external signs of disease such as swelling and hardness of the affected gland(s) or clots or discoloration of the secretion are present. Nevertheless, the subclinically infected quarter has a lowered milk yield, altered milk composition and excretes the infecting organism. Subclinical mastitis is a major element in the world-wide economic loss associated with mastitis, which exceeds £½ billion annually.

Dynamics of herd infection

Figure 21.1 illustrates the dynamics of udder disease within the herd. The mammary glands can be placed in one of three categories: uninfected, subclinically infected or clinically infected. The relative proportions of animals in these categories varies between herds. Pathogen type also influences the dynamics. For example, coliform infections tend to become rapidly clinical while *Staphylococcus aureus* infections often persist as subclinical infections for weeks or months. Clinical mastitis will usually be given antibiotic therapy and the clinical cure rate is generally high (>90 per cent). Elimination of the infection is however rarer, particularly with staphylococcal infections. The mammary gland has a range of defence mechanisms of which phagocytosis of invading organisms by polymorphonuclear leucocytes is probably the most important. Spontaneous elimination of infection by these mechanisms will occur. The rates of spontaneous elimination are low for staphylococcal infections (<20 per cent),

Table 21.1 Species of micro-organism frequently isolated from clinical bovine mastitis

Staphylococcus aureus	*Escherichia coli*
Streptococcus agalactiae	*Klebsiella pneumoniae*
Streptococcus dysgalactiae	*Enterobacter* sp.
Streptococcus uberis	*Proteus* sp.
Actinomyces (Corynebacterium) pyogenes	*Pseudomonas aeruginosa*
Bacillus cereus	
Mycoplasma bovis	Prototheca
Mycoplasma californicum	Fungi
Mycoplasma canadense	

Table 21.2 Distribution of clinical coliform mastitis cases with stage of lactation when first found

Lactation stage when found (weeks)	Number of coliform cases	Percentage	Cases/week
0–1*	86	20.8	86.0
2–5†	94	22.9	23.5
6–10	48	11.6	9.6
11–20	58	14.1	5.8
21–30	51	12.4	5.1
31–40	33	8.0	3.3
>40	41	10.0	–

* Uninfected at drying-off.
† Uninfected at calving.

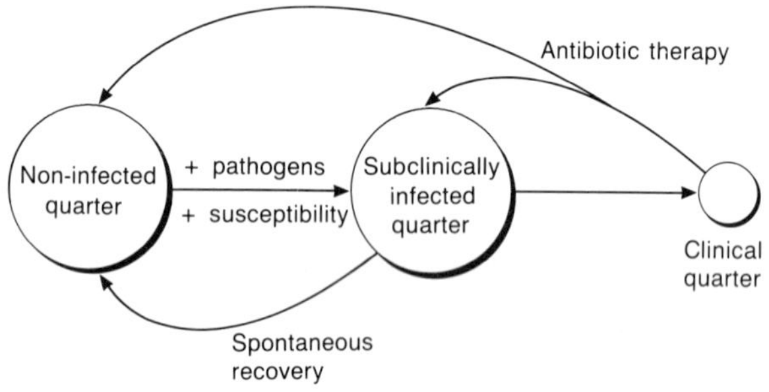

Fig. 21.1 Pattern of intramammary infection and clinical mastitis in a dairy herd.

high for *Escherichia coli* (>70 per cent) and intermediate for streptococcal infections.

Effects of lactation age and stage

Udder infection may develop when the cow is lactating or dry. Infection rates are highest in the early dry period although these infections often do not persist or develop into clinical mastitis until the next lactation. Clinical mastitis is most common at calving and in the first weeks of lactation. The incidence of clinical disease and new infection increases with lactation number. An example for coliform mastitis is shown in Table 21.2.

The precise reasons for these effects of age and stage are not known. The high incidence of mastitis around calving is largely a consequence of high new infection rate in the dry period and a periparturient suppression of host defences. Increasing disease with age is probably not due to increased intramammary susceptibility but to increasing ease of penetration of the teat duct by pathogens.

Teat duct

The teat duct is the usual portal for microbial invasion and, conversely, the major barrier to infection. The bovine teat duct varies in length from 4 to 18 mm, with a median of 12 mm. It has a heavily keratinized surface and the keratin lining is crucial to the maintenance of its barrier function (Plate 21.1). Removal of keratin by mechanical means increases susceptibility to bacterial colonization and invasion. The barrier function has both physical and chemical elements. Antibacterial lipids and basic proteins have been identified within the keratin lining of the teat duct (Williams & Mein, 1985).

The diameter of the canal and the depth of the keratin layer have been shown to be positively and negatively correlated with infection respectively. Certain defects in machine milking operation can adversely affect the defensive properties of the teat duct, increasing mastitis incidence (see section on machine milking, p. 294 and Chapter 24). Colonization or infection of the streak canal, particularly adjacent to the teat orifice, is common with pathogens such as *Staph. aureus* or *Streptococcus agalactiae*. Such colonizations may persist for long periods in the absence of intramammary infection but are largely prevented or eliminated by postmilking teat disinfection. Other organisms are often present within the teat duct including *Corynebacterium bovis* and coagulase-negative staphylococci and there are reports of the isolation of anaerobes. The environmental organisms, such as coliforms and *Strep. uberis* rarely colonize the teat duct and this difference is important in the pathogenesis of infection.

Transmission, sources and control of udder pathogens

Broadly, the micro-organisms causing bovine mastitis can be classified into two groups.

1 Organisms with a reservoir of infection associated with intramammary infection. These are best represented by *Staph. aureus*, *Strep. agalactiae* and, to some extent, *Strep. dysgalactiae*. Transmission arises largely at milking time, although infections will occur in the dry period. These organisms survive well on the teat skin, colonize teat ducts and lesions. Good control can be achieved by the application of hygiene at milking, particularly postmilking teat disinfection. Antibiotic therapy plays a valuable role both by reducing levels of herd infection and by infection prophylaxis. Careful application of control measures based upon teat disinfection and dry-cow antibiotic therapy will eradicate *Strep. agalactiae* over the course of one to two years provided infected animals are not introduced into the herd. Levels of *Staph. aureus* and *Strep. dysgalactiae* will also fall to low levels. In some herds, poor elimination rates of staphylococcal infection by therapy will require the heavy culling of chronically infected animals to achieve rapid progress.

2 Organisms with reservoirs independent of intramammary infection. Many species of mastitis-causing micro-organisms fall into this category but the most commonly encountered examples are the coliforms, aesculin-hydrolysing streptococci (predominantly *Strep. uberis*) and *Pseudomonas aeruginosa*. These organisms exist in various sites on the cow including the gut, genital tract and tonsils and can multiply in cattle litter or water to reach high populations. Consequently, teat challenge occurs in the milking interval or when cows are not milked. Although there is potential for interquarter transfer at milking time it appears not to be the predominant infection mechanism. Postmilking teat disinfection does not prevent infection. Antibiotic therapy has no beneficial effects on coliform mastitis prevention but does reduce the rate of new dry-period infection with *Strep. uberis*.

As control measures are more effective in controlling the initial category of infections their prolonged use leads to a reduced mastitis incidence and to a change in pattern, in which the second category of 'environmental organisms' predominate.

Diagnosis of clinical mastitis

The detection of clinical mastitis depends upon the examination of the mammary gland and its secretion. The affected gland may show swelling, heat, hardness and, in chronic infections, areas of fibrosis may be palpated. The secretion may be clotted, serous or, occasionally, bloodstained (Plate 21.26). In acute cases systemic signs of disease may also be present including pyrexia, anorexia and occasionally recumbency. Examples are shown of the clinical changes in Plate 21.2.

Clinical disease is most commonly seen in lactating animals, particularly in early lactation, but may develop in the non-lactating gland also. Because the dry animal is rarely closely scrutinized these cases often remain undetected until calving. 'Summer mastitis' is an acute disease of the non-lactating mammary gland and may afflict cows, heifers or young calves. Characteristically, it is caused by mixed infection with *Actinomyces pyogenes* and anaerobic bacteria, commonly *Peptococcus indolicus*. The disease is prevalent in northern Europe over the summer months and the incidence varies markedly within quite small areas. Clinically, the first signs are often a distended and swollen teat, sometimes with high fly populations feeding on it. This progresses in an ascending fashion to a severe hard swelling of the gland (Plate 21.2c) and the elaboration of large quantities of foul smelling, thick yellow secretion, occasionally blood-tinged. Systemic signs of disease are common. The animal will often be pyrexic, anorexic and dull. Swelling of the legs and joints are common and abortion or death may follow (Plate 21.2d). In the lactating cow, acute clinical mastitis is most commonly associated with coliform infection in early lactation. In these cases systemic signs may be detected before any local signs of mastitis are detected. Pyrexia, anorexia and recumbency are often present caused by the release of endotoxin within the mammary gland. In general, the clinical signs of mastitis are inadequate for a confident diagnosis of the likely aetiology. This poses significant problems for the selection of a suitable antibiotic therapy and leads to the prescription of broad-acting antibiotics.

It is important (and in many countries statutory) that dairy cows are examined before each milking for signs of clinical mastitis. This allows abnormal milk to be discarded and the affected animal to be given therapy as rapidly as possible, thereby reducing tissue damage and minimizing the risks of infection transfer. An alternative to examination of the foremilk for clotting during preparation for milking is to use in-line filters, installed in the long milk tube to screen the total milk yield. Disadvantages of this approach are that (i) the affected quarter(s) have to be identified by an additional examination of the strippings milk and (ii) the abnormal milk may have passed to the bulk supply prior to detection, particularly in direct-to-pipeline milking systems. Palpation of the udder after milking also aids clinical mastitis detection but the increase in cows milked per man hour and the provision of automatic cluster removers have precluded this process in many parlour operations. Some milking equipment contains sensors to aid the detection of abnormal milk and this is likely to become more common.

Diagnosis of subclinical mastitis

A range of tests can be applied to milk to detect subclinical mastitis (Schultze, 1985). These tests generally detect either the infecting organism (either directly or indirectly) or the changes to the secretion as a consequence of inflammation. These changes are both cytological and biochemical. Most tests are laboratory based although the California Mastitis Test (CMT) and electrical conductivity measurements can be used at the cow side. Tests can be placed in three categories and applied either alone or in combination.

Bacteriological examination

The secretion from a normal mammary gland is sterile although it may acquire bacteria from a colonized teat duct during collection. Therefore, the detection of a pathogen in an aseptically collected milk sample is indicative of infection. The numbers of organisms excreted per millilitre of milk from an infected gland fluctuates widely; hence the recovery of even low numbers of bacteria can be regarded as meaningful if the sample has been taken with adequate care and is not contaminated with adventitious bacteria. Bacteriological examinations have the advantage of being positive or negative, whereas most other tests require the imposition of a threshold value which varies between animals and herds (Bulletin, 1987a).

A suitable sample is required for bacteriological examination, most commonly foremilk although strippings samples can also be employed. A stream of milk should be discarded prior to thorough disinfection of the teat surface using pledgets of cotton wool soaked in 70 per cent alcohol (ethanol, methylated spirit or isopropanol). Cleaning should involve a hard scrub of the surface and is not adequate until the pledget remains clean. If the teat surface is washed prior to sampling, which is advisable only if soiled, then it should be dried prior to alcohol cleaning. If this care is not taken the bacteriological analysis of the sample is not dependable. A sample of 10–20 ml should then be collected into a sterile, preferably wide-mouthed, container. After collection samples should be examined with the minimum delay. If this is to exceed 90 minutes the sample should be refrigerated at <4 °C. Samples can be frozen (−20 °C) prior to examination although this reduces pathogen numbers (particularly Gram-negatives) and precludes cytological and some biochemical examinations. The bacteria most commonly causing bovine mastitis will grow aerobically on blood agar. Anaerobes, *Mycoplasma* spp. and *Leptospira* spp. require more specialized techniques not appropriate to the practice laboratory. The inclusion of 0.1 per cent aesculin in the blood agar is useful in the differentiation of *Strep. uberis* from other streptococci. A volume of milk (10–50 μl) is spread over the surface of the agar plate, which should be incubated for 24–48 hours at 37 °C. An advantage of a bacteriological examination is that the causative organism can be identified and provides a possibility for antimicrobial sensitivity testing. Disadvantages include cost, complexity and time delay. Detailed methods for the collection and bacteriological examination of milk samples for infection are available (Bulletin, 1981).

Cytological examination (see Chapter 23)

Milk from a healthy, uninfected bovine mammary gland contains somatic cells comprising macrophages, neutrophils and lymphocytes. The number of these is usually <250 000 cells/ml milk. When mastitis is present the cell count increases, primarily as a consequence of neutrophil infiltration. Subclinically infected quarters usually have cell counts in excess of 250 000 cells/ml but, because of the dynamic nature of the disease, this value can vary considerably and will sometimes fall below this threshold (Table 21.3).

During clinical episodes the cell count will be elevated, counts in excess of 5 000 000 cells/ml being commonplace. The cell count is detectable by a microscopic count or by electronic means. Detailed description of the methods employed are available (Bulletin, 1984). An indirect estimate of cell counts can be made using a variety of tests such as the CMT or Whiteside test. These tests are based upon a gelling reaction between the nucleic acid of the cells and a reagent, either a

Table 21.3 Variation in the cell count of a mammary gland infected with *Staph. aureus*

Day sampled	Bacteria/ml	Cells/ml ('000)
1	2 800	880
2	6 000	144
4	7 000	104
5	10 000	896
13	>10 000	152
14	1 200	1 000
15	>10 000	168

detergent (CMT) or sodium hydroxide (Whiteside). The reactions are categorized from 0 to 4. Reactions of 3 and 4 have a high probability of infection being present. Many countries employ cell counting of herd bulk-milk as an estimate of herd mastitis levels. Individual cow milk cell count services are available in many countries as an intermittent or regular service (e.g. the Milk Marketing Board in England and Wales and the Dairy Herd Improvement Association in the USA). A consistently high bulk milk cell count is characteristic of a high level of subclinical infection in the herd. Herds with counts <250 000 cells/ml generally have little economic loss associated with subclinical disease. Such herds may however still suffer significant costs due to a high incidence of clinical mastitis, associated with short-duration infections such as *Strep. uberis* and coliforms.

Biochemical and other tests

Inflammation of the mammary gland leads to a variety of compositional changes in milk either because of local effects or because of an increase of serum components entering the milk. Some of these changes can be used to screen for subclinical mastitis.

Significant changes in ionic composition occur with both Na^+ and Cl^- levels increasing, K^+ decreasing. The individual ions can be directly determined but more commonly the net change in ionic composition is used, measured as an increase in electrical conductivity. Both laboratory and farm-based meters exist and milking equipment incorporating electrodes to measure milk conductivity during milking is marketed in some countries. However, as for the majority of the milk parameters, the conductivity values of normal and infected quarters overlap and conductivity values vary between herds. These facts make the application of threshold values for diagnosis inaccurate. A fall in lactose concentration is also usual and has been employed diagnostically but has poor discrimination.

Enzymatic changes also occur. Some of the enzyme changes are associated with the increase in cell count (e.g. catalase), others with secretory cell damage (e.g. part of *N*-acetylglucosaminidase (NAG) increase) or with increased permeability (plasmin). The use of NAG has been widely tested and found to correlate well with cell count and infection and offers promise as a cow-side test.

As serum components leak into the mastitic gland they can be employed as indicators of inflammation. The most studied have been antitrypsin and bovine serum albumin (BSA). Automated methods for the

Table 21.4 Changes in milk composition associated with mastitis (examples of 'typical values')

	Somatic cells (1000)	
	Normal <20–750	Mastitic 100–>10 000
Sodium (mg/100 ml)	57	104
Chloride (mg/100 ml)	100	200
Potassium (mg/100 ml)	170	150
Conductivity (mM NaCl)	<50	>56
Lactose (mg/ml)	48	44
Catalase		increased 20-fold
NAG		increased 6-fold
BSA (mg/ml)	0.25	>0.6

NAG, *N*-acetyl glucosaminidase; BSA, bovine serum albumin.

detection of antitrypsin have been developed and the test is more sensitive than BSA. Table 21.4 summarizes the major compositional changes in milk due to udder infection and inflammation. For more detail of these tests and their application the reader is referred to Schultze (1985).

Use of individual cow or quarter sampling in herd investigations

Mastitis control relies upon the application of effective control measures to the herd rather than identification or special treatment of individual animals. However, bacteriological or other diagnostic tests can be employed to identify the nature of a herd problem or individual animals for segregation or culling. As payment of milk on the basis of cell count becomes more common then the emphasis placed on these systems tends to increase.

If the aetiology of clinical mastitis is to be determined then a microbiological analysis is needed. Such analyses provide information on the patterns of the disease within a herd since there will be delay between sampling and diagnosis during which therapy will usually have begun. Often a broad-spectrum antibiotic is employed to cover the range of possibilities. However, the pattern of disease may be helpful in determining the attention needed to remedy the herd problem. The isolation of *Strep. agalactiae* indicates either that teat disinfection and dry-cow therapy are not being employed effectively or infected animals have been introduced. A pattern of high herd cell count, repeated clinical cases and the frequent isolation of *Staph. aureus* would be typical of poor elimination of infection by lactation or dry-period therapy. This might prompt the use of bacteriological analysis of samples taken after treatment or at drying-off and calving.

Individual cow cell count or other diagnostic tests can be used to identify chronically infected animals for culling although such animals might be identifiable via an examination of clinical records. In the majority of herds the records are unfortunately inadequate for such a purpose. When using individual cow cell counts or other indirect tests the variation in inflammation should be remembered. Confident diagnosis on a single sample is inaccurate. The changes in these measures due to lactation stage and yield are also relevant. Cell counts in colostrum and in dry-cow secretion are naturally elevated and diagnostically unreliable. As lactation declines and yield falls cell count and electrical conductivity increase slightly. Milk composition and cell count may remain permanently altered or elevated in glands that have suffered severe secretory tissue damage, even if the causative organism has been successfully eliminated (see Chapter 23).

Cattle housing and mastitis

In many countries climatic conditions require that cattle are housed for at least part of the year with consequences for mastitis. Housing increases mastitis because the confinement of the animals and the multiplication of micro-organisms in various litters elevate teat challenge, and consequently mastitis. Prominent among these are bacteria are the coliforms, *Strep. uberis* and faecal streptococci.

The relationship between housing and mastitis is most clearly established for coliform mastitis. Coliform bacteria have been shown to multiply readily in organic litters, particularly sawdust, reaching counts of >100 million/g. These numbers often exceed those found in bovine faeces and impose a risk of infection. Sawdust has been shown to act as a source of *Klebsiella pneumoniae*, particularly if not kiln-dried, and can lead to severe mastitis problems. Some outbreaks have been controlled by switching from sawdust to sand, which tends to harbour lower numbers of coliforms and reduces the risk of disease.

Streptococcus uberis colonizes the bovine gut and is excreted in faeces and consequently contaminates cattle litter. In straw, multiplication of the organism often occurs leading to high levels of teat challenge and increased infection rates (Bramley, 1982). Since *Strep. uberis* is particularly infectious for the non-lactating or parturient udder this can be a particular problem if dry-cow or calving accommodation is not adequately cleaned and bedded.

Since multiplication in the litter is a crucial factor in increasing challenge to the teat surface regular removal and replacement of bedding offers the soundest basis for reducing it (Fig. 21.2; Dodd *et al.*, 1984).

The climate within cattle housing is also important since high humidity favours the survival and multiplication of micro-organisms. It has been found that cattle litter generally appearing to be clean and dry can harbour high numbers of micro-organisms and this can pose significant problems when giving advice over herd mastitis problems.

The design and size of yards and cubicles influence cow cleanliness and thus milk bacteriological quality and mastitis. Cubicles that are too short will leave cows' udders lying in the alleyway while those which are too long will lead to dunging on the cubicle surface itself. Obviously, the correct dimensions vary depending upon breed and age. Improper placement of access gates and water troughs in yards will lead to excessively dirty lying areas. Use of dung channels and grids can increase the incidence of damaged teats, etc.

These and other ways in which the environment influences mastitis are the subject of a review by the International Dairy Federation (Bulletin, 1987b). Detailed information on suitable dimensions and designs for cattle housing are also available (Sumner, 1981).

Machine milking and mastitis

There is unequivocal evidence that the events occurring at milking time influence the incidence of mastitis. These influences may be via the hygiene practised at milking time or because of effects of the milking machine *per se*.

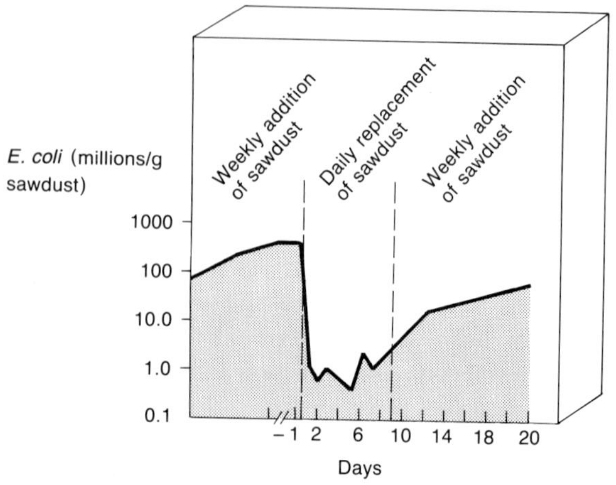

Fig. 21.2 Controlling coliform contamination of sawdust in cubicles by daily removal and replacement.

Milking time hygiene

The milk secreted by infected cows contains varying numbers of pathogenic micro-organisms. Herd milking provides opportunities for the transmission of these bacteria between udder quarters and cows via the milking machine itself, the milker's hands or cloths.

Various techniques can be employed at milking time to reduce transmission including:
1 using disinfected water for teat washing;
2 employing individual paper towels or cloths for teat drying;
3 wearing rubber gloves;
4 applying a suitable disinfectant to the teat surface after milking; and
5 disinfecting or heat treating the cluster between milking cows.

In addition, segregation of infected animals from the healthy herd can be used although it is impractical in most herds and incurs the cost of a diagnostic procedure. The use of measures such as those described above can reduce infection rates by about 50 per cent, effects being greatest against *Staph. aureus*, *Strep. agalactiae* and *Strep. dysgalactiae* (Fig. 21.3). The measures are relatively ineffective against coliforms and *Strep. uberis* infection because of their wider distribution in the environment.

Of the various measures to prevent new intramammary infections among milking cows, postmilking teat disinfection is the most valuable. Various disinfectants are used, most commonly iodophors, chlorhexidine and hypochlorite. Emollients are often added to promote good skin condition and rapid healing of lesions. These disinfectants will rapidly destroy bacteria reaching the teat surface during milking and will prevent colonization of the teat duct and the infection of teat lesions.

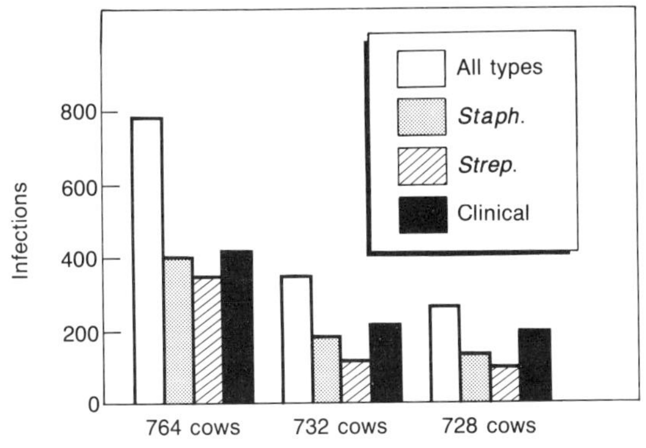

	Exp. control	Partial hygiene	Full hygiene
Pasteurizing teatcup liners	–	–	✓
Paper udder cloths	–	✓	✓
Disinfect hand dipping	–	✓	✓
Disinfect teat dipping	–	✓	✓

Fig. 21.3 Effect of milking time hygiene on new udder infections.

The importance of premilking hygiene in the production of milk of high bacteriological quality should be emphasized. Data show that effective washing of the teat followed by drying significantly reduces the bacterial content of bulk milk. Washing without drying has no benefit compared with not washing and may increase hazards of infection as contaminated material from the wet teats and udder runs into the liner mouthpiece during milking. Ideally, a suitable concentration of an approved disinfectant (usually iodine or chlorine) should be included in the wash water supply. There have been examples of coliform and *Pseudomonas* mastitis problems associated with contaminated udder wash water supplies. These are unlikely where mains water is in use although uncovered water storage tanks may become contaminated with faeces or carcasses of small animals and provide a source of infection. For a review of this subject see Bramley & McKinnon (1990).

Milking machine-induced infection and mastitis

During machine milking changes in pressure occur beneath the teat as a consequence of the changes in volume occurring as the liner opens and closes. Additional pressure changes may result from adventitious admissions of air as clusters are put on, taken off, slip, etc. These changes are called vacuum fluctuations and their extent and severity will be influenced by complex interactions of milking machine design and operation and by the capacity of the vacuum reserve. Low vacuum reserve will exacerbate the changes.

If the vacuum beneath the teat end is higher than the vacuum in the claw then milk and air will move towards the teat. The more extreme the pressure difference and the narrower the bore of the tubes the greater the velocity of the movement. These movements of milk can be sufficiently violent to implant material through the teat duct into the teat sinus, leading to mastitis. The placement of an interceptor plate or shield helps to protect from these infections. Further refinements have included the construction of claws that isolate the individual quarters by valves, partitions or diaphragms, etc. Vacuum fluctuations can be reduced by ensuring that milking machines are constructed to the relevant international standards, regularly maintained and tested. Various field experiments indicate that 10–20 per cent of lactation infection is due to vacuum fluctuation but the variation between herds is high.

The effective collapse of the liner on the teat end is also important in ensuring that machine milking does not increase mastitis. If pulsation is absent, of short duration (<0.31 s) or if the liner is too short for the teat then increased rates of new infection will result. For many years overmilking has been believed to be a major factor in increasing mastitis. Numerous experiments have failed to establish a relationship, even when extreme overmilking has been employed. It is probable that overmilking will exacerbate problems if other malfunctions are present and it does increase teat end eversion (see p. 326).

Incomplete milking and certain designs of liner have also been found to increase the incidence of clinical mastitis although apparently not increasing new infection rate. The mechanisms are not well understood but probably relate to the efficiency of the removal of bacteria, their toxins and the products of inflammation.

A review of the influence of machine milking on mastitis has been published (Bulletin, 1987c).

Aetiology of mastitis

It has already been stated that mastitis is a consequence of intramammary infection with one or more micro-organisms of many different genera. The following section provides information on the most common or important of the different mammary infections.

Staphylococcus aureus (see p. 343)

In most countries this organism is the predominant cause of subclinical mastitis but is also isolated from clinical disease. The important sources of infection are infected udders, teat ducts or teat lesions. Extramammary sources do exist, notably the vagina and tonsils but do not appear important in the pathogenesis of infection. It has proved possible to eradicate staphylococcal mastitis from individual herds by the application of hygiene at milking time and culling. The major limitation to more effective control of staphylococcal mastitis remains its poor response to antibiotic therapy. There are a variety of reasons for this of which antibiotic resistance plays only a minor role. *In vitro* demonstration of sensitivity of staphylococci to an antibiotic is no guarantee of therapeutic success. The ability of the bacteria to survive inside polymorphonucleocytes (PMN), macrophages and epithelial cells, protected from antibiotic action, may significantly contribute to their therapy resistance. Additionally, the pathological changes, notably granulomata and fibrosis, induced in chronic staphylococcal infections renders chronically infected cows essentially incurable. Most commonly staphylococcal udder infection is chronic, acute mastitis being less common than with other bacteria. However, acute gangrenous staphylococcal infections can arise in which uncontrolled growth of the organism occurs elaborating large quantities of α toxin. Such infections are probably not due to strains of increased virulence but rather to a failure by the host to mount an effective defence. Workers in California showed the critical role of the PMN in this defence since subclinically infected cows, made neutropenic, rapidly developed acute gangrenous staphylococcal mastitis (Schalm *et al.*, 1976) (for therapy see p. 839).

Streptococcus agalactiae (see p. 348)

The sources of *Strep. agalactiae* are similar to those of *Staph. aureus*, namely the teats and udder. Consequently, milking time hygiene is an effective means of preventing infection during lactation. Since *Strep. agalactiae* is much more easily eliminated by intramammary antibiotic therapy than staphylococci it is eliminated from herds employing teat disinfection and dry-cow therapy effectively and routinely. Additional sources are humans, many of whom carry Group B streptococci, and pigs. However, the widespread eradication of *Strep. agalactiae* indicates that these sources are relatively unimportant. The cross-species pathogenicity of human and bovine strains has been debated and remains unclear but, broadly speaking, bovine strains should be regarded as pathogenic for man. Human strains are able to infect cattle. The disease may exist as an acute clinical mastitis or persist as a subclinical infection. The duration of infection is shorter than staphylococci, primarily because of the better response to therapy. Outbreaks of *Strep. agalactiae* are indicative of poor hygiene and therapy and are usually solved by careful attention to procedures. More rapid elimination of *Strep. agalactiae* can be achieved by diagnosis and treatment of infected animals although the economic basis for this is doubtful (for therapy see p. 838).

Streptococcus dysgalactiae (see p. 347)

Very good control of lactation infections can be achieved by teat disinfection indicating that cow-to-cow transfer is an important mechanism. However, infection in the dry period and in heifers is commonplace, particularly among animals not protected by dry-cow therapy. Outbreaks of clinical mastitis with *Strep. dysgalactiae* frequently follow a breakdown in herd hygiene practices or increases in teat lesions. The incidence of teat lesions can increase rapidly following failures in pulsation, excessive milking vacuum or adverse housing or climatic conditions. In such outbreaks the machine should be given a thorough examination by an expert and the teats closely inspected for damage. The inclusion of a high level of a suitable emollient in the teat dip can promote rapid healing of lesions and prevent their colonization.

Clinical *Strep. dysgalactiae* mastitis can be acute with anorexia and pyrexia in addition to the local signs. However, the response to therapy is usually rapid and elimination rates with penicillins are similarly high to *Strep. agalactiae*. *Streptococcus dysgalactiae* is also encountered in mixed culture with other organisms, notably *A. pyogenes* and *P. indolicus* in summer mastitis. The bacteria can be isolated from bovine tonsils and the bovine genital tract and these sources, allied to the ability of the organism to infect and colonize lesions, may be important in the pathogenesis of dry-period infections.

Streptococcus uberis **and other aesculin-hydrolysing streptococci**

These organisms are an important cause of bovine mastitis and, in some herds, are the major cause of clinical udder disease. Several species can be involved but the predominant one (>70 per cent) is *Strep. uberis*. Others include *Strep. bovis*, *Strep. faecalis* and *Strep. faecium*. Infection with these organisms is not controlled by postmilking teat disinfection although dry-cow antibiotic therapy reduces infection rates by about 50 per cent. However, *Strep. uberis* remains the commonest cause of infection in the dry period and susceptibility to infection has been shown to increase following drying-off (Marshall *et al.*, 1986). In untreated dry cows the highest rates of infection occur in the initial two weeks following drying-off while in animals given antibiotic therapy at drying-off infection tends to be periparturient. The high infection rates in the dry period and the failure of teat disinfection to control disease emphasize the independence of milking and transmission. The bacteria are widely disseminated on the cow, are present in low numbers in cattle faeces and multiply in bedding materials, particularly straw, to reach high levels. Deep straw yards for housing dry cows seem to pose a particular risk factor. Not all strains are virulent for the lactating gland and a capsular layer is often elaborated conferring resistance to phagocytosis. Susceptibility of the lactating gland to infection may be influenced by the lactoperoxidase system, which in turn can be affected by feeding regimens altering milk thiocyanate levels. Although *Strep. uberis* is sensitive *in vitro* to a range of antibiotics, intramammary therapy often is ineffective and chronic infections are common in some herds. Under these circumstances cow-to-cow transmission may become more important (for therapy see p. 839).

Coliforms (see pp. 339, 342)

The coliform species most commonly implicated in mastitis are *E. coli*, although other species including *Enterobacter aerogenes*, *Ent. oxytoca*, *K. pneumoniae* and *Citrobacter* spp. are also encountered. Infection is more common among housed cows and occurs particularly around calving. Subclinical infection is uncommon and peracute mastitis occurs frequently. A small proportion of these animals (around 5 per cent) may die as a consequence of endotoxaemia. This can be treated by prompt use of supportive therapy, notably administration of large volumes (>20 l) of isotonic fluids. The use of anti-inflammatory drugs, particularly non-steroidal anti-inflammatories, may also be helpful. The dry gland is relatively resistant to coliform infection (cf. *Strep. uberis*, p. 297) due to the antibacterial activity of the iron-binding protein lactoferrin. Transmission between cows is unimportant in pathogenesis and the use of postmilking teat disinfection and dry-cow therapy does not reduce infection rates. The primary source of infection is bovine faeces although secondary multiplication of the bacteria to high numbers in cattle litter is often a factor (see section on cattle housing and mastitis, p. 294).

Infection with coliform bacteria leads to a rapid development of inflammation and often the influx of neutrophils eliminates the infection (Hill *et al.*, 1979). In some animals, particularly in early lactation and in high-yielding cows, this is not effective possibly because the rate of neutrophil diapedesis is poor. Recent research indicates that low levels of selenium may be implicated in the process (Erskine *et al.*, 1989) (for therapy see p. 839).

Actinomyces (Corynebacterium) pyogenes (see Chapter 22)

This bacterium is often involved in suppurative conditions in cattle, including mastitis. It is most frequently encountered as one of the mixture of pathogens responsible for 'summer mastitis' in northern Europe. This acute clinical disease of the non-lactating animal has been described in the section on diagnosis (see p. 291). *Actinomyces pyogenes* may also infect the lactating cow, or infection may be carried over from the dry period. Infection in the lactating cow is usually associated with teat damage.

The epidemiology of summer mastitis has been much studied because of its epidemic and destructive nature. The disease has been associated with fly-borne transmission and the sheep head fly *Hydrotaea irritans* has been shown able to carry *A. pyogenes*, *Strep. dysgalactiae* and the anaerobic peptococci responsible for the disease. With one exception transmission experiments with infected flies have proved unsuccessful but data do reveal that the use of insecticides or barriers (surgical tape, Stockholm tar, etc.) reduces the disease incidence. The most effective control measure is the prophylactic use of dry-cow therapy. A review of the epidemiology, transmission and pathogenesis has been published (Thomas *et al.*, 1987).

Mycoplasmas (see p. 342)

In recent years several species of *Mycoplasma* have been recognized as important causes of bovine mastitis. The most common cause is *Mycoplasma bovis* but other species implicated include *M. bovigenitalium*, *M. canadense*, *M. californicum* and *M. alkalescens*.

Characteristically, infection with *Mycoplasma* leads to a mastitis, often involving multiple quarters, which is refractory to antibiotic treatment. The secretion may remain normal at the onset although a granular or flaky deposit is recognized on standing. In the later stages a purulent or thick secretion, without offensive smell is often reported. Swelling and firmness is common but after a few days the mammary gland may reduce in size. Milk secretion is severely reduced. Swelling of the supramammary lymph nodes occurs and there may be pyrexia, transient malaise and arthritis. Secretion of mycoplasmas in the milk frequently lasts for two months and often for longer. Intermittent shedding is common. Clearly, such cows constitute an infection risk for the herd. Most reports relate to infection in lactating cows but outbreaks among dry cows, notably with *M. californicum*, do occur (Jasper, 1982).

Diagnosis requires the application of specific microbiological and serological tests in specialist veterinary diagnostic laboratories. These involve culture from milk onto selective media and a range of serological tests, often growth inhibition, to identify the species.

The most severe problems with this disease have occurred in large dairy herds in California and Florida. There is strong circumstantial evidence that careless use of bulk sources of antibiotic in these herds may have significantly contributed to the outbreaks. Nevertheless, it should be considered as highly infectious and affected animals either removed or isolated within the herd. Examination of bulk milk has proved a useful screening method for affected herds. If a herd is suspected of having a problem with *Mycoplasma* mastitis then specialist advice should be rapidly sought. For further information the reader is referred to detailed reviews (Boughton, 1979; Jasper, 1982) (for therapy see p. 890).

Leptospira infection (see also p. 570)

Increasing concern has arisen over leptospirosis for a variety of reasons. Most importantly organisms of the hebdomadis subgroup are pathogenic for man. The organism most involved is *Leptospira hardjo* and this is responsible for the so-called 'milk drop syndrome' and is also associated with abortion in affected herds. The characteristic milk drop appears initially as a mastitis, usually with the milk yield of all four quarters falling to zero within 24 hours. Pyrexia is common and the udder secretion is thickened or clotted and occasionally bloody. The udder remains flaccid and the condition usually resolves within seven to fourteen days. Cases may be restricted to a few animals or up to 50 per cent of animals may become affected over a period of two to three months (Jackson & Bramley, 1983). Antibiotic therapy with tetracyclines or streptomycin may aid the resolution of the clinical phase and reduce carriers although immunity develops following infection. A vaccine is available, which requires an annual booster to ensure adequate protection. Infection of man may occur via infected urine droplets, particularly in herringbone milking parlours and leads to a febrile illness characterized by severe headaches. In a proportion of cases this can lead to complications including meningitis and encephalitis.

Coagulase-negative staphylococci and *Corynebacterium bovis*

Several species of coagulase-negative staphylococci are commonly isolated from aseptically collected milk samples. These include *Staph. epidermidis*, *Staph. simulans* and *Staph. xylosus*. Most of these organisms are of low virulence although some isolations are associated with clinical disease. These organisms generally produce a slight elevation of somatic cell count, which may increase resistance to infection with major pathogens.

Similarly, *Corynebacterium bovis* is not usually associated with clinical disease and primarily colonizes the distal teat duct. It is rapidly eliminated by antibiotic therapy and its spread is prevented by effective teat disinfection. In the absence of such measures it may be isolated from >70 per cent of aseptically collected milk samples. Growth on blood agar requires incubation for 48 hours, preferably at 30 °C, and stimulation by fatty acids supplied either by the milk or by additions to the media such as Tween 80.

Recommendations for control of mastitis

In the USA, UK and Australasia and many other parts of the world there is a recommended mastitis control scheme based upon the '5-point plan'. The elements in the scheme are as follows.

1 Apply an approved teat disinfectant after every milking.
2 Treat clinical cases of mastitis.
3 Infuse long-acting antibiotic into all quarters at drying-off.
4 An annual milking machine test and appropriate maintenance.
5 Cull cows showing repeated cases of clinical mastitis.

These measures were the basis of controlled experimentation in many countries and have been widely employed since the 1970s. Teat disinfection is to reduce rates of new infection rate during lactation, the dry-cow therapy serves to eliminate a high proportion of subclinical infections present at the end of lactation and to prevent many new dry-period infections. Treatment of clinical mastitis assists the elimination of infection and in the resolution of clinical signs of disease

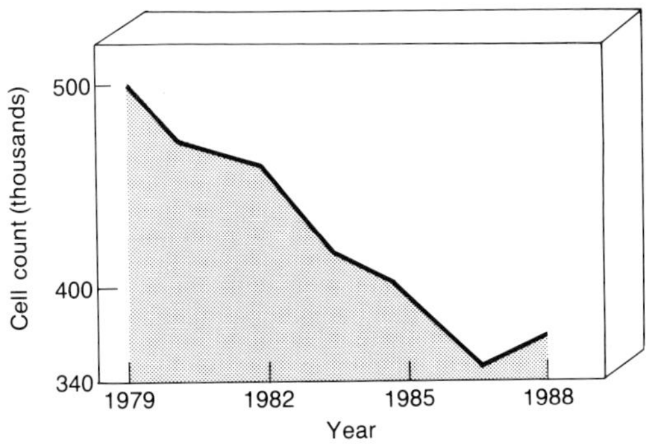

Fig. 21.4 Reduction in bulk milk cell count in England and Wales between 1979 and 1988.

and culling is employed to remove chronically affected cows. Finally, the milking machine maintenance is intended to ensure efficient milking and prevent machine-induced infections as described above (therapy for mastitis is dealt with in Chapter 55).

A review of the progress in mastitis control following the introduction of these techniques has been described by Booth (1988). This shows major reductions in clinical mastitis incidence and in the reduction of bulk milk cell count (Fig. 21.4). The present status of improving mammary gland immunity is described in Chapter 27.

References

Booth, J.M. (1988) 1. Control measures in England and Wales. How have they influenced incidence and aetiology? *British Veterinary Journal*, **144**, 316–22.

Boughton, E. (1979) *Mycoplasma bovis* mastitis. *Veterinary Bulletin*, **49**, 377–87.

Bramley, A.J. (1982) Sources of *Streptococcus uberis* in the dairy herd. I. Isolation from bovine faeces and from straw bedding of cattle. *Journal of Dairy Research*, **49**, 369–73.

Bramley, A.J. & McKinnon, C.H. (1990) The microbiology of raw milk. In *Dairy Microbiology*, Vol 1 (ed. by R.K. Robinson). Academic Press, New York.

Bulletin (1981) Laboratory methods for use in mastitis work. International Dairy Federation Bulletin 132, Brussels.

Bulletin (1984) Recommended methods for somatic cell counting in milk. International Dairy Federation Document 168, Brussels.

Bulletin (1987a) Bovine mastitis. Definition and guidelines for diagnosis. International Dairy Federation Bulletin 211, Brussels.

Bulletin (1987b) Environmental influences on mastitis. International Dairy Federation Bulletin 217, Brussels.

Bulletin (1987c) Machine milking and mastitis. International Dairy Federation Bulletin 215, Brussels.

Dodd, F.H., Higgs, T.M. & Bramley, A.J. (1984) Cubicle management and coliform mastitis. *Veterinary Record*, **114**, 522–3.

Erskine, R.J., Eberhart, R.J., Grasso, P.J. & Scholz, R.W. (1989) Induction of *Escherichia coli* mastitis in cows fed selenium-deficient or selenium-supplemented diets. *American Journal of Veterinary Research*, **50**, 2093–2100.

Hill, A.W., Shears, A.L. & Hibbitt, K. (1979) The pathogenesis of experimental *Escherichia coli* mastitis in newly calved dairy cows. *Research in Veterinary Science*, **26**, 97–101.

Jackson, E.R. & Bramley, A.J. (1983) Coliform mastitis. *Veterinary Record* (In Practice Suppl., Vol. 5, No. 4) 135–46.

Jasper, D.E. (1982) The role of *Mycoplasma* in bovine mastitis. *Journal of the American Veterinary Medical Association*, **181**, 158–73.

Marshall, V.M.E., Cole, W.M. & Bramley. A.J. (1986) Influence of the lactoperoxidase system on susceptibility of the udder to *Streptococcus uberis* infection. *Journal of Dairy Research*, **53**, 507–14.

Schalm, O.W., Lasmanis, J. & Jain, N.C. (1976) Conversion of chronic staphylococcal mastitis to acute mastitis after neutropenia in blood and bone marrow produced by an equine anti-bovine leukocyte serum. *American Journal of Veterinary Research*, **37**, 885–94,

Schultze, W.D. (1985) Development in the identification of diseased udder quarters or cows. Proceedings International Dairy Federation Seminar *Progress in the Control of Bovine Mastitis. Kieler Milchwirtschaftliche Forschungsberichte*, **37**, 319–28.

Sumner, J. (1981) Housing systems and mastitis In *Mastitis Control and Herd Management*, pp. 223–36. Technical Bulletin 4. National Institute for Research in Dairying, Shinfield, Reading, Berks.

Thomas, G., Over, H.J., Vecht, U. & Nansen, P. (eds) (1987) *Summer Mastitis*. Martinus Nijhoff, The Netherlands, 1–224.

Williams, D.M. & Mein, G.A. (1985) The role of machine milking in the invasion of mastitis organisms and implications for maintaining low infection rates. Proceedings International Dairy Federation Seminar *Progress in the Control of Bovine Mastitis. Kieler Milchwirtschaftliche Forschungsberichte*, **37**, 415–25.

Further reading

Bramley, A.J. & Dodd, F.H. (1984) Mastitis control — progress and prospects. *Journal of Dairy Research*, **51**, 481–512.

Schalm, O.W., Carroll, E.J. & Jain, N.C. (1971) *Bovine Mastitis*. Lea & Febiger, Philadelphia, 1–360.

Chapter 22: Summer Mastitis

by J.E. HILLERTON

Summer mastitis is an acute or peracute multifactorial infection of the non-lactating bovine mammary gland although clinical signs are often not obvious until parturition. The disease is reported from all four continents where dairy cattle are herded. It is, however, most prevalent in northern Europe and particularly common in some European cattle such as the Friesian/Holstein breeds, being rare in the Zebu.

Aetiology (see p. 343)

Bacteriological analysis of summer mastitis secretion shows a complex infection. Usually *Actinomyces* (*Corynebacterium*) *pyogenes* predominates and the severity of the infection is related to toxin production from synergistic growth with other bacteria that are anaerobic (see p. 302). *Peptococcus indolicus* is the most common anaerobe but *Bacteroides melaninogenicus* and *Fusobacterium necrophorum* are often found. An undescribed microaerophilic coccus, the Stuart–Schwann coccus is also found. It is a commensal rarely growing in pure subculture. *Streptococcus dysgalactiae* is also common and believed by some to be a primary agent predisposing to *A. pyogenes* infection.

Much of the reported variation in bacterial culture, and especially isolation of anaerobes, probably results from suboptimal collection and transport of samples, allowing anaerobes to die out.

Epidemiology

Summer mastitis is considered to be epidemiologically most severe in northern Europe. It is also prevalent in Japan, and parts of the USA, as well as being reported from Greece, Australia, Zimbabwe and Brazil. The incidence varies greatly from country to country, as does the severity of the infection. Most cases in Florida are recognized when heifers calve with a non-functional quarter from which the causative bacteria can be recovered, whilst in Japan systemic illness is more common.

The incidence of summer mastitis varies locally. It is greater in the more intensive dairy areas but does not just depend on the density of cattle. It is only in the dairy industry that the importance of the disease is well recognized. It can be prevalent in beef cattle but loss of function of one-quarter is not so important economically in the suckler cow. The Dutch, Germans and Danes believe that summer mastitis is associated with sandy soils, but these correlate well with the best grassland. The high humus content, open structure and free-draining of sandy soils are particularly suitable for foraging, soil-dwelling insect larvae.

The disease is most common in summer and early autumn but can also occur in spring. As well as season, it is particularly associated with calving pattern. In Eire, with many spring-calving herds, the spring incidence is marked. The black and white dairy breeds seem most susceptible and in the absence of preventive measures the incidence is greatest in older cows.

Transmission

It is a long and widely held belief, although supported only by circumstantial evidence, that flies transmit summer mastitis.

The peak incidence of disease in Europe occurs in July, August and September when flies are most abundant on cattle. The sheep headfly (or plantation fly), *Hydrotaea irritans*, is the most frequent visitor to the teats of dry cows and heifers. Flies around pastured cattle have been shown to carry the summer mastitis pathogens even in the absence of disease in the herd. The disease prevalence is coincident with the geographical distribution of the fly in Europe. Control of flies on cattle reduces the incidence of summer mastitis. Some 60 per cent of infections occur in the front quarters, which, it has been suggested, flies can reach more easily.

However, summer mastitis is common outside the fly season, although rarely with the same epidemiological distribution of cases within the herd. The disease occurs geographically where neither *Hydrotaea irritans* nor a readily identifiable substitute occurs. Numerous attempts in Britain, Germany, Denmark and The Netherlands to transmit the disease using flies have failed despite earlier reports of success.

Initial cases of summer mastitis in an outbreak probably occur by chance. Increased incidence will depend on the density of animals at risk; hence there is a peak incidence in spring-calving herds simply because more animals are challenged when they are most susceptible. Probably the role of the fly is to increase the challenge. It therefore is involved in secondary transmission. The fly may also contribute by stressing animals. Fly pestering can reduce milk yields by inducing gross behavioural changes. Susceptibility to infection during late gestation when there are other environmental and husbandry stressors, especially poor forage and heat, may increase with fly challenge.

Pathogenesis

Damage to secretory tissue is caused primarily by toxin from *A. pyogenes*, with other virulence factors including a haemolysin, a coagulase and a hyaluronidase. The activity and quantity of these is enhanced in mixed culture with *P. indolicus*.

The route of invasion of the udder by a mixture of bacteria is unknown but it seems unlikely that simultaneous invasion by up to five species of bacteria occurs. It is possible to isolate one or more of these pathogens from the udder of the lactating or dry bovine in the absence of overt clinical signs so it is likely that some predisposing factor(s) is needed to cause clinical disease.

Evidence for the teat route of invasion in natural infections comes from the frequency of summer mastitis following teat-end damage. It has been possible to produce infections following surface contamination of the teat with *A. pyogenes* alone. There is, however, no unequivocally accepted mechanism. Possibilities, each with proponents, include colonization of the teat skin or orifice spreading through the teat duct into the gland, bacteria entering the gland by draining via a supramammary lymph node from another site and invasion by haematogenous spread. All of the pathogens are ubiquitous on the bovine, easily recoverable from mucous membranes and various lesions, and so a number of routes of invasion may occur naturally.

Clinical disease

Diagnosis of the later pathogenic stages of summer mastitis is relatively easy and requires little experience. Early stages are more difficult to distinguish from other infections.

The infection is more commonly ascending so the primary sites are in the teat or in lactiferous tissue near the base of the teat. Initially, there is local inflammation and oedema. Expression of udder secretion may reveal a foul smell indicative of anaerobic bacteria. In summer months the teat may be attractive to flies and if the animal is housed the hind legs attract biting flies. Slightly later, behavioural changes in the animal related to toxaemia become apparent. The animal may be lethargic, inappetant, stop cudding and will become detached from the herd. These signs are easy to recognize at pasture. In newly calved and housed animals the first signs are often tenderness in the quarter, which can be confused with excessive intramammary pressure, and local temperature. The secretion will be discoloured, thick and creamy, rather than colostral, perhaps very clotted in a serous fluid, and frequently foul smelling.

In addition to the extreme mastitis, in later stages pyrexia and lethargy develop. If the infection remains local there may be rupture of mammary abscesses to the exterior. More commonly, the animal becomes systemically ill with progressive lameness from the hind legs, swelling of joints and an elevated temperature. The bacteraemia/toxaemia may be fatal in a few per cent of cases; similarly there may be abortion. Perinatal death is substantially increased and many calves, often born prematurely, fail to thrive.

The infection develops rapidly after the initial recognizable signs so confirmation of summer mastitis by bacteriology is rarely quick enough. Attempts have been made to develop cow-side diagnosis of anaerobic involvement based on specific metabolites but no practical technique is available. The time delay for confirmation is impractical. Recent evidence showed that

80 per cent of diagnoses of summer mastitis were correct (Hillerton *et al.*, 1987). The other infections would also respond readily to the same therapy so unless drastic action, such as teat amputation or immediate culling, is indicated misdiagnosis in favour of summer mastitis has no economic or welfare disadvantages.

Treatment

A number of different approaches to treatment can be taken. The one selected will depend on the anticipated outcome of the case, which in turn depends on the clinical severity of the infection. In a small number of cases the only recommendation is for immediate culling. Less drastic is to treat the infection purely as an abscess; to amputate the teat and drain. This is practised commonly on the European mainland with non-pregnant younger animals, which are often then reared for beef.

In cows and heifers near to or at parturition the prognosis depends on the speed of diagnosis. In most cases in dry cows the infection is sufficiently well developed that destruction of secretory function is virtually complete. A clinical cure can sometimes be achieved but rarely a bacteriological cure. The prognosis is much better if the infection is diagnosed early, and therapy started immediately.

The pathogens are susceptible to a wide range of antibiotics including penicillin/streptomycin preparations. However, there is a poor cure rate when the only therapy is infusion into the udder. This is because the tissue destruction is extensive locally and so diffusion of the antibiotic is limited. A greater success has been claimed for erythromycin, which diffuses more readily. Success has also been claimed for anti-anaerobe preparations containing metronidazole. Chlortetracycline can be useful in the lactating animal but should not be used in the dry gland as all secretory function will be lost.

Claims have been made for a variety of other preparations including proteolytic enzymes mixed with antibiotics but controlled studies are rare. Usually, the most successful outcome follows a coordinated effort: frequent stripping of the quarter combined with parenteral intramuscular antibiotics and an intramammary infusion. This conventional approach, although labour intensive, affords the best prognosis for the udder. If systemic involvement is established then treatment of clinical signs to secure the health of the animal is all that can be achieved as the function of the infected quarter has been lost.

The patient should be quarantined as it is a source of further infection.

Control

Summer mastitis is so destructive and expensive that considerable investment in time and materials is made by the 40 per cent of farmers in England and Wales who regularly experience losses. Preventive measures are neither simple nor foolproof and usually are damage-limiting rather than totally preventive. The basic aims are to limit exposure to infection from the herd, to prevent colonization of lesions and to prevent spread of bacteria to the mammary tissue.

Assuming that summer mastitis infections will arise anyway it is important to recognize these early and segregate the infected animal to limit direct transfer of bacteria via, for example, bedding systems and indirect transfer by flies. *Hydrotaea irritans* do not pester housed cattle, so separate housing of infected animals is good practice.

The epidemiological spread of infection is related to the density of susceptible animals and the abundance of vectors. Reducing the density of late gestation cattle by spreading the calving pattern and completely avoiding the fly season of July, August and September in northern Europe are likely to be highly effective.

Considerable effort is spent on fly control but this is the least effective method of disease control as persistent presence of insecticide on teats is hard to achieve. The synthetic pyrethroids now in common use are applied in ear-tags or as pour-ons to the back and probably spread by diffusion in sebum. However, the teats lack hair and sebaceous glands are sebum deficient, so limiting spread. Effective fly control on teats is only achieved by direct application or frequent reapplication of insecticide, or by the use of two ear-tags per animal.

Frequently, summer mastitis follows infected lesions on or near the teats. These can be prevented or limited by use of surgical tapes, ensuring that the teats are cleaned first and not bandaged too tightly, or by frequent application of teat disinfectant. Many farmers teat dip dry cows and heifers daily. This allows frequent inspection, trains the heifers to the milking parlour and ensures good teat condition. Prevention of teat lesions may reduce greatly the attractiveness for flies.

The best tested and most effective means of reducing the incidence of summer mastitis is the general application of prophylactic antibiotic infused into the teat at drying-off. Following administration of synthetic penicillins in a long-acting base, summer mastitis rarely occurs within three weeks. Longer effects are achievable with some preparations. Where the incidence of disease warrants extra investment it is advisable to repeat the application of antibiotic after three weeks.

The main problem is avoiding milk contamination after an early calving. All the evidence available shows a significant reduction of summer mastitis following use of dry-cow therapy. It can also be applied to heifers if the antibiotic is introduced gently into the teat duct.

Attempts to produce a vaccine against summer mastitis have met with little success. This remains a long-term goal and will become more likely as multivalent vaccines are developed.

Reference

Hillerton, J.E., Bramley, J.A. & Watson, C.A. (1987) The epidemiology of summer mastitis: a survey of clinical cases. *British Veterinary Journal*, **143**, 520–30.

Chapter 23: Cell Counts and Mastitis Monitoring

by D.J. O'ROURKE AND R.W. BLOWEY

Cell counts

What is a somatic cell count?

Somatic cells are white blood cells. They are found throughout the body and their main function is to protect against disease. When large numbers accumulate they are visible as pus. The measurement of the number of somatic cells in milk is known as a somatic cell count.

Factors affecting the somatic cell count

MASTITIS

Inflammation in the udder is in no way different from inflammation in other tissues. The cardinal signs of inflammation, namely swelling, redness, heat, pain and loss of function, may not always be of recognizable intensity in mastitis. Signs of clinical mastitis are grossly visible but subclinical mastitis will go unnoticed. The majority of mastitis cases are bacterial in origin. One of the basic host responses to a bacterial infection is the infiltration of white blood cells from the blood into the udder. This is accomplished through the processes of diapedesis and chemotaxis. The degree and the nature of the cellular response is likely to be proportional to the severity of the infection. In addition to bacterial infections, there are certain other factors, some of which are physiological, that affect the cellular content of milk.

STAGE OF LACTATION

The somatic cell count is high during the first week of lactation, then soon decreases and remains low for several weeks after which a gradual increase occurs until the end of lactation. As the milk volume decreases in the latter part of lactation, an apparent increase in cell numbers occurs from mere concentration of cells in a smaller volume of milk. The presence of high cell numbers in colostrum may probably be due to an excessive desquamation of epithelial cells in a small volume of milk in a gland resuming functional activity after a dormant period (Schalm *et al.*, 1971).

LACTATION AGE

The somatic cell count increases with the lactation age of the cow. (Fig. 23.1) (Blackburn, 1966). On the basis of histopathological examination of udders, the increase in the average number of polymorphonuclear leucocytes with advancing lactation age was attributed to an increase in the extent of subacute inflammation of the ducts as well as an increase in the severity of lobular lesions.

STRESS

A sudden upset in the cows' routine, for example a herd blood test or coming indoors in the autumn, can cause a raised cell count for a day or two.

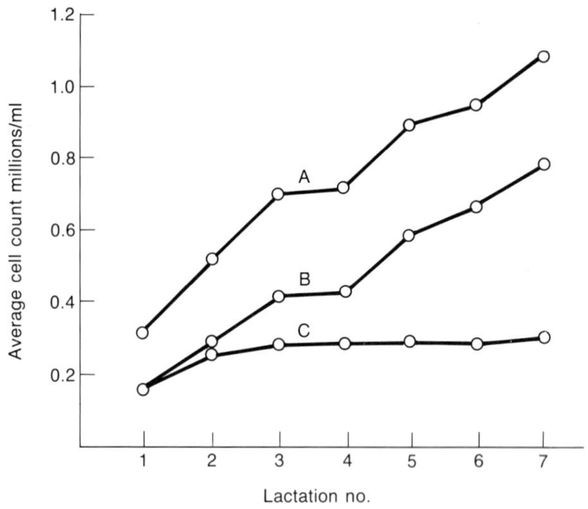

Fig. 23.1 Average cell count for each of seven lactations. A, total cell count; B, polymorphonuclear leucocyte count; C, count of cells other than polymorphonuclear leucocytes. Source: Blackburn (1966).

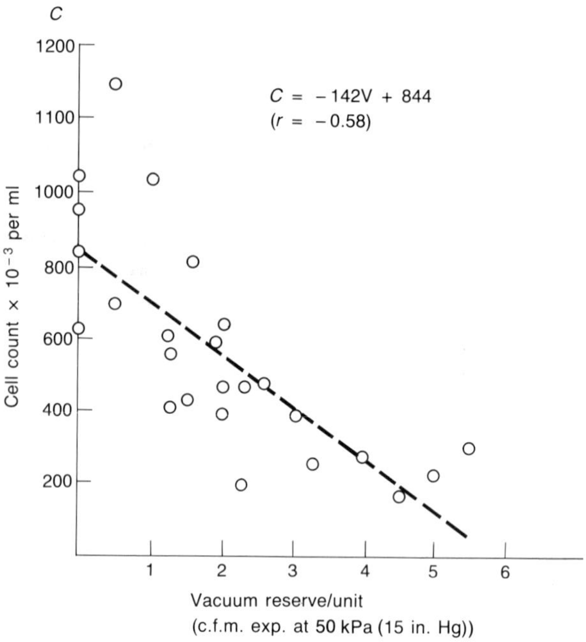

Fig. 23.2 Relationship between mean cell count of herd bulk milk (C) and vacuum reserve per unit (V). Source: Nyhan & Cowhig (1967)

OESTRUS

Bulling cows tend to have increased cell counts that are probably stress related.

MILKING INTERVAL

Irregular milking intervals will influence the somatic cell counts in milk. Comparisons of somatic cell counts in milk have generally shown higher counts for shorter milking interval. This variation in cell numbers is explained on the basis of total volume of milk secreted leading to a greater dilution of somatic cells during the longer milking interval (Schalm *et al.*, 1971).

MILKING MACHINE

A significant correlation between cell counts and milking machine reserve air was observed by Nyhan & Cowhig (1967) in a survey of milking machine efficiency and mastitis in a random sample of 26 dairy farms (Fig. 23.2). Six of the herds were milked with machines that had a vacuum reserve of more than 0.11 m^3/min free air (4 ft^3/mm free air) and these were the only herds with a mean bulk milk cell count of <300 000 cells/ml. However, more recent work in Australia (Olney *et al.*, 1983) concluded that in the absence of mastitis infections vacuum fluctuations, vacuum level, overmilking or varying pulsator rates will not cause stress or irritation that will lead to an increase in somatic cell counts.

Determination of cell content of milk

REFERENCE METHOD: MICROSCOPIC COUNTING (Heeschen, 1975)

The method of microscopic counting of cells in a dry stained smear has been available for many years now although it has some possible errors. The optical and manual operations involved are tedious, especially in the case of serial tests, and the following sources of error must not be overlooked.

1 Distribution of cells in the smears may not be homogeneous. The decision as to whether the stained structures observed are actually cells may be difficult in some cases and must be made subjectively.

2 To estimate the cell content every microscopic field examined must be multiplied by a relatively large factor, and this can be a source of considerable error.

Consequently, the primary object of microscopic counting is the screening of other counting techniques.

ELECTRONIC PARTICLE COUNTING

This can be carried out by the following methods.

Coulter counter (International Dairy Federation (IDF, 1981))

With the aid of the Coulter counter it is possible to determine rapidly and accurately the number of particles over a certain size in a suspension. Prior to the determination of the number of cells, the milk is treated as follows.

1 Cells are stabilized to make them resistant to further treatments.

2 The milk to be examined is diluted with an electrolyte.

3 The fat globules are dispersed to well below the Coulter counter threshold.

The treated milk is passed through a 100 µm aperture located between two electrodes. When a particle passes through the aperture, a small quantity of highly conductive liquid in the circuit is displaced by a particle of lower conductivity. The increased resistance raises the voltage, producing a voltage pulse proportional to the volume of the particle. The number of pulses indicates the number of particles passing through the aperture. The pulses are fed into a threshold circuit so that only those exceeding a particular threshold value (T) are counted.

Fossamatic (IDF, 1981)

This instrument is an automatic microscope for counting cells in liquids. Cells are stained with ethidium bromide and are then excited with a high-energy lamp, causing them to emit light at a characteristic wavelength. The emitted light energy is detected electronically, the result being displayed and printed out for each successive sample.

ACCURACY OF THESE METHODS

The precision obtained in the Fossamatic instrument is comparatively high. However, it is not essentially different from that obtained in the Coulter counter. In practical operation, the Fossamatic instrument has proved to be superior to other methods tested. This applies to the rate of samples as well as the handling of the instrument (Heeschen, 1975).

In an International Dairy Federation (IDF) questionnaire in 1983 on the cell counting methods 20 countries indicated they used Fossamatic, 17 used Coulter counter and two used the microscope method.

Table 23.1 Distribution of cow and quarter infections shown against cell count ranges. Source: Pearson & Greer (1974)

Cell count ranges ($\times 10^3$ cells/ml)	No. of herds	Infections	
		In quarters (%)	In cows (%)
219–490	12	9.61	25.8
535–789	12	17.76	42
1005–1700	5	29.54	54.4

Interpretation of somatic cell counts

Somatic cell counts can be carried out both on (i) herd bulk milk and (ii) individual cow's milk.

HERD BULK MILK

The seasonal variation in bulk milk cell count (BMCC) is well recognized, although perhaps not fully explained by stage of lactation effects. It is generally assumed that a herd's BMCC will be assessed over a 12-month period, but this will not be the case if the whole herd is dry for a time, as frequently occurs in countries that produce milk almost exclusively from grass. Cell counts carried out only during the mid-lactation period of production, which occurs in some areas, will inevitably be lower (Booth, 1985).

Monthly cell counting has been shown to provide a fair estimate of the subclinical mastitis status of a herd; furthermore, the annual mean can be updated on a rolling basis by substituting the current month's count of the same month of the previous year (Booth, 1985).

A herd of cows with physiologically normal quarters could expect a BMCC of <200 000 cells/ml. Herds with cell counts below this figure do exist (12.4 per cent of herds in England and Wales; Booth, 1988) but evidence shows that even in these herds there is some subclinical infection (Tables 23.1 and 23.2). A BMCC of 250 000 cells/ml is considered to be a realistic upper limit for herds with mastitis under control (Table 23.3).

The prevalence of quarters infected clinically, and perhaps more importantly subclinically, with major pathogens such as *Staphylococcus aureus* or *Streptococcus agalactiae* and to a lesser extent *Streptococcus dysgalactiae* and *uberis*, is the most important factor affecting the BMCC. Gram-negative organisms such as *Escherichia coli* are usually rapidly eliminated from the udder and do not tend to cause subclinical infections. Unless milk from clinical cases reaches the bulk tank, infections of this type do not tend to influence the BMCC significantly; BMCC, therefore, is a poor indication of Gram-negative infections (David & Jackson, 1984).

Both monthly and annual rolling mean figures must be examined to detect trends over a period of time rather than figures for a single month. Where subclinical infections with major pathogens like *Staph. aureus* are not well controlled it is possible to see a gradual

Table 23.2 Herds, by bulk milk cell counts, and prevalence of infection with major pathogens. (Source: Wilson & Richards (1980)

Bulk milk cell count (× 103 cells/ml)	Percentage of quarters in herd affected					
	5	5–10	10–20	20–30	>30	Total
<300	28* (53)	12 (23)	12 (23)	1 (2)	0	53 (100)
301–500	48 (27)	56 (32)	52 (30)	12 (7)	7 (4)	175 (100)
501–750	23 (16)	25 (17)	61 (43)	15 (11)	18 (13)	143 (100)
751–1000	10 (14)	10 (14)	23 (33)	15 (21)	12 (17)	70 (100)
>1001	2 (4)	4 (8)	13 (25)	14 (26)	20 (38)	53 (100)
Total	111 (22)	107 (22)	161 (33)	58 (12)	57 (12)	494 (100)

* indicates number of herds. Numbers in parentheses are percentages.

Table 23.3 Guidelines for interpretation of bulk milk cell counts

Bulk milk cell count ($\times 10^3$ cells/ml)	Estimate of mastitis problem
<250	Slight
250–499	Average
500–750	Above average
750–1000	Bad
>1000	Very bad

increase in BMCC over a period of time, rather than a sudden explosive increase. A sudden spectacular rise in the BMCC where the levels have been consistently <250 000 cells/ml could indicate an outbreak, with mastitis milk reaching the bulk supply due to faulty mastitis detection.

Sixteen countries reported BMCCs carried out at approximately monthly intervals in the 1983 IDF survey, four reported twice monthly counting and two at variable intervals (Booth, 1985).

Table 23.4 summarizes the national mean cell counts of 12 of the 13 countries that were able to provide data in this survey; the thirteenth country provided a percentage figure only.

INDIVIDUAL COW'S MILK

Several countries now carry out monthly cell counts on the milk samples taken from cows for milk recording purposes. No cost–benefit analysis has been carried out and it seems unlikely that the information obtained from these counts every month is economic for herd management purposes. They may however provide a rather more detailed monitor of the herd mastitis situation than that provided by the monthly BMCC.

Table 23.4 National mean cell counts in 1982. Source: Booth (1985)

Country	Cell count ($\times 10^3$/ml)	Mean*
Switzerland	164	G*
Finland	193	A
Sweden	227	G
Germany (FR)	235	Median
Norway	246	A
Austria	280	G
Denmark	280	G
Canada	325	A
New Zealand	428	A
Australia	433	A
Belgium	437	A
United Kingdom	456	G

* A, arithmetic; G, geometric.

Table 23.5 Relationship between the bulk milk cell count and individual cow cell counts. Source: MMB (1985)

Bulk milk cell count ($\times 10^3$ cells/ml)	Percentage of cows with counts ($\times 10^3$ cells/ml)		
	<250	250–500	>500
<300	49	36	15
300–500	33	33	34
500–700	19	31	50
>700	10	22	67

Individual cow cell counts on an occasional basis can be of value to farmers and their veterinary surgeons for the following reasons.

1 To estimate the proportion of cows in a herd that are infected.

2 To screen the herd in order to identify cows with high cell counts for bacteriological examination.
3 To identify cows for possible culling (but at least two samples at monthly intervals are required).
4 As a guide to the effectiveness of dry cow treatment.
5 In a herd with high total bacterial count (TBC) where the equipment has already been checked, as a first step in identifying the cows that may be the cause of the high TBCs.

Samples are normally of whole milk, taken from the recorder jar or bucket or, less frequently, from each quarter.

Table 23.6 Interpretation of individual cow milk cell count.

Count (thousand cells/ml)	Interpretation
Less than 250	Probably uninfected
250 to 500	Suspicious: possibly infected in one quarter
Over 500	Infected in at least one quarter

Stage of lactation will have some effect; counts are high in the first week after calving and tend to rise slightly in the last few weeks of lactation. First calvers that have never been infected will normally have counts of 100 000 cells/ml or less.

Data from the Milk Marketing Board (MMB, 1985) has shown that, where the whole herd is sampled, up to two-thirds of the cows could be infected at that time if the bulk milk count is over 700 000 cells/ml (Table 23.6). Even with a bulk milk count between 300 000 and 500 000, on average one-third of the cows may be infected.

Mastitis monitoring

Introduction

There are few conditions in dairy cows that lend themselves to such a detailed objective numerical monitoring as mastitis. Mastitis is still a significant problem in dairy herds in all countries and many of the factors leading to a high incidence are associated with hygiene and husbandry, i.e. they are under the direct control of the farmer or stockman. It is therefore vital that there is a constant monitoring to ensure that all parties involved are made aware immediately a problem starts to develop.

One of the largest British surveys, starting with 45 000 cows in 378 herds, was completed in 1983 (Wilesmith *et al.*, 1986). Defining a 'case' of mastitis as one quarter affected and with a separate case commencing if seven days had elapsed since the disappearance of clinical signs, they found an incidence of 54.6 cases per 100 cows in 1980, declining to 41.2 cases per 100 cows by 1982. This is in broad agreement with the data of Blowey (1986), reporting a much smaller survey of 22 herds monitored by a veterinary practice, where the incidence of mastitis fell from 51.0 cases in 1979 to 31.8 cases per 100 cows in 1985 (Table 23.7).

Recording systems

The precise system used by the farmer to keep mastitis records is not particularly important, provided:
1 it is used accurately and kept up to date;
2 all information is recorded, namely date, cow identity, quarter affected, treatment used and results of bacteriological samples (if taken);
3 the records are in a form that is acceptable and usable for the person compiling them; and
4 they are regularly reviewed by both the farmer and his veterinary adviser and any necessary action is taken following this review.

An analysis of data needs to be carried out at least every six months. Intervals longer than this would fail to achieve the aims of the monitoring (detailed later in this section, p. 311). It is also important to be seen to be using the data, thereby maintaining the interest and enthusiasm of the herdsman for continuing with the

Table 23.7 The average performance of the 22 herds monitored (Blowey 1986)

Period of records	Number of herds being recorded	Herd size	Rolling mean herd milk cell count ($\times 10^3$/ml)	Annual milk sales (l)	Percentage cows affected	Mastitis cases/ 100 cows	Intramammary tubes used per cow	Intramammary tubes used per case treated	Percentage cases which recurred
Oct. 1979–Sept. 1980	22	91.7	346	6011	26.5	51.0	2.6	5.1	25.0
Sept. 1980–Aug. 1981	24	105	302	5820	25.4	49.6	2.7	5.8	16.3
March 1981–Feb. 1982	22	101	310	5921	25.8	45.9	2.4	5.6	14.9
April 1982–March 1983	16	123.7	302	5949	27.2	49.3	2.5	5.0	16.1
April 1983–March 1984	16	123.8	255	5651	23.6	42.7	1.9	4.2	13.1
April 1984–March 1985	23	111.5	243	5479	19.6	31.7	2.1	7.1	10.3

Table 23.8 A 'league table' derived from mastitis data analysis

Herd number	Number of cows	Rolling mean cell count ($\times 10^3$)	Mean herd yield (annual sales) (l)	Percentage cows affected	For whole herd: Cases per 100 cows	For whole herd: Tubes used Per cow	For whole herd: Tubes used Per case	For mastitic cows: Average number of cases	For mastitic cows: Percentage which recurred	For mastitic cows: Quarters per cow
1	65	321	5800	38	60	3.5	5.7	1.6	15	1.4
2	81	745	6000	21	30	0.9	2.9	1.5	12	1.3
3	46	275	5850	19	40	4.1	9.4	2.2	45	1.2
4	134	267	5178	21	30	1.2	4.6	1.2		1.2
6	95	346		29	70	9.8	13.5	2.5	33	1.6
7	110	333	6500	27	70	2.7	3.8	2.6	40	1.6
8	132	272	6036	28	60	1.8	2.9	2.2	29	1.6
9	50	441		30	70	2.1	3.1	2.2	36	1.4
10	60	210		18	60	1.7	2.8	3.4	35	2.2

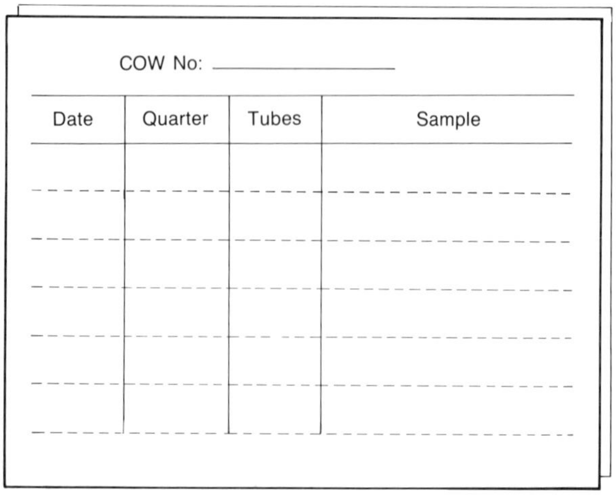

Fig. 23.3 A page from a herdsman's mastitis recording book. This is kept during the life of the cow.

recording. Wall charts are the simplest method of recording; computers may be used, while others provide a specific mastitis recording booklet, with a page for each cow (Fig. 23.3; Blowey, 1983). This has the advantage that a cow's lifetime mastitis history is readily available. Whatever system is used, it must be capable of producing information on previous disease, to assist with decisions on culling.

Analysis of information

Regular checks must be carried out by analysing the recorded information in order to:

1 assess the incidence of mastitis on each farm and hence the efficacy of the control procedures in use;

2 compare the performance of the farm with 'standard targets' or with the herds of other members of the group being monitored.

The wide variety of criteria that can be used to monitor mastitis are shown in Table 23.8, which is part of a 'league table' taken from a herd recording programme (Blowey, 1984). Bulk milk cell count is clearly the traditionally used parameter, but this is mainly a reflection of subclinical *Staph. aureus* or *Strep. agalactiae* contagious mastitis. It provides relatively little information on the incidence of environmental mastitis. The percentage of cows affected gives the proportion of cows in the herd that have been clinically affected by mastitis during a 12-month recording period. Any one of these cows may have had mastitis in one or more quarters and any one quarter may have had two, three or more mastitis incidents over a 12-month period. Defining a case as one quarter affected once, and a remission of clinical signs for six days or more being needed before a new case commences, then the *case* incidence of mastitis can be calculated. As far as the farmer is concerned, this will be a more accurate reflection of the 'amount of mastitis' occurring in the herd. If a herd has a low percentage of cows affected, but a high number of cases per 100 cows (for example herd 7,

Table 23.9 Case incidence and tube usage over a 3-year recording period. Source: Wilesmith *et al.* (1987)

	1980	1981	1982
Cases/100 cows	54.6	49.8	41.2
Tubes used/100 cows	280 (33–1032)	273 (23–1112)	259 (19–1003)
Tubes used/clinical case	6.1 (1.1–29.4)	6.1 (0.9–53.5)	5.8 (0.9–19.5)

Table 23.8), then that herd has a problem with either (i) a large number of down-calving cases, with maybe all four quarters affected at the same time or (ii) a proportion of 'chronics' in the herd, which have had repeated attacks of mastitis in one or more quarters over the lactation. This can be expressed as the proportion of treated cases that recurred and is clearly very high for herd 7.

These two situations can be separated by monitoring the percentage that recurred, namely the proportion of treated quarters that required a second or subsequent treatment during a 12-month recording period. Additional information can be obtained by calculating indices for the cows affected, namely for 'mastitic cows' (Blowey, 1984). For example, in this category (i) cases per mastitic cow gives an indication of the average frequency with which a cow gets mastitis during a 12-month period and (ii) quarters per mastitic cow then gives a further indication of whether it is one quarter being regularly affected, or all four quarters affected at once.

In many instances, intramammary antibiotic tube usage is obtained from different sources, e.g. the veterinary practice, or other sales invoices. This has the advantage in that it provides a check on the accuracy of the data being supplied by the farmer. For example, if it is calculated that 10 tubes are used for each case treated, there are several possible explanations.

1 The cases treated are very slow to respond, either because the wrong antibiotic is being used, or because there is an unusually resistant organism, or because treatment is not instigated until the case is quite well advanced.

2 Tubes are being used at a rate well in excess of the manufacturer's recommendations.

3 Tubes are being used for purposes other than the treatment of mastitis.

Table 23.10 Targets for herd mastitis incidence. Source: Blowey (1986)

	Target	Interference level
Percentage cows affected per annum	20	25
Cases/100 cows per annum	30	35
Milking cow antibiotic tubes/ affected cow per annum	1.7	2.0
Percentage cases requiring a repeat treatment during a 12-month period	10	15
Percentage dry cows affected per annum	1.0	2.5

4 Not all cases of mastitis are being recorded. This is the most likely cause of an extremely high tube usage per case.

The mean tube usage per cow in the herd and per case treated as recorded by Wilesmith *et al.* (1986) (Table 23.9) was slightly higher than that recorded by Blowey (1986) (Table 23.7). However, on individual farms Wilesmith *et al.* (1986) found that average tube usage over a 12-month recording period varied from 0.9 to 53.5 tubes per case treated and it was for this reason that they concluded that tube usage was not a reliable indicator of mastitis incidence within a herd. However, coincident with a decrease in mastitis incidence from 54.6 to 41.2 cases per 100 cows per annum, there was a decline of 280 to 259 tubes used per 100 cows. Similarly, in the data of Blowey (1986) (Table 23.7), tube usage fell from 260 to 210 tubes used per 100 cows in a period when mastitis incidence declined from 51.0 to 31.7 cases per 100 cows per annum. Tube usage would therefore appear to give some indication of mastitis incidence, although it is not a figure that should be used in isolation.

Target figures

Targets for mastitis incidence have been suggested by some authors and are shown in Table 23.10. These can be used by an individual farmer to assess the progress of a control scheme.

Uses of mastitis monitoring

Most points have been referred to already, but an appraisal of the uses of recording makes a useful summary of the subject.

1 Monitor the progress of an individual cow. Any cow that has had four or more cases in one quarter during a 12-month period should be considered for culling, or at least for special treatment, for example repeat dry-cow therapy.

2 Monitor herd status. Is mastitis incidence acceptable or should more effort be put into control? The surveys of both Blowey (1986) and Wilesmith *et al.* (1986) showed a marked decrease in mastitis incidence over the recording period and it is likely that the simple discipline of recording, leading to an increased awareness of the problem, will lead to improvements.

3 A recording system provides an opportunity for greater veterinary involvement in on-farm advice and discussion. Recording in itself often provides the herdsman with greater motivation in mastitis control, and this is particularly the case if league tables are supplied, indicating how well a specific herd compares with the others being monitored.

4 If problems occur, an analysis of the records can sometimes indicate the likely epidemiology of the organism(s) involved and hence the control measures required. For example, a herd with a high percentage of cases requiring repeat treatments is likely to be affected by staphylococcal or streptococcal cow-to-cow transmitted mastitis. Alternatively, because a heavily contaminated environment tends to expose all cows to the same level of infection, a high incidence of environmental mastitis would be seen in the records as a high percentage of cows affected, almost an equal number of cases per 100 cows, but only low numbers of cases per mastitic cow and a low percentage of cases recurring.

References

Blackburn, P.S. (1966) The variation in the cell count of cow's milk throughout lactation and from one lactation to the next. *Journal of Dairy Research*, **33**, 193–8.

Blowey, R.W. (1983) Data recording and analysis in dairy herds. Proceedings of the Society of Epidemiology and Preventive Medicine, pp. 19–28.

Blowey, R.W. (1984) Mastitis monitoring in general practice. *Veterinary Record*, **114**, 259–61.

Blowey, R.W. (1986) An assessment of the economic benefits of a mastitis control scheme. *Veterinary Record*, **119**, 551–3.

Booth, J.M. (1985) Bulk milk somatic cell counting: Methods in use and a proposal for the standard presentation of data. In *Proceedings of the International Dairy Federation Seminar Progress in the Control of Bovine Mastitis*, Kiel, F.R. Germany, pp. 274–81.

Booth, J.M. (1988) Progress in controlling mastitis in England and Wales. *Veterinary Record*, **122**, 299–302.

David, G.P. & Jackson, G. (1984) The collection and interpretation of herd mastitis data. *British Veterinary Journal*, **140**, 107–14.

Heeschen, W. (1975) Determination of somatic cells in milk — technical aspects of counting. In *Proceedings of the International Dairy Federation Seminar on Mastitis Control*, Reading, England, pp. 79–92.

International Dairy Federation (IDF) (1981) Recommended methods for somatic cell counting in milk. Document 132, pp. 5–16.

Milk Marketing Board of England & Wales (MMB) (1985) The use of mastitis cell counts on individual cow milk samples. Leaflet no. ICCCS/VS/885.

Nyhan, J.F. & Cowhig, M.J. (1967) Inadequate milking machine vacuum reserve and mastitis. *Veterinary Record*, **81**, 122–4.

Olney, G.R., Scott, G.W. & Mitchell, R.K. (1983) Effect of milking machine factors on somatic cell count of milk from cows free of intramammary infection. *Journal of Dairy Research*, **50**, 135–52.

Pearson, J.K.L. & Greer, D.O. (1974) Relationship between somatic cell counts and bacterial infections of the udder. *Veterinary Record*, **95**, 252–7.

Schalm, D.W., Carroll, E.J. & Jain, N.C. (1971) *Bovine Mastitis*. Lea & Febiger, Philadelphia.

Wilesmith, J.W., Francis, P.G. & Wilson, C.D. (1986) Incidence of clinical mastitis in a cohort of British dairy herds. *Veterinary Record*, **118**, 199–203.

Wilson, C.D. & Richards, M.S. (1980) A survey of mastitis in the British dairy herd. *Veterinary Record*, **106**, 431–5.

Chapter 24: The Milking Machine

by D.J. O'ROURKE

How it works

A milking machine installation consists of a pipework system linking various vessels and other components, which together provide the flow paths for air and milk. The forces necessary to move air and milk through the system arise from the fact that the system is maintained at a vacuum. Thus it is atmospheric pressure that forces air, and intramammary pressure that forces milk, into the system and the combination of these forces causes flow.

A milking machine has five basic components and any machine, no matter how big, can be broken down into these components (Figs. 24.1 and 24.2).

1 Vacuum pump: to supply the vacuum.
2 Regulator: to control vacuum level.
3 Pulsators: to open and close the liners.
4 Clusters: to attach to the cow.
5 Containers: to store milk.

Figure 24.1 shows diagrammatically the flow of air and milk through a bucket milking machine. Milk enters the teatcups and travels through the short milk tubes to the claw where air is admitted to break up the columns of milk and improve milk flow away from the claw. The milk and air travel along the long milk tube to the container (bucket). A pulsator is normally situated on the lid of the container and this admits air, which aids in the collapse of the liners during the closed phase of pulsation. Air is also admitted through the regulator, which is situated on the vacuum pipeline.

The flow pattern is similar in the milking pipeline machine except that the milk and air from each claw flow through the milk pipeline to a common receiver where air and milk are separated (Fig. 24.2). Depending on the type of milk pump used air may be admitted when milk is released from the receiver and pumped to the bulk tank.

The flow pattern of the recorder type machine is similar to the milking pipeline machine except that air admitted at the claw is separated from the milk at the recorder jar (Fig. 24.3). Air has to be admitted at this point through a special inlet or through the teatcups at the end of each milking operation to force the milk from the recorder jar to the receiver jar (which is under vacuum). Some air may pass along with the milk as the jar empties especially if the controls are not expertly handled. This air is separated from the milk at the receiver.

Functions of main components of a milking machine

Vacuum pump. To extract air and maintain the machine under vacuum.

Interceptor. To prevent the ingress of foreign matter into the vacuum pump.

Sanitary trap. To prevent milk vapour from entering the pulsators.

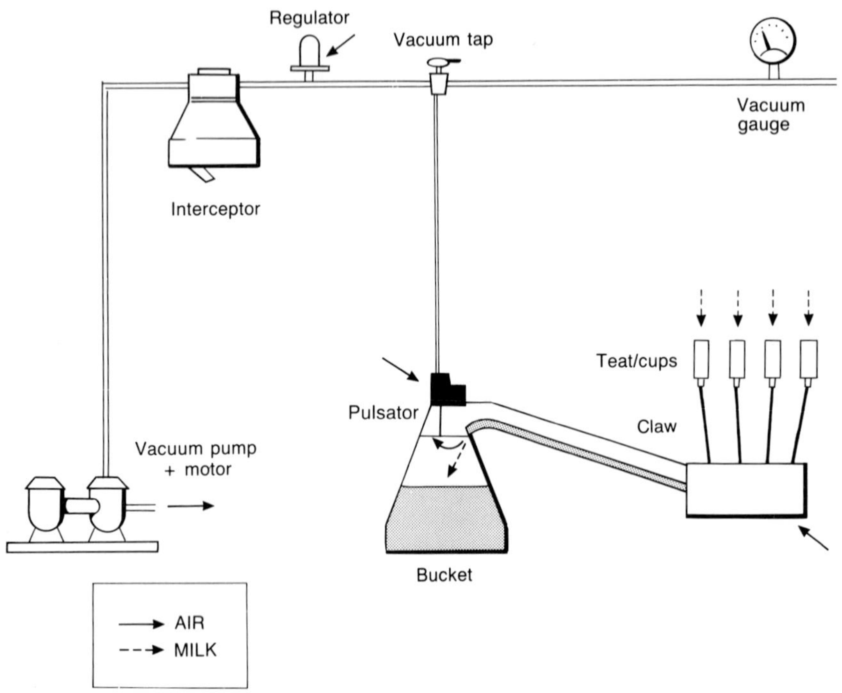

Fig. 24.1 Bucket milking machine.

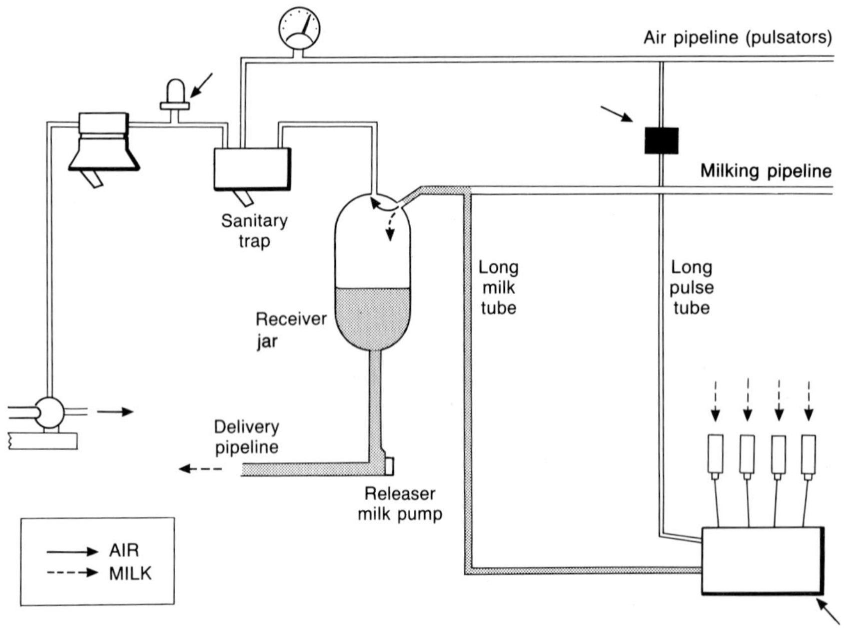

Fig. 24.2 Milking pipeline machine.

Vacuum regulator. To maintain a constant vacuum level. It limits the maximum level by admitting air into the plant when a predetermined vacuum level has been reached. When the vacuum level drops, the regulator closes; this stops admission of air and the vacuum level rises until the present level of vacuum is reached at which time the regulator opens again and admits air.

Pulsation. This causes the liner to open and close: when there is vacuum in the pulsation chamber the

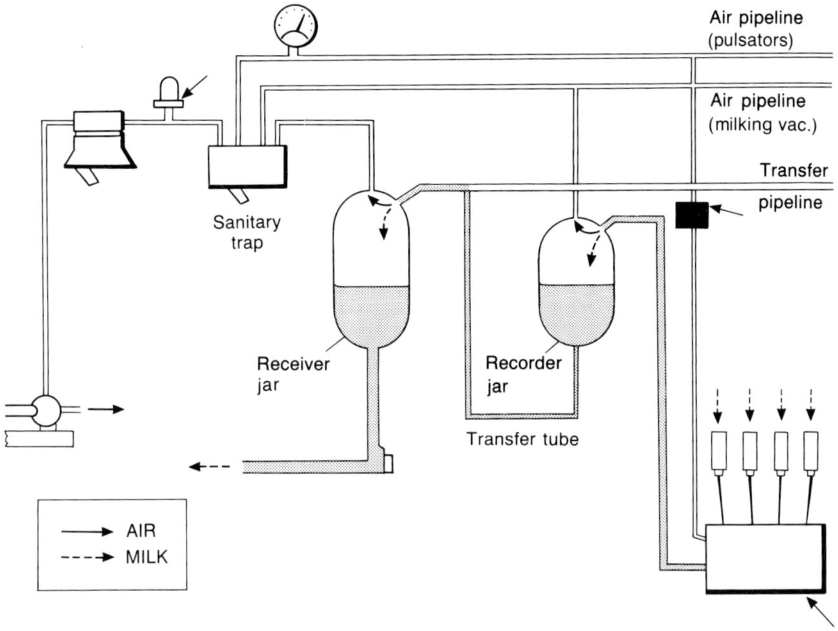

Fig. 24.3 Recorder milking machine.

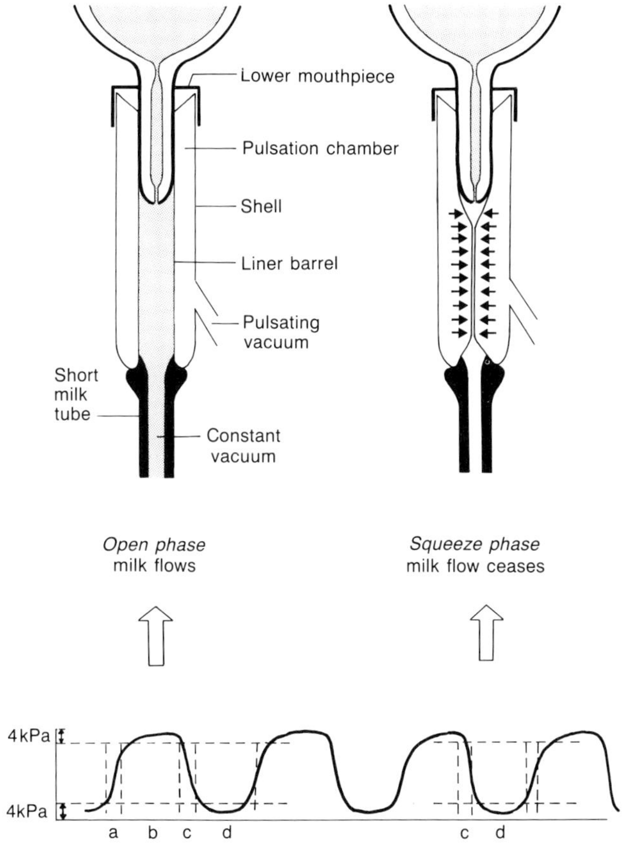

Fig. 24.4 Pulsation chamber waveform.

liner opens and milk flows; when air is admitted into the pulsation chamber the liner collapses, milk flow stops and the teat is massaged. In fact, milk generally flows when the liner is more than half open. The exact function of pulsation has not been established but is now thought to be relief of congestion around the teat orifice. Figure 24.4 shows a typical pulsation chamber waveform containing the four phases: (i) a phase, liner opening; (ii) b phase, liner fully open; (iii) c phase, liner closing; and (iv) d phase, liner fully closed.

Liners. The performance of liners is related to various dimensions of liners and various other physical properties of the liner. The liner is the major determinant of milking characteristics (O'Shea, 1982).

Milking machine testing

Milking machines are tested to assess whether they are in good mechanical condition and conform to working standards laid down by the standards institution of that country where used.

Static test

This type of test has been carried out for many years. It is basically an engineer's test to check correct functioning of the components of the machine. The machine is set for milking and plastic bungs placed in the liner mouthpieces. No milk flows and therefore the test will only give an indication of how the machine will perform in the hands of a milker.

There are three measurements to look for when interpreting a static test report.

1 *Effective reserve*. As pointed out earlier, vacuum within the plant is created by the vacuum pump. Air is used by the pulsators, air holes in the claws, and leaks in the plant, etc. The spare vacuum capacity left after compensating for these leakages is called the effective reserve. This effective reserve is used to compensate for additional leakages during cluster application and removal and cluster fall-offs.

2 *Pulsation*. Table 24.1 shows the recommendations for pulsation characteristics.

3 *Leakages*. The static test will measure the air consumption of the major components in the machine and there are a set of standards for the maximum they are allowed. It is worth checking that results of the test are within the normal range.

PRACTICAL TIPS

As a veterinary surgeon in practice there are two simple ways of checking the effective reserve of a machine.

1 Put the plant in the milking position and plastic bungs in the liners. For every five units, open one and let air in. If the effective reserve is sufficient the vacuum level, as read at the vacuum gauge, should not drop by more than 2 kPa (about $\frac{3}{4}$ inch Hg) (O'Shea, 1982).

2 Again put the plant in the milking position and plastic bungs in the liner. By letting air into the plant drop the vacuum to 33 kPa (10 inches). Close off the air leakage. The vacuum should return to 50 kPa (15 inches) within 3 seconds (Mein, 1984).

Dynamic test

Dynamic testing was only indicated in 1 per cent of herds (O'Callaghan *et al.*, 1982) where there was a mastitis problem and the static test had revealed no faults. At that time, equipment was either very sophisticated and expensive (UV recorder) or crude (pulsation pen recorder). In recent years, with the advent of computer technology, new recording machines specially designed for dynamic testing have been developed.

In dynamic testing the vacuum level is measured at the clawpiece and other areas of the machine, e.g. the recorder jar, throughout the milking of a number of cows. This allows the determination of what is happening when milk and air are flowing in the machine and also assessment of the ability of the milker to use the machine properly.

There are three measurements to look for when interpreting a dynamic test reading.

1 *Cyclic fluctuations*: generated within the claw as a result of pulsation (Fig. 24.5).

2 *Irregular fluctuations*: occur as a result of changes in air flow during milking, which leads to a drop in vacuum (Fig. 24.6).

3 *Liner slip*: sudden air admission between the liner and the teat (Fig. 24.7). A problem exists if more than five slips or falls per 100 cows milked require correction by the milker(s) (Mein, 1984).

Table 24.1 Recommendations for pulsation characteristics. Source: O'Shea (1982)

Parameter	Acceptable range	Acceptable range in any one plant
Rate	53–63 c/min	6 c/min
Ratio	55–70%	8 percentage points
d-value	Not less than 15%	Not less than 15%

Milking machines and mastitis

The milking machine can act as a vector in three ways: (i) cow-to-cow transfer of bacteria via contaminated clusters; (ii) internal flow between clusters within the plant; and (iii) quarter-to-quarter transfer within the cow via the claw.

A farm survey in Ireland in 1967 showed a highly significant regression of bulk milk cell count on effective reserve of the milking plant, i.e. as effective reserve decreased cell count increased (Nyhan & Cowhig, 1967). Subsequent work showed that unstable vacuum (a combination of large irregular fluctuations and moderate cyclic fluctuations) caused higher new infection rates than stable vacuum.

Further work carried out at the National Institute for Research in Dairying at Reading in the early 1970s (Cousins, 1972; Cousins *et al.*, 1973; Thiel *et al.*, 1973) found that large irregular fluctuations or large cyclic fluctuations *per se* did not increase new infection rates. However, any combination of large irregular fluctuations with substantial cyclic fluctuations caused a large increase in new infections. The results also suggested that infections were most likely to be initiated towards the end of milking.

During the late 1970s research workers at Moorepark in Ireland (O'Callaghan *et al.*, 1976; O'Shea *et al.*,

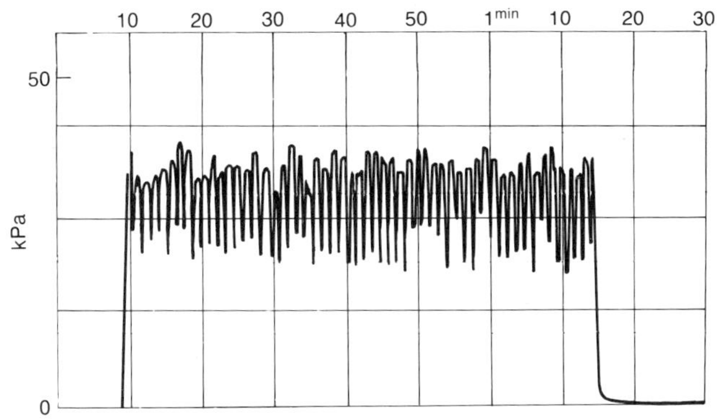

Fig. 24.5 Vacuum changes (cyclic fluctuations) at the teat end during milk flow.

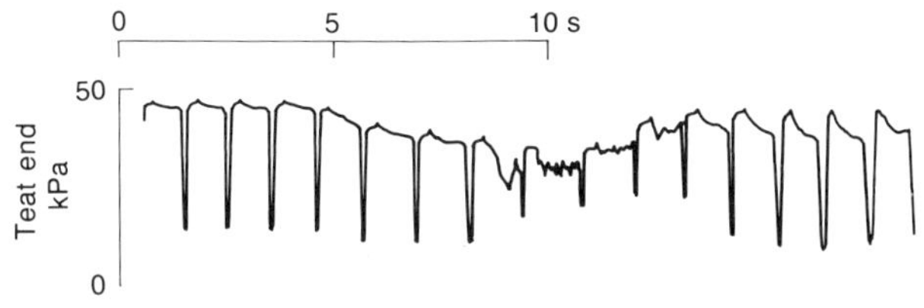

Fig. 24.6 Vacuum changes (irregular fluctuations) at the teat end during milk flow. Source: Nyhan (1968).

1976, 1979, 1981; O'Shea & O'Callaghan, 1978, 1982) showed that plant vacuum stability *per se* had little effect on new infection rate. It was suggested that the effect of generalized vacuum instability is mediated via increased liner slip, i.e. sudden air admission between the liner and the teat. Liner slip, in turn, is largely a function of liner design and also of vacuum stability.

When slip occurred in one quarter, impacts of milk

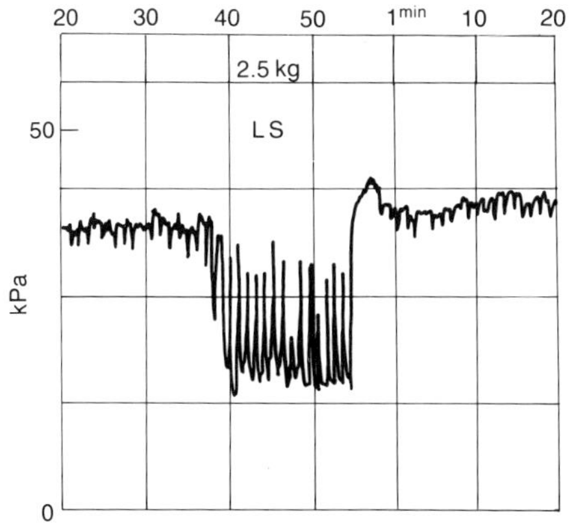

Fig. 24.7 Liner slip at the teat end during milk flow. LS, liner slip; 2.5 kg, flow rate of 2.5 kg/min.

droplets were detected in other quarters connected by the claw to the teat in which the slip occurred and a high number of new infections occurred in these impacted quarters.

This liner slip theory is compatible with many other results. Liner slips are more frequent at fore teats, the infections are more often seen in hind teats (Rabold & Pichler, 1980). Slip frequency is most common at morning milkings and at high flow rates and infections are most frequent in cows with high milk flow rate (O'Shea *et al.*, 1980).

Further work carried out on simulated liner slips at Moorepark in the early 1980s (O'Shea *et al.*, 1981) yielded the following results.

1 There were equal numbers of new infections with inaudible and audible liner slips.

2 Liner slips at the start of milking or the end of milking only, or during the total milking period caused almost equal numbers of new infections.

3 Liner slips increased new infections when teats were heavily contaminated with environmental bacteria (*Escherichia coli* and *Streptococcus dysgalactiae*).

Liner slip is now considered to be the major mechanism of spread of mastitis at milking.

Developments in milking machine technology

Shields

During the late 1970s research workers at Reading developed shields (deflector plates) in the teat cup chamber between the short milk tube and the teat end (Fig. 24.8). Trials on 15 herds in England and 16 herds in Australia showed that the shields prevented about 10 per cent of quarters from becoming infected (Griffin *et al.*, 1980a).

Ball claw

In the early 1980s research workers at Reading developed a cluster to prevent the transfer of pathogens between teats during milking (Griffin *et al.*, 1980b). It was a simple practical modification of the clawpiece to contain one-way valves within the clawpiece for each of the four short milk tube connectors (Fig. 24.9). Field trials showed an overall 14 per cent reduction in new infection rate due to the clawpiece (Griffin *et al.*, 1982). However, there was an unexpected larger reduction (17 per cent) in new infection rates from environmental sources of exposure (*Streptococcus uberis*, coliforms and others) than those (8 per cent) transmitted mainly at milking time within the udder or on teat sores

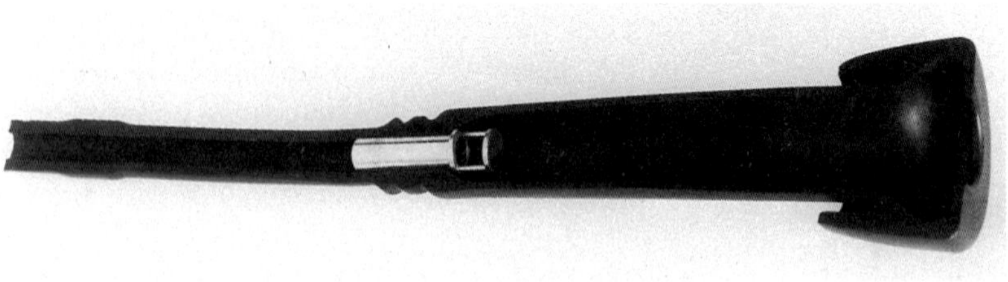

Fig. 24.8 Shielded liner. Photo courtesy Institute of Animal Health (IAH), Compton.

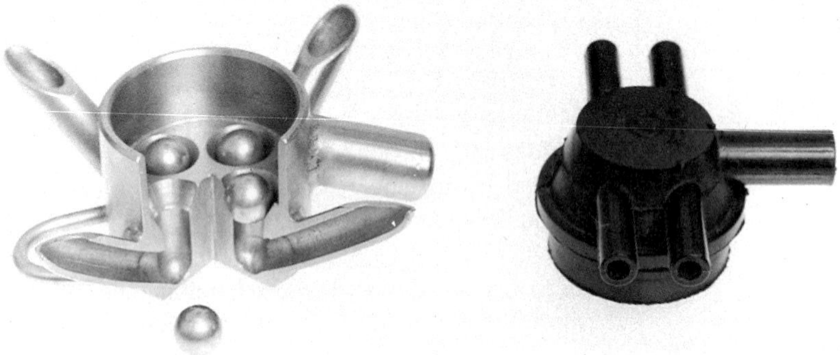

Fig. 24.9 Ball claw cluster. Photo courtesy IAH, Compton.

(*Staphylococcus aureus*, *Strep. agalactiae* and *Strep. dysgalactiae*).

Hydraulic milking

Following research on the ball claw, Griffin and Grindal carried out an experiment to ascertain the effects of blocking the air bleed on new infections. Initial results were promising and this new method of milking was christened 'hydraulic milking'. Research at Compton on the ball claw under hydraulic milking conditions has shown that as the liner starts to open high vacuum levels (up to 90 kPa) are generated beneath the teat (Grindal, 1987). Although high vacuum levels have been shown to increase teat damage during conventional milking (Smith & Peterson, 1946) further trials with hydraulic milking have not shown them to be a problem. Trials on the effect of hydraulic milking on new infection rate are ongoing at the moment.

Two other products, mimicking the effect of the ball claw, appeared on the market in 1985 and claimed to carry all the benefits of hydraulic milking at a fraction of the cost of the ball claw.

In the first of these a ball was put in the short milk tube. Research workers in Australia stated that they did not recommend the use of these one-way valves in the short milk tube as they were concerned that the valves might increase mastitis if the air admission hole in the clawpiece became blocked (G.A. Mein, pers. comm.).

The second of these was where the ball was placed in the liner. Results, so far, with this product have only shown a reduction in total bacterial count.

Large-bore pipelines

These have come from the USA where it is not uncommon to see milk lines of 75 mm (3 inches) in diameter. At present, there are standards recommended for sizes of pipelines by the International Dairy Federation group (Table 24.2).

At a National Mastitis Council Meeting in the USA, it was stated that the American standards for 38 mm (1½ inches) and 50 mm (2 inches) pipes are reasonable while the 62 mm (2½ inches) and 75 mm (3 inches) may not have been thoroughly evaluated (Spencer, 1981).

Isolator claw

This claw was developed in the early 1980s in New Zealand to counter the problem of mastitis cross-

Table 24.2 Recommendations for sizes of milking pipelines. Source: O'Callaghan *et al.* (1982)

Number of units	Minimum bore of milking pipeline (mm)
2–5	31
6–8	38
9–20	50

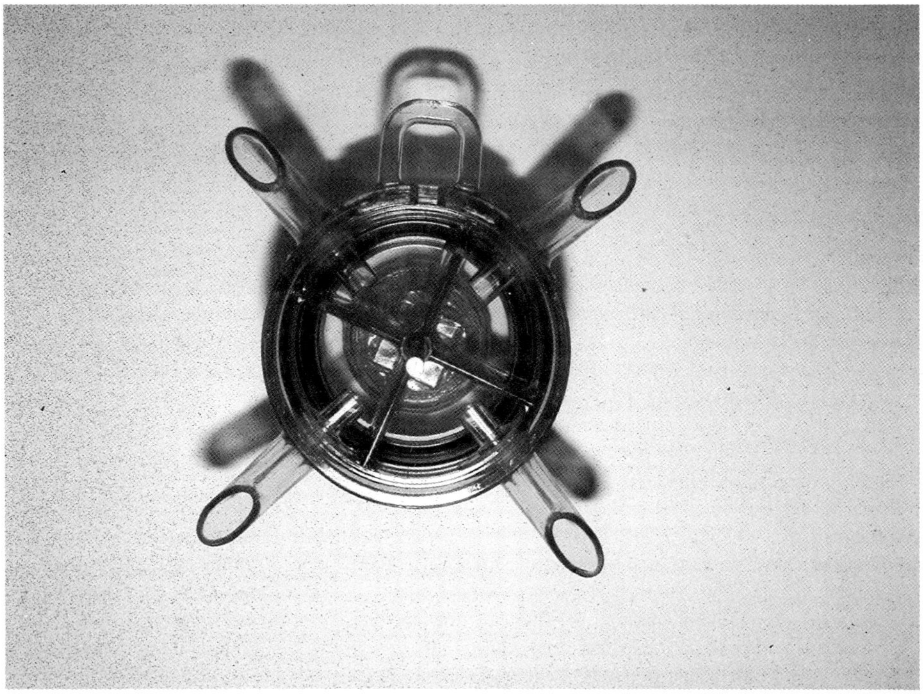

Fig. 24.10 Isolator claw.

infection. The isolator body has internal plastic walls that divide it into four individual sections, so there is no mixing with milk from the other three quarters (Fig. 24.10). A trial carried out on identical twin first-lactation heifers, where one twin was milked with a conventional claw and one with the isolator claw, showed that those milked with the isolator claw had lower cell counts and produced an average of 9 kg of fat more than their twins milked with the conventional claw. A claimed feature of the isolator claw is its ability to offer vacuum balancing, and thus reduce liner slip (Leitch, 1986).

Control measures

The milking machine is only one component that can be involved in mastitis. Mastitis control involves continual implementation of each of the recommendations in the five-point control programme. Changing some of the components in the milking machine may help in the short term but only a concerted effort in carrying out the full programme will control mastitis in a herd in the long run.

The following points are recommendations that should help to reduce mastitis resulting from the milking machine.

1 Maintain proper vacuum levels.
2 Attach and remove clusters properly to minimize massive changes of vacuum and entry of air into the clawpiece.
3 Make sure clusters are attached properly on each cow.
4 Select liners with low slip characteristics.
5 Dry teats before attaching clusters in order to reduce the numbers of bacteria.
6 Have the machine tested at least once a year.

References

Cousins, C.L. (1972) *The relationship between the milking machine and new intramammary infection.* PhD Thesis, University of Reading.

Cousins, C.L., Thiel, C.C., Westgarth, D.R. & Higgs, T.M. (1973) Further short-term studies of the influence of the milking machine on the rate of new mastitis infections. *Journal of Dairy Research*, **40**, 289–92.

Griffin, T.K., Mein, G.A., Westgarth, D.R., Neave, F.K., Thompson, W.H. & Maguire, P.D. (1980a) Effect of deflector shields fitted in the milking machine teat cup liner on bovine udder disease. *Journal of Dairy Research*, **47**, 1–9.

Griffin, T.K., Bramley. A.J. & Dodd, F.H. (1980b) Milking machine modifications in the control of bovine mastitis. In *Proceedings of the International Workshop on Machine Milking and Mastitis*, Moorepark, pp. 19–29.

Griffin, T.K., Grindal, R.J., Staker, R.T., Shearn, M.F.H., Bramley, A.J., Simpkin, D.L. Higgs, T.M. & Westgarth, D.R. (1982) Development and evaluation of control techniques for bovine mastitis. Control of intramammary infection by

modification of the design of the milking machine. Report of the National Institute for Research in Dairying, Reading, pp. 37–8.
Grindal, R.J. (1987) Efect of ball-valve milking clusters on udder disease. *Veterinary Record*, **121**, 250–2.
Leitch, J. (1986) In isolation. *Dairy Farmer*, **33**, 30–1.
Mein, G.A. (1984) Simple 'on-farm' checks of a milking installation. Interpretation of machine test report forms. Seminar for Veterinarians on Machine Milking and Mastitis, Werribee, Australia.
Nyhan, J.F. (1968) The effect of vacuum fluctuations on udder disease. In *Proceedings of the Symposium on Machine Milking*, Reading, pp. 71–82.
Nyhan, J.F. & Cowhig, M.J. (1967) Inadequate milking machine vacuum reserve and mastitis. *Veterinary Record*, **81**, 122–5.
O'Callaghan, E., O'Shea, J., Meaney, W.J. & Crowley, C. (1976) Effect of milking machine vacuum fluctuations and liner slip on bovine mastitis infectivity. *Irish Journal of Agricultural Research*, **15**, 401–17.
O'Callaghan, E., O'Shea, J., Kavanagh, A.J. & Doyle, H.J. (1982) Machine milking and milking facilities. An Foras Taluntais, p. 24.
O'Shea, J. (1982) Milking machines — the function and performance of components. *Irish Veterinary Journal*, **36**, 78–87.
O'Shea, J. & O'Callaghan, E. (1978) Milking machine effects on new infection rate. In *Proceedings of the International Symposium on Machine Milking and Mastitis*, 17th Annual Meeting of the National Mastitis Council, Louisville, Kentucky, pp. 262–8.
O'Shea, J. & O'Callaghan, E. (1982) The effect of liner slip on mastitis infection rates. In *Proceedings of the Conference on Dairy Production from Pasture*, Hamilton, New Zealand Society of Animal Production, pp. 77–8.
O'Shea, J., O'Callaghan, E., Meaney, W. & Crowley, C. (1976) Effects of combinations of large and small irregular and cyclic vacuum fluctuations in the milking machine on the rate of new udder infection in dairy cows. *Irish Journal of Agricultural Research*, **15**, 377–99.
O'Shea, J. O'Callaghan, E. & Meaney W.J. (1979) Relationship between milking machine and the incidence of mastitis in dairy cows. *Irish Journal of Agricultural Research*, **18**, 225–35.
O'Shea, J., O'Callaghan, E. & Lenoard, R.O. (1980) Milking performance of commercial clusters with standard pulsation. In *Experiments on Milking Machine Components at Moorepark, 1976–1979*, pp. 40–64.
O'Shea, J., O'Callaghan, E. & Meaney W.J. (1981) Incidence of new infection in dairy cows subjected to solenoid-induced air blasts during milking. *Irish Journal of Agricultural Research*, **20**, 163–83.
Rabold, K. & Pichler, D. (1980) Some environmental influences on mastitis of cow herds in South Germany. In *Proceedings of the International Workshop on Machine Milking and Mastitis*, Moorepark, pp. 121–7.
Smith, V.R. & Peterson, W.E. (1946) The effect of increasing the negative pressure and widening the vacuum release ratio on the rate of removal of milk from the udder. *Journal of Dairy Research*, **29**, 45–53.
Spencer, S.B. (1981) Sizing milking systems — a review. Annual Meeting of the National Mastitis Council, pp. 141–6.
Thiel, C.C., Cousins, C.L., Westgarth, D.R. & Neave, F.K. (1973) The incidence of some physical characteristics of the milking machine on the rate of new infection. *Journal of Dairy Research*, **40**, 117–29.

Chapter 25: Skin Infections of the Bovine Teat and Udder and Their Differential Diagnosis

by J.K. SHEARER, T. TESOPGONI AND E.P.J. GIBBS

Introduction

Teat lesions in milking cattle are due to a variety of causes, infectious and non-infectious. Viral skin infections of the bovine teat and udder are principally due to pseudocowpox virus, bovine herpesvirus 2 and papillomavirus, but, on occasions, teat lesions may occur in association with a generalized viral infection, such as foot-and-mouth disease, vesicular stomatitis, or mucosal disease. Although the vernacular use of 'cowpox' to describe any teat infection is common, cowpox (as caused by cowpox virus) is an unusual disease and has been recognized only in Europe.

There are several bacterial and non-infectious skin conditions of the teats and udder (as will be summarized later, see p. 327) that can be equally as troublesome as viral infections. Irrespective of cause, when teat infections occur in a milking herd they predispose cattle to secondary bacterial infection by *Staphylococcus aureus*, *Streptococcus dysgalactiae* and other bacteria. Cows, particularly newly calved heifers, become difficult to milk and the milking time may be prolonged by as much as 50 per cent.

Currently, there are no vaccines in use to protect cattle from any of the viral diseases and treatment is palliative. Differentiation of the diseases affecting the teats and skin of the udder is important, however, for reasons of public health and exotic disease control; cowpox and pseudocowpox are zoonotic diseases causing skin infections that can affect herdsmen and any vesicular lesions on the teats should always raise suspicion of foot-and-mouth disease.

In this chapter, particular attention is given to pseudocowpox and bovine herpes mammillitis, the two diseases that cause greatest concern to dairy farmers in the industrial nations of the world.

Infectious lesions of the teat (see Table 25.1)

Bovine herpes mammillitis

Aetiology

Bovine herpes mammillitis (BHM) is caused by bovine herpesvirus 2 and is closely related, if not identical, to Allerton virus, the causative agent of pseudo-lumpy skin disease; it is unrelated to bovine herpes virus 1, the aetiological agent of infectious bovine rhinotracheitis (see p. 256).

The genome is linear double-stranded DNA, 220 kbp. The virus produces intranuclear inclusions and syncytia in infected cells.

Epidemiology

Also known as bovine ulcerative mammillitis, BHM was first recognized in Scotland. The virus has since

Table 25.1 Infectious conditions of the teat and udder skin of cattle

Cowpox and vaccinia
Pseudocowpox
Bovine herpes mammillitis
Bovine papillomatosis (warts)
As part of generalized disease, e.g.
foot-and-mouth disease
rinderpest
lumpy skin disease
mycotic dermatitis

been isolated from affected cattle world-wide in countries such as the USA, Australia and Brazil.

In the northern hemisphere, BHM commonly occurs as a seasonal disease between August and December. In a completely susceptible herd, the disease spreads quickly with nearly all cows developing infection over one to two months. In other herds, only the newly calved heifers introduced into the milking herd for the first time are affected. Recrudescence of clinical disease is unusual, even though latent infections do occur. Whether latently infected older cattle are the reservoir of infection from which the newly calved heifers become infected is conjectural. It is thought that susceptible pregnant cows may become infected some time before parturition, but do not develop lesions until calving.

The method of transmission of the virus between farms with closed herds is unknown, although biting flies have been incriminated as possible vectors.

Clinical signs and lesions

Bovine herpes mammillitis is a disease initially characterized by a painful oedematous teat swelling. The incubation period ranges from three to seven days. The disease is generally more severe than either cowpox or pseudocowpox and the lesions are ulcerative rather than proliferative. Newly calved heifers are usually the most severely affected, particularly if they have postparturient oedema of the udder. Initial lesions are followed by the development of an irregularly shaped vesicle (0.5–5.0 cm in diameter) (plate 25.1). Within 24 hours, the vesicles rupture, leaving an ulcerated surface that exudes copious serum (plate 25.2). Upon drying this exudate forms a thick, dark reddish-brown scab (plates 25.3 and 25.4). In the absence of secondary infection, healing is complete in three weeks by granulation and regrowth of the epithelium (plates 25.5–8). Lesions on the udder may coalesce with those of the teat and may extend to the perineum resulting in vulvovaginitis as a sequel to infection of the skin of the mammary gland.

Differential diagnosis

Bovine herpes mammillitis usually occurs in summer and autumn. The oedema of teats, vesication and ulceration and extensive scab formation over most of the teat surface is strongly suggestive of BHM. Epidemics of BHM can occur in a region, which can lend support to the diagnosis.

Pseudocowpox

Aetiology

Initially confused with cowpox virus, it was not until 1963 that it was demonstrated in the USA that pseudocowpox virus was a member of the genus *Parapoxvirus*. Pseudocowpox virus is closely related to the virus of orf (contagious ecthyma, contagious pustular dermatitis) of sheep, and also to the bovine papular stomatitis virus (see p. 216).

The virus contains a linear double-stranded DNA, 130 kbp, and produces intracytoplasmic inclusions in infected cells.

Epidemiology

Referred to in the past as false cowpox, varicella, waterpox, udderpox and natural cowpox, pseudocowpox occurs in most countries of the world. It is the most common cause of teat lesions in North America and the UK. Lesions of pseudocowpox may be seen in a herd during any season of the year. The immunity is short-lived, lasting four to six months; thus, pseudocowpox is commonly seen as a chronic problem in most herds. Nevertheless, it may occur as an acute herd problem, which spreads rapidly affecting a majority of the cows in the herd. Lesions in such primary outbreaks are frequently more extensive.

Clinical signs and lesions

After an incubation period of about six days, localized erythematous and oedematous areas appear on the teats. These lesions are painful, making cows difficult to milk. Within 48 hours, a small orange papule develops, followed by the formation of an elevated small dark red scab (2–3 mm) (plate 25.9). In some cases, a vesicle will form in the centre of the papule, but this is rare with pseudocowpox in contrast to bovine herpes mammillitis. The progressive enlargement of the edges of the lesions leads to umbilication of the central scab (plate 25.10). Healing of the lesion is centrifugal and the primary scab is often shed after 10 to 12 days, leaving the classical raised 'horseshoe' or 'ring' lesion, which is pathognomonic for pseudocowpox (plate 25.11). As adjacent lesions enlarge, they may coalesce to form linear scabs extending the entire length of the teat (plate 25.12). Pseudocowpox lesions are primarily found on the teat; however, 5–10 per cent of affected animals develop lesions on the udder. Healing usually occurs within four to five weeks, leaving no scars. In herds where 'teat chaps' are common, pseudocowpox virus can be detected in many of the lesions.

In man, pseudocowpox virus causes a localized infection on the fingers or hands, commonly called 'milker's nodule'. These nodules are painful and may extend to the entire arm of the person affected.

Differential diagnosis

In contrast to BHM, pseudocowpox is a chronic problem in most herds. Lesions are proliferative, progressing to small 'ring' or 'horseshoe' type lesions rather than ulcerative. Atypical lesions (plates 25.13–16) may be observed and confused with warts or mild traumatic injuries to the teats and udder but, in general, a careful examination of the herd will allow the clinician to differentiate pseudocowpox from other diseases. It must be remembered that pseudocowpox is often present in herds where the major problem may be due to BHM or even cowpox.

Cowpox

Aetiology

Cowpox virus shares with Jenner a central role in the development of vaccines and the control of smallpox in man. The current use of vaccinia virus (the derivative virus used for protection of man from smallpox) in a new role as a recombinant vaccine vector for many diseases, maintains attention on cowpox. Few people realize that cowpox was considered an unusual disease even in Jenner's time. Occasional outbreaks of cowpox still occur in cattle in Europe, but from the perspective of the dairy industry they are of little importance.

The causative agent of cowpox is an orthopoxvirus, very similar to, but distinguishable from, vaccinia virus by its biological properties in laboratory animals and its larger genome (220 kbp compared with 185 kbp for vaccinia virus). The virus produces intracytoplasmic inclusions in affected cells.

Epidemiology

The epizootiology of cowpox is unknown. Cowpox virus has been isolated from skin infections in man and carnivores in which no direct contact with cattle could be established. It is currently thought that a reservoir exists, possibly rodents.

Once infection is present within a herd, however, the disease appears to spread by the milking machine and the hands of milkers. Between and within herds, biting insects may also be responsible for mechanical transmission. At present, the disease is confined to western Europe. In other areas of the world, outbreaks of teat lesions, clinically indistinguishable from cowpox but caused by vaccinia virus from an uncovered vaccination site in an attendant, have been reported. Since the eradication of smallpox in 1979, most countries have discontinued vaccination against smallpox, although military personnel in the USA are still vaccinated. Currently, there is little likelihood of vaccinia infections occurring naturally on the teats of cattle in most parts of the world, but if widespread use of vaccinia recombinants becomes popular, either in man or domestic animals, a resurgence in vaccinia mammillitis in cattle is conceivable.

Clinical signs and lesions

The incubation period is approximately five days, after which an irregular prodromal fever and tenderness of the teats is noticed. A roseolar erythema occurs at the side of future pock development: oedema may be localized to the area of the erythema, or may involve the whole teat. A vesicle forms three to four days after the initial onset of signs (plate 25.17) and rapidly progresses to a pustule, which subsequently ruptures and suppurates (plate 25.18). The classical development of a thick red scab ranging in size from 1 to 2 cm in diameter and said to be pathognomonic for cowpox may now form (plate 25.19), but more frequently an ulcerated surface is observed (plate 25.20). Healing is centripetal and, in uncomplicated cases, takes place within three weeks. Immunity to re-infection is said to be lifelong.

Laboratory diagnosis

SAMPLE COLLECTION

An accurate laboratory diagnosis depends upon the quality of the samples submitted. Whenever a viral aetiology is suspected, the clinician should remember the following points.

1 During the early stages of the disease, the titre of virus is the highest at the affected sites.
2 Viruses only replicate in living cells and light exposure, desiccation, disinfectants and extreme pH are likely to inactivate them.
3 Samples taken at the later stages of the disease are often contaminated by bacteria.

Skin scrapings should be collected from animals with early lesions and should be kept on cold packs during submission to the laboratory. Samples intended for virus isolation should be collected into virus transport medium.

DIAGNOSTIC TECHNIQUES

Electron microscopy

Skin scrapings for electron microscopy should be submitted in a sterile bottle without additive. Direct observation of virus by electron microscopy is rapid and has the advantages of detecting combined virus infections and non-viable virus.

Tissue culture

Isolation of virus in tissue culture may be used when electron microscopy is not available. Vesicular fluids, early scabs and scrapings from the underlying raw surface of lesions are appropriate samples. Some strains of pseudocowpox fail to grow *in vitro*. Tissue culture has the advantage that vaccinia virus can be distinguished from cowpox virus.

Histological identification

Collecting a biopsy of a teat lesion is seldom easy. If one is collected, the tissue should be preserved in 10 per cent formol saline or preferably Bouin's solution. Each of the infections discussed above has a characteristic histopathology if an early lesion is sampled.

Paired serum samples

Blood should be collected during the acute stage of the disease and again 14 days later for serological diagnosis. A fourfold rise in antibody can be demonstrated for cowpox and BHM infections, but no serological response is generally detected to pseudocowpox.

Treatment

There is no specific treatment for viral skin infections of the teat and udder; treatment is palliative and symptomatic. Topical corticosteroids can reduce the inflammation of BHM and topical anaesthetic ointment will alleviate the pain, but treatment is expensive and difficult to justify for an entire herd. Antibiotics may be necessary to control secondary bacterial infection.

Prevention and control

When practical to do so, new animals should be examined and quarantined 14 days prior to their introduction into the herd. Infected cows should be isolated and milked last. Effective fly control should be instituted to minimize mechanical transmission. Teat cups of the milking machine as well as the milker's gloves should be disinfected between cows. These measures should help to reduce the spread of the virus within and between herds. Premilking and postmilking teat dipping and wearing of gloves by milkers are probably the most effective approaches.

Non-infectious lesions of the teat end
(see Table 25.2)

Introduction

In addition to infectious lesions of the bovine teat are those caused by traumatic events, chemical injury, environmental conditions, insects and the milking machine. As discussed earlier, teat lesions, regardless of cause, are frequently colonized by staphylococci and *Strep. dysgalactiae*. Consequently, high new infection rates and increased numbers of clinical cases of mastitis are common sequelae in herds where teat lesions are prevalent (plate 25.21).

Teat trauma

Traumatic lesions of the teat are most commonly the result of the cow stepping on her teats or wire cuts.

Table 25.2 Non-infectious conditions of the teat and udder skin of cattle

Traumatic, e.g.
barbed wire
grazing kale
mud
'treads'
Irritant chemicals, e.g.
incorrect strength disinfectants
any corrosive agent
Photosensitization
Excessive postparturient oedema

They are a troublesome problem for the veterinarian as well as the dairyman. Histologically, the teat wall contains an abundance of elastic connective tissue that provides for expansion and contraction of the teat as it fills and evacuates milk in the lactating cow. The near constant movement associated with these physical dynamics of the teat combined with milking preparation procedures and milk collection complicate the normal process of healing.

The dairyman's challenge is in getting cows with teat lesions milked. Because these lesions are generally painful and cows resist preparation and milking procedures they are difficult if not hazardous to milk.

A further complication is mastitis. Teat lesions are readily colonized by bacteria and thus serve as an important reservoir of infection. Udder preparation cloths, hands of the milker and milking machine components facilitate the transfer of infectious organisms between quarters of the same cow and can be responsible for cow-to-cow transmission as well. Emphasis on milking hygiene procedures becomes crucial in control of new infections whenever teat lesions are present.

Depending on severity and the period of time prior to discovery, teat lacerations may be repaired surgically. Fresh superficial lacerations of the teat skin (within 12 hours of occurrence) in which the vascular supply has not been significantly damaged have the best prognosis. These are generally amenable to surgical closure. If, on the other hand, such lesions go unnoticed for a couple of days and become heavily contaminated, cleansing in mild disinfectant solution and removal of the skin flap tissue are likely to be the best therapeutic approach.

Teat lacerations that extend into the teat cistern are of greater concern and generally carry a more guarded prognosis. The exposed edges of the cistern lining must be sutured using a suture pattern that will turn the edges inward creating an impervious seal. If this is not achieved healing cannot occur and draining fistulae develop. The teat wall muscle layers and the skin may be closed separately or individually. Most advise intramammary and/or systemic therapy for four to five days as a precaution against the development of mastitis. A protective bandage allowing access to the teat end for milking is recommended. Milk should be retrieved from the gland through the use of teat cannulas.

Pastured cattle have a lower incidence of teat trauma than confined cattle. Housing factors of primary importance are associated with the amount of space available to the cow for resting and rising. Further, individual cow characteristics and conformation increase the potential for teat trauma in some cows.

Chemical injury

Teat lesions resulting from chemical injury most often occur as a result of the application of a defective teat-dip product. Iodophor-based teat dips, possibly because of their widespread use, are frequently the offenders. However, the problem has been observed with quaternary ammonium dips, chlorhexidine-based dips, dodecyl benzene sulfonic acid and hypochlorite teat dips. Lesions appear as dry, roughened, proliferative regions around the teat end that are usually discoloured by the teat dip. This discolouration may be present on 40–50 per cent of the teats in the affected herd. Changing to a dip with better conditioning properties will result in the rapid improvement of teat skin health.

In the case of iodophor dips, problems have arisen secondary to inadvertent freezing of the dip on-farm or in transit. When these solutions freeze they separate sending emollients to the bottom of the container and leaving excessive amounts of the active ingredients in a layer suspended above. The subsequent application of this concentrated iodine causes teat irritation and lesions. Depending on the degree of insult these lesions can be quite severe.

The mistaken use of a concentrated udder wash solution in place of a teat dip causes a more severe type of lesion and often affects up to 80–90 per cent of the herd. The lesion is characterized by scab formation over the distal portion of the teat exposed to the dip solution.

On occasion the addition of lime or other chemicals to the bedding material will result in teat skin and udder irritation. Lesions tend to be worse on the lateral sides of the teats and may extend onto the sides of the udder.

Environmental injury

TEAT CHAPS

Teat chapping is a common problem in the more temperate regions of the world where climatic conditions favouring dampness and cooler temperatures prevail. Activities associated with milking such as udder preparation, the milking process and postmilking teat dipping all exacerbate chapping problems. Chaps usually occur as horizontal cracks in the teat skin. Serum exudates from these cracks result in the formation of linear scabs (plate 25.22). The surrounding teat skin may appear dry or leather-like and flake.

The primary significance of chaps is that they are readily colonized by staphylococci and *Strep. dysgalactiae* and thus constitute a threat to individual cows affected as well as the herd. Drying of the teats and udders before cows leave the milking parlour, particularly during inclement weather conditions, is an important preventive measure. Further, the use of teat-dip products containing hydroscopic skin softening agents such as glycerine or lanolin are helpful in controlling chapping problems.

FREEZING OR FROST-BITE

Initially, frozen teats will appear reddened or pale. If severe the lesion progresses to the state where a scab forms over the distal half of the teat. In time, usually several days, this scab will loosen and fall off exposing a raw denuded teat end. As a second scab begins to develop the duct becomes occluded. Milking becomes difficult and may require opening of the streak canal surgically.

In less severe cases, scab formation does not occur and cows become receptive to milking after only a few days. Cows immediately leaving the milking parlour with wet teats (from dip or milk) to areas with inadequate protection during cold weather may develop frost-bite on the teat ends. Freezing of the droplet on the teat end confines the lesion to the teat-end orifice area. The result is as described above for frozen teats.

Treatment consists of attempts at keeping the teat duct patent and preventing the development of mastitis. Severely affected cows may need to be culled. Drying of the teats and udder prior to exit from the milking parlour and providing adequate wind breaks and shelter for milking cows is essential. The suspension of teat dipping procedures should be considered during extremely cold weather.

SUNBURN

Severe reddening and drying of the teats and udder are observed in sunburn conditions, when severe blisters may form. The application of moisturizers, ointments, and salves to the affected areas are advised for treatment.

PHOTOSENSITIZATION (see p. 686)

This condition occurs when photodynamic agents are eaten in their preformed state. Upon exposure to sunlight, the unpigmented skin areas develop an erythema and oedema, which results in severe lesions that most commonly appear on the lateral aspects of the teats and udder (plate 25.23). These lesions are highly susceptible to secondary bacterial infection.

Milking machine-induced teat lesions

Malfunctioning milking equipment can result in damage to the teat. This damage may be by direct trauma to the teat or indirect, occurring over an extended period of time through the induction of degenerative changes in the teat. These changes in teat tissue health are primarily associated with circulatory disturbances. Proper pulsation is essential for the circulation of blood and lymph in the teat. When normal circulation is disrupted teat-end health diminishes.

Direct damage to the teat may be caused by excessive milking vacuum, inadequate pulsation, and careless use by the operator. Subcutaneous haemorrhages in the teat epithelium and prolapses of teat duct tissue are possible consequences with severe malfunctions of milking equipment or its use.

Insect-induced teat lesions

Summer mastitis is an acute suppurative disease of the non-lactating mammary gland. First described in Europe, in recent years it has been reported in the USA and other countries as well. It occurs sporadically throughout the year in Europe with annual incidences in England and Wales estimated to be around 2 per cent of heifers and dry cows. In the USA some estimate incidences of 5–6 per cent on certain farms during the summer months.

While some questions remain, in both the USA and Europe epidemics of summer mastitis have been coincident with periods of greatest fly challenge. Further, data indicate that effective fly control reduces disease incidence. These findings support the possibility of insect involvement. European data suggest that biting flies are responsible for the initial damage to the teat end and implicate the cattle fly, *Hydrotaea irritans*, as the infection vector in summer mastitis (see Chapter 22).

Differential diagnosis of skin lesions of the bovine teat

The following is an aid to the diagnosis of lesions of the udder and teats in severely affected milking herds (see Table 25.3). With the exception of teat chapping, the aetiology of which appears to be complex, most outbreaks of teat lesions in cows are due to three types of virus: (i) cowpox, (ii) pseudocowpox and (iii) BHM.

Accurate diagnosis is important for various reasons. A major factor is the zoonotic potential of cowpox and pseudocowpox. Secondly, there is the need to differentiate foot-and-mouth disease as occasionally vesicles

Table 25.3 The clinical appearance and diagnostic procedures for teat conditions (other than BHM, cowpox, bovine vaccinia mammillitis and pseudocowpox)

Condition	Clinical appearance	Confirmatory diagnostic procedure
Blackspot (plate 25.27)	Scabby infection of teat orifice with *Fusiformis necrophorus* but often other organisms	Isolation of *F. necrophorus* (often unsuccessful)
Chaps (teat) (see Plate 25.22)	Skin fissures often through dermis. Haemorrhage may occur with scab formation at the fissure edge. Often horizontal lesions	None. Parapex virus particles may be found but their importance unknown. Heavy bacterial contamination of lesion common
Folliculitis and impetigo	Pustule with surrounding erythema	Isolation of *Staphylococcus aureus*
Foot-and-mouth disease (see Plate 25.24)	Vesiculation of teat, buccal and interdigital mucosae. Pyrexia	Presence of virus. *Notifiable* in most countries
Mud abrasion (plate 25.28)	Abrasions on lateral surface of the udder	
Photosensitization (see Plate 25.23)	Lesion progresses from erythema, oedema to serous exudation through skin. There is then necrosis, ulceration and scab formation. Pigmented areas of teat unaffected	
Ringworm (plate 25.29)	Typical grey crusty lesions	Isolation of *Trichophyton verrucosum*
Theleitis and serous exudate from udder skin in peracute mastitis (plate 25.30)	Teat swollen, painful with udder skin involved. Cow febrile and toxic	Isolation of bacteria
Vesicular stomatitis	Vesiculation of teat, buccal and interdigital mucosae	Virus isolation. As similar to foot-and-mouth may need to notify
Warts		
Filiform (plate 25.31)	Pedunculated attachment to teat	
White nodule (plate 25.32)	Broad attachment to teat. Variable in size. Some warts intermediate between filiform and nodule	

occur on the teats before their appearance in the mouth and foot (plate 25.24).

When investigating an outbreak it is best to examine as many cattle as possible because the lesions in a single cow may not be typical. Often mixed disease occurs (plates 25.25 and 26) and an assessment of the development of lesions rather than just examination of the most severely affected cattle helps in the diagnosis.

On occasions the clinical appearance of the lesions can be modified by environmental factors, thereby making recognition of the condition difficult. Such factors include the teat cluster, mud or coloured teat dips. In these problems laboratory diagnosis becomes essential, although it is advisable in all disease investigations.

Further reading

Farnsworth, R.L. & Seiber, R.L. (1978) Relationship of teat end lesions to intramammary infections. *Proceedings of the National Mastitis Council*, pp. 17–24.

Francis, P.G. (1984) Teat skin lesions and mastitis. *British Veterinary Journal*, **140**, 430–6.

Gibbs, E.P.J. (1984) Viral diseases of the skin of the bovine teat and udder. *Veterinary Clinics of North America. Large Animal Practice*, **6**, 187–202.

Gibbs, E.P.J. & Rweyemamu, M.M. (1977) Bovine herpesvirus, 1, 2 & 3. *Veterinary Bulletin*, **47**, 317–43, 411–25.

Gibbs, E.P.J., Johnson, R.H. & Osborne, A.D. (1970) The differential diagnosis of viral skin infections of the bovine teat. *Veterinary Record*, **87**, 602–9.

Sieber, R.L. & Farnsworth, R.J. (1978) The etiology of bovine teat lesions. *Proceedings of the National Mastitis Council*, pp. 5–15.

Sieber, R.L. & Farnsworth, R.J. (1984) Differential diagnosis of bovine teat lesions. *Veterinary Clinics of North America. Large Animal Practice*, **6**, 313–21.

Chapter 26: Factors Affecting Milk Quality

by R.W. BLOWEY

Introduction

Most countries with a developed dairy industry now pay producers on the basis of both total volume sold and compositional quality and with the slowly increasing move for a larger proportion of milk to be used for manufacturing, this trend is likely to continue. In addition, many countries also have a milk quota system and to maximize profitability, a farmer must produce a specified amount of milk of optimum quality. Much attention has therefore been paid to factors affecting milk quality the most important aspects of which are reviewed in this chapter. The composition of average Friesian/Holstein milk is given in Fig. 26.1. Feeding has by far the greatest impact on milk quality and as such will be discussed first.

Feeding and milk composition

This is an extremely complex area to study, since it is often difficult to differentiate the separate effects of, for example, plane of nutrition, system of allocation of food, frequency of feeding and feed composition. Superimposed on this are effects of feeding before and after calving and the problem of differentiating between compositional values and overall yield. For example, in a high-yielding cow the milk fat content (g/kg milk) may be reduced, but the overall fat production (kg/day) may be increased.

Feeding before calving

Severe underfeeding, leading to cows calving down in condition score 2 (overall scale 1–5, see p. 16) or less, will reduce milk yield, fat, protein and lactose and although these effects are greatest in early lactation, they will persist throughout it. The extent of the depression is approximately 20 g/kg (0.2 per cent) in milk fat and 10 g/kg in protein. Less severe underfeeding has little effect on milk protein, and provided that high quality diets are provided after calving, some of the effects on milk quality can be eliminated (Garnsworthy & Topps, 1982).

Very fat cows have an increased fat content in their milk, and it has been estimated that milk fat increases by 2 g/kg for each 1.0 unit rise in condition score. This effect lasts for the first five to six weeks of lactation only. It would appear that it is the overall degree of fatness at calving that affects milk quality: the level of feeding and rate of liveweight change prior to calving seems to have relatively little effect.

Feed constituents (see p. 87)

The greatest effect arises from the forage : concentrate ratio in the ration and its influence on milk fat content. Milk fat is synthesized from the fatty acids acetate and butyrate, products of the ruminal fermentation of forage and other feeds containing fibre. As the level

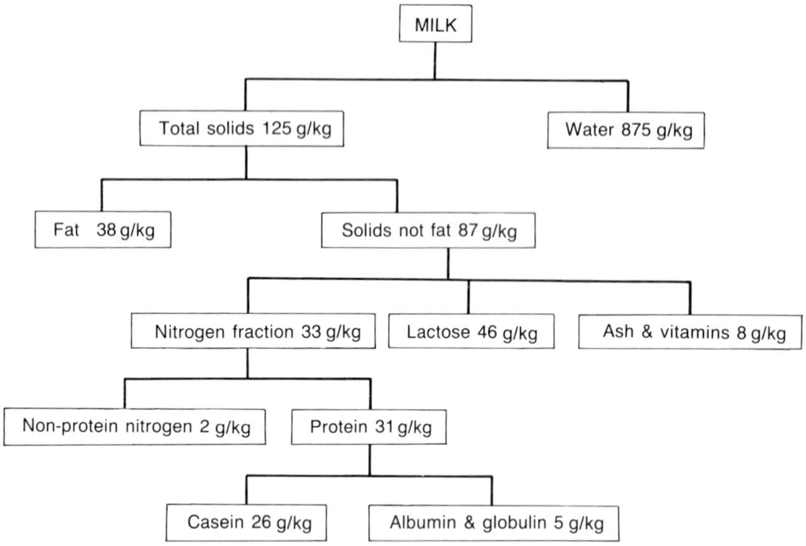

Fig. 26.1 The compositional quality of milk.

of concentrates in the ration increases, the proportions of acetate and butyrate fall and that of propionate rises. There is also a decrease in ruminal pH and a depressed activity of cellulolytic degradation, which can eventually result in depressed dry matter (DM) intake. The extent of the depression varies with the materials being fed, but as an approximate guide, forage : concentrate ratios should not be allowed to fall below 60:40. For example, Sutton (1986) calculated that milk fat fell by 5 g/kg (0.05 per cent) for every 100 g/kg decrease in the proportion of hay in the diet, even when the overall energy content of the ration remained constant. However, there was a good deal of variation and probably a better way of estimating dietary effect is to express the overall fibre content of the diet on the basis of acid detergent fibre (ADF). Milk fat has been shown to fall when overall dietary ADF drops to below 200–250 g/kg DM. This is equivalent to approximately 450 g long forage/kg dietary DM, although on much higher forage diets, milk yield could be depressed. The type of concentrate also has an effect. The energy fraction of a concentrate can be derived from four main sources, namely:

1 sugar, for example molasses;
2 starch, for example barley and maize;
3 digestible fibre, for example sugar-beet pulp, cotton seed, citrus pulp, etc.;
4 fats and oils.

Table 26.1 (Sutton *et al.*, 1985) shows that concentrates containing a high level of digestible fibre cause less depression of milk fat and produce an overall higher fat yield (kg/day), even though total milk volume is reduced due to lack of starch. This was particularly noticeable at the higher levels of concentrate feeding.

Table 26.1 Effect of proportion and type of concentrate in a mixed diet on milk production in early lactation. Source: Sutton *et al.* (1985)

	600 (g/kg diet)		700 (g/kg diet)	
	Starchy concentrate	Fibrous concentrate	Starchy concentrate	Fibrous concentrate
Consumed (kg air dry feed/day)				
Hay	7.2		3.5	
Concentrates	10.8		14.0	
Dietary ADF (g/kg DM)	192	231	136	180
Milk yield (kg/day)	26.3	26.5	32.0	25.5
Fat concentration (g/kg)	41.5	42.9	22.6	36.2
Fat yield (kg/day)	1.09	1.12	0.73	0.91

ADF, acid detergent fibre

It is, of course, the amount of starch in the ration and its conversion into propionate and glucose that is one of the main determinants of the volume of milk produced. The energy in digestible fibre products such as sugar-beet pulp is derived from cellulose and hemicelluloses and is slowly fermented. Maize is also slowly fermented and as such causes less depression of milk fat, compared with other more rapidly fermented starch sources such as barley. Uncooked ground maize will, to a certain extent, pass through the rumen and into the small intestine. This possibly explains why maize-based concentrates give an overall lower level of yield than conventional barley products. Both features are particularly noticeable at higher concentrate intakes. Root crops, e.g. fodder beet, have most of their energy stored as the sugar sucrose. Generally, they produce better levels of fat but lower yields than a comparable amount of starch.

The effect of diet on milk protein is almost the opposite to that seen with milk fat. On high-forage diets, increasing the proportion of concentrate in the ration (especially high-starch concentrate) will increase milk protein, but only up to a level of 50–60 per cent of concentrate in the diet. Beyond this, milk yield may rise and milk fat concentration will fall, but protein levels will remain constant. The net effect is an overall rise in protein yield. These changes are represented diagrammatically in Fig. 26.2. Clearly, within a quota system, there will be an optimal level for a farmer, both in terms of milk yield and milk quality, but this will depend on the economic milk price : concentrate cost ratio prevailing at the time, and a full discussion is well outside the scope of this review.

Of course, low forage intakes may not occur intentionally. Poor quality fodders such as very wet, very acid or very butyric silages will depress intakes and thereby increases the concentrate : forage ratio. A more common problem is probably inadequate access. Self-feeding consolidated silage, particularly behind an electric wire, may depress intakes of even good quality material by as much as 5–10 per cent and could further exacerbate the problem.

There is no requirement for 'long fibre' in the basal ration to maintain milk quality, and diets containing long fibre length generally give the same milk quality as finely chopped silage (Thomas, 1984). However, there is some evidence that silage diets give better milk quality than rations of equal metabolizable energy intake based on hay. Fine grinding of forage will depress milk fat when used as the sole ration, but if used as a supplement to conventional forage it has no effect (Thomas, 1984).

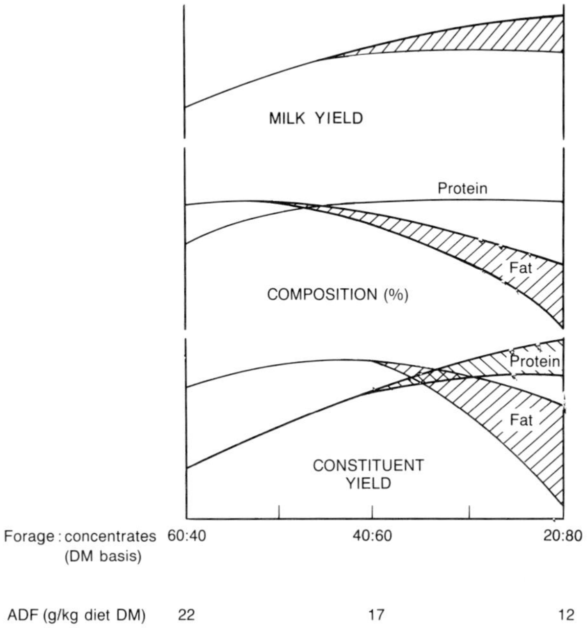

Fig. 26.2 The relationship between forage : concentrate ratio or acid detergent fibre (ADF) and milk yield and composition.

Dietary fat

Manufacturers may increase the energy content of a concentrate by adding fat, either directly into the product or by fat-spraying the outside of the cubes. Fat 'prills' may also be added to the ration, e.g. a complete diet, as a separate constituent. Provided that saturated (or 'hard') fats such as tallow, coconut or palm kernel oil are used, and only to a maximum of 5–6 per cent, this will increase the fat content of the milk. However, milk protein content will be slightly depressed, but as milk yield is likely to increase, overall milk protein yield remains constant. Levels of fat above 7 per cent interfere with ruminal function, leading to a depression of both total milk yields and the fat and protein contents. Increased levels of unsaturated ('soft') fats, such as maize, cotton seed, groundnut and especially fish oils, should not be used because they will coat the surface of fibre particles in the rumen, thereby depressing fibre digestion and leading to a fall in the milk fat content. If the fat can be made to bypass the rumen, e.g. by 'protecting' it with formaldehyde treatment, then there is no depression of fibre digestion and the long-chain fatty acids can be utilized more fully and overall milk fat rises. Protected fat will produce a depression of milk protein, especially if used at high levels. Certain feed components can be used to increase milk fat. For example, expelled palm kernel cake (6–8 per cent oil in DM) contains a high proportion of short-chain (C_{14}) fatty acids and when added to the diet at 1–2 kg/day will often boost butterfat. Palatability can sometimes be a problem however.

Dietary protein (see p. 84)

The effects of dietary protein on milk quality, including milk protein, are less well defined. It is the energy content of the ration that has the major effect on milk protein, particularly at high forage intakes. Severe dietary protein deficits will depress milk protein, although this may be partly because the requirements of the ruminal micro-organisms have not been met and as such total dry matter intake, and therefore the overall dietary energy intake, are inadequate.

Feeding systems

It is possible to overcome some of the effects of high concentrate, low forage diets by feeding the cows more frequently. In a series of experiments at the National Institute for Research in Dairying (Sutton, 1986), cows were given concentrate diets varying from 600 to 900 g/kg (namely 60 per cent to 10 per cent forage) fed either twice daily or up to six times daily. The results are given in Table 26.2 and show that for all levels of concentrate feeding, milk fat was higher with a greater frequency of daily feeds. As one might expect, the differential was greatest at the highest level of concentrate feeding, where twice daily feeding had produced a severe depression of milk fat. The concentrate used was a standard material containing high levels of starch. Had a highly digestible fibre product been used, it is unlikely that the depression of milk fat would have been so great — hence the response to more frequent feedings would also have been considerably less. It is generally assumed that diets leading to high propionate and low acetate in the rumen will reduce milk fat. However, increasing the frequency of feeding does not seem to depress propionate concentrations sufficiently to account for the full benefit to milk fat synthesis. It would appear that high plasma insulin concentrations are the main factor depressing milk fat and that the release of insulin is stimulated by peaks of propionate production, such as occurs after a large feed of concentrate, rather than the steady supply of propionate that will be a feature of more frequent feeding. The effect of increased levels of insulin is to promote lipogenesis in adipose rather than mammary tissue.

Table 26.2 Effect of number of daily meals of starch-based concentrates on milk yield and composition. Source: Sutton (1986)

Concentrates				
(kg/day)	10.0	11.5	12.8	14.0
(g/kg diet)	600	700	800	900
ADF (g/kg diet DM)	192	162	124	99
Milk yield (kg/day)				
2 meals	19.3	19.7	20.6	23.0
6 meals	20.8	20.2	24.5	21.4
Milk fat (g/kg)				
2 meals	34.3	32.6	31.6	17.9
6 meals	36.2	39.2	35.3	29.7
Milk protein (g/kg)				
2 meals	31.4	33.2	31.7	32.0
6 meals	31.8	34.1	31.2	33.2

Table 26.2 shows that milk protein is unaffected by frequency of feeding, or by the level of concentrate fed at these high levels of concentrate : forage ratio.

Complete diets (see p. 95) offer an opportunity for even feeds of concentrate throughout the day. When milk fat is low, due to depression by an excessive concentrate : forage ratio, feeding the same constituents in a complete diet will lead to an increase in the fat content. Milk protein may also increase on complete diets, but this is thought to be due to the effects of an increased dry matter intake, rather than any particular effect on frequency of feeding.

Since the introduction of milk quotas in the UK (see p. 20), there has been a greater tendency to feed forage and concentrates have been fed on a 'flat-rate' basis, rather than the more traditional system of a basic allocation for maintenance and an increasing quantity of concentrate depending on yield. Provided that good quality forage is available *ad libitum* (and this is essential to the success of the system), there is no significant effect on milk quality throughout the lactation. Since high levels of 'starchy' concentrates promote high yields, cows calving onto a 'flat-rate' system tend to 'peak' at a lower level in early lactation and hence the 'dilution' effect of high yields depressing milk quality is not seen. Any reduction in milk quality on a flat-rate system is compensated for by slightly higher quality later in lactation. If access to forage is restricted, then clearly decreasing concentrate in early lactation will depress milk protein.

The depression of milk fat caused by high-concentrate diets can also be counteracted by the use of buffers. The most commonly used compound is sodium bicarbonate, fed at 12.5–15 kg/t, or 100–125 g/cow/day. The extent of the improvement depends on the original level of milk fat, the response being greatest in herds where butterfat is already low due to high levels of starchy concentrate being fed twice daily. Feeds such as sugar-beet pulp also have a good buffering capacity (sometimes also known as the cationic exchange capacity), whereas others, such as maize gluten, can lead to a more acid fermentation. It is interesting to speculate on the effects of the increasing use of sulphuric acid as a silage additive. This is a 'strong' acid, thus requiring a greater buffering, and could exacerbate milk fat problems in a way that formic or lactic acids would not.

Non-nutritional factors

Age of cow

Heifers generally have the highest milk quality, there being a fall of about 3 g/kg (0.3 per cent) in fat and 7 g/kg (0.7 per cent) in solids not fat (SNF) per lactation thereafter. The rate of decline continues until approximately the fifth lactation, after which it becomes more gradual. The decline in SNF is primarily due to a decline in lactose and mainly occurs during the first three lactations. Protein declines by approximately 1.0 g/kg (0.1 per cent) per lactation over this period.

Stage of lactation

Milk quality is, of course, very high at calving (colostrum has at least double the dry matter content, i.e. 25 per cent, of normal milk, see p. 177), but then declines as yield increases, reaching a minimum at about 50–70 days after calving. Milk fat may drop by as much as 10 g/kg (1.0 per cent) and protein by 3 g/kg (0.3 per cent) over the period. This depression is partly due to a 'dilution' effect of high yields and partly to the inherent inability of the early lactation cow to consume sufficient energy to meet the demands of production. Feeding high levels of 'starchy' concentrates and, in so doing, boosting the volume of milk produced, can in some circumstances exacerbate the decline in milk quality. Both milk fat and protein tend to increase after 70 days, but milk protein only rises significantly if the cow becomes pregnant and the rapid rise in both fat and protein that occurs in later lactation (e.g. six months after calving) is greater in the pregnant animal. Farms practising 'block calving', for example from August to October, often experience a marked fall in milk quality two to three months later (e.g. November to February) due to the fact that a large number of cows are at peak yield and relatively few are pregnant.

Changes in lactose follow an opposite pattern. The lactose content of colostrum is low, but rises rapidly after calving to reach a peak by two weeks into lactation. This level is maintained until six weeks, but there is then a steady fall, the rate accelerating towards the end of lactation. Changes in lactose are therefore a mirror image of changes in fat and protein.

Season of the year

In the UK there is a sharp fall in milk fat at the end of winter, when cows are turned out to grazing. This can be partly offset by providing access to hay or straw, although intakes of such forages are often poor when highly palatable grass is available and, if only 1–2 kg are consumed, this will have little benefit. To overcome the situation (and to improve grassland management and conservation), a system of 'storage' or 'buffer' feeding has been introduced, whereby cows are kept in at night on silage. Experiments carried out at Crichton Royal Farm (Table 26.3) showed that this significantly improved butterfat and although yields were marginally lower, overall fat yield was increased. However, protein yields were lower.

Often there is also a fall in milk protein during the winter housing period, (November to March in the UK), probably due to a lower energy content of the diet at this time of the year and also to a stage of lactation effect. Protein levels then rise rapidly in April and May, following turnout to spring grazing. There is very little seasonal change in lactose concentrations.

Disease

Liver fluke (see p. 238) can depress both milk fat and milk protein and this depression in milk quality may be seen in the absence of any other clinical signs of fluke. Heavy infestations of lice (see p. 250) and gastrointes-

Table 26.3 The effect of silage feeding at grazing on milk quality. Source: Phillips & Leaver (1983)

	Grazing	Restricted grazing and silage
Milk yield (kg/day)	19.9	18.9
Milk composition		
Fat (g/kg)	35.6	39.4
Protein (g/kg)	35.1	34.8
Solids yield		
Fat (g/day)	708	745
Protein (g/day)	698	657

Table 26.4 Approximate breed variations in milk yield and quality. Source: MMB (1983)

	Milk yield (kg)	Milk fat (g/kg)	Protein (g/kg)
Ayrshire	4988	39.0	33.8
British Friesian	5610	37.8	32.6
British Holstein	6292	37.3	32.0
Guernsey	4017	46.4	36.3
Jersey	3876	51.9	38.5

tinal worms (see p. 231) may also reduce milk quality, but these are unlikely in adult milking cows.

Mastitis (see Chapter 21) leads to a reduction in yield, lactose and butterfat. For example, a herd with a cell count of 750 000 cells/ml could be losing 750–900 l/cow/year, 50 g/kg (0.5 per cent) lactose and a smaller amount (30 g/kg, 0.3 per cent) of milk fat. Milk protein levels will increase slightly with mastitis.

Genetic variation

It is well known that Channel Island cattle such as the Jersey and Guernsey have higher milk quality than other breeds. Approximate breed values are given in Table 26.4. Of course there are large variations between individual animals within a breed, and this is the basis of genetic selection. The selection of animals on the basis of yield alone could lead to a decrease in fat and protein contents and care should be taken to ensure that bulls with a high improved contemporary comparison (ICC) for both fat and protein are selected. There is less genetic variation within breeds for protein and lactose than for fat and hence the greatest rate of genetic progress will be made by selecting for fat. For example, the range of fat content within a breed is over 20 g/kg, whereas genetic variation for protein is only approximately 10 g/kg (Crabtree, 1984). The genetic variation for lactose is even lower.

Management factors

Milking intervals would appear to have an effect on milk quality in that on twice daily milking, the fat content is higher in the afternoon. This is entirely due to a 'carryover' effect (Dodd, 1984). At the end of milking, some 10–20 per cent of the milk present remains in the udder and cannot be removed. The fat content of this milk is very high, 150 g/kg (15 per cent) or higher and it is withdrawn at the next milking. If there is an uneven interval between milkings, milk produced after the shorter interval will have a higher fat content because of the reduced 'dilution' effect of the additional milk produced. The total daily fat production remains constant, irrespective of the variation in milking interval and therefore of fat content. Increasing the frequency of milking to three or even four times daily does not alter milk quality significantly, although yields may rise by 10–15 per cent.

References

Crabtree, R.M. (1984) Milk compositional ranges and trends. In *Milk Compositional Quality and its Importance in Future Markets* (ed. by M.E. Castle & R.G. Gunn), pp. 35–42. BSAP Occasional Publication No. 9. Edinburgh
Dodd, F.H. (1984) Herd management effects on compositional quality. In *Milk Compositional Quality and its Importance in Future Markets* (ed. by M.E. Castle & R.G. Gunn), p. 77. BSAP Occasional Publication No. 9. Edinburgh
Garnsworthy, P.C. & Topps, J.H. (1982) The effect of body condition of dairy cows at calving on their food intake and performance when given complete diets. *Animal Production*, **35**, 113–19.
Milk Marketing Board (1983) *United Kingdom Dairy Facts and Figures*, pp. 1–208. The Federation of United Kingdom Milk Marketing Boards, Thomas Ditton.
Phillips, C.J.C. & Leaver, A.D. (1983) The effect of offering silage to set-stocked dairy cows. *Animal Production*, **36**, 507.
Sutton, J.D. (1986) In *Principles and Practice of Feeding Dairy Cows*, pp. 203–18. NIRD Technical Bulletin No. 8.
Sutton, J.D., Bines, J.A. & Napper, D.J. (1985) Composition of starchy and fibrous concentrates for lactating dairy cows. *Animal Production*, **40**, 533.
Thomas, C. (1984) Milk compositional quality and the role of forages. In *Milk Composition Quality and its Importance in Future Markets* (ed. by M.E. Castle & R.G. Gunn), pp. 69–76. BSAP Occasional Publication No. 9. Edinburgh

Chapter 27: The Enhancement of Mammary Gland Immunity Through Vaccination

by K. KENNY, F. BASTIDA-CORCVERA AND N.L. NORCROSS

Introduction

The examination of immunological methods to increase resistance of the dairy cow to the pathogens that cause mastitis has been ongoing for almost a century. Yet, even now, this area of bovine immunity generates enormous controversy. There are two opinions on the role of immunological intervention in mastitis control programmes. The first believes that it is not possible to generate protective immunity in the mammary gland and that control measures will have to be directed towards management, therapeutic strategies and genetic selection (Mellenberger, 1977; Anderson, 1978). The second opinion voices that vaccination has a role in a mastitis control programme (Colditz & Watson, 1985). This latter view is derived from an improved knowledge of the bovine immune system and from research reports which indicate that heightened resistance to certain pathogens can be generated. It is necessary to state that there are many unsolved problems in bovine mammary immunity and that there are also conflicting results and unsubstantiated reports. The pathogens that account for over 99 per cent of bovine clinical mastitis have one common feature. This is the lack of a commercial vaccine to prevent disease caused by members of the same bacterial genera in humans.

Anatomy of the mammary gland (see also Chapter 20)

The bovine udder is comprised of four mammary glands. The main arterial supply is from the bilateral external pudendal arteries while the venous return is via the external pudendal veins and the subcutaneous abdominal veins. There are two lymph vascular systems, a superficial and a deep set. The superficial set drain the cutaneous area and the teat walls while the deep set is associated with the finer branches of the arteries and veins. The lymphatics drain into the superficial inguinal (supramammary) lymph nodes. There is variation in the development and number of the superficial inguinal lymph nodes. Typically there is one large node quite superficially placed and one smaller node that is in a deeper location. The large node measures 7–10 cm in length, 4–6 cm wide and is 2–3 cm thick. The lymph node is composed of a cortex that is rich in B cells, a paracortex containing T cells and antigen presenting cells and a medulla where there are B cells, T cells and plasma cells. The efferent vessels pass to the deep inguinal node. The lymph then passes through the medial iliac nodes, enters the lumbar trunk which runs cranially to the cisterna chyli and then to the thoracic duct.

The mucosa of the teat or streak canal is arranged in longitudinal folds and is lined by stratified squamous epithelium, which constantly undergoes keratinization.

A slightly projecting fold marks the proximal end of the teat canal, the so-called Furstenberg's rosette. The teat cistern (sinus) is the cavity directly proximal to the teat canal, and this continues into the parenchyma of the udder as the gland cistern (lactiferous sinus), which possesses a two-layered columnar epithelium. The secretory tissue is divided into lobes that are comprised of lobules and there is an extensive duct system. The secretory epithelium is typically one cell thick ranging from low cuboidal to tall columnar depending on the stage of lactation. No mucus is present in the mammary gland of the cow. Furstenberg's rosette is infiltrated with lymphocytes. Lymphocytes are also found in the connective tissue of the lamina propria of the mucosa and the predominant cell is the IgA plasma cell. Some workers say that the IgG cell predominates.

Defence mechanisms of the gland

Non-specific and specific defence mechanisms exist in the bovine mammary gland. Non-specific factors include teat and teat duct shape and structure, teat duct patency and teat duct keratin. Teat duct keratin owes its protective properties to fatty acids and basic proteins. Lysozyme, an enzyme that can cleave certain bacterial cell walls, is present at very low concentrations in bovine secretions. Lactoferrin can bind iron and reduce the availability of iron to micro-organisms; however, citrate can inhibit this protein. The lactoperoxidase/thiocyanate/hydrogen peroxide system has activity against micro-organisms. Complement can be activated by bacterial cell wall components such as lipopolysaccharide (LPS) of Gram-negative organisms and can cause lysis of these bacteria by the alternate pathway.

There are four specific mechanisms operative in the gland. These are mediated by antibodies, directed against epitopes of the pathogens or their toxins, and work in concert with phagocytic cells and complement. The mechanisms include prevention of bacterial adherence to epithelial cells, neutralization of toxins elaborated by micro-organisms in the mammary gland, opsonization of pathogens and direct lysis of pathogens. The key role of humoral immunity is based on the fact that mastitis pathogens are extracellular organisms. A role for cellular immunity has not yet been established.

To increase resistance there are two avenues that can be taken. Firstly, to increase non-specific protection, which would be widely effective against all pathogens. Secondly, to increase or develop specific immunity to each mastitis pathogen. The latter is difficult since there is a great number of species and strains of bacteria each with characteristic virulence factors. The challenge is to characterize the virulence factors and identify protective epitopes of mastitis pathogens. The next step is to establish whether one can stimulate and maintain sufficient protective antibody in milk.

Immunoglobulin in lacteal secretions (see p. 286)

The concentration of immunoglobulin in serum and colostral secretions is shown in Table 27.1.

Four classes of antibody have been described in the bovine (Butler, 1986). They are IgA, IgE, IgG and IgM. Two subclasses of IgG have been recognized and they are IgG_1 and IgG_2. IgG_2 has now been divided into two sub-subclasses IgG_{2a} and IgG_{2b}. Antibody can be derived from local synthesis or from serum via selective transport or transudation. The half-life in serum of IgA, IgM, IgG_1 and IgG_2 respectively is 3, 5, 17 and 22 days. Serum IgA of cattle is probably synthesized by bronchial or gut-associated lymphoid tissue, while IgM and IgG are most likely synthesized by the spleen and peripheral lymph nodes.

The literature indicates that from 50 to 100 per cent of milk IgA is produced locally. Plasma derived IgA is selectively transported into most mucosal secretions by vesicular transport following its binding to secretory component on epithelial cells. IgA is the major immunoglobulin in most bovine secretions, but not in milk. There are conflicting reports concerning the origin of milk IgM with one author indicating it is entirely serum derived while another group indicate that 75 per cent is locally synthesized. Most milk IgG_1 is serum derived. About 90 per cent of IgG_2 found in milk is locally produced. The acinar epithelial cells have binding sites for IgG_1 and IgG_2. Near parturition new binding sites appear that have a high affinity for IgG_1 and these transfer enormous quantities of IgG_1 to colostrum, which serves as a source of immunoglobulin for the calf. It is evident that to increase specific IgG_1 in milk the serum level of specific IgG_1 must be increased whereas for IgA appropriate plasma cells in the lamina propria must be generated.

Table 27.1 Concentration of immunoglobulins in serum and colostral secretions (values are expressed in mg/ml)

	IgG_1	IgG_2	IgM	IgA
Serum	11.2	9.2	3.0	0.37
Colostral whey	48.2	4.0	7.1	4.6
Milk whey	0.5	0.06	0.08	0.08

Biological activity of antibody

Antibody molecules can be considered as having two components. Firstly, the two antigen binding sites (Fab fragments) recognize and bind antigen. Secondly, the Fc portion of the molecule is considered the effector part since it is involved in fixing complement components and interacting with specific Fc receptors on phagocytic cells. It is established that for certain protective effector functions, antibody must not only be directed against a particular epitope but must be of the correct isotype.

Secretory IgA serves to protect mucosal surfaces from colonization and penetration by undesirable micro-organisms. In the bovine upper respiratory tract IgA is important in defence against infectious bovine rhinotracheitis and parainfluenza infections. IgA-mediated protection from bacterial disease may involve agglutination, inactivation of toxins or opsonization. IgA has been reported to be opsonic only in the presence of complement. Traditionally, this antibody is believed to be unable to activate the classical complement pathway; however, one report suggests it can. Opsonization could also occur through FcR-mediated mechanisms. Fc receptors for IgA exist on the surface of monocytes and polymorphonuclear neutrophils (PMN) in other species but have not been described in the cow. Secretory IgA can augment the bacteriostatic effects of lactoferrin. Porcine IgA can lyse *Escherichia coli* in the presence of lysozyme and complement. There is minimal lysozyme in bovine milk. Lacteal IgA is largely associated with milk fat globules.

IgM is 10–20 times as effective as IgG in complement fixation. This ability to fix complement may explain why IgM is bacteriocidal for Gram-negative pathogens. In this manner it can also opsonize micro-organisms for uptake by phagocytic cells. One report describes the presence of receptor for this isotype on bovine neutrophils but not on macrophages. This antibody can agglutinate bacteria and permit them to be flushed out at milking. It can also neutralize toxins.

IgG_1 and IgG_2 are efficient at fixation of complement. They have been shown to be able to neutralize toxins from bacterial pathogens. Cytophilic antibodies are capable of attaching to certain cells in such a way that these cells are subsequently capable of specifically absorbing antigen. It has been shown that IgG_2 is cytophilic for bovine blood neutrophils and for ovine mammary neutrophils. This phenomenon remains to be demonstrated for bovine milk neutrophils. When macrophages were examined *in vitro*, it was found that they were capable of binding both IgG_1 and IgG_2. The capacity of these isotypes to prevent adherence is unknown.

Complement

The complement system is a collective term for a series of proteins which, when activated, can opsonize micro-organisms or cause cell lysis. It consists of a classical pathway, an alternate pathway, a common amplification method and a common terminal pathway. The ability of specific antibody to bind to a micro-organism and fix complement promotes uptake of that micro-organism since phagocytes (neutrophil, macrophage) possess a receptor for the C3b component of complement. It was found that the guinea-pig rather than the ovine erythrocyte is most suitable to the measurement of bovine complement. In lacteal secretions complement levels are highest as lactation ends, in the dry period and in the early part of lactation. Milk does contain anticomplementary activity, which is believed to be due to casein or other proteins. When a sensitive radioactive marker was employed, levels of complement were demonstrated throughout lactation. The classical pathway is activated by antibody while the alternate pathway is activated by lipopolysaccharides or polysaccharides, which can bind C3b and prevent its degradation. Products of the reaction include C3a and C5a, which are chemotactic for leucocytes.

Cells of the mammary gland (see also Chapter 23)

In dry and lacteal secretions the predominant cell type is the macrophage while in colostrum the polymorphonuclear neutrophils (PMN) serves this role. Ductal epithelial cells may be found in milk. The cellular composition of gland secretions is shown in Table 27.2 (Lee *et al.*, 1980).

The number of cells/ml in dry-period secretion is 30 times that of normal milk with 4000 times as many actual lymphocytes. Using sensitive markers and flow cytometry these *lymphocytes* have been characterized as shown in Table 27.3 (Duhamel *et al.*, 1987).

Previous studies indicated higher numbers of B cells with values of 20 per cent quoted. There is a higher

Table 27.2 Percentage of cellular composition of gland secretions

	PMN	Macrophage	Lymphocyte	Epithelial
Milk	3	80	16	2
Colostrum	62	35	4	0
Dry gland secretion	3	89	7	1

Table 27.3 Lymphocytes of gland secretions and blood

	B cell	T cell	Null
Peripheral blood lymphocytes	21.2	66.4	9.4
Dry secretion	2.8	88.1	5.4
Colostrum	3.5	89	15.1

percentage of T cells in mammary secretions than in blood. In the month before parturition gland secretions contain 1 million cells/ml with macrophages and lymphocytes in equal numbers. These lymphocytes respond to mitogens. However, these responses are lower than those of the peripheral blood lymphocytes from the same animal. Macrophages and T cells are involved in antigen presentation. T cells can produce cytokines, which can affect PMN recruitment into the gland.

The *macrophage* has received less attention than the PMN. The macrophage in the mammary gland functions in phagocytosis and killing, it eliminates fat in the involuting gland and plays a role in local immunity through antigen processing and presentation. A considerable population of macrophages exists beneath the alveolar and ductal epithelium. Bovine mammary macrophages have receptors for both IgG_1 and IgG_2. It has been found that the goat mammary macrophage was not a terminal cell but was capable of division with 2–6 per cent of the population dividing. Macrophages can phagocytose *Staphylococcus aureus* but a percentage survive intracellularly. Mammary macrophages produce chemotactic activity for neutrophils after they have phagocytosed and killed *Staph. aureus*, *E. coli* or after exposure to endotoxin.

The pool of mature *polymorphonuclear neutrophil* leucocytes present to fight infection numbers about 100 billion. In the circulation this pool consists of circulating granulocytes both in the central stream of blood vessels and in the marginal pool. The half-life of the cell in the bloodstream is about 9 hours. There is a substantial number developing in the bone marrow. The marginal pool moves slowly along the vascular endothelium and passes between endothelial cells to enter the perivascular space. Attraction of neutrophils to inflammatory sites is a corner-stone of host defence against invading bacteria. Chemotaxis describes the reaction by which the direction of locomotion of cells is determined by the substances in their environment. Products of the complement pathway such as C5a and C3a are chemotaxins. Phagocyte-bound antibody may allow antigen-specific chemotaxis to occur. There are three types of granules present within the bovine neutrophil and they contain peroxidase, digestive enzymes, lactoferrin and basic proteins.

Milk from normal uninfected glands contains 10 000–300 000 cells/ml and the predominant cell is the macrophage. Subclinically infected quarters contain 750 000 cells/ml, while the secretion of infected quarters contains millions of cells per millilitre and in these instances the predominant cell is the PMN, which is attracted into the gland by chemotactic stimuli. A pre-existing leucocytosis confers increased resistance to infection; however, increased amounts of serum factors in the milk typically accompany this leucocytosis. A concentration of 200 000–500 000 cells/ml prevent *Aerobacter aerogenes* from multiplying sufficiently to cause acute mastitis and also prevents infection with *Streptococcus agalactiae*. When intramammary devices increase cell counts to 900 000/ml in strippings, protection against environmental pathogens is achieved. Field trials in Israel with intramammary devices indicated a marked reduction in clinical mastitis and an increase in milk yield.

Upon infection of the gland, PMNs respond by adhering to the endothelium and passing through it by diapedesis. They then migrate down chemotactic gradients and upon contact and recognition of the pathogen, ingestion occurs and the pathogen is exposed to the microbicidal system of the PMN. Both oxygen dependent and independent pathways exist within neutrophils to kill ingested microbes. Antibody and complement exert their effect at the stage of contact and recognition and promote ingestion through opsonization. Phagocytic cells may also recognize general physicochemical characteristics of foreign micro-organisms. Non-immune recognition can occur. Bacterial toxins can damage the PMN and phagocytosing PMNs can cause damage to mammary epithelium.

Phagocytosis by mammary PMNs is much less efficient than that by blood PMNs; PMN function in the mammary gland is impaired by milk fat globules, casein and the lower glycogen content of milk PMNs compared with blood PMNs. Casein micelles can coat the surface of the neutrophil and inhibit the antibacterial systems, whereas fat globules are ingested and exhaust the contents of the cytoplasmic granules of the PMN. Cows vary in both the ability of their PMNs to phagocytose and in the ability of their milk to support phagocytosis. In non-vaccinated animals it requires almost 24 hours for a leucocytosis to develop in milk following infection. Antigen-specific inflammatory response can be established in the gland by parenteral immunization and one of the effector inputs of vaccination is the more rapid response of the PMN to infection.

One apparent discrepancy is that despite the presence of high levels of phagocytic cells in the gland during the dry period, the gland is very susceptible at this time to new infection. This may be the result of poor phagocytic efficiency of these cells or the non-lactating gland is an unfavourable environment for them. It has been shown that colostrum and dry secretion compromise PMN function by blocking their Fc receptors. To increase the efficacy of phagocytosis one could increase and maintain a high level of opsonin in milk through immunization, decrease PMN mobilization time in response to pathogen invasion and select for cows with superior phagocytosis. One could also increase and maintain a high PMN concentration in milk, although this may adversely affect milk quality. It is necessary to stress the limitations of PMN function since once an infection is established a leucocytosis may be insufficient to clear the infection as evidenced by chronic infections occurring in the face of a high somatic cell count (SCC). With *Mycoplasma* a massive leucocytosis may not provide protection from infection.

Intramammary infection and pathogenicity

To induce mastitis a pathogen must first pass the teat canal to enter the gland, survive the bacteriostatic and bactericidal mechanisms and multiply. Milk is an ideal medium for bacterial growth. *Colonization* of the gland depends on the adherence capacity of the pathogen. The ability of mastitis pathogens to adhere to ductular epithelial cells has been examined. *Streptococcus agalactiae* and *Staph. aureus* adhered readily and in large numbers while *Strep. dysgalactiae* and *Strep. uberis* adhered moderately. In contrast *E. coli, Klebsiella* spp. and *Actinomyces pyogenes* adhered poorly. Attachment to ductular epithelial cells is an important stage in the pathogenesis of mastitis caused by *Staph. aureus, Strep. agalactiae* and other streptococci. Milk from an infected quarter can inhibit this adherence, which is probably protein mediated. In coliform mastitis the organisms grow in secretions and there is little tissue invasion. Bacteria that colonize mucosal surfaces must not only adhere but also multiply at a sufficiently rapid rate to replenish newly exposed epithelial cell surfaces, as old epithelial cells along with adherent bacteria are flushed away. Because surface epithelial cells are shed, colonization of a mucosal surface *in vivo* requires continual re-attachment. Damage to the gland typically reflects toxin production by the micro-organism and the beneficial effects of vaccination with staphylococcal toxoids are a reduction in the clinical signs of infection.

New infections are commonest at drying-off and at parturition; 20–50 per cent of infections occur during the dry period due to the ease with which bacteria can penetrate the streak canal and gain access to the teat sinus. When lactation ceases the flushing of milk through the teat canal stops, teat dipping ceases and a build-up of pressure can occur within the udder. Almost 100 per cent of clinical mastitis occurs during lactation with 60 per cent taking place in the first 40 days. The outcome of infection depends on the rate of growth of the organism, the production, absorption and activity of toxins and the immune status of the host. The increase in infection with advancing age was a result of re-infection and persisting infection and that the incidence of new infections did not change with the age of the animal.

The immune response against the major pathogens will now be discussed.

Escherichia coli (see also p. 297)

Teat dipping and other control measures effective against staphylococci and streptococci have decreased the somatic cell count and made quarters vulnerable to coliform infection. Coliform mastitis is an opportunist infection. In one study 290 *E. coli* isolates were examined and 81.7 per cent could be grouped into 63 O-serogroups with the remainder being untypable. In the UK it was found that mastitis strains did not possess the virulence factors associated with invasive or enteropathogenic strains of *E. coli* and that serum resistance was the key feature of clinical isolates. It was found that 75 per cent of strains were capsulated but the contribution of a capsule is unclear since most unencapsulated strains were serum resistant. Capsulation may increase serum resistance. Serum sensitive strains are killed rapidly, with over 90 per cent killed in 15 minutes by freshly collected 10 per cent normal bovine serum. For *Ae. aerogenes* bactericidal activity is a property of IgM and IgG_1 but not of IgG_2.

The Gram-negative cell wall consists of an inner cytoplasmic membrane and a cell wall that is composed of mucopolysaccharide–peptidoglycan, phospholipid protein and (LPS). Resistance to the bactericidal activity of normal serum is attributable to the O-antigen of the LPS. Lipopolysaccharide from serum-resistant strains are relatively enriched in long-chain O-antigen LPS subunits, compared with serum-sensitive strains, and these O polysaccharides may mask lipid A, which could activate the alternate complement pathway. If the longer polysaccharide chains do bind C3b, the distance from the outer membrane of the bacteria is too far for insertion of the complement membrane attack complex.

Lipopolysaccharide is composed of three distinct subunits. The outermost O polysaccharide is linked to the core polysaccharide, which is covalently bound to the lipid A. The O polysaccharides are made up of a series of identical repeating oligosaccharide units containing three to five sugars each. This is the immunodominant part of the molecule. The O polysaccharide displays great diversity in length and sugar constituents whereas the core polysaccharide is conserved. Because of the great diversity of the O polysaccharides of LPS, a search for shared epitopes on other parts of the molecule has been undertaken in an effort to find an antigen that could be used for active immunization. There are 160 types of O polysaccharide in *E. coli* alone and 90 capsular types. Lipopolysaccharide is known to act as a B cell mitogen, a polyclonal B cell activator and a T cell independent antigen.

Escherichia coli does not adhere to mammary epithelial cells. When serum-resistant strains gain access to the lactating gland they start to multiply. The pathogenic effects of *E. coli* mastitis are believed to be mediated by the release of LPS (endotoxin) from the bacterial cell wall. The host reaction to endotoxin can be overexuberant and this exaggerated response is often responsible for the severity of this mastitis. Fever, disseminated intravascular coagulation, hypotension, shock, complement activation and death can occur. Macrophages are the principal method by which endotoxins are removed and in the presence of LPS the macrophages become activated and secrete the cytokines interleukin 1, interleukin 6 and tumour necrosis factor, which mediate endotoxic events and are responsible for the clinical signs. These factors cause an influx of PMN. Antibiotics, other than colistin and polymixin, have little effect on endotoxin-induced pathology and may actually exacerbate the clinical condition due to their causing the release of additional endotoxin from the bacteria during killing. Some authors propose that a cytotoxic factor other than endotoxin is responsible for the damage to mammary tissue.

In *E. coli* mastitis, the lesions are confined to the superficial layer of the teat and lactiferous sinus. The lactiferous sinus possesses a two-cell thick epithelium. Infection with *E. coli* results in an influx of large numbers of subepithelial PMNs, which migrate into the lumen of the gland. In early coliform mastitis the PMNs adhere together and attach to the epithelium. There is extensive sloughing and necrosis of epithelial cells of the lactiferous and teat sinus. The reaction is centred on the ductular tissue; secretory tissue is not involved. Endotoxin induces an initial neutropenia as neutrophils shift from the circulating to the marginal pool and are destroyed. There is then a neutrophilia as mature neutrophils are released from the bone marrow reserve.

The dry gland is much less responsive to endotoxin than the lactating gland and mild histopathological changes are noted following infusion. *Escherichia coli* is not capable of establishing itself permanently in the gland in the first half of the dry period. One experiment revealed that in the 30 days before parturition the bacteria maintained infection in 14 of 37 inoculated quarters and all these quarters had peracute toxic mastitis after parturition. Thus the response of the cows to *E. coli* infection of the mammary gland differs depending on the stage of lactation. The inflammatory response is a function of the physiological state of the gland and that the influx of neutrophils is correlated with blood flow. Following infusion of 500 colony forming units (c.f.u.) of *E. coli*, newly calved cows mobilize PMNs slowly since they appear to be refractory to the presence of irritants in the udder. This permits great bacterial replication and a large subsequent release of endotoxin, which is often fatal.

Killing of some *E. coli* strains within the udder requires a neutrophilia only, whereas for others up to 30 per cent serum products are required. A leucocytosis of 200 000–500 000 cells/ml prevents an infusion of *Ae. aerogenes* multiplying sufficiently to cause acute mastitis. For virulent strains a PMN response and opsonin are typically required. The severity of the disease may be influenced by the presence or absence of a capsule. In decomplemented non-immune serum, colostrum and whey the main opsonin for *E. coli* is IgM and that there is no absolute requirement for complement in the opsonization of *E. coli* by the adult dairy cow. This IgM may be natural antibody derived from natural exposure and may act via a receptor for IgM on neutrophils. Later work found IgG_2 from immune bovine serum or whey will opsonize *E. coli*. Hill showed that the dominant immunogen responsible for the opsonic response is the capsule since strains sharing the same K85 capsule were also opsonized (Hill *et al.*, 1983). To protect against coliform mastitis it is important to stimulate antibody with maximal antibacterial and opsonic properties.

Following local and intramuscular administration of killed *E. coli* there was an increase both in specific IgA and total IgA in the respective quarter of the mammary gland. The actual biological activity of this sIgA is unknown. It is known that porcine sIgA has bactericidal activity for *E. coli* when in the presence of complement and lysozyme, but the lysozyme content of bovine lacteal secretions is minimal. Intramuscular injection of endotoxin into cows induces endotoxin pyrogenic tolerance and an increase in the rate with which serum killed *E. coli*. Hill *et al.* (1983) showed that *E. coli* B117, an encapsulated strain, stimulates long-lasting opsonic activity following infusion of 300 c.f.u. into a quarter.

It is clear that immunity to coliforms revolves around antibody and PMN. The PMN can have a negative or positive impact on the outcome of coliform infection of the gland. An initial leucocytosis will protect against acute mastitis since the bacteria will be killed rapidly. If the bacteria gain entry to the gland and replicate the subsequent influx of PMNs will cause a massive release of endotoxin from the bacteria and acute clinical signs will be evident. When a neutropenia was induced in the cow by horse anti-bovine leucocyte serum and cows were inoculated with *Ae. aerogenes*, the neutropenia was found greatly to decrease the inflammatory response in the gland.

With the multiplicity of O-serogroups and the many capsular types associated with mastitis isolates the possibility of generating wide ranging protective immunity appears to be very difficult. For immunological prevention of Gram-negative infection to be a possibility three requirements must be met. A common antigenic structure must exist, and this must function as an immunogen. The response to this immunogen must generate protective antibodies. Antibody to the O polysaccharide antigen or LPS affords protection against homologous challenge. Gram-negative core antigens have immunologic homology across bacterial species. Typically, these antigens are masked by the immunodominant O polysaccharide. In contrast to smooth organisms, rough mutants, so-called because of their colonial morphology, have incomplete synthesis of O polysaccharide side chains, and consequently have varying amounts of the core glycolipid exposed. The *E. coli* J5 strain is an Ra mutant of *E. coli* O11 : B4. It is a uridine diphosphogalactose 4-epimerase deficient mutant that has an LPS devoid of O antigen. Animals immunized with killed mutant bacteria are able to make antibodies to the core region and are protected from challenge with heterologous live organisms. Human recipients vaccinated with an *E. coli* J5 preparation had reduced mortality from Gram-negative septicaemia.

Studies in California of IgG_1 antibody titres to the core antigens of J5 showed that titres of less than 1 : 240 were associated with 5.33 times the risk of clinical coliform mastitis. In a field trial, 246 cows received three doses of J5 killed cells (7.5 billion bacteria/dose) in Freund's incomplete adjuvant, twice in the dry period and once after calving; 240 unvaccinated cows served as controls. Six cases of clinical mastitis occurred in vaccinated cows with 29 occurring in control cows. There was concern that the toxic effects of lipid A could cause vaccination reactions but this did not appear to be so. This vaccine is now licensed for use in the state of California.

There is controversy concerning what are the protective factor(s) that vaccination induces. There is good evidence that it is antibody to core glycolipid; however, it is possible that vaccination also causes polyclonal stimulation of IgG and IgM specific for O polysaccharide. Antibodies to core glycolipid show highly variable cross-reactivity with heterologous strains of *E. coli*. Recent studies indicated that the protective ability of antibodies to core glycolipid induced by J5 vaccination may reside in their ability to bind to released LPS. This release would occur after antibiotic therapy, phagocytic destruction or complement-mediated lysis. Two laboratories have shown that J5 antibody binds to invading bacteria at a time when the core antigens are most exposed, i.e. early in their growth phase. This antibody may have bactericidal activity, opsonic properties or it may neutralize the toxic effects of lipid A. Bacterial LPS can induce enhanced non-specific resistance to bacterial, viral and parasitic infections and it remains to be determined if the above vaccination scheme achieves this. Hyperimmune serum from J5 vaccinated cows may have some therapeutic value in coliform mastitis.

***Klebsiella* spp.** (see also p. 297)

Klebsiella spp. are environmental pathogens and opportunist invaders of the bovine mammary gland. It is similar to *E. coli* in this regard and immune mechanisms active against *E. coli* may exert an effect on *Klebsiella* spp. There are two types of cell surface polysaccharides to note. Firstly, the O-antigen side chains of LPS and secondly the capsular polysaccharides. The genus *Klebsiella* has been classified serologically into at least 77 capsular or K types and there have been eight somatic types or O groups described; 33 capsular types of *Klebsiella pneumoniae* were isolated from cows belonging to 12 herds and within individual herds up to 13 types could be found. *Klebsiella* spp. may be serum sensitive or serum resistant. The primary feature of pathogenic strains is their ability to withstand the bactericidal effects of normal serum and following infusion of small numbers of serum-resistant bacteria into normal mammary glands a severe mastitis is evident. This mastitis is prevented by a pre-existing leucocytosis or by the presence of specific antibody, thus indicating the role of these components in the prevention of infection by this organism. Complement is believed to be responsible for the rapid killing of serum-sensitive *K. pneumoniae*.

Cell wall O-antigens are responsible for this resistance to serum bactericidal activity. The majority of *Klebsiella* isolates possess a well-defined capsule that confers resistance to phagocytosis in the absence of specific antibody. Antibodies specific for O-antigens can penetrate the capsule and, if the antibody is exposed at the surface, opsonize some encapsulated strains. Certain encapsulated strains mask these antibodies and in such instances no opsonization occurs. Capsular polysaccharide protects against phagocytosis and serotype-specific anticapsular antibodies cause opsonization via complement or Fc receptors on phagocytes, explaining why type-specific protection can be achieved by vaccination with the homologous capsular polysaccharide. In human medicine a 24-valent capsular polysaccharide vaccine has been used to stimulate specific antibody, which promotes the uptake and killing of invading bacteria. This vaccine generates antibody considered to be protective against 72 per cent of *Klebsiella* spp. blood isolates and 82 per cent of all typeable bacteraemic strains. A polyvalent vaccine containing the common capsular polysaccharides could be prepared for dairy cows and examined in appropriate field trials. Such a vaccine would mesh with antibodies to the core glycolipid induced by vaccination with the J5 mutant of *E. coli*.

***Mycoplasma* spp.** (see p. 298)

Mycoplasmas lack a cell wall and are surrounded by a membrane that is similar to the cytoplasmic membrane of bacteria. Several species of *Mycoplasma* cause mastitis but *Mycoplasma bovis* is most prevalent. *Mycoplasma* mastitis can cause severe economic losses since many animals can be affected, often in multiple quarters. Antibiotics have little success and after a prolonged time cows may recover. There have been clinical data, re-infection trial data and field vaccination intervention observations that immune prophylaxis may be possible. Consider an udder with an infected quarter that resolved. Up to two months after infection all quarters of the gland are resistant to challenge. Quarters that recovered from infection are immune for up to six months while over one year after infection all quarters are susceptible to re-infection. Studies of *M. bovis* specific immune response have failed to differentiate between resistant and susceptible animals. In experimental infection IgM is predominant up to 57 days after which IgG takes over. Daily IgA and IgG production is higher in those quarters in which infection had resolved. The immunity may be based on locally produced IgA and IgG with a cellular input.

Cows in all stages of lactation are susceptible, those in early lactation suffering more severely. A pre-existing leucocytosis does not prevent cows from challenge. The presence of serum components and PMN does not affect the continuation of replication and spread by *Mycoplasma*. Mycoplasmas can attach to neutrophils and macrophages in the absence of specific antibody and persist and even multiply on the cell surface. Resistance to killing by serum is a virulence determinant. This killing is performed by the alternate complement pathway. The surface of certain strains may be an activating factor for this pathway. The killing of *M. bovis* has been examined and IgG_2 were more efficient for PMN while IgG_1 and IgG_2 were effective for macrophages. Neutrophils are not capable of killing *M. bovis* unless specific antibody is present, IgG_1, IgG_2 and IgM specific for *M. bovis* did not kill *Mycoplasma* on their own. *Mycoplasma* may have a suppressive effect on lymphocyte function.

Formalin-inactivated protein (1 mg) from *M. bovis* has been used as antigen. It was given by the subcutaneous and intramammary route. Vaccination generated specific IgM, IgG_1 and IgG_2 antibody in serum but no IgA. Infection with *M. bovis* gives high IgM, IgG_1 and IgG_2 in serum with a specific IgA also. In the whey the vaccinated cows had a specific IgG_1 only. In a challenge trial seven of eight quarters of vaccinated cows became infected but cleared while of six of eight infected control quarters, four remained infected with two clearing. (Boothby *et al.*, 1986). There is little additional evidence that vaccination with killed organisms will prevent mammary infection with mycoplasmas and systemic antibody does not seem to protect against infection. Possibly IgA is needed and this isotype is not stimulated by killed vaccine. No attenuated strains have been identified despite one strain being passaged on artificial media for 10 years. Vaccination may produce an immune response that can result in cellular inflammation.

The predominant cell in the secretion of cows with *Mycoplasma* mastitis are neutrophils but one report indicates that, in field episodes, initially eosinophils were in the alveoli and they were joined by mononuclear cells. *Mycoplasma bovis* produces an inflammatory toxin, which is a polysaccharide. It increases vascular permeability and has received minimal attention since its first description. It is clear that immunity to *Mycoplasma* mastitis is poorly understood and that vaccination is not a realistic possibility in the near future. The interaction of *M. bovis* with antibody and complement is worthy of further investigation as is the inflammatory toxin. IgA is an important factor in the resolution of *Mycoplasma*-induced respiratory disease in humans as is the T lymphocyte. Their significance in the cow remains to be determined.

The summer mastitis complex (see also Chapter 22)

There are conflicting views on what is the causative organism(s) of summer mastitis and how these organisms spread and invade the gland. Summer mastitis typically affects the non-lactating gland of heifers or dry cows. Mixed bacterial infections are involved in the aetiology of summer mastitis. *Actinomyces* (*Corynebacterium*) *pyogenes*, *Peptococcus indolicus*, a microaerophilic coccus and *Strep. dysgalactiae* are the pathogens believed to have a role in this condition. Summer mastitis has been induced in heifers with *Ac. pyogenes* and *P. indolicus* or with these two organisms and the microaerophilic coccus of Stuart *et al.* (1951). It appeared that the cultures were more virulent if grown together and infused rather than grown separately and then mixed for infusion. Some studies show that *P. indolicus* and the microaerophilic coccus may not be required though this view has fallen out of favour.

Glands were challenged in either mid-lactation, one week prior to drying-off, at drying-off and when dry with either *P. indolicus* or *A. pyogenes*. Dry-period infections with *A. pyogenes* were more severe and were rarely eliminated even with antibiotic therapy. Infections during lactation were eliminated naturally or with antibiotics. Intermittent recovery from the lactating gland without clinical signs of infection was possible for up to three months after challenge. *Actinomyces pyogenes* does not adhere to mammary epithelial cells and this may explain why summer mastitis is typically associated with the non-lactating gland. *Peptococcus indolicus* established itself in the gland when infused one week before (66 per cent) or at drying-off (100 per cent). This bacteria was eliminated at calving or early in the lactation. Combined infections were more severe, often with systemic involvement. In the dry gland, an acute mastitis similar to summer mastitis could be established if the two bacteria were inoculated together or if quarters shedding *P. indolicus* were inoculated with *A. pyogenes*. *Peptococcus indolicus* and to a lesser extent the microaerophilic coccus stimulated the growth and the hemolysin production of *A. pyogenes*. Of six precipitin types of *P. indolicus* occurring in cattle, type B seems to occur most commonly in healthy cattle. This type is widespread in healthy cattle. Contamination of teat surfaces with *A. pyogenes* or *Strep. dysgalactiae* leads to intramammary infection, but does not with *P. indolicus*, posing the question of whether this organism reaches the gland from another route.

The aerobes may create an environment with low oxygen tension and facilitate growth of the anaerobic coccus and production of toxins. *Peptococcus indolicus* is unable to grow when the oxygen tension reaches 0.5 per cent. *Actinomyces pyogenes* grows best in milk when the pH is greater than 7, as in the dry gland. *Actinomyces pyogenes* produces haemolysin and proteases. The toxin is lethal to mice on intravenous administration and the toxin can be formal toxoided. *Peptococcus indolicus* produces peptocoagulase, and the microaerophilic coccus produces hyaluronidase and deoxyribonuclease.

Early vaccines were composed without regard to the complex nature of the aetiology, typically containing *Ac. pyogenes* with or without haemolysin and the results were poor. Sorenson showed that *A. pyogenes* alone had no protective effect but that a triple bacterin preparation composed of *A. pyogenes*, *P. indolicus* and the microaerophilic coccus was worthy of further study after preliminary encouraging results (Sorensen, 1972). An *A. pyogenes* toxoid preparation stimulated antibodies in cattle and offered mice a significant degree of protection to the challenge of 150 million bacteria intraperitoneally.

There is a marked lack of data on the immune response of the cow to these pathogens and very little is known on how these bacteria interact with phagocytic cells and the requirements for killing. This situation means that approaches to vaccination will be quite empirical for some time. In the interim, additional field trials with this triple bacterin are warranted. Infections with *A. pyogenes*, *P. indolicus* and the microaerophilic coccus generated antibodies to surface antigens of these bacteria and these antibodies were shown to reside principally in the IgG_2 subclass. The antigens secreted into the extracellular fluid by *P. indolicus* appear to be the antigens against which the cow directs an immune response.

Watson indicates that *A. pyogenes* is susceptible to the bactericidal activities of bovine neutrophils *in vitro* and complement did not play a role in this killing, but antibody did (Watson, 1989). The bactericidal activity of neutrophils incubated with milk was positively correlated with titres of IgG_2 and IgM but not IgG_1 or IgA. Complement again was not involved.

Staphylococcus aureus (see also p. 296)

Staphylococcus aureus has been described as a persistent pathogen of the gland due to the failure of therapy during the lactating period to achieve bacteriological cures. An intracellular location within phagocytes may offer *Staph. aureus* a survival mechanism from the effect of antibiotics during chronic infection. It is a contagious pathogen and infusion of less than 10 c.f.u. into the teat sinus can cause mastitis. Teat dipping and dry-cow therapy have made some inroads into the incidence of mastitis caused by this pathogen.

The value of immunization with staphylococcal antigens has generated controversy. Early attempts at vaccination were unsuccessful and these failures can be explained to a degree by the low numbers of bacteria used and the culture of these bacteria in conventional media, which causes the loss of surface polysaccharides that are important virulence factors. Later work demonstrated a limited protection against homologous strains along with a reduction in the severity of clinical infection due to antitoxins and a reduction in spread of *Staph. aureus* mastitis in vaccinated herds. More recently, there have been reports that generate cautious optimism on the value of immunization in protecting against challenge or natural exposure to heterologous strains.

The cell wall is composed of peptidoglycan, teichoic acid and protein A. At one time peptidoglycan was considered to be the key cell surface component involved in promoting opsonization of *Staph. aureus* by both heat-labile and heat-stable factors in normal serum. However, it was noted that the majority of staphylococci from bovine mammary glands produce exopolysaccharide and that this antigen is an important virulence factor, which is rapidly lost on subculture on conventional laboratory media. The precise nature of this substance is unclear with debate on whether it is a slime layer, a microcapsule or a pseudocapsule. Some researchers believe that this surface antigen has some similarity between isolates while others believe that this surface antigen can be classified into a capsular type in the same manner human strains have been classified. The latter scheme was employed in one study and capsular types 5 and 8 accounted for almost 70 per cent of bovine isolates. But a smaller study found that bovine isolates were not typeable by this method. Eleven capsular types have been identified in human strains. This area requires clarification since if this is so a vaccine containing the appropriate capsular types should be examined.

This surface polysaccharide does not interfere significantly with the binding of opsonins to the bacterial surface but rather with the exposure of opsonic factors in the proper configuration on the true external surface of the microbe and in this manner inhibits complement and opsonin-mediated phagocytosis. Thus antibody and complement may bind to peptidoglycan but they are unable to interact with receptors located on phagocytes. Increased virulence associated with the polysaccharide is related to a delay in chemotaxis and phagocytosis. Specific antibody is necessary for opsonization of these strains.

Staphylococcus aureus has a number of virulence factors. Attachment to ductal epithelial cells is an important step in colonization and surface epitopes are likely to be involved. Specific antibody has been shown to prevent this adherence. Protein A is a component of the cell wall. Strains with the highest amounts of protein A are phagocytosed at a slower rate because protein A is antiphagocytic since it depletes complement and can bind to the Fc portion of IgG molecules. Protein A has high affinity for IgG_2 and lesser affinity for IgG_1. This may be critical if IgG_2 is an effector molecule of importance since protein A secreted by the bacteria could tie up this antibody. *Staphylococcus aureus* expresses a large amount of extracellular slime when grown in modified media.

Staphylococcus aureus produces around 30 extracellular proteins some of which have been shown to be virulence factors. Alpha toxin is believed to be responsible for much of the tissue damage seen in staphylococcal mastitis and beta toxin has been shown to cause inflammation of the gland. Toxins such as leucocidin may compromise gland defences by damaging phagocytes or lymphocytes. During chronic staphylococcal mastitis the recruitment or proliferation of specific B lymphocytes into plasma cells is impaired. Neutralizing antibodies can be induced through vaccination and these lessen the damage to secretory tissue. Gudding showed that *Staph. aureus* adhered to epithelial cells and toxins released caused lesions of ulceration and erosions in the epithelial layer throughout the ductal system (Gudding *et al.*, 1984). This damage permits staphylococci to bind to such subepithelial components as type II collagen, fibrinogen and fibronectin. Fibronectin is a large glycoprotein found in the extracellular matrix of connective tissue, and in humans the expression of fibronectin binding sites correlates with the invasiveness of the organism and may mediate adherence by *Staph. aureus*.

It is evident that protective antibodies should be directed against the exopolysaccharide to prevent adherence and promote opsonization while toxin neutralizing antibodies would lessen clinical damage and protect the cellular defences of the gland. In a field trial with a staphylococcal bacterin–toxoid preparation encouraging results were obtained. Fewer new infections, less culling and lower somatic cell counts were evident in vaccinated cows as opposed to controls. The bacterin was composed of two strains of *Staph. aureus* whose exopolysaccharides showed cross-reactivity with 90 per cent of bovine mastitis isolates of *Staph. aureus*. Each dose of bacterin contained over 10 billion c.f.u. The toxoid component contained α and β haemolysins. The protective mechanism of this vaccine is under investigation.

Australian workers believe that killed vaccine stimulates IgG_1 and that the protection afforded by vaccination with live bacteria is due to the generation of specific IgG_2 that is cytophilic for PMNs. It is believed that PMNs can respond faster to infection of the gland and that these PMNs may enter the gland carrying IgG_2 on their membrane. Cows deficient in IgG_2 are very likely to succumb to peracute gangrenous mastitis following infection with *Staph. aureus*. Vaccination with live bacteria poses a problem and consequently killed bacteria have been used with dextran sulphate as an adjuvant to stimulate specific IgG_2 antibody. In challenge studies in sheep, the incidence of peracute gangrenous and acute clinical mastitis and the decrease in milk yield is lower in the vaccinated animals. It would be encouraging if other researchers confirmed these results. The role of the PMN in defence against *Staph. aureus* became apparent when antibovine leucocyte serum converted a chronic staphylococcal mastitis to an acute gangrenous type. Macrophages from the dry bovine gland phagocytose *Staph. aureus* readily but kill them very slowly. In normal glands there is a 24-hour lapse between entry of bacteria into the gland and the accumulation of 500 000 PMN/ml and this delay allows infection to become established. Vaccination can decrease this lag period to six hours. The decreased response time of PMNs to staphylococcal infection following local vaccination is related to mononuclear cell function. Local immunization of the gland with staphylococcal vaccines stimulate IgA and IgM and provides a good degree of protection. Immunity to coagulase-negative staphylococci will be similar in terms of surface antigens but the coagulase-negative staphylococci do not secrete the same array of toxins.

Streptococci (see also p. 296)

STREPTOCOCCUS AGALACTIAE (GROUP B STREPTOCOCCI)

Streptococcus agalactiae is an obligate parasite of the bovine mammary gland and this should allow this pathogen to be eliminated from a herd through culture and therapeutic means. This easy step should take precedence over the task of generating protective antibody. Group B streptococci can be divided into five distinct serotypes based on the presence of type-specific antigens. Types Ia, Ib, II and III have distinct carbohydrate determinants that are capsular antigens. Type Ic strains have the type Ia carbohydrate determinant and a protein determinant called the Ibc protein, which is also shared with type Ib strains and some type II strains. Type I strains also share an additional determinant called the type Iabc carbohydrate. Type-specific antigens are located on the surface of the bacterium and induce protective antibodies. The group-specific polysaccharide is common to all strains and is composed of rhamnose, *N*-acetylglucosamine and galactose. There are two additional protein antigens called R and X. X is often associated with bovine mastitis isolates. Recently two additional serotypes, IV and V, were described. Efforts to type the isolates characterized as non-typeable by the conventional scheme have been undertaken resulting in the description of NT1, NT2 and NT3 antigens. Streptococci are composed of peptidoglycan and group-specific antigens. The group-specific antigens may be either polysaccharides or teichoic acids. The former are attached to the peptidoglycan while the teichoic acid group antigens are found in greater amount beneath the cell wall than in it. The type-specific polysaccharide may form a part of the cell wall or form a surface layer.

In New York state dairy herds, three types of Group B streptococci were found: Ia (69.6 per cent), II (16.7 per cent) and III (10.1 per cent). Within a single herd one type predominates with only slight incidence of other types. In Denmark type III is the most common. The protein antigen X is also widespread. No M protein antigens have been identified in bovine streptococci. Increase in the sialic acid moiety occupying the terminal side chains of the group antigen increases virulence. Streptococci of group B have also been phage typed.

Streptococcus agalactiae is an obligate parasite of the mammary gland and attachment to epithelia is a prerequisite for colonization. *Streptococcus uberis* and *Strep. dysgalactiae* are not obligate udder pathogens and can survive on other parts of the cow and in the environment. A leucocytosis of 200 000–500 000 cells/ml prevents infection with *Strep. agalactiae*. This bacteria colonizes the milk ducts. It does not bind significant amounts of fibrinogen, fibronectin or type II collagen. Surface lipoteichoic acid may aid in the attachment to mucosal surfaces. In humans, it has been shown that virulent Group B streptococci contain five times more lipoteichoic acid than non-virulent strains but the significance of this in relation to bovine mastitis is unknown. Extracellular proteins of Group B streptococci include hyaluronidase and deoxyribonucleases. Group B streptococci produce a CAMP factor the significance of which is unknown, but cows with experimentally induced Group B streptococci mastitis show rises in neutralizing titres. CAMP factor is lethal for rabbits and mice. The extracellular type-specific antigen may be important, since it can bind and exhaust specific antibody. Invasive isolates show an increased capacity for synthesis of the polysaccharide and a shift towards less encapsulation was observed during *in vitro* passage, emphasizing the necessity for careful selection and production of strains as immunogens.

Antibody to the capsular polysaccharides and Ibc protein protect mice against lethal challenge but antibody directed against the group-specific carbohydrate does not. The polysaccharides are non-toxic in mice, guinea-pigs and rabbits and like other T independent antigens are weakly immunogenic in mice, rabbits or primates. It is worth noting that in humans there is a good immune response to these polysaccharides if there are pre-existing levels of antibody present (2–3 μg/ml). This may equate with the natural opsonins seen in dairy cows. However, non-immune people respond poorly to the vaccine.

In cattle, most opsonizing antibody is directed to the weakly immunogenic type-specific polysaccharide located on the cell wall. This antibody is a more efficient opsonin if it binds complement. The sera of cows contains low levels of natural opsonin. Cows vaccinated with killed *Strep. agalactiae* contain specific antibody in their whey. Following infection high levels of serum and whey antibodies are generated. The bactericidal activity of neutrophils for *Strep. agalactiae* is dependent on both antibody and complement. Intramammary vaccination with killed or live *Strep. agalactiae* type Ia resulted in a significant production of specific IgA, IgM, IgG_1 and IgG_2. The actual amount of IgA was higher in vaccinated than in non-vaccinated glands. In a mouse protection assay IgA and IgM were more protective than IgG_1.

Cows have been hyperimmunized with *Strep. agalactiae* and challenged with either 2–5 c.f.u. or 120 c.f.u. The two cows challenged with low numbers had no clinical signs and no positive culture, while controls had both. The two given 120 c.f.u. had positive culture but no clinical signs (Norcross *et al.*, 1968). This would suggest that under field conditions with low levels of exposure a degree of protection can be achieved. Mackie showed that heifers became systemically hyperimmune following vaccination by the subcutaneous and intravenous routes but despite high titres there was little real difference between the hyperimmune and non-vaccinated heifers following challenge with *Strep. agalactiae*, and concluded that antibody produced locally may be critical. It is necessary to point out that the intramammary challenge was carried out with an average of 40 million bacteria. It has been shown that antibody to *Strep. agalactiae* could be produced locally in the udder. The antibody response following infusion of live *Strep. agalactiae* into a quarter is biphasic with IgA peaking after 24 hours and then declining, with IgG_1 appearing by 72 hours, peaking at 144 hours and then declining. In non-infected quarters the IgA response is absent. It is possible that the IgA is of serum origin due to its rapid appearance and arises because of changes in vascular integrity. Bactericidal activity is confined to the first phase and opsonic activity is associated with IgA only (Mackie *et al.*, 1986).

A second dose of vaccine was necessary to produce a measurable IgG_1 response to type Ia antigen. Adjuvants were compared for their effect on the immune response of lactating cows to a bacterin–toxoid preparation of *Staph. aureus*, *Strep. agalactiae* and staphylococcal alpha toxoid. Freund's incomplete adjuvant was superior to aluminium hydroxide and a metabolizable emulsion. If further immunological studies are done in the cow it is likely that conjugates of type-specific carbohydrate and proteins will be prepared since these conjugates induce high levels of antibodies to both the protein and the carbohydrate antigens in contrast to the poor immunogenicity of carbohydrate or polysaccharide antigens alone. One protein carrier could be the protein X of *Strep. agalactiae* since antibodies to this protein have recently been shown to have some protective properties against infection with this bacterium. CAMP factor may be a suitable protein for further examination.

STREPTOCOCCUS UBERIS (see p. 297)

Streptococcus uberis has been examined serologically, biochemically and by studies of its DNA and enzymes. It does not fit into the Lancefield classification since 25 per cent of strains type as group E and a few fit into other groups. A similar percentage of strains are CAMP positive and some authors state that this bacterium produces a haemolytically active product also, called the uberis factor, which exerts lethal effects when administered parenterally to rabbits and mice.

When examined for its ability to bind to extracellular matrix proteins, *Strep. uberis* was found to bind low levels of fibronectin, fibrinogen and type II collagen. *Streptococcus uberis* is relatively slow growing in the mammary gland and attachment may be an important step in infection with this organism. The susceptibility of the dry mammary gland to infection with *Strep. uberis* increases with time and in the second half of the dry period all quarters are susceptible. This may relate to low levels of lactoferrin at this stage. In an experiment, two strains were examined, one resistant to killing by PMNs resuspended in milk, the other readily killed; 250–500 c.f.u. were infused into lactating and dry cows. In non-lactating cows both strains caused disease in 6 of 10 quarters. In lactating cows the resistant strain causes clinical mastitis in 16 of 18 quarters, whereas the susceptible strain affected only 2 of 18 quarters. The quarters that resisted this strain did so without apparent inflammatory reaction.

Hill has shown that quarters previously infected with *Strep. uberis* are significantly protected from subsequent infection by the same bacteria (Hill, 1988). A protein antigen common to many strains of *Strep. uberis* has been characterized but its protective capacity has not been examined. The hyaluronic acid capsule of this organism is being closely examined to see if specific antibodies for this capsule can be generated that are opsonic. There is some indication that immunological activity against this pathogen can be stimulated in the gland. However, until more is understood on the protective antigens that are common to this species it is unlikely that any immunity which could cover most isolates could be generated.

STREPTOCOCCUS DYSGALACTIAE (see p. 296)

Streptococcus dysgalactiae is a member of the Group C streptococci and possesses a hyaluronic acid capsule. The group C antigen is a carbohydrate composed of rhamnose and *N*-acetylgalactosamine and three type-specific antigens have been identified, IIa, IIb and IIc. This bacterium is able to cause mastitis on its own and is one of a number of pathogens involved in the aetiology of summer mastitis. Strains of highest infectivity are those that can adhere to mammary epithelial cells the best. *Streptococcus dysgalactiae* binds high levels of fibronectin, low levels of collagen and moderate amounts of fibrinogen. Protein G is present in the cell walls of some Group C streptococci strains and in one study *Strep. dysgalactiae* was able to bind 40 per cent of bovine IgG_1 and 75 per cent of bovine IgG_2. Non-specific binding of immunoglobulin by this organism may protect it from the defence mechanism of the gland. Some strains produce fibrinolysin specific for bovine fibrin. Group C streptococci produce hyaluronidase and deoxynuclease.

Cows develop protective antibody following immunization. Cows hyperimmunized with this organism also showed a degree of resistance to challenge exposure of 5–10 c.f.u./ml of the homologous strain (Stark & Norcross, 1970). This bacterium has been neglected in terms of protective immunity for the past 20 years and with the development of new techniques in immunology and bacteriology it would be prudent to examine the immune response of the cow to this pathogen again and further evaluate its virulence factors. Stark & Norcross concluded that there was no cross-reactive protective epitopes shared by the three groups of mastitis streptococci.

Mucosal immune system

The concept of a common mucosal immune system was proposed following the observation that subsequent to intestinal exposure to antigen, specific immunity was evident at distant mucosal sites. Immunocompetent cells (specific lymphocytes) can migrate from Peyer's patches or mesenteric lymph nodes to distant sites, become resident and respond to sensitizing antigen. This does not seem to be true for ruminants since it appears that there is no selective migration of lymphocytes between the mammary gland and the gut of the cow. Labelled lymphocytes from the supramammary lymph node recirculated to the prescapular and supramammary lymph node, whereas labelled iliac mesenteric lymphocytes were recovered from intestinal mesenteric nodes. It was concluded that lymphocytes do not migrate efficiently between the gut and mammary gland of the cow. Studies in sheep have indicated the existence of two major groups of recirculating lymphocytes, a peripheral and an intestinal pool. Local administration of antigen to the mammary gland would stimulate lymphocytes in the lamina propria to expand clonally and some of these cells would traffic to the supramammary lymph node. Following local immunization, lymphocytes may emigrate from the gland or antigen may reach other lymphatic tissues and generate specific cells. Oral administration in the cow stimulates IgG_1, and the presentation of antigen to the intestine results in an increase in specific IgG in both the serum and mammary secretions.

Generation of immune response

Immune responses designed to protect the bovine mammary gland from infection can be generated by three methods. Parenteral immunization can be performed by the intramuscular, subcutaneous or intravenous route. This method will generate serum antibody but systemic immunization has a poor ability to affect the immune status of the gland. It is known that when mammary epithelium becomes inflamed sizeable amounts of circulating antibody pass into the lacteal secretions from the serum by transudation. There will always be a lag time before such antibody can exert effects on an invading micro-organism.

Direct injection of antigens into the udder stimulated both a local and systemic response. The cells necessary for an immune response, namely the macrophage or antigen presenting cell, the T lymphocyte and the B lymphocyte are all present in the mammary gland. Local infusion of killed antigen into the dry gland can give rise to the production of local antibody and this production can persist well into lactation. Levels of IgA and IgG_1 in milk can be increased by local antigenic stimulation of the udder. This is not noticed if antigen is given to the lactating gland. Antigen-stimulated lymphocytes may migrate to other quarters or antigen may be transferred to other quarters, leading to the secretion of specific antibody in the secretion of these quarters. Also, if systemic immunization is carried out at drying-off, a booster infusion shortly before parturition allows the gland to give a heightened and prolonged response through the next lactation. It has been shown that administration of antigen followed by local infusion recruits cells from systemic lymphoid tissue that have been primed by intraperitoneal immunization.

Vaccination in the region of the draining lymph node of the mammary gland appears to stimulate serum antibody and promote the production of local antibody. This may be due to the trafficking of lymphocytes from the gland. The superficial inguinal lymph node can increase threefold in size in cases of clinical mastitis but antibody has its greatest effect when it is present in lacteal secretions before infection is established.

What are the important components of successful immunization of the bovine mammary gland? It is important to identify protective *antigens* of pathogens and to elucidate the mechanisms of host–pathogen interaction that lead to mastitis. It is evident that antigens produced from bacteria that have been extensively passaged in the laboratory may bear little resemblance to those being expressed by the micro-organism in the cow. The numbers of bacteria required to stimulate a protective response is much greater than was previously thought.

The *route* of immunization is important. The J5 *E. coli* vaccine is given subcutaneously and affords some protection to coliform mastitis. However, in general the administration of antigen in the region of the draining lymph node with or without local infusion is likely to have greatest impact on the generation of antibodies in the lacteal secretions. The *time* of vaccination is another important factor since most infections occur at drying-off, during the dry period and in the periparturient period. Vaccination should be designed to offer maximum protection at these times.

Adjuvants are substances that act in a non-specific manner to augment the immune response to an antigen. The magnitude, duration and isotypic composition of the response can be affected. The mechanism of action of adjuvants is not fully understood but the following are involved.

1 Adjuvant immobilizes the antigen in a depot and permits its slow release to the immune system, or maintains a reservoir of antigen within macrophages.

2 They can alter lymphocyte recirculation and promote both lymphocyte trapping and antigen localization in draining lymph nodes.

3 Macrophages may be stimulated to secrete interleukin 1 and other cytokines that promote antigen presentation and lymphocyte proliferation.

Adjuvants may be able to stimulate antibody to poorly immunogenic substances and may also be able to stimulate antibody of the most effective isotype to promote a protective function such as opsonization.

Limitations of vaccination

The scientific literature contains numerous reports documenting the failure of vaccination to protect against intramammary challenge with a pathogen. Such reports account for the two opposing views concerning the role of vaccination in future mastitis control programmes. Challenge studies often have consisted of infusing millions of bacteria into the teat sinus, which is not an accurate reflection of natural infections in which only a few organisms will traverse the teat duct and reach the cistern to multiply. A better way to examine immunization schemes for efficacy would be to do field trials in herds where exposure to the pathogen will occur, with half the herd receiving vaccine and half receiving placebo. The evaluation of clinical inflammation, persistence of leucocytosis and of bacterial shedding and the effect on milk production are important parameters to record in any trials. The excess extrapolation of results obtained using laboratory animals has caused confusion with regard to what actually happens in the bovine mammary gland.

The dairy cow undergoes periods of severe stress in each lactational cycle and there is increasing evidence to support the theory that immune dysfunction occurs at certain times. Immunosuppression can occur during pregnancy, lactation and parturition. Much interest has been directed to the four-day period prior to and subsequent to parturition, the so-called periparturient immunosuppression. The immune dysfunction may be due to immunoregulatory proteins produced during pregnancy, by suppressor cells or by the influence of hormones such as prolactin.

Secretion taken just after drying-off and at parturition has an inhibitory effect on blastogenic responses to mitogens. Proliferative response to mitogens by blood and milk lymphocytes is low for one week before parturition and lowest on the day before calving (Kehrli *et al.*, 1989). This may relate to the high incidence of clinical mastitis and intramammary infection that occurs at calving and up to 30 days after calving. It is believed that colostrum contains cytotoxic factors that can block the FcRs of phagocytes. Neutrophils showed increases in certain parameters two weeks before parturition and decreased dramatically by the first week after parturition. The ingestion capacity remained steady but chemotaxis was defective. By the first week after parturition lymphocyte blastogenosis was significantly impaired and this postpartum impairment can affect neutrophil function by the release of or failure to release cytokines.

Since the concentration of PMNs is used to assess milk quality and a major defence component of the gland will involve a leucocytosis with specific antibody, some authors have become tied up in the semantics of whether protection afforded by such a leucocytosis is by definition mastitis. It is clear that such a protective response can be interpreted in this manner. But one cannot ignore the mounting evidence that indicates that, for certain pathogens, appropriate immunization strategies can reduce the number of clinical cases, reduce the number of new infections, improve the response to therapy and decrease the severity of clinical mastitis. If this involves a transient leucocytosis, it is likely that people will accept the benefits.

The mammary gland of the cow has limited defensive capabilities with regard to PMN function and level of opsonins. In developed countries, good cows yield on average 25 l of milk for each day of their lactation. To maintain levels of antibody in this volume of secretion requires an enormous synthetic rate. Immunization does not confer absolute protection and at best will complement good husbandry and other mastitis control procedures. For certain mastitis pathogens there is little prospect for immunological intervention in the next decade or two. For *E. coli* and *Staph. aureus* it appears that vaccination may become a component of a mastitis control programme.

References

Anderson, J.C. (1978) The problem of immunization against staphylococcal mastitis. *British Veterinary Journal*, **134**, 412–20.

Boothby, J.T., Jasper, J.E. & Thomas, C.B. (1986) Experimental intramammary inoculation with *Mycoplasma bovis* in vaccinated and unvaccinated cows: effect on the mycoplasmal infection and cellular inflammatory response. *Cornell Veterinarian*, **76**, 188–97.

Butler, J.E. (1986) Biochemistry and biology of ruminant immunoglobulins. *Progress in Veterinary Microbiology and Immunology*, **2**, 1–53.

Colditz, I.G. & Watson, D.L. (1985) Immunophysiological basis for vaccinating ruminants against mastitis. *Australian Veterinary Journal*, **62**, 145–52.

Duhamel, G.E., Bernoco, D., Davis, W.C. & Osburn, B.I. (1987) Distribution of T and B lymphocytes in mammary dry secretions, colostrum and blood of adult dairy cattle. *Veterinary Immunology and Immunopathology*, **14**, 101–22.

Gudding, R., McDonald, J.S. & Cheville, N.F. (1984) Pathogenesis of *Staphylococcus aureus* mastitis: bacteriologic, histologic, and ultrastructural pathologic findings. *American Journal of Veterinary Research*, **45**, 2525–31.

Hill, A.W. (1988) Protective effect of previous intramammary infection with *Streptococcus uberis* against subsequent clinical mastitis in the cow. *Research in Veterinary Science*, **44**, 386–7.

Hill, A.W., Heneghan, J.S., Field, T.R. & Williams, M.R. (1983) Increase in specific opsonic activity in bovine milk following experimental *Escherichia coli* mastitis. *Research in Veterinary Science*, **35**, 222–6.

Kehrli, M.E., Nonnecke, B.J. & Roth, J.A. (1989) Alterations in bovine lymphocyte function during the periparturient period. *American Journal of Veterinary Research*, **50**, 215–20.

Lee, C.-S., Wooding, F.B.P. & Kemp, P. (1980) Identification, properties and differential counts of cell populations using electron microscopy of dry cows secretions, colostrum and milk from normal cows. *Journal of Dairy Research*, **47**, 39–50.

Mackie, D.P., Meneely, D.J., Pollack, D.A. & Logan, E.F. (1986) The loss of opsonic activity of bovine milk whey following depletion of IgA. *Veterinary Immunology and Immunopathology*, **11**, 193–8.

Mellenberger, R.W. (1977) Vaccination against mastitis. *Journal of Dairy Science*, **60**, 1016–21.

Norcross, N.L., Dodd, K. & Stark, D.M. (1968) Use of the mouse protection test to assay streptococci antibodies in bovine serum and milk. *American Journal of Veterinary Research*, **29**, 1201–5.

Sorensen, G.H. (1972) Sommermastitis. Den mulige beskyttende virkning af to forskellige vacciner overfor eksperimentelle infektioner. *Nordisk Veterinar Medicin*, **24**, 259–71.

Stark, D.M. & Norcross, N.L. (1970) Response of bovine to immunization against *Streptococcus dysgalactiae*. *Cornell Veterinarian*, **60**, 604–12.

Stuart, P., Buntain, D. & Langridge, R.G. (1951) Bacteriological examination of secretions from cases of summer mastitis and experimental infection of non-lactating bovine udders. *Veterinary Record*, **63**, 451–3.

Watson, E.D. (1989) *In vitro* function of bovine neutrophils against *Actinomyces pyogenes*. *American Journal of Veterinary Research*, **50**, 455–8.

Further reading

Craven, N. & Williams, M.R. (1985) Defences of the bovine mammary gland against infection and prospects for their enhancement. *Veterinary Immunology and Immunopathology*, **10**, 71–127.

Gonzalez, R.N., Cullor, J.S., Jasper, D.E., Farver, T.B., Bushnell, R.B. & Oliver, M.N. (1989) Prevention of clinical coliform mastitis in dairy cattle by a mutant *Escherichia coli* vaccine. *Canadian Journal of Veterinary Research*, **53**, 301–5.

Hill, A.W. (1979) The pathogenesis of experimental *Escherichia coli* mastitis in newly calved dairy cows. *Research in Veterinary Science*, **26**, 97–101.

Newby, T.J., Stokes, C.R. & Bourne, F.J. (1982) Immunological activities of milk. *Veterinary Immunology and Immunopathology*, **3**, 67–94.

Nickerson, S.C. (1985) Immune mechanisms of the bovine udder: an overview. *Journal of the American Veterinary Medical Association*, **187**, 41–5.

Lameness

Chapter 28: Foot Lameness

by D.J. PETERSE

Introduction

Lameness is a common and important economic problem, often seen on a herd basis. The severity of lameness in a herd and its degree of acceptance by the farmer varies. In most cases it originates in the hoof and the area directly connected to it. Lameness caused by disorders in other parts of the locomotor system is less frequent and is usually restricted to individual animals (see Chapter 29).

In Denmark, the economic loss can be expressed per case of lameness or per cow as shown in Table 28.1.

A British survey concluded that 5.5 per cent of cows in the national herd received veterinary attention for lameness (Russel *et al.* 1982). This did not include the many other cows that would have received farmer treatment. The cost to the national dairy herd was estimated at £36 million, or £9.20 for every cow affected and non-affected. Leg disorders accounted for only a small proportion (12 per cent) of the total, most of which were calving injuries. Foot lesions accounted for 88 per cent of cases, the majority of which (84 per cent of foot lesions) were in the hind feet, and more specifically (64 per cent) in the lateral claw of the hind feet. A secondary survey, carried out using on-farm data, indicated that whereas 6.3 per cent of the total herd were treated by veterinary surgeons for lameness, the overall incidence, including farmer treatment, was 25 per cent per annum (Whittaker *et al.* 1983).

A number of disorders occur, not all of which are fully understood. Depending on the category of cattle, namely dairy cows, young stock or fattening steers, different diagnoses may predominate. Feeding, management, housing systems and immune status determine which claw disorder may occur in a given instance.

Generalized infections producing clinical signs in the claw, e.g. foot-and-mouth disease, will not be dealt with in this chapter.

Importance of conformation and its interaction with the environment

One of the most striking characteristics of nearly all lameness cases, both infectious and non-infectious, is the predominant involvement of the hind feet. In the case of infectious disorders the hind feet are often exposed to faeces and urine to a greater extent, which makes the predisposition understandable. However, even in free housing systems, where the chance of infection in both hind and front feet is equal, hind feet are more frequently involved. This observation has prompted several studies of the anatomical basis for the predisposition. External examination of legs and claws has consistently failed to quantify any specific factors. Much more precise measurements of the claws and legs

Table 28.1 Economic costs of lameness

	Cost per case(£)	Cost per cow(£)
Loss of production	20.00	4.50
Loss of weight	3.50	1.00
Loss if culled	155.00	3.00
Costs of treatment	12.00	6.00

indicate that there is an association between sole ulcers and, for example, the length of the dorsal wall, the angle of the dorsal wall with the ground surface and the heel depth. In general, a steep claw seems less prone to sole ulcer. However, it has to be realized that the association may illustrate a predisposition to sole ulcer or simply indicate two signs of the same condition.

The shape of the claw is dependent on the environment. Tied systems or free housing systems, full concrete floors or slatted floors each have their effect on claw shape. Depending on the way the animal moves, different parts of the claw are more or less loaded with the cow's weight and so more or less abraded. On slatted floors a cow has a short step and the hind feet are not brought far forward under the body. The result is a steep claw with high heels. It appears that the cow does not enjoy moving on such a surface. In experiments where choice is offered, walking is restricted to movement to and from the feeding and lying area.

Analyses have been made of the cow's movement, the loading of the claws and their interaction with specific floor conditions, especially their smoothness and slipperiness. By measurement it can be shown that a general pattern exists. Thus during the contact of the claw with the ground there is initially a braking force and sequentially a driving force. Forces to the lateral wall, to the sole and a small amount of rotation can be registered. Due to variation between animals and the technical constraints of examining large numbers, it is not yet clear how this information can be incorporated into understanding the lameness problem. Analysis of weight distribution between the lateral and medial hind claw indicates overloading of the lateral claw in all adult cows. In addition, during small movements of the standing animal there is more extensive load variation on the lateral than on the medial claw. This higher degree of stretching of the tissues between the horny capsula and the third phalanx could be the triggering factor. Exostoses found on the solar surface of the lateral claw bone probably result from this stretching. The reason for overloading of the lateral hind claw in adult cattle could be the result of a vicious circle. Even in two-year-old cattle, both pregnant and non-pregnant, a small overload on the lateral claw can be measured. During the initial stages of damage to the lateral claw pododerm the cow will try to reduce weight on the affected site and move with care, thus less wear will occur. However, the affected tissue reacts by repair and horn production will be stimulated, leading to a greater heel depth in the lateral compared with the medial claw. This in turn leads to the lateral claw being further overloaded and makes it even more prone to further damage or delayed repair.

Treatment of a sole ulcer by reducing the depth of the lateral heel stimulates recovery, and paring the feet to distribute weight more equally between lateral and medial claws can help prevent sole ulcers. The primary factor in this sequence of events could be the difference in position of the hind phalanges in the lateral and medial claws. In the lateral claw the third phalanx rests partly on the sole, while in the medial claw it is more firmly attached to the wall, thus reducing the pressure on the tissues between the posterior side of the claw bone and the horny capsula.

The stretching and depressing forces that deform the horny capsula during each step are also thought to be responsible for the favoured site of the white line in lameness. Friction between stretching and compression is concentrated on the posterior part of the lateral hind claw wall, halfway between the coronet and sole. However, in the front feet, there is a clear predisposition for the medial claw to be affected. No valid reason has been found for this phenomenon. These predispositions cause an animal lame on all four feet to adopt a very characteristic stance. The front feet are placed against each other or even crossed, while the hind feet are positioned wide apart and the cow is often cow-hocked, as the claws are turned laterally.

Horn production

The horn is a product of the stratum germinatinum. The wall is produced by the coronet. This horn wall is attached to the underlying corium by primary folds. The secondary folds, as in the horse, are missing. On the stratum germinatinum, papillae produce tubules. Histologically, the wall of the tubules, their centre and horn between the tubules can be distinguished. The number of tubules and the thickness of their wall are a factor determining horn strength. Another field where attempts have been made to qualify the claw horn is that of the chemical composition. Chemically, horn consists of keratins. These proteins are linked together by sulphydryl bridges. The number of sulphydryl bridges differs in various parts of the horny capsula, the hardest horn containing the highest numbers. Black pigment has a good reputation for being harder but it is questionable whether this is based on overall breed differences in lameness or whether the presence of melanin does provide additional strength to the horn. The horn-producing process can be influenced by a large number of factors such as nutrition, both total energy intake as well as availability of the more specific sulphur-containing amino acids, copper, zinc, biotin; and also by the degree of abrasion, ambient temperature, claw disorders and age. On average the dorsal wall horn production is 5 mm/month. In the heel region horn production is greater. Correction of the shape of the hind claws by trimming means particularly removing horn from where the horn growth is greatest. Thus in decreasing sequence most paring is of the lateral heel, followed by lateral toe region and medial toe region. The medial heel needs hardly any paring.

Diminishing capillary diffusion due to low ambient temperature or in cases of laminitis will interrupt the horn production of the stratum germinatinum, which is demonstrated by a groove in the horny capsula. Research has concentrated on supplying extra methionine, zinc or biotin rather than producing convincing experimental data that these dietary constituents are lacking and thereby justifying their extra provision.

Horn wear depends on hardness of the horn and thus its water content. Wet conditions underfoot have a dramatic effect on the hardness of horn. This is clearly demonstrated when attempting to pare feet in very dry weather. The detachment of water from the horn by using products such as formalin or copper sulphate diminishes the wear rate. The physical qualities of the floor have a strong effect on abrasion. It needs several weeks to establish the equilibrium between horn production and abrasion.

Typical cattle with overworn soles are reluctant to move. Most wear is in the toe region. Since the wall horn production starts at the coronet any damage in that region will be noticeable in the horn wall, and is most apparent in the heel area. Skin infections and injuries just along the coronet product an interruption in the horn wall. Sandcracks, sometimes hardly visible vertical fissures, may result. They are painful, slow to heal and often relapse.

Disorders in the hooves

In today's dairy herds few totally sound hooves can be found, especially during the winter housing period. Manifestations of the important claw disorders vary from slight signs to serious lameness. Thus when examining lameness cases one has to realize that some mild signs of a particular claw disorder may be present that are not the cause of lameness, and that often signs of two disorders occur together. Also it has to be accepted that in really complicated and long-standing cases the primary disorder may no longer be recognizable. In this complex field it is helpful when analysing problems to use the scheme in which primary disorders are separated from secondary signs. Besides the common English names for the various conditions, the Latin names proposed by an international working party will be used.

Interrelationship of the digital disorders

Primary claw disorders can be divided into infectious causes and those of a metabolic–traumatic origin. All signs in diseased claws can be described as more or less separate entities although they can also be examined for their similarities. The flow chart (Fig. 28.1) presents an outline of the main claw disorders in which their various interrelationships is suggested. It also enables a wide range of signs to be concentrated into a few basic diagnoses. These diagnoses, based on examination of several animals in a herd, allow for prevention and treatment to be more effective. Thus the veterinarian's work is not just restricted to treatment of the most lame animals.

Although some signs can be a sequel of different disorders, a close inspection in most cases gives an indication of the condition, e.g. whether an interdigital overgrowth is a sequel of interdigital phlegmon or interdigital dermatitis. Thus in the first case the overgrowth is often in the middle of the interdigital space and in the second case it is sited away from the centre near the wall of the lateral claw. Sole ulcers originating from a laminitic process are found under the proximal edge of the claw and often there is separation from the sole by haemorrhage (plate 28.1). Extension to the axial surface is especially noticeable in heifers. The ulcer caused by heel horn erosion is a part of the heel horn erosion as, for example, under the edge of the cleft. Thus these ulcers tend to be located in the heel area. In the same way sole ulcers originating from laminitis or interdigital dermatitis can be differentiated, as can heel horn erosion caused by interdigital or digital dermatitis. Thus heel horn erosion resulting from interdigital dermatitis gradually develops from the proximal axial part of the heel over a wide area. This results in extensive underrunning of the heel horn. In cases of digital dermatitis these erosions are more focal and restricted to the affected area of the coronet or pododerm.

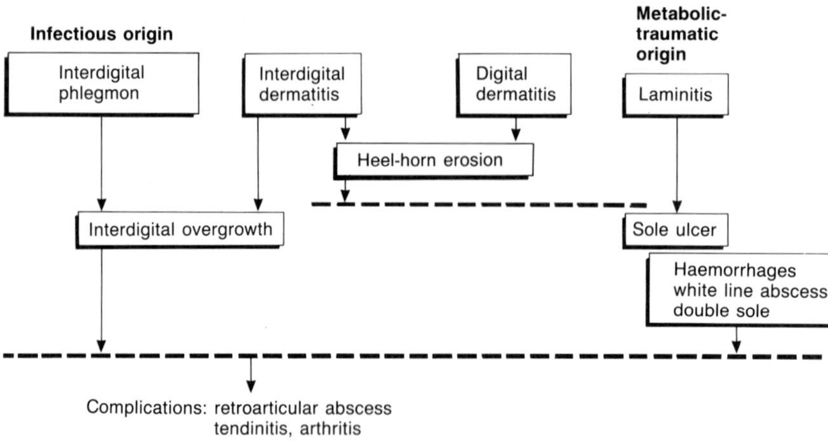

Fig. 28.1 Outline of the main claw disorders

Infectious claw disorders

Introduction

A number of bacterial species are incriminated in foot disorders, such as *Bacteroides*, *Fusobacterium*, spirochaetes and *Campylobacter*. It is usually accepted that combinations of these bacteria are responsible for the disorders. The question then arises as to what extent some are essential for disease and which of the isolated species belong to the normal interdigital flora. It is characteristic for these groups of bacteria that they grow under anaerobic or facultative anaerobic conditions. Their volatile fatty acid production causes a specific smell by which each infection can be recognized. The infections are described as separate entities, but often they are mixed together and in consequence very complex clinical pictures can result.

Interdigital phlegmon (foul of the foot, interdigital necrobacillosis)

This disorder is an acute painful inflammation of the interdigital subcutaneous tissues. Swelling may be seen at the dorsal area of the digit, but most frequently the plantar side of the pastern is thick and painful. The affected animal shows a rise in body temperature, some distress and is severely lame.

Even in the first stage of infection the interdigital skin remains intact. However, in later stages, and if treatment is delayed, a purulent diphtheritic necrosis can be seen in the interdigital skin. Complications such as inflammation of the tendons and a pedal arthritis are possible. In these cases a deformed thickened digit can be the end result. Interdigital overgrowth (hyperplasia) is another common sequel to infection.

Interdigital phlegmon is the most common cause of lameness in young stock and fattening units, either in individual animals or as small outbreaks. In dairy herds with older cows the incidence is less and cases are often restricted to young heifers recently introduced into the herd. The hind claws are more frequently involved than the front claws both at pasture and in loose housing systems. Adverse conditions described vary from dry hard ground to very wet and muddy areas. Anything that damages the skin and anything encouraging crowding of the animals favours the disease. The incidence in loose housing systems is similar to that in cattle grazing outdoors.

Fusobacterium necrophorum is generally considered to be the cause, and different biotypes with varying virulence can be differentiated. It is accepted that the bacteria invade through traumatic dermal injuries and also after superficial inflammation of the skin. *Bacteroides melaninogenicus*, another normal environmental bacterium, may play an essential role in the pathogenesis of the condition.

Affected animals probably acquire a local immunity as a digit is seldom affected twice. Thus in experimental infection a cow's foot can only be used once for a challenge with the causal agent. Sometimes interdigital phlegmon-like signs can be observed but the onset of the condition is slow and the response to antibiotic therapy is poor. This may be another infectious claw disorder that has been complicated by a *F. necrophorum* infection.

Treatment

In the early stages, treatment with oral sulphonamides (e.g. sulphanilamide) is effective. However, better results can be expected from the parenteral administration of sulphonamides (sulphanilamide or sulphadimidine) or antibiotics (e.g. penicillin or tetracyclines). It may be necessary to continue treatment for three days. In general the response to therapy is good, but when necrotic areas are present local disinfection and wound treatment are necessary. Complicated cases, in which the inflammation has extended to the tendons or the joint, require concentrated surgical treatment and prognosis is much more guarded.

Prevention

Although *F. necrophorum* is part of the normal environmental flora, and eradication is therefore impossible, use of a foot bath containing 3 per cent formalin solution can reduce the number of cattle affected in an outbreak. In fattening units with slatted floors low pressure hosing of the solution onto the feet (and slats) is useful, while it has been claimed that in straw yards the use of paraformaldehyde crystals reduces incidence. Reduction of the incidence by using food additives has also been tried. Ethylenediamidedihydroiodide (EDDI, 0.25 mg/kg body weight daily for two weeks) as a feed additive is useful in beeflot units. A decrease in incidence of 30 per cent has been observed. However, its use can be complicated by a depression of the immune system, resulting, for example, in signs of respiratory distress.

Dermatitis interdigitalis (plate 28.2)

In the nomenclature used for claw diseases the diagnosis interdigital dermatitis should be reserved for a superficial inflammation of the interdigital skin, especially in the area between the bulbs. *Bacteroides nodosus* is considered to be the causal agent, similar to the aetiology of dermatitis contagiosa interdigitalis (footrot) in sheep. However, *F. necrophorum* increases the severity of infection. *Bacteroides nodosus* can be subdivided into different strains by tests of antigen structure and the presence or absence of proteolytic enzymes. It is probable that sheep and cattle have their own distinct types. *Bacteroides nodosus* strains isolated from cattle seem to have less elastase activity and in experiments cattle strains were only able to evoke benign footrot (scald) in sheep. In practice it is thought that cross-infection between species probably does not play an important role in disease spread.

Bacteroides nodosus can survive for only a few weeks in the animals' environment. As it is not a part of the natural flora of cattle and sheep the eradication of the bacterium on a farm should be possible. The inflammation of the interdigital epidermis is not particularly extensive but the area is usually sensitive to touch. The odour produced by the anaerobic flora is characteristic. Commonly both hind feet are affected. Although the initial eczema seems to have this rather benign character, it is the next step in the pathogenesis that causes problems. Inflammation of the epidermis at the heel results in disturbances of local horn production with the onset of erosion and underrunning of the heel horn (plates 28.3 and 4). In severe cases the heel horn may disappear totally and a deep cleft will result. Mild attacks produce several smaller clefts. These affected claws become deformed. As a reaction to the inflammation, horn growth will be stimulated and at the same time the cow reduces floor contact with the sensitive parts of the foot so that abrasion and wear diminishes. In the long term, affected cows can be distinguished by their sensitive gait, cowhocked stance and oversized lateral claws when compared with the medial claws.

In such cases the lateral hind claw may be overloaded with up to 75 per cent of the total weight. Thus a sole ulcer can easily develop and if so it is often localized to the cleft under the hard edge of horn produced by the continuing dermatitis.

Certain circumstances favour this infection, such as a warm and wet environment. Where tied systems are in operation, the incidence in the second half of the housing period is high but it is also common in free-stall systems, especially those with wet floors. In situations where the claws are 'washed' by a mixture of dung, urine and water, the eczema on the interdigital skin may not be noticed and only the secondary changes in the heel horn indicate the diagnosis. During the pasture period the severity of the signs and the infection rate diminish. Only in zero-grazing systems and where the cattle are housed at night does the infection continue into the spring and summer. The diagnosis is made on clinical signs. Isolation of *B. nodosus* requires an experienced laboratory as the organism is extremely fragile in culture. A fluorescent antibody technique is an easier confirmation of the diagnosis.

There are, however, many other hypotheses concerning the aetiology of sole ulcers. Some consider ulcers to result from contact with environmental bacterial flora, together with erosive chemical components from urine and dung combined with an increased susceptibility due to an insufficient supply of zinc. In the UK it is commonly accepted that excessive standing, leading to bruising of the solar corium, is an important factor. In support of this, surveys have shown a lower incidence of sole ulcers in straw yards than in cubicle housed (free stall) systems. This is said to be because straw yards are more comfortable, and cows spend longer lying down, thus reducing trauma on the corium between the pedal bone and solar horn. A cow should spend approximately 14 hours each day lying down. If cubicles are uncomfortable, either because of their design or because inadequate bedding is used, then cows are reluctant to lie in them. They then spend longer standing and an increased incidence of sole ulcers results. Freshly calved heifers are a particular problem. They are often reared at pasture and/or in loose housing. Following introduction into the milking herd, not only do they have to compete at the bottom of a new social dominance, and become accustomed to a new feeding system (during which they may develop ruminal acidosis), but they also often have to find and learn how to use cubicles. The consequences of these three factors is often extremely soft soles in heifers, followed one to two months later by sole ulcers.

Treatment

The superficial inflammation of the interdigital skin can be treated by contact with a 3 per cent formalin solution. Often this is practised by means of a foot bath, but it can be sprayed by low pressure equipment or used in a claw boot or as an ointment under bandages. It must be realized that re-infection is to be expected; thus in tied systems the standing has also to be disinfected and in free stall systems regular use of the foot bath is necessary. Formalin cannot be used in complicated cases where the deeper-lying tissues are exposed as it delays healing. Use of an antibiotic/gentian violet aerosol for treatment of individual cases is also effective.

The secondary signs of heel horn erosion and sole ulcers need precise paring of the claw. The pressure on the area of inflamed pododerm has to be removed, and the whole claw remodelled so that most of the weight is shifted onto the medial claw. In severe cases a block can be fixed by glueing, nailing or screwing to the medial claw. This contributes enormously to a fast recovery. Secondary interdigital overgrowths may also need treatment. Mild disinfectants like washing soda (sodium carbonate) in a claw sack for some hours followed a few days later by 3 per cent formalin solution can be applied to shrink the overgrowth. Paring the central medial edge of each claw, thus increasing the space between the digits and reducing secondary trauma on the overgrowth, will help considerably in mild cases. Surgical removal is easily carried out on larger lesions. Unfortunately relapses often occur.

Prevention

The prevention of interdigital dermatitis is based primarily on regular use of a formalin foot bath during the risk period. The bathing has to satisfy certain standards:

1 The skin/solution contact has to be sufficient, thus the bath has to be long enough (2.5–3 m); the claws should not be too muddy, and the concentration must remain between 3–5 per cent formalin (formalin = 37 per cent formaldehyde).

2 The skin/solution contact has to be long enough; the formalin film will remain for 30 minutes if not removed by dung, mud or grass. The formalin on the skin must reach the temperature of the skin, which is normally above 20 °C.

3 The skin/solution contact must be repeated twice a day for four successive days, and in an infected area this treatment has to be repeated monthly; if the animals are to be moved to a clean area or barn, one hour in a foot bath is a useful preventive measure at the start of the housing period.

Foot bathing before milking has to be avoided because of the formalin smell for the milker and because its irritant properties will make the cows fidgety. In addition to its disinfectant properties, formalin has a hardening effect on the stratum corneum. This layer becomes thicker and may be a better barrier against the penetration of *B. nodosus*. Other disinfectants such as creolin (2 per cent) and copper sulphate (5–10 per cent) have less effect than formalin and other disadvantages such as the penetrating smell and potential environmental pollution. Zinc sulphate (10 per cent) is used in the treatment of footrot in sheep and is the best alternative. Zinc can be absorbed by skin and horn and may contribute to hoof quality. Experiments have produced variable results however.

Dermatitis digitalis (plate 28.5)

Dermatitis digitalis has been described as a cause of herd outbreaks of lameness in Italy, England and The Netherlands. Its signs, including its smell, seem to be quite distinctive from other infections. In the initial phase, probably two to three weeks after infection, a circumscribed area 1–2 cm^2 diameter appears on the skin just above the coronet, with an intensely painful exudative superficial inflammation. Although the lesion is not proliferative, the surface has a strawberry-like appearance. The pastern is occasionally a little swollen but this is not a consistent feature. The predominant infected areas are the skin at the dorsal and especially plantar end of the interdigital cleft, but it can also be found on an interdigital overgrowth, in a sole ulcer and around the dew-claws. In longer standing cases the affected area expands, the directly adjacent heel horn disappears, longer hairs grow around the area and sometimes affected skin reacts by producing elastic filaments. In the long term some cases resemble dermatitis verrucosa.

The cows are often affected in both hind claws and their intense pain and suffering is evident. In housed cattle the infection spreads easily especially where stocking density is high and hygiene in suboptimal. Herds are often initially infected by purchased animals. Until now no common causal agent has been isolated. Material from infected claws can sometimes produce lesions in uninfected cattle, but transmission is not easy, indicating that environmental or other predisposing factors must be important. Spontaneous recovery is seldom observed.

Treatment

Therapy involves treatment of the affected area with a tetracycline spray combined with gentian violet. Unlike the parenteral treatment, one topical application without further dressing results in nearly 100 per cent recovery with a second treatment seldom necessary. All efforts to treat the wounds with disinfectants or non-antibiotic medicaments have failed. Once a herd is infected it needs a continuous control programme. The number of affected cows can be so large that individual care is not possible and then a herd treatment is necessary. In these cases a foot bath with a tetracycline solution (1 g/l) and bathing for four successive days can be practised. Ten days after the tetracycline baths a strong solution of 5 per cent formalin in a foot bath may be used to harden the skin. However, others have considered that excessive use of formalin may exacerbate digital dermatitis. Intensive use of antibiotic solutions induces resistance.

Mud and frost eczema

Under very cold and wet conditions a dermatitis in the area from the coronet to the dew claws can occur. Initially, an exudative eczema develops, but this stage is often missed. The exudate then dries among the hairs, crusts are formed, and the swollen skin hardens and cracks following movements of the joints. Deep horizontal skin fissures occur at the pastern and along the coronet and lameness can be severe.

Several bacterial species and moulds have been isolated from the wounds but no causal agent has been identified. The condition is mainly seen in one to two-year-old stock housed on slatted floors during the winter, but it also occurs in animals at pasture during rainy periods in the summer and autumn. Several animals may become infected over a short period. A change in environment should prevent further spread. Lesions slowly resolve even without treatment. Mild disinfectants such as teat dips and oily ointments assist recovery.

Differential diagnosis

The differential diagnoses of digital skin infections include signs of general infections such as foot-and-mouth disease (see p. 537) and the mucosal form of bovine virus diarrhoea (see p. 660). Signs of local disorders must also be considered, such as solanin (potato) poisoning, chemical irritations from use of over-strong solutions in a foot bath and chorioptic mange (see p. 683). A good history and the signs presented generally enable a clear diagnosis to be made.

Claw disorders of metabolic–traumatic origin

Introduction

The adjectives 'metabolic' and 'traumatic' are combined here in order to meet a compromise. It is logical that a purely traumatic injury (e.g. a nail through the sole) will result in pododermatitis. On the other hand, it is generally agreed that a pododermatitis also develops after acute laminitis (pododermatitis aseptica). However, many cases of pododermatitis result from the combination of a weakened pododerm and horn caused by laminitis together with claws stressed by weight or physical trauma from the environment. Current concepts concerning the aetiology of pododermatitis, and whether metabolic or traumatic factors receive most attention, depend on the personal experience of the protagonist as well as local management and circumstances. There have been only a limited number of experiments concerning pododermatitis and their results have seldom provided convincing support for any specific theory. The laminitic process in the horse is similar to laminitis in cattle and may be used because it is a greater source of researched information.

According to herd records and questionnaires, clinical cases of acute laminitis are responsible for a very low percentage of all lamenesses in cattle. However, sole ulcers and white line lesions originating from this laminitic process are a very important part of the non-infectious lameness incidence. The most susceptible cattle are heifers in the period around calving. In young stock the disorder (and sole ulcers) are seldom noticed with the exception of fattening bulls. In these animals it is known that sudden changes in the ration, especially when there is a restricted forage supply, may induce laminitis. Conditions that predispose to laminitis include stress by transport, moving to new herds, sudden changes in ration, no opportunity to adapt to concrete floors, a protracted calving or dystokia with complications such as retained fetal membranes or mastitis. In many management systems several of these activating factors are concentrated around calving. It is thus understandable that lameness is often linked with calving. Less frequent are cases for which the possible source of the disorder is a toxic component in the ration, e.g. a specific mould in silage or a factor in barley.

Sometimes young heifers show sensitivity of their hooves and reluctance to move when the housing period starts. The clinical signs are likely to be those of laminitis, and often result from excessive standing following sudden introduction onto concrete and a cubicle-housed system.

Pododermatitis aseptica (Laminitis: clinical, subclinical, acute, chronic)

In the diagnosis of pododermatitis aseptica all attention is focused on the pododerm, but it must be realized that the local dysfunction is part of a more generalized disorder that affects other organs of the animal. The origin of the disorder is localized to the claw only when the laminitis is primarily traumatic. Pododermatitis aseptica may also be initiated in the digestive tract or, less frequently, by the occurrence of a serious inflammatory process elsewhere in the body. Commonly, more than one factor is involved, for example a combination of trauma and diet. The laminitic process varies from clinical to subclinical, and the course of the disorder may be acute, subacute or chronic. Classifications are often rather confusing, depending on one's conception of the aetiology and pathogenesis of the condition. If the laminitic process is restricted to a generalized condition that causes perfusion problems in the claw, the duration of acute laminitis will be short. However, the consequences may be longer term. Thus a solar ulcer may become visible a long time after the initial process has resolved. If local changes in the claw are considered to be an essential component of the laminitic process, the duration from start to the appearance of clinical signs in the claw may vary from just a few days in very serious cases, to a few months. In less serious cases of longer duration the classification acute, subacute and chronic seems most suitable. Awareness of these two distinguishable classification systems for laminitis may be important for treatment when it has to be decided whether it is the initial or the secondary process (or both) which can be controlled.

Clinical signs

The initial phase of laminitis can be clinical as well as subclinical. In the clinical form generalized distress may be observed. The animal has an arched back stance with its legs under the body; sometimes the front legs are crossed and the hind legs wide apart. The cow shifts her weight from one foot to another and is reluctant to move. Walking is evidently painful and lying times are lengthened. Pulse and respiratory rates are increased and appetite is reduced or absent. In the common volar artery the pulsation becomes palpable and visible, while the veins, especially on the lateral hind legs just above the hock, are engorged. The coronet may have a swollen appearance. The hooves are normal in shape but are warm and sensitive on palpation. At a later stage, painful walking and reluctance to move are the most dominant signs. In very serious cases loosening of the horny sole can be seen during careful searching with the hoof knife. Exudate and haemorrhagic transudate may seep out. In less serious cases haemorrhages become visible at the toe, white line and sole–heel junction after one or two months. These local signs may be seen after two to three months in sole ulceration or white line ulceration and even later in underrun sole.

It is noticeable that the lateral hind claws are the most seriously affected and there exists a clear symmetry between the left and right sides in severity and the area on the sole and the time when signs become noticeable. These observations make it unlikely that accidental trauma was responsible for the damage. Later the claw wall shows scars in the form of a ridge and groove in the dorsal side. This mark moves distally with growth of the horn. A total horizontal fissure may occur in severe cases. At the end of the lactation most minor sole ulcers have resolved and the signs in less serious cases will have disappeared previously. Deformity of the hoof may be present for a longer period although recovery without visible deformity is possible. However, internal weaknesses, caused by scars in the pododerm, make these animals much more susceptible to relapses in subsequent lactations. Often the local signs are noticed but the initial phase has been missed or considered to be part of the usual puerperal weakness. Pathological examination of the claws reveals a primary injury of the capillary endothelium that has caused decreased blood perfusion, with leakage of blood from the capillary walls and degeneration of the stratum germinatinum. The latter leads to horizontal fissures. In older cases thrombi, haemorrhages and fibrosis in the corium can be observed. Rotation of the pedal bone is less evident than in laminitic horses.

Aetiology

Although other starting points for laminitis cannot be excluded, the digestive tract seems to be the most important. Overloading of the rumen with easily fermentable carbohydrates, sugars and starch is often connected with cases of laminitis. In dairy farming this overload may happen in the first fortnight after calving, when the total feed intake is hardly 75 per cent of the potential maximum, but the amount of concentrates fed is already at a maximal level. This results in a roughage : non-roughage ratio well below the advised minimum of 1 : 3. In the rumen the pH decreases below 5.5 and the production of several potentially toxic agents is possible. In the literature, histamine, D-lactic acid and bacterial endotoxins are mentioned. However, in experiments under conventional management conditions none of these agents has been proven to play a role and only extreme overdosing has been successful in inducing the disorder. In addition, in natural disorders it is seldom that pathological concentrations of these toxic compounds are found in the blood. Although the production of pathological quantities of the above agents in the rumen is recognized, their absorption through the intact wall of the digestive tract is not so easily acceptable. However, it is possible that micro-lesions develop. Usually after absorption, detoxification occurs in a well functioning liver but in freshly calved animals fatty livers are often found under today's management systems and this could result in persistence of the toxicity. Thus toxic agents that pass these alimentary and hepatic barriers will be spread by the circulation and can affect all organs. The performance of the animal, in terms of milk production, will not be optimal. However, the reaction of the tissues in the claw is the most predominant problem because of the weight stress on these tissues. The possibility of short-circuiting of the local blood circulation by a system of arteriovenous shunts can result in capillary wall damage, which will be exaggerated locally due to the slow removal of toxic agents and the presence of hypoxia.

Our ignorance of the basic causal mechanisms means that all hypotheses about the pathways of activity of locally released mediators in the inflammation and perfusion processes are speculative. Generally, the accepted hypothesis is that the primary lesions occur in the capillary circulation, while the stratum germinatinum is involved in a second stage and there are then signs of degeneration due to hypoxia. On the other hand there is the concept that a specific, but as yet unknown, factor primarily affects the stratum germinatinum and makes it unable to produce normal healthy horn. The histochemical construction of the horn changes with the decreased incorporation of sulphydryl bridges. Although this may be due to the suboptimal local blood supply, a deficiency of sulphur-containing amino acids could also be the cause of this phenomenon.

Diagnosis

The approach to the herd that is suspected from clinical signs to have lameness due to laminitis is carefully to examine the cattle and also their management. Adverse observations include the following.

1 Dry cows that are too fat.
2 Freshly calved animals without well-filled rumens.
3 Too little feeding space per cow.
4 Little forage in the feed trough or forage with a low fibre content.
5 Very rough floors.
6 Inadequate or poorly bedded, uncomfortable lying areas leading to excessive standing.

In a disease outbreak there may be herd information of a high incidence of indigestion, inappetance, displaced abomasa, acetonaemia or milk fever. In the individual cow, milk production data, especially fat and protein contents in the first week of lactation, may give an indication. Thus low fat (<4.0 per cent) and high protein (>3.4 per cent) content, which are due to the high-energy intake from offering high levels of concentrate ration, can be replaced by high fat (>4.5 per cent) and low protein (<3.0 per cent) levels, which in turn will lead to disappointing production. With a decreasing forage intake, the acidosis that is induced by the high concentrate feed may develop into acetonaemia. Analysis of precalving and postcalving nutrition management and judgement of the quality of the products offered will often provide an explanation as to the cause of the problem. However, disappointingly, experience has shown that sometimes no satisfactory explanation can be found for laminitis cases either individually or on a herd basis. Provision of adequate housing, encouraging freshly calved cows to spend less time standing, can be an important factor. If cubicles are used, they should be well-bedded and of adequate dimensions, and ideally heifers should spend at least part of their rearing life becoming accustomed to the cubicle system.

Treatment

In the very early stages of the disorder attempts can be made to alter the initial process and thereby regulate digestion in the digestive tract if this seems to be the source of the problem. If infection such as mastitis or endometritis is the primary cause of the toxaemia, antibiotics are recommended. At the same time therapy should stimulate the circulatory supply to the feet. Pain-reducing drugs such as phenylbutazone and flunixin meglumine, which inhibit prostaglandin synthesis and thereby prevent capillary vasoconstriction, could be tried in acute cases. In horses heparin has been tried to prevent thrombosis. Movement onto a soft bed and bathing in warm water may also help stimulate the circulation. In cattle the use of antihistamines has been replaced by corticosteroids, although there is a warning that if used later than 24 hours after onset the latter may have an adverse effect.

In the later stages attention is mainly focused on the comfort of the patient. Thorough corrective trimming of the claws prevents an extreme weight load being placed on vulnerable areas. A soft bedding produces equal distribution of the weight over all eight claws, avoids local damage of the sole and encourages the animal to lay down. It also helps prevent progression to secondary complications like (peri)tarsitis.

Often the ration has to be balanced to the feed intake of the animal. It is claimed that an extra supply of sulphur-containing amino acids protected against ruminal digestion has a positive effect, but at present there are no convincing data to support this. If the signs are restricted to haemorrhages in the sole or sole ulcers, symptomatic treatment by paring is often sufficient. Bandages and antibiotics are only advised in exceptional complicated cases. The fixation of a wooden or rubber block by glue or nails under the sound medial claw will assist in pain relief and improve recovery rates.

Prevention

Prevention of laminitis partly concerns the prevention of acidosis by avoiding rations with highly fermentable carbohydrates. In practice it requires reduction of concentrate intake on a dry matter basis so that the concentrate : roughage ratio at all stages of the lactation is not greater than 1 : 3. The roughage provided must have adequate fibre length and content and the sugar/starch content of the concentrates must not be excessive. High levels of concentrates (10 kg) increase the risk of ulcers, particularly if suddenly introduced to the ration. The addition of buffers (for example, 12.5 kg sodium bicarbonate/t of concentrate) may help prevent acidosis, but usually they have a variable effect or laminitis. In addition, provision of the total concentrate ration in small quantities over the day does not have much effect unless there is free access to a high digestible fibre forage. The stress of transport, the new social dominance following entry of freshly calved cows and heifers to the herd and also weight stress have to be avoided. Animals that have been adapted before calving to their postcalving management, housing system and nutrition are best fitted to avoid laminitis.

Vertical claw fissures

Vertical fissures occur primarily in front feet. Mostly they are restricted to isolated cases. An animal may be severely lame due to a pus-forming inflammation even though the fissure is hardly visible. Another clinical form is the rough vertical fissure, which can persist for long periods without any indication of recovery. There seems to be an inborn weakness and often both front feet are affected. In early cases antibiotic treatment is successful but in chronic cases trimming and removing pressure by a foot block beneath the sound claw will be necessary. Environmental circumstances like hard floors and dry sandy conditions leading to loss of superficial perioplic horn seem to predispose to the condition.

Fracture of the third phalanx (pedal bone)

A fracture of the pedal bone is considered, like a sandcrack, to be the result of trauma caused by hard floors. The front feet are most commonly involved. The animal is severely lame and hardly uses the affected claw. The diagnosis can be proven by an X-ray. Although in most instances a single animal is affected, herd problems have occurred in cases of fluoride intoxication due either to industrial pollution or concentrates polluted by fluorine-containing mineral salts.

General prevention

It is advisable to locate a foot bath where daily use is possible without causing difficulties for the stockmen.

Cows passing through the bath have to be kept on floors that allow time for the fluid to work so that it is not immediately removed by grass, mud or dung. The solution requires time to take effect. Foot bathing is practised in several ways: walking through baths, stationary foot bathing for an hour, and sometimes a low pressure sprinkling system. Solutions that can be used in this connection include formalin (3–5 per cent), zinc or copper sulphate (5–10 per cent), sodium chloride (10 per cent) and creolin (2 per cent). Formalin gives the best results but has the disadvantage of its penetrating smell and so is unpleasant to work with. Zinc and copper sulphate may contribute to local environmental pollution and the dairy industry does not appreciate contamination of milk with copper. It is claimed that zinc penetrates skin and horn and contributes to the health of the hoof.

Regular hoof trimming is commonly practised in modern dairy farming. If hoof trimming is restricted to the seriously lame animals, it is then only a form of treatment. However, if at-risk animals are trimmed when not lame, claw disorders can be treated at a very early stage and aggravation may be prevented. Also correction of weight distribution between the lateral and medial hind claw decreases the susceptibility to sole ulcers.

As the animals are most prone to claw disorders in the period around and just after calving, the best period for routine trimming by the stockman is at drying-off. In cases where trimming of the whole herd is carried out by professionals and no clear calving season exists, there is no preferable time to do this. In intensive zero-grazing systems, twice yearly trimming may be necessary. An easily managed foot trimming crush on the farm encourages the stockmen to treat animals at an early stage.

Soft bedding such as deep litter with sand, straw or sawdust ensures that in lame animals there is less risk of secondary injuries to the legs, such as peritarsitis, than if on hard surfaces such as concrete or rubber mats. Soft comfortable beds also encourages cows to lie down, thus reducing the incidence of traumatic laminitis.

Aspects of breeding have been considered and several approaches have been made. An indirect selection criterion has been sought in the chemical or histological composition of the claw horn. Also claw measurements can be used. Direct criteria are the presence of signs of claw disorders or the number of treatments required per animal. However, the indirect parameters have a rather low relationship to the occurrence of claw disorders. A disadvantage of these parameters is the uncertainty as to whether they are predisposing factors for, or the sequelae of, the disorders. Secondly, it discounts the suggestion that susceptibility to claw disorders may not be localized within the claw itself. Consequently, the repeatability of these parameters is often very disappointing.

It is preferable that the occurrence of claw disorders be considered in the criteria for breeding purposes. When incorporated in inspection systems they can contribute to improvement of the claw quality. However, the recording of treatments, e.g. by veterinarians, farmers, etc., sometimes provides insufficient information because of a lack of uniformity in diagnosing conditions and differences between individuals in their involvement with lameness cases.

There are, however, a few disorders described with a clear genetic component. Examples are a hereditary laminitis in Jerseys but from which they do not recover, and epithelia keratogenesis imperfecta, an inability to produce a normal hoof. Many also consider that deformed claw shape, as in cork-screw claws, has a genetic background.

References

Russel, A.M., Rowlands, G.J., Shaw, S.R. & Weaver, A.D. (1982) Survey of lameness in British dairy cattle. *Veterinary Record*, **111**, 155–65.

Whittaker, D.A., Kelly, J.M. & Smith, E.S. (1983) Incidence of lameness in dairy cows. *Veterinary Record*, **113**, 60–2.

Chapter 29: Lameness Above the Foot

by A.D. WEAVER

Nerve paralyses

Introduction

Nerve paralyses of the forelimb include the suprascapular, brachial plexus and radial. The main hindlimb involvement is with the femoral, obturator, tibial, peroneal and sciatic. The usual common aetiological component is trauma. The typical age of affected individuals varies from neonate to mature cow. The treatment in all forms involves careful nursing and supportive care (e.g. oral fluids), and management of the primary lesion (e.g. fracture). Sometimes multiple nerve injuries occur as in the downer cow syndrome, which is considered separately (p. 368).

Suprascapular paralysis

Aetiology and pathology

The suprascapular nerve originates from cervical 6 and 7 roots. It may be involved in brachial plexus injuries (see p. 365). The nerve supplies the supraspinatus and infraspinatus muscles. It has no sensory component. It is occasionally injured by blunt trauma in calves butted by others at mangers and troughs when the vertical bar barrier bruises the scapular region. Associated injuries can include fractures of the scapular neck or acromium.

Clinical signs and diagnosis

Suprascapular paralysis causes few clinical signs initially. The shoulder joint may be slightly abducted and the forward phase of the stride shortened. After one week muscular atrophy causes increased prominence of the scapular spine ('sweeney').

Treatment

Treatment is purely palliative. Vitamin B complex may be given systemically. The prognosis is usually good.

Brachial plexus

Aetiology

Trauma, as from sudden caudal ventral displacement of the shoulder and entire forelimb, together with abduction can lead to separation of any group of the nerve roots C6 to T2. The nerves mainly affected are the radial, median and ulnar. Occasionally, the nerves are damaged by penetrating injury in the axilla with extensive additional damage to the vasculature. More frequently, the plexus is injured during traction in dystokia and severe abduction of the forelimb.

Pathology

The nerves are avulsed close to the spinal cord and result in a complete loss of motor supply to the forelimb. Occasionally, the cranial segments of the network (supplying the suprascapular and axillary nerves) are spared.

Clinical signs and diagnosis

The forelimb is non-weight bearing and is maintained in flaccid extension, with a tendency for the digits to be dragged. Sensation is absent from the level of the elbow distally. Muscular atrophy is evident after seven days.

Differential diagnosis includes radial paralysis (dropped elbow, more localized loss of skin sensation) and humeral shaft fracture with or without radial nerve injury (see p. 373), and forelimb dislocation.

Treatment and prevention

Since brachial plexus avulsion has a very poor prognosis, treatment is not usually justified. In calves with partial brachial plexus avulsion, anti-inflammatory drugs and limb support are suggested. Affected cattle should be confined to a well-bedded stall and care should be taken to avoid the development of decubital damage to the analgesic lower limb.

Radial paralysis

Aetiology and pathogenesis

The nerve (roots C7–T1) is damaged in its distal portion secondarily to humeral shaft fractures, which tend to be spiral, comminuted and to have sharp protruding spikes of bone. Radial nerve paresis frequently occurs following a long (one to two hour) period of general anaesthesia in lateral recumbency when the primary damage is a compressed vascular compartment. While partial paralysis is more common, complete radial paralysis can result from brachial plexus injuries or severe trauma.

Clinical signs and diagnosis

The main signs are a dropped elbow due to triceps paralysis, knuckled fetlock and an inability to advance the limb (Fig. 29.1). If the limb is placed in its usual position, the fetlock flexes as an attempt is made to

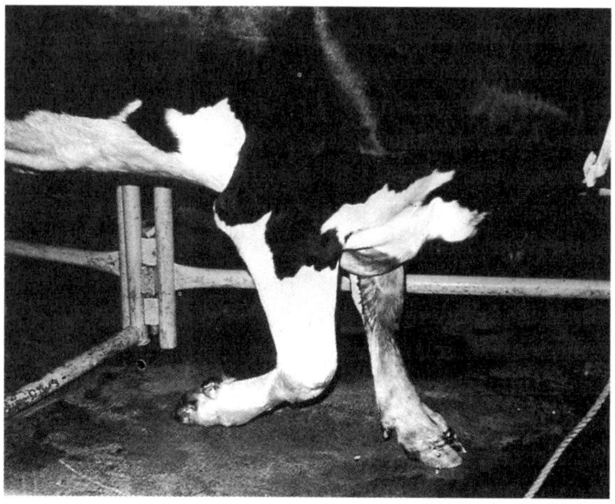

Fig. 29.1 Radial paralysis of right foreleg of six-year-old Friesian cow. Paralysis was present on standing following 120 minutes in right lateral recumbency for surgery of a septic parotiditis under general anaesthesia. Total recovery took 48 hours. The classical signs are present: dropped elbow, flexed carpus and inability to extend forelimb for weight bearing.

bear weight. Sensory loss can be detected over the elbow and lateral aspect of the forearm.

Differential diagnosis includes humeral fracture with or without radial paralysis.

Treatment and prevention

The prognosis is good if the nerve has not been sectioned by humeral bone fragments. Treatment is supportive, keeping the animal on soft bedding and on non-slip surfaces. The fetlock should be bandaged to prevent iatrogenic trauma. Anti-inflammatory drugs and vitamin B complex may be given systemically. Cattle maintained in lateral recumbency under general anaesthesia should have soft supporting surfaces and the down forelimb should be extended forwards to reduce the pressure on the vasculature to the lower parts of the limb. Also, the upper foreleg should not be roped tightly down against the table, whereby it would increase pressure on the lower leg.

Femoral paralysis

Aetiology and pathology

The femoral nerve (L4–6 spinal nerve roots) has a short course, ramifying in the iliopsoas and quadriceps muscles. It is liable to damage in the oversized fetus of large-framed breeds (Simmental, Charolais, Holstein) at delivery when presented in the 'hiplock' or 'stifle lock' position, which tends to cause femoral hyperextension as forced traction is exerted. The femoral nerve, usually unilaterally, is drawn against the pubic brim at the pelvic inlet. The injury can occur in either anterior or posterior presentation. The lesion is sometimes a rupture of the nerve, but more frequently involves very severe perineural haemorrhage and oedema. In other cases, the quadriceps femoris muscle is severely stretched and incurs damage to its vascular and nerve supply. The resulting quadriceps atrophy presents with typical clinical signs.

Clinical signs and diagnosis

The animal, usually a neonate, is unable to maintain the stifle in extension due to quadriceps dysfunction. The joint is flexed and the digit rests with minimal weight bearing. Usually, hock and digital joints are also flexed, though the toe is not dragged. A small area of loss of skin sensitivity may be detectable lateral and proximal to the stifle joint. Quadriceps atrophy within 10 to 14 days results in a triangular depression in the lateral cranial part of the thigh. Fibrosis of the remaining quadriceps muscle mass develops later. The stifle joint may become unusually prominent. Differential diagnosis involves dorsal or lateral patellar luxation, septic gonitis, femoral fracture or growth plate separation, hip dislocation and quadriceps rupture.

Treatment and prevention

The prognosis is guarded or poor. Recovery is unlikely in calves with femoral nerve rupture. The recovery time for regeneration was about four months in an experimental study when a 5 mm ($\frac{1}{2}$ inch) length of femoral nerve was resected surgically (Buchthal *et al.*, 1984). Treatment is primarily careful supportive nursing care. Calves should receive colostrum by bottle within 6 hours of birth if the injury has prevented rising to suck. Clean and dry bedding is essential. The calf should be frequently turned. Analgesics, anti-inflammatories, and vitamin E and selenium preparations should be given.

Obturator paralysis

Aetiology and pathology

Obturator paralysis classically involves unilateral or bilateral damage to the nerve, usually in heifers during dystokia due to fetal oversize or maternal immaturity, when the nerve (L4–L6 nerve roots) is damaged by fetal pressure on its course along the medial aspect of the ileum or along the pelvic floor. Experimental section of the nerve, which innervates the adductor muscles (gracilis, pectineus, adductor and external obturator), has caused mild abduction of one or both hind limbs but experimental animals have been able to rise without difficulty (Vaughan, 1964; Cox, 1981). A common synonym for obturator paralysis, 'calving paralysis', is considered a misnomer since the latter is usually associated with the 'downer cow' syndrome (Cox & Onapito, 1986) (see p. 368). Many clinical cases of so-called obturator paralysis have a more complex aetiology involving branches of the sciatic nerve or primary muscle damage.

Clinical signs and diagnosis

Abduction of the hindlimb (unilateral) or a straddled gait (bilateral) are the classical signs. Confusion clinically may result from the stance adopted by a heifer with an oedematous and overstocked udder and with pelvic fractures. Rectal and vaginal examination may reveal minor pelvic damage associated with the paralysis. Some cattle are recumbent and such recumbency is rarely due to simple unilateral obturator injury. Cattle are liable to slip with gross hindlimb abduction, giving rise to hip luxation. Skin sensation remains unimpaired. Diagnosis is based on the history of possible injury at parturition and on the characteristic stance and gait.

Treatment and prevention

The animal should be kept on non-slip surfaces to avoid possible hip luxation or femoral neck fracture. The hocks and hind feet should be kept close together by a figure of eight pattern of rope above the hocks on fetlocks. The distance between these joints should not exceed 30 cm (12 inches), which permits the animal to rise. Supportive care should be continued for several days. Breeding management should be reviewed to avoid a high incidence of dystokia in heifers and to prevent damage during forced extraction of the fetus.

Tibial paralysis

Aetiology and pathology

Tibial paralysis is rare. It is associated with iatrogenic damage following deep infections in the caudal thigh musculature or lacerating injuries in the medial aspect of the hock with associated damage to related tendons.

Clinical signs and diagnosis

Tibial paralysis results in hock flexion from inability primarily to cause gastrocnemius contraction, which would result in hock extension. It also causes hyperextension of the digits in that the weight is borne more on the heels. Skin sensation is absent over the caudal aspect of the metatarsus and digits. Differential diagnosis includes peroneal paralysis and gastrocnemius and flexor tendon rupture.

Treatment and prevention

Treatment is symptomatic, involving confinement and vitamin B complex injections.

Peroneal paralysis

Aetiology and pathology

As with the tibial nerve, the peroneal nerve is a major branch of the sciatic nerve (L6–S2 nerve roots). Its common site of damage is over the lateral aspect of the stifle joint where the nerve lies relatively close to the skin surface. It is liable to injury following sudden (falls) or chronic pressure (prolonged recumbency).

Clinical signs and diagnosis

The hock is hyperextended, and fetlock and digits are flexed (knuckled over) (Fig. 29.2). The foot can be placed in its normal position. Skin sensation is lost dorsally from the fetlock distally to the coronary band. Diagnosis is easily made on the clinical signs and sensory loss. Differential diagnosis involves tibial paralysis and painful digital diseases.

Treatment and prevention

The prognosis is good with recovery usually evident in a few days. Self-induced trauma to the fetlock is minimized by application of a soft bandage or a light resin cast to the fetlock.

Sciatic paralysis

Sciatic nerve paralysis involves the nerve that originates from three ventral roots (L6, S1–2). Damage to L6 root may be an important component of 'calving paralysis' or obturator paralysis (Cox, 1981) (see p. 366). The sciatic nerve is liable to damage unassociated directly with parturition but in prolonged unilateral recumbency. The site is usually close to the medial aspect of the femoral greater trochanter and may be associ-

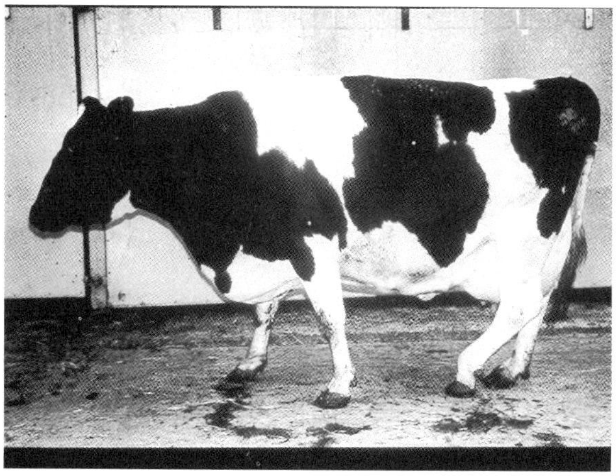

Fig. 29.2 Peroneal paralysis in six-year-old Friesian cow showing extended hock and knuckling of fetlock. Two days previously the digit had also been flexed. Some weight is now borne on claw normally. Total recovery took another three days.

ated with struggling. Such circumstances can involve partial recovery from milk fever or postparturient hypocalcaemia, as the cow struggles to rise on a slippery surface (e.g. concrete) (Cox & Onapito, 1986). Rarely, sciatic paralysis is secondary to femoral neck or pelvic fracture (pubis, ischium), or iatrogenic in origin from septic infection arising from intramuscular injections.

Clinical signs and diagnosis

The limb is entirely non-weight bearing. Sensation is lost from the limb distal to the stifle except for a strip on the medial aspect of the thigh distal to the mid-metatarsal region, which is supplied by the saphenous branch of the femoral nerve. Differential diagnosis should include femoral fracture, the signs of which will include crepitus, possibly swelling and abnormal mobility, and septic gonitis and tarsitis.

Treatment and prevention

The prognosis is usually hopeless. Many cases are presented as 'downer cows'. It is vital that this paralysis be recognized early, so that long-term nursing measures will not be instituted. Early slaughter is advisable.

Downer cow syndrome (see p. 594)

Defined as 'a cow down in sternal recumbency for unknown reasons', the syndrome usually affects high-yielding dairy cows in the first 48 hours postpartum. The condition has a multiple aetiology including traumatic, metabolic, neurological and toxic infectious causes. The following are examples.

1 Traumatic: sacroiliac luxation and subluxation, bilateral or unilateral coxofemoral luxation, pelvic fracture.
2 Metabolic: non-responsive hypocalcaemia, hypokalaemia.
3 Neurological: lymphosarcoma infiltration into thoracic or lumbosacral spinal canal.
4 Toxic infectious: septic metritis, acute coliform mastitis (p. 291).

The primary recumbency, whether due to dystokia (46 per cent of cases), milk fever (38 per cent), or other causes (16 per cent) (Chamberlain, 1987), is followed by secondary recumbency. The usual explanation for the development of a downer syndrome in a cow, which is unsuccessfully treated for clinical signs diagnostic of hypocalcaemic parturient paresis or milk fever, is that the hypocalcaemia has been treated too late and that unrecognized traumatic injury has already taken place. Half of all 'downer cows' develop within 24 hours of parturition. Affected cows tend to be high producers. The incidence is higher in winter. Survey data indicate a considerable range (3.8–28.2 per cent) in the incidence of downer cows as a percentage of cases of milk fever (Cox, 1988). In one USA study, 33 per cent of downer cows recovered, 23 per cent were slaughtered, and 44 per cent died or were euthanized (Cox *et al.*, 1982).

Pressure damage causes ischaemia of muscles and nerves. Following a variable period of struggling, further skeletal injury such as gastrocnemius muscle rupture may occur. The differential diagnosis is often difficult since frequently a non-responsive milk fever cow does not appear to have any further specific abnormality.

The aetiology of this pressure damage involves effects resulting from the 'compartment syndrome' (Cox, 1988). Increased pressure develops within an osteofascial compartment following external pressure or internal filling of the compartment with blood or oedematous fluid, or both. External pressure results in ischaemia, 'leaky' vessels, and a postcompression swelling. The effects of the crush syndrome, which refer to the systemic results of muscle damage, involve largely the absorption of muscle breakdown products.

One specific cause of the downer cow syndrome is pressure damage to the hindquarters following a period of prolonged recumbency (3–6 hours or more), resulting both in extensive muscle damage and reversible or irreversible changes in the sciatic nerve caudal to the proximal end of the femur and to the peroneal nerve.

Consideration of the aetiology and pathology of traumatic factors is reviewed in other sections (see Fractures, p. 370; Dislocations and subluxations, p. 375; Muscle and tendon injuries, p. 380).

Clinical signs and diagnosis

By definition the animal is recumbent. The cow is usually alert, eats, and can defecate and urinate. Affected cows make little or no attempt to rise in the hindlimbs. Some alert cows move around using the forelimbs and have been termed 'creeper cows'. Cows confined to a stanchion do not have facilities to demonstrate this movement, which may appear after the animal is transferred to a well-bedded stall or box. Dull or comatose and anorectic cows may be 'downers' due to systemic toxic factors (coliform mastitis, severe metritis). Occasionally, downer cows are hyperexcitable due to hypomagnesaemia or hypocalcaemia (see Chapter 39).

Rectal palpation is crucial to evaluate various traumatic aetiologies: sacroiliac (sub)luxation, pelvic fracture, severe, intrapelvic, soft tissue injury and coxofemoral luxation, as well as to check the state of the uterus (puerperium). External assessment includes palpation of the spine for abnormal angulation, swelling, or crepitus (fracture), musculature of the hindlimbs, especially the adductor group medially (muscle rupture), manipulation of the upper hindlimb and pelvis for evidence of fracture or dislocation, and determination of possible loss of skin sensation. The possibility of acute coliform mastitis should be investigated. The cow should be turned to the opposite side for similar examination of the other hindlimb. Cows usually prefer to lie with the more painful hindlimb uppermost.

Downer cows have variable changes in blood mineral levels, some showing a persistent hypocalcaemia, hypophosphataemia, and possible hypomagnesaemia. The role and significance of hypokalaemia is disputed. The release of potassium from damaged muscle cells does not necessarily cause hyperkalaemia because the usual coexisting hypocalcaemia has a tendency to cause hypokalaemia. All cases show an elevated creatine kinase (CK), which is specific for muscle injury. In one study (Chamberlain, 1986), CK peaked at 24 hours after onset of recumbency in cows that recovered to stand, and at 48 hours in cows that became permanent 'downers'. Plasma or serum CK values reflect the total mass of injured muscle, but CK half-life is such that it is of doubtful value as a prognostic indicator several days after initial recumbency, when little further active muscle damage may be occurring.

Plasma aspartate aminotransferase (AST) is elevated in animals with muscle damage. This enzyme is also released in cardiac myopathies, but postpartum increases in downer cows are almost invariably related to the muscle component.

In cows recumbent for over 48 hours (at the time of second clinical examination), clinical pathology can be re-assessed. Urinalysis may now reveal proteinuria indicative of myoglobinuria (from muscle breakdown), ketonuria and bilirubinuria (from partial anorexia).

If the aetiology of the persistent recumbency remains in doubt, a repeat complete clinical examination should bear in mind less common causes (e.g. infiltration of lymphosarcoma into the spinal canal). A careful recheck of the history may aid diagnosis at this stage.

Treatment and prevention

The downer cow should be moved to a well-bedded loose box not later than 24 hours after the onset of recumbency. Ample food and water must be provided in low, wide-based containers.

The primary aim is to raise the cow. Any attempt should be made on a relatively non-slip surface. Personnel should be ready to assist with tail support following provocative stimulation (e.g. electric goad). Hip clamps, e.g. Bagshaw hoist, may be applied to the wings of the ilium for a maximum of 20 minutes. Usually, the ability of the cow to bear weight is obvious. While slung in this manner, the hindquarters should be checked for symmetry and the opportunity taken to flex and extend each hindlimb to check for fractures. Other devices for elevation include air cushions or bags and webbing slings. Some cows that can stand following hoisting require to be hobbled above the hocks or hind fetlocks to prevent abduction of the hindlimbs.

Hip clamps may be repeatedly applied for a few minutes of forced elevation of the hindquarters to improve circulation. When lowered, the cow should be placed with the previously dependent side uppermost.

The most important component of treatment is good nursing. The cow must be made comfortable. Owners should be observant for the possible development of a toxic (e.g. coliform) mastitis during recumbency. Rapid loss of weight, signs of systemic toxicity, and anorexia are grave prognostic indicators. Soft bedding is essential for effective nursing in all downer cows, which should be turned several times daily.

Parenteral treatment includes repeated injection of solutions containing calcium–phosphorus–magnesium with glucose and potassium. Additional potassium should only be given by stomach tube (e.g. 50 g KCl daily). Fresh water should be available alongside a bucket containing a commercial electrolyte solution. Tripelennamine hydrochloride given as 12 ml solution i.v. is an effective stimulant and antihistaminic that makes a downer cow appear more alert (Chamberlain, 1987). Analgesics such as phenylbutazone and flunixine meglumine should be restricted to cows with obvious signs of pain.

The prognosis is good in well-nursed 'creeper cows' with some voluntary hindlimb movement and cows that are capable of a short period of weight bearing when hoisted or slung. The prognosis is poor in animals with no hindlimb movement. Proprioceptive reflexes should be repeatedly checked in such cows.

Generally, excellent nursing, a consistently good appetite, and some spontaneous movement should encourage owners to persist and practise patience.

Valuable prognostic indicators for survival in a limited British survey of 64 downer cows were as follows.

1 On day 2 of recumbency: body condition score, quality of nursing care, absence of hypocalcaemia, relative hypomagnesaemia, and lower AST and CK enzyme levels.

2 On day 4 of recumbency: survival was associated with little further rise of CK and with continued good nursing.

A recent postal survey in the USA of 15 veterinarians' experience with slings used on 145 cows showed a recovery rate of 52 per cent (Cox, 1988).

Prevention depends primarily on the avoidance of parturient paresis associated with milk fever (see Chapter 39). Calving should take place in properly designed areas with good footing. Many farms will benefit from stalls with 30 cm (12 inches) clean sand as bedding. On problem farms, successful reduction of the incidence of downer cows has been primarily attributed to closer observation for the initial signs of milk fever and its prompt treatment.

Periparturient cows should be placed onto a minimal slip surface and sand is excellent for this purpose if straw-bedded calving boxes are not available.

A high incidence of downer cows in first-calf heifers, where hypocalcaemia can be ruled out, may be due to dystokia. Breeding policies may require modification such as use of a smaller breed bull or later first service dates for heifers.

Fractures

Introduction

In the assessment of bovine fractures, several factors require consideration in each clinical situation.

Economics

With some exceptions, economic consideration is a vital factor. Many cattle not used for breeding, e.g. steers, are best slaughtered at once, since treatment would be costly. Young potentially valuable breeding stock fall into a different category, where slaughter value is negligible in comparison with the potential value following fracture healing.

Size, age and sex

Young cattle respond well to restrictions imposed during fracture immobilization. They tend to rise easily despite external fixation and to be less liable to develop decubital lesions. The soft thin cortices of long bones in calves make plate and screws generally an unsuitable means of internal fixation.

Disposition

An advantage of fracture healing in cattle compared with horses is their tolerant disposition making handling easier.

Location and character

Generally, the more proximal the fracture, the more difficult is its anatomical reduction and rigid fixation. Thus humeral and femoral fractures have notoriously low recovery rates, while metatarsal and metacarpal fractures usually heal well. Fracture of the distal phalanx, in which displacement is minimal, is discussed elsewhere (see Fracture of distal phalanx, p. 362).

Comminuted fractures are the rule in cattle. Many fractures are closed initially but become open following inappropriate handling such as movement to a stall. The prognosis for open fractures, especially proximal fractures (humerus, tibia, femur), is guarded. Soft tissue damage is often limited to haematoma and oedema resulting from the original insult and movement of the fractured bone ends. In certain instances, significant nerve damage (e.g. to radial nerve in a spiral humeral shaft fracture) may be an important consideration in the prognosis.

Most fractures tend to be oblique or spiral in cattle. Maintenance of reduction while external or internal fixation is applied tends to be more difficult than with transverse fractures.

Duration of fracture

Unlike small animals and horses, the duration of a bovine fracture before presentation can often be 12–24 hours, a consequence of the relatively casual methods of husbandry practised on some farms. The result is invariably a greater degree of soft tissue injury than in a freshly presented fracture. One effect of a longer duration of movement at a fracture site is an open fracture.

First aid

Fractures should be immobilized on the farm premises as soon as possible. Suitable materials include padding with old towels or sheeting, and splinting with polyvinyl chloride tubing, or stiff rods such as broomsticks placed at 90° to each other (e.g. cranial and lateral surfaces of the forelimb to stabilize metacarpal fracture) and fixed in position with duct tape. The joints above and below the fracture should be immobilized. This technique is impossible in femoral, tibial and humeral fractures. In tibial fractures, a Robert Jones bandage comprising layers of cotton wool firmly bound by cotton bandage can achieve adequate immobility if sufficient bulk is applied.

Fracture repair

In certain fractures (e.g. rib) spontaneous healing is the rule. In others (e.g. external angle of ilium) repair usually takes place but a sequestrum may form. The sequestrum generally is only a cosmetic blemish but sometimes becomes infected and requires removal.

Most fractures require treatment by methods of external or internal fixation, or both, if recovery is to take place.

Long bone fractures: external fixation

External fixation of fractures is usually satisfactory if the site is distal to the humerus or proximal tibial metaphysis. A minimum of equipment is required, and extensive experience is unnecessary. External fixation is unsuitable for more proximal sites, in open fractures with gross contamination and fractures occurring in two limbs simultaneously. Young cattle develop osteomyelitis following open long bone fractures more frequently than older cattle. Careful examination of the fracture site, preferably after clipping of the skin, is essential to avoid missing an open fracture. External fixation alone may be contraindicated in very heavy animals.

Choice of materials and technique for external fixation

Immobilization techniques include the splint or cast, the modified Thomas splint, and both methods together.

Casting materials available today include plaster of Paris (one form of which is rapid-setting), thermoplastic polyester polymers (Hexcelite), and polyurethane resin incorporated into woven material of polyester (Cuttercast, Baycast) or fibreglass (Deltalite/Scotchcast). Casts should always be applied over a layer of padding. The depth of padding should be considerably greater if soft tissue swelling is anticipated at the fracture site and also should be generous over bone prominences. The padding should extend beyond the intended proximal point of the cast. The cast should immobilize the joints proximal and distal to the fracture site. Thus, in a one-month-old calf with a distal metacarpal shaft fracture, the cast should extend at least 8 cm (3 inches) proximal to the radiocarpal joint and similarly distal to the fetlock.

Positioning is very important in applying a cast. General anaesthesia is rarely necessary; xylazine is usually adequate for restraint and analgesia. The limb must be forcibly extended for fracture reduction and then maintained immobile until the cast has set. Traction on the distal part of the limb may be aided by inserting wire through holes drilled in the toes.

The advantages of a lightweight cast include increased comfort and ease of rising, and are achieved by fibreglass (e.g. Vetcast, Deltalite, Scotchcast), which has a strength five times greater than plaster of Paris. Weight reduction is also possible using several layers of plaster overlaid by fibreglass casting tape, once the plaster has hardened. Strength combined with lightness are the results.

Some fractures require radiography before reduction and immobilization to determine the extent and severity of bone damage. Fractures may also be radiographed two to three weeks after immobilization to assess the degree of healing. Removal of the cast at this time is often unnecessary. The radiolucency of cast materials varies, plaster of Paris being poor, Deltalite/Scotchcast fair with some mottling, and Cuttercast/Baycast is excellent.

Extension bars have sometimes been incorporated into external casts. These U-shaped metal stirrups have the curved part of the U distal to the toes, so that weight is borne by the bar and transferred proximally to the cast, into which the two arms of the extension bar are buried during cast application. Such a device is only useful if there is a specific indication to avoid weight bearing by the digits. The effective increase in limb length makes standing up and ambulation more difficult. A modification is the hanging cast. This device comprises one or more intramedullary pins that are drilled through the proximal fracture fragment, and onto which a U-shaped bar is fitted after the usual external immobilization has been applied. When weight is borne, it is transferred proximally to load bearing by the proximal fracture site, so that the fracture site is not stressed.

Thomas extension splints may be put on either forelimb or hindlimb. Good padding is essential both at the points (axilla, inguinum) where maximal pressure will be applied, as well as at any contact points more distally. The Thomas extension splint must be 'made to measure' for the individual case (e.g. circumference of proximal and distal rings, length of cranial and caudal longitudinal bars). In growing stock the length should be slightly greater (e.g. 5 cm or 2 inches) than necessary to permit growth. Some materials have expansion clamps or rings on the longitudinal bars to allow continual modification.

The bottom ring should be wired to the foot to maintain the leg in extension. Bandages and padding should be placed around the limb at potentially exposed areas before they are taped to the longitudinal bars. In the hindlimb, the metatarsus may be fixed to the caudal bar, the tibial (gaskin) area to the cranial bar. The extension splint should be checked carefully for fit and effective immobilization of the fracture site before release of the patient. Many cases will benefit from combination of an external cast (e.g. fibreglass) and a Thomas extension splint.

Cattle up to 350 kg (800 lb) will generally adapt well to Thomas splintage. Patients should be confined to a stall with relatively little straw bedding. Assistance to rise may be needed initially. The cast or splint should be checked daily for skin abrasions, cast fracture or slackness.

Neonatal and other calves less than a month old with simple fractures and rapid callus formation may require external support for two weeks only (Fig. 29.3). Other young cattle should be checked for progress at three weeks by removing the cast with an oscillating saw. Sometimes the same splint may be re-applied (e.g. with Deltalite, Cuttercast).

Humeral fractures in cattle aged two and a half months to three years can heal four to six weeks following Thomas splintage (Wintzer, 1961). In other cases, immobility has been unsatisfactory and non-union has resulted despite massive callus formation.

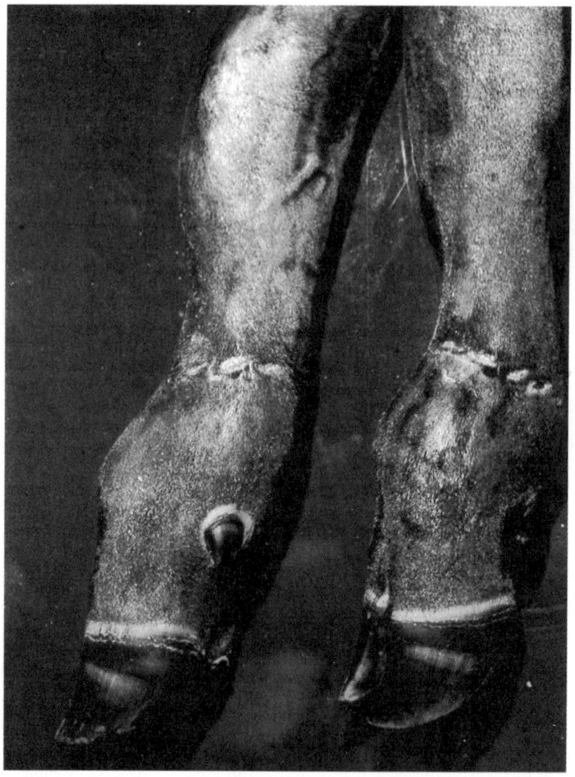

Fig. 29.3 Bilateral distal metacarpal fractures in a one-day-old Saler calf. Circular lesions result from pressure of obstetrical chains applied during forced extraction. In the absence of percutaneous infection (seen here) external immobilization from mid metacarpal to coronary level is indicated.

Open fractures, at sites where external fixation is practical, require particular attention. The presence of skin perforation should carry the presumption of an open fracture even if bone cannot be seen or palpated through the injury. The wound is cleansed and carefully explored. Any free bone fragments should be removed. Larger wounds require debridement. It may be useful to take tissue samples or a blood clot for microbiological culture in the case of valuable cattle. Wounds should be copiously irrigated with a polyionic solution (isotonic balanced electrolyte with neutral pH). The value of adding a 0.1 per cent povidone-iodine solution (1 : 100 dilution of povidone-iodine 10 per cent solution) has not been established in cattle.

Antibiotics should be given parenterally in all open fractures in cattle. Natural and synthetic penicillins are the first choice. Systemic antibiotics should be continued for seven to ten days. Antibacterial sensitivity patterns may be checked via samples taken at an early stage and before antibiotics are given. Samples should preferentially be taken from infected bone at surgery rather than from discharging sinus tracts where contamination with surface pathogens will complicate interpretation of laboratory results. Antibiotic therapy should be instituted as soon as possible following identification of an open fracture. Small wounds may be covered with a sterile protective dressing, but any external support of the fracture site should be removed after three to five days to permit quick assessment of the wound. Young cattle develop osteomyelitis following open fractures more frequently than adults. The reason may be a richer blood supply in the damaged area.

Long bone fractures: internal fixation

Introduction

Economic factors are often important in considering internal fixation of bovine long bone fractures. Expertise in the discipline is also essential for successful reduction and rigid support under aseptic surgical conditions.

Anatomical factors mean that long bone repair by internal fixation is most frequently required in humeral, femoral and tibial fractures. Young calves have very thin cortical bone and screws are liable to loosen or be stripped during insertion. Failure is the common result.

Both access to the fracture site and reduction are much simpler in the calf than adult.

In adult cattle, where the cortex is thick and dense, the major problems are associated with general anaesthesia (e.g. regurgitation, rumen tympany, compromised ventilation), the soft tissue mass through which the fracture site is approached, and the initial difficulty of anatomical reduction, when muscle spasm compounds the degree of overriding of the fragment ends.

Specialist texts should be consulted for details of internal fixation of specific bovine fractures (Ferguson, 1985).

Humeral fractures

Animals up to yearling size (e.g. 250 kg, 550 lb) are amenable to internal fixation unless the fracture is severely comminuted. Such fractures are usually oblique and spiral. There is often severe overriding, making reduction difficult. Intramedullary pinning (or stack-multiple-pinning) combined with cerclage wiring is often the technique of choice.

Humeral fractures are difficult to plate due to their short length and spiral configuration. Multiple bone fragments often necessitate the use of lag screws.

In older and heavier cattle, internal fixation is less successful due to greater mechanical forces. Often long-term Thomas splintage is adopted.

Femoral fractures

Femoral shaft fractures are relatively common in calves. No form of external immobilization is helpful. Internal pinning (Steinmann) rarely achieves sufficient immobility of the fracture site. The technique of choice is usually plate and screws, possibly double plating, with two plates placed at about 90° to each other (lateral and cranial).

Similar techniques may be attempted in older cattle. Resolution presents major problems. The huge mechanical force acting at femoral fracture sites makes bending of the plates or loss of screws common. Some femoral shaft fractures eventually heal with some months of stall rest alone.

Tibial fractures

Tibial shaft fractures are amenable to a variety of fixation techniques since exposure is relatively easy. Problems arise with severely comminuted or multiple fractures extending into the proximal and distal metaphyses. As alternatives to plate and screws, and additional support by a Thomas splint, some tibial fractures may be immobilized by cerclage wire with external support. Yet others lend themselves to transfixation pinning. In this method at least two Steinmann pins are placed through both cortices of both proximal and distal segments under strict asepsis, the protruding ends are cut to protrude about 2.5–5 cm (1–2 inches) from the skin, and a resin bridge is placed over these protrusions to immobilize the fracture site. The sites of skin puncture should be carefully covered with dressings to reduce the chance of infection tracking along the pins and causing osteomyelitis, which is the primary complication of this technique.

Growth plate and other injuries

Separation of the growth plate is a common complication of forced traction in dystokia. The usual site is the distal metacarpus or metatarsus (Fig. 29.4). Non-weight bearing swelling and crepitus are major clinical signs. Cases must be distinguished from distal metacarpal/metatarsal shaft fractures and fetlock dislocation

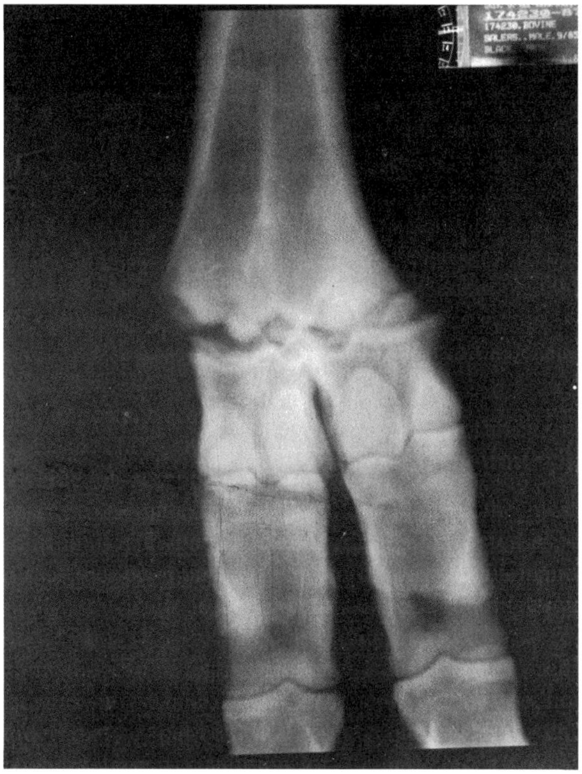

Fig. 29.4 Separation and displacement of distal metacarpal growth plate in 15-month-old Limousin bull. Complete recovery followed manipulation and traction reduction (over 1000 kg pull) and four weeks immobilization in resin cast.

or subluxation. Most cases respond to manual reduction and some weeks' immobilization in a cast.

Other sites of growth plate separation include the distal femur, distal tibia and distal radius. Apart from external support, cross and Rush pinning are suitable methods of immobilization. The pins in the first method traverse the epiphysis obliquely to emerge through the opposite metaphysis. In Rush pinning, the pin is directed from the epiphysis to slide in a sledge-runner fashion proximally along the internal surface of the opposing diaphysis. Although such pins are liable to displace rather easily, healing is rapid and the success rate is high.

A specific and difficult orthopaedic problem is fracture of the femoral neck and separation of the proximal femoral physis. Most cases result from dystokia. Diagnosis is difficult as precise localization of the fracture requires radiography. The differential diagnosis includes proximal femoral shaft fracture and pelvic fracture involving the acetabulum. The simplest method of treatment is confinement, which has a low success rate. Alternatively, the femoral head may be resected to permit development of a pseudoarthritis, but lameness usually persists along with obvious muscle atrophy and compensatory conformational changes in the contralateral limb. Finally, internal fixation by Knowles pins or lag screws has been successful (Ferguson, 1982) but requires intraoperative radiography to ensure the correct direction of insertion from the lateral aspect of the greater femoral trochanter.

Vertebral fractures

Aetiology and pathology

Elsewhere in this chapter, reference is made to long bone fractures and growth plate separation (p. 373) resulting from excessive traction during dystokia. But vertebral fractures due to forced traction usually in an exotic beef breed such as Charolais can lead to fracture and/or luxations in the caudal thoracic or cranial lumbar region (preferentially T12–L3). The common form is a fracture of the caudal physis of T13 (Schuh & Killeen, 1988).

Post-mortem changes include perirenal and perivertebral haemorrhage, fractured ribs, cord compression, severed cord, subdural haemorrhage, and myelomalacia.

Clinical signs and diagnosis

The calf is alive before traction is applied in dystokia, but following delivery the calf is weak, usually recumbent, with a swollen head, dyspnoea, and spinal deviation. These calves usually die within 24–48 hours from neurogenic shock (pain, trauma, hypoxia).

The normal rigidity of the spine in the affected thoracolumbar region invariably cannot tolerate the spinal curvature induced during typical traction on forelimbs of a fetus in anterior presentation when these dorsal structures become stretched and convex. When fetal hips lock on entering the maternal pelvis, the thoracolumbar region is approximately level with the maternal vulva. If the fetal body is then twisted and bent from side to side, acting as a pivot, a considerable risk of excessive shearing or traction forces can develop.

Treatment and prevention

The magnitude of traction forces in dystokia should be appreciated. Two men can exert a 350 kg pull for 30 seconds. A calf-puller machine can produce over 500 kg traction. Adequate lubrication of the birth canal and an instinctive reluctance to use more than manual pressure are the two most important preventive measures, since treatment is useless. A greater willingness to adopt caesarean section in oversized viable fetuses will help prevent further accidental injuries.

Pelvic fractures

Aetiology and pathology

Pelvic fractures are rare in cattle. Trauma is almost always involved. The most common pelvic fracture involves the tuber coxae, which is damaged during passage through a narrow doorway or in a sudden fall laterally onto hard ground (Fig. 29.5). Unlike other pelvic fractures, the tuber coxae fragment may be pulled ventrally by the fascia lata, becoming a sequestrum from an inadequate blood supply and may develop a septic draining tract to the exterior.

Another specific aetiology is separation of the pubic symphysis, resulting from excessive traction on a fetus in the pelvic canal of an immature heifer.

Osteoporosis is a predisposing factor to pelvic fracture in some high-yielding dairy herds.

Other pelvic fractures involve the wing or shaft of the ilium, tuber ischii, and the acetabular margin. The ilial fractures usually involve massive trauma, such as falls down cliffs. Tuber ischii damage may result from road traffic accidents in which the impact is caudal. Acetabular margin fracture chips often involve traumatic hip luxations.

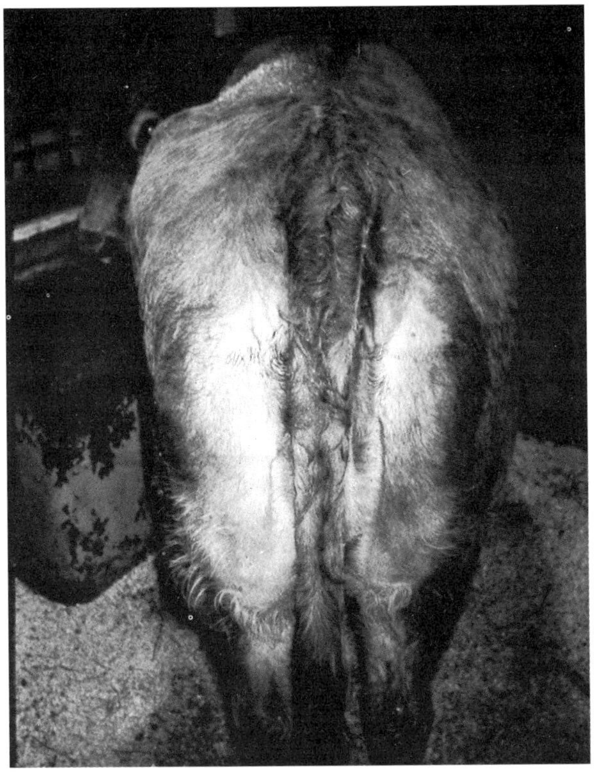

Fig. 29.5 Fracture of right wing of ilium in adult cow, showing asymmetry relative to the greater femoral trochanter and ischial tuberosity.

Clinical signs and diagnosis

The degree of lameness varies considerably from nil (tuber coxae) to severe and even to recumbency (pubic and ilial shaft fractures). The external bony landmarks are frequently asymmetrical. Crepitus may be obvious as the animal walks. Rectal palpation will often permit localization of the crepitus and an appreciation of surrounding soft tissue injury. One useful technique is palpation during lateral rocking of the hindquarters. Fractures of the ilial shaft, pubis and cranial ischium can be appreciated on such rectal exploration. Vaginal palpation should be performed in mature cows and recently calved heifers.

Clinical diagnosis of acetabular fractures, which tend to involve the dorsal rim, is difficult as the localized crepitus must be distinguished from coxofemoral dislocation (in which the greater femoral trochanteric position is abnormal) and femoral neck or physeal fractures (which may be suspected from the increased mobility of the hip region in the affected limb). Radiography is essential for diagnosis in some cases, but, due to size and equipment constraints, is rarely feasible.

Other differential diagnoses include pelvic bruising leading to haematoma formation and pelvic abscessation. Haematomas rarely cause lameness, while abscesses tend to have a more gradual onset and a protracted course. Several sites of pelvic fractures can lead to nerve trunk (sciatic, femoral, obturator) and blood vascular damage (middle uterine artery, internal pudendal, internal iliac arteries and veins).

Fractures of the bodies of the ischium and pubis invariably involve the obturator foramen, usually also the obturator nerve, and are serious in that marked pain and discomfort tend to cause prolonged periods of recumbency and a reluctance to stand. Commonly, both bones are fractured, making the pelvis unstable, and healing is then unlikely. In some cases, healing is liable to be accompanied by excessive callus formation. This sometimes extends to produce hip osteoarthritis and a persistent lameness.

Degenerative osteoarthritis of the hip in older bulls and cows leads to considerable peripheral new bone formation. Sometimes, following minor trauma, small portions of the new acetabular dorsal rim are chipped off (pathological fractures), leading to a sudden increase in severity of the lameness. Often such fracture chips will heal by fibrous tissue, but lameness persists.

Treatment and prevention

Surgery is indicated in few cases of pelvic fracture, e.g. tuber coxae sequestrum. The only useful treatment is generally rest in a well-bedded stall. Use of hip clamps (e.g. Bagshaw hoist) to raise animals is contraindicated. Few cattle become acclimatized to slings, which often appear to increase the discomfort caused by the fracture. Cases of pelvic fracture should be re-assessed after three to four weeks of good nursing, and, in the absence of obvious improvement, most cases should be salvaged.

Dislocations and subluxations

Hip joint

Aetiology

Coxofemoral luxation is sporadic, occurring mostly in two to five-year-old cattle. It has an association with parturition and the early postpartum period. At this time, ligamentous relaxation is maximal and obturator or other nerve injury during dystokia may predispose cattle to abduct the hindlimbs and to slip the feet laterally resulting in a splayed-leg collapse.

Hip dislocation can occur in various directions, craniodorsal being most frequent (about 80 per cent of total), and cranioventral and caudoventral being less common.

Pathology

The gross pathological changes in luxation include rupture of the joint capsule and of the ligament of the femoral head (teres ligament), loss of articular cartilage and surrounding soft tissue, haemorrhage and oedema.

Clinical signs and diagnosis

A sudden onset of lameness is the only consistent sign. Other so-called typical signs refer only to the common craniodorsal luxation, when the leg is held rotated outwards, the hock medial, and stifle more lateral than normal. The leg may appear shortened and the greater femoral trochanters are asymmetrical, the affected side being relatively more dorsal. Movement of the limb is somewhat restricted and painful. Crepitus may be appreciated on limb abduction and flexion. Rectal palpation aids localization of crepitus to the hip. It will also help to differentiate the less common directions of luxation. In cranioventral luxation, abnormal movement may be appreciable cranial and lateral to the pelvic inlet when the cranial border of the pubis is followed. In caudoventral luxation into the region of the obturator foramen, movement may be noted as the leg is abducted, flexed and extended, released, taking the femoral head out of and back into the margin of the foramen.

Diagnosis may be confirmed in smaller cattle on ventrodorsal radiographs. Differential diagnosis includes femoral neck fractures, physeal separation, pelvic (acetabular) fractures, and greater femoral trochanteric fractures.

Treatment

Manipulative reduction should be attempted in all uncomplicated cases of craniodorsal luxation seen within 24 hours of the onset. The chance of successful manual reduction decreases markedly thereafter. Cases of caudoventral dislocation, which are often recumbent, perhaps due to additional obturator damage, have a poorer prognosis.

The common craniodorsal luxation is treated by careful positioning of the patient so that the body is fixed while the affected upper leg can be extended in various directions. Deep sedation (xylazine) is advisable. The leg is forcibly circumrotated in ever-increasing circles by an assistant to loosen up the periarticular soft tissues, which may be in spasm. A large firm block is placed between the ground and the medial femoral region to act as a fulcrum when medial pressure is exerted on the stifle, tending to cause hip abduction. The limb is subject to controlled traction along an imaginary line from the greater trochanter to the femoral head. The veterinarian should concentrate on distal pressure on the greater trochanter. The amount of femoral head movement usually increases with time, and manipulation should not be quickly abandoned. Reduction is usually very obvious, and traction should be stopped at once, otherwise a caudoventral luxation may be produced. Once replaced, the limb is circumrotated slowly and carefully in an attempt to remove blood and other debris from the acetabulum. The animal should not be permitted to stand at once, since spontaneous reluxation is liable. The hindlimbs should be shackled above the hocks or fetlocks for 24–48 hours. A good non-slip surface should be beneath the cow when standing up and, if available, a hip hoist is a useful aid.

Recently, a high success rate has followed open surgery for reduction of hip dislocations (Tulleners *et al.*, 1987). In this series few cases responded to manipulation. As experienced by others, caudoventral and cranioventral dislocations present special problems since limb traction cannot be exerted in the correct direction. The standard surgical approach is medial and cranial to the greater trochanter through the gluteal musculature. Care should be taken to avoid the sciatic nerve. The femoral head is mobilized and moved appropriately with a combination of manipulation by a non-sterile assistant handling the hock, which can be easily rotated slightly or, at will, abducted, and moved by appropriate instrumental leverage. Toggling through the femoral head and acetabulum to produce an artificial intra-articular ligament was unsuccessful in a long-term study.

Recumbency following hip dislocation and for a period after successful reduction means that careful watch should be kept on the possible development of acute severe mastitis, since many cases have recently calved. Excellent nursing in good comfortable surroundings is essential for recovery.

Apart from a surgical series (Tulleners *et al.*, 1987) in which many animals were immature and, therefore, better surgical candidates, most cases have a guarded prognosis for craniodorsal dislocation and a poor prognosis for any other direction. Recumbency at presentation makes recovery less likely.

Hip dislocation is the clinical diagnosis in a certain proportion of 'downer cows' (see p. 368).

Sacroiliac luxation and subluxation

Aetiology

Sacroiliac displacement involves a partial or complete separation of the fibrocartilaginous joint surfaces. The aetiology usually involves excessive ligamentous flaccidity around parturition, when most cases occur. Some cases involve a degree of dystokia. A condition of sacroiliac distortion is recognized when there is no displacement, but excessive mobility of the joint surfaces is detectable. In true luxation considerable haemorrhage and soft tissue damage occurs in the joint space and peripherally (haematoma formation).

Clinical signs and diagnosis

Signs of sacroiliac luxation are characteristic. The lumbosacral spine is dropped relative to the sacral tuberosities of the ilium, which are correspondingly prominent. Cows initially prefer recumbency and show slight ataxia, hindquarter weakness, and some knuckling of the hind fetlocks. These signs are attributed to associated bruising of the ventral nerve roots of L5–S2. Crepitus can be easily elicited from the sacroiliac region. The dropped spine may develop over two to three days and be preceded by evidence of localized pain. Rectal palpation of luxation reveals the sacral promontory has been pushed caudally and depressed, so reducing the dorso-ventral diameter of the pelvic inlet. Very severe cases may be unable to stand as a result of spinal nerve trauma.

In cases of subluxation and distortion, the signs are relatively mild. Some hindlimb ataxia and weakness may appear. Crepitus may be noted during rectal palpation as the cow is walked forwards, and localized swelling over the ventral part of the joint is diagnostic when the history indicates a sudden onset.

Differential diagnosis includes coxofemoral osteoarthritis, pelvic fractures, obturator or other nerve damage, lumbar spondylitis and progressive hindlimb paralysis (spinal abscess, lymphoma).

Treatment and prevention

The prognosis is favourable for cases of distortion and subluxation that are confined to a well-bedded stall for a few days. More severe, recumbent cases of luxation or subluxation have a guarded or poor prognosis. A sacroiliac luxation never undergoes spontaneous reposition and manual reduction is impossible. However, some cows can survive for years with sacroiliac luxation despite the bizarre appearance of the hindquarters.

In nursing affected cows, no forcible attempt (hip clamp, electric goad) should be made to make them stand. Analgesics (phenylbutazone) every second day for one week may increase comfort.

Stifle joint: femoropatellar

Aetiology and pathology

Patellar luxation may occur dorsally, medially and laterally. Dorsal displacement (fixation) is seen in mature cattle as an intermittent condition, unassociated with any known trauma. Medial patellar displacement is rare and is usually congenital. Anatomical defects predisposing to medial luxation have not been clearly identified, though in newly calved heifers with large udders the abducted hindlimb posture may lead to temporary medial patellar luxation.

Lateral patellar luxation is occasionally seen as a specific entity in mature cattle and young calves. This luxation in calves may sometimes be secondary to quadriceps atrophy resulting from femoral paralysis (see p. 366). In calves that first show signs at three months (Weaver & Campbell, 1972) without history of femoral paralysis, no predisposing factors have been identified.

Clinical signs and diagnosis

In dorsal patellar luxation or fixation, the first sign may be initial hindlimb stiffness followed by a jerky action in which the limb remains extended caudally longer than usual, and is then pulled forwards and upwards in a movement resembling equine stringhalt (Fig. 29.6). This action may be intermittent and separated by several normal strides, or it may be repeated. If the cow is pushed backwards, the hindlimb may become fixed temporarily in extension. This extension may persist, whereby the foot is dragged along the ground (permanent upward fixation). Palpation reveals the patella to be more prominent and dorsal than usual, and the patellar ligaments are unusually easily felt. The patella is now resting partly in the supratrochlear fovea, while the medial patellar ligament is felt to be fixed around the medial trochlear ridge.

Both medial and lateral patellar fixation are associated with a characteristic posture. The stifle is markedly flexed, and the limb collapses on weight bearing, exactly as in femoral paralysis (p. 366). Bilaterally affected

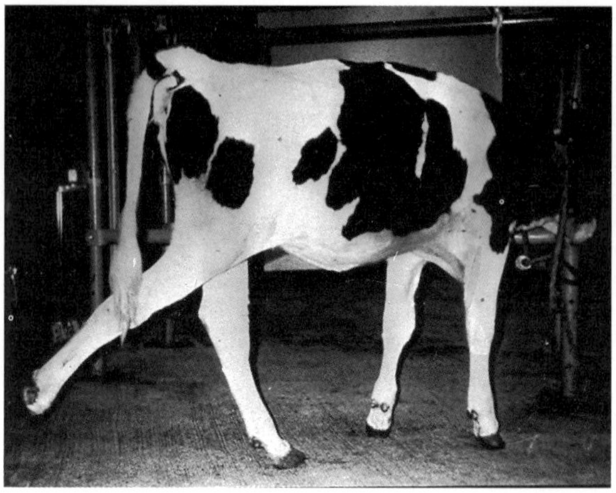

Fig. 29.6 Upward patellar fixation in 15-month-old Canadian Holstein heifer. The degree and duration of caudal extension were unusual. Heifer recovered following medial patellar desmotomy.

calves prefer recumbency. The patellar position is obvious visually and on palpation. It can usually be replaced on to the femoral trochlea but may immediately reluxate. Radiography can confirm the abnormal position but is a superfluous procedure. Differential diagnosis includes femoral nerve paralysis, quadricep muscle rupture, gonitis and distal femoral epiphyseal separation.

Treatment and prevention

Dorsal patellar luxation should be treated by medial patellar desmotomy if signs persist for more than a week. Surgery is preferably carried out in the standing cow as an aseptic procedure following sedation and local analgesia. A large udder or a difficult temperament makes recumbency (affected side down) necessary in some cases. The surgical site is superficial to the most distal palpable point of the medial patellar ligament, close to its insertion into the tibial tuberosity. A 3 cm ($1\frac{1}{4}$ inch) long vertical skin incision is made cranial to the ligament. A tenotome is inserted just deep to the ligament with the blade in a vertical position. A Hey Groves knife, with a blunt rounded point, is ideal for this surgery. The conventional disposable scalpel blade and (Bard) handle are unsuitable since slight movement easily results in breakage and loss of the blade. The cutting edge is rotated through 90° towards the skin and the medial patellar ligament is sectioned without damaging or entering the joint cavity. A single non-absorbable skin suture achieves adequate wound apposition. The operated cow should walk normally at once. No deleterious long-term pathology has been reported in operated cattle.

Both medial and lateral patellar luxation are treated by a joint overlap procedure. In lateral luxation the femoropatellar joint is incised longitudinally about 1 cm ($\frac{1}{2}$ inch) medial to the patella, which is replaced in the trochlea. The capsule is closed by vertical mattress sutures in a joint capsular overlap procedure. Sometimes this technique fails to maintain the patella in position. The fascia of the thigh may then be split dorsally to permit replacement. Bilateral cases should be operated with a one week interval. In medial patellar luxation, the overlap procedure is carried out lateral to the patella.

Stifle joint: femorotibial

Aetiology and pathology

Complete femorotibial luxation is rare and incurable. Subluxation is relatively common and is typically seen in the mature cow or bull as a result of primary cranial cruciate injury (see p. 383). Predisposing factors include heavy weight and sudden twists and falls as when mounting or being mounted by cows in oestrus. The cranial cruciate ligament is partially or completely ruptured (Fig. 29.7). Damage to the caudal cruciate is less

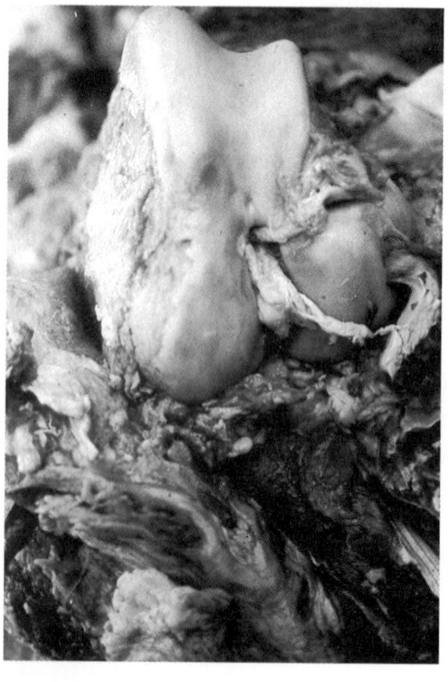

Fig. 29.7 Degenerative osteoarthritis of stifle of aged beef cow showing ruptured cranial cruciate ligament, massive osteophyte proliferation along margins of femoral trochlea and cartilaginous loss on femoral condyles.

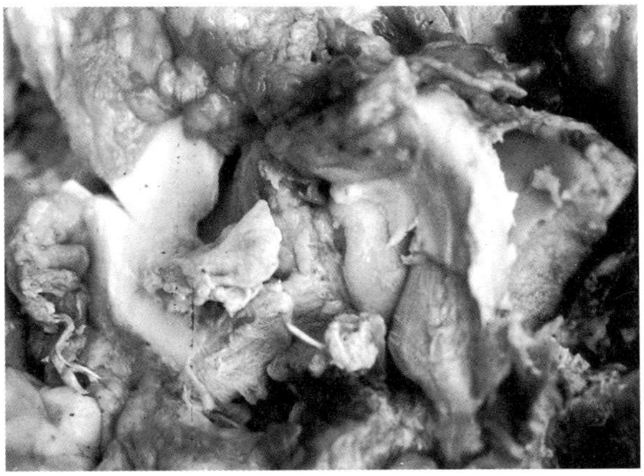

Fig. 29.8 Degenerative osteoarthritis of stifle joint of aged cow exposing damaged menisci and tibial condyles. Menisci are eroded and partially detached, allowing partial eburnation of the underlying tibial condyles. Surrounding musculature is pale due to extensive fibrosis.

likely. One or both tibial menisci are often torn and displaced at the time of rupture (Fig. 29.8). Secondary osteoarthritic changes quickly develop with initial loss of articular cartilage from the femoral condyles, followed by exposure and erosion of subchondral bone and peripheral osteophyte proliferation at the joint margins.

Clinical signs and diagnosis

A sudden onset of a medium degree lameness is characteristic of femorotibial subluxation due to cruciate injury. There is generalized soft tissue swelling and crepitus may be spontaneous or may be induced by rotating the point of hock laterally and medially to produce some rotation of the tibial joint surfaces. The tibial tuberosity may be unusually pronounced and a 'drawer-forward' sign may be demonstrable initially. The animal, placed in lateral recumbency with the affected limb uppermost, has the stifle put into moderate extension. The clinician then attempts to move the proximal tibial region cranially, relative to the femoral condyles. Sometimes this movement is even appreciable as the animal walks. If not diagnostic on palpation, and if radiographic facilities are available, lateral views of the stifle may demonstrate significant (approximately 2.5 cm (1 inch)) cranial displacement of the tibial plateau relative to the femoral condyles. In some cattle, arthrocentesis is advisable to rule out septic gonitis and to demonstrate the presence of cartilaginous debris and blood in the femorotibial joint. Other differential diagnoses include collateral ligamentous injuries, patellar fracture, and, in young cattle, proximal tibial epiphyseal separation.

Treatment and prevention

Although radical surgery involving replacement of the ruptured cranial cruciate ligament by skin or synthetic material has occasionally been successful, these cases have either been experimental animals in which the ligament has been sectioned, or smaller animals in which surgery has been done very soon after the original injury. Most cases have lacked adequate long-term follow-up studies.

Fetlock joint: metacarpophalangeal and metatarsophalangeal

Aetiology and pathology

Dislocation is rare. It invariably involves rupture of both collateral ligaments as well as the intra-articular structures. Trauma is usually so severe that massive soft tissue injury exposes the joint surfaces. Subluxation either in a medial–lateral or cranial–caudal direction is seen sporadically.

Clinical signs and diagnosis

Clinical signs include a non-weight bearing stance, swelling, obvious gross displacement and crepitus on manipulation of the distal extremity. Diagnosis is usually easy. Differential diagnoses include epiphyseal separation in calves, and distal metacarpal, metatarsal and proximal phalangeal fractures. Subluxation presents with similar signs of gross swelling but crepitus may be hard to elicit. Subluxations can be successfully reduced following sedation and extension. A support bandage or cast should be applied subsequently.

Treatment and prevention

Treatment is usually hopeless. If the joint surfaces can be replaced to be congruent, a synthetic collateral ligament may be inserted by utilizing steel wire anchored to screws drilled into each epiphysis. Alternatively, the ligaments may be replaced with polypropylene material. It is usually impossible effectively to suture together the ruptured ends. In young calves the synthetic material may require later removal to permit normal growth of the epiphysis, otherwise the material is left *in situ*.

Muscle and tendon injuries

Introduction

The muscles most liable to rupture include the gastrocnemius, the adductor group and the cranial tibial (peroneus tertius). All three types are particularly liable to damage when a heavy cow is struggling to rise postpartum (see Downer cow syndrome, p. 368).

Specific muscles

The gastrocnemius is particularly exposed to damage as a primary extensor of the hock. Prolonged recumbency, excessive weight, and possibly mineral imbalance leading to a degree of osteomalacia can predispose to gastrocnemius rupture.

The common site is the tendon–muscle junction. The rupture is usually complete and leads to considerable swelling due to extravasation of blood and the development of oedema. The hock is dropped and weight bearing is minimal. Diagnosis is rarely in doubt since the clinical picture is typical.

Gastrocnemius muscle rupture is treated by stall rest and maintenance of the hock in extension by means of a Thomas splint. In yearling animals, compression screws can be drilled from the caudal surface of the calcaneus into the distal portion of the tibial shaft to immobilize the tarsus for some weeks so that fibrous repair at the rupture site can take place.

Cranial tibial (peroneus tertius) rupture is also traumatic, resulting from falls or from excessive traction upwards of the hindlimb by ropes strung over an overhead beam and followed by severe struggling. The animal has a characteristic gait. While the hock is abnormally extended, the stifle remains flexed, in other words, the reciprocal stifle–hock action is lost. When standing, any abnormality may be hard to detect. The limb can be extended caudally so that the metatarsus and tibia form a straight line while the stifle remains flexed. The gastrocnemius tendon is then slack. The site of muscle rupture varies from its origin in the extensor fossa of the femur to the insertion and to the muscle belly itself. Some area of painful swelling is apparent and most cases respond to stall rest over a period of one to four weeks.

Adductor muscle damage has been briefly discussed under downer cow syndrome (see p. 368).

Ventral serrate rupture is spectacular due to loss of its normal anatomical function of supporting the chest in the form of a sling between the forelegs. The scapular cartilage projects above the level of the thoracic spine and is readily palpated subcutaneously. The prominence varies in degree, being more obvious when weight is borne and less obvious in the forward swing of the limb. Colloquially termed 'loose shoulder', Channel Island breeds, especially the Jersey, appear to be predisposed. This feature may reflect a smaller muscle mass relative to body weight. The aetiology in young cattle is possibly related to muscular dystrophy (vitamin E and selenium deficiency). Pathological examination of chronic cases in adult cattle reveals severe muscle degeneration, fibrous tissue proliferation and serous infiltration. While mild cases may recover completely, complete rupture is incurable, but animals move around well and emergency slaughter is rarely necessary.

Contracted flexor tendons

Aetiology and pathology

Contracted digital flexor tendons are the commonest congenital abnormality in cattle. The name 'contracted tendons' is a misnomer, as the primary abnormality is an arthrogryposis or articular rigidity, usually in flexion (Fig. 29.9). Most cases are mild and self-correcting as the calf moves around to an increasing extent. Some are more severe and sometimes associated with other congenital defects such as cleft palate and arthrogryposis.

Contracted tendons usually affect both deep and superficial flexors, and sometimes the suspensory ligaments. The condition is bilaterally symmetrical in the forelimbs. Sometimes the hindlimbs have abnormal hock extensor rigidity and fetlock flexion.

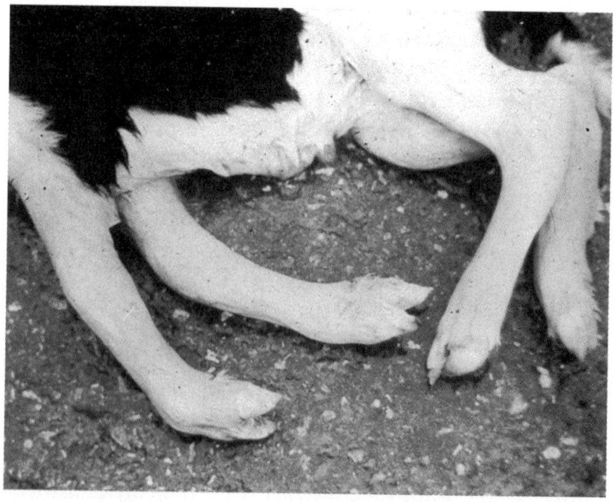

Fig. 29.9 Contracted flexor tendons (forelimb) and flexed hocks in a neonatal Holstein calf, which was unable to stand. Synonyms: arthrogryposis or articular rigidity.

Some breeds (e.g. Belgian Blue) have a very high incidence in which a relationship is suspected between relatively excessive fetal size and abnormal intra-uterine posture. Dystokia is almost invariable in such cases. Akabane virus and the ingestion of various toxic plants (e.g. *Lupinus* species and locoweed) have been alleged in other high incidence outbreaks.

Clinical signs and diagnosis

Mild cases show about 10–20° excessive flexion of the carpus and fetlocks. Forced extension discloses the tautness in the flexor tendons and suspensory ligament. The abnormality is generally symmetrical. Some calves may have a split palate and arthrogryposis of the carpi and tarsi. Joints are not swollen and extension is not unduly painful. When moved, mild degrees of abnormal flexion will result in calves moving on the pastern, but, in severe cases, the calf is totally recumbent or will walk on the distal skin of the fetlock and rapidly develop abrasions and cellulitis, perhaps allowing secondary infection to establish itself and bring the risk of a septic arthritis.

Treatment and prevention

In milder cases, splinting of the leg is normally sufficient. A half-section of a 5 cm (2 inch) diameter polyvinyl drainpipe may be placed on a well-padded limb to immobilize the flexed joints in maximum extension. Such a splint in a neonatal calf must be checked by weekly removal and replacement. The toes should be left exposed to encourage weight bearing and walking. If the stance is not corrected in four weeks, surgery is indicated.

More severe cases will only respond to surgery, which should be undertaken at two to three weeks old, after the immediate neonatal stress period. Correction of carpal flexion is possible at the mediopalmar side of the carpus by an initial longitudinal incision through the retinaculum flexorum, exposure of the superficial part of the superficial flexor, and by complete transection of the retinaculum flexorum, which also involves section of the radial carpal flexor. If normal extension is not achievable, the deep flexor and deep part of the superficial flexor are transected, preserving carefully the neurovascular bundle of median artery, vein and nerves. Finally, the palmar carpal ligament may be sectioned. The wound is closed by sutures and then bandaged and cast for five weeks.

Correction of fetlock flexion is similarly a multistep procedure. The skin incision is at the mediopalmar aspect of the metacarpus, and the superficial portion of the flexor tendon is transected. The deep flexor and deep part of the superficial tendon may be sectioned similarly for adequate extension. Small stab incisions may be made in the suspensory ligament. Bandaging and cast immobilization of the limb are again necessary.

Surgery is likely to be unsuccessful in very severe cases of contracted tendons where abnormal flexion creates an angle of $<90°$ between radius and metacarpus.

Prevention of the primary aetiological stimulus is difficult as arthrogryposis leading to contracted tendons may result from infectious agents (Bovine virus diarrhoea (BVDV), Akabane virus) or toxic plant material.

Joint diseases

Osteochondrosis

Aetiology and pathology

Osteochondrosis is seen primarily in young fast-growing beef cattle on a high calorie intake. Normal endochondral ossification is disturbed at the cartilaginous endplate of the epiphysis and at the metaphyseal growth plate, and is associated with a failure of vascular invasion. The thickness of articular cartilage increases as a result of continued growth and lack of wear, whereupon the failure of adequate nutrient diffusion causes a degeneration of the chondrocytes. The result is a characteristic cleft formation, producing cartilaginous flaps that undergo endochondral ossification. Another process is the formation of cyst-like lesions in the subchondral bone.

It is not yet known to what extent the changes are generalized, as most surveys have only examined specific joints (e.g. stifle, carpus or atlanto-occipital). Changes tend to be symmetrical. Sometimes the joint surfaces of several forelimb bones are normal, while significant changes occur in their physes. Osteochondrosis has been reported in the coxofemoral, femoropatellar, femorotibial and tibiotarsal joints of the hindlimbs, and in the scapulohumeral, humororadial radiocarpal, and metacarpophalangeal joints of the forelimbs.

Clinical signs and diagnosis

Steers and young bulls are predominantly affected. Some lesions cause no clinical signs, while others produce a mild progressive lameness. Some lesions heal following production of fibrocartilage. This accounts for the larger percentage of lesions in autopsies than in clinical series of lame cattle. Other lesions progress

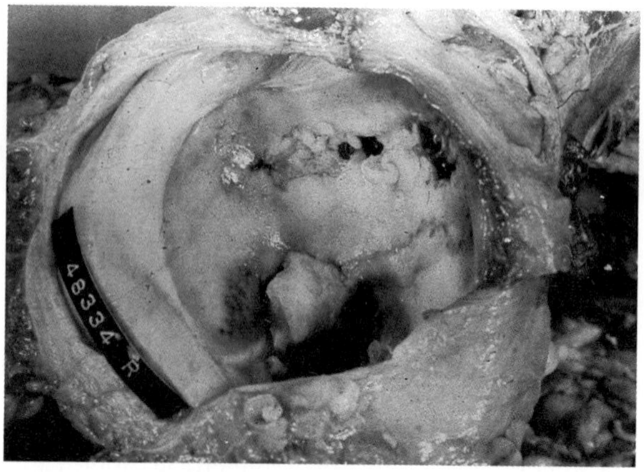

Fig. 29.10 Severe hip dysplasia seen in right acetabulum of nine-month-old Hereford bull. Severe fissuring and loss of cartilage and erosions in subchondral bone.

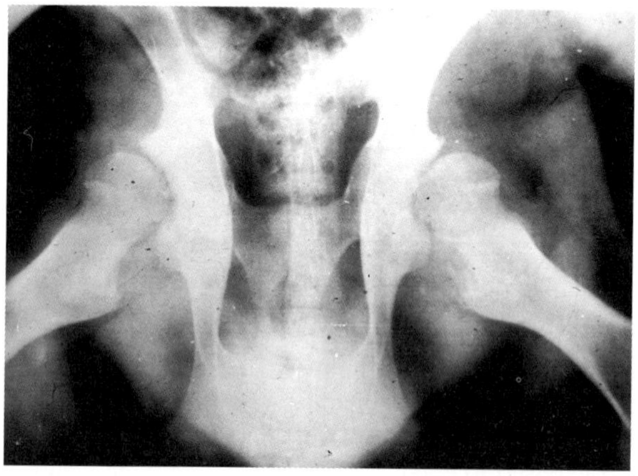

Fig. 29.11 Severe hip dysplasia evident in ventrodorsal radiograph of pelvis of five-month-old Angus bull that had experienced progressive hindlimb lameness for two months. Both femoral heads are subluxated and severe secondary osteoarthritis affects the acetabular rims.

to become a secondary degenerative osteoarthritis or degenerative joint disease (DJD). Exacerbations of a mild slight lameness have been attributed to additional joint trauma. If warranted, a doubtful case may be radiographed. cartilaginous defects are unlikely to be demonstrated unless pneumoarthography is performed. Suspicious evidence of osteochondrosis is the presence of a free calcified body within the joint ('joint mouse').

Treatment and prevention

Theoretically, as in the horse and dog, removal of the cartilaginous flap and curettage of the underlying bone is indicated. Surgical treatment has, however, not been adopted in cattle for economic and anatomical reasons. Management measures in high-incidence situations include a more restricted calorie intake and transfer to a softer bearing surface to reduce concussion. Lame steers should be confined. Osteochondrosis in a bull should stimulate consideration of its conformation as a possible predisposing factor.

Hip dysplasia

Aetiology and pathology

Hip dysplasia is seen in bulls of various fast-growing beef breeds, predominantly the Hereford and Aberdeen Angus, though isolated cases have been reported in numerous other breeds. In the Hereford breed, particular families have been alleged to have a high incidence. The condition is probably a sex-linked heritable characteristic. Although some cases are observed in the neonate, most develop in calves four to twelve months old with erosion of the acetabular cartilage close to the attachment of the accessory cartilage, which normally functions to extend the effective articulating surface (Fig. 29.10). The femoral articular cartilage usually undergoes a shallower but more extensive erosion.

Later changes include traumatic synovitis, fraying of the intra-articular ligament, and a tendency to subluxation. Secondary degenerative joint disease follows in a few weeks.

Clinical signs and diagnosis

Lameness develops slowly and is preceded by a period in which abnormal lateral swinging of the hindquarter is seen. The bull calf spends increased periods in recumbency. Feed intake is reduced and hindquarter atrophy starts. Unilateral or bilateral crepitus is detectable in the hip region and may be localized more precisely if rectal palpation is feasible. The development of subluxation is recognizable from demonstration of the Ortolani sign: with the hand resting on the skin over the greater femoral trochanter, when weight is taken off the hind leg, a distinct 'plop' is felt as the femoral head drops into the acetabulum from its previous position on the dorsal acetabular rim.

In smaller calves, ventrodorsal pelvic radiographs may demonstrate secondary joint changes and a tendency to subluxàtion (Fig. 29.11). Any radiographic suggestion of shallowness of the acetabulum is usually the result of the secondary changes and not a primary anatomical feature.

Differential diagnosis is important in apparently unilateral cases. Stifle disease, acetabular and other pelvic fractures, hip luxation and slipped femoral epiphysis are all to be considered. A confirmed bilateral hip lameness in young bulls is usually diagnostic of hip dysplasia.

Treatment and prevention

No successful treatment has been reported. Affected bull calves and yearlings should be slaughtered. The hip joints should be retained for pathological confirmation of the clinical diagnosis.

Degenerative arthritis

Aetiology and pathology

Degenerative arthritis (degenerative joint disease, DJD) is attributed to a 'wear-and-tear' phenomenon. This chronic non-infectious disease involves primary degeneration of articular cartilage, generally accompanied by secondary sclerosis and eburnation of subchondral bone, peripheral osteophyte formation and surrounding soft tissue proliferation.

Though a common incidental finding at slaughter, its primary clinical significance is as a cause of progressive debilitating lameness involving major weight-bearing joints. In one study of the stifle and hip joints of cattle disease, atrophy frequently led to partial condemnation at slaughter (Weaver, 1977). Other studies have shown the frequent involvement of the hock and carpal joints. Overweight and straightlegged cattle may be predisposed to early DJD but control studies are lacking. An inherited DJD of the stifles of Holstein cattle has been reported (Kendrick & Sittmann, 1966). Nutritional imbalance leading to osteochondrosis (see p. 381), which can lead to secondary DJD, is another aetiological possibility.

Subchondral bone cysts were the most frequent cause of stifle lameness in a Canadian survey (Ducharme *et al.*, 1985). The lateral tibial condyle was most frequently affected, followed by the opposing femoral condyle. The age range was six to eighteen months.

Early fibrillation of articular cartilage leads to necrotic and degenerative chondrocytes, which results in decreased proteoglycan production in the cartilaginous matrix. The cartilage becomes soft and somewhat yellowish. Chondrocyte destruction causes release of lysosomal enzymes, especially cathepsin D. Fibrillated cartilage withstands stress relatively poorly, and fissuring, thinning, or cartilaginous erosion follows.

Pain in DJD originates from the exposed subchondral bone and from the associated capsulitis and synovitis. Clinically, the joint enlarges partly as a result of the increased volume of synovia.

Clinical signs and diagnosis

A progressive lameness with gradual muscle atrophy and weight loss is commonly seen. The affected limb, usually hind, tends to be dragged as flexion of the affected joint is reduced. Movement of the stifle or hock results in palpable joint enlargement. In the stifle, proliferative changes (osteophyte formation, periarticular fibrosis) affect both femoropatellar and femorotibial compartments, and crepitus may be noted. Some cases of stifle DJD reflect a secondary response to cranial cruciate rupture or meniscal injury. In the hock, major changes are usually seen craniomedially, affecting the intertarsal and tarsometatarsal joint space (similar to equine 'spavin'). Relatively rarely do changes extend proximally to the tibiotarsal joint. Degenerative joint disease of the hip can be suspected in older cows where the more distal parts of the limb are normal clinically and where crepitus can be detected over the gluteal region and confirmed on rectal palpation.

Subchondral bone cysts can only be diagnosed on radiographic examination. Cases of DJD, ligamentous rupture and septic arthritis show ranging radiographic features. Degenerative joint disease of the stifle and hock shows the extent of the proliferative reaction. Lateral radiographs of the stifle in rupture of the cranial cruciate ligament have the 'drawer-forward' features seen in dogs. Septic arthritic cases on radiography demonstrate soft tissue swelling and distension of the joint capsule in early cases, and when more advanced the radiographic changes include loss of subchondral bone.

Synovial fluid analysis is only justified when the differential diagnosis includes infectious arthritis or when fluid is withdrawn prior to injection of a local analgesic solution to assess whether lameness is lessened. Synovia in DJD is clear or slightly turbid, increased in volume, does not clot, has a low (<10 per cent) polymorphonuclear lymphocyte count, a slightly elevated protein (about 3 g/dl), and a near-normal mucin precipitate (Greenough *et al.*, 1981).

Differential diagnosis, apart from infectious forms of arthritis, includes fluorosis as a primary cause of DJD, osteoporosis, rickets and osteoarthritis deformans, all three of which occur in young growing animals, and osteomalacia. A sudden onset of lameness sometimes represents an exacerbation of a non-clinical DJD following a periarticular fracture (e.g. caudal surface of tibia in femorotibial DJD).

Treatment and prevention

Treatment is purely palliative. Affected cattle should be rested (p. 862). Phenylbutazone may be given (initially 10 mg/kg orally, then 5 mg/kg) every second day for its analgesic and anti-inflammatory properties. Aspirin (100 mg/kg orally b.i.d.) is an alternative regimen. Flunixin meglumine has few obvious advantages over either phenylbutazone or aspirin for arthritides and is considerably more expensive. Prolonged low-dosage therapy with phenylbutazone in cattle with painful arthritides has not led to any demonstrable deleterious effects such as gastrointestinal ulceration or renal papillary necrosis. Corticosteroids and dimethyl sulphoxide (DMSO) have also been advocated. The majority of young cattle with stifle lameness due to subchondral bone cysts formation recovered following conservative treatment (Ducharme *et al.*, 1985). Preventive measures include attention to the conformation of further breeding stock, especially bulls, to avoid a hindlimb conformation that is liable to lead to excessive concussive forces in progeny.

Infectious (septic) arthritis

Introduction

Infectious arthritis in this context is synonymous with septic arthritis. The rare primary septic arthritis develops from direct joint penetration by a contaminated foreign body. This section considers secondary septic arthritis resulting from spread of pathogens from an adjacent localized focus, and tertiary septic arthritis resulting from systemic or haematogenous spread from a focus elsewhere in the animal.

Septic arthritis: joint ill in neonate

Aetiology and pathology

Joint ill in calves is classified as a tertiary septic arthritis. The primary infection is in the umbilicus, often as an umbilical abscess with extension along the umbilical veins towards the liver. Otherwise, spread is from a primary enteric infection. Common pathogens isolated are *Escherichia coli*, *Streptococcus* and *Staphylococcus* spp., *Actinomyces pyogenes Erysipelothrix insidiosce* and *Salmonella* spp. Usually, more than one joint is affected, most commonly the carpus, tarsus and femorotibial joints. The route of haematogenous spread is through metaphyseal or epiphyseal vessels or, alternatively, to the synovial membrane. Establishment of foci of infection is naturally favoured by the slowed flow rate of blood through a network of venous sinusoids in the metaphyseal vessels.

Pathological changes start with an intense polymorphonuclear inflammatory response in the synovial membrane, the permeability of which is increased, permitting protein leakage into the synovial fluid. Later release of lysosomal and other enzymes into the synovia causes degeneration of the articular cartilage, which is weakened by defective nutrition due to an overlying fibrin deposit. The result is extensive loss of articular cartilage, acute synovitis, thickening of the joint capsule, and sepsis in the growth plate and metaphysis (particularly associated with salmonella infection).

Clinical signs and diagnosis

The first sign is lameness. Later, joint swelling (Fig. 29.12) and pain are apparent. The joint capsule may be distended from an increased synovial volume. The polyarthritis is rarely symmetrical. Not all cases are associated with either gross umbilical sepsis or with severe enteritis. Calves that are immune depressed as a result of low gamma globulin levels (inadequate colostral intake) are at higher risk. Lameness becomes severe after a few days.

Radiology is not a great aid to diagnosis, as the only initial abnormality is the soft tissue swelling. After two to three weeks, changes suggestive of joint destruction are apparent.

Arthrocentesis is a more valuable aid to diagnosis in early cases. Apart from an increased volume, synovial fluid in a calf with joint ill is turbid, clots, and has a loose flaky character in the mucin precipitate. The protein content is 6–8 g/dl and a Giemsa smear reveals an almost pure (98 per cent) and massive population of polymorphonuclear lympocytes. Taken aseptically, synovial fluid may be submitted for culture, which is often problematical with this particular material.

Differential diagnosis must be made from physeal and intra-articular fractures.

Treatment and prevention

Early and vigorous treatment is essential in joint ill. High therapeutic levels of systemic antibiotics should be given for two to three weeks. Intra-articular antibio-

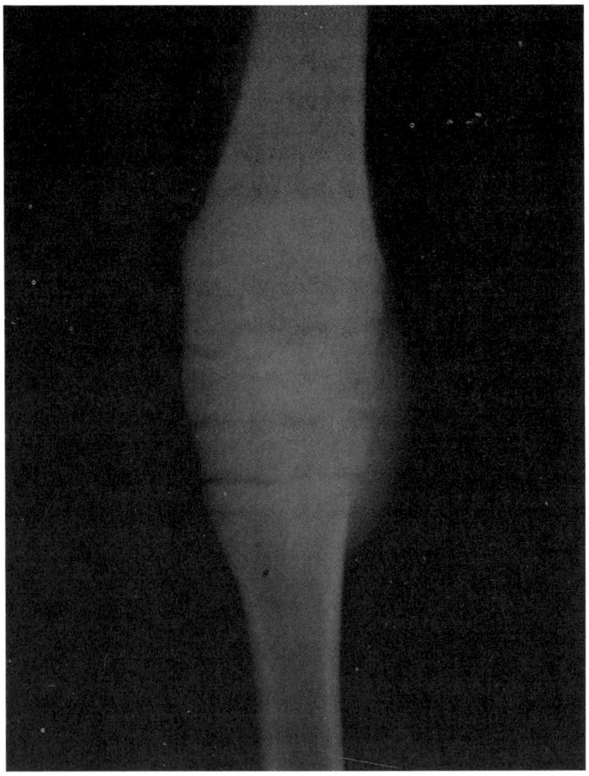

Fig. 29.12 Extensive soft tissue swelling of lateral aspect of left carpal region in a six-month-old Hereford calf. Bone lysis is evident in the distal part of the radial carpal and fused second and third carpal bones. Lysis resulted from transverse fracture of the proximal surface of the distal component of the joint. Recovery followed removal of the bone fragment, curettage and irrigation.

tic medication is contraindicated, as the blood supply ensures adequate concentrations are obtained in synovia following systemic injection. Suitable antibiotics include penicillin, ampicillin and tetracyclines.

Joint lavage with a sterile polyionic solution or physiological saline is helpful. Generally, an in–out, through-and-through system using two 14 gauge needles is effective. Open arthrotomy with removal of the fibrin clots and purulent material has been successful in some series and appears more useful in less complex joints such as the stifle rather than in carpus or tarsus.

Supportive care is important. Bandaging for support reduces discomfort and so maintains the appetite. Low level oral dosage with phenylbutazone can improve the general attitude (p. 847). Some calves also require management of the enteritis by fluid therapy (see p. 175) and others require drainage of an umbilical abscess. Inadequate levels of gamma globulins may, with difficulty due to the large volumes, be corrected by giving intravenous plasma.

Septic arthritis: older cattle

Aetiology and pathology

The main site of septic (infectious) arthritis in mature cattle is the distal interphalangeal joint resulting from secondary spread from a focus in the sensitive solar laminae or from complications of interdigital necrobacillosis (see pp. 360 and 356).

Septic digital arthritis is fully discussed elsewhere (p. 357). Other joints liable to be affected by septic arthritis include the fetlock, either by extension along the digital flexor sheath from a digital focus, or by direct trauma from a deep wound (Fig. 29.13). The major hindlimb weight-bearing joints, the tarsus, stifle and hip are occasionally involved as a result of haematogenous spread such as pyaemic vegetative endocarditis

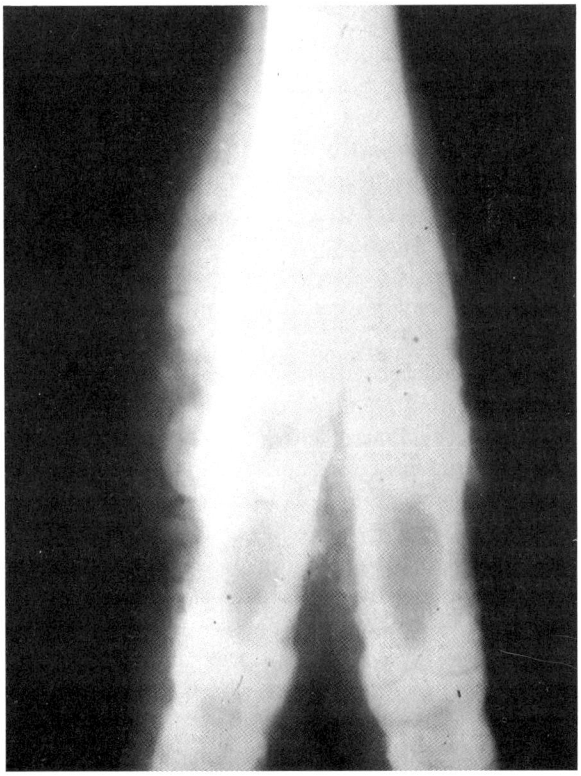

Fig. 29.13 Massive periosteal proliferation of fetlock region (metatarsophalangeal joint) of a four-year-old Holstein cow resulting from sepsis of the joint originating from an ascending septic tenosynovitis.

(e.g. from primary reticuloperitonitis) or in the tarsus from contiguous spread from an infected subcutaneous bursitis.

Organisms commonly recovered from septic arthritis in adult cattle include *A. pyogenes*, *E. coli*, *Staphylococcus* and *Streptococcus spp.*, *Fusobacterium necrophorum* and *Bacteroides melaninogenicus* (anaerobe) have occasionally been reported. The major problem is *A. pyogenes*. Once infection is in the synovial fluid, joint destruction involves the same processes as described for DJD. The difference lies in the speed of destruction. The synovia is usually turbid or frankly purulent.

Three recent reports from the UK (Bracewell & Corbell, 1979; Wyn-Jones *et al.*, 1980) and USA (Madison *et al.*, 1989) have described an idiopathic, acute suppurative gonitis with severe lameness and synovitis. Articular erosions were evident radiographically on the lateral tibial plateau. Much evidence indicates the likelihood that *Brucella abortus* vaccination may be the cause of the idiopathic gonitis.

Clinical signs and diagnosis

Septic arthritis in a major weight-bearing joint causes a rapidly progressive disease with severe lameness, swelling and localized pain. In contrast to DJD, the animal may be anorexic and milk yield can drop abruptly in dairy cattle. Crepitus is not usually apparent. Arthrocentesis reveals a flocculent or purulent fluid that clots. It has a high leucocyte count of which over 90 per cent are polymorphs. The protein content often exceeds 8 g/dl and the mucin precipitate is abnormally flocculent.

A category 'suspect septic' refers to an early septic process associated with obvious lameness but apparently normal yellow synovia. The presence again of a high percentage of neutrophils in a dense leucocyte population is confirmation of early septic arthritis. Radiography in early (<10 days duration) septic arthritis is usually unhelpful. From 14 days onwards, subchondral bone destruction and a peripheral periostitis are suggestive of joint sepsis.

Culture of synovial fluid is frequently negative in terms of isolation of pathogens, especially if antimicrobial therapy has already started. It is helpful if synovia is immediately inoculated into a diphasic culture bottle with sodium polyanetholsulphonate to enhance recovery of the organism. Culture of synovial biopsy material is usually more rewarding but is frequently impractical.

Treatment and prevention

The prognosis for septic arthritis is guarded or poor. Early aggressive treatment is essential. Parenteral antibiotic therapy should be initiated as soon as possible. Until sensitivity, based on synovial cultures, is available 48 hours after sampling, penicillin or ampicillin is the drug of choice for most pathogens. Penicillin is most likely to be effective *in vivo* against all common pathogens except *Staphylococcus aureus* (where erythromycin, lincomycin, gentamicin, or cephalosporin may be better) and coliforms (gentamicin or trimethoprim–sulphadiazine).

The joint should be irrigated and drained (through-and-through lavage) through two wide-bore inflow–outflow portals produced by 14 gauge needles. Alternatively, small arthrotomy incisions may be made for the same purpose. Irrigation should be done with large volumes (>5 l) of polyionic solutions, physiological saline, or with dilute (0.1 per cent) povidone-iodine solution.

Radical surgery also has a place if suitable facilities exist for the maintenance of asepsis and for general anaesthesia. Radical surgery comprises opening the joint following section of collateral ligaments and incision of joint capsule, evacuation of purulent material, curettage of infected cartilaginous surfaces, restoration of joint stability by suturing capsule and ligaments, and immobilization of the area, if in the distal limb, to prevent ankylosis. Such surgery has been more successful in the fetlock, carpus and tarsus than in the stifle, elbow, or shoulder joints.

Idiopathic gonitis (Bracewell & Corbell, 1979; Wyn-Jones *et al.*, 1980; Madison *et al.*, 1989) carries a good prognosis for recovery, regardless of the method of treatment. Heifers were treated successfully with a variety of antimicrobials, including procaine penicillin G, neomycin and ampicillin, and, in some cases, with through-and-through needle lavage with a polyionic solution. Lateral patellar arthrotomy with curettage of lytic areas on the lateral tibial plateau may be useful adjunct therapy.

There is no place for intra-articular antibiotics. Drainage of infective material from a poorly vascularized area is important, whereas systemic antibiotics adequately penetrate the well-vascularized joint capsule. Antibiotics should be given for at least two weeks. Preferred antibiotics are usually penicillin G, ampicillin, centiofur and gentamicin. Non-steroidal anti-inflammatory drugs should be given if pain is severe and persistent. The dosage is as for cases of DJD (see p. 384).

Miscellaneous neuromuscular diseases

Spastic paresis

Aetiology and pathology

Spastic paresis is a progressive condition of the hindlimbs of unknown origin. It is characterized by contraction of the gastrocnemius muscle and tendon and of other associated calcanean tendons and muscle bellies. This spasm leads to severe extension of the hock. The condition has been observed in numerous breeds, but the highest incidence in dairy and beef cattle respectively is probably in the German and Dutch Friesian and the Aberdeen Angus.

It is hypothesized that an overactive stretch reflex is the major mechanism (De Ley & De Moor, 1977). Selective deafferentation of the gastrocnemius muscle by resection of the dorsal root fibres containing afferent nerve fibres (L5–6) abolished clinical signs. Plasma SGOT is reduced, and alkaline phosphatase is increased in affected calves, which also show a decreased P, Ca, and homovanillic acid concentration in CSF. The last-named effect indicates a lowered metabolic rate of CNS dopamine (De Ley & De Moor, 1975).

Clinical signs and diagnosis

The typical clinical signs are characteristic, and difficulty only arises in very early cases. Signs may start at six weeks to six months, rarely later. Cases encountered in adult cattle are best considered to be forms of progressive hindlimb paralysis, likely to involve spinal cord pressure resulting from vertebral exostoses.

The affected hindlimb is extended so that the hock angle is approximately 180° (normal is about 140°). The calf walks with a tendency to drag the toes. The limb may jerk intermittently at rest. It is advanced in a pendulum-like style. Later, less weight is taken and the calf may hop forward. Palpation reveals a very firm gastrocnemius muscle and tendon. The hock can be flexed manually without causing pain. On release the hock immediately adopts the original extended position (Fig. 29.14).

Lateral radiographs of the hock of calves affected for several weeks show several features indicative of the chronic overextension. The distal part of the tibial metaphysis is abnormally curved caudally; the distal tibial and tuber calcanei growth plates are widened; exostoses are present around the distal tibial growth plate, along with some osteoporosis. Often the most striking feature is a cranial curvature of the proximal part of the calcaneus.

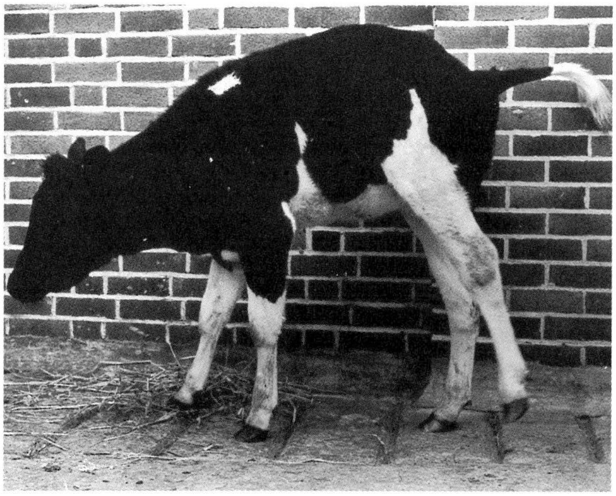

Fig. 29.14 Severe spastic paresis of left hindlimb of a four-month-old Friesian heifer, showing overextension of hock joint. Note spasm and elevation of the tail, and arched back as calf attempts to put more weight on the forelimbs.

In early cases, differential diagnosis includes dorsal patellar luxation, septic or non-infectious gonitis or tarsitis, fracture dislocation of the calcaneus, joint ill and luxation of the biceps femoris muscle.

Treatment and prevention

Since spastic paresis has a hereditary predisposition, breeding animals should be salvaged. Surgery can successfully alleviate the condition by either tenotomy or neurectomy.

Tenotomy has traditionally involved section of the gastrocnemius tendon and partial section of the superficial flexor tendon a little proximal to the point of the hock in the standing animal under local anaesthetic infiltration. A 6 cm ($2\frac{1}{2}$ inch) vertical skin incision is made caudally over the Achilles tendon to expose the two tendons. After section, the skin is sutured and the immediate surgical effect is usually pronounced hock flexion, with the joint initially close to the ground. Initial results have been consistently favourable, but a gradual recurrence of the abnormal posture is frequently seen, especially in older (six to ten-month-old) calves. Bilaterally affected calves should have the second leg operated four weeks following initial surgery.

It has been claimed that this classical operation ignores the fact that a second, deeply situated, tendon of insertion of the gastrocnemius muscle is left untouched. The modified operation, therefore, involves a lateral approach just cranial to the Achilles tendon, which is dissected to isolate the caudal component of the gastrocnemius tendon, from which a 2 cm (1 inch) length is resected. The superficial flexor tendon is left untouched. The cranial tendon of the gastrocnemius is identified and a similar tenectomy performed. In some cases, the dense fascia caudal to the distal end of the tibia is transected (Pavaux *et al.*, 1985).

Neurectomy of the tibial nerve or of its gastrocnemius branches is the alternative to tenotomy. Clinical results have been better than with tenotomy. Since identification of the multiple (seven or more) branches of the tibial nerve innervating the gastrocnemius muscle is awkward, complete tibial neurectomy has been advocated (Boyd & Weaver, 1967). Surgery is performed under sedation and epidural block, or general anaesthesia. The site is the lateral thigh, between the two heads of the biceps femoris muscle. The tibial and peroneal nerves are identified by stimulation by forceps or by electrical means. Tibial nerve stimulation causes hock extension and fetlock and digital flexion. The tibial nerve should have a 2 cm (1 inch) portion removed at its most proximal point. Complications following this surgery are uncommon.

Spastic syndrome

Aetiology and pathogenesis

This chronic progressive disease, which initially is characterized by clonic–tonic spasms of the hindlimb musculature, is also known as 'crampy', 'stretches' or progressive hindlimb paralysis. The aetiology is unknown despite several attempts to find significant pathological lesions in the brain or spinal cord. Idiopathic muscular cramps is one current proposed explanation for the signs (Wells *et al.*, 1987).

The condition occurs in mature cattle of many breeds, both dairy (e.g. Holstein, Friesian and Guernsey) and beef (Hereford, Angus). The incidence in at least one breed (Danish Red) is significantly higher in bulls than cows. Many affected cattle have straight rear legs and poor hock conformation. Many bulls with spastic syndrome have spinal spondylosis. A single recessive gene with incomplete penetrance may be the mode of inheritance.

Clinical signs and diagnosis

Sudden episodic spasmodic contractions affect the muscles of both hindlegs, and sometimes also the back, neck and forelegs. The animal appears normal during recumbency. Signs are evident soon after rising. The individual appears normal between episodes.

The onset of the syndrome is slow, then signs may appear for a few months only to disappear for several weeks. The hindlimbs are hyperextended caudally in a fixed manner that may persist for several minutes. Spasms may extend forward to the forelimbs and neck muscles. The head is extended and the forefeet advanced with the back arched. If then forced to move, the gait is stiff and ungainly, and episodic raising of the hindlimbs may also be seen during forward movement.

Animals generally spend considerable periods recumbent when the condition is advanced.

Other conditions that may confuse an initial diagnosis are relatively few but include bilateral DJD affecting the stifle or hock, and severe spinal spondylosis.

Treatment and prevention

The spastic syndrome is incurable. Palliative treatment has included vitamin D, bone meal and sedatives. Phenylbutazone has provided temporary relief in some cases. Affected bulls and apparently normal bulls that sire affected progeny should be culled from any breeding programme.

Diseases of skin and subcutis

Skin wounds are more liable around the limbs than the trunk and head. Their nature and treatment are adequately discussed in textbooks of general surgery. One unusual problem is the constricting foreign body, usually rubber or wire, which slides over the foot to the level of pastern or metacarpus or metatarsus where it slowly becomes embedded in a mass of granulation tissue, which presents as a circumferential wound (Fig. 29.15). Such wounds require careful investigation because the band may be very deep and contacting bone.

Two specific disorders are discussed below. Generally, damage to skin and subcutis is more liable over pressure points such as the lateral aspect of the stifle, elbow and hock. Loss of the integument permits low-grade infection to become established. In a very contaminated environment such damage, which results from pressure points and poor vascularity, may result in localized abscessation and pyaemic spread to the lungs, liver, kidneys and heart. The common organism is *A. pyogenes*.

Affected cattle should be put out on soft bedding, the wounds should be cleansed with chlorhexidine hy-

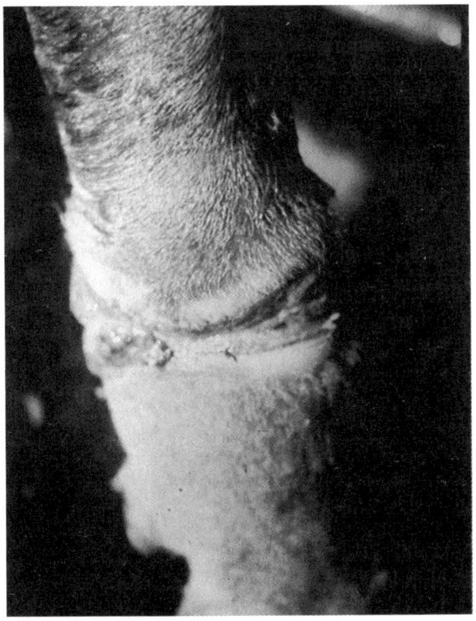

Fig. 29.15 Circumferential wound of metatarsal soft tissues. This two-year-old crossbred Hereford steer had a wire embedded deep to the soft tissues, resulting in mild lameness. Wound healed in four weeks following removal of foreign body.

drochloride, and systemic antibiotics should be injected for five to seven days to prevent systemic spread. The prognosis for healing is good if appetite is maintained along with a satisfactory body score unless clinical signs of involvement of other organs (e.g. heart) are apparent.

Tarsal cellulitis

Aetiology and pathology

Almost all cases of hock enlargement result from repeated trauma against concrete surfaces in stanchions or loose housing. Typically, soft tissue swelling over the lateral aspect of the tarsus may be a false or acquired bursitis. Medial swelling of the joint is minimal unless the lateral enlargement is pronounced. Lameness is rarely seen unless the fluid distension becomes massive, when a mechanical restriction of joint flexion causes stiffness, or a low-grade infection arises. Radiographs have repeatedly shown the absence of bone changes.

The swelling is usually symmetrical. Hair loss and skin excoriation are evident. Usually the skin is not broken. Occasionally, a central area of skin sloughs, permitting a dirty red–brown material to escape. At this time, septic infection can supervene and a purulent discharge may be noted for several days before granulation tissue fills the cavity of the false bursa.

Clinical signs and diagnosis

The distribution of the swelling and absence of lameness are almost characteristic (Fig. 29.16). An infectious tarsitis causes a more diffuse swelling and obvious lameness, as will a tarsal bone fracture. Tarsal hydrarthrosis first causes a preferential synovial distension of the joint capsule cranially and medially, then both medial and lateral to the caudal border of the tibiotarsal bone, and cranial to the base of the calcaneus. Tarsal hydrarthrosis is a cosmetic blemish and causes no lameness.

Treatment and prevention

The seasonal occurrence of tarsal bursitis, becoming increasingly severe during the housed period and disappearing in the summer grazing months, is evidence that tarsal bursitis is related to the specific environment. Errors and deficiencies usually can be found in the lying-in areas of loose-housed herds. Some cows may refuse to use cubicles and remain out on the slurry-covered concrete. They often have problems rising from the slippery surface, during which the wet skin of the lateral part of the hock is repeatedly abraded. Other cows suffer injury when they rise awkwardly in poorly designed or badly bedded cubicles. Standings that are up to 30 cm (12 inches) too short for the particular breed and neck rails placed 5 cm (2 inches) too

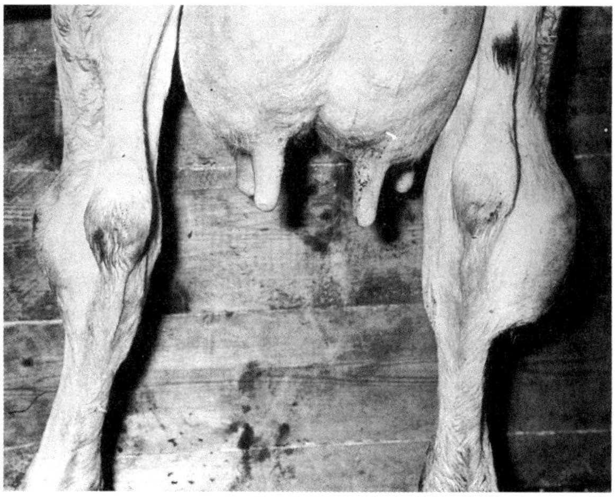

Fig. 29.16 Right tarsal bursitis in a five-year-old Holstein cow with digital problems resulting in prolonged recumbency. Left supratarsal skin shows evidence of previous injury.

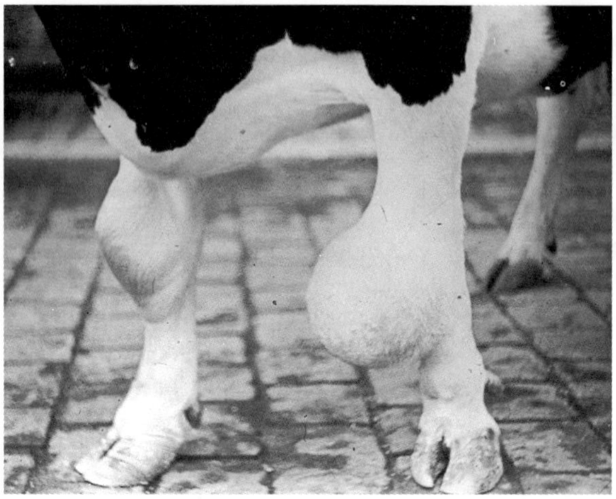

Fig. 29.17 Severe bilateral carpal bursitis in an eight-year-old Friesian cow associated with *Br. abortus* infection (Czechoslovakia).

low may force cows to stand with the hind feet in the passageway. Careful observation (e.g. during oestrous detection) will usually disclose the specific problem.

Treatment should be conservative and medical. It should never involve a long incision to drain fluid from the false bursa, neither should one attempt radically to dissect out this bursa. Most cases are best left untreated in the absence of lameness. If lameness eventually occurs as a result of a low-grade tarsal infection, systemic antibiotics (oxytetracyclines) rapidly reduce the size of the swelling. Corticosteroids are usually ineffective. Infected cases may be bandaged daily and be irrigated with warm water, but the response tends to be incomplete. A cluster of cases indicates a need to check the loafing areas and cubicles.

Carpal bursitis

Aetiology and pathology

Carpal bursitis or carpal hygroma involves the skin, subcutaneous precarpal bursa and adjacent soft tissues. Very rarely does infection extend into the joint. Repeated contusion from contact points of the stanchions, stalls, or floor in housed cattle is the main predisposing factor. The condition is similar to tarsal cellulitis in that the swelling recedes in cattle when spending most of the time at pasture. Some cases have been associated with *Br. abortus* infection (Fig. 29.17).

Clinical signs and diagnosis

A soft penetrating and painless swelling develops on the dorsal aspect of the carpus, usually with evidence of skin contusion. It tends to be symmetrical and no breed or age predilection is recognized. Minor swellings are merely a cosmetic blemish. The exceptional large grapefruit or melon-sized mass may cause a slight mechanical lameness but no pain. The fluid appears to be synovia-like, yellow and clear, but less tenacious. It is produced by the bursal lining. The cavity tends to be multilocular. Differential diagnosis from a precarpal abscess or septic carpitis, both of which are painful and cause lameness, is simple.

Treatment and prevention

Surgical drainage is rarely necessary. Such drainage (as in tarsal bursitis, p. 389) is fraught with the risk of introducing infection into a sterile site. The skin is more liable to contamination every time the animal lies down. It is hard to protect the area with a bandage. Most cases respond if placed in a well-bedded straw yard (winter) or put to pasture (summer), i.e. into surroundings where predisposing trauma can be avoided.

Drainage is only needed when gait, feed intake and production are affected. The drainage should be done as an aseptic procedure. A mixture of antibiotic and corticosteroid solution should be instilled into various sections of the collapsed cavity and such injection should be repeated at weekly intervals.

Radical surgical removal of the bursa and excessive skin is possible, but is a haemorrhagic and time-consuming process despite the presence of a tourniquet proximal to the carpus. General anaesthesia is usually required as adequate local infiltration of the bursal wall is impractical.

Destruction of the bursal lining with an astringent (copper sulphate) or irritant disinfectant (tincture of iodine) is not advisable, as a severe local reaction is produced, and dissection, curettage and repeated irrigation of the wound are essential steps before secondary healing eventually occurs.

Prevention involves careful attention to the housing system for the existing herd. Multiple cases of carpal bursitis should lead to modification of the lying accommodation, such as lengthening of the stalls, adjustment of head or neck stalls or mangers, and change of or increase in the bedding. Problem cows should be put into straw yards before the swellings cause a clinical problem.

Ankylosing spondylitis

Aetiology and pathology

Defined as an acquired fusion of the ventral aspects of the bodies of the caudal thoracic and lumbar vertebrae, sufficient pressure may be exerted on the ventral and lateral spinal cord tracts or the ventral nerve roots to cause some hindlimb weakness, ataxia or paralysis. Exostoses develop on the ligaments of the caudal 2–3 thoracic and cranial 2–3 lumbar spinal bodies first (T11–L3). Degenerative changes in the intervertebral discs may predispose to exostosis formation. The new bone may extend into the spinal canal as 'replacement bone'. Sometimes, possibly resulting from a fall or a violent ejaculation, part of the exostosis may fracture, the fracture line extending through the vertebral body. Fluid exudate (blood, oedema) from the fracture may cause pressure on the spinal cord.

Clinical signs and diagnosis

An early sign may be a reluctance or difficulty in mounting cows, attributable to the mechanical effects of a relatively inflexible thoracolumbar spine. Usually there are no premonitory signs and the bull suddenly has difficulty in rising and may adopt a 'dog-sitting' position or may be completely paraplegic, dragging the digits caudally. Sometimes marked ataxia suddenly develops.

The site of trauma can rarely be accurately defined due to problems of size. Crepitus is rarely elicited. Swelling of the back musculature is not seen. On rectal examination, exostoses may be palpable dorsal to the aortic bifurcation, but such exostoses are a normal feature of mature and older bulls. In one extensive series of bulls followed to slaughter, severe signs of tail and hindlimb paralysis were only seen in two cases, though all bulls had varying degrees of ankylosing spondylitis.

Differential diagnosis includes other causes of spinal cord compression such as aberrant migrating larvae and infiltrating neoplasms, as well as hindlimb degenerative joint disease.

Treatment and prevention

The prognosis depends on the degree and extent of nerve damage. In the progressive ataxic or paraplegic case, it is poor. Mild cases may improve following rest and use of corticosteroids and diuretics to reduce the oedema. Animals should be bedded on deep straw to prevent the development of decubital lesions. Many mild cases relapse following partial recovery. Slaughter on humane grounds is often the action of choice.

Mineral imbalance-related lameness: rickets, osteomalacia (see also p. 217)

Aetiology and pathology

Mineral, indeed nutrient, imbalance can result in lameness from calfhood through the growing yearling stage to maturity and old age. The pattern almost invariably involves an imbalance or deficiency of two or more factors.

During growth the important elements in normal development of healthy bone collagen, which is the framework for provisional calcification of the zone of hypertrophied cartilage, are vitamin D, copper, protein and energy. Mineralization of the cartilaginous matrix results in deposition of much calcium, phosphorus and carbonate, with lesser amounts of sodium, magnesium and fluoride. Vitamin D, calcium and phosphorus are essential to the formation of this bone mineral.

In the prenatal period, identified deficiency diseases resulting in abortion or the birth of progeny with skeletal defects include lupinosis (congenital arthrogryposis), manganese (contracted tendons), and zinc and vitamin A deficiencies (multiple defects).

Vitamin D deficiency in calves leads by a complex pathway involving the parathyroid gland, kidney and intestine to deficient calcification of long bones and of the cartilaginous matrix. The result in calves is rickets. The zone of provisional calcification is widened but the new osteoid is not mineralized. In adults, the same deficiency causes osteomalacia, which is rare except in northern Australia and South Africa. Usually a calcium : phosphorus imbalance is also involved. Vitamin D-deficient diets may be identified on some farms where feed is home-mixed.

Clinical signs and diagnosis of rickets

Calves have swelling of the metaphyses and growth plates of the long bones, especially the distal metatarsus and metacarpus, fetlock and pastern. The swellings are rather painful to pressure. The costochondral junction exhibits the classical 'rickety rosary' in calves. Radiographic changes include a widened area of radiolucency at the growth plate with flaring of the distal metaphyses, usually in the carpus, pastern and fetlock.

The diagnosis rests on the soft tissue swelling at characteristic sites, lameness, and in cases of doubt, feed analysis. Serum or plasma may reveal depressed levels of calcium, phosphorus and an elevated alkaline phosphatase.

Differential diagnosis includes physeal dysplasia and joint ill (polyarthritis).

Clinical signs and diagnosis of osteomalacia

The relative or absolute phosphorus deficiency, usually acquired from low phosphorus pastures, is classically associated with the development of pica and osteophagia, variable degrees of lameness including pathological fractures of long bones, weight loss, stiffness and recumbency. Deficiency tends to be exaggerated in cows due to the demands of pregnancy and lactation. Fertility may be severely reduced. Hypophosphataemia is accompanied by normal blood levels of calcium. The condition must be distinguished from DJD.

Vitamin D-deficient osteomalacia in grazing animals is seen in temperate climates with a shortage of sun-cured hay and affects cattle stressed by the demands of pregnancy and lactation. The clinical manifestation resembles the phosphorus-deficient form.

Treatment and prevention

In rickets, increased vitamin D in the ration coupled with restoration of a normal Ca : P ratio with adequate intake brings a rapid response.

Osteomalacia in adult cattle is treated by dietary supplementation with rations high in phosphorus.

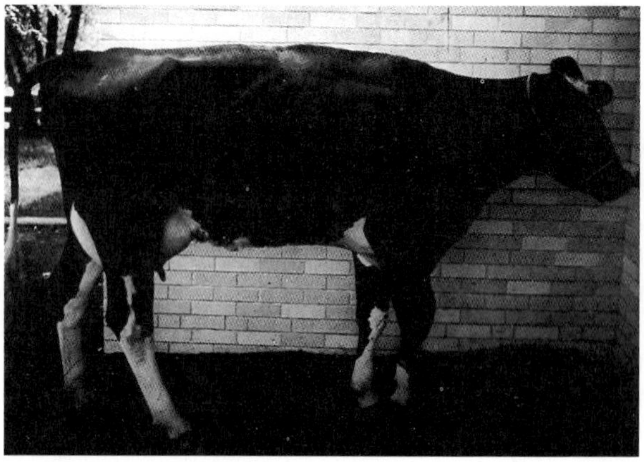

Fig. 29.18 Distal right radial septic physitis in two-year-old Holstein heifer. Weight bearing is minimal due to severe pain and soft tissue swelling. The aetiology, in the absence of penetration, was probably haematogenous.

Osteomyelitis

Aetiology and pathogenesis

Osteomyelitis of the limb bones in cattle occurs in two forms, one in growing cattle, the other in adults.

A haematogenous form is seen in calves six to twelve months old as a result of *Salmonella* infection, which localizes in the metaphysis, physis and epiphysis of long bones such as the metacarpus (Kersjes *et al.*, 1966; Gitter *et al.*, 1978). Blood flow through the metaphyseal sinusoids is slow, facilitating easy bacterial deposition and proliferation. Many clinical cases are multifocal and cause rapid destruction of bone. Other organisms in calves include *A. pyogenes* and *E. coli*. In older, growing cattle, less than two years old, a growth plate osteomyelitis may involve the distal metatarsus or distal tibia. Common bacterial isolates are *A. pyogenes* and *Salmonella* spp. (De Kesel *et al.*, 1982). Periarticular soft tissue swelling is prominent (Fig. 29.18). The radiographic extent of bone destruction is very variable and appears to be unrelated to the involvement of epiphysis and metaphysis, which are equally likely to be affected. Many cases have infected sequestra in the osteomyelitic focus.

In adult cattle, osteomyelitis of long bones is a sporadic isolated phenomenon. The aetiology may again involve haematogenous spread, or may arise following direct trauma. Open long bone fractures are an obvious example (see p. 370). Less obviously, saucer fractures of the diaphysis may lead to formation of a sequestrum. Sequestra in long bones of cattle are related to common sites of lacerating wounds, notably the proximal half of the dorsal aspect of the metatarsus (Firth, 1987). This author hypothesizes that severe contusion alone may produce sufficient subcutaneous soft tissue damage to render the area susceptible to infection and subsequent adjacent bone sequestration.

A specific form of osteomyelitis is Brodie's abscess, which is a circumscribed abscess lined with a granular membrane surrounded by sclerotic bone (Weaver, 1972). Synonyms are chronic fibrous osteomyelitis and chronic bone abscess. Though the lining is histologically a definite pyogenic membrane, bacteriological culture may be sterile. Both *F. necrophorum* and *A. pyogenes* have been involved in cases of Brodie's abscess in three and six-months-old calves (Weaver, 1972).

Clinical signs and diagnosis

Osteomyelitis usually causes severe, continuing pain with local swelling. These signs relate to the active process such as long bone infection following an open fracture when, if left untreated, purulent material, sometimes with bone spicules, is discharged to the exterior. Cellulitis may be severe and additional sinuses may form.

Osteomyelitis in calves where infection is in and surrounding the epiphysis presents differently. Localization of the lameness may be difficult due to the absence of local swelling. Local pain is usually evident.

Chronic osteomyelitis may not cause lameness when the infected focus is effectively walled off by dense sclerosed bone (involucrum). Sometimes, in such cases, lameness suddenly develops as infection flares up once more.

Osteomyelitis rarely extends to involve joints except in the digit and any resentment to joint flexion is usually due to extension from the diaphyseal or metaphyseal focus.

Systemic effects of osteomyelitis include lassitude, mild fever and a reduced appetite. Radiology is indicated in most cases to confirm the diagnosis, to determine the extent of the pathological process, and to assess the possibility of useful surgical intervention. Osteoporosis results from the loss of bone by erosion and its replacement by infected granulation tissue. Periosteal new bone is often evident and is variable in amount. Initially, the periosteum is elevated over an osteomyelitic focus with an underlying loss of cortical density. Later, in animals where a sequestrum forms, new subperiosteal bone is deposited while sclerosis is evident around the sequestrum.

Differential diagnosis of osteomyelitis with an open wound involves determining the primary lesion. Some cases of wounds may not involve the periosteum and lameness may reflect pain due to subcutaneous abscessation, septic myositis or extensive intramuscular abscessation. Open wounds should, therefore, be explored with a sterile probe.

Osteomyelitis of long bones without evidence of skin trauma must be differentiated from fissure fractures, subperiosteal haematoma, subcutaneous abscesses and rare bone tumours. In calves, haematogenous bacterial infection of metaphysis, growth plate and epiphysis must be distinguished from joint ill, epiphyseal separation and metaphyseal fractures.

Treatment and prognosis

Cattle with systemic involvement (pyrexia, anorexia) should be given parenteral antibiotics for three to five days. Many cases respond to this therapy. Non-responsive cases should be considered for surgery. This applies particularly to cases of Brodie's abscess and incision should be made over the metaphysis to attempt aspiration of the contents of the abscess if subperiosteal in position. In other cases a sinus tract through the cortex may be enlarged to evacuate the contents and to permit curettage of the adjacent necrotic bone and pyogenic membrane.

Cattle with open long bone fractures and osteomyelitis should have sequestra removed and check radiographic films taken. Treatment then depends on the type of fracture and extent of osteomyelitis. The options are discussed elsewhere (p. 371).

Calves with bacterial infection of the metaphysis sometimes respond to parenteral antibiotics alone, otherwise local debridement and irrigation of the focus is justified.

Physeal dysplasia

Aetiology and pathology

Physeal dysplasia, also loosely termed epiphysitis (though the epiphysis is not involved in an inflammatory process), is primarily a defective development of one or more growth plates, which later may become necrotic and inflammatory and later may still be purulent. The problem usually affects the lower limb, especially the carpal and fetlock joints. The pathogenesis apparently involves a reduced blood supply to the growth plate as a result of uneven or excessive mechanical pressure. The metaphyseal side, dependent on an adequate blood supply for calcification and ossification, is more affected than the epiphyseal surface. The pathological process has not been thoroughly investigated in cattle, but necrosis of the ground substance, resulting from folding of the cell columns and loss of continuity, has been noted histologically in housed fattening cattle. Poor-quality, uncomfortable floor surfaces predispose rapidly fattening cattle with limited exercise space to physeal dysplasia.

Gross pathology reveals some subcutaneous oedema and red or red–grey discoloration around the growth plate, which is either necrotic or, in severe cases, purulent. In its most severe form the growth plate undergoes separation.

Copper deficiency or a combined copper–molybdenum deficiency (see pp. 218, 263) has also been associated with physeal dysplasia as a result of defective collagen formation. The abnormal collagen does not permit normal mineralization. The result is stiffness and lameness in calves with a characteristic distal metatarsal swelling. Another result is an increased incidence of long bone fractures.

Clinical signs and diagnosis

The swellings are usually symmetrical, and hindlimbs are affected more often. The enlarged area in the lame calf or yearling is painful. Weight loss is rapid in beef cattle aged nine to eighteen months. Occasionally, several animals in a group of cattle are affected simultaneously following violent exercise, for example at turning out to pasture from confined housing. Isolated cases may result from trauma on slats.

In the copper-related form the limbs may be bowed either laterally or medially, the gait is stilted, and the swellings tend to be symmetrical. However, other signs of copper deficiency are present, including unthriftiness, a rough discoloured hair coat and diarrhoea.

Radiographic features include rarefying lesions with an increased width of the growth plate with irregularity and fragmentation, but with an absence of reactive change around the metaphyseal margin. The radiographic changes are more severe in cattle with physeal separation and secondary repair. Milder radiographic changes are evident in many cattle of the same group that do not show lameness.

The list of differential diagnoses includes rickets, traumatic separation of the growth plate, bacterial ostitis, septic arthritis and fractures. Radiography is necessary to permit this differentiation.

Treatment and prevention

Only the copper-related syndrome is responsive to treatment by an appropriate diet change. Mild non-copper-related cases respond to rest and external support by lightweight casting. Most cases of such lameness should be salvaged before there is further weight loss.

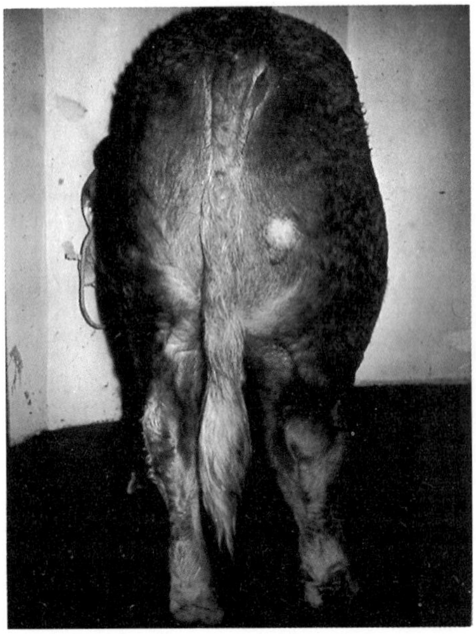

Fig. 29.19 Massive septic myositis in right hindquarters of two-year-old Saler bull. The light area (shaved) shows the site of exploratory needle puncture. Abscess cavity contained 12 l of pus. *Actinomyces pyogenes* was recovered in pure culture. Severe oedema extends down to the hock. Recovery followed drainage and irrigation.

Lameness of iatrogenic origin

Some forms of upper limb lameness may be the result of treatment for disease or injury. Various entities have been discussed elsewhere: radial paralysis from prolonged lateral recumbency during anaesthesia (p. 365), neonatal long bone fractures and physeal separations resulting from excessive traction in dystokia (p. 372), and traumatic injury and transection of the gastrocnemius tendon (p. 380). Another form of iatrogenic damage is that following intramuscular injections. Occasionally, particularly in calves, the sciatic nerve may be injured. More frequent is the development of an abscess following a subcutaneous injection, which rarely causes lameness and remains a cosmetic blemish. When a non-sterile preparation, or a dirty syringe and needle are used for an intramuscular injection, the results may be more serious. As a rule, infection is sealed off by fibrous tissue with no ill-effects. Sometimes the result is a massive abscess, which causes lameness and requires prompt surgical drainage and daily irrigation to prevent recurrence (Fig. 29.19).

References

Boyd, J.S. & Weaver, A.D. (1967) Spastic paresis in cattle. *Veterinary Record*, **80**, 529–30.

Bracewell, C.D. & Corbell, J. (1979) An association between arthritis and persistent serological reactions to *Brucella abortus* in cattle from apparently brucellosis-free herds. *Veterinary Record*, **106**, 99–101.

Buchthal, F., Rosenfalk, A. & Behse, F. (1984) Sensory potential of normal and diseased nerves. In *Peripheral Neuropathy* (ed. by P.J. Dyck), p. 995. W.B. Saunders, Philadelphia.

Chamberlain, A.T. (1986) Prognostic indicators in the downer cow. In *Proceedings of the British Cattle Veterinary Association*, pp. 57–68.

Chamberlain, A.T. (1987) The management and prevention of the downer cow syndrome. In *Proceedings of the British Cattle Veterinary Association*, 20–30.

Cox, V.S. (1981) Understanding the downer cow syndrome. *Compendium of Continuing Education for the Practicing Veterinarian*, **3**, 47–53.

Cox, V.S. (1982) Pathogenesis of the downer cow syndrome. *Veterinary Record*, **11**, 76–9.

Cox, V.S. (1988) Nonsystemic causes of the downer cow syndrome. *Veterinary Clinics of North America. Food Animal Practice*, **4**, 413–33.

Cox, V.S. & Onapito, J.S. (1986) An update on the downer cow syndrome. *Bovine Practice*, **21**, 195–9.

Cox, V.S., Marsh, W.E., Steuernagel, G.R. *et al.* (1982) Downer cow occurrence in Minnesota dairy herds. *Prev. Vet. Med.* **4**, 249–55.

De Kessel, A., Verschooten, F., De Moor, A., Steenhaut, M. & Wouters, L. (1982) Bacteriele Osteitis–Osteomyelitis ter Hoogte van Groeiplaten bij het Rund. *Vlaams Diergeneesk. Tijdschr.*, **51**, 397–422.

De Ley, G. & De Moor, A. (1975) Bovine spastic paresis: cerebrospinal fluid concentrations of homovanillic acid and 5-hydroxyindolacetic acid in normal and spastic calves. *American Journal of Veterinary Research*, **36**, 227–8.

De Ley, G. & De Moor, A. (1977) Bovine spastic paresis: results of selective desafferation of the gastrocnemius muscle by means of spinal dorsal root resection. *American Journal of Veterinary Research*, **38**, 1899–1900.

Ducharme, N.G., Stanton, M.E. & Ducharme, G.R. (1985) Stifle lameness in cattle at two veterinary teaching hospitals (42 cases). *Canadian Veterinary Journal*, **26**, 212–17.

Ferguson, J.G. (1982) Management and repair of bovine fractures. *Compendium of Continuing Education for the Practicing Veterinarian*, **4**, S128–S136.

Ferguson, J.G. (1985) Principles and application of internal fixation in cattle. *Veterinary Clinics of North America. Food Animal Practice*, **1**, 139–52.

Ferguson, J.G. (1985) Special considerations in bovine orthopedics and lameness. *Veterinary Clinics of North America. Food Animal Practice*, **1**, 131–8.

Firth, E.C. (1987) Bone sequestration in horses and cattle. *Australian Veterinary Journal*, **64**, 65–9.

Gitter, M., Gray, C., Richardson, C. & Pepper, R.T. (1978) Chronic salmonella infection in calves. *British Veterinary Journal*, **134**, 113–21.

Greenough, P.R., MacCallum, F.J. & Weaver, A.D. (1981) *Lameness in Cattle*, 2nd edn. Wright Scientechnica, Bristol 1–41.

Kendrick, J.W. & Sittmann, K. (1966) Inherited osteoarthritis of dairy cattle. *Journal of the American Veterinary Medical Association*, **149**, 17–21.

Kersjes, A.W., Frik, Y.F. & Van de Watering, C.G. (1966) Bacteriele osteitis bij rundereen. *Tijd. Diergeneesk.*, **91**, 1537–47.

Madison, J.B., Tulleners, E.P., Ducharme, N.G. *et al.* (1989) Idiopathic gonitis in heifers: 34 cases (1976–1986). *Journal of the American Veterinary Medical Association*, **194**, 273–7.

Pavaux, C., Sautet, J. & Lignereux, J.Y. (1985) Anatomie du muscle gastrocnemien des bovins appliquée à la cure chirurgicale de la paresie spastique. *Vlaams Diergeneesk. Tijdschr.*, **54**, 296–312.

Schuh, J.C.L. & Killeen, J.R. (1988) A retrospective study of dystocia-related vertebral fractures in neonatal calves. *Canadian Veterinary Journal*, **29**, 830–3.

Tulleners, E.P. (1986) Metacarpal and metatarsal fractures in dairy cattle: 33 cases (1979–1985). *Journal of the American Veterinary Medical Association*, **189**, 463–8.

Tulleners, E.P., Nunamaker, D.M. & Richardson, D.W. (1987) Coxofemoral luxations in cattle: 22 cases (1980–1985). *Journal of the American Veterinary Medical Association*, **191**, 569–74.

Vaughan, L.C. (1964) Peripheral nerve injuries: an experimental study in cattle. *Veterinary Record*, **76**, 1293–1301.

Weaver, A.D. (1972) Chronic localised osteomyelitis of the bovine limb. *British Veterinary Journal*, **128**, 470–6.

Weaver, A.D. (1977) An investigation into condemnations for hind limb disease in slaughtered cattle with particular reference to the stifle and hip joints. *Veterinary Record*, **100**, 172–5.

Weaver, A.D. & Campbell, J.R. (1972) Surgical correction of medial and lateral patellar luxation in calves. *Veterinary Record*, **90**, 567–9.

Wells, G.A.H., Hawkins, S.A.C., O'Toole, D.T. *et al.* (1987) Spastic syndrome in a Holstein bull: a histologic study. *Veterinary Pathology*, **24**, 345–53.

Wintzer, H.J. (1961) A possible method of treating long bone fractures in cattle. *Dtsch. Tierarztl. Wschr.*, **68**, 226–8.

Wyn-Jones, G., Baker, J.R. & Johnson, P.M. (1980) A clinical and immunopathological study of *Brucella abortus* strain 19-induced arthritis in cattle. *Veterinary Record*, **107**, 5–9.

Fertility

Chapter 30: Reproductive Physiology in Cattle

by P.J. HARTIGAN

Introduction

Reproductive efficiency in a cattle enterprise is a function of good management. Therefore, it is important that the help and advice provided to management by the veterinarian should be based upon a sound appreciation of the physiological mechanisms that control the principal reproductive events.

The essential numerical data on reproduction in cattle are well known: puberty in bulls and heifers at 10–15 months of age; normal oestrous cycles of 18–24 days (mean = 21 days); normal oestrus lasts 12–24 hours (mean = 18 hours); ovulation occurs about 24 hours after the LH peak at the beginning of oestrus; normal gestation lasts 278–293 days (mean = 280 days); the interval from parturition to first ovulation can be as short as 15 days. The physiological control of each of these events is exerted by a system of interdependent endocrine organs that form the hypothalamic–pituitary–gonadal axis, an important limb of the neuroendocrine system.

The primary purpose of this Chapter is to provide a succinct outline of the salient features of the neuroendocrine system as it affects reproduction. Why is it considered necessary to do this in a text addressed primarily to clinicians? Essentially, because we believe that it will enhance the reader's understanding of the pathogenesis of many of the reproductive problems encountered in practice and, as a consequence, it will foster a more methodical and perceptive approach to diagnosis and treatment. Underpinning that belief is the knowledge that efficient reproductive performance in the female is dependent on an integrated and precisely-timed sequence of hormonal changes that are regulated by the hypothalamus in response to changes in the external and internal environments. Of course, this means that the sequence and timing of the hormonal changes are vulnerable to a great variety of stresses and noxious agents. Many of these deleterious factors have been recognized — and will be mentioned later in the relevant sections — but it is likely that many more remain to be discovered, in particular subtle but significant stresses associated with modern developments in cattle husbandry. The individual best placed to identify 'new causes' of reproductive inefficiency is the informed clinician working with problem herds; however, such insights are less likely if the investigator is not fully alert to the central role of the neuroendocrine mechanisms and their sensitivity to the effects of dietary and metabolic factors, hormone imbalances, stressors, drugs, age, and many other influences.

The hypothalamus

In the neuroendocrine system the dominant role is played by the hypothalamus, which acts as a relay station where neural and hormonal messages are decoded and translated into appropriate signals to ensure

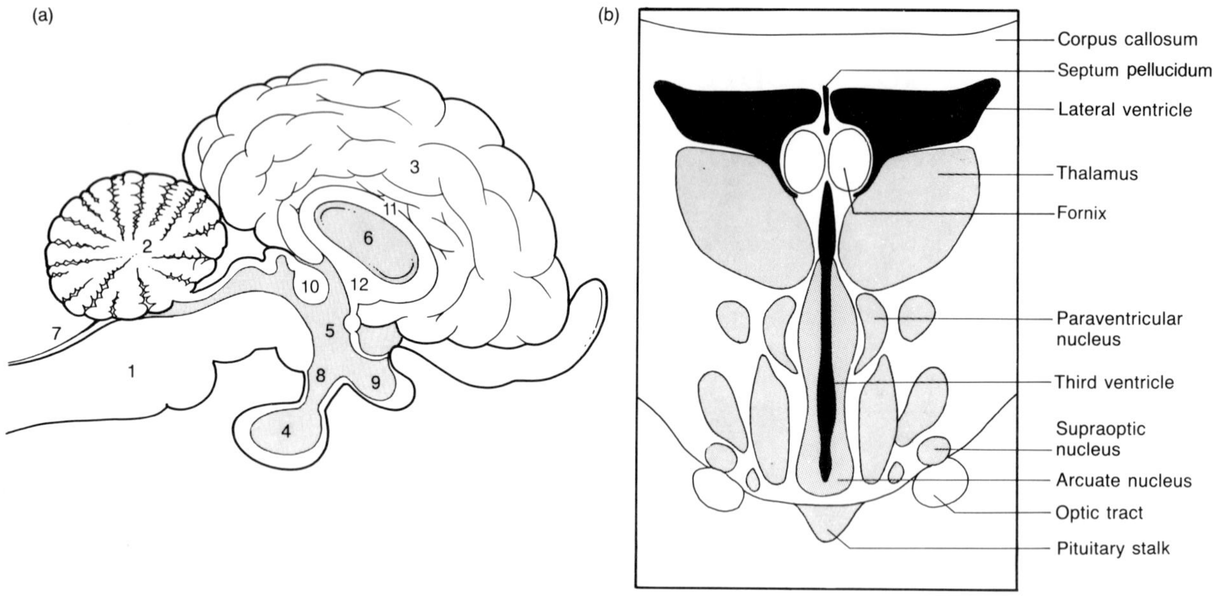

Fig. 30.1 Diagrams of bovine brain. (a) Saggital section. (b) Frontal view through hypothalamus and pituitary stalk along the plane shown in (a). 1, Medulla oblongata; 2, cerebellum, 3, cerebrum; 4, pituitary gland; 5, third ventricle; 6, septum pellucidum; 7, fourth ventricle; 8, hypothalamus (forming lateral wall of third ventricle); 9, optic nerve; 10, thalamus; 11, corpus callosum; 12, fornix.

the cooperation of the endocrine system with the nervous system in regulatory activities (Fig. 30.1). It is able to do so because it contains many neurones that are capable of forming and releasing peptide hormones (neurohormones) that regulate the functions of various organs, principally via the pituitary gland.

These regulatory peptides are synthesized and packaged into granules in the cell body of the neurone before they are transported down the axon to the nerve terminals where they are stored pending release. The peptidergic neurones retain the electrophysiological properties of nervous tissue and they use their electrical activity to release the peptides.

A typical peptidergic neurone (Fig. 30.2) has many hundreds of synapses and through these it receives neural inputs (information) from most parts of the brain. (It also receives information from humoral inputs; we shall return to this topic later). The neural and humoral inputs may be stimulatory or inhibitory; at any one moment the response of the peptidergic neurone will reflect its assessment of the current interplay between the synergistic and conflicting stimuli. When the stimulatory inputs exceed a critical threshold an action potential is generated, the nerve impulse passes down the axon and it causes the release of the (stored) peptide at the nerve terminals. Usually, the nerve terminals are in close apposition to capillaries with highly fenestrated walls that allow the peptide molecules to enter the vascular circulation promptly on release.

The most appropriate example to illustrate the physiological phenomena just described is the milk ejection reflex (Fig. 30.3). This reflex depends on a suckling-induced release of oxytocin. Oxytocin is produced by peptidergic neurones whose cell bodies are located (principally) in the paired paraventricular nuclei in the hypothalamus and whose axons pass through the pituitary stalk into the posterior pituitary gland. Suckling evokes sensory impulses that travel via the spinal cord to the brain where they converge on the paraventricular nuclei and generate the impulses in the peptidergic neurones that lead to the release of oxytocin from the nerve endings in the posterior pituitary gland. The reflex is completed when the oxytocin in the blood perfusing the mammary gland induces 'let down' of milk. Conceptually, this is neuroendocrine regulation at its simplest: the neurone that 'reads' the afferent sensory message also produces and releases the effector hormone. This is possible only because the posterior pituitary gland, which arises as a downgrowth of neural tissue from the floor of the third ventricle, retains a direct neural link with the hypothalamus.

The anterior pituitary gland

The anterior pituitary gland (adenohypophysis) arises as an upgrowth from the roof of the primitive mouth

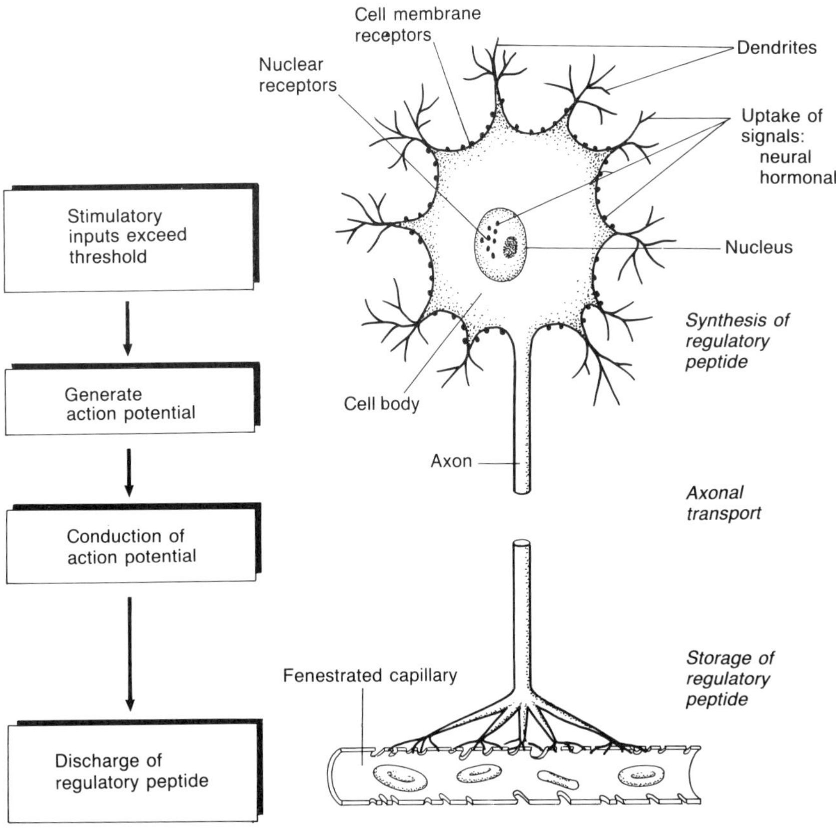

Fig. 30.2 This diagrammatic representation of a typical peptidergic neurone depicts: (i) the uptake of neural signals by dendrites; (ii) the uptake of endocrine signals by specific receptors located either in the cell membrane (for large and water-soluble hormones) or in the nucleus (for lipid-soluble hormones); (iii) the endocrine response to signals (synthesis, transport and storage of regulatory peptide); (iv) the neural response to signals (generation and conduction of action potential, which is responsible for the discharge of the regulatory peptide).

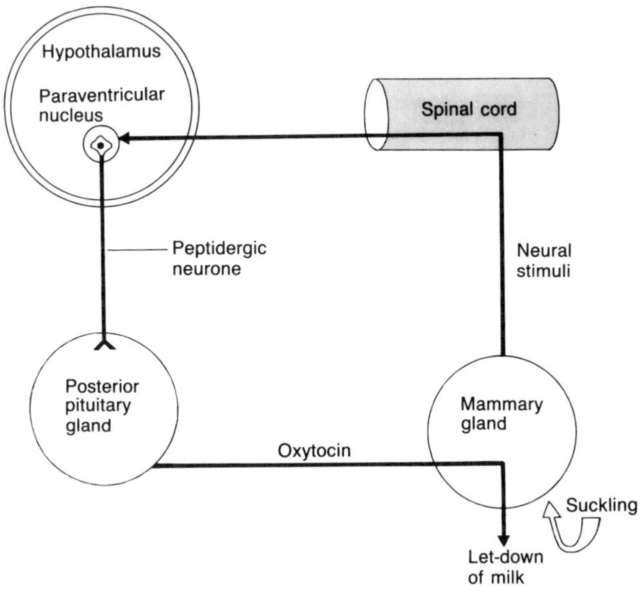

Fig. 30.3 Diagrammatic representation of the suckling reflex, in which neural stimuli elicit an endocrine response.

and, therefore, it does not have a direct neural link with the hypothalamus. A vascular route has to be used to bring the regulatory peptides from the hypothalamus to the adenohypophysis. A specialized arrangement of the vasculature, the hypothalmo-hypophyseal portal system, has evolved for that purpose. In contrast to the normal sequence of arterioles, capillaries and venules, a portal system begins and ends with capillaries. In this instance, the superior hypophyseal artery gives rise to a plexus of capillaries (the primary plexus) in the region of the median eminence at the top of the pituitary stalk. From this the blood is drained by the hypophyseal portal veins, which pass down the pituitary stalk to end in a secondary plexus (the sinusoidal capillaries) within the anterior pituitary gland (Fig. 30.4). From there the blood returns to the general circulation via the anterior hypophyseal vein.

In contrast to the posterior pituitary gland, which does not produce the hormones it releases, the anterior lobe actually synthesizes the trophic hormones it releases into the circulation, including the gonadotrophins: follicle stimulating hormone (FSH) and lu-

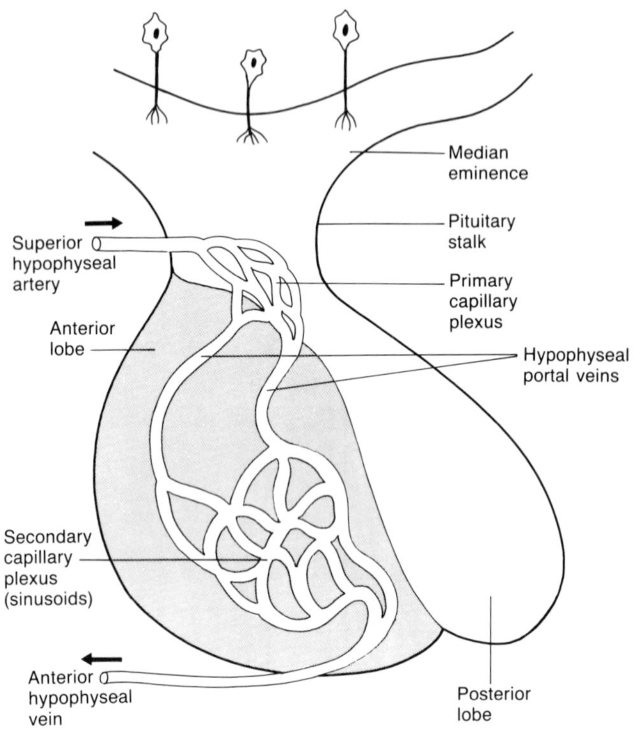

Fig. 30.4 The primary capillary plexus, the hypophyseal portal veins, and the secondary capillary plexus form the hypothalamo–hypohyseal portal system that intervenes between the superior hypophyseal artery and the anterior hypophyseal vein. This is the route taken by GnRH which is synthesized by neurones whose cell bodies lie within the arcuate nucleus of the hypothalamus and whose axons ab onto the external walls of the capillaries in the primary plexus.

teinizing hormone (LH). However, the release of the trophic hormones is governed by stimulatory or inhibitory peptides produced in the hypothalamus. For instance, the secretion of FSH and LH is controlled by a gonadotrophin-releasing hormone (GnRH), which is synthesized by peptidergic neurones in the hypothalamus and is brought to the anterior pituitary gland via the hypothalamo-hypophyseal portal system. The axons of the neurones that produce GnRH end in the median eminence, in close apposition to the fenestrated capillaries of the primary plexus. When a nerve impulse induces a discharge of GnRH from the nerve terminals, this hypothalamic factor is transported via the primary plexus, the hypophyseal portal veins and the secondary plexus to the secretory cells of the anterior lobe. It stimulates the release of the gonadotrophins, which enter the general circulation via the draining anterior hypophyseal vein. Other hypothalamic factors may exert inhibitory actions in the anterior pituitary gland, e.g. prolactin inhibitory factor.

Neuroendocrine links

Since the peptidergic neurones form the functional links between the neural and endocrine systems, they need to be able to receive, decipher and react to signals generated by either system in response to changes in the internal and external environments. Neural signals from other regions of the brain converge on the hypothalamus bringing important cues from the special senses (sight, sound, smell), various exteroceptors (suckling, mating, pain), interoceptors (stimulation of the cervix and uterus) and stress (physical, emotional, overcrowding). The peptidergic neurones also respond to humoral signals, especially to hormones acting through feedback loops. Again, the input may be stimulatory (positive feedback) or inhibitory (negative feedback). Although there are some important positive feedbacks, e.g. oestrogen prior to ovulation, the majority of feedback loops are negative.

Feedback

In its simplest form a negative feedback loop (Fig. 30.5a) is a closed system in which hormone A stimulates the production and release of hormone B which, in turn, has an inhibitory effect on the cells that produce hormone A. Such a loop provides a very efficient mechanism by which circulating hormones are maintained within stable normal limits while retaining their responsiveness to the immediate needs of the body. For instance, when the concentration of hormone B in the circulation rises towards its upper normal limit it exerts negative feedback on its trophic hormone. Thus, hormone A is prevented from exceeding its upper normal limit; the concentration of A in the circulation declines and, of course, so does the activity of its target cells. The resultant decline in hormone B attenuates the negative feedback inhibition (Fig. 30.5b) and the secretion of hormone A is enhanced before it falls below its lower normal limit.

In a positive feedback loop (Fig. 30.6a) hormone B stimulates rather than inhibits the production of more hormone A. This is an inherently unstable system in that it is liable to generate ever-increasing quantities of each of the hormones (Fig. 30.6b); in other words, it lacks the checks and balances of a negative feedback system. However, it is ideal for situations that call for short-term but self-limiting responses. The positive feedback loop may be a purely hormonal phenomenon; for example, the brief but highly significant period of positive feedback by oestrogen that elicits the pre-ovulatory surge of LH. Other important positive feedback mechanisms are initiated by neural stimuli from

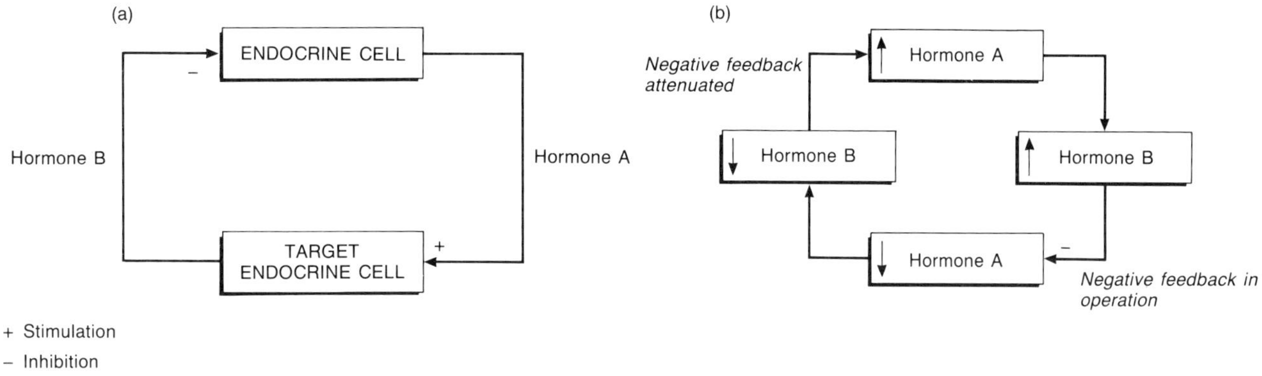

Fig. 30.5 Negative feedback. Example: hormone A, FSH; hormone B, oestrogen. (a) FSH stimulates the production of oestrogen by the granulosa cells of the ovarian follicle; (b) the oestrogen exerts an inhibitory effect on the release of FSH by the pituitary gland.

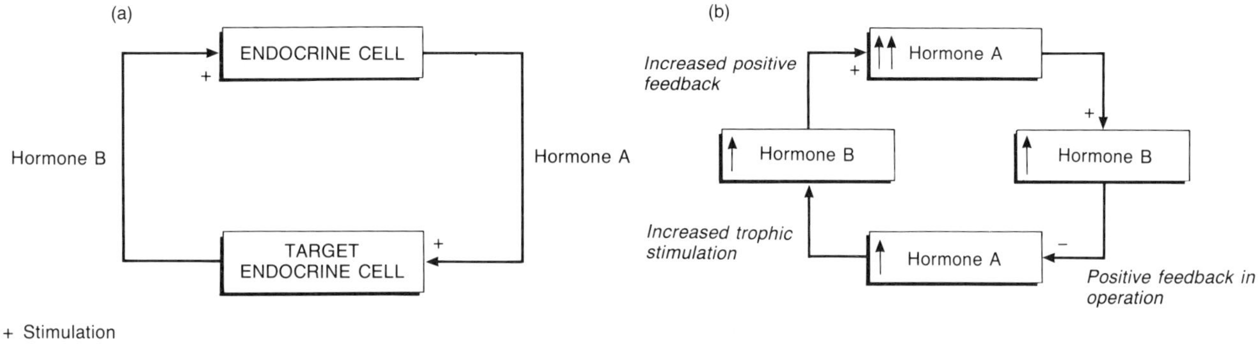

Fig. 30.6 Positive feedback. Example: the gonadotrophins FSH and LH (hormone A) stimulate the secretion of oestrogen (hormone B) by the granulosa cells of the preovulatory ovarian follicle (see Fig. 30.24). The rapidly rising concentration of oestrogen (the 'oestrogen surge') stimulates the hypothalamus and the pituitary gland to release a surge of gonadotrophins that is responsible for ovulation.

exteroceptors, e.g. the suckling reflex, or interoceptors, e.g. stretch receptors in the cervix and vagina during the second stage of parturition, that induce reflex release of oxytocin. These two reflexes are excellent examples of self-limiting responses; removal of the physical stimulus terminates the reflex response almost at once.

The feedback mechanisms involved in the control of the reproductive tract are complex and involve several sets of secretory cells in series (Fig. 30.7). For descriptive purposes, three types of complex feedback loops are recognized:

1 Long loop: for example, gonadal hormones acting at the level of the brain or pituitary gland (Fig. 30.8).
2 Short loop: for example, pituitary gonadotrophins acting at the level of the hypothalamus (Fig. 30.9).
3 Ultra-short loop: hypothalamic peptides acting at the level of the hypothalamus (Fig. 30.10).

The feedback effect of a particular hormone is not an intrinsic property of the molecule itself; for instance, although oestrogen is inhibitory (negative long loop feedback) during most of the oestrous cycle it exercises an essential stimulatory effect (positive long loop feedback) shortly before ovulation. Clearly, a single hormone can vary the message it conveys to the hypothalamus. This raises a crucial question: how do the gonadal steroids, the pituitary gonadotrophins and the hypothalamic peptides encode the signals that constitute the feedback messages? By definition, feedback depends on the ability of the target tissues to detect changes in hormone concentrations in the circulation, and to induce the appropriate re-adjustments (further changes). Hence, the system depends on fluxes rather than constancy as the means of communication.

Endocrine signals: generation and reception

Two basic types of endocrine signals are used: pulses and surges (Fig. 30.11). A *pulse* of a particular hormone is a discrete burst of secretion of relatively short duration and modest amplitude. A *surge* occurs when a sequence of frequent pulses, often of high amplitude, produces a massive increase extending over a period of 12–24 hours. The precise message read by the target

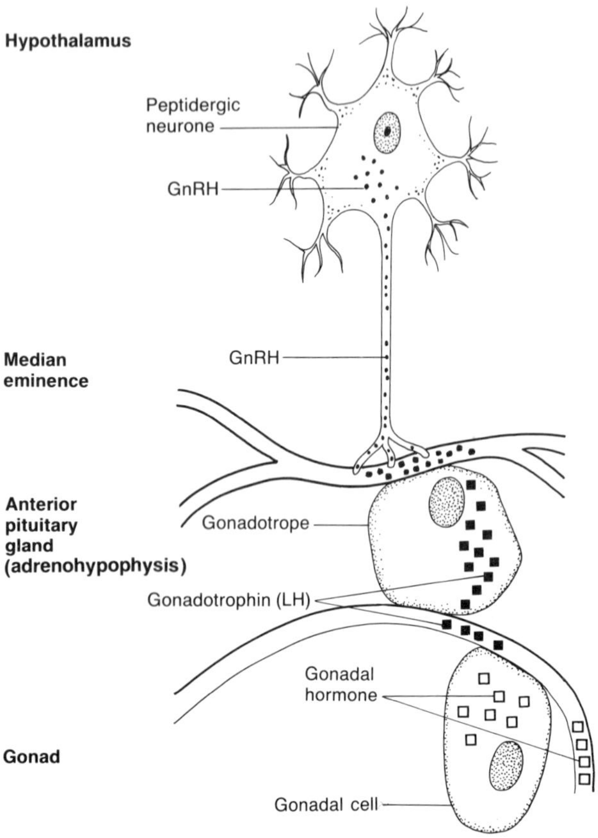

Fig. 30.7 Secretory cells in series: peptidergic neurone secretes GnRH; gonadotrope secretes LH, FSH; gonadal cell secretes testosterone, progesterone or oestrogen.

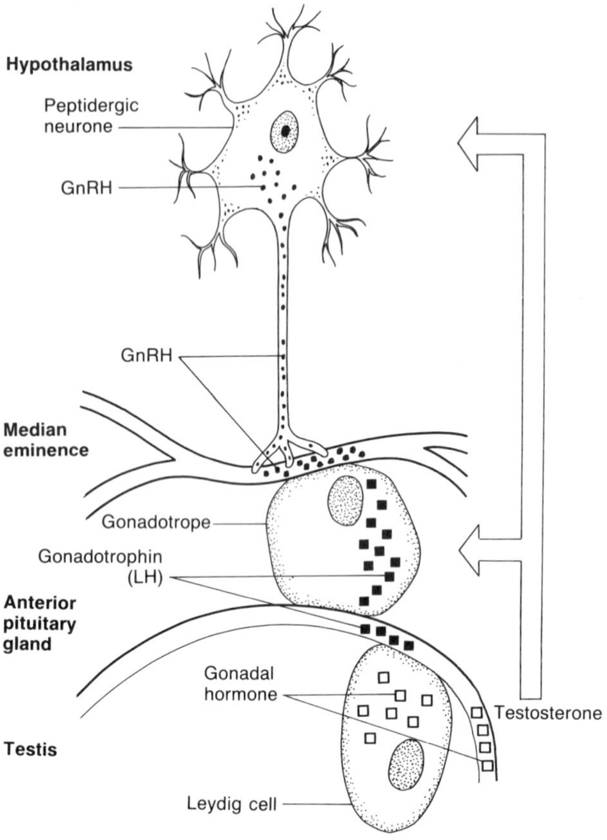

Fig. 30.8 Long loop negative feedback. LH induces Leydig cells to secrete testosterone; testosterone exerts so-called long loop feedback (i) on adenohypophysis (suppressing secretion of LH) and (ii) on hypothalamus (suppressing secretion of GnRH).

tissue depends on the characteristics of the signals: their amplitude, duration, frequency and form.

Endocrine signals are detected only by cells that have specific receptors to which a particular hormone will bind. The receptors may be located in the cell membrane or within the cell, mainly in the nucleus (see Figs. 30.2 and 30.12). The polypeptide hormones, e.g. GnRH, and the glycoprotein hormones, e.g. LH, FSH, bind to receptors in the cell membrane (Fig. 30.12a), whereas the lipid-soluble gonadal steroids can diffuse through the cell membrane to react with intracellular receptors (Fig. 30.12b). The location of the specific receptors determines the mechanism by which the target cells express their characteristic responses to a hormone and, in turn, the different mechanisms determine the speed at which the final response is elicited. When a gonadal hormone binds to its specific receptor in the nucleus of a target cell, it initiates a series of biochemical reactions that takes several hours to produce the new proteins that elicit the characteristic response to that hormone (Fig. 30.12b). By contrast, when a gonadotrophin binds to its receptor in the cell membrane, it elicits the final response much more rapidly because the resultant cascade of enzymatic activity utilizes enzymes that exist already within the cell. Binding of the hormone (the 'first messenger') to the receptor activates an enzyme within the cell membrane that acts as a catalyst in a reaction that produces a 'second messenger', e.g. cyclic AMP, that, in turn, alters the activities of the enzymes that produce the final and characteristic response by the cell (Fig. 30.12a).

The sensitivity of a target tissue to a particular hormone will vary depending upon the number of specific receptors it has available for binding that hormone. At any time, the number of receptors depends on the balance between degradation and synthesis of receptors. A hormonal stimulus may increase the sensitivity of a target tissue by increasing the rate of synthesis of the specific receptors; a good example of this 'up regulation' is the increase in LH receptors induced in the granulosa cells of the preovulatory follicle by FSH (see p. 417). Alternatively, the hormone stimulus may de-

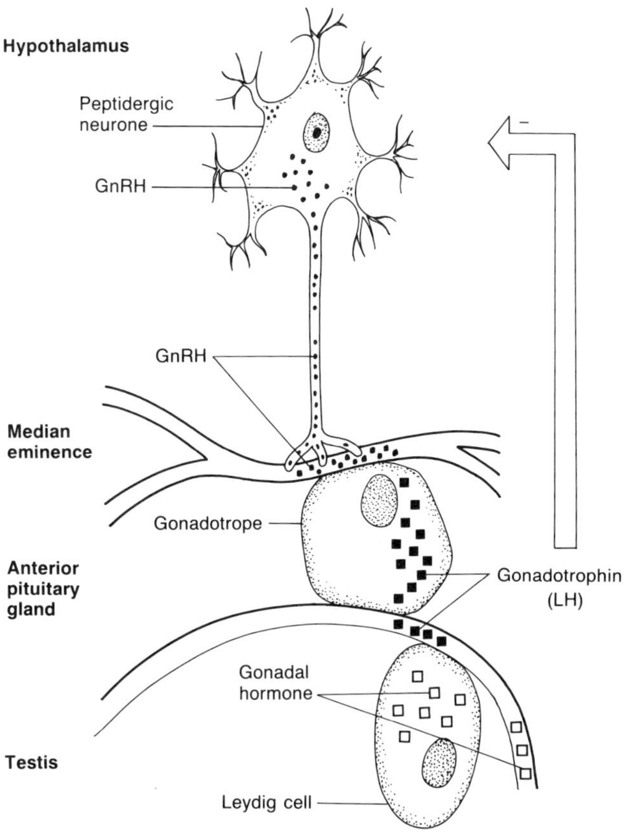

Fig. 30.9 Short loop negative feedback. GnRH induces the gonadotropes to secrete LH; LH exerts negative feedback on the release of GnRH by the hypothalamus.

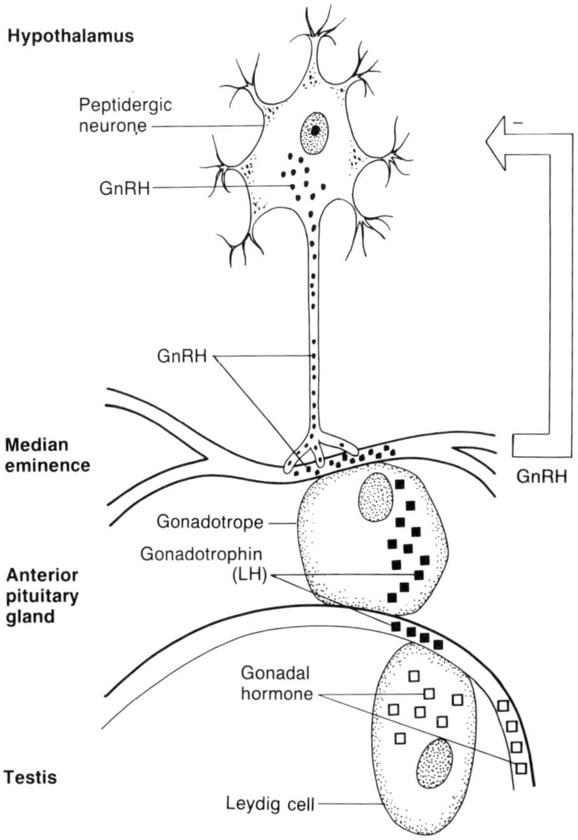

Fig. 30.10 Ultra-short loop negative feedback. The hypothalamic hormone (GnRH) regulates its own secretion.

crease the sensitivity of the target tissue because it increases the degradation and/or decreases the synthesis of receptors; for instance, GnRH can 'down regulate' its own receptors in the adenohypophysis, especially when the gonadotropes are subjected to constant stimulation rather than pulsatile stimulation by the releasing hormone (see p. 419).

The inherent mode of secretion of hormones in the neuroendocrine system is pulsatile and it is controlled by an oscillator or pulse generator in the hypothalamus. The activity of the pulse generator can be modulated both by neural inputs and by feedback signals from the median eminence, the pituitary gland and the gonads. In turn, the pulse generator will seek to ensure that the characteristics of the signals emanating from the pituitary gland and the gonads are altered so as to elicit the appropriate responses from target tissues in the reproductive tract. In that way the hypothalamus exercises fine tuning as well as gross control over reproductive events such as puberty, oestrus, gametogenesis, pregnancy, parturition and lactation.

Puberty

Puberty, the process by which animals become capable of producing offspring, is often given a very restricted definition. According to Short (1984), 'we generally refer to puberty as that moment at which the female first comes into oestrus and ovulates, or the male first produces spermatozoa in his ejaculate'. The trouble with this widely-held perception of puberty is that it concentrates exclusively on the apparent endpoint of a protracted and complex physiological process and suggests that puberty is a discrete event that can be assigned to a particular day (or moment!). There is the additional problem that the apparent end-point (first release of the gametes) is not necessarily conclusive evidence that the animal has now reached the stage at which it can reproduce itself; for instance, it is clear that many heifers may not be capable of doing so until well after first ovulation (see review by Moran *et al.*, 1989).

In fact, the onset of puberty is a gradual process

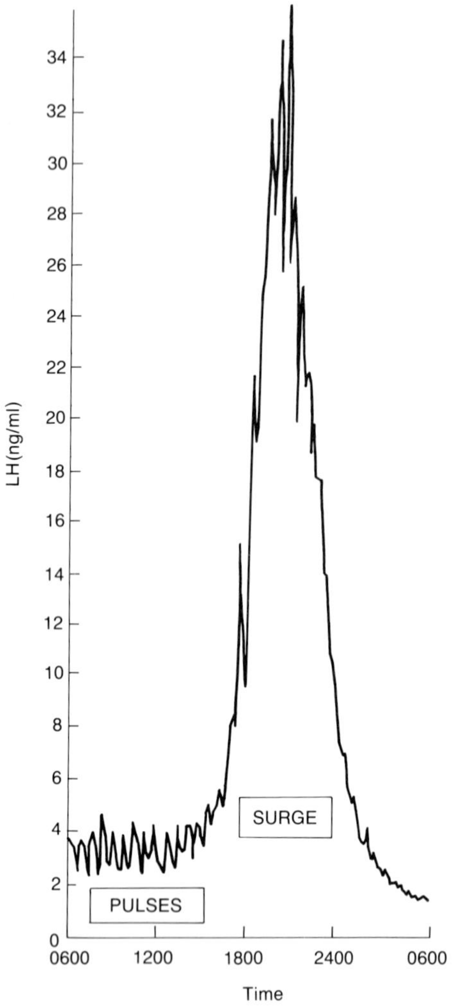

Fig. 30.11 Preovulatory surge of LH on day 18 of the oestrous cycle in a cow. Redrawn, with permission, from Rahe *et al.* (1980) *Endocrinology* **107**, 498–503.

that is in train for several months during which there are significant morphological, physiological and behavioural responses to the progressive expression of both the steroidogenic and gametogenic activities of the gonads. The essential feature of the process is the maturation of the brain–hypothalamic–pituitary–gonadal axis, which culminates in the adult pattern of reproductive activity. The components of the hypothalamic–pituitary–gonadal axis are present before birth and, even at that stage, each component is capable of responding to appropriate hormonal signals. During gestation, steroid hormones released from the placenta have an inhibitory effect on the fetal hypothalamus that suppresses the activities of the axis. After birth the axis becomes an independent regulatory system that secretes increased amounts of gonadotrophins and gonadal steroids. However, the system is restricted to a relatively low level of activity (juvenile level); for instance, in the female the level of activity is well below that required for ovulation or cyclic ovarian activity. The restraint is due partly to fine sensitivity of the GnRH pulse generator to negative feedback by gonadal steroids and partly to inhibitory inputs from the neural circuits that control the hypothalamus.

The transition to sexual maturity is brought about by progressive changes in the neuroendocrine activities of the axis in response to a variety of internal and environmental factors. The 'gonadostat' hypothesis postulates that the essential change during the transition to sexual maturity is a progressive decrease in sensitivity of the hypothalamus to the negative feedback effects of gonadal steroids (Fig. 30.13) so that the frequency of GnRH pulses is increased progressively. This leads to an increase in the sensitivity of the pituitary gonadotropes to GnRH and to an increase in the responsiveness of the gonads to the gonadotrophins (Fig. 30.14). Greater quantities of gonadotrophins are released from the pituitary gland and, in turn, greater quantities of steroids are released by the gonads. For instance, in the female the sensitivity of the hypothalamus to the negative feedback effect of oestrogen declines progressively and, as it does so, the increasing quantities of oestrogen from the ovaries can no longer hold the axis within the juvenile pattern of activity. There is a gradual movement of the regulatory system towards the adult pattern (Figs 30.13 and 30.14). Eventually, the ovaries produce a surge of oestrogen that exerts a positive feedback effect on the surge generator in the hypothalamus (Fig. 30.14) and this induces a surge of LH that leads to ovulation.

As our knowledge of these changes expands, there is increasing evidence that sexual maturity is regulated to a considerable extent by changing patterns of neural control over the hypothalamus. These alterations in intrinsic neural activity do not appear to be dependent on gonadal hormones; however, they play a crucial role in that they gradually release the GnRH pulse generator from the restraints exercised by the central nervous system during the juvenile period, thus enabling it to respond to the gonadal steroids in the adult manner. It is evident that the classical 'gonadostat' hypothesis does not furnish an entirely satisfactory explanation of the onset of puberty in all its details. Nevertheless, it does provide a conceptual framework that is adequate for the purposes of this text.

The first ovulation is likely to be silent; it appears that the hormonal requirements for the expression of oestrus are small quantities of progesterone from a

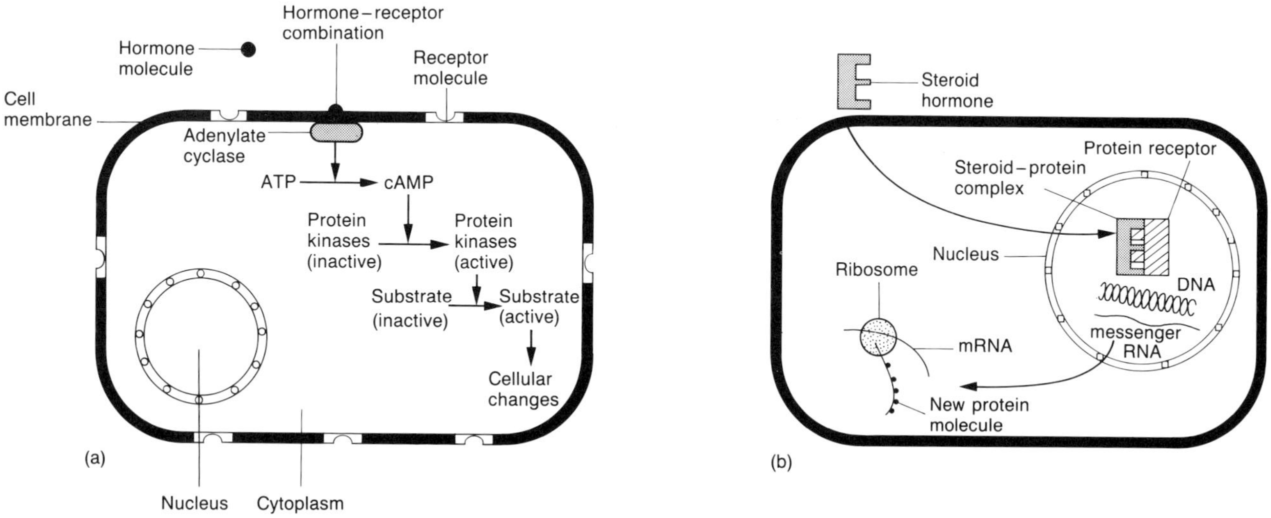

Fig. 30.12 Interaction of hormones with target cells. In (a) a glycoprotein ('the first messenger') binds with receptors in the cell membrane and activates adenylate cyclase in the membrane. Adenylate cyclase converts ATP to cyclic AMP ('the second messenger') which, in turn, activates various protein kinases. The resultant cascade of enzymatic activity produces the characteristic cell response to the endocrine signal. In (b) a steroid hormone enters the nucleus where it binds to its receptor. The receptor–hormone complex binds to a particular region of DNA and activates particular genes. The activated genes promote the synthesis of particular messenger RNA molecules that pass from the nucleus to the cytoplasm where they induce the synthesis of proteins (mainly enzymes) that are responsible for the characteristic actions of that hormone in that cell type.

regressing corpus luteum followed by a surge of oestrogen from the preovulatory follicle — a sequence that is absent at the time of first ovulation. Thus, the first oestrus observed by the stockperson indicates that the process of puberty is well advanced but it does not provide a precise date for the 'moment' of puberty.

The earliest possible maturation of the individual components of the reproductive axis (and, therefore, of the axis itself) is determined by genes, i.e. there are inherent breed variations in the onset of puberty. However, in all breeds this process is subject to delays caused by a variety of endogenous and exogenous influences, some of which can be manipulated by the stockperson to ensure that the heifer is ready for breeding at the desired time. The principal environmental factors that influence the onset of puberty are: season of birth, level of nutrition, growth rate, photoperiod, high ambient temperatures, intercurrent diseases, and presence of the male.

Specific reference to these factors will be made in the clinical segment of the text. For the moment, suffice it to say that, as a general guideline, the stockperson should devise a management strategy in the knowledge that the onset of puberty is a labile process that is conditioned by competition between the reproductive system and the other body systems of the growing animal for energy and specific nutrients. Reproduction, particularly in the female where it involves pregnancy followed by lactation, is an energy-consuming process to which Nature assigns a relatively low priority for the prepubertal animal. Evidence is accumulating from work on a number of species that inadequate intake of energy or nutrients can depress or abolish the activities of the GnRH pulse generator in the juvenile animal. This has been attributed, variously, to deficiencies in body weight, in rate of growth, in fat content or in fat : lean ratio. There is no agreement on the particular cue(s) that inhibit(s) the pulse generator but there is general acceptance of the thesis that the function of the generator is closely coupled with energy balance and that it is allowed to progress from the juvenile to the adult level of activity in the female only when the energetic status appears to be adequate to sustain pregnancy and lactation.

Selective culling is an integral part of efficient management of the dairy herd. It can be practised successfully only when the stockperson has available an adequate number of high-quality heifers due to calve down at the appropriate time. This requires careful management of the prepubertal animal to ensure that the reactivation of the hypothalamic pulse generator is not delayed unduly by environmental influences, principally nutritional factors and subclinical diseases.

Similarly, young bulls intended for breeding purposes require careful management during the juvenile period because the onset of puberty in the male is also

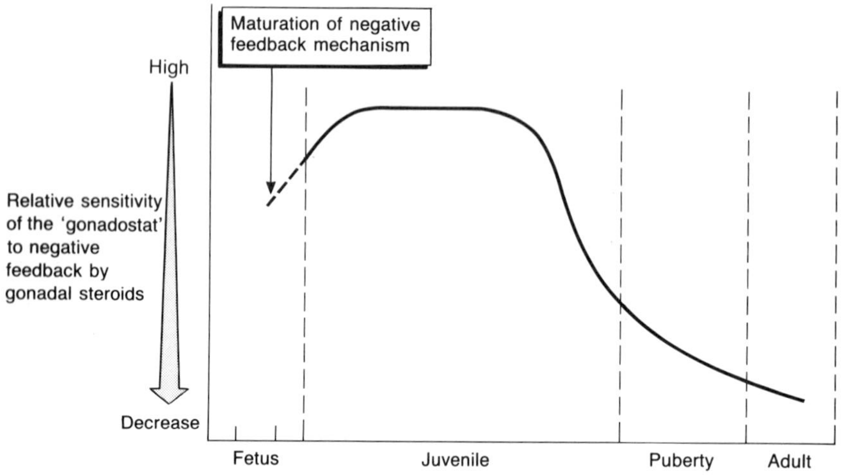

Fig. 30.13 Maturation of the negative feedback system and changes in set point of the hypothalamic gonadostat extending from the fetal life through puberty to adulthood (modified from Grumbach *et al.* (1974) *Control of the onset of puberty*, p. 158).

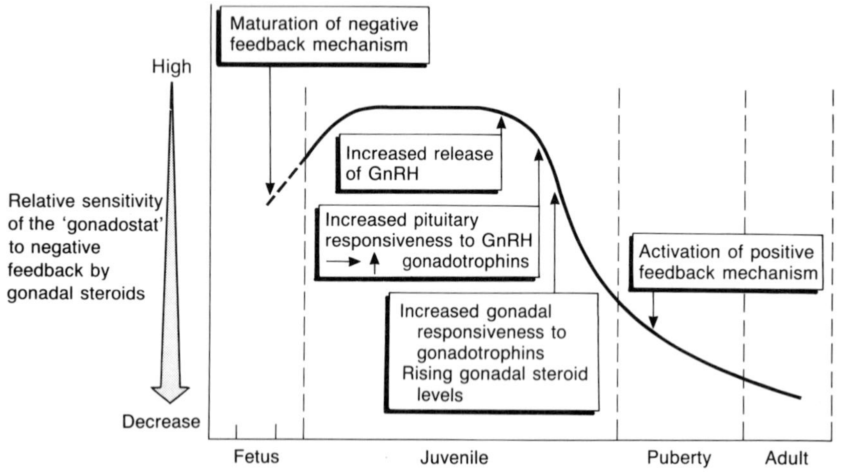

Fig. 30.14 The change in set point of the hypothalamic gonadostat (denoted by the dashed and solid lines) and the maturation of the negative and positive feedback mechanism from fetal life to adulthood (from Grumbach *et al.* (1974) *Control of the onset of puberty*, p. 158).

influenced by a variety of factors (including breed, season of birth, energy intake and liveweight gain) that affect the reactivation of the hypothalamic GnRH pulse generator.

Male physiology

In the male, puberty is associated with changes in the pattern of LH secretion, a gradual increase in the concentration of testosterone in the blood, rapid growth of the testes and the initiation of spermatogenesis. In essence, the adult pattern of GnRH release is attained and the testes proceed to fulfil two primary functions: the synthesis and release of androgens (*steroidogenesis*) and the production of spermatozoa (*gametogenesis*). In most male mammals, these functions are performed best at temperatures somewhat lower than body core temperature.

In the bull the testes are located in the pendulous scrotum, where they are attuned to function at 3–4°C below core temperature. The three principal mechanisms by which the scrotal temperature is reduced are as follows.

1 Precooling of the arterial blood supply as it passes through the vascular cone in the spermatic cord. The vascular cone consists of a coiled segment of the spermatic artery that is surrounded by the pampiniform plexus of the spermatic vein. Because of this anatomical arrangement the arterial blood and the venous blood are flowing in parallel but in opposite directions; this allows for an efficient countercurrent exchange of heat between the two vessels. The net result is that the arterial blood delivered to the testes is several degrees below body core temperature.

2 Sweating from the many sweat glands in the scrotal skin.

3 Physical contact with cold ground or other cold objects.

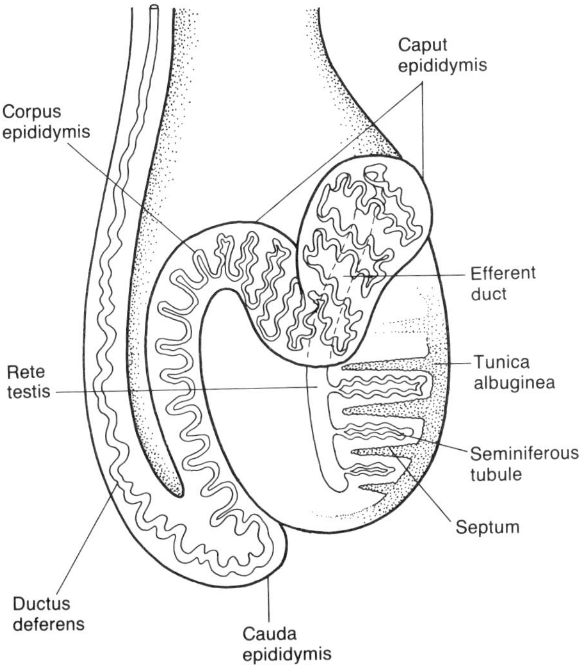

Fig. 30.15 Outline morphology of the testis.

In very cold weather, the temperature at the base of the scrotum may be up to 7°C below core values but the bull can attempt to curtail the drop in temperature by drawing the scrotum closer to the (relatively) warm body wall by contracting the cremaster and dartos muscles.

The gametogenic function of the testes is much more heat sensitive than the steroidogenic function; for instance, a retained testicle in a cryptorchid animal ('rig') may secrete androgens but the seminiferous tubules will remain infantile in structure and they will not produce spermatozoa. The retained testicle has a propensity to develop neoplasms.

Morphology of the testis

The testis is surrounded by a thick fibrous capsule, the tunica albuginea, from which septa project inwards to divide the substance of the testes into lobules (Fig. 30.15). Each lobule contains one to four highly convoluted seminiferous tubules and interstitial tissue that fills the spaces between the convolutions.

The interstitial tissue contains blood vessels, lymphatic vessels, nerves and the steroid-secreting Leydig cells.

The seminiferous tubules are about 200 μm in diameter and they may be up to 70 cm long; they open at both ends into the rete testis (Fig. 30.15). The tubules contain two populations of cells: (i) a fixed population of non-proliferating somatic cells, the Sertoli cells, and (ii) a migratory population of proliferating, differentiating germ cells (Fig. 30.16).

SERTOLI CELLS

The Sertoli cells have been described as the 'backbone' of the tubule. They are columnar cells that rest on the basement membrane and extend the full depth of the epithelial layer; they envelop the developing germ cells in deep recesses in their lateral walls and, ultimately, in their luminal surfaces. The Sertoli cells continually alter shape to accommodate the morphological changes in the germ cells during their migration from the base to the luminal surface. The plasma membranes of adjacent Sertoli cells form specialized interepithelial tight junctions that extend entirely around the circumference of each cell (Fig. 30.17). These junctions constitute the epithelial component of the blood–testis barrier that precludes the passage of many substances from the blood or interstitial fluid into the lumen of the seminiferous tubule. They also divide the intercellular spaces into two compartments: the basal compartment that contains the undifferentiated germ cells and the adluminal compartment that provides the appropriate microenvironment for the more differentiated germ cells (see below).

The basal surface of the Sertoli cell has specific receptors for FSH. The cells respond to the gonadotrophin by secreting (i) a nutrient fluid that sustains the germ cells in the intercellular spaces, (ii) androgen-binding protein that binds and transports testosterone to the epididymis, and (iii) inhibin that modulates the secretion of FSH by negative feedback at the pituitary gland (Fig. 30.18). Sertoli cells also have receptors for androgens; it is known that testosterone can maintain the functional integrity of the Sertoli cell when FSH is withdrawn.

Sertoli cells are resistant to relatively high levels of heat, ionizing radiation and many toxins, e.g. cadmium, nitrofurans, cytotoxins, that destroy differentiating germ cells.

GERM CELLS

A detailed description of the process of spermatogenesis (see Table 30.1) is beyond the scope of this text. Suffice it to say that the spermatogonia are the stem cells and that they begin the process by undergoing a number of mitotic divisions in the basal compartment. These divisions produce a pool of cells that are joined to each other by intercellular bridges (Fig. 30.19).

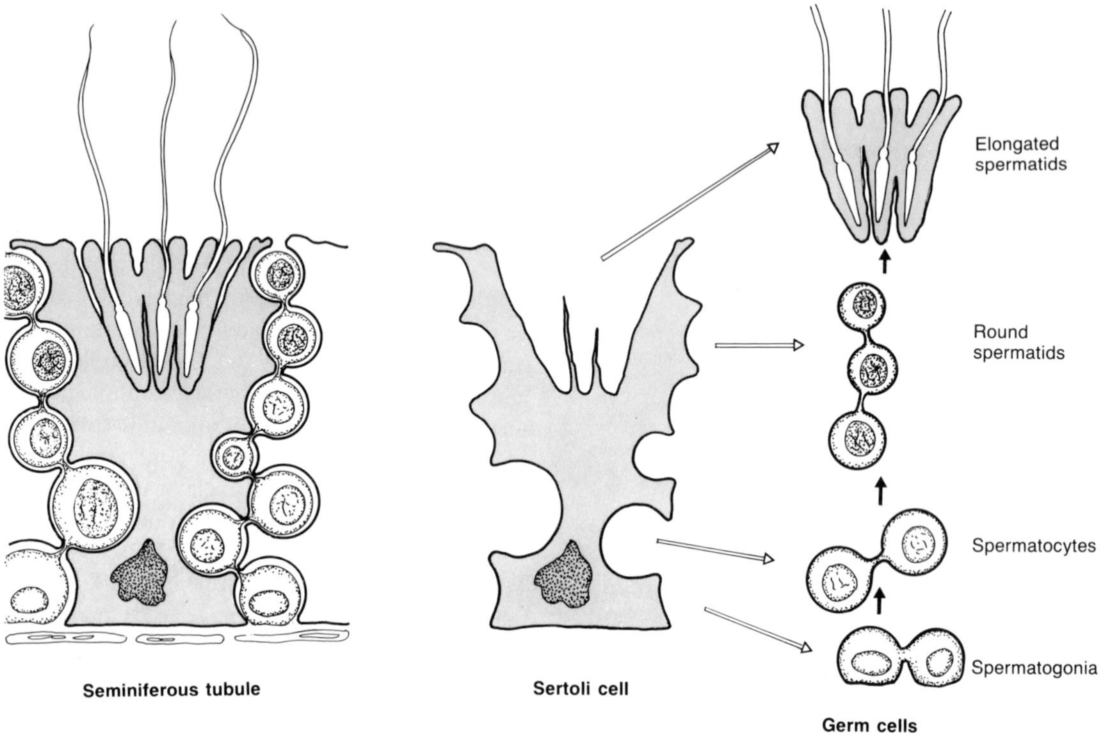

Fig. 30.16 The histology of the seminiferous tubule. The diagram depicts the Sertoli cell and the germ cells in intimate contact as they are *in vivo* and, also, separately to show the outlines of the individual cells. (Adapted from Bloom & Fawcett (1968) *A Textbook of Histology*, 10th edn. p. 813.)

Table 30.1 Principal stages in the development of spermatozoa (spermatogenesis)

Cell type	Number of chromosomes
Spermatogonium	2n
Primary spermatocyte	2n
Secondary spermatocyte	n
Spermatid	n
Spermatozoon	n

Cohorts of spermatogonia from this pool are moved to the adluminal compartment while one spermatogonium from the group remains behind in the basal compartment. It enters a resting phase during which it is highly resistant to ionizing radiation and toxic agents. This will be the stem cell from which the next cycle of spermatogenesis will begin (two weeks later). In the mean time, the newly arrived cells at the base of the adluminal compartment proceed to undergo meiosis as primary spermatocytes (first meiotic division) and secondary spermatocytes (second meiotic division). The haploid secondary spermatocytes are still attached to each other by intercellular bridges and after a short period each of them divides to yield two spermatids. As the process of spermatogenesis proceeds the germ cells move progressively towards the lumen of the tubule, still attached to the Sertoli cell; the final stages take place at the luminal surface. The conversion of the spermatid to the spermatozoon does not involve cell division, merely morphological reorganization (referred to as *spermiogenesis*). The principal changes are condensation of the nucleus and acquisition of the acrosome in the head region, reorganization of the mitochondria in the middle piece, development of the tail and loss of excess cytoplasm that moves caudally and is shed as the residual body, which is phagocytosed by the Sertoli cell. The intercellular bridges are lost with the residual bodies and each spermatozoon now is a separate cell, that soon escapes from the luminal surface of the Sertoli cell (*spermiation*). When the fully developed spermatozoon is released into the lumen of the seminiferous tubule it is non-motile. It is transported passively from the tubule into the rete testis and thence to the epididymis. Motility is acquired during passage through the epididymis.

In summary, during spermatogenesis the germ cells advance through three major processes:

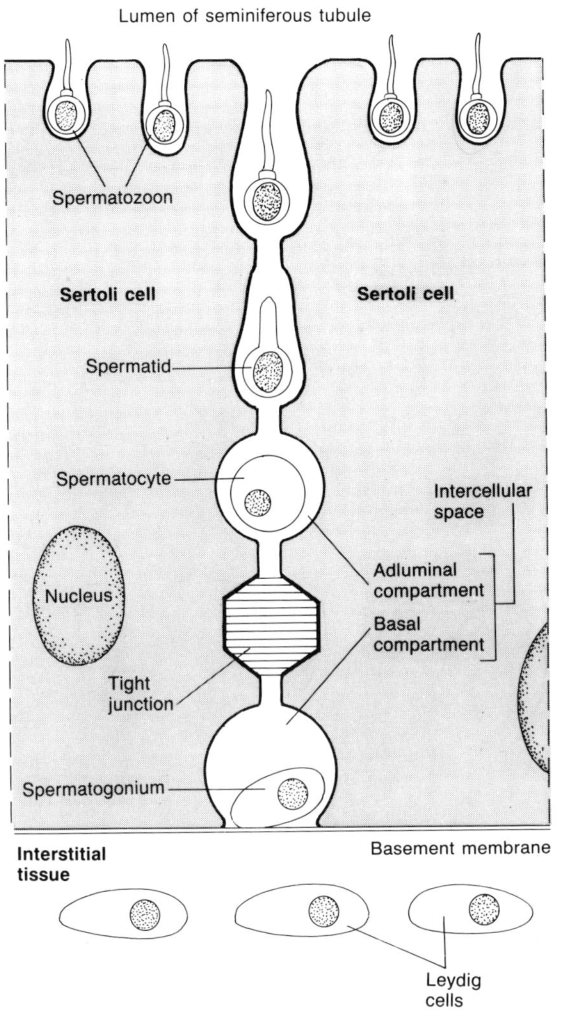

Fig. 30.17 The relationship between the germ cells and Sertoli cells during spermatogenesis. (After Berne & Levy (1988) *Physiology*, 2nd edn., p. 993).

1 Proliferation of stem cells by mitosis in the basal compartment.
2 Reduction of the chromosome number by meiosis in the adluminal compartment.
3 Morphological transformation of a conventional cell (the spermatid) into the very specialized structure of the spermatozoon (spermiogenesis) in the adluminal compartment.

This sequence of mitotic, meiotic and packaging events requires 56 days for completion in the bull. It is a very orderly sequence in which each of the component cells has a fixed lifespan so that cellular differentiation proceeds at a fixed rate. The spermatogonium that reverts to the resting phase remains quiescent in the basal compartment for 14 days (equivalent to 25 per cent of the entire cycle) before it enters mitosis and begins the next

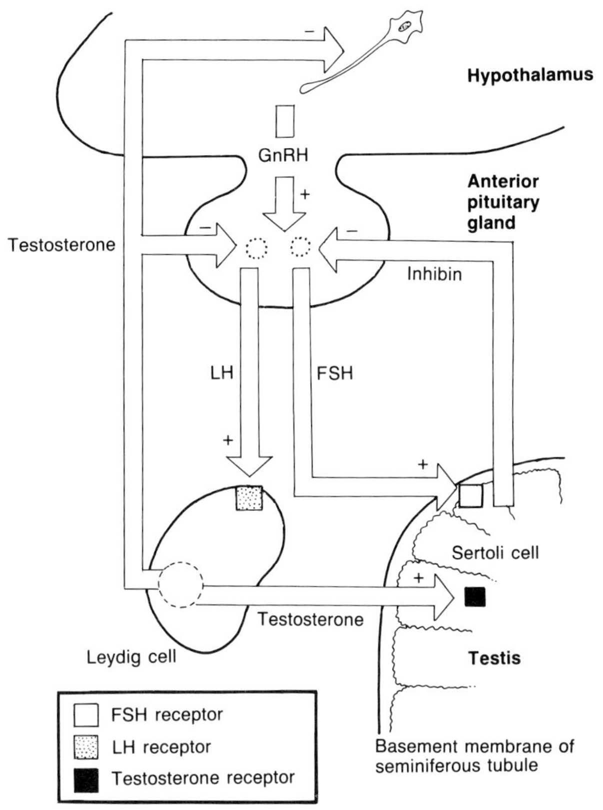

Fig. 30.18 Hormonal interactions in the hypothalamic–pituitary–testicular axis.

spermatogenic cycle. The cells derived from the new cycle advance in a similar orderly fashion behind the cells from the previous cycle as they move progressively towards the luminal surface. In fact, this arrangement means that four successive cycles of spermatogenesis will be in train in the seminiferous epithelium at any moment. Furthermore, since both the intervals between the commencement of the cycles and the rates of progress of the cells through spermatogenesis are constant, a histological examination of a cross-section of a seminiferous tubule will reveal a characteristic set of cell associations at any one time. In most mammals the same set of cell associations is seen at all points in the circumference of the tubule (this represents the 'cycle of spermatogenesis'); however, adjacent segments of the tubule tend to have a different set of cell associations, each either in advance of or behind its neighbours (this constitutes the 'wave of spermatogenesis').

Some of the progeny of the original spermatogonia do not complete the full course; large numbers (perhaps 20 per cent) of differentiating germ cells die without reaching maturity and these are removed by the Sertoli cells.

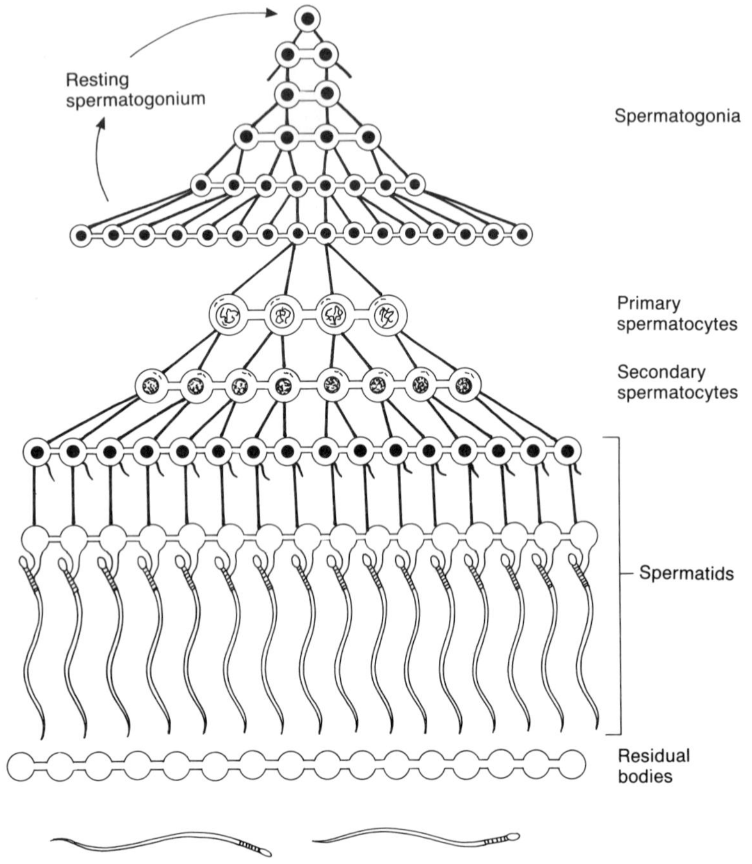

Fig. 30.19 The process of spermatogenesis. (Reproduced, with permission from Bloom & Fawcett (1968) *A Textbook of Histology*, 10th edn. p. 834.)

The spermatozoon

The essential features of the mammalian spermatozoon are depicted in Fig. 30.20. Only one structure warrants further comment at this juncture: the acrosome, an organelle that undergoes significant morphological change as an essential prelude to fertilization. The acrosome contains a number of lytic enzymes (particularly hyaluronidase, neuraminidase and acrosin); it has been described as a modified lysosome and, like all lysosomes, it has a bilaminar structure. The inner acrosomal membrane is adherent to the nuclear membrane, while the outer acrosomal membrane underlies the cell membrane. When the ejaculated spermatozoon undergoes the acrosome reaction in the female genital tract, the outer acrosomal membrane forms point fusions with the cell membrane creating a sequence of vesicles over the head of the sperm and allowing the lytic enzymes to escape through the resultant pores (see p. 421).

Neuroendocrine control

The steroidogenic functions and the gametogenic functions are segregated anatomically: androgen synthesis by the Leydig cells in the interstitial spaces and spermatogenesis within the seminiferous tubules (Fig. 30.17). Both functions are controlled by the pituitary gland through the secretion of the gonadotrophins. Luteinizing hormone binds to specific receptors on the cell membranes of Leydig cells and they respond by secreting androgens (principally testosterone), which in turn inhibit LH secretion by negative feedback. When the concentration of testosterone in the blood declines sufficiently the 'brake' on LH secretion is released and the resultant rise in LH in the circulation induces the Leydig cells to secrete testosterone (Figs 30.18 and 30.21). The negative feedback effect of testosterone on LH secretion is exercised at the level of the hypothalamus (influencing the secretion of GnRH) or at the pituitary gland (modulating the responsiveness of the gonadotropes to GnRH). In this manner the hypothalamic–pituitary–Leydig cell axis maintains the concentration of testosterone in the general circulation within normal limits.

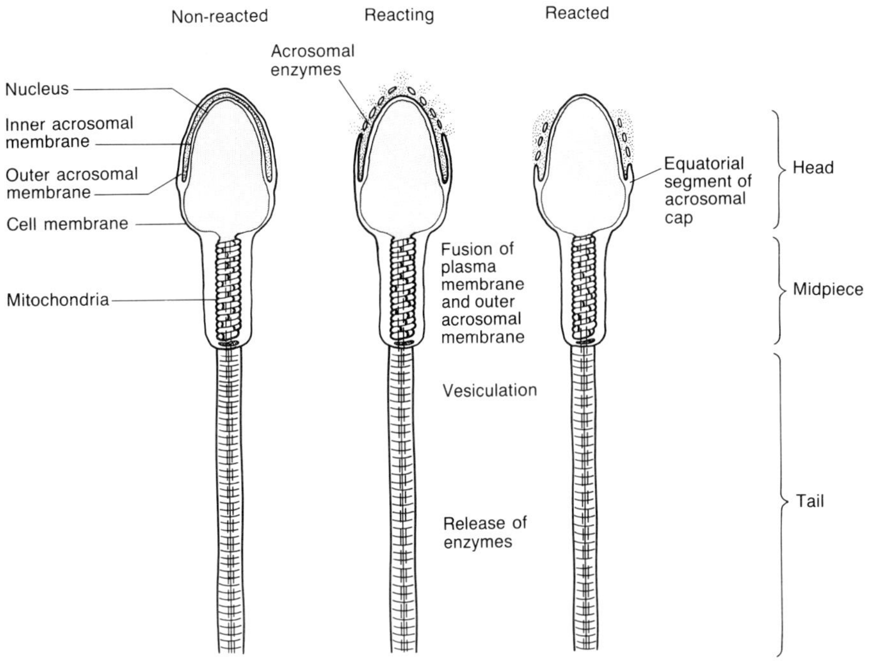

Fig. 30.20 The spermatozoon undergoing the acrosome reaction.

Sertoli cells respond to FSH by secreting fluids and proteins that sustain the differentiating germ cells. Follicle stimulating hormone is absolutely essential for the initiation of spermatogenesis in immature animals but once the normal germinal epithelium has been established FSH does not appear to be essential for the start of each successive spermatogenic cycle. Another action of FSH is to stimulate the conversion of testosterone to oestradiol by the Sertoli cells. The Sertoli cells also secrete inhibin, a polypeptide that inhibits the release of FSH by the pituitary gland (Fig. 30.18).

There is no doubt that an intact hypothalamic–pituitary–testicular axis is essential for normal testicular function; however, apart from the fact that FSH is essential for the initiation of the process in immature animals, it is unclear what specific roles in the process of spermatogenesis are played by the individual hormones that constitute the axis. On the basis of information available in the literature, the following deductions have gained wide acceptance:

1 Differentiating germ cells lack hormone receptors and, therefore, they are not affected directly by the hormones.
2 Sertoli cells have specific receptors for FSH and for androgens but not for LH.
3 Testosterone is required for the first mitotic division of the stem cell in the basal compartment.
4 Testosterone is necessary for the reduction division of the primary spermatocyte.
5 FSH is essential for the final steps in the maturation of the spermatids.
6 There is controversy as to whether or not testosterone is required for the earlier steps in the maturation of the spermatids.
7 It is likely that all the other steps in spermatogenesis can proceed without the specific intervention of a particular hormone.

Thus, FSH and testosterone exercise direct actions on the seminiferous tubules, while LH does so indirectly via the production of testosterone.

It should be noted that even where specific hormonal stimulation is essential, the hormone serves to ensure that the event occurs but it does not alter the *rate* of progress of spermatogenesis, which is a feature that is determined by genes rather than hormones.

The epididymis

When spermatozoa are transported from the rete testes through the efferent ducts to the initial segment of the epididymis they are neither motile nor capable of fertilization. They acquire these attributes during passage through the epididymis.

The epididymis is a highly convoluted tubule lined by specialized epithelium and surrounded by connective tissue, which incorporates concentric layers of smooth muscles that increase in thickness from the initial segment to the terminal segment. Anatomists describe the epididymis as consisting of three parts

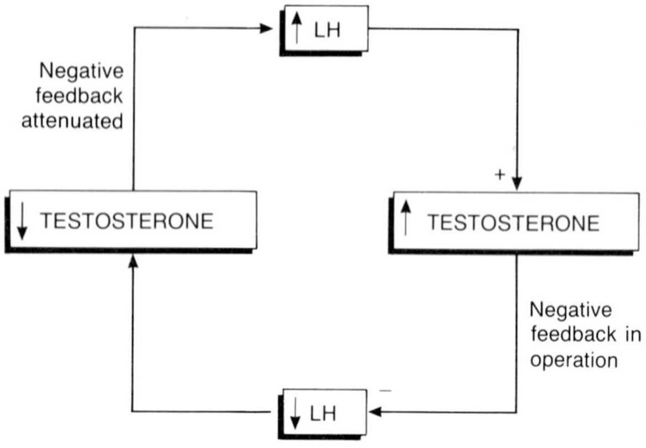

Fig. 30.21 The reciprocal relationship between the concentrations of testosterone and LH in the general circulation.

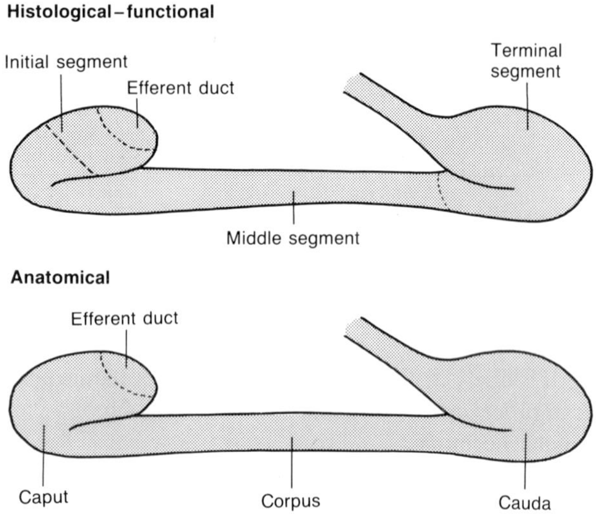

Fig. 30.22 The regions of the bovine epididymis.

(Fig. 30.15): the caput (head), the corpus (body) and the cauda (tail). A more recent histological–functional classification has designated at least eight regions in the epididymis of the bull but for the purposes of this text it is sufficient to refer to the three principal segments used in that scheme: the initial segment, the middle segment and the terminal segment (Fig. 30.22). The efferent ducts empty into the initial segment, which is specialized for the bulk reabsorption of water and electrolytes. The middle segment, which includes most of the caput and corpus, is responsible for the sperm maturation. The terminal segment, largely the cauda, stores the mature spermatozoa pending ejaculation.

In many species the initial segment is the principal site for absorption of water from the luminal fluids. The bull is an exception in that the bulk of the water has been absorbed by the efferent ducts before the contents reach the epididymis. The secretions from the epithelial cells of the initial and middle segments induce significant alterations in the functions and composition of most of the component parts of the spermatozoon. The principal functional changes are the acquisition of progressive motility and the ability to fertilize an egg. Fine structural changes have been observed in the plasma membrane, the acrosomal membranes, the nucleus and the tail. Changes in the composition of the plasma membrane appear to be central to the process of maturation of the spermatozoon as it passes through the epididymis; in particular, its protein composition is altered either by adsorption of components from the epididymal fluid or by modification or loss of existing components in response to enzymatic activity of the epididymal fluid. It is important to note that these biochemical changes are associated with the acquisition of the ability to fertilize but they do not complete the process of maturation — this will occur only after the ejaculated spermatozoa have been capacitated within the female genital tract (see p. 421).

Ejaculated spermatozoa have species-specific receptors that bind to the zona pellucida of the egg. The spermatozoa acquire these receptors in the epididymis, under the influence of testicular androgens.

The ability of the epididymis to facilitate maturation of the spermatozoa and to maintain the viability of the mature spermatozoa in the cauda is critically dependent on testicular androgens. Obviously, some of the testosterone reaches the epididymis in the arterial blood but it is probable that most of it comes via the efferent duct system bound to androgen-binding protein. The epithelial cells of the epididymis have androgen receptors and they rapidly convert the testosterone to dihydrotestosterone, which then regulates epididymal functions. It has been clearly established that the maturation of spermatozoa is regulated by dihydrotestosterone rather than by testosterone.

Movement of spermatozoa through the middle segment is by continuous peristaltic contractions of the smooth muscles that surround the epididymal tubule. The rate of transport in this segment is not influenced by ejaculation and in the bull it is estimated to take two to three days. It follows that the fertility of sperm should not be depressed even when the bull is ejaculating frequently. By contrast, the muscles surrounding the terminal segment are relatively inactive except when they are stimulated to contract during ejaculation; it follows that frequency of ejaculation can have a significant effect on the duration of storage of potentially fertile spermatozoa and on the numbers of fertile sperm available for ejaculation at a particular time.

Seminal plasma

The fluid portion of the ejaculate is called the seminal plasma. It consists of the testicular and epididymal secretions in which the spermatozoa are suspended when they pass from the cauda epididymis into the vas deferens plus the secretions from the various accessory glands, which are added as the spermatozoa are propelled along the vas deferens and the urethra during ejaculation.

The bull ejaculates 1–15 ml of semen containing $0.8–2.0 \times 10^9$ spermatozoa/ml.

Female physiology

Oestrous cycle

From a neuroendocrine perspective, the oestrous cycle is controlled by the secretory activities of three principal components: peptidergic neurones in the hypothalamus, gonadotropes in the adenohypophysis and steroid-secreting cells in the ovaries. It is clear that ultimate control is exercised by the hypothalamus through characteristic cyclic changes in the pattern of GnRH release, which are reflected in the circulating levels of FSH, LH, oestrogens and progesterone. Nevertheless, from the perspective of the practising veterinarian — who generally has to base his decisions on the history of behavioural oestrus, findings at rectal examinations and, perhaps, results of assays of steroid hormones — it would appear as if it is the ovary that times the events of the oestrous cycle. The following description of the physiology of the oestrous cycle will attempt to relate that clinical perspective to the underlying neuroendocrine mechanisms. It will begin with a description of the endocrine background to behavioural oestrus, proceed to an outline of the morphological changes in the ovaries during the oestrous cycle, followed by an account of the relationship between this ovarian cycle and the activities of the hypothalamic–pituitary–ovarian axis and, finally, it will highlight the physiological mechanisms that can be manipulated in the artificial control of the oestrous cycle.

OESTRUS

By definition, the oestrous cycle is the interval between the onset of two successive periods of sexual receptivity (oestrus). Both the expression of oestrus and the duration of the cycle are the result of cyclic changes in the ovaries that involve two temporary endocrine structures (the Graafian follicles and corpora lutea) and their principal secretions (oestrogens and progesterone).

It has been shown that behavioural oestrus results from exposure of the anterior hypothalamus to *both* progesterone and oestrogen in physiological concentrations and in the proper temporal sequence. Progesterone on its own inhibits oestrus. Furthermore, in the absence of priming by progesterone, physiological concentrations of oestrogen fail to elicit the signs of oestrus; thus, in the pubertal heifer the first preovulatory follicle produces a surge of oestrogen that feeds back positively on the pulse generator and induces an effective ovulatory surge of LH but it does not induce behavioural oestrus. In the adult cow the normal sequence is a high concentration of progesterone (P_4) for 10–14 days followed by a rapid decline in P_4 and an immediate increase in oestrogen from the growing preovulatory follicle (Fig. 30.23). This sequence results in behavioural oestrus that appears to be coupled with the preovulatory surge of LH so that ovulation occurs approximately 24 hours after the onset of oestrus. Thus, the behavioural action of oestrogen is primed by the high concentrations of progesterone in mid-cycle and it is facilitated by the relatively rapid decline in circulating progesterone at the end of the cycle.

The duration of oestrus may vary from 8 to 30 hours and the behavioural signs may recur frequently throughout the period or they may be evident during two shorter periods at the beginning and end with a quiescent period between them ('split oestrus').

OVARIAN MORPHOLOGY DURING THE OESTROUS CYCLE

The cow is a polyoestrous animal and, if she is not pregnant, she will tend to return to oestrus repeatedly throughout the year at intervals of 18–24 days (mean = 21 days). By convention, the day of oestrus is designated day 0 and the length of the cycle is calculated from that baseline.

There can be considerable variation (within the normal range) in the length of the oestrous cycle: even successive cycles in the same cow may vary by several days. Most of this variation is due to differences in the duration of the luteal phase of the ovarian cycle, i.e. in the functional lifespan of the individual corpus luteum. According to Hansel & Snook (1970), luteal regression may begin as early as day 15 or as late as day 19 of normal (20–24 day) cycles. The early stages of luteal regression are not detectable by rectal palpation.

The clinician has a further problem in the assessment of ovarian morphology due to recurring waves of fol-

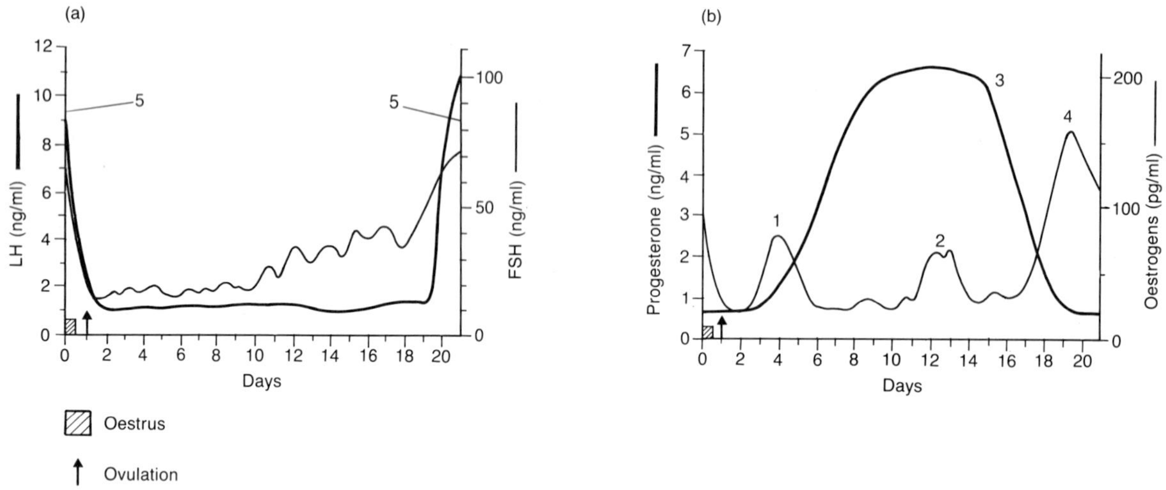

Fig. 30.23 Changes in concentrations of gonadotrophins (a) and ovarian steroids (b) in peripheral plasma during a 21-day oestrous cycle in the cow. During most of the cycle progesterone (P_4) secreted by the corpus luteum (CL) is the dominant hormone, exercising strong negative feedback on the hypothalamic-pituitary axis. However, the tonic concentrations of gonadotrophins released during the luteal phase induce two waves of palable follicles that are associated with small peaks of oestrogen (1, 2). When the CL regresses, the concentration of P_4 declines (3) and oestrogen concentration climbs to a peak, the oestrogen surge (4) which triggers a surge of gonadotrophins (5) that induces ovulation.

licular growth that occur throughout the cycle, even during the peak of the luteal phase. The cow has at least three waves of development of palpable follicles during each cycle: one between days one and six that culminates in one or more large (up to 12 mm in diameter) non-ovulating follicles at days nine to 11, another between days 12 and 16 that produces one or more even larger follicles, and a third that begins after luteolysis and culminates in ovulation. Marion & Gier (1971) reported that the follicle destined to ovulate is less than 10 mm in diameter when the corpus luteum begins to regress and that it grows to 16–20 mm over the next four or five days. Thus, the follicles that are palpable during the first two waves of growth undergo atresia during the luteal phase but once luteolysis occurs, a dominant follicle can grow to ovulatory size within a few days. However, it is not possible to distinguish between dominant follicles that will become atretic and preovulatory follicles by rectal examination. It is obvious that the functional corpus luteum plays a primary role in the control of the oestrous cycle, a fact that is central to all therapeutic regimes that aim to control the cycle.

HORMONAL CHANGES DURING THE OESTROUS CYCLE

The structural changes that occur during the oestrous cycle are accompanied by the secretion of hormones that take part in the ordered sequence of inhibitory and stimulatory signals that modulate the activities of the hypothalamic–pituitary–ovarian axis. During the luteal phase both progesterone from the corpus luteum and oestrogen from the non-ovulatory follicles restrain the hypothalamic–pituitary axis by negative feedback. The frequency of the pulse generator is reduced to one pulse of GnRH every four–eight hours and the concentrations of gonadotrophins in the peripheral circulation are restricted to basal levels. As a result, the dominant follicles in the first two waves of folliculogenesis do not ovulate but undergo atresia. Luteolysis, which is required to remove this inhibition, occurs spontaneously when the uterus, under the trophic influence of progesterone followed by oestrogen and oxytocin, produces sufficient prostaglandin $F_{2\alpha}$ ($PGF_{2\alpha}$) to kill the corpus luteum (see p. 418). The resultant fall in progesterone concentrations releases the GnRH pulse generator, which increases its frequency to one pulse every hour (approximately). The concentrations of FSH and LH rise in the peripheral circulation and the third wave of folliculogenesis proceeds to ovulation of the dominant follicle.

Follicular phase

The growing dominant follicle contains two populations of steroid-secreting cells: theca interna cells and granulosa cells. The cells of the theca interna have specific receptors for LH and they respond to this gonadotrophin by synthesizing androgens (androstenedione and testosterone) that diffuse across the basement membrane into the granulosa cell layer. During the early stages of folliculogenesis the granulosa cells have receptors for FSH and they respond to this gonadotrophin by converting the thecal androgen to oestrogen (Fig. 30.24). As the follicle grows under the trophic influences of both FSH and oestrogen, the granulosa cells acquire increased numbers of FSH receptors and oestrogen receptors and the follicular fluid gains increasing concentrations of both FSH and oestrogen. Follicular oestrogen passes into the circulation and eventually reaches sufficiently high concentrations to constitute the oestrogen surge that exerts a positive feedback on the hypothalamic–pituitary axis (Fig. 30.25). The frequency of the GnRH pulse generator increases, the sensitivity of the adenohypophysis to GnRH is increased by a self-priming action of the GnRH, and the pituitary gland releases the preovulatory surge of LH. By now, FSH has induced the appearance of LH receptors on the cell membranes of some of the granulosa cells close to the basement membrane of the follicle and they respond to the LH surge. The response to LH is both morphological (ovulation, formation of the corpus luteum) and secretory (progesterone).

This switch from negative feedback by progesterone and oestrogen to positive feedback by oestrogen is the crucial hormonal event that leads to ovulation. The timing and rate of change of the oestrogen surge are critical: any significant deviation in either factor can result in delayed ovulation or anovulation.

Luteal phase

Luteinizing hormone is the principal luteotrophin in the cow; under normal circumstances, tonic secretion of LH maintains the functional corpus luteum until $PGF_{2\alpha}$ from the uterus causes luteolysis at the end of the cycle. It is important to realize that 'normal circumstances' include the correct antecedent hormonal pattern: specifically, serum progesterone at luteal phase concentrations for a few days before it subsides and is followed by serum FSH at normal preovulatory concentrations. Failure of this sequence or inappropriate serum concentrations of either hormone seem to affect the lifespan of the corpus luteum (short luteal phase) and/or its capacity to secrete progesterone (inadequate luteal phase), phenomena that are common after the first ovulation at puberty or postpartum. It is not known how the (prefollicular phase) progesterone exerts its influence on the activities of the next corpus luteum;

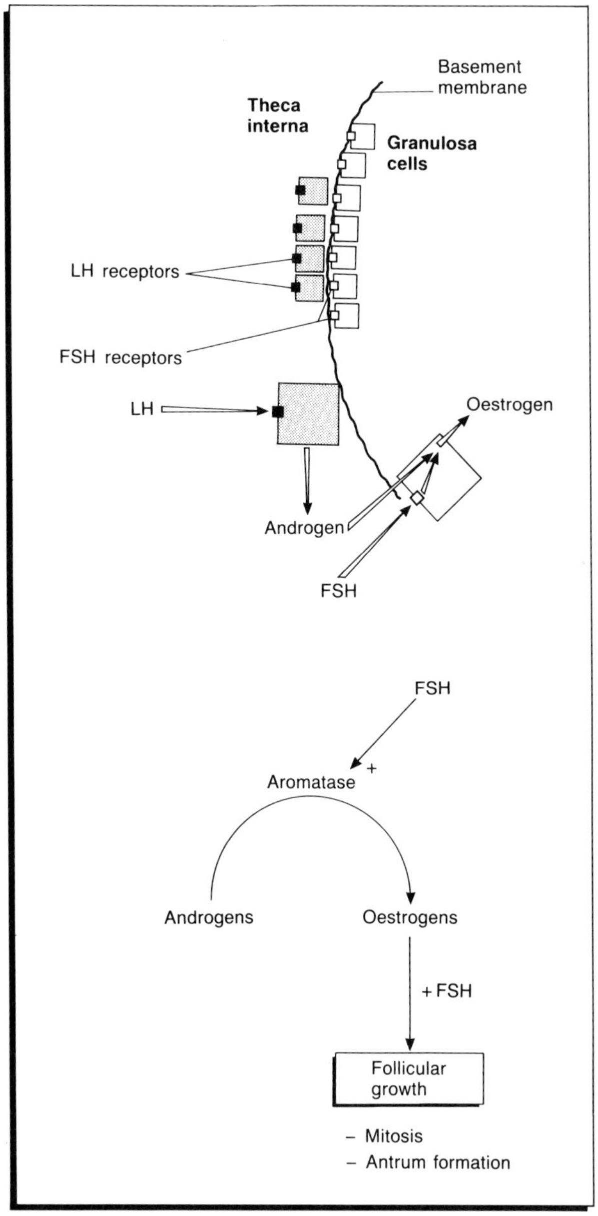

Fig. 30.24 Formation of oestrogen by ovarian follicle.

the FSH could do so through its role in the induction of LH receptors on the granulosa cells of the preovulatory follicle.

After ovulation the granulosa cells and the theca internal cells differentiate into luteal cells that secrete progesterone. The corpus luteum grows progressively in size until days 16–18 of the oestrous cycle. Histologically, the mature corpus luteum is seen to contain two morphologically distinct populations of parenchymal cells: small luteal cells (10–20 µm) and large luteal cells (20–35 µm). All of the small cells are derived

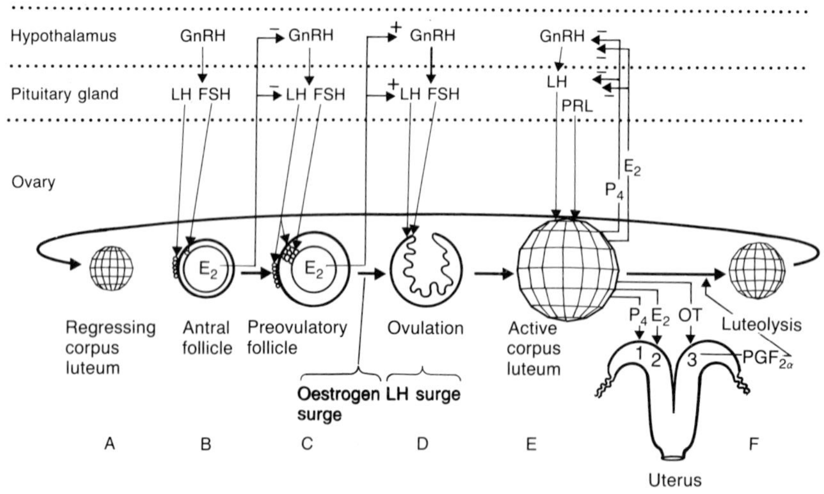

Fig. 30.25 Inter-relationships between the hypothalamus, pituitary gland, ovary and uterus during the oestrous cycle. When the corpus luteum (CL) regresses at the end of a cycle (A), the hypothalamus and pituitary gland are released from the strong negative feedback exerted by progesterone (P_4) throughout the luteal phase of the cycle. FSH and LH stimulate the growth and secretory activity of a dominant ovarian follicle (B) that secretes increasing quantities of oestradiol (E_2). The initial low concentrations of E_2 have a negative feedback effect until the preovulatory follicle produces a surge of oestrogen (C) that exerts a positive feedback and results in a surge of LH that causes ovulation (D). A new CL develops under the trophic influence of both LH and prolactin (PRL). It secretes P_4 and E_2 that re-assert a strong negative feedback effect on the hypothalamic-pituitary axis. In addition, the P_4 causes an accumulation of fatty acid precursors in the endometrium (1). After day 10, E_2 induces the synthesis of prostaglandin from the stored precursors (2). Finally, oxytocin (OT) causes the release of the $PGF_{2\alpha}$(3), which is transferred from the uterus to the ipsilateral ovary by a countercurrent mechanism (see Figure 30.25) and induces luteolysis (F). [See Figure 30.23 for changes in concentrations of the hormones in the peripheral plasma].

from thecal cells and, until the sixth day of the oestrous cycle, nearly all of the large cells are derived from the granulosa cells. After day six, some small luteal cells differentiate into large luteal cells, so that the large cells are of mixed origin and the proportion of large cells increases as the corpus luteum matures (from less than 2 per cent at days three to five to almost 5 per cent at days 10 to 18).

It is significant for the clinical management of the oestrous cycle to realize that the small luteal cells and the large luteal cells differ in their abilities to respond to the recognized luteotrophin (LH) and luteolysin ($PGF_{2\alpha}$). Receptors for LH are numerous on the small cells but they are scanty or absent on the large cells. Therefore, LH stimulates the small cells to secrete progesterone but it has no such effect on the large cells. Despite this and the numerical predominance of small luteal cells throughout the luteal phase, it is generally agreed that most of the progresterone is secreted by the large luteal cells. Progesterone is secreted as pulses at a frequency that is different from that for LH. This does not diminish the importance of LH as the principal luteotrophin in the cow: LH does not have direct control over the quantities of progesterone secreted by the large cells but it does exert an important indirect control by regulating the differentiation of small cells into large luteal cells, a process during which the steroidogenic activities of the cells seem to be turned on fully and permanently. On the other hand, receptors for $PGF_{2\alpha}$ are numerous on large luteal cells but are absent from the small cells. Since the young corpus luteum (days three to five) is composed almost entirely of small cells, it is not surprising that it is refractory to the luteolytic action of $PGF_{2\alpha}$. The luteolysin becomes effective when the large luteal cells assume responsibility for most of the secretory activity.

It is well known that during the first four or six days of the oestrous cycle exogenous oxytocin can inhibit the growth of the corpus luteum and block its secretory activity. This is possible because the small luteal cells have specific receptors for oxytocin and interaction between the receptors and the peptide leads to inhibition of the LH-stimulated secretion of progesterone by the small cells. In the mature corpus luteum the large luteal cells synthesize oxytocin and it has been suggested that this peptide may play a significant role in local 'large-cell-to-small-cell communication' during prostaglandin-induced luteolysis.

Prostaglandin $F_{2\alpha}$ is formed in the endometrium. It leaves the uterus in the uterine vein and most of it is transported in the venous blood to the lungs where it is degraded rapidly into its inactive metabolite, PGFM. However, some $PGF_{2\alpha}$ is brought directly from the

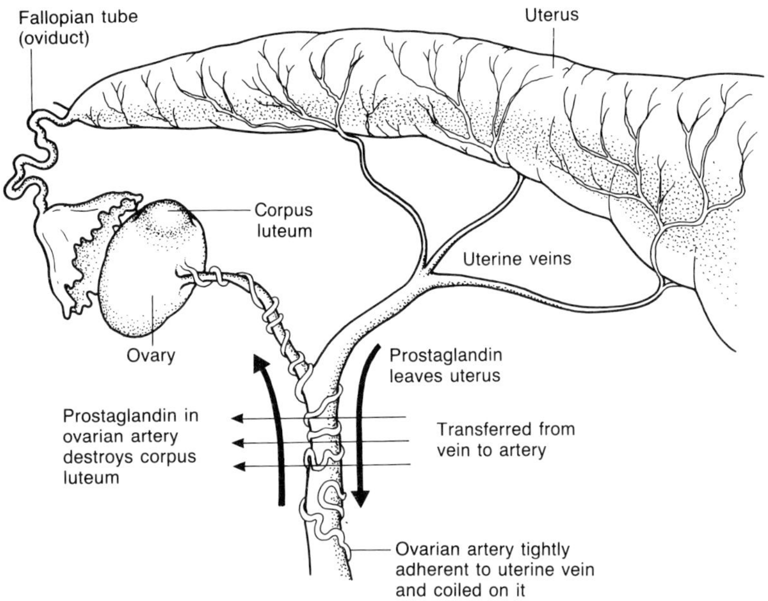

Fig. 30.26 The transfer of $PFG_{2\alpha}$ from the uterus to the ovary by a countercurrent mechanism (after Baird, 1984).

uterus to the adjacent ovary by means of a countercurrent mechanism (Fig. 30.26) that transfers the luteolytic agent from the uterine vein to the ovarian artery. Prostaglandin $F_{2\alpha}$ is released from the uterus in pulses and there is evidence that the minimum requirement for normal regression of the corpus luteum at the end of the oestrous cycle (i.e. effective luteolysis by endogenous $PGF_{2\alpha}$ is a pulse lasting 1 hour repeated about every six hours over a period of 24–30 hours. (By contrast, after day five of the oestrous cycle the corpus luteum can be removed by a single injection of exogenous luteolysin, in an appropriate dose.)

The timing and magnitude of $PGF_{2\alpha}$ release from the uterus is determined by the sequential interactions of progesterone, oestradiol and oxytocin with the endometrium. During the early part of the oestrous cycle the endometrial cells have many receptors for progesterone and coupling of the steroid with its receptors effectively blocks the production of $PGF_{2\alpha}$; however, it causes an accumulation of fatty acid precursors in the endometrium. After about 10 days the action of progesterone on the endometrium declines (possibly due to progesterone-induced loss of its own receptor: 'down regulation'), and oestradiol from developing ovarian follicles promotes the formation of endometrial receptors for oestradiol and oxytocin. Coupling of oestradiol with its receptors increases the synthesis of $PGF_{2\alpha}$ from the fatty acid precursors, while coupling of oxytocin (principally from the corpus luteum) with its receptors in the endometrium leads to immediate secretion of $PGF_{2\alpha}$. It is probable that the duration of the pulses is determined by the rapid 'down regulation' of oxytocin receptors (within 1 hour) and that the frequency of the pulses reflects the regeneration time of the oxytocin receptors in response to oestradiol (6 hours).

The precise mechanism by which $PGF_{2\alpha}$ induces luteolysis has not been established. It causes a significant reduction in luteal blood flow and it couples with specific receptors on the large luteal cells. However, the other steroidogenic cells, the small luteal cells, do not have receptors for $PGF_{2\alpha}$ and it has to be assumed that some type of intercellular communication between the large cells and the small cells is involved in terminating the LH-induced secretion of progesterone by the small luteal cells. Oxytocin, which is formed in the large luteal cells and has specific receptors on the small luteal cells, is an obvious candidate messenger.

In any case, the corpus luteum is insensitive to $PGF_{2\alpha}$ during the first four days of the cycle but between day five and day sixteen the administration of $PGF_{2\alpha}$ or an analogue will cause rapid luteolysis followed, within a few days, by oestrus and ovulation.

PHARMACOLOGICAL REGULATION OF THE OESTROUS CYCLE

The pharmaceutical industry has provided an array of natural and synthetic hormones — GnRH, gonadotrophins, steroids, prostaglandins — that can be used to regulate the oestrous cycle. The use of these agents for specific purposes will be described when we deal with the clinical conditions in which they have been found to be effective. Nevertheless, it is appropriate at this juncture to emphasize a few basic principles that should be borne in mind when the clinician is contemplating the use of reproductive hormones for therapeutic purposes.

The GnRH generator imposes a pulsatile mode of secretion on the hypothalamic–pituitary–ovarian axis. The component parts of the axis respond to hormonal signals that are encoded in the frequency and, to a lesser extent, the amplitude of the pulses. However, these target tissues may not be able to decode a hormonal stimulus that is either non-pulsatile or pulsatile at non-physiological frequencies. As an example, repeated small pulses of exogenous GnRH will induce pulsatile releases of gonadotrophins and these responses will be enhanced by the self-priming action of GnRH. On the other hand, continuous infusion of GnRH or intermittent infusions of GnRH at markedly non-physiological frequencies will soon lead to complete refractoriness of the pituitary gland to the continued stimulation (see p. 405). Therapeutic regimes should be planned with due recognition of these observations. A single bolus of exogenous GnRH is likely to be effective only when a preovulatory follicle is present already.

During the luteal phase of the oestrous cycle the corpus luteum acts as an effective 'brake' on the pulse generator: pulse frequency is reduced so that circulating gonadotrophins are maintained at tonic concentrations and the dynamic surges required to cause ovulation cannot occur. Luteolysis removes the brake, the pulse frequency increases and ovulation occurs within four or five days. Hence, there are two methods by which control over the length of the cycle and ovulation can be achieved: the use of a luteolytic agent to kill the corpus luteum of the current cycle or of a progestogen to create an 'artificial' luteal phase, which will be followed by ovulation shortly after withdrawal of the progestogen. These methods can be used separately or in combination. Since prostaglandin does not kill the very young corpus luteum (less than five days after ovulation), the usual recommendation is to give two injections 11 days apart.

The ovarian hormones create conditions in the tubular genital tract that facilitate the transport and survival of the gametes and the conceptus. The appropriate muscular activity, secretions and flow of fluids in the female tract are governed by oestrogen and progesterone released from the ovaries in the correct concentrations, at the correct times and in a specific sequence. Therefore, any therapeutic agent that alters the delicate balance of ovarian hormones during the follicular and early luteal phases of the oestrous cycle is a potential hazard to pregnancy, even when a normal fertile cow is bred to a highly fertile bull. In addition, the ovarian hormones influence the responses of the female genital tract to infectious agents. For instance, the uterus has a higher degree of susceptibility to bacterial infection during the luteal phase than it has during oestrus. This is because the migration of neutrophils into and through the endometrium is inhibited by progesterone, which also depresses the phagocytic activity of the cells once they have arrived in the endometrium. Therefore, the clinician should exercise great care to avoid the introduction of contaminated or irritant material into the uterus during the luteal phase.

Pregnancy

TRANSPORT OF GAMETES IN FEMALE GENITAL TRACT

Fertilization takes place in the oviduct, close to the junction of the isthmus and the ampulla (Fig. 30.27). Transport of the ovum from the ovary is achieved by muscular and ciliary activity and flow of fluids in the ovarian bursa and ampulla of the oviduct. After natural mating, spermatozoa have to traverse the cervix, the uterus and the uterotubal junction. Again, muscular activity and flow of fluids are largely responsible for the transport of the male gametes. The appropriate muscular activities, secretion and flow of fluids in the female genital tract are regulated by the ovarian hormones (oestrogens and progesterone) released in the correct concentrations and in the proper sequence. Therapeutic procedures that significantly alter the relative concentrations or sequence of the hormones can disrupt the transport mechanisms, which in some instances may cause the loss of gametes or of the conceptus.

The transport of spermatozoa is not an entirely passive process: the motility of the male gametes makes a significant contribution to the successful completion of the hazardous voyage from vagina to oviduct during which the vast majority of the spermatozoa are lost, partly as a result of phagocytosis but largely by expulsion to the exterior in cervical mucus. It appears from the literature that two distinct populations of spermatozoa arrive in the oviduct:

1 those that are transported rapidly but are incapable of fertilizing the ovum; and

2 those that are transported more slowly to the functional sperm reservoir and are capable of fertilization.

Spermatozoa have been recovered from the ampulla of the oviduct within 3–5 minutes after mating. This rapid transport is due to muscular contractions in the female genital tract. During oestrus the contractions begin at the cervix and move towards the oviduct; at the end of oestrus the direction of the contractions is

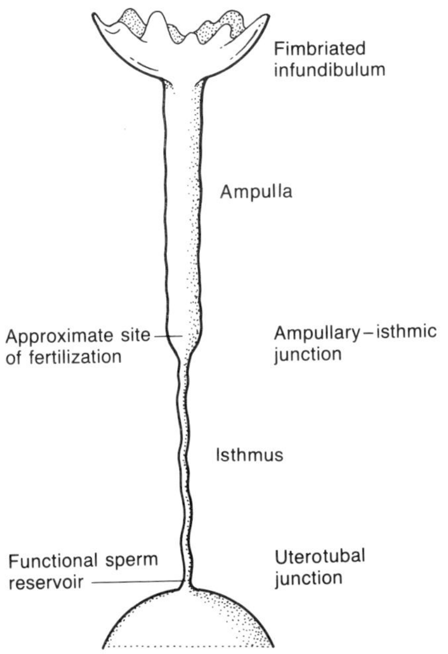

Fig. 30.27 Schematic diagram of the uterine tube (oviduct, Fallopian tube).

reversed. Most of the spermatozoa that reach the oviduct during the initial rapid transport phase are damaged or dead and they do not include the sperm that fertilizes the ovum. It has been suggested that these non-viable spermatozoa may play a significant physiological role, by releasing products that elicit local muscular and secretory responses that facilitate transport and sustenance of the gametes.

According to Hunter & Wilmut (1984), viable spermatozoa are transported more slowly: heifers mated early in oestrus took 8–12 hours to establish an adequate population of viable spermatozoa in the oviduct. Then, the gametes were sequestered, in a relatively quiescent state, in the caudal 2 cm of the isthmus for a further 18–20 hours before they began a progressive migration towards the site of fertilization. Thus, the caudal isthmus served as the functional sperm reservoir, the immediate source of viable spermatozoa at the time of ovulation. It is known that both the temperature and the oxygen tension are lower in that segment of the isthmus than they are in the ampulla and it is thought that these factors may be responsible for the depressed motility of the spermatozoa in the reservoir up to the time of ovulation. At ovulation, the temperature and oxygen tension are elevated in the lumen of the caudal isthmus, the sequestered spermatozoa begin to exhibit activated motility (hyperactivation) and they migrate to the site of fertilization. Hyperactivation is in response to the 'pick-up' of follicular fluid and the ovum by the oviduct.

CAPACITATION AND THE ACROSOME REACTION

The spermatozoa deposited in the female reproductive tract are not immediately capable of fertilizing an ovum. During transport through the tract they undergo physiological changes that make them competent to penetrate the zona pellucida and fuse with the ovum, i.e. they undergo *capacitation*. It is thought that during capacitation the spermatozoon loses some proteins it has acquired, by adsorption or incorporation into the plasma membrane, during exposure to epididymal fluid or seminal plasma. This does not cause any visible change in the morphology of the spermatozoon but it does alter the physical and chemical properties of the plasma membrane permitting an influx of calcium ions required for the induction of the hyperactivated form of motility and of the acrosome reaction. The hyperactivated motility endows the capacitated spermatozoa with strong thrusting power that facilitates migration from the isthmus to the ampulla and subsequent passage through the zona pellucida. The acrosome reaction is an essential prerequisite for fertilization — a spermatozoon with an intact acrosome cannot penetrate the ovum.

The acrosome reaction (Fig. 30.20) involves multiple point fusions between the plasma membrane and the outer acrosomal membrane over the front half of the sperm head. The fusions give rise to a series of small vesicles formed by fragments of both membranes. The vesicles are separated by small pores through which the acrosomal enzymes escape. There is controversy as to whether or not the escaping enzymes aid the passage of the spermatozoa through the cumulus oophorus in the cow. As the reaction proceeds, the pores enlarge at the expense of the vesicles so that the vesicles have been lost by the time the sperm penetrates the zona pellucida. When one of the advancing spermatozoa reaches the perivitelline space, it fuses with the plasma membrane of the ovum and its genetic material is incorporated into the conceptus at fertilization.

The fusion of the egg and the sperm triggers a series of reactions that prevent polyspermy by making both the zona pellucida and the plasma membrane of the ovum impenetrable to other spermatozoa.

It is often stated that capacitation requires a 6-hour sojourn in the female tract. However, Bedford (1983) suggested that it is unlikely that the processes would be synchronized to ensure that all the surviving spermatozoa would have been capacitated at a fixed minimum time after deposition in the female tract. Asynchrony in the time to capacitation would appear to be more advantageous in that it would allow for small populations of potential fertilizing spermatozoa to be available

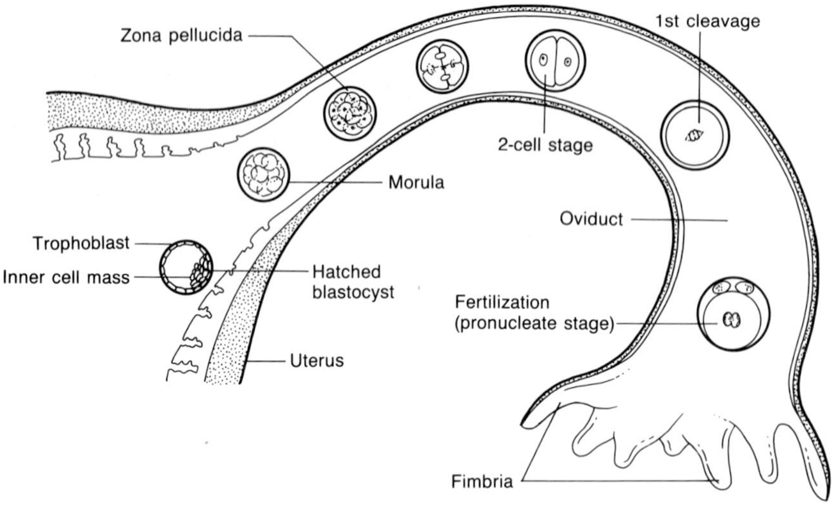

Fig. 30.28 Schematic diagram to illustrate the changes in the conceptus during transport down the uterine tube and into the uterine lumen (after McLaren (1984) In *Reproduction in Mammals*, 2nd edn. (ed. by C.R. Austin & R.V. Short), Book 3, p. 21).

sequentially over a period spanning several hours before and after ovulation. Indeed, there is evidence that only 10–20 per cent of bovine spermatozoa have undergone capacitation and the acrosome reaction within 3 hours of insemination, while other spermatozoa do so several hours later.

Again, the inappropriate use of exogenous hormones may hamper capacitation and the acrosome reaction.

MATERNAL RECOGNITION OF PREGNANCY

Normally, the conceptus enters the uterus about 72 hours after ovulation, at the 8–16 cells stage. The cells (blastomeres) form a solid mass (morula) still contained within the zona pellucida. By day seven or eight, fluid secreted by the blastomeres accumulates in a central cavity (blastocoele) and the zygote is now called a blastocyst. The cells have been arranged into two distinct populations (Fig. 30.28).

1 The flattened trophoblast cells that form the wall of the blastocyst and ultimately will form the chorion.

2 A group of cells that form the inner cell mass at one pole beneath the trophoblast cells and are destined to form the fetus.

The blastocyst hatches from the zona pellucida on day 9 to 11 and on day 13 it begins to elongate so that during the third week it occupies most of the pregnant (ipsilateral) horn and a portion of the non-pregnant (contralateral) horn. The process of attachment begins at day 19 or 20 when there are definite areas of adhesion between the trophoblastic epithelium of the conceptus and the endometrial epithelium; implantation is completed between days 35 and 42. The conceptus plays an important role in prolonging the functional lifespan of the corpus luteum, an essential requirement for the maintenance of pregnancy. The critical period for the extension of the lifespan of the corpus luteum in the cow is between day 15 and day 17; if there is a conceptus present at that time the mother will 're-cognize' that she is pregnant and the luteolytic pulsatile pattern of $PGF_{2\alpha}$ release from the endometrium will be attenuated or abolished. Since maternal recognition of pregnancy precedes the physical attachment of the conceptus to the endometrium, it is evident that the utero-ovarian regulatory mechanisms that 'rescue' the corpus luteum are responding to a biochemical dialogue between the conceptus and the maternal tissue that is initiated by a variety of signal factors released into the uterine lumen by the preimplantation conceptus.

The bovine conceptus can synthesize a number of products (steroids, prostaglandins, peptides, proteins) that may interact with the maternal utero-ovarian axis. There is evidence to suggest that the conceptus releases different signal factors at different times and that the relative importance of each of these factors may change during these early days of pregnancy. A hypothesis consistent with current information is that the bovine conceptus initiates both antiluteolytic and luteotrophic activities. Regression of the corpus luteum is prevented by a group of proteins secreted by the conceptus between days 16 and 26 of pregnancy. The term bovine trophoblast protein-1 (bTP-1) has been used to identify these proteins, which have been shown to be structurally related to alpha interferons; bTP-1 exerts this antiluteolytic effect by inhibiting the synthesis of $PGF_{2\alpha}$ in the endometrium. Putative luteotrophic factors include a lipid-like substance released

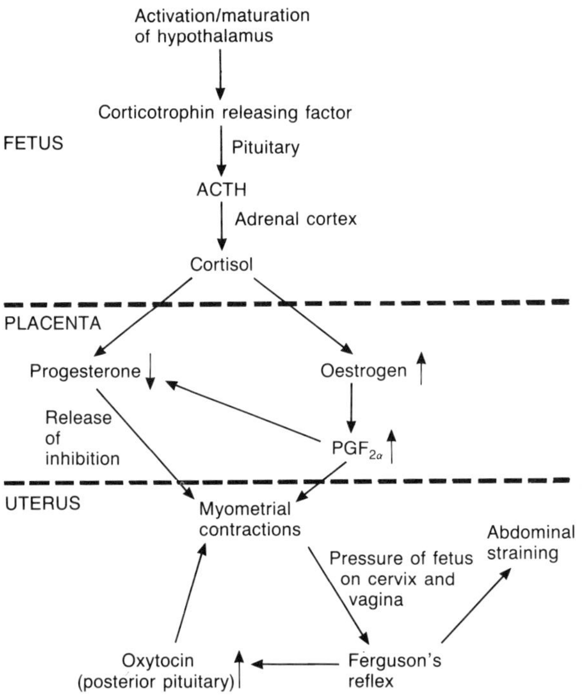

Fig. 30.29 The endocrine control of parturition (Reproduced with permission from Peters, A.R. & Ball, P.J.H. (1987) *Reproduction in Cattle*, p. 109. London, Butterworth's).

by the conceptus between day 13 and day 18 of pregnancy and, possibly, PGE_2 from the endometrium.

MAINTENANCE OF PREGNANCY

Once the normal conceptus–endometrial–ovarian regulatory axis of pregnancy has been established, the uterus comes under long-term control by progesterone. In the cow, a fully functional corpus luteum is essential to maintain pregnancy up to day 235; thereafter, the adrenal glands seem to be able to secrete sufficient progesterone to maintain pregnancy in ovariectomized cows. The placenta contributes little to the circulating concentrations of progesterone at any time during pregnancy. The principal luteotrophin appears to be LH, assisted by prolactin. The corpus luteum maintains the plasma progesterone concentration above 10 ng/ml from the second week of gestation until term. Progesterone plays a dominant role in the maintenance of pregnancy. It exercises a 'block' on the uterine muscle in that it depresses the amplitude of contractions, suppresses the reactivity to oxytocin and $PGF_{2\alpha}$, and prevents the development of synchronous coordinated contractions that might expel the fetus prematurely. It does not abolish the spontaneous contractility of the myometrial cells.

PARTURITION

Since parturition depends on coordinated rhythmic contractions of the myometrium as well as involuntary contractions of the abdominal muscles and 'softening' of the birth canal, the final preparation for delivery of the fetus must involve removal of the progesterone block. This is achieved by significant changes in the hormonal profile coupled with the acquisition of gap junctions by the myometrial cells.

The hormonal changes are initiated by the fetus, triggered by the recognition of 'stress' by the fetal hypothalamic–pituitary axis (Fig. 30.29). This results in the release of ACTH that stimulates the fetal adrenal to release increased amounts of cortisol. The cortisol induces the placenta to release increased quantities of oestrogens into the maternal circulation, and both the cortisol and the oestrogens act on the endometrium to increase the output of $PGF_{2\alpha}$, which causes luteolysis. Thus the oestrogen : progesterone ratio has been switched strongly in favour of oestrogen and the inhibitory effect of progesterone on the uterine muscle has been abolished. The oestrogens promote uterine contractility by stimulating the synthesis of contractile protein and of receptors for both oxytocin and $PGF_{2\alpha}$, and by facilitating the formation of gap junctions between adjacent myometrial cells. Gap junctions are intercellular structures that link cells and allow them to exchange ions and electrical impulses. In the parturient uterus they provide the routes through which electrical activity is propagated; in other words, they provide the structural basis for a functional syncytium that permits synchronization of myometrial contractions. Thus, the switch to oestrogen domination at full term enables the uterine muscle to develop spontaneous rhythmical contractions. The more powerful contractions during parturition are generated in response to $PGF_{2\alpha}$, augmented during the second stage of labour by oxytocin. Both of these hormones influence smooth muscle activity by regulating the concentration of calcium ions in the myometrial cells. A deficiency of calcium in a pregnant female at full term is associated with atony of the uterine muscle and a tendency to prolapse of the uterus.

Softening of the birth canal is achieved by the cascade of hormones: a rise in oestrogen concentrations followed by the activities of relaxin and $PGF_{2\alpha}$. Parturition can be induced after about day 255 of gestation by a single injection of a synthetic glucocorticoid that simulates the effects of fetal cortisol, or after 270 days by $PGF_{2\alpha}$. Retained placenta can be a problem with either method.

Tocolysis

Drugs that stimulate β_2-adrenoceptors of the myometrial cells cause relaxation of the uterine muscle. They have been used for this purpose in non-pregnant cows undergoing embryo transfer and in pregnant cows at full term to delay parturition (tocolysis) or to facilitate obstetrical operations such as fetotomy, caesarean section or replacement of uterine prolapse. The duration of the tocolysis depends on the pharmacological effects of the agent and on the position of the fetus at the time of treatment. For instance, clenbuterol causes an outflow of calcium ions from the myometrial cells and that renders the cells unresponsive to oxytocin for some hours. When a single therapeutic dose of clenbuterol is given early in stage one of labour it can delay parturition for 5–8 hours, but if it is given in stage two after the cervix has been fully dilated the delay may be as short as an hour or two. It has been reported that when uterine contractility returns, the treated animal tends to have an 'easier' calving; it is suggested that this is due to greater widening and softening of the birth canal.

Physiology of the postpartum period

During pregnancy the high concentrations of progesterone and oestrogen in the circulation exert a prolonged negative feedback on the maternal hypothalamic–pituitary–ovarian axis. The principal long-term effect of this inhibition is a progressive decline in the amount of LH in the pituitary gland. This appears to be due to inhibition of the synthesis of LH by the gonadotropes, largely due to negative feedback by the high concentrations of oestrogens towards the end of gestation. The depletion of the pituitary stores of LH means that as pregnancy progresses the response of the pituitary gland to GnRH is greatly diminished, the concentration of LH in the circulation is low and the ovaries are relatively quiescent. Immediately after calving, the cow has a period of anoestrus, the length of which can be influenced by age, season, nutritional status, dystokia, milk yield, suckling, uterine pathology or subclinical disease.

In the days immediately after parturition the hypothalamic–pituitary–ovarian axis is no longer functioning as a highly integrated tripartite regulatory system: the non-cyclic (anoestrous) ovaries have become sleeping partners. Before breeding can begin, the ovaries must be re-activated and re-instated as fully active members of the axis. This will involve adjustments in the activities of all three components plus the uterus, which influences the activities of the ovaries via a local utero-ovarian axis.

RE-ACTIVATION OF THE HYPOTHALAMIC–PITUITARY–OVARIAN AXIS

The mechanisms for the synthesis and release of GnRH by the hypothalamus and those for the release of the gonadotrophins by the pituitary gland appear to remain intact and functional throughout pregnancy. Secretion of FSH requires minimal stimulation by GnRH and FSH is not considered to be a major limiting factor in the resumption of cyclic ovarian activity. In the recently calved cow, FSH is secreted at an average frequency of one pulse every 2 hours and plasma concentrations reach a peak within five days after parturition before reverting to the levels found in the normal oestrous cycle. Therefore, the core of the problem for the postparturient cow is the need to restore the pituitary stores of LH to their normal levels so that the pituitary gland can respond to pulses of GnRH by releasing pulses of LH of sufficient amplitude to stimulate follicular maturation.

Nett (1987) reviewed the literature and proposed that the re-activation of the hypothalamic–pituitary–ovarian axis during the postpartum period is a two-phase process. In the first phase, which may last for two to five weeks after calving, the frequency of the GnRH pulse generator is low (one pulse every 4–8 hours) but it is adequate to stimulate the biosynthetic machinery in the gonadotropes; the rate of synthesis of LH is increased. Each pulse of GnRH releases a relatively small pulse of LH but the amplitude and frequency of these LH pulses is insufficient to stimulate the growth of large follicles in the ovaries. Because the pulses of GnRH are sufficiently spaced only a small portion of the newly synthesized LH is released into the circulation and, gradually, the pituitary replenishes its stores of LH. Eventually there is enough LH to provide pulses of sufficient amplitude to stimulate the growth of large follicles. This marks the beginning of the second phase. The growing follicles begin to secrete more oestradiol which, in the early stages, reaches the hypothalamic–pituitary axis in the low concentrations that stimulate the formation of oestrogen receptors in the hypothalamus and anterior pituitary gland. This increases the sensitivity of these tissues to feedback effects of oestrogen. The growing follicles produce relatively small pulses of oestrogen that exert a positive effect on the GnRH-induced release of LH. Thus, the hypothalamic–pituitary axis has re-established active functional links with the ovaries and the extended axis has initiated the cascade of hormonal and morphological changes that will culminate in a preovulatory surge of LH and ovulation.

OESTROUS CYCLES IN POSTPARTUM COWS

The first ovulation may or may not be associated with oestrus; estimates of silent ovulation range from 40 to 70 per cent. Frequently, oestrus is not observed until the end of the first full-length oestrous cycle. The first preovulatory surge of LH may be followed in some cows by a complete cycle with a normal luteal phase. However, other cows may have an initial cycle of normal duration but with reduced concentrations of progesterone. Another group that may constitute approximately 50 per cent of either the dairy herd or the beef herd has been reported to have a short luteal phase of five to ten days duration during which the corpus luteum secretes reduced amounts of progesterone (Lamming *et al.*, 1981). These corpora lutea are not killed by the usual luteolytic process: their ability to synthesize progesterone is lost prematurely. The transient low levels of progesterone after the first ovulation may have a significant (but, as yet, unidentified) effect on hypothalamic function and they almost certainly play a role in ensuring that oestrus is expressed before the second ovulation.

As mentioned above, a variety of factors can delay the onset of oestrous cycles. Nett (1987) suggested that the first phase of the recovery process, i.e. the events leading to normal stores of LH in the pituitary gland, is relatively independent of the suckling stimulus and environmental stressors but that the second phase, i.e. events leading to an increased frequency of LH pulses, is susceptible to inhibition by such factors.

In general, milked dairy cows ovulate earlier in the postpartum period than do suckling dairy cows or beef cows. For instance, Lamming's group at Nottingham has reported that milk progesterone profiles on 505 milked dairy cows indicated a mean calving-to-first-ovulation interval of 24 days compared with approximately 60 days for 365 suckled beef cows. Suckling depresses the frequency of LH pulses, probably because it induces a release of endogenous opioids that inhibit the normal pulsatility of the hypothalamic–pituitary axis. There are high concentrations of prolactin in the circulation of lactating cows but, according to Lamming *et al.* (1981), there is no evidence that hyperprolactinaemia plays a significant role in the suckling-induced inhibition of ovarian activity. The potency of the suckling stimulus declines with time after parturition. The duration of the period of inhibition can be influenced by other environmental factors, such as poor nutrition or season at calving (photoperiod?). For instance, cows that calved during January to June took significantly longer to resume ovarian activity than did those that calved during July to December (Lamming *et al.*, 1981).

The primary objective of the neuroendocrine adjustments in the early postpartum period is to reinstate the ovaries as fully functional components of the hypothalamic–pituitary–ovarian axis.

UTERINE INVOLUTION

It should be emphasized that the uterus exercises some control over the activities of the ovaries by way of a local utero-ovarian axis and that uterine pathology can put a brake on the ovarian contribution to the larger neuroendocrine axis. Synthesis and metabolism of $PGF_{2\alpha}$ are elevated in the bovine uterus during the early postpartum period and this is reflected in the presence of a major metabolite (PGFM) in the blood at that time. There is accumulating evidence that ovarian function does not resume until the concentration of this metabolite has fallen below a critical threshold. There appears to be a significant negative correlation between the duration of elevated concentrations of PGFM after calving and the time required for completion of uterine involution (Lindell & Kindahl, 1983). Persistent uterine infections prolong the period of high concentrations of PGFM and the time to uterine involution. A problem may arise in the infected cow that ovulates very early in the postpartum period because these continuously elevated concentrations of prostaglandin are not sufficient to induce luteolysis and a mutual interdependence between the infection and the corpus luteum may be established, thus rendering the cow liable to develop pyometra. However, the majority of cows do not ovulate until after the postpartum infections have been eliminated from the uterus, a process that may be enhanced by the fluctuating levels of oestrogens released from the follicles that begin to grow in the ovaries in response to FSH released by the pituitary throughout the early weeks after parturition.

During the second week after parturition the pool of antral follicles in the ovaries is increased both in dairy cows and in beef cows. The increase in numbers is largely due to the development of medium-size follicles (4–8 mm in diameter), particularly in the ovary contralateral to the previous pregnancy. This predominance of the contralateral ovary seems to persist for about four weeks, with the result that the majority of first ovulations are from the contralateral ovary. It has been suggested that a very early ovulation from the ipsilateral ovary in an infected cow may increase the risk of development of pyometra (Hartigan *et al.*, 1974).

It is perfectly 'normal' for bacteria to invade the bovine uterus during the first few days after parturition. Bacteriological studies have revealed that a very wide range of micro-organisms, both pathogens and commensals, gain entry but repetitive sampling showed that when parturition was uncomplicated the contamination of the uterus was transient and that the isolates varied from one sample to the next. At the end of the fourth week postpartum only 30 per cent of the cows had bacteria in the uterus, mostly non-pathogens (Griffin *et al.* 1974). Under optimal conditions, most cows have eliminated the pathogenic contaminants before cyclic ovarian activity begins. On the other hand, cows that experience dystokia, traumatic damage to the endometrium or retention of placental membranes are less efficient in dealing with pathogens. There is a significant reduction in the efficiency of phagocytic cells in the endometrium and uterine lumen and, as a result, potential pathogens may persist and induce endometritis or metritis. Again, in the majority of cows the endometritis tends to be short-lived; the combination of phagocytosis, local antibody production and myometrial contractions that are normal features of the involutionary period effect clearance of the micro-organisms and resolution of the endometritis. However, it is important to stress that infusion of irritants (antibiotics, iodine) that inhibit phagocytosis, extensive intra-uterine manipulation that damages the endometrium or an early ovulation that causes the onset of a precocious luteal phase may permit a pathogenic micro-organism to become established within the uterus, particularly if the concentration of PGFM is still high. In such circumstances the prostaglandin produced by the uterus is inadequate to cause luteolysis. The result is that the defense mechanisms of the host are depressed by the progesterone from the corpus luteum and the pathogens cause continuing damage to the endometrium, thus preventing the release of a luteolytic dose of prostaglandin. At this stage, the pathogen and the corpus luteum have established a mutual interdependence that predisposes to the development of pyometra. The vicious circle can be broken by exogenous prostaglandin. The important point is that inappropriate medication early in the postpartum period can interfere with the physiological progress of involution and induce long-term pathological consequences.

If purulent endometritis/metritis develops it does not abolish ovarian activity immediately and totally. Initially, it causes prolonged cycles, usually with silent ovulations for some months before anoestrus supervenes. Obviously, the best prospects of full recovery to fertility will depend on diagnosis and treatment before the hypothalamic–pituitary axis ceases to function.

References

Baird, D.T. (1984) In *Reproduction in Mammals*, 2nd edn (ed. by C.R. Austin & R.V. Short), Book 3, p. 104. Cambridge University Press.

Bedford, J.M. (1983) Significance of the need for sperm capacitation before fertilization in eutherian mammals. *Biology of Reproduction*, **28**, 108–20.

Bloom, W. & Fawcett, D.W. (1968) A Textbook of Histology, 10th edn., p. 824, Saunders, Philadelphia.

Genuth, S.M. (1988) In *Physiology* (eds R.M. Berne & M.N.C. Levy) 2nd edn., p. 993, Mosby, St. Louis.

Griffin, J.F.T., Hartigan, P.J. & Nunn, W.R. (1974) Non-specific uterine infection and bovine fertility I and II. *Theriogenology*, **1**, 91–106 and 107–14.

Grumbach, M.M., Roth, J.C., Kaplen, J.L. & Kelch, R.P. (1974) In *Control of the onset of puberty* (eds M.M. Grumbach, G.D. Grove & F.E. Meyer) p. 158. Wiley, New York.

Hansel, W. & Snook, R.B. (1970) Pituitary ovarian relationships in the cow. *Journal of Dairy Science*, **53**, 945–61.

Hartigan, P.J., Langley, O.H., Nunn, W.R. & Griffin, J.F.T. (1974) Some data on ovarian activity in post-parturient dairy cows in Ireland. *Irish Veterinary Journal*, **28**, 236–41.

Hunter, R.H.F. & Wilmut, I. (1984) Sperm transport in the cow: peri-ovulatory redistribution of viable cells. *Reproduction Nutrition Development*, **214**, 597–608.

Lamming, G.E., Wathes, D.C. & Peters, A.R. (1981) Endocrine patterns in the post-partum cow. *Journal of Reproduction and Fertility*, Supplement **30**, 155–70.

Lindell, J.O. & Kindahl, H. (1983) Exogenous prostaglandin $F_{2\alpha}$ promotes uterine involution in the cow. *Acta Veterinaria Scandinavica*, **24**, 269–74

Marion, G.H. & Gier, H.T. (1971) Ovarian and uterine embryogenesis and morphology of the nonpregnant female mammal. *Journal of Animal Science*, **32** Supplement 1, 24–47.

McLaren, A. (1984) In *Reproduction in Mammals*, 2nd edn. (eds C.R. Austin & R.V. Short) book 3, p. 21. Cambridge University Press, Cambridge.

Moran, C., Quirke, J.F. & Roche, J.F. (1989) Puberty in heifers: a review. *Animal Reproduction Science*, **8**, 167–82.

Nett, T.M. (1987) Function of the hypothalamic–hypophyseal axis during the post-partum period in ewes and cows. *Journal of Reproduction and Fertility*, Supplement 34, 201–13.

Rahe, C.H., Owens, R.E., Fleegen, J.L., Newton, A.J. & Harms, D.G. (1980) Pattern of plasmaluteinizing hormone in the cyclic cow: dependence upon the period of the cycle. *Endocrinology*, **107**, 498–503.

Short, R.V. (1984) In *Reproduction in Mammals*, 2nd edn. (eds C.R. Austin & R.V. Short) book 3, p. 139. Cambridge University Press, Cambridge.

Chapter 31: Problems After Calving

by H. BOYD

This chapter deals with the important diseases of the two-week period after calving, the puerperium. Various problems occur at this stage including forms of trauma and prolapse, acute metritis, necrotic vaginitis and retained fetal membranes.

What happens at, and after, calving is the basis for subsequent efficient reproduction. This is clearly demonstrated by the adverse effect of all the abnormalities listed above on return to cyclicity and to pregnancy rates. Postparturient metabolic diseases, such as parturient paresis, have a similar effect. The foundations for successful herd fertility are:

1 good 'general' health;
2 adequate nutrition before, and after, calving; and
3 good reproductive health at, and after, calving.

There have been some advances in this field in the last few years but much of the basic knowledge is well established and to avoid lengthy description and discussion of conditions well known to every bovine practitioner, only the main features of the important conditions and recent developments will be listed.

Manifestation

Reproductive abnormalities that occur in the puerperial period include the following.

Retained fetal membranes. A common condition that is defined as non-separation of the fetal membranes by 24 hours (or 12 hours by some workers) after calving. The incidence varies from study to study but tends to be about 11 per cent (Wetherill, 1965; Arthur *et al.*, 1989); in a survey of >160 000 calvings in The Netherlands the average incidence was only 6.6 per cent (Joosten *et al.*, 1988). The manifestation is self-apparent, the major variable being the effect of the condition on the cow's health. In many cases health is unaffected. However, possibly the majority of cows are off colour with mild disturbances of appetite, respiration and body temperature. In a small number of cows, acute metritis develops and the cow is very ill, with typical signs of toxaemia and septicaemia. Without effective treatment this condition can be fatal.

Acute puerperal metritis is relatively rare. Acute inflammatory changes occur in the endometrial, myometrial and peritoneal layers of the uterus within a few days of calving. A fetid, reddish discharge flows from the vulva and abdominal straining is noted. Septicaemic and toxaemic signs are present.

Traumatic lesions of the birth canal and to pelvic nerves sometimes follow dystokia. Problems include penetrating wounds of the uterus or vagina, tearing of the cervix, rectovaginal fistula, tearing of the vulva and prolapse of the uterus or vagina.

Necrotic vaginitis can be caused by trauma and excessive pressure. It is a painful condition manifested by straining, raised tail and discharge of purulent material and necrotic tissue from the vulva. On occasion, infection spreads to the uterus causing metritis.

Periparturient metabolic diseases are dealt with elsewhere in this book (see Chapter 39).

Aetiology

Retained fetal membranes. Fetal membrane retention has been reviewed by Paisley *et al.* (1986). There are two main ways in which retention occurs.

1 Interference with the separation of the fetal villi from the maternal caruncles. This can be associated with the following.

(a) Premature calving (induced or spontaneous) without the normal histological preparation for separation.
(b) Prolonged gestation resulting in excessive growth of the dam's caruncles.
(c) Trauma with oedema of the villi, which occurs after caesarean section, torsion of the uterus and other dystokias.
(d) Infectious conditions (with or without abortion) result in inflammatory changes that bind together the maternal and fetal tissue in the placentome.
(e) Hyperaemia of the placentomes.
(f) Necrosis of the villi.

2 Lack of uterine contractions. Observations on uterine contractions after calving suggest that in many cases of retained fetal membranes, their frequency and amplitude are greater than in cows that released the membranes normally. However, on some occasions retention is associated with uterine atony: for instance after over-extension of the myometrium as in cases of hydrops allantois, or prolonged labour, or in hypocalcaemic cows.

Acute puerperal metritis. In all cows during and after calving the uterus is exposed to infection from the surrounding environment. Studies of the bacterial population of the uterus in the week after calving have resulted in reports that vary from claims that 'all or nearly all cows' have a large polymicrobial population in the uterus to statements that 'less than half' of the cows examined are infected. Some of this variation may be due to timing of sampling. Under normal circumstances the natural defence mechanisms will have eliminated all the injurious bacteria about two to four weeks after calving and the isolate will be largely non-pathogenic contaminants.

Why then should a relatively small number of cows become seriously ill with acute metritis? The physiology of the response to normal postpartum infection suggests that there are two main factors that lead to a pathological result.

1 The uterus is exposed to an unusually high polymicrobial challenge that includes some of the more pathogenic organisms.

(a) Two common factors that increase the burden of infection on the uterus are dystokia, with resultant trauma inside the uterus, and the use of dirty calving boxes.
(b) After delivery of an emphysematous calf the uterus may be heavily infected with anaerobic organisms.
(c) Retained fetal membranes increase the level of infection.
(d) There is evidence of synergistic action between infectious agents, such as *Actinomyces (Corynebacterium) pyogenes* and anaerobic organisms (*Fusobacterium necrophorum* and *Bacteroides melaninogenicus*), which is believed to be aetiologically important (Olson *et al.*, 1984).

There is no evidence that high exposure to non-pyogenic organisms necessarily results in invasion of the uterus nor that the strains of pathogens that do cause metritis are inherently more pathogenic than those that are eliminated by the majority of cows.

2 The natural defence mechanisms are less effective than normal. Important factors that cause this include the following.

(a) Dystokia.
(b) Manipulation within the uterus after calving.
(c) Lack of uterine contractions.
(d) Concomitant infection with immunosuppressant organisms such as IBR virus.
(e) The effect of diet before calving is unresolved; it is possible that excess energy intake leading to fatty liver, insufficient protein and micromineral deficiency may impair the uterine defence mechanisms.

Traumatic lesions. The aetiology of most of these is self-apparent. Necrotic vaginitis is initiated by trauma of the vagina during parturition, often as the result of pressure from delivery of a relatively oversized calf or by calving ropes or instruments. Infection with *F. necrophorum* or *Clostridium* species results in a locally severe reaction and serious systemic illness.

Diagnosis

In many cases presented immediately after calving, diagnosis is quite simple, for example, retained fetal membranes or prolapse of the uterus. However, a cow that is acutely ill just after calving could be suffering from a variety of conditions including acute metritis and, therefore, a systematic approach to diagnosis is necessary both for differential diagnosis and to ascertain the seriousness of the condition.

History. The history will not aid diagnosis very much in individual cases but may aid in the understanding of the aetiology so that appropriate herd preventive measures may be advocated.

Conditions and events before calving. This covers whether the cow was ill before calving, either illness not related to reproduction or conditions that are obviously related, such as pathological vaginal discharge.

Information about feeding and management before calving should be gathered, with the object of finding whether the diet predisposed to metabolic diseases, including fatty liver.

Conditions and events at, and after, calving

1 The place where the cow calved should be inspected to assess the level of environmental hygiene during calving.

2 The farmer should be asked if the calving was assisted and, if so, how much and what help was given, by whom and what hygienic precautions were taken.

3 Details of treatment given by the client have to be recorded, in particular antibiotics and treatment for milk fever.

4 The clinician should find out if the condition is common in the herd.

General examination. A thorough general clinical examination must be undertaken.

Specific reproductive examination

1 *Rectal palpation*. In cases of acute metritis the local examination should be as gentle as possible. Rectal examination will indicate the size of the uterus and if it is inflamed; however, rectal examination contributes very little to the diagnosis. Handling should be kept to the minimum because there is a danger of causing exudation from the mesometrium and producing adhesions. In acute metritis the uterus is friable and easily damaged. Rectal examination is not indicated in cases of retained fetal membranes.

2 *Vaginal examination*. A careful, gentle manual exploration carried out with due hygienic precautions and lubrication will reveal local damage to the vagina, and if it causes straining will demonstrate the nature of the fluid in the uterus.

3 *Intra-uterine examination*. There is no real indication for this. Manipulation inside the uterus should be minimal as it can reduce the uterine defence mechanism by curtailing phagocytosis. In acute metritis it is contraindicated because of tissue damage and the distress to the animal. If the veterinarian intends to remove retained fetal membranes manually it is necessary to examine the strength of attachment by intrauterine palpation but this will be done when treatment is attempted.

4 *Laboratory examination*. Microbiological examination can be used to identify the causative organisms and assess their sensitivity to different antibiotics. In acute cases that require immediate treatment the knowledge acquired is of little immediate value but can be useful if a change of treatment is indicated and for understanding the aetiology.

If it is possible, a swab is introduced via a sterile speculum to minimize contamination. Samples should be cultured aerobically and anaerobically. The method of storing and transporting the sample to the laboratory should be discussed beforehand with microbiologists at the laboratory.

There is little point in sampling for bacteriology in cases of retained fetal membrane because, inevitably, there will be a variety of incidental micro-organisms.

Treatment

Retained fetal membranes. Veterinarians have been arguing over the need for manual removal of retained fetal membranes for decades. It should be borne in mind that although theoretical considerations and the results of some field trials tend to favour non-removal there are also arguments in favour of manual removal, which include the following.

1 It removes a major source of infection and putrefying protein.

2 It removes the unpleasant smell, which can taint the milk, and physical presence of the retained membranes.

3 The cow may be less likely to develop systemic illness.

4 The cow may be less likely to have disturbed fertility later.

5 The cow may be less likely to suffer from reduced milk yield.

Perhaps the most powerful argument in favour of manual removal is that a small number of conservatively treated cows become very ill and require life-saving treatment.

Those in favour of manual removal claim that the danger of reproductive or general disease is greatly reduced, with gentle handling, a willingness to stop manual removal where the attachment is firm and the use of local or systemic antibiotics.

The technique has been described in a number of standard text books (e.g. Arthur *et al.*, 1989).

The arguments used against manual removal of the retained fetal membranes include the following.

1 The cow just after calving is ready to deal with the large amount of infected material and decomposing necrotic caruncles that are sloughed off into the uterus in the normal course of events; the need to get rid of fetal membranes as well presents no insurmountable problem to most cows.

2 Intra-uterine manual intervention should be avoided because it interferes with the natural defence mechanism by reducing phagocytosis for several days.

3 Manual removal of the membranes is never complete and numerous villi and remnants of placenta are left attached.

4 Manual removal causes trauma and adds to the likelihood of persisting local infection.

5 If the cow is ill, systemic treatment is sufficient to deal with the problem and manual removal may make the cow even more ill.

Some advocates of conservative treatment may intervene only if the animal develops signs of systemic disease, in which cases the treatment is systemic administration of a broad-spectrum antibiotic. Other veterinarians simply cut off the part of the membranes that is visible to reduce the smell and only apply other treatment in those (few) cases that become ill.

Prostaglandin $F_{2\alpha}$ or analogues has been administered systemically to encourage the removal of fetal membranes. Similarly, oxytocin used up to 36 hours after calving may increase myometrial contractions and hasten expulsion of the membranes. Oestrogen alone has also been used (but is likely contraindicated).

While there is argument about the best treatment at the time of retention, there is general agreement that it is important to examine cases of retained fetal membranes about 18–30 days after calving to identify and treat those cows that have developed chronic metritis or pyometra.

Acute metritis. The major concern in treating a case of acute metritis is that the cow is seriously ill and that death is a real danger. The cow should be moved to a well-bedded, comfortable box and encouraged to eat and drink. Nursing is important. As these cases are septicaemic and toxaemic they should be treated as described elsewhere (Chapter 38). Systemic antibiotic treatment applied in the correct dose and maintained over the full recommended course is essential. Choice of antibiotic will be influenced by the clinician's experience and local knowledge. For follow-up treatment, antibiotic sensitivity tests will help in the correct choice of antibiotic.

Uterine infusion and drainage is to be avoided while the cow is systemically ill. On the other hand, after the acute phase of the disease a technique of gentle flushing and fluid withdrawal, as described by Arthur *et al.* (1989) reduces the quantity of infected material in the uterus and facilitates myometrial contractions.

Many clinicians introduce antibiotics into the uterus after systemic treatment but the following points, discussed by Paisley *et al.* (1986), should be borne in mind in connection with the intra-uterine infusion of antibiotics.

1 Pus and organic debris can inhibit sulphonamides, aminoglycosides and nitrofurazone.

2 Enzymes that inactivate some antibiotics (e.g. penicillinase) may be produced by some of the organisms found in the uterus.

3 The anaerobic (or partially anaerobic) environment of the uterus interferes with the action of those antibiotics that require oxygen to work (gentamicin, kanamycin, streptomycin, neomycin).

4 Many antibiotic preparations are in media that are irritant to the endometrium and therefore may increase absorption of toxins from the lumen.

Traumatic lesions. These are treated according to general principles of wound treatment. In the case of necrotic vaginitis emollient fluids are applied locally along with an appropriate systemic antibiotic.

Prognosis

Retained fetal membranes. Moller *et al.* (1967) describe a large clinical trial in which the results of a wide variety of treatments were studied. They pointed out that cows that are ill and cows with metritis must be treated but they concluded that the evidence did not indicate a need to treat cases of uncomplicated placental retention. In fact it appeared that any type of drug therapy for this condition tended to depress subsequent pregnancy rates, whereas cows that were not treated (that is membranes not removed, no drug therapy administered) had pregnancy rates that were not significantly different from those achieved by cows that passed the membranes at the proper time. The use of an oestrogen in cases of retained fetal membranes was contraindicated.

The effect of retained fetal membranes on subsequent fertility depends on whether metritis develops or not, which in turn may be affected by the therapy employed; unfortunately this information is usually absent from reports.

In an extensive field study with cows that retained the placenta for at least 48 hours, Leslie *et al.* (1984) reported that 14 per cent of the cows developed pyometra and 15 per cent developed chronic endometritis. In four herds in which a conservative approach to treatment was employed, metritis developed in 40 of 73 cases of retained fetal membranes (Sandals *et al.*, 1979). From study of days to service, days to conception and services per conception these authors concluded that the condition of retained fetal membranes alone has little effect on subsequent fertility. In a large field study (Halpern *et al.*, 1985) 45 per cent and 41 per cent of primiparous and pluriparous cows with retained fetal membranes developed metritis. In the heifers there was no significant adverse effect of retained fetal membranes on fertility. In adult cows with no subsequent metritis, retention for five or more days caused poorer pregnancy rates than controls. Retention for more than seven days caused a long calving-to-service interval and poor pregnancy rate.

Rowlands & Lucey (1986) reported that the lactation yield following retained fetal membranes was 7 per cent lower than expected.

Acute metritis. With acute metritis prognosis refers to the possibility of death, adverse effect on health, yield and future reproductive function. Most of these cases make a fairly slow recovery as regards body condition, milk yield and return to cyclicity and pregnancy.

Rosenberger & Tillman (1960) reported that mortality in treated cases was 1 per cent milk yield was reduced to about 75 per cent of expected quantity; and about 30–40 per cent of cases exhibited subsequent infertility with 25 per cent of these being eventually culled as infertile. Sandals *et al.* (1979) reported 2 (7 per cent) deaths in 29 cases with retained fetal membranes complicated by acute metritis. After recovery there may be adhesions affecting the uterus, the oviducts and bursal area, resulting in reduced fertility.

Traumatic lesions. Response to treatment of vaginal lesions is usually good and the signs will disappear within about 10 days. In these cases there is no interference with future reproduction. In a few cases the infection spreads and affects the uterus with resultant poor prognosis for fertility. Scar tissue may cause narrowing of the birth canal and interference with the next calving.

Concerning nerve damage, reference should be made to Chapter 29 or to obstetrical text books.

Prevention

The most important way of reducing puerperal problems is to avoid dystokia. Where dystokia does occur it is essential that it is dealt with correctly at an early stage and that any developing problems observed after calving are also treated as soon as possible. Attention to all aspects of hygiene is also a basic requirement.

Dystokia. If it were a purely veterinary matter it would be relatively simple to reduce the incidence of dystokia in the majority of herds. However, the measures required may not be acceptable to the farmer. Simple modifications such as improved supervision of calving and better housing may be judged to be too expensive. The breed of bull that gives least dystokia, such as Aberdeen Angus, may not produce the type of calves wanted. The farmer may want to use a breed, such as Charolais, that may produce many dystokias.

Particular consideration has to be given to the possible effect of embryo transfer of large, dystokia-prone breeds, into unsuitable recipients.

The consequences of several synergistic adverse effects tend to be particularly serious. Therefore, if a client choses to use a breed or bull that is liable to produce a high rate of dystokia it is particularly important to avoid any other factor that predisposes to dystokia.

Application of the following precautions will reduce the incidence of dystokia in a herd.

1 Selection of sires that produce calves of suitable size and conformation for the dams concerned. This refers to the breed and to the individual bull within the breed. Special care is needed for first calvers.

2 Induction of premature calving, if the fetus is likely to be too large at full term for a normal calving.

3 Control of energy intake and avoidance of macromineral imbalances.

(a) Do not let the dams get too fat, as the perirectal and perivaginal fat will narrow the birth canal, the dam may be less capable of forceful labour, and the calf may also be larger. This is also an important way of avoiding necrotic vaginitis and other damage to the vagina. At calving a condition score of 2.5 (p. 16) is advised.

(b) Avoid undernutrition as cows in very poor condition have more problems of dystokia.

4 Assuring a suitable environment, especially for cows that calve inside or in a restricted area. This should be clean, well bedded, with a good water supply, properly lit and with enough space to get at the cow if need be and to allow observation without disturbing the cow.

The farm staff should be in reasonably comfortable surroundings while observing and assisting the cows.

5 Avoid stress and disturbance of the calving cow (Hindson, 1976).

6 Suitable supervision and timely intervention at calving will reduce the severity of those cases of dystokia that do occur (Hodge *et al.*, 1982). Too precipitate intervention has also to be avoided.

7 Proper training of the farmer and stockworkers in how to assist at calving. This training should be supplied either by the veterinarian or in a suitable course (Blowey, 1988).

8 When veterinary assistance is needed, the farmer and his staff must decide at an early stage to call for help. It is important that the veterinarian and the farmer should agree before the start of the calving season how these problems will be dealt with and at what stage the farmer will call for professional help.

Treatment of cows after calving. Attempts to prevent retained fetal membranes by routine treatment of all cows at calving are generally ineffective and impractical because of the relatively low incidence and morbidity of the condition. The incidence of retention is increased greatly when parturition is induced with corticosteroids and there is evidence that prostaglandin $F_{2\alpha}$ can be an effective therapeutic agent in such cases. Gross *et al.* (1986) used dexamethasone to induce parturition in 66 cows; they injected prostaglandin $F_{2\alpha}$ into 40 cows within 1 hour of delivery and treated 26 cows with saline (controls). The incidence of retention in the prostaglandin $F_{2\alpha}$ treated cows was 8.8 per cent compared with 90.5 per cent in the controls.

The value of treatment with prostaglandin $F_{2\alpha}$ or an analogue soon after full-term calving is still a matter for discussion. Results obtained by Herschler & Lawrence (1984) and Studer & Holtan (1986) suggest that routine treatment 8–14 hours after parturition with an analogue of prostaglandin $F_{2\alpha}$ can reduce the incidence of metritis in cases with retained fetal membranes.

Oxytocin injection 3–6 hours after calving does not appear to be very effective in preventing retained fetal membranes (Miller & Lodge, 1984).

All cows that are assisted at calving should receive a course of systemic antibiotic treatment starting as soon as they calve.

Metabolic diseases, such as milk fever, should be dealt with appropriately and if these cases are common, investigation into their causes is essential. This aspect of bovine medicine is dealt with elsewhere in this book (p. 577).

References

Arthur, G.H., Noakes, D.E. & Pearson, H. (1989) *Veterinary Reproduction and Obstetrics (Theriogenology)*, pp. 1–641. Baillière Tindall, London.

Blowey, R.W. (1988) *A Veterinary Book for Dairy Farmers*, p. 1–456. Farming Press, Ipswich.

Gross, T.S., Williams, W.F. & Moreland, T.W. (1986) Prevention of the retained fetal membrane syndrome (retained placenta) during induced calving in dairy cattle. *Theriogenology*, **26**, 365–70.

Halpern, N.E., Erb, H.N. & Smith, R.D. (1985) Duration of retained fetal membranes and subsequent fertility in dairy cows. *Theriogenology*, **23**, 807–13.

Herschler, R.C. & Lawrence, J.R. (1984) A prostaglandin analogue for therapy of retained placentae. *Veterinary Medicine and Small Animal Clinica*, 822–6.

Hindson, J.C. (1976) Retention of the fetal membranes in cattle. *Veterinary Record*, **99**, 49–50.

Hodge, P.B., Wood, S.J., Newman, R.D. & Shepherd, R.K. (1982) Effect of calving supervision upon the calving performance of Hereford heifers. *Australian Veterinary Journal*, **58**, 97–100.

Joosten, I., Stelwagen, J. & Dijkhuizen, A.A. (1988) Economic and reproductive consequences of retained placenta in dairy cattle. *Veterinary Record*, **123**, 53–7.

Leslie, K.E., Doig, P.A., Bosu, W.T.K., Curtis, R.A. & Martin, S.W. (1984) Effects of gonadotrophin releasing hormone on reproductive performance of dairy cows with retained placenta. *Canadian Journal of Comparative Medicine*, **48**, 354–9.

Miller, B.J. & Lodge, J.R. (1984) Postpartum oxytocin treatment for prevention of retained placentas. *Theriogenology*, **22**, 385–8.

Moller, K., Newling, P.E., Robson, H.J., Jansen, G.J., Meursinge J.A. & Cooper, M.G. (1967) Retained fetal membranes in dairy herds in the Huntly district. *New Zealand Veterinary Journal*, **15**, 111–16.

Olson, J.D., Ball, T., Mortimer, R.G., Farin, P.W., Adney, W.S. & Huffman, E.M. (1984) Aspects of bacteriology and endocrinology of cows with pyometra and retained fetal membranes. *American Journal of Veterinary Research*, **45**, 2251–5.

Paisley, L.G., Mickelsen, W.D. & Anderson, P.B. (1986) Mechanisms and therapy for retained fetal membranes and uterine infections of cows: A review. *Theriogenology*, **25**, 353–81.

Rosenberger, G. & Tillmann, H. (1960) *Tiergeburtshilfe*. Paul Parey, Berlin and Hamburg.

Rowlands, G.J. & Lucey, S. (1986) Changes in milk yield in dairy cows associated with metabolic and reproductive diseases and lameness. *Preventive Veterinary Medicine*, **4**, 205–21.

Sandals, W.C.D., Curtis, R.A., Cote, J.F. & Martin, S.W. (1979) The effect of retained placenta and metritis complex on reproductive performance in dairy cattle — a case control study. *Canadian Veterinary Journal*, **20**, 131–5.

Studer, E. and Holtan, A. (1986) Treatment of retained placentas in dairy cattle with prostaglandin. *Bovine Practitioner*, No. 21, 159–60.

Wetherill, G.D. (1965) Retained placenta in the bovine: a brief review. *Canadian Veterinary Journal*, **6**, 290–4.

Chapter 32: Oestrus and Oestrous Cycles: Problems and Failures

by H. BOYD

Manifestation

Normal oestrous cycles, clear oestrous expression and efficient and accurate detection of oestrus are essential for the successful management of reproduction in cattle.

Failure to observe oestrus or lack of oestrus adversely affect the efficiency of production and profitability by interfering with the reproductive markers shown in Table 32.1.

Inaccurate oestrous detection, i.e. identification of a cow as being in oestrus when she is not, leads to cows being served when fertilization is not possible because there is no ovulation at the expected time after insemination.

Considerable economic loss is caused by missed services that result in longer than planned intervals from calving to first service. A missed oestrus will cause a delay of about 21 days until the next chance for service and this loss in milk production time and delay in producing a calf results in a loss of income. Assessment of the real loss (litres of milk/year; calves/100 cows/year) and the economic loss is complex (James & Esslemont, 1979), particularly in times of overproduction of milk. It has been suggested that in the UK a loss of up to £3/day occurs for every day over planned calving interval at the present time (1990). An American estimate in 1986 was $2.50/day (Bartlett *et al.*, 1986). In beef cows, delay in achieving pregnancy results in a similar loss; this is partly due to management problems but also because at weaning the calf is younger and therefore weighs less.

Clients present individual cases of cows that have not been seen in oestrus when due or overdue for service but mostly the problem is seen on routine fertility visits when postservice anoestrus is also detected. The problem, which is most serious when it occurs on a herd or group basis, is often picked up on herd record analysis.

Heifers. Delayed puberty may affect targets for breeding age or date. It occurs mainly as a group problem because heifers are handled and fed in groups and the cause of anoestrus is nearly always related to the environment or to the management, particularly feeding. Occasionally, anoestrus is manifested in a group of heifers after natural service, which the farmer erroneously thought was successful because of lack of returns to service.

Cows after calving. An extended interval between calving and first service, calculated on a herd basis, is the most important manifestation of dysfunction of cyclicity and oestrus. A farmer with a serious problem may not be aware of it because of poor records or good ones that are not used properly. In the example given in Table 32.2, in 15 herds that were not in fertility control programmes, the target for calving interval was 12 months and to achieve this target, cows should have had their first services 56–76 days after calving. The distribution of days from calving to first service for the 1595 cows served in these herds shows that about half of the cows were first served after the target date (Boyd & Munro, 1980).

On the best farm, 67 per cent of the cows were served within 77 days of calving and on the worst farm only 21 per cent of cows reached that target.

The situation in this group of herds is quite typical of the results obtained in many surveys carried out in different countries and demonstrates the seriousness of

Table 32.1 Aspects of reproduction affected by failure to observe, or lack of, oestrus

Heifers
Age at first calving
Season of first calving
Cows
Interval from calving to first service (and thus calving to conception)
Timely observation of returns to service

Table 32.2 Percentage of cows with various calving-to-first-service intervals in days

	Calving-to-first-service interval (days)			
	0–55	Target 56–77	78–99	>100
Per cent cows	15.9	32.2	24.7	27.1
Cumulative per cent	15.9	48.1	72.8	99.9

Table 32.3 Percentage of cows with various intervals between services in days (Warren, 1984)

	Inter-service interval (days)					
	1–17	18–24	25–35	36–48	49–90	91+
Per cent cows	6	37	13	18	18	8

the problem. Within herds the incidence of the problem is quite variable at different times and there may be periods of four to six weeks when a high proportion of cows appear to stop cycling or exhibit poor oestrus signs.

The number of cows treated by veterinarians for anoestrus and suboestrus is much lower. Saloniemi *et al.* (1986) gave the incidence as 5.2 per cent of cows, falling from first calvers (6.3 per cent) to older cows (3.7 per cent). Markusfeld (1987) diagnosed inactive ovaries after two rectal examinations in 8.5 per cent of 7751 lactations.

Another manifestation of absence of oestrus is the cow that starts cycling and then stops, a situation recorded in 5.2 per cent of cases in a survey based on progesterone assays by Bulman & Lamming (1978). In a similar study (Kassa *et al.*, 1986), cyclicity started and then stopped in four (3.2 per cent) of 125 lactations.

Cows after service. Analysis of data from approximately 35 000 cows in 255 British herds (Warren, 1984) showed that 26 per cent of interservice intervals were greater than 48 days (Table 32.3).

These results are similar to the results obtained in other surveys. For example, in the 15 herds discussed above (Table 32.2), 25 per cent of the returns to service were after a delay greater than 48 days and in Boyd & Reed's study (1961) in smaller herds at a time when management was less intensive, 23 per cent of returns were greater than 48 days.

In Warren's (1984) report the average interservice interval was 39 days, i.e. delayed return to service is 39−21 days = 18 days. This is almost exactly the same delay as was recorded by de Kruif (1975) in smaller herds in Holland. In some other surveys there were rather fewer very long intervals, possibly due to different culling patterns or more efficient heat detection. In contrast, Moller *et al.* (1986) in New Zealand reported that only 8.6 per cent of return-to-service intervals were greater than 36 days.

While survey data do not explain why a cow has not been served, discussion with farmers makes it clear that in the majority of cases the reason is that the cow has not been seen in season. In conclusion, failure to have cows served because they have not been seen in season is a widespread and important condition.

Aetiology

The aetiology of anoestrus in the cow and heifer is complex because as presented to the veterinarian it includes several different conditions as shown in Table 32.4.

Because there is a wide range of types of anoestrus there is also a wide range of causes, some unknown. Moreover, there is a variety of management and environmental factors that contribute to poor oestrous detection rates.

Physiological anoestrus. It is important to bear in mind that during certain phases of the reproductive cycle, the absence of oestrus is physiological. These are prior to puberty, during pregnancy, and for at least two weeks after calving.

Table 32.4 Aetiology of anoestrus

Physiological anoestrus: prepuberty, pregnancy, puerperium
True anoestrus: no cycle, blocked cycle (pyometra)
Silent oestrus: ovarian cycles but no behaviour
Weak oestrus: very short oestrus, poor expression
Unobserved oestrus: oestrus normal, human error

It is not uncommon for a cow that is pregnant to be presented to the veterinarian as a case of anoestrus. This occurs if there is unknown access to a bull, or unrecorded insemination, or misidentification of the cow inseminated.

In dairy cows, from which the calves are removed a day or so after birth, ovulation rarely occurs earlier than 15 days after calving. In cows that are suckling, usually beef cows, the duration of non-cyclicity may be extended. The effect of suckling of one or more calves is to inhibit the return to cyclicity via neurohormonal routes, which can be modified by nutritional factors. This is demonstrated by the observation that some well-fed, well-managed beef suckler herds achieve a tight calving pattern at the same season each year, which requires an early return to cyclicity while the cows are still suckling their calves. Dairy cows are sometimes given several calves to suckle and if their feeding level is reduced at the same time, ovarian cycles are likely to stop.

The seasonal effect, which results in a delayed return to cyclicity after calving in the spring (see pp. 437), is most marked in suckling cows.

For a list of factors that affect the onset of puberty see chapter 30.

True anoestrus. The major causes of true anoestrus are summarized in Table 32.5.

1 In heifers, bilateral gonadal aplasia, which causes permanent anoestrus and sterility, occurs in the common condition of freemartinism, found in the majority of female calves that are co-twins with males. It is also observed in bilateral ovarian hypoplasia, a rare inherited condition, in which the genes are passed on through fertile individuals with unilateral gonadal hypoplasia. Poor nutrition is important and discussed below.

Table 32.5 Major causes of true anoestrus

Heifers
Freemartinism
Ovarian hypoplasia
Inactive ovaries (poor nutrition)
Cows
Dystokia and postpartum problems
Delayed involution (inactive ovaries)
Pyometra (persistent corpus luteum)
Cystic ovarian disease
Poor nutrition, especially first calvers
Age-related factors

2 In cows a variety of abnormalities at or around calving, such as dystokia, retained fetal membranes and milk fever have been shown to be followed by delayed return to cyclicity.

These conditions tend to delay involution of the uterus and predispose to metritis. The uterus produces prostaglandin during involution (Garcia, 1982) and delayed involution results in a longer duration of prostaglandin production. Initiation of cycles is delayed until prostaglandin levels are basal, which may explain why delayed involution results in late return to cyclicity.

It is also possible that the factors which cause the initial perinatal problems also cause delayed involution and delayed return to cyclicity. It has been suggested, for example, that excess feeding, particularly of concentrates, prior to calving results in metritis after calving and also independently lengthens the time from calving to cyclicity. This complex subject has been reviewed by Sejrsen and Neimann-Soerensen (1982) and Smidt and Farries (1982).

Another serious consequence of abnormalities around calving is metritis. Metritis, among other adverse effects, will delay involution. Worse still metritis may develop into pyometra, possibly in the following way. When ovulation and the development of a corpus luteum occur in a cow in which the uterus is still infected after calving, the resultant progesterone reduces the normal uterine defence mechanism against purulent infection, causes the cervix to close tightly and reduces myometrial contractions. These then change the purulent metritis, in which the pus drains out of the uterus via the patent cervix, into a pyometra, in which the pus accumulates in the uterus. One effect of pyometra is to interfere with luteolysis, which would normally be brought about by release of prostaglandin $F_{2\alpha}$ from the endometrium. The condition of pyometra may then persist for many weeks until the corpus luteum regresses spontaneously. This is followed by oestrus, opening of the cervix and escape of pus.

3 Ovarian cysts are quite commonly recorded in cases of anoestrus and in fact the majority of cows with cystic ovarian disease exhibit anoestrus. The likely hormonal mechanism of cystic ovarian disease is failure of the preovulatory luteinizing hormone (LH) surge. In some cases there may be failure of the ovary to respond to LH at the start of oestrus (Brown *et al.*, 1986). Cystic ovarian disease is a very complex condition and in many cases, the cyst produces a mixture of steroids. Absorption of the steroid from the cyst into the general circulation is also very variable. Cysts are often classified as either follicular (about 70 per cent) or luteal and it is easy to understand why the cow with the luteal cyst,

Table 32.6 Causes of silent and weakly expressed oestrus

Social
Pain and fear
Weight loss
Genetic factors

which is predominantly progesterone producing, does not exhibit oestrus, though it is less clear why she fails to cycle. However, follicular cysts with oestrogen production are also found in cases of anoestrus. This may be due to the low level of the steroid produced in some cases while in other cases it may result from the negative effect on the behavioural centre of high levels of oestrogen circulating more or less continuously. Another explanation for the lack of oestrus in cows with follicular cysts is that the behavioural centres in the brain, which control the expression of oestrus, respond better to oestrogens if they have been primed by progesterone. However, the cause and effect relationship is not clear-cut. In the postpartum period, particularly during the first six weeks, some cows experience ovulation failure followed by the development of palpable but functionally transient cystic structures that do not interfere with subsequent cyclicity. In a small number of cows these cysts are persistent and delay return to cyclicity. Towards the end of this period many farmers become concerned about lack of oestrus and so the cow is presented for veterinary examination. By about six weeks after calving an ovarian cyst should be regarded as pathological.

Factors associated with the occurrence of cystic ovarian disease are discussed in Chapter 33.

4 The role of nutritional deficiencies in anoestrus is relatively straightforward in heifers but is complex in adult dairy cows.

(a) In heifers it has been shown in many field trials that low energy intake that causes slow growth rate is associated with delayed puberty. Onset of puberty tends to be related to body weight rather than age. The mechanism is discussed in Chapter 30.

(b) In adult lactating dairy cows it is not clear how feeding affects return to cyclicity after calving, even when only energy is considered. Factors that have been listed as putative causes include the feeding levels before and after calving, particularly the ratio of forage to concentrate; the body condition at calving and its changes after calving; the actual milk yield; and the potential milk yield. One method to try to take into account these many interacting factors is to measure the body condition of cows at calving and the change in body condition until service and conception. There is, however, no unanimity about the role these various yield- and feed-related factors play in reproduction.

5 Several studies have shown that cows in their first lactation exhibit a disproportionally high incidence of true anoestrus, with featureless ovaries. A variety of explanations for this have been put forward, including the possibility that this is a physiological age effect. One suggestion is that this is mainly the result of the high incidence of dystokia that occurs in first calvers (de Kruif, 1975).

Age effect, however, is not consistently disadvantageous for young animals, and it should be borne in mind that retained fetal membranes (p. 427), milk fever (p. 577) and to a lesser extent postpartum metritis (p. 427) are more commonly found in older animals than in first calvers, and these too are factors that tend to delay return to ovarian cyclicity.

The high incidence of anoestrus in first calvers is often attributed to nutritional and environmental factors. Excessive weight loss and very poor body condition result in cessation of ovulation and cyclicity, presumably through hypothalamic–pituitary dysfunction. Cows continue to grow until their second or third lactation and therefore young animals have to carry out the tasks of milk production, growth and reproduction simultaneously, at a time when adult dentition has not been fully developed. In dairy cows it is also the time when the young, smaller cow is introduced to the highly competitive environment of a herd, which, particularly during the housing period, makes it difficult for small animals to compete for food.

In many cases first calvers may be introduced to concrete floors for the first time in their lives just after calving and, when associated with high protein feeding, this may result in laminitis (p. 360) and lameness. Lameness (Chapters 28, 29) is a cause of weight loss that can result in true anoestrus and also, because of the associated pain, can cause poor oestrous expression in animals that are cycling.

6 Among miscellaneous causes of persistent corpus luteum is the rare condition of uterus unicornis, in which one horn of the uterus is absent. Ovulation on the side without a uterine horn results in a corpus luteum that is not exposed to locally produced prostaglandin and therefore does not regress after 16 or 17 days.

Silent and unobserved oestrus. Once cycles have been established, silent oestrus is not a common phenomenon, as was clearly demonstrated by Williamson *et al.* (1972) who carried out continuous observation of 107 cows for 21 days and concluded that four demonstrated silent oestrus. This has been confirmed by others in field trials in herds in which silent oestrus was thought to be a problem. Generally, when oestrous detection methods are improved, there is a corresponding reduction in the number of cases regarded as silent oestrus. Many cases previously diagnosed as silent oestrus are in fact unobserved oestrus.

Incidence figures are most reliable when based on serial progesterone assays as in the study of 1400 cows by Ball & Jackson (1984) in which 21 per cent of the cows had ovulated but had not been seen in oestrus. This level of non-detected oestrus is in agreement with other studies.

To what extent delayed return to service is due to unobserved oestrus is not clear but Humbolt (1982) using milk progesterone assays calculated that only 29 per cent of delayed returns were due to embryonic death and that 73 per cent were due to anoestrus (including true, silent and unobserved oestrus).

However, ovulation without the accompanying signs of oestrus (that is, silent oestrus) does occur. The best documented situation relates to the first ovulation after calving, particularly if it occurs within the first 20 days. Otherwise it is almost impossible to distinguish between silent and unobserved oestrus. Some instances of oestrus are so weak or last for such a short time that detection by conventional observation is a matter of chance.

Standing oestrus lasts for about 8–12 hours in cows and 6–8 hours in maiden heifers. However, 20 per cent of heats last less than 6 hours (Esslemont *et al.*, 1985).

The causes of silent oestrus, weak oestrus and short oestrus are not well understood but those considered to be the main ones are presented in Table 32.6.

1 Social factors within the group of cows, the size of the group and the reproductive status of the rest of the group, all play a role in oestrous behaviour and in the frequency of mounting (Britt, 1987). Mounting requires that there is both a cow in oestrus and cow that is willing to mount.

Cows that are usually bullied or are low in the pecking order are less likely to stand to be ridden when they are in oestrus than more dominant cows.

A small group of cows, say fewer than four or five, may be less effective at stimulating mounting behaviour than a larger group.

Cows at different stages of the reproductive cycle vary in their likelihood of trying to mount a cow in oestrus. The most likely to jump are those in or near oestrus, followed by non-pregnant cows in the luteal phase followed by pregnant cows. At the end of an intensive breeding season when most cows are pregnant the remaining cows to be served may be more difficult to detect because of the absence of cows willing to mount.

The presence of a bull inhibits cow-to-cow interaction but this may be made up for by the bull's own sexual monitoring of the herd. However, a bull may not choose to serve all cows in oestrus if several are in season at the same time.

2 Pain and fear. As oestrus is a behavioural phenomenon that is subject to psychological influences, it can be inhibited by discomfort, pain or fear. Severe adverse weather conditions such as driving rain and cold reduce cows' interest in sexual behaviour. Slippery flooring produces fear of falling and may inhibit oestrous behaviour. The pain caused by lameness inhibits oestrus expression.

3 Weight loss. It has been suggested that weight loss is associated with an increase in silent heats.

4 Genetic factors are almost certainly involved. The subjective nature of the measurement of oestrous expression makes it difficult to gather enough reliable data to evaluate the hereditary influence. Reports from progeny testing stations, where large groups of daughters from bulls under test were kept, showed that different daughter groups exhibited oestrus in characteristic ways. Bane (1964) has described differences between breeds in expression of oestrus.

Epidemiological data. In a study of 70 775 lactations in Finnish Ayrshire cows in which only cases treated by veterinarians were analysed (Saloniemi *et al.*, 1986) it was noted that the chance of a cow being presented to the veterinarian as anoestrus was affected by parity (highest risk in first calvers), calving season (highest risk in cows that calved from September to February), herd milk yield (highest incidence in high-yielding herds) and the occurrence of metritis (Chapter 31), mastitis (Chapter 21) and ketosis.

Diagnosis

A systematic approach to diagnosis is essential and the clinician should follow the steps outlined in Table 32.7.

If the anoestrous cow is in a herd in which the veterinarian is running a fertility control programme

Table 32.7 The diagnosis of anoestrus

History (including records)
General clinical examination (including condition score)
Special examination of the reproductive system
Rectal
Vaginal
Aids to diagnosis
Laboratory tests

involving regular visits, diagnosis will be both easier and more reliable because there will be historical information available and it will be simpler to introduce routine sampling where this is indicated.

There are two separate but overlapping aspects of diagnosis.

1 *Stage 1.* Assessment of ovarian status to determine whether the case is:

(a) true anoestrus, in which there is no ovarian cyclicity, or in which cyclicity has been blocked; or

(b) silent or unobserved oestrus, in which ovarian cycles are taking place.

2 *Stage 2.* Assessment of the causes of the condition.

Stage 1. Assessment of ovarian status. Since the word 'cycle' implies repetition, theory would dictate that assessment of whether or not a cow is cycling necessitates repeated examinations over an interval that should allow the observation of two oestrous periods. Under practical conditions it is usually assumed that the animal is cycling if it is possible to prove that ovulation has taken place recently. Another common assumption concerns a group of animals. It is usually considered that the group as a whole is cycling if two-thirds of the cows are in the luteal phase, i.e. the same fraction of the oestrous cycle that the luteal phase occupies. Furthermore the description of the 'luteal phase' given in Chapter 30 presents some difficulties in connection with diagnosis. This is because a corpus luteum is unlikely to be palpable until several days after it has become functional. Progesterone assay of milk or plasma will only produce a definite, recognizable rise after a similar delay. At the other end of the cycle, a corpus luteum is palpable after it is no longer functional. Use of ultrasound may help to overcome these difficulties.

Accordingly, for clinical purposes 'luteal phase' is defined as from day 5 to day 17 and the normal 'period of low progesterone' is expected to be from day 18 through oestrus (day 0) to day 4. This definition applies to the majority of cows in a normal population and is needed to form a basis for rational diagnosis but its use should be tempered by the realization that no definition will fit all cases (Bloomfield *et al.*, 1986).

The first step is to take a history of the case. Relevant information, required for both stages of diagnosis, is shown in Table 32.8.

The next step is to find out if there is functional luteal tissue present in the ovaries. The traditional way to do this is to palpate the ovaries per rectum but there are now several choices. One is to carry out a single or a series of milk progesterone assays, which gives a quick, reliable result. Another is ultrasound scanning, which allows the user to observe luteal tissue in the ovary (Figs. 32.1, 32.2) (Omran *et al.*, 1988).

Table 32.8 History taking for anoestrus cows

Date of calving
Any abnormality at and after calving
Has the cow been seen in oestrus since calving?
Could the cow be pregnant?
Oestrous detection methods in the herd
Are there other cows in the herd with similar problems?

The choice of method will depend on circumstances as each method has advantages and disadvantages. Rectal palpation is immediate, simple, requires little restraint of the cow and, if part of a routine visit, relatively cheap. It also allows other observations to be made on both other parts of the reproductive tract and the animal's general condition. There is minimal risk of misidentification of the animal, a danger always present when samples are taken for analysis. On the other hand it is a less accurate indicator of luteal function than a progesterone assay. Real-time ultrasound scanning is a valuable tool that, in experienced hands, is capable of giving a very accurate picture of ovaries and uterus (Figs. 32.3, 32.4, 32.5). The main disadvantage is the cost, the time required for a good result and the possible incompatability of sophisticated equipment with the dirty, wet, cow housing environment (Hughes & Davies, 1989).

Dawson (1975) compared the findings made by rectal palpation shortly before slaughter with the post-mortem observations. He identified accurately 125 (89 per cent) of 141 ovaries with corpora lutea. The errors were mainly in cows with small corpora lutea and also some with cysts or follicles.

On the basis of progesterone milk assays (which were assumed to be correct) Ott *et al.* (1986) summarized their own and other workers' results as shown in Table 32.9).

The use of progesterone assays has the advantage that they can be incorporated into a fertility control

Table 32.9 The accuracy of diagnosis by rectal palpation based on comparison with progesterone milk assay

	Corpus luteum	
	Present	Absent
Number of cases	244	158
Accuracy (%)	82	70

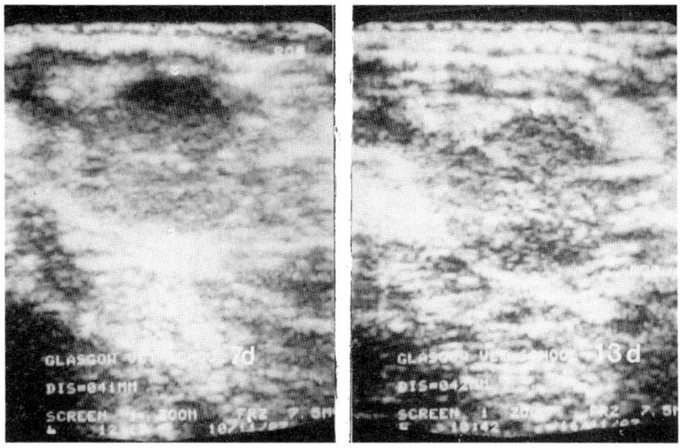

Fig. 32.1 Corpus luteum (7 and 13 days).

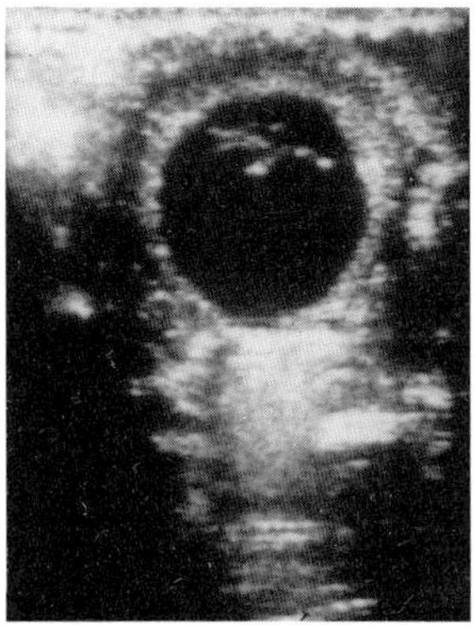

Fig. 32.2 Luteinising follicular cyst.

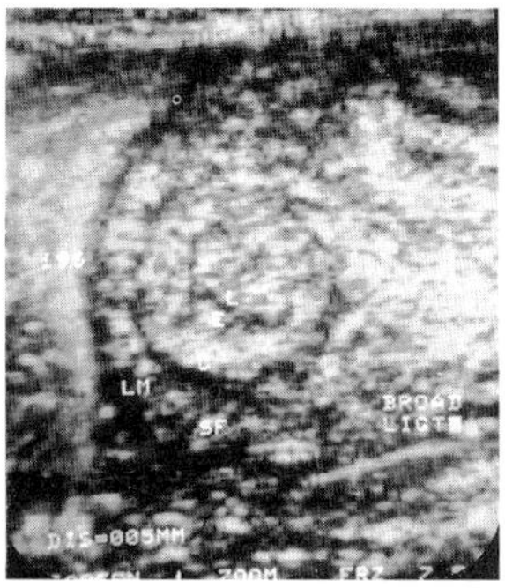

Fig. 32.3 Non-pregnant uterine horn.

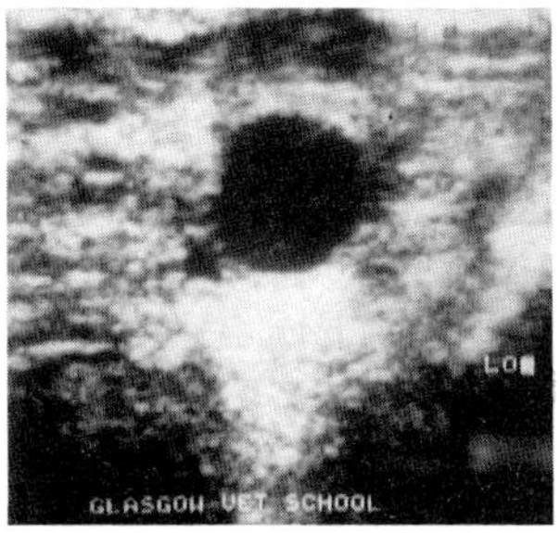

Fig. 32.4 Pre-ovulatory follicle within the ovarian stroma.

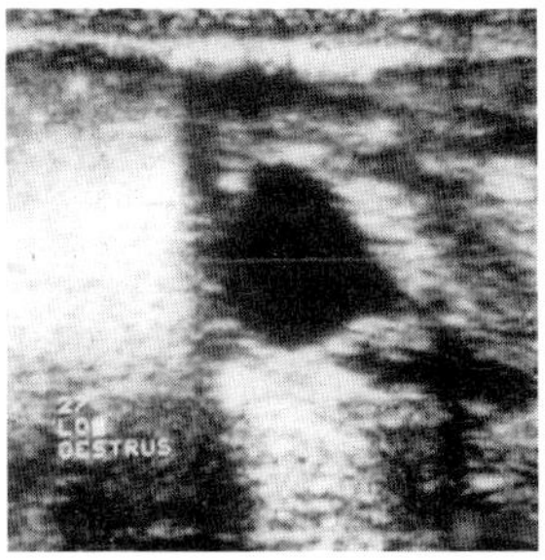

Fig. 32.5 Ovulatory follicle.

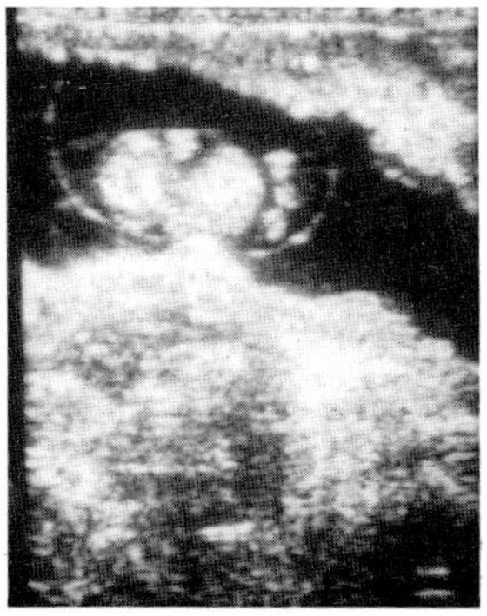

Fig. 32.6 44-day pregnancy.

programme and used prior to a visit, so that the clinician has information available before the examination of the animal. They can also be used after the visit to give extra information about the case. There may be slight problems in deciding the level of circulating progesterone that can be taken as indicative of luteal function.

If there is evidence of functional luteal tissue, the possibilities shown in Table 32.10 exist.

The simplest way to decide whether the animal is pregnant or has a pathological condition is to carry out rectal palpation of the ovaries and genital tract, plus in some cases a vaginal examination. This will, however, fail to reveal very early pregnancy. This is a situation for the use of ultrasound equipment, which allows the positive detection of a conceptus as early as 20 days after service and the recognition of changes in the uterus associated with pregnancy even earlier. For the sake of clarity Fig. 32.6 shows an ultrasound image of a 44-day pregnancy.

The most common finding is that ovaries and uterus appear to be normal and these cases are usually regarded as normal cycling cows.

The accuracy of diagnosis of a luteal cyst has been investigated by Booth (1988) and the clinical finding of luteal cysts was confirmed by progesterone assay in only 54 per cent of cases.

If initial examination shows there is no functional luteal tissue, there are also the various possibilities shown in Table 32.11.

When the initial examination reveals no luteal function and apparently normal ovaries and tract, the cow's ovarian status is unresolved. If she is cycling normally and in the low progesterone phase of the cycle, a corpus luteum will become palpable in the ovary within nine days, at most, from the first examination. A second examination at 10 days after the first will detect this corpus luteum. This second examination must not be delayed too long as some cows (those at day 5) will go into the low progesterone phase again in about 12 days after the first examination. These calculations can be upset by the considerable variations in cycle lengths and progesterone patterns that occur in a normal population of cows, as detailed by Bloomfield *et al.* (1986).

Table 32.10 Likely reasons for the presence of functional luteal tissue

Cycling (days 5–17 inclusive)
Pregnancy
Ovarian pathology (luteal cyst)
Uterine pathology (pyometra with persisting corpus luteum)

Table 32.11 Likely reasons for no luteal tissue being present

True anoestrus
Cycling (day 18 through oestrus to day 4)
Ovarian pathology
Freemartin: heifer
Cystic ovarian disease

If a second examination or sampling is required it is best done 10 days after the first. It is even better if serial sampling for progesterone assays can be arranged. It is necessary to work out a satisfactory regime of sampling. This involves making a compromise between the biological ideal, which might be daily samples, and what is acceptable to the farmer because of the cost, labour and interference with the milking routine. For example, a sampling regime of two samples per week, which will give a useful picture of the oestrous cycle but is not frequent enough to time oestrus exactly, may be unacceptably frequent for a farmer.

It is also very useful in these cases to carry out a vaginal examination (described on p. 429) at the time of the initial examination, as the presence of copious, clear mucus is strongly indicative of the peri-oestral stage of the cycle. In this way vaginal examination may allow a diagnosis to be made without the need for a second progesterone assay or a second rectal palpation.

Detection of Graafian follicles in the ovary, the observation of uterine tone and assays for oestrogens are all of limited value because they do not give clear indication of ovulation and cycling. There are a number of aids to detection of oestrus that can aid diagnosis (Boyd, 1984, see also p. 445).

The veterinarian now knows whether the cow or group of cows is exhibiting true anoestrus or is undergoing ovarian cycles. If a conclusion of anoestrus has been reached an important question is whether (i) the cow is in 'deep' anoestrus, which means that she is not likely to start cycling soon and is not likely to respond to treatment, or (ii) whether she is in 'shallow' anoestrus and liable to begin cycling soon and be responsive to therapy. Unfortunately, it is almost impossible to predict accurately the depth of anoestrus. However, if the cow is in extremely poor condition and if she has small hard ovaries she is likely in deep anoestrus.

Detect of the LH peaks that occur in the cow about to start cycling and are absent in those in deep anoestrus requires a series of samples taken at short intervals. At present (1991) LH assays cannot be done in a practice laboratory.

Stage 2. Assessment of the cause of anoestrus or silent oestrus. This section deals with the difficult question of how to find out what has caused the abnormal ovarian status or the problem of oestrus expression or detection. This may become an increasingly important matter if farmers use the new techniques that are available to monitor cyclicity without veterinary help. In these circumstances the veterinarian would be called in to deal with the problem after ovarian status had been determined.

To some extent procedures followed for diagnosis of ovarian status also give the clinician an understanding of the causes of the ovarian dysfunction. Examples of these are listed in Table 32.12.

Three of the causes of inactive ovaries, delayed involution, concomitant disease and nutritional deficiency present some problems in diagnosis.

In cases of delayed involution, usually the enlarged uterus and particularly the enlarged cervix, which involutes more slowly, makes the diagnosis of the immediate cause easy. However, on some occasions, by the time the cow is examined the uterus may well have returned to normal size and the veterinarian will have to depend on a history of periparturient problems and possibly of abnormal vaginal discharges noted by the farmer.

The clinician should see if there is any other disease condition in the cow examined for anoestrus. Especially important is any disease that causes loss of body condition or pain.

There is a complicated series of factors, such as actual and potential milk yield, feeding before and after calving and weight change after calving, which are very difficult to assess. Body condition of the cow should be noted at the time of examination for anoestrus, but this deals with only part of the problem (Anon., 1984). If body condition is poor or if there are many cases of inactive ovaries, feeding should be investigated. Feeding analysis and metabolic profiles are discussed elsewhere in this book (see Chapters 7 and 40).

On occasion there is no clear reason for the occur-

Table 32.12 Causes of dysfunction of the ovarian cycle

Freemartinism (congenital)
Ovarian hypoplasia (inherited)
Uterus unicornis (congenital)
Pyometra (periparturient problems)
Some cases of inactive ovaries
Nutritional
Systemic disease
Delayed involution

rence of inactive ovaries, either in the individual cow or when the condition affects a group of animals.

When investigating silent oestrus and unobserved oestrus, the veterinarian should find out about the following.

1 Organization of oestrous detection.
2 Layout of the buildings.
3 State of the floors.
4 The way the cows are handled, moved around and assigned to groups.
5 Amount of knowledge of oestrus and oestrous cycle among the people who are detecting oestrus.
6 Motivation for oestrous detection.
7 Time made available.
8 Personalities of the people involved.

Treatment (see Chapter 58)

When using proprietary products, the clinician should consult the data sheets, produced by the manufacturers, for details of use, contraindications and other guidance. Successful treatment, i.e. oestrus, service and pregnancy, depends not only on veterinary therapy but on husbandry and breeding management, some aspects of which are described in the data sheets and also on p. 53. Different manufacturers of apparently similar products often give slightly different advice about their use and users should be aware of the major differences between some of these products, as very clearly expressed by Lewis (1987). Some of the drugs used in therapy are dangerous for humans and some could cause return to service and abortion in cows and therefore the veterinarian must handle them responsibly.

Where drugs that result in oestrus are used, efficiency will be enhanced if the client is told to increase the time for oestrus detection and aids to oestrous detection are used, such as tail paint.

True anoestrus: no functional luteal tissue. Two things should be remembered when dealing with these cases.

1 All healthy, reasonably well-fed cows will start cycling some time after calving.
2 There must be an underlying reason for the occurrence of this type of true anoestrus and an attempt should always be made to find what the cause is and deal with it. Where the cause appears to be nutritional, improved feeding should be part of the treatment of the affected individual and also should be considered for recently calved cows.

At present there are two main hormonal treatments for inactive ovaries, (i) administration of gonadotrophin-releasing hormone (GnRH) and (ii) insertion of a progesterone-releasing intravaginal device (PRID).

Administration of an adequate dose of GnRH results, in the majority of cases, in luteinization of ovarian follicles followed by a period of progesterone production that can first be identified about five days after treatment. The duration of this progesterone phase is very variable, ranging from one or two days to the normal cyclic corpus luteum's life span and therefore the interval from treatment to oestrus is very variable, about 8–22 days. It is desirable to follow up these cases to ensure that luteinization has taken place, which may be done by rectal palpation, by progesterone assay or by ultrasound scanning.

If there is luteal tissue present at the follow-up examination, it is useful to treat the animal with prostaglandin $F_{2\alpha}$ or an analogue as this will make detection of the resulting oestrus easier. Routine fertility control visits are often at fortnightly intervals and this is a suitable period between the initial and follow-up treatment.

If, on the follow-up examination, there is no luteal tissue the cow should be dealt with as a new case.

The use of a PRID also mimics the progesterone rise before first ovulation. The PRID is left in the vagina for 12 days and the animal should be served at the oestrus that occurs in many cases about two or three days after withdrawal. Fixed-time insemination 48 and 72 hours (or a single insemination at 56 hours) after withdrawal is recommended. If oestrus is observed later another insemination should be carried out. Avoid stress and drastic change of diet at and after treatment.

Rather more complex treatment regimes have been applied (for example, Galloway *et al.*, 1987). Other treatments include intra-uterine irrigation using various stimulants or systemic treatment with pregnant mare serum gonadotrophin or follicle stimulating hormone (FSH) or oestrogens. Many farmers believe that rectal palpation of the ovaries and uterus initiates oestrus.

True anoestrus: functional luteal tissue. The therapeutic approach is to cause luteolysis by systemic injection of prostaglandin $F_{2\alpha}$ or an analogue followed by insemination at observed oestrus. In the case of pyometra, the client should be advised to delay service until it appears that the infection has cleared up, as indicated by an oestrus at which the mucus from the vulva is free of pus. It is advisable that the veterinary surgeon should examine these cases at a follow-up visit.

Practically all cases of uterus unicornis will be culled, but if one is treated, the veterinarian should check the side of subsequent ovulation compared with the absent horn.

Silent oestrus/unobserved oestrus: corpus luteum present. There are two standard approaches in these cases, the choice being between (1) the induction of luteolysis using prostaglandin $F_{2\alpha}$ or an analogue and (2) leaving the animal untreated to be observed when she comes in season. The method chosen will depend on many variable factors, such as the season, the time since calving, the herd calving pattern and the inclination of the client, and therefore the decision has to be made individually for each case.

Treatment with prostaglandin $F_{2\alpha}$ or an analogue should, in the majority of adult cows, result in oestrus in two to seven days' time, with the peak period being days 3 and 4 after treatment. Service should be at observed oestrus and aids to oestrus detection should be used.

Cows that are not seen in oestrus after treatment should be re-examined after 14 days (Young, 1989) with a view to treating with prostaglandin $F_{2\alpha}$ or an analogue, if appropriate.

Conservative treatment is preferred in the first instance by some clients who would rather leave the animal untreated, are content to know that she is cycling and hope to observe the next oestrus. In these cases aids to heat detection should be used and the animal re-examined if she is not seen in season within the next two weeks.

Silent oestrus/unobserved oestrus: no corpus luteum present. These cases do not require drug therapy but call for improvement in husbandry, i.e. heat detection and, possibly, feeding.

Because diagnosis is uncertain until the second examination, it is questionable whether these cows should be treated at the first visit. The veterinarian, however, may decide that the case for treatment before final diagnosis is strong because otherwise the chance of loss of production time is increased.

If there is no corpus luteum on the second examination, the condition is to be regarded as true anoestrus and dealt with accordingly.

Prognosis

In considering prognosis, primary attention has to be paid to return to cyclicity, which can be measured either by observation of oestrus or, more reliably, by one or more progesterone assays at planned times after treatment.

The outcome of treatment is influenced by both the veterinarian and the client (and perhaps also by the cow) as presented in Table 32.13.

Factors influenced by the veterinarian, which affect the outcome of treatment for anoestrus, are as follows.

1 The accuracy of diagnosis is the basis for correct treatment. There is good evidence that identification of a corpus luteum by palpation by experienced veterinarians is about 80 per cent accurate (p. 438) and that differentiation between follicular and luteal cysts is much less accurate (p. 439).

2 Selection of cases for treatment has an important influence on the outcome. For example, the corpus luteum early in the cycle is less responsive to prostaglandin $F_{2\alpha}$ or an analogue than is the mid-cycle corpus luteum. Accurate assessment of the stage of the cycle will aid in the correct selection of animals for treatment. Similarly, if treatment is confined to cases in which corpora lutea are positively diagnosed, better results will be obtained than if less critical selection of cases is undertaken, which may well be justifiable, for example towards the end of a tight seasonal breeding period.

Other factors that influence the success of luteolysis and whether the cow comes in season after successful luteolysis are not well documented. However, it is possible that nutritional factors are involved in the subsequent expression of oestrus.

3 The choice of the particular commercial product used for treatment may influence the outcome, as not all products that superficially appear to be the same are equally effective. There are differences between commercial products in their luteolytic efficiency and none achieve 100 per cent luteolysis (Ball & Jackson, 1984; Martinez & Thibier, 1984).

4 Re-examination and retreatment in good time of all cases that do not respond to the initial treatment will affect the time from initial treatment to oestrus, service and conception.

The farmer also affects the outcome of the treatment in important ways.

1 The efficiency of detection of oestrus in the herd is crucial to the effectiveness of treatment when measured by the number of cases that come into season within a certain number of days.

Table 32.13 Contribution of farmer and veterinary surgeon to influencing prognosis

Prognosis influenced by veterinarian
Accuracy of diagnosis
Selection of cases
Product used
Follow-up examination
Prognosis influenced by farmer
Oestrous detection
Herd pregnancy rate
Culling rate

2 The first-service pregnancy rate in the herd, which is to some extent under the control of the farmer, will have a great effect on the success rate as measured in time to conception.
3 High culling rate and willingness to cull may result in apparently good results because the failures are culled.

Heifers. Freemartins and cases of bilateral ovarian hypoplasia are sterile and will never cycle or become pregnant.

Groups of heifers with delayed puberty due to low energy intake will return to cyclicity after restoration of a suitable energy intake level and other correction of the feeding. How long this will take depends on many things. Under the best possible circumstances, i.e. where the animals are in not excessively poor condition and where there is no complicating disease factor, it will take approximately two months of good feeding before most of the group start cycling (Imakawa *et al.*, 1986).

True anoestrus after calving in cows. In cases of pyometra with a corpus luteum, the failure to cycle is very effectively dealt with by using prostaglandin. Ott & Gustafsson (1981) reported that more than 80 per cent of treated cows emptied the uterus and came in season a few days after treatment. If one treatment fails to produce luteolysis, then a second injection almost certainly will be successful. The problem is one of restoring the uterus to normal function and this will be dealt with later.

Inactive ovaries are treated with either GnRH or a PRID, and some indication of the results that can be obtained were shown in a field study (Ball & Lamming, 1983) involving 62 acyclic cows, as shown in Table 32.14.

There were two main differences between the two methods. Firstly, ovarian response to the PRID was better. Secondly, after the PRID, fixed-time insemination resulted in 59 per cent conceptions (measured by milk progesterone) whereas after GnRH, a number of cows that responded successfully were not seen in heat so that only 26 per cent of the cows treated became pregnant at the ovulation after treatment. One problem with GnRH is that the luteal tissue produced has a very variable lifespan with the result that ovulation can be from eight to about 20 days after treatment. Occasionally, cows come into oestrus two or three days after treatment with GnRH and this may either be the result of treatment or due to treating an animal that was just about to start cycling spontaneously.

In all reports on treatment of inactive ovaries there are some animals that do not respond to conventional treatment. It is obvious that cows that are still under the influence of the original aetiological factors (such as poor condition) are unlikely to respond well. Similarly, cows in deep anoestrus, i.e. animals that have not started producing intermittent LH surges, will not respond satisfactorily to hormonal treatment. It appears that cows with small hard ovaries respond poorly to treatment.

Table 32.14 The efficacy of two different methods of treating true anoestrus (after Ball & Lamming, 1983)

Treatment	Per cent ovulated	Per cent pregnant to intended ovulation	Failure in oestrous detection
PRID plus fixed time AI	89.7	59	–
GnRH plus AI at observed oestrus	73.9	26	22

In considering the outcome of treatment of cows with cystic ovarian disease associated with anoestrus there are a number of relevant points to note.
1 With the important exception of cases seen within six weeks of calving, spontaneous resolution of these cases is not to be relied on (Garcia & Larsson, 1982).
2 The condition tends to recur after treatment unless the animal becomes pregnant.
3 To the extent that there is a familial predisposition to cystic ovarian disease, the use of offspring from affected dams for breeding purposes is not advisable. This is likely less critical for cases with anoestrus than with return to service.
4 Results have to be looked at in two stages. The first stage is the resolution of the cystic condition and the induction of normal oestrus and ovulation. The second is getting the affected cow pregnant.

Where diagnosis is correct and appropriate treatment is given the return to ovarian normality is good. The majority of luteal cysts respond to prostaglandin $F_{2\alpha}$ or an analogue; in one study (Booth, 1988) 79 per cent of cows had low levels of circulating progesterone within seven days. In the same field trial 73 per cent of cases with follicular cysts that were treated with GnRH or human chorionic gonadotrophin (HCG) plus progesterone had functional luteal tissue by 14 days after treatment.

The pregnancy rate achieved again depends very much on the ability of the farm staff to detect oestrus and have the cow served at the correct time. This, plus the difficulty in accurate diagnosis of the type of cyst present, means that on many farms an unacceptably high percentage of cows with cystic ovarian disease are eventually culled as being not pregnant in time.

Silent and unobserved oestrus after calving in cows. Prognosis for unobserved oestrus is good and pregnancy rate is not greatly different from that for cycling cows in the same herd that have been observed in oestrus. Seguin (1981) compiled results from six trials in which 886 cows were treated; 67 per cent were in oestrus after treatment and pregnancy rate to service at that oestrus was 54 per cent. Seguin also cited trials in which controls and treated cows had the same pregnancy rate, whereas O'Farrell & Hartigan (1984) obtained a statistically significantly poorer pregnancy rate in the suboestrus cows treated with an analogue of prostaglandin $F_{2\alpha}$ than in controls. This latter finding is supported by an analysis of more than 10 000 cases of unobserved oestrus in Israel and 30 000 normal controls (Mayer *et al.*, 1987). First-service pregnancy rate for unobserved oestrus cows was 35.2 per cent compared with 60.3 per cent for the controls.

In an interesting study (Ball & Jackson, 1984) in which non-detected oestrus cows were treated with an analogue of prostaglandin $F_{2\alpha}$ and monitored by observation and progesterone assays, 84 per cent of the cows had complete luteolysis after a correctly timed injection. Of all the cows treated 42 per cent were seen in oestrus within four days of treatment and 60 per cent within 14 days.

One factor that makes prognosis difficult is the effect of the age of the corpus luteum on the response to prostaglandin $F_{2\alpha}$ or an analogue. Luteolysis is unlikely to occur in cows treated before day 5 of the cycle and it may be day 7 before maximum effect results. Even when luteolysis occurs, the time from treatment to ovulation varies greatly depending, in a complex manner, on the day of the cycle on which the cow is treated (MacMillan, 1983), which is likely to be dependent on the pattern of follicular development in the ovary.

Prognosis is improved if the veterinarian actively follows up all cases, both those treated and those left untreated, within two weeks.

Long interservice interval. Prognosis in these cases is similar to preservice cases but because of the longer time since calving the urgency to get the cow re-served is greater.

Prevention

The economic importance of prevention of anoestrus in all its forms can hardly be overstated. The cost-effective application of preventive measures, however, calls for careful consideration, and a balance has to be achieved between undue intervention in cows that would resume normal cycles spontaneously and unnecessary loss of time due to leaving intervention too late. For example, the majority of cows that are not cycling by six weeks after calving will be coming in season by eight weeks, i.e. in time for service within the target period. On the other hand, cows that are left without examination and treatment until the end of the target period for first service, say 11 weeks after calving, will lose a great deal of production time.

Heifers. Prevention of delay in the onset of puberty depends on good nutrition and the avoidance of diseases that interfere with growth rate.

The first step is establishment of clear targets. The farmer should decide at what age, or at what time of the year, the heifers should have their first calves. It is a simple calculation from that target to decide when the service period should start, so that the majority of the heifers calve within the planned period. The exact timing for the start of the service period will depend on how critical both the beginning and the end of the calving period is held to be. If conditions are good, such as a healthy, fertile young bull running with well-grown, healthy, cycling heifers, more than 80 per cent of heifers should be in calf after six weeks of the service period and practically all by nine weeks.

To ensure that the majority of the heifers are cycling at the beginning of the service period it is necessary to aim for a growth rate that achieves the appropriate body weight, taking account of the breed involved. Table 32.15 is an example of targets for cattle in the UK.

The veterinarian has a number of roles to play. Initially, it is necessary to make the farmer aware of the need to plan for a specific calving season or age and what this implies in terms of growth rates. Thereafter, the job is mainly to give advice and to make sure that the client monitors the growth rate of the heifers and onset of puberty. The farmer should consult the veterinarian at an early stage if it looks as though not enough animals are starting to cycle at the expected time.

Avoiding disease conditions that will interfere with growth is also the veterinarian's responsibility and is described elsewhere in this book. This should not only assist the attainment of the target for age at puberty but should also help to reduce the high mortality rate that occurs between birth and puberty.

Most farmers are aware that female calves born twin to a bull calf are very likely to be sterile freemartins. Few realize that measurement of the vagina in the very

Table 32.15 Target body weight (kg) for heifers at service and calving

	Friesian	Ayrshire
Weight at service (15 months)	330	285
Weight precalving including conceptus (24 months)	510	450

Table 32.16 Factors likely to prevent postpartum anoestrus

Normal calving or treated if dystokia
Disease-free puerperium or treated in time
Suitable pre- and postpartum feeding
Efficient oestrous detection

young calf and comparison with a normal calf can be used to decide if a suspect calf is a freemartin. Alternatively, blood sampling from six weeks of age from both twins for cytogenetic analysis will usually clarify the issue and allow early culling if desired.

Prevention of anoestrus in adult cows after calving. The foundations for early return to normal cyclicity and getting cows served are listed in Table 32.16.

All these factors are very much under the farmer's control, although the veterinarian has an important part to play in ensuring that the husbandry is up to standard; that intervention, if required, at and after calving is timely and appropriate; and that cyclicity is monitored and aberrations are treated.

1 *Prevention of dystokia and postpartum abnormalities* is a basic requirement for optimal cyclicity and fertility and has been discussed on p. 431.

2 *Routine veterinary postpartum examination and treatment* can effectively limit the adverse effect of abnormalities around calving and delayed involution. It is essential to examine all cows that experienced dystokia or postpartum problems by not later than 28 days after calving. Many veterinary practitioners incorporate routine examination of all cows two to four weeks after calving, as this allows them to deal with problems early.

There is an attractive concept that by routinely administering prostaglandin $F_{2\alpha}$ or an analogue, GnRH or both in the early postpartum period it is possible to improve return to cyclicity and pregnancy rate.

It is clear that GnRH given before day 20 after calving will initiate early cycles and prostaglandin $F_{2\alpha}$ or an analogue given a little later increases the number of cycles in the first six weeks after calving (Benmrad & Stevenson, 1986).

The effect of these treatments on calving-to-first-service interval and pregnancy rate is less well defined. Table 32.17 shows results obtained in several field trials. The numbers of cows in the groups range from 29 to 79.

These treatments applied routinely to normal cows do not appear to confer any benefit in terms of reproductive efficiency and there is the danger that induction of a corpus luteum in a cow that still has an infected uterus after calving can lead to pyometra. Selected treatment of cows with uterine or ovarian pathology is on the other hand entirely justified.

3 *Nutrition.* For normal reproductive function it is vitally important that nutritional levels before and after calving are correct. It has been suggested that condition score (see p. 16) at calving should be 3.0 and 2.5–3.0 at service (Anon., 1984).

Oestrous detection. Once the foundation for good fertility has been established it is essential to ensure that oestrous detection is as good as humanly possible.

Before discussing how oestrous detection can be improved it is worth asking the question — why is oestrus detection inefficient? After all most of the stockworkers who carry out this task have worked with cows for most of their lives and know very well the signs of oestrous.

The answer is that good oestrous detection requires accurate observation and recording of behavioural events several times a day over months on end and is therefore a very demanding task. It is made more difficult because of the short duration of oestrus exhibited by many cows, the time of the night or day when oestrus occurs, the weak and indefinite nature of signs shown by some cows when in season and the fact that some animals not in season exhibit some of the signs of oestrus. Veterinarians who wish to educate dairyworkers on heat detection would be well advised

Table 32.17 Effect of various treatments on interval from calving to first service

Calving–service interval (days)				Reference
$PGF_{2\alpha}$	GnRH	Both	None	
–	81	–	77	Langley & O'Farrell (1979)
–	88/89	–	83	Nash *et al.* (1980)
–	72/74	–	73	Nash *et al.* (1980)
–	–	61	63	Richardson *et al.* (1983)
92	108	85	84	Etherington *et al.* (1984)
61	67	64	58	Benmrad & Stevenson (1986)
73	–	–	69	Young & Anderson (1986)

* $PGF_{2\alpha}$, prostaglandin $F_{2\alpha}$

to attempt to carry out heat detection themselves, so that they may understand the practical difficulties.

The stockworker's dilemma occurs when a cow exhibits signs of oestrus just short of actually standing to be ridden and the decision is taken to have the cow inseminated. If the cow is not in season this decision is criticized. However, if the cow is not inseminated, a cow in season has been missed. In a large herd these critical decisions have to be made many times a year.

Good heat detection is based on the following facts.

1 The definitive sign of oestrus is standing freely to be ridden. It has been proposed that a cow which mounts onto another cow's head is in oestrus. Cows in oestrus, of course, also mount other cows.

2 There may be an interval of as much as 30 minutes between bouts of riding.

3 Oestrus rarely lasts for more than 18 hours and in many cases for less than 6 hours.

4 Oestrous often starts during the night.

5 Oestrous expression is greatest during quiet times of the cow's day and night. This means oestrus is seen less often around milking times and when cows are fed.

6 As well as a willingness to stand on the part of the cow in oestrus, it is necessary to have a cow that wants to mount and as discussed above (see aetiology, p. 434), this can cause particular problems late in the breeding season when most cows are pregnant.

7 When cows are loose housed there is often a particular area that cows prefer to use for oestrus expression.

8 Stalled cows may have reduced physical expression of oestrus (Claus *et al.*, 1983).

A rational system of oestrous detection should be based on these facts and the following points are required for a good heat detection system.

1 Observe the cows three times per day for 30 minutes each time. The periods of observation should be when the herd is peaceful after milking and feeding. Often these times are:

(a) briefly before collecting the cows for morning milking;

(b) in mid-morning;

(c) before the evening milking; and

(d) late in the evening, a very good time for detection of oestrus.

2 Make sure the housing conditions are suitable for cows and observer. Good non-slippery floors on which the cows must feel secure are essential. The observer must be able to see all the cows clearly, should be comfortable, and should have a paper and pen to write down details of the cows' behaviour. Good lighting is required.

3 The cows must be clearly identified.

There are many aids to heat detection and there is at present (1991) one substitute for detection, i.e. progesterone assays (review by Boyd, 1984).

Aids to heat detection either detect unobserved standing to be ridden or depend on the fact that cows in oestrus are likely to behave in ways that, although not unique to oestrus, occur with greater frequency during oestrus. Increased frequency of bellowing, increased restlessness, reduced milk yield, change in routine behaviour such as order of coming into the milking parlour for milking, and increased body temperature are non-specific, oestrus-related events. There are also a number of physical changes in the genitalia related to oestrus that can be measured, such as change in electrical resistance of the mucus in the vagina.

Marking systems fixed on the cow's pelvic region to detect standing to be ridden when the cows are not being observed can be valuable in suitable circumstances. Examples are tail paint, tail chalk and detectors that contain dye which is squeezed out under sustained pressure from another cow. All of these suffer from the defect that they may be triggered off by rubbing or pressure that is not caused by the cow standing freely to be ridden.

Television cameras with video recording have also been used to observe cows continuously and can be viewed later, at increased speed. There are problems of identity (very big numbers on shoulders and rumps are needed) and replaying the recordings is a tedious chore.

Milk progesterone assays, which can be used either as an aid to or as a replacement of oestrous detection, are discussed later.

The difficulty is to develop practical systems to measure and interpret at least some of these changes, all of which can be useful to a varying extent. The following system is purely hypothetical but possible. An ideal system would detect and record these changes automatically, followed by automatic analysis and interpretation. As many herds have out-of-parlour feeding systems in which each cow is identified electronically and the feed intake recorded by computer, it is not difficult to envisage an extension of this system. At each milking restlessness measured by a pedometer, order of milking, milk temperature (measured in the milking machine) and milk yield would be recorded automatically. These data would be plotted on a chart for each cow on which other information such as calving date, last oestrus, date for start of the service period, results of progesterone assays and other relevant information would be included. From this information the computer could assess the likelihood that the cow was in or coming into oestrus, and alert the stockworker.

Anoestrus after service. In the majority of cases, delayed return to service is due to unobserved oestrus, as has been shown in the reduction in the number of long return-to-service intervals when oestrus detection is improved. One problem, in a case where the return-to-service heat signs are indefinite, is that the result of inseminating a cow that has been served and could be pregnant may be loss of the conceptus.

Improved efficiency by using aids to heat detection is particularly suitable in these cases because the service date can be taken as the start of the oestrous cycle. Clearly, in those cases where insemination takes place in the luteal phase this starting point is erroneous, a fact that will become clear to the stockworker as heat detection aids and substitutes are used.

Use of a three-week calendar and the application of a marker such as tail paint shortly before expected return to service can help efficiency of observation.

Systematic use of milk progesterone assays at about the expected time of return to service can help in overcoming problems of long interservice intervals. High progesterone followed by two successive days of low progesterone is an indication that service should be carried out on the next day. Eddy & Clark (1987) demonstrated, in four large dairy herds, that the efficiency of heat detection after service could be improved greatly by using milk progesterone assays. The preferred sampling regime was every second day from days 18 to 24 after service. The financial benefit to cost ratio was 7.5 : 1. Some veterinarians report improvements based on a single progesterone assay on day 19 after service. For good results it is necessary for the stock personnel to understand the test and to be willing to carry out the extra work carefully and conscientiously. Very poor pregnancy rates result if progesterone assays are used as the only basis for insemination without the active incorporation of oestrous detection (Foulkes & Goodey, 1988).

Acknowledgement

The ultrasound images are reproduced with kind permission from Professor J.S. Boyd, University of Glasgow Veterinary School.

References

Anon. (1984) *Dairy Herd Fertility*. Ministry of Agriculture, Fisheries and Food, Reference Book 259, p. 1–80. HMSO, London.

Ball, P.J.H. & Jackson, P.S. (1984) The use of milk progesterone profiles for assessing the response to cloprostenol treatment of non-detected oestrus in dairy cattle. *British Veterinary Journal*, **140**, 543–9.

Ball, P.J.H. & Lamming, G.E. (1983) Diagnosis of ovarian acyclicity in lactating dairy cows and evaluation of treatment with gonadotrophin-releasing hormone or a progesterone releasing intravaginal device. *British Veterinary Journal*, **139**, 522–7.

Bane, A. (1964) Fertility and reproductive disorders in Swedish cattle. *British Veterinary Journal*, **120**, 431–41.

Bartlett, P.C., Kirk, J.H., Wilke, M.A., Kaneene, J.B. & Mather, E.C. (1986) Metritis complex in Michigan Holstein–Friesian cattle: incidence, descriptive epidemiology and estimated economic impact. *Preventive Veterinary Medicine*, **4**, 235–48.

Benmrad, M. & Stevenson, J.S. (1986) Gonadotrophin-releasing hormone and prostaglandin $F_{2\alpha}$ for postpartum dairy cows: estrous, ovulation and fertility traits. *Journal of Dairy Science*, **69**, 800–11.

Bloomfield, G.A., Morant, S.V. & Ducker, M.J. (1986) A survey of reproductive performance in dairy herds. Characteristics of the patterns of progesterone concentrations in milk. *Animal Production*, **42**, 1–10.

Booth, J.M. (1988) The milk progesterone test as an aid to diagnosis of cystic ovaries in dairy cows. *Veterinary Record*, **123**, 437–9.

Boyd, H. (1984) Aids to oestrus detection — a review. In *Dairy Cow Fertility* (ed. by R.G. Eddy, & M.J. Ducker), pp. 60–7. British Veterinary Association, London.

Boyd, H. & Munro, C.D. (1980) Experience and results of a herd health programme — rectal palpation and progesterone assays in fertility control. In *IX International Congress on Animal Reproduction and AI*, Vol. 2, pp. 373–80.

Boyd, H. & Reed, H.C.B. (1961) Investigations into the incidence and causes of infertility in dairy cattle. Fertility variations. *British Veterinary Journal*, **117**, 18–35.

Britt, J.H. (1987) Detection of oestrus in cattle. *Veterinary Annual*, **27**, 74–80.

Brown, J.L., Schoenemann, H.M. & Reeves, J.J. (1986) Effect of FSH treatment on LH and FSH receptors in chronic cystic-ovarian-diseased dairy cows. *Journal of Animal Science*, **62**, 1063–71.

Bulman, D.C. & Lamming, G.E. (1978) Milk progesterone levels in relation to conception, repeat breeding and factors influencing acyclicity in dairy cows. *Journal of Reproduction and Fertility*, **54**, 447–58.

Claus, R., Karg, H., Zwiauer, D., von Butler, I., Pirchner, F. & Rattenberger, E. (1983) Analysis of factors influencing reproductive performance of the dairy cow by progesterone assay in milk fat. *British Veterinary Journal*, **139**, 29–37.

Dawson, F.L.M. (1975) Accuracy of rectal palpation in the diagnosis of ovarian function in the cow. *Veterinary Record*, **96**, 218–20.

Eddy, R.G. & Clark, P.J. (1987) Oestrus prediction in dairy cows using an ELISA progesterone test. *Veterinary Record*, **120**, 31–4.

Esslemont, R.J., Bailie, J.H. & Cooper, M.J. (1985) *Fertility Management in Dairy Cattle*, pp. 1–143. Collins, London.

Etherington, W.G., Bosu, W.T.K., Martin, S.W., Cote, J.F., Doig, P.A. & Leslie, K.E. (1984) Reproductive performance in dairy cows following postpartum treatment with gonadotrophin releasing hormone and/or prostaglandin: a field trial. *Canadian Journal of Comparative Medicine*, **48**, 245–50.

Foulkes, J.A. & Goodey, R.G. (1988) Fertility of Friesian cows on the second, third and fourth days of low milk progesterone concentration. *Veterinary Record*, **122**, 135.

Galloway, D.B., Brightling, P., Malmo, J., Anderson, G.A., Larcombe, M.T. & Wright, P.J. (1987) A clinical trial using a regimen which includes a norgestomet implant and norgestomet plus oestradiol valerate injection as a treatment for anoestrus in dairy cows. *Australian Veterinary Journal*, **64**, 187–9.

Garcia, M. (1982) Reproductive functions during the post partum period in the cow. A review of the literature. *Nordisk Veterinaer Medicin*, **34**, 264–75.

Garcia, M. & Larsson, K. (1982) Clinical findings in post partum dairy cows. *Nordisk Veterinaer Medicin*, **34**, 255–63.

Hughes, A.E. & Davies, D.A.R. (1989) Practical uses of ultrasound in early pregnancy in cattle. *Veterinary Record*, **124**, 456–8.

Humbolt, P. (1982) Respective incidence of late embryonic mortality and post insemination anoestrus in late returns to oestrus in dairy cows. In *Factors Influencing Fertility in the Postpartum Cow* (ed. by H. Karg, & E. Schallenberger), pp. 298–304. Nijhoff, The Hague.

Imakawa, K., Day, M.L., Garcia-Winder, M., Zalesky, D.D., Kittok, R.J., Schanbacher, B.D. & Kinder, J.E. (1986) Endocrine changes during restoration of oestrous cycles following induction of anestrus by restricted nutrient intake in beef heifers. *Journal of Animal Science*, **63**, 565–71.

James, A.D. & Esslemont, R.J. (1979) The economics of calving intervals. *Animal Production*, **29**, 157–62.

Kassa, T., Ahlin, K.-A. & Larsson, K. (1986) Profiles of progesterone in milk and clinical ovarian findings in postpartum cows with ovarian dysfunctions. *Nordisk Veterinaer Medicin*, **38**, 360–9.

Langley, O.H. & O'Farrell, K.J. (1979) The use of Gn-RH to stimulate early resumption of oestrous cycles in dairy cows. *Irish Journal of Agricultural Research*, **18**, 157–65.

Lewis, C.L. (1987) Prostaglandin reaction. *Veterinary Record*, **120**, 423–4.

MacMillan, K.L. (1983) Prostaglandin responses in dairy herd breeding programmes. *New Zealand Veterinary Journal*, **31**, 110–13.

Markusfeld, O. (1987) Inactive ovaries in high-yielding dairy cows before service: Aetiology and effect on conception. *Veterinary Record*, **121**, 149–53.

Martinez, J. & Thibier, M. (1984) Fertility in anoestrous dairy cows following treatment with prostaglandin $F_{2\alpha}$ or the synthetic analogue fenprostalene. *Veterinary Record*, **115**, 57–9.

Mayer, E., Francos, G. & Neria, A. (1987) Eierstocksbefunde und Fertilitaets-Parameter bei Kuehen mit 'unbeobachteter Brunst'. *Tieraerztliche Umschau*, **42**, 506–9.

Moller, K., Lapwood, K.R. & Marchant, R.M. (1986) Prolonged service intervals in cattle. *New Zealand Veterinary Journal*, **34**, 128–32.

Nash, J.G., Ball, L. & Olson, J.D. (1980) Effects on reproductive performance of administration of GnRH to early postpartum dairy cows. *Journal of Animal Science*, **50**, 1017–21.

O'Farrell, K.J. & Hartigan, P.J. (1984) The treatment of non-detected oestrus (NDO) in dairy cows with cloprostenol. *Irish Veterinary Journal*, **38**, 23–8.

Omran, S.N., Ayliffe, T.R. & Boyd, J.S. (1988) Preliminary observations of bovine ovarian structures using B-mode real time ultrasound. *Veterinary Record*, **122**, 465–6.

Ott, R.S. & Gustaffson, B.K. (1981) Therapeutic application of prostaglandins for post partum infections. *Acta Veterinaria Scandinavica*, Suppl. 77, 363–90.

Ott, R.S., Bretzlaff, K.N. & Hixon, J.E. (1986) Comparison of palpable corpora lutea with serum progesterone concentrations in cows. *Journal of the American Veterinary Medical Association*, **188**, 1417–19.

Richardson, G.F., Archbald, L.F., Galton, D.M. & Godke, R.A. (1983) Effect of gonadotropin-releasing hormone and prostaglandin $F_{2\alpha}$ on reproduction in postpartum dairy cows. *Theriogenology*, **19**, 763–70.

Saloniemi, H., Groehn, Y. & Syvaejaervi, J. (1986) An epidemiological and genetic study on registered diseases in Finnish Ayrshire cattle. II. Reproductive disorders. *Acta Veterinaria Scandinavica*, **27**, 196–208.

Seguin, B.E. (1981) Use of prostaglandins in cows with unobserved oestrus. Acta Veterinaria Scandinavica (Suppl.) **77**, 343–53.

Sejrsen, K. & Neimann-Soerensen, A. (1982) Nutritional physiology and feeding of the cow around parturition. In *Factors Influencing Fertility in the Postpartum Cow* (ed. by H. Karg & E. Schallenberger), pp. 325–57. Nijhoff, The Hague.

Smidt, D. & Farries, E. (1982) The impact of lactational performance on post-partum fertility in dairy cows. In *Factors Influencing Fertility in the Postpartum Cow* (ed. by H. Karg & E. Schallenberger), pp. 358–83. Nijhoff, The Hague.

Warren, M.E. (1984) Biological targets for fertility and their effects on herd economics. In *Dairy Cow Fertility* (ed. by R.G. Eddy & M.J. Ducker), pp. 1–14. British Veterinary Association, London.

Williamson, N.B., Morris, R.S., Blood, D.C. & Cannon, C.M. (1972) A study of oestrous behaviour and oestrus detection methods in a large commercial dairy herd. 1. The relative efficiency of methods of oestrus detection. *Veterinary Record*, **91**, 50–8.

Young, I.M. (1989) Dinoprost 14-day oestrus synchronisation schedule for dairy cows. *Veterinary Record*, **124**, 587–8.

Young, I.M. & Anderson, D.B. (1986) First service conception rate in dairy cows treated with dinoprost tromethamine early post partum. *Veterinary Record*, **118**, 212–13.

Chapter 33: Return to Service

by H. BOYD

Manifestation

Return to service or detection of non-pregnancy are the ways in which poor pregnancy rate is presented and can have a major economic impact in any herd, particularly noticeable where a tight seasonal calving pattern is sought.

Interservice intervals. The interval in days that has elapsed between the unsuccessful service and the next oestrus is part of the manifestation of the condition of return to service. The concept of normal and abnormal interservice intervals has been discussed in connection with postservice anoestrus (p. 437). While the distribution of interservice intervals varies greatly between herds, reflecting in part the management efficiency in the herd, in many cattle populations fewer than 50 per cent have an interservice interval of 18–24 days.

Observable abnormality. Another manifestation of return to service is the normality or otherwise of the cow at the return oestrus. Certain deviations from normality in these cows can be observed by the farmer, in particular the presence of a purulent discharge from the vulva. Aberrant sexual behaviour will also be reported by the farmer. In relevant cases, the observant client may notice some of the changes associated with cystic ovarian disease, such as slackening of the pelvic ligaments and voice change. In general, however, the cow that returns to service presents an apparently normal oestrus both as regards behaviour and visible signs.

The way in which return to service is presented by the client affects the clinician's response to the problem. It is presented either as an individual cow problem or as a herd (or group) problem; and it is presented with or without evidence of past or present pathology.

Individual cows. Individual cases are presented in two quite different ways, which influence how they are dealt with.

1 Some cows are presented to the veterinarian that have been served only two or three times and are still not pregnant.

To understand these cases properly they have to be considered within the context of the entire population of cows and heifers in the herd. In any group of apparently normal cows served correctly by a fertile bull or inseminated properly with good semen, either for the first time after calving or at a repeat service, a considerable number will return to service. Most of these animals are only temporarily infertile and the majority will become pregnant within an acceptable time. Although there is some understanding of the stage at which these losses occur, i.e. whether there is fertilization failure or embryonic death, the aetiology is known to only a limited extent. For this reason these returns appear to happen at random.

Field studies show that about 12 per cent of cows are still not pregnant after three services as is demonstrated in Table 33.1, which is taken from a population of 5744 cows with a first insemination pregnancy rate of 60.6 per cent (Boyd & Reed, 1961a). 'Actual results' are compared with the 'expected results' that would have occurred if all subsequent inseminations had had a pregnancy rate of 60.6 per cent.

Farmers often wait until a cow has had three unsuccessful services before presenting her to the veterinarian and Table 33.1 shows that (with certain reservations)

Table 33.1 The percentage of cows that required various numbers of inseminations for pregnancy with a first insemination pregnancy rate of 60.6 per cent

Number of inseminations required for pregnancy	Actual results		Expected results	
	Per cent	Cumulative per cent	Per cent	Cumulative per cent
1	60.6	60.6	60.6	60.6
2	20.4	81.0	23.9	84.5
3	7.2	88.2	9.4	93.9
>3 or culled	11.8	100.0	6.1	100.0

about half of these cows, 6.1% versus 11.8%, are not pregnant because of the same (unknown) factors that establish the level of the first insemination pregnancy rate. It is therefore to be expected that half of these cows will not exhibit any diagnosable cause of return to service and that their expectation of pregnancy at the next service is about the same as that for first insemination.

Warren (1984) cites published data from four different cattle populations in which pregnancy rates to first service ranged from 47 to 57 per cent. Within these populations, however, the herd pregnancy rates would vary widely.

2 Other cases, for which the term 'chronic repeat breeder' might be used are presented because they have returned to service repeatedly over a long period of time. These cases have been differentiated into apparently normal repeat breeders and those with abnormalities on the basis of cycle length, sexual behaviour and detectable abnormality, a differentiation of limited clinical value. These chronic repeat breeders require a different approach from the cases discussed in (**1**) above because they are generally cows that the owners regard as particularly valuable and therefore the clinician can devote more time and cost to them. Prognosis in chronic repeat breeders is inevitably poor because they have been given so many opportunities to become pregnant without success.

It is animals of this type that are hospitalized in teaching and research institutions where they are given expensive diagnostic and therapeutic treatment.

There is no realistic incidence figure for chronic repeat breeders because their retention in the breeding herd is dependent on extraneous factors but clearly is unlikely to be more than 6 per cent of the breeding population, though it may be higher in individual herds.

Herd or group problems. Return to service may affect many animals in the herd in which case the client is very worried about the extent of the problem and the serious effect it will have on production and profits. For an assessment of the condition it is necessary to analyse the breeding records to determine pregnancy rate (or other measure of the success rate of services) and interservice intervals.

The range of incidence of return to service is very wide. In a population of herds with any given mean herd pregnancy rate there is a tendency for the herd averages to be distributed at random round this mean, as demonstrated in Table 33.2. The overall herd first insemination pregnancy rate in the 191 herds was 59.9 per cent (Boyd & Reed, 1961a). Although not demonstrated here, it is usual for the distribution to be skewed towards the lower end of the scale. Similar data have been reported in more recent surveys.

It is helpful to think of the pregnancy rate for any individual herd as dependent on the combined effects of the following factors.

1 The random variation round the mean of the population of herds.

2 The background effect, which is dependent on management and environmental factors that are liable to be constant over a long period. Examples, any of which individually would tend to result in low herd pregnancy rates, are inaccurate oestrus detection, unsatisfactory feeding, and a high incidence of purulent metritis due to bad calving conditions.

3 Specific pathogenic causes, such as a subfertile bull or campylobacteriosis.

4 The incidence of chronic repeat breeders, which to some extent relates to (**2**).

Aetiology

There are three main stages at which failure to achieve or maintain a pregnancy can occur. Although it is often not possible to assign an individual case to one of these stages this knowledge is useful in understanding the aetiology of return to service. The stages are shown in Table 33.3.

In addition there are cases of return to service that cannot be attributed to a particular stage.

Table 33.2 Distribution (%) of herd average first insemination pregnancy rates on 191 dairy herds

Herd first insemination pregnancy rate							Total
<31	31–40	41–50	51–60	61–70	71–80	>80	
3.1	3.7	16.2	25.1	27.2	19.4	5.2	99.9

Table 33.3 Reasons for unsuccessful services

Stage 1	Ovulation failure
Stage 2	Fertilization failure
Stage 3	Loss of the conceptus

Table 33.4 Definition of cystic ovarian disease

Persisting, steroid-secreting follicles >2.5 cm in diameter
No functional corpus luteum
Abnormal sexual cycle (anoestrus, nymphomania, virilism)
More than six weeks after calving

Stage 1. Failure of ovulation after oestrus. The most important condition in which there is oestrus without ovulation is cystic ovarian disease. It is important to define 'cystic ovarian disease' because not all cases of ovarian cysts are pathological (see Table 33.4). Also, when studying aetiology the conclusions reached are affected by which animals are included as clinical cases. For example, cows identified as having cystic ovarian disease at routine preservice veterinary examination will form a different population from cystic ovarian disease cases detected in repeat breeder cows.

Histological and biochemical examination of ovarian cysts demonstrate that cysts are complex structures. On clinical examination and gross anatomical inspection, however, there appears to be two main types of cysts: follicular cysts, which are like large follicles, and luteal cysts in which obvious luteal tissue produces a thick cyst wall. A corpus luteum with a central lacuna is not pathological if it contains enough luteal tissue for physiological function (Okuda *et al.*, 1988).

It is well known that follicular cysts occur during the first few weeks after calving in some cows that then return to regular cyclicity, and this can be regarded as part of the physiological process of return to normal cyclic ovarian function (Artmur *et al.*, 1989). It is often suggested that cows with cystic follicles up to six weeks after calving should be regarded as normal unless they are nymphomaniac or show other signs of abnormality.

Guenzler & Schallenberger (1980) point out that 'our understanding of the mechanisms contributing to the formation of ovarian cysts in cattle is still very limited'. Table 33.5 is hypothetical but should act as a reminder that there are several possible routes that can result in cystic ovarian disease.

Table 33.5 The possible pathogenesis of cystic ovarian disease

Insufficient luteinizing hormone (LH) release: hypothalamic–pituitary dysfunction (commonest cause)
Insufficient production of LH by the pituitary (rare)
Failure of the ovary to respond to LH (perhaps about 20% of cases)

There have been many studies of the causes of cystic ovarian disease and factors that predispose to the condition are listed in Table 33.6. There is lack of unanimity about causes, which may reflect differences between the populations of cattle selected for investigation as well as variations in the definition of cystic ovarian disease.

1 *Heredity.* A familial predisposition to cystic ovarian disease through sire or dam has been recognized for many years (Bane, 1964). Other studies have produced less clear-cut results or even failed to detect an hereditary effect at all (Dohoo & Martin, 1984a). It is possible that this difference is partly due to the stage at which diagnosis is carried out. If the incidence is assessed at routine preservice checks most of the detected cysts are likely to be attributed to environmental factors rather than heredity; on the other hand one might expect considerably more evidence of hereditary predisposition if the assessment is made on a sample of repeat breeders.

While most veterinarians are generally aware that there is an hereditary component in cystic ovarian disease, their clients want to know to what extent breeding a replacement heifer from a cow with cystic ovarian disease will increase the risk of that daughter having the disease. It is not easy to answer this because cystic ovarian disease may not occur in a daughter until she has had several calves and so field studies take many years and involve complex statistical analysis.

Studies carried out by Henricson (1957) helped to answer the question. He analysed data from two artificial insemination (AI) centres of cases presented at the time of insemination, and classified cows as:

(a) having cystic ovarian disease on more than one occasion in a service period;
(b) having only one observation of cystic ovarian disease; and
(c) without cystic ovarian disease.

Table 33.6 Factors that predispose to or cause cystic ovarian disease

Heredity
High yield
Age
Exogenous oestrogens
Season of the year
Dystokia and periparturient disease

Table 33.7 Dam effect on incidence of cystic ovarian disease (COD) in daughters

Number of times COD diagnosed in dam in one service period	Average frequency of COD in daughters	
	Centre 1	Centre 2
>1	0.255	0.228
1	0.170	0.158
0	0.143	0.116

The effect of age was taken into account and the results expressed as an average frequency of the condition, where 1.00 is equivalent to an incidence of 100 per cent (Table 33.7).

Henricsson (1957) also studied the effect of the sire and noted that the average frequency of cystic ovarian disease in individual bulls' daughters ranged from 0.00 to 0.258.

Whether the low incidence of cystic ovarian disease in beef breeds is directly due to hereditary factors, to the lower milk production or to some other factor is not known.

2 *High milk yield.* Cystic ovarian disease may be related to high milk yield. It occurs most frequently at the peak of lactation and at the age when the cow has reached her full milking potential which is why it is more common in pluriparous cows than in first calvers. There is a secondary peak of cases late in lactation; presumably these are cases that have been picked up on the examination of repeat breeders. Bartlett *et al.* (1986a) discussed, without coming to a conclusion, whether high milk yield causes cystic ovarian disease, cystic ovarian disease causes high yield or there is a common cause of both! Saloniemi *et al.* (1986) think that the relationship between cystic ovarian disease and ketosis was due primarily to high milk yield, leading to greater energy demands that in turn resulted in both ketosis and intereference with LH production or release.

Some workers have been unable to find an adverse effect of high milk yield on the occurrence of cystic ovarian disease (e.g. Dohoo & Martin, 1984a).

3 *Age.* It is widely accepted that cystic ovarian disease is rare in heifers before their first calving, not common in first-lactation cows and then increasingly observed in mature cows, with possibly some slight fall off in old animals.

4 *Exogenous oestrogens.* Administration of oestrogens will cause a premature LH peak. If this is done shortly before natural oestrus the cow may not be able to produce a second LH peak and consequently the ovulation expected after the natural oestrus does not occur. This may be one explanation why a single large dose of an oestrogen for therapeutic purposes may be followed later by cystic ovaries.

An analogous situation may arise when oestrogenic substances, such as those found in mouldy brewers' grains, are eaten.

5 *Seasonal effect.* There is a very definite seasonal effect reported by many authors with most reports indicating that the incidence is highest in winter (Dohoo *et al.*, 1984; Saloniemi *et al.*, 1986). The effect can be so great that Bane (1964) stated that it is meaningless to talk of an incidence figure for cystic ovarian disease if details of season (and age) are excluded. The range in his data was from 2.23 per cent for cows that calved in May to 9.68 per cent for October calvers. The relative frequency of severe cases was higher in autumn calvers. Some authors (Bartlett *et al.*, 1986a) reported high levels in summer and autumn.

The causes of the seasonal effect are not clear but obviously could include the hours of daylight, temperature extremes and feeding.

6 *Dystokia and periparturient disease.* Some information suggests that dystokia and periparturient diseases may predispose to cystic ovarian disease. It is possible that preparturient factors that cause the postpartum conditions also affect the incidence of cystic ovarian disease, for example overfeeding leading to fatty liver (Reid *et al.*, 1979). However, it has been demonstrated experimentally that damage to the endometrium can prolong the existence of cystic follicles and so inhibit spontaneous recovery (Fathalla *et al.*, 1978).

7 *Other causes.* It is possible that gross adhesions can so tightly bind the ovary that ovulation does not take place but this must be a rare phenomenon. Of much greater importance is the concept that in cows which had other reproductive disorders there were possibly more than expected numbers of cystic ovarian disease (Jasko *et al.*, 1984).

Reviews of the literature show that incidence ranges from about 6 to nearly 20 per cent (Kesler & Gaverick, 1982; Bartlett *et al.*, 1986a). However, diagnostic methods affect the reported incidence figure, for example Coleman *et al.* (1985) found that the single most important factor which influenced the incidence was the veterinarian who made the diagnosis! Selection of cases is also important as has been discussed already.

It is generally agreed that follicular cysts make up about two-thirds of recognized cases of cystic ovarian disease (Nakad *et al.*, 1983; Booth, 1988).

Table 33.8 Causes of fertilization failure

Interference with egg transport
Interference with sperm transport
Delayed ovulation
Insemination at wrong time in relation to ovulation
Service too soon after calving
Poor-quality spermatozoa
Failure to serve the cow
Metritis and salpingitis
Vaginitis cervictis

Table 33.9 Causes of ovarian and bursal adhesions

Trauma
Rectal palpation
Enucleation of corpus luteum
Caesarean section
Ascending infection
Postpartum metritis
Therapeutic infusion of uterus
Descending infection
From peritoneum
Specific infections, e.g.
Ureaplasma sp.
Mycoplasma sp.
Leptospirosis

Stage 2. Fertilization failure. To achieve fertilization a number of events in the cow (oestrus, ovulation, gamete transport) and in the bull (spermatozoa production, insemination) have to take place and must synchronize with each other. Failure of any one of these events to occur correctly or at the right time will almost certainly result in fertilization failure. The causes of fertilization failure will be discussed under the headings shown in Table 33.8.

The first two causes, interference with gamete transport, are relatively rare occurrences.

1 *Interference with egg transport.* After ovulation the egg has to be transported to the site of fertilization in the oviduct. Adhesions affecting the ovary and bursa and blockage of the oviduct will prevent this happening. Factors that cause adhesions, which are fairly rare, are listed in Table 33.9. The ease with which fluids and small objects can be transported spontaneously up or down the oviduct is demonstrated in two techniques used to investigate oviduct patency. In one of these tests, dye is introduced into the uterus and ascends spontaneously through the oviduct into the peritoneal cavity and in the other test starch granules deposited in the bursa descend through the oviduct into the uterus and vagina.

Transport in the oviduct is under hormonal control and can be affected by abnormal variations in steroid hormone production and by oxytocin but the role of these factors in field conditions is not known.

As transport of the egg depends on secretory and ciliary activity in the oviduct, salpingitis will interfere with transport of both eggs and spermatozoa, even when the lumen remains patent.

2 *Interference with transport of spermatozoa.* Adhesions in the female tract that block egg transport, and have been discussed above, will generally interfere with transport of spermatozoa. There are rare anatomical abnormalities such as White Heifer disease (segmental aplasia of the paramesonephric ducts), which results in blockage of the tubular genitalia at various levels.

Poor AI technique, such as insemination in the anterior vagina or caudal half of the cervix will result in the majority of cases in the loss of much of the inseminate by reflux through the vulva. In contrast, in natural service the ejaculate is deposited in the anterior vagina and on the external os of the cervix but the volume of the ejaculate and the enormous number of spermatozoa allow loss by reflux while sufficient spermatozoa are transported to the oviduct. Returning to AI, a rough operator could damage the uterus with the insemination pipette. While it is unlikely that bad insemination technique is much of a problem with a technician inseminator service, it is very likely that the range of expertise among stockworkers who inseminate their own cows is so great that some gross technical errors are made.

3 *Delayed ovulation.* Delayed ovulation is a condition in which the interval from the onset of oestrus to ovulation is so much longer than normal that service at the recommended time does not result in fertilization because of the ageing of the spermatozoa. While many authors are of the opinion that the condition is rare, there are a number of papers that suggest that it occurs quite commonly (Hancock, 1948; Nakao *et al.*, 1984). Watson and MacDonald (1984) studied events around insemination using rectal palpation and assays for progesterone and oestradiol-17β. They concluded that in cows with a follicle in the ovaries on the day after insemination (possibly delayed ovulation) this was due to erroneous timing of insemination in relation to the onset of oestrus and not to delayed ovulation.

As the condition is so difficult to study ideas about its aetiology must be theoretical. There is, however, a general view that there is an abnormality of the LH surge. It has been hypothesized that deficiency of energy intake may be involved aetiologically.

The role of stress is also speculative but it is interesting that corticosteroids can block LH release (Wagner & Li, 1982); also the fact that the adrenal cortex under the influence of adrenocorticotrophic hormone (ACTH) can produce some progesterone may be significant (Watson & Munro, 1984).

A little understood condition called long low progesterone was described by Jackson *et al.* (1979) as affecting 18 per cent of cows treated with an analogue of prostaglandin $F_{2\alpha}$ and also about 18 per cent of control cows. After oestrus there was an excessively long period of low progesterone, followed by a rise which semed to indicate that ovulation took place eventually. The herd incidence ranged from 7 to 33 per cent and appeared to be low in herds with adequate nutrition. Other surveys have not revealed such a high incidence. Some workers think long low progesterone is most commonly associated with treatment with prostaglandin $F_{2\alpha}$ or an analogue.

4 *Insemination at wrong time in relation to ovulation.* Service during the luteal phase is only a minor problem with natural service but a major one with AI. In natural service, a cow restrained in a service crate may be mated when she is not in oestrus.

Artificial insemination at the wrong time is an important cause of fertilization failure. Progesterone assays of milk or blood taken on the day of insemination will detect insemination during the luteal phase of the cycle but will fail to pick up inseminations that are one or two days too early or too late. The reported incidence of luteal phase progesterone levels on the day of insemination is variable. The incidence of 5.2 per cent in well-run herds reported by Claus *et al.* (1983), with over 20 per cent in problem herds, is typical of several other trials. Laitinen *et al.* (1985) in a large field study reported that the lowest incidence of luteal phase inseminations occurred in the summer. Oltner & Edqvist (1981) observed that in herds with a high incidence of wrongly timed inseminations, even inseminations apparently at the correct time resulted in low pregnancy rates, presumably because of other aspects of poor management.

The reasons are misidentification of a cow that actually is in season or misinterpretation of sexual behaviour, such as jumping another cow, which is thought incorrectly to indicate oestrus. The stockworkers are often under considerable pressure to get all cows served by a target date and are criticized by veterinarians, and others, that cows in oestrus are missed too frequently. This can result in error through an over-enthusiastic determination to increase the oestrous detection rate.

Incorrect timing of insemination in relation to onset of oestrus also occurs. Watson *et al.* (1987) confirmed that insemination 24 hours or more after the cow is first seen in oestrus results in marked reduction in pregnancy rate. It is likely that insemination very early in oestrus also causes reduced fertility. There is a long-established, successful rule of thumb about the ideal time for insemination (Trimberger, 1948). Cows first seen in the morning should be inseminated late that afternoon. Cows first seen in the afternoon or evening should be inseminated next morning. Cows still in oestrus 24 hours after first being seen should receive a second insemination. This pragmatic recommendation takes account of the relatively short lifespan of both spermatozoa and ova within the female tubular tract (about 24 hours), the apparent need for capacitation of bull spermatozoa (about 6 hours) and the interval from the onset of oestrus to ovulation (about 25 hours) (see p. 420).

Incorrect timing within oestrus is of little significance with natural service in which the service is usually early in oestrus. The large quantity of the ejaculate and the great numbers of spermatozoa deposited in the anterior vagina ensure that there is a long-lasting supply of fertile spermatozoa in the oviduct at the site of fertilization.

5 *Service too soon after calving.* It has been known for many decades that service within six weeks of calving results in very poor pregnancy rate. The reasons are likely of both ovarian and uterine origin so most likely in some cases the cause is fertilization failure and in others embryonic death. Return to normal cycle length and levels of circulating ovarian steroids takes some weeks after calving. Elimination of infection and restoration of endometrial structure and function after calving also requires time. On average, by about eight weeks after calving, pregnancy rate reaches a plateau.

6 *Poor-quality semen.* Poor semen quality may result in either low pregnancy rate or no pregnancies at all, mainly through fertilization failure but also to some extent through embryonic death. Again there are marked differences between natural service and AI. Because of laboratory control of the semen and follow-up of the results of insemination it is very unlikely that semen supplied by a reputable AI organization will give poor pregnancy rates without this information being available to the user, or at least the supplier. By contrast a bull used for natural service may be of low fertility or even sterile and serve a number of cows before the owner realizes that something is wrong. Farmers are often not aware that a bull that has been fertile may become infertile or lose libido.

Schemerhorn *et al.* (1986) found that a technician

inseminator service gave rather better results than farmer insemination. If AI technique is satisfactory poor results with farmer inseminations could possibly be related to mishandling of the semen.

Where fresh diluted semen is used, semen that is stored too long will give poor results.

7 *Failure to serve the cow.* In certain circumstances when a bull is used to serve the cows, a cow in oestrus is not served. Bulls can develop abnormalities of the penis that prevent normal service, and lack of libido is not uncommon (p. 484). When animals are running freely, such as heifers or beef cattle, it is essential to include an adequate number of bulls in the group. If there are too few bulls for the number of cows, some cows in oestrus may not served. The required cow to bull ratio depends on the type of terrain, the age and libido of the individual bulls (see p. 484).

8 *Vaginitis, cervicitis, metritis and salpingitis.* Infection of the tubular genitalia may interfere with the survival of the spermatozoa in transit and so reduce the chance of fertilization. Metritis is common but in addition a number of species of organisms have been recovered from the oviducts and may cause salpingitis or directly affect fertilization, as for example reported by Grahn *et al.* (1984), in connection with fertilization failure with BVD infection. Infectious agents in the oviduct include *Leptospira hardjo*, *Ureaplasma* sp., *Mycoplasma bovigenitalium* and *Acholeplasma laidlawii*.

Stage 3. Embryonic death. The stage of the embryo lasts from fertilization of the egg until about day 42 after conception by which time the organ systems have been laid down and placentation has been established.

In any group of breeding cattle, however normal they appear, there will occur a considerable amount of embryonic death, most of it within the first three weeks after fertilization (Sreenan & Diskin, 1986). Knowledge of the aetiology of this important condition is still very limited but it is possible to produce a list of factors that have been shown to cause embryonic death or are at least very likely involved (Table 33.10). In the vast majority of cases the actual cause is not known.

Table 33.10 Factors that cause embryonic death

Extreme environmental temperatures
Specific and non-specific endometritis
Aged gametes
Local trauma
Genetic factors
'Biological filter'

1 *Extreme environmental temperatures.* Controlled experiments have demonstrated that cattle that are mated in a high environmental temperature and kept there after service exhibit a high rate of embryonic death. In work in which cows were exposed to hot summer sunshine without shade in Florida, possible causes of the heat-induced embryonic death have been identified as high uterine temperature, decrease in the blood flow to the uterus, and slight change in the amounts of progesterone and oestrogen about the time of oestrus (Thatcher and Collier, 1986).

Poor pregnancy rate is a problem when European cattle are introduced into hot countries where they are exposed to temperatures above 30 °C; it is quite likely that increased embryonic death is part of the reason. There is little doubt that genetic factors are involved in this as in other aspects of heat tolerance. Crosses between indigenous heat tolerant breeds and European breeds are more heat tolerant than the imported animals and they are more fertile. The improved fertility appears to be the result of the dam's enhanced ability to control body temperature rather than to an inherited ability of the embryo itself to tolerate high body temperature in the dam.

The position is less clear with extreme cold but there are indications that a corresponding adverse effect occurs. In countries with very cold winters cattle are housed in well-insulated buildings and so are not exposed to the rigours of very low temperature. The problem could arise during unusually cold periods in temperate climates where housing tends to provide cover rather than warmth.

2 *Metritis.* Metritis in varying degrees of intensity is a common condition causing infertility in cattle. Where caused by infection it can be divided into *non-specific*, exemplified by *Actinomyces (Corynebacterium) pyogenes* infection, and *specific*, typified by *Campylobacter (Vibrio) fetus* infection. There are a number of infections that are difficult to classify such as infectious bovine rhinotracheitis (IBR), *Ureaplasma* sp. and *Haemophilus somnus*.

Non-specific metritis is the result of either massive infection or of the infective organisms taking advantage of a deficient uterine defence mechanism usually caused by damage at and after calving. Non-specific infection can be facilitated by synergic action of different organisms, for example *A. pyogenes* and *Fusobacterium necrophorum*.

The incidence of non-specific endometritis depends partly on how intensively the herd is studied. Andriamanga *et al.* (1984) cite studies that show a 10 per cent incidence but observed in two herds an incidence of 34.7 per cent. Bartlett *et al.* (1986b) reported that in 18 per cent of lactations metritis occurred. The variation between herds is great.

Specific infections colonize the undamaged uterus. Two important specific infective agents are *C. fetus* and *Trichomonas foetus*. Campylobacteriosis is spread venereally and causes a mild endometritis in infected females that have not had previous experience of the condition. It has been shown in slaughter experiments that in infected animals fertilization rate is normal and that the infertility is due in the main to embryonic death within three weeks after conception. Loss of the embryo is likely due to interference with the uterine environment. Trichomoniasis, a parasitic venereal disease that still occurs in some countries (Clark *et al.*, 1986), is similar to campylobacteriosis with one major difference, the occurrence of pyometra in a number of cases.

Other infectious agents that are introduced from the vagina into the uterus at insemination, but not at natural service, are *Ureaplasma* (Doig *et al.*, 1979), which cause a purulent metritis and infertility. *Haemophilus/Histophilus* also causes vaginitis and reduced fertility. For detailed discussion of a wide range of infectious agents see Morrow (1986).

Infectious conditions can cause infertility in three ways.

(a) The febrile reaction raises the temperature of the uterus. Blue tongue is an example of a disease that causes a high temperature resulting in loss of the embryo at about the time of hatching from the zona pellucida, about day 8 after service.

(b) The organism infects the uterus and causes metritis, which presumably interferes with embryo nutrition and may also infect the embryo. Examples are IBR virus (p. 256) and *Chlamydia* infections. It is likely that, in general, mild endometritis causes embryonic death whereas in cases of purulent metritis there may be interference with spermatozoa survival and thus fertilization failure.

(c) Infection of the conceptus can cause its death. The thought that embryo transfer could transmit infectious diseases from the sire or the dam is worrying. In theory bacterial and fungal infections are less likely than viral infections to be carried by embryos. From experimental studies with many different viruses it appears to be the case that if the zona pellucida is intact and if the embryo is washed properly, there is little danger of the transmission of viral infections by embryo transfer (Singh, 1987).

(d) Endotoxins produced by Gram-negative infections can increase prostaglandin $F_{2\alpha}$ production and interfere with luteal function (Fredriksson, 1984).

3 *Aged gametes*. Fresh chilled semen ages after several days and the inseminated cows have a lower pregnancy rate, the mechanism almost certainly being both through reduced fertilization rate and increased loss of embryos. There is no evidence of adverse effects from ageing of frozen semen stored in liquid nitrogen. Fertilization of ageing eggs is also likely to result in an increased amount of embryonic death.

4 *Local trauma*. This cause of loss affects the late embryo and early fetus. One source of local trauma to the pregnant uterus is the hand of a person carrying out pregnancy diagnosis, or some other palpation of the uterus. In one study the average loss was 2.82 per cent of cows diagnosed pregnant (Beghelli *et al.* 1986). Franco *et al.* (1987) reported a fetal loss rate of 9.5 per cent in cows diagnosed pregnant on days 42–46. The technique, which was carried out on two days, involved palpation of fetal fluid, identification of the amniotic vesicle and slipping of the chorioallantoic membranes.

In a very large field study in which they used milk progesterone assays, Laitinen *et al.* (1985) estimated that 1.8 per cent of cows that returned to service were pregnant at the time of re-insemination. When a pregnant cow is inseminated, the conceptus must be at risk either through trauma or by the introduction of infection into a progesterone-dominated uterus. An experienced inseminator may be able to feel the difference in the cervix and avoid deep insemination.

5 *Genetic factors*. Mention has been made of the variable breed susceptibility to high environmental temperature that causes embryo death.

In some cattle, in the process of cell division, translocation of parts of certain chromosomes without loss of genetic material has taken place, a condition that is passed on to future generations. These individuals can be identified by cytogenetic examination of leucocytes. When semen from bulls with translocation is used for insemination there is a slight increase in the incidence of return to service, which is believed to be the result of embryonic death, presumably because of lack or excess of some genetic material due to abnormal division at meiosis.

Some epidemiological studies demonstrate that there can be hereditary differences in fertility measured in several different ways but opinions differ. It is obviously not possible to extrapolate from 'infertility' to embryonic death.

6 *'Biological filter'*. One unproven but attractive hypothesis is that some embryonic death may represent a form of biological filter by which means abnormal embryos are lost as early as possible and the dam can return to normal breeding (Bishop, 1964).

Stage 4. Stage of failure not known. It should be clear from the limited number of factors listed as known to cause embryonic death, that in the majority of cases the cause is unknown. Some factors that result in return to service can affect different stages, for example late insemination can result in fertilization failure in some cases and embryonic death in others. There is a very large grey area concerning the aetiology of return to service, particularly where groups of affected animals are concerned. The difficulty concerning the relationship between (possible) aetiological factors and return to service is twofold.

Some factors almost certainly cause an increased return to service via an unknown mechanism. An example is the aetiological relationship between loss in body condition from calving to service and associated poor pregnancy rate. When this occurs it is presumably mediated hormonally but it is not known whether the cause is fertilization failure or embryonic death.

To complicate matters further, additive effects of two or more types will produce low pregnancy rates. Two or more independent minor adverse factors that occur at the same time will produce a poor result. For example, Boyd & Reed (1961b) observed that variations in three factors (calving-to-first-service interval, age of cow and age of fresh semen) caused a range of pregnancy rates from 22 to 70 per cent. As mentioned above, synergistic action of two or more adverse aetiological factors, for example *A. pyogenes* and *F. necrophorum*, can result in a more severe pathological condition than either singly.

Many of the putative causes of return to service are far from being proven but they cannot be simply dismissed for that reason. Amongst these possibly adverse factors are the following.

1 Short-term change in feeding and environment particularly at turnout in the spring and at housing in the autumn.
2 Stressful effect of disputes about dominance among cows that are subject to frequent change of groups in dairy herds.
3 Sudden very cold environment.
4 Non-reproductive systemic illness.
5 Deficiencies and imbalances in minerals and vitamins (almost impossible to generalize because of very local effect of feeding practices, local soil deficiencies and many other variables).
6 Very high milk yield.
7 Lameness.

There are various reasons why there is so much uncertainty in a field where numerous workers have gathered observations and data for several decades. Because expected pregnancy rate is about 50 per cent, the random variation in fertility in groups is great and this necessitates large, properly controlled groups in trials in order to give reliable results. The possibility of erroneous conclusions from any single trial is so great that only results which are consistently repeated in different populations can be regarded as reliable.

In recent years there have been a number of epidemiological studies of a highly statistical nature on the relationships between various aspects of management and production, disease and reproduction. Because of the complexity of interrelationships very large numbers of observations are needed and these reports are based on data from populations that range from about 2000 to >70 000 lactation records.

While there are considerable differences between the findings certain concepts are emerging.

1 Reproductive diseases at and after calving up to conception tend to occur in an interrelated complex.
2 Some diseases that are not directly related to reproduction appear to have an adverse effect on reproduction.
3 There is disagreement on the effect of high yield on fertility.
4 There is disagreement on the effect of hereditary factors on fertility.

As an example, data from the very large study by Saloniemi *et al.* (1986) showed the consequential effects (i.e. an effect must follow a possible cause) described in Table 33.11.

For details, which are complex, the reader is referred to the original texts, some of which are listed here: Andersson & Emanuelson (1985): hyperketonaemia and fertility; Bartlett *et al.* (1986a): cystic ovarian disease; Bartlett *et al.* (1986b): metritis; Curtis *et al.* (1985): metabolic, reproductive mastitis; Dohoo & Martin (1984a): age, season and sire; Dohoo & Martin (1984b): mastitis, ketosis, reproduction; Dohoo *et al.* (1984): disease, production, culling; Fulkerson (1984): various on reproduction; Rowlands *et al.* (1986): interrelationship of diseases; Saloniemi *et al.* (1986): reproductive diseases.

Diagnosis

Although a herd consists of many individuals, diagnosis of a return-to-service problem that affects a large part of a herd requires a different approach from that taken to investigate the cause in an individual animal. For this

Table 33.11 The consequential effects of management and disease on problems of fertility (from Saloniemi *et al.*, 1986)

Cause	Consequential effect			
	Retained fetal membranes	Metritis	Anoestrus/ suboestrus	Ovarian dysfunction
Winter calving	No	Yes	Yes	Yes
Highest herd milk yield	Yes	Yes	Yes	Yes
Parturient paresis	Yes	Yes		
Mastitis		Yes	Yes	
Ketosis		Yes	Yes	Yes
Retained fetal membranes		Yes		
Metritis			Yes	Yes

Table 33.12 The systematic diagnosis of return to service

History
General clinical examination and body condition
Examination of the reproductive tract (rectal, vaginal and suitable aids)
Appropriate laboratory tests
Analysis of records

reason the individual will be dealt with first, followed by the herd fertility problem.

Diagnosis of the individual repeat breeder cow. One problem with diagnosis is that by the time the cow is recognized as being a repeat breeder the situation that prevailed at the time of reproductive failure may well have changed.

The clinician should take a history and carry out a systematic clinical examination to find out if any of the factors that are likely to cause return to service are present. The fullness of the investigation will depend to a large extent on the value of the animal.

A systematic approach to diagnosis is essential and the following procedure is suggested (Table 33.12).

1 *History.* The history covers various points as shown in Table 33.13.

2 *General examination.* The clinician should carry out a brief general examination looking at the following points:

(a) body condition;

(b) signs of non-reproductive disease;

Table 33.13 The main factors to be covered in history taking

Date of calving
Dystokia and puerperal diseases
Postpartum reproductive disease
Other diseases (e.g. lameness, metabolic)
Service details
  Dates
  Bull used
  Natural or AI
  Inseminator service or farmer insemination
Major management or environmental changes
Is this a herd or individual cow problem?

(c) signs of vaginal discharge or dried pus or mucus on the tail; and

(d) other signs, for example raised tailhead.

3 *Rectal examination.* The technique of rectal palpation of the genital tract is fully described in various textbooks, as are the characteristics of the various normal and abnormal structures in the ovaries and tract. The purpose of carrying out a rectal examination is to assess:

(a) the state of the ovaries;

(b) the condition of the bursae and oviducts;

(c) uterine abnormality or status (e.g. metritis, adhesions, pregnancy);

(d) internal slackness of the pelvic ligaments;

(e) absence of fat inside the pelvis (body condition);

(f) vulval discharge (stimulated by palpation).

The accuracy of diagnosis is important, and because of the availability of simple hormone assays, has been assessed for some ovarian structures. Data concerning accuracy of diagnosis of the corpus luteum is given on p. 438 and below for diagnosis of cystic ovarian disease.

Accuracy of diagnosis of cystic ovarian disease by rectal palpation. There are obvious difficulties in trying to assess the nature of a cyst without rupturing it. A large, soft corpus luteum with no palpable ovulation papillum can be mistaken for a cyst. Some authors are very sceptical about the accuracy of diagnosis of cystic structures, for example Guenzler & Schallenberger (1980) and Stolla *et al.* (1980).

Table 33.14 demonstrates the accuracy of diagnosis by rectal palpation of the type of cyst with accuracy being assessed by progesterone assay (Leslie & Bosu, 1983; Ax *et al.*, 1986; Booth, 1988).

As has been already mentioned, variations in diagnosis between veterinarians is great (Coleman *et al.*, 1985).

Accuracy of diagnosis of endometritis. Clinical diagnosis of metritis is based on assessment by palpation of

Table 33.14 The accuracy of rectal palpation in diagnosis of cystic ovarian disease

Diagnosis based on rectal examination	Number	Apparently correct	Per cent correct	Reference
Follicular cyst	72	42	58.3	Ax *et al.* (1986)
Follicular cyst	140	117	84	Booth (1988)
Luteal cyst	32	32	100	Leslie & Bosu (1983)
Luteal cyst	59	32	54	Booth (1988)

* All cysts were diagnosed as follicular.

the size and condition of the uterus and by the observation of a purulent discharge. It is extremely difficult to assess the accuracy of these techniques in the absence of a simple, cheap objective test. Uterine biopsies are easy to take but require skill, experience and time to interpret; the technique for the collection of uterine swabs for microbiology is demanding in skill and requires special equipment and needs subsequent processing and interpretation (Studer & Morrow, 1978; Noakes *et al.*, 1989). Many more cases are identified by laboratory methods than by clinical. In addition, confusion may occur in herds with purulent vaginitis caused by *Haemophilus somnus* (Stephens *et al.*, 1986) where the discharge of pus is not associated with metritis.

4 *Vaginal examination.* There is a choice of two methods of vaginal examination on the farm. These are manual or visual using a vaginal speculum. In both cases the perineal region and vulva is thoroughly cleaned and the veterinarian uses fresh plastic gloves. With manual examination mucus in the anterior vagina is gathered and on withdrawal of the hand examined visually. Minimum lubrication is used to avoid confusion between the mucus and the lubricant. The cervix and vaginal wall is palpated for lesions and abnormalities. The vaginal speculum should be introduced with care and when fully inserted will give a clear view of the cervix. With both techniques the clinician may have difficulty in passing the vulvo-vaginal junction, which is the narrowest part of the tract at this level. Table 33.15 shows the factors that should be checked in a vaginal examination.

5 *Selection of samples for laboratory examination.* Selection of the appropriate laboratory examinations and the frequency of sampling depends very much on circumstances, including the value of the cow. The items listed in Table 33.16 should be considered.

To extend the physical examination beyond what is possible by palpation, dye tests to check the patency of the *oviducts* can be carried out using the technique developed by Coulthard described briefly in Arthur *et al.* (1989).

If the cow is hospitalized, sequential sampling is facilitated and rectal palpation can be carried out daily. In addition, observation for sexual behaviour should be carried out three times per day, or by other means such as TV camera with a video recorder.

6 *New technological aids to diagnosis.* In recent years advances in biochemistry, electronics and fibre optics, along with skills and materials developed for embryo transfer, have opened up new diagnostic possibilities. There is every reason to believe that new equipment and concepts will continue to be produced, which presents problems as well as opportunities for the veterinarian. Most of the new techniques do not require specifically veterinary skills and so may be used by a wide range of operators, although for best effect

Table 33.15 Factors to be checked by vaginal examination

Anatomical abnormalities
Heifer
Damage
Dystokia
Sadistic human interference
Type and quantity of mucus
Purulent
Clear oestrous mucus

Table 33.16 Types of samples required for various laboratory tests

Single milk progesterone assay: confirms or partially replaces rectal palpation
Serial milk progesterone assays: monitor events around service, confirm diagnosis, monitor treatment
Other hormonal analysis (LH): a series of samples needed at short intervals
Oestrone sulphate from milk, blood (specifically from the placenta: indicates live calf)
Blood for cytogenetic analysis
Blood for serology
Purulent material from the uterus: aerobes and anaerobes, antibiotic sensitivity
Uterine biopsy for histology
Samples from the cervix and uterus for serology and cytology

knowledgeable interpretation is needed. Choices have to be made about the lasting value of each new step forward as investing capital and training in inappropriate technology is unproductive.

The relatively new aids to diagnosis can be classified as:

(a) quick, cheap and, in some cases, automated hormone analysis;
(b) non-invasive (or acceptably invasive) examination of internal organs: ultrasound, hysteroscopy, endoscopy;
(c) automatic or semiautomatic recording of physical and behavioural changes that are related to the animal's reproductive status, such as body temperature, restlessness and changes in milk composition;
(d) computer analysis of data: compilation over time of various measurements in the individual and analysis of herd records.

Diagnosis of a herd problem. It is necessary to approach the diagnosis of a herd fertility problem systematically. It is not practical to lay out in any detail a series of steps to be followed because as the investigation develops the information obtained guides the continued course of the investigation.

The four main causes of herd problems are poor fertility management, infertile male, nutritional errors and deficiencies, and infectious conditions. In general terms the steps required are shown in Table 33.17.

1 *History.* The object of history taking is to acquire information on the factors shown in Table 33.18.

2 *Analysis of the records.* It is useful, if possible, to examine the breeding records before visiting the herd. If there are no records then establish a recording system. The objectives of record analysis in connection with a herd fertility problem are the following.

(a) To assess the current level of fertility in the herd to determine the seriousness of the condition.
(b) To look for clues to aetiology, by looking at the fertility of subgroups within the herd:
   (i) bull, semen or inseminator;
   (ii) age group;
   (iii) yield group;
   (iv) seasonal effect;
   (v) familial effect;
   (vi) relevant infectious disease: non-specific metritis after calving, specific metritis with signs of venereal spread.
(c) After a cause of the infertility has been suspected, a valuable technique is to group the records of all animals that are influenced by the suspect factor and compare these with the records from all other cows.

It can be difficult to identify the cause of a problem where farmer insemination is associated with poor pregnancy rate. In these cases there may be no comparative data on the bull's fertility, the problem could be due to poor insemination technique or to improper semen handling.

3 *Examination of the animals.* It is very useful to examine as many cows as possible to get a current picture of the herd, to observe the condition of the cows and to detect the incidence of obvious reproductive abnormalities. It also reveals the (in)accuracy of the information supplied by the farmer or farm staff. Advice should be given about culling of individuals that have a very poor prognosis.

By this stage the clinician should have a good idea of the type of problem and how the investigation then develops is a matter of common sense which cannot be detailed further.

Table 33.17 Steps required to diagnose a herd fertility problem

History
Analysis of records
Breeding
Health
Production
Selected clinical examinations and sampling
Conclusion

Table 33.18 History taking in determining herd fertility problems

General aspects of the herd and farm
Number of breeding stock (male and female)
Number of hectares for the cattle
Type of housing
Details of grazing
Targets for reproduction and production
Other enterprises
Information about the stockworkers
Definition of the problem
Anoestrus
Return to service
Vaginal discharges
Other manifestations
Duration of problem
Proportion of herd affected
Reproductive management
Calving management
Service management: cows and heifers (heat detection, timing of AI)
Bulls
Feeding

Treatment (see Chapter 58)

The veterinarian is faced with some difficulties when having to decide on appropriate and effective treatment for cows that are presented as infertile. This is partly because of the complex aetiology of return to service but also because of the time that has passed since the factors that initiated the problem were present. When using pharmaceutical products the reader is advised to consult the manufacturers' data sheets for details of treatment, dangers and contraindications. Wherever possible the treatment should be followed up to see whether it has been successful or not and, if need be, repeated or changed.

Ovulation failure. The most important cause of ovulation failure is cystic ovarian disease. Treatment is based on whether the cyst has been diagnosed as follicular or luteal. In most cases the condition is caused by hypothalamic–pituitary dysfunction and it is, therefore, logical to treat the condition systemically. There is little or no benefit in rupturing the cyst manually, which also involves a slight risk of causing ovarian adhesions. Nor does there appear to be any benefit from administration of drugs directly into the cyst.

Many cystic structures found less than 42 days after calving are transient and benign, and in general these do not require to be treated. Only if abnormal behaviour indicates that they are pathological or if there is some pressing management need should they be treated.

For follicular cysts the three drugs of choice are human chorionic gonadotrophin (HCG), which may be used with or without progesterone, gonadotrophin-releasing hormone (GnRH) and a progesterone-releasing intravaginal device (PRID). They all work in different ways to achieve the same end, i.e. to put the animal under the influence of progesterone. One effect of this is to allow a build-up of LH in the pituitary so that enough endogenous LH is available when spontaneous oestrus and physiological release of GnRH takes place after removal of the progesterone (via natural luteolysis or by removal of the PRID). This leads to normal ovulation, and in all cases the cow should be served at the first heat after treatment. Delay in getting the cow pregnant may result in recurrence of the condition.

Human chorionic goradotrophin has an LH-like direct action on the ovary to produce luteinization of the cyst or follicles. GnRH stimulates the release of LH from the pituitary to achieve the same result. In both cases the lifespan of the luteal tissue produced is variable, ranging from about six days to about 18 days, and oestrus can be expected about 8–22 days after treatment. It is desirable to examine the treated cows about 10–14 days after treatment for the presence of luteal tissue. If there is luteal tissue, treatment with prostaglandin $F_{2\alpha}$ or an analogue is a suitable way of increasing the predictability of the following oestrus. Service should be at that oestrus and aids to oestrus detection should be used. If there is no satisfactory response to the first treatment, the cow should be re-examined and treated again.

For cysts with functional luteal tissue injection of prostaglandin $F_{2\alpha}$ or an analogue followed by insemination at observed oestrus is the most suitable treatment.

An alternative treatment, suitable for both types of cystic ovarian disease, is the insertion of a PRID, which can be left in position for 12 days, and after withdrawal the cow should be served, either at fixed time or preferably at observed oestrus. Administration of prostaglandin $F_{2\alpha}$ or an analogue either on the day of withdrawal or the day before has been reported and may tighten up the time to ovulation. In some reports prostaglandin $F_{2\alpha}$ or an analogue is given before the introduction of the PRID to ensure that there is no endogenous progesterone at PRID withdrawal. As the corpus luteum is not always responsive to prostaglandin $F_{2\alpha}$ or an analogue and a PRID is not reliably luteolytic, the latter approach does not seem to be logical. If fixed time insemination is used and oestrus is observed later the animal should be inseminated again.

Fertilization failure

1 *Delayed ovulation.* For many years one of the standard ways of treating apparently normal repeat breeders on the farm has been to administer HCG or, more recently, GnRH on the day of service. The theory behind this is that many of these cases were thought to be due to delayed ovulation. An alternative approach is to inseminate the cow again 24 hours after the first insemination.

Alternatively, conservative treatment, i.e. recommending that the cow be served at the next oestrus without further treatment, is an approach for cases of possible delayed ovulation in which no abnormality has been detected.

2 *Interference with transport of egg or spermatozoa.* When this is due to bilateral blockage of the oviducts (or other parts of the female tract), there is no simple treatment. In some cases the diagnostic dye test may remove a minor blockage and attempts have been made to achieve this by adding antibiotics and corticosteroids to the dye, which is introduced into the oviduct end of

the uterus under gentle pressure using a cuffed catheter. In very valuable animals the use of embryo transfer techniques could be considered.

Other factors that can cause failure of fertilization are: (i) service at the wrong time, (ii) poor-quality semen, (iii) infertile bull, (iv) problems with artificial insemination. These are dealt with elsewhere under Prevention, in Chapter 35 on the bull, or by common sense.

Embryonic death. Although the aetiology of early embryonic death is listed under six headings (p. 455) only two are suitable for conventional treatment: non-specific metritis (already dealt with under purulent metritis on p. 431) and specific metritis caused by *C. fetus* and a variety of other infections. All the other conditions should be corrected by management improvements or are dealt with in different chapters of this book.

Because *C. fetus* subsp. *fetus* infection (vibriosis) is a venereal disease, treatment has to be thought of in terms of the herd.

In the bull, in which infection is limited to the surface of the prepuce and penis, spontaneous cure does occur but is erratic and unreliable. Moreover, if the bull continues natural service of infected cows he will be re-infected as the superficial nature of the infection does not stimulate an immune response in the bull.

The common treatment of the bull is preputial lavage with a mixture of penicillin and streptomycin in an oily medium (Melrose *et al.*, 1957). It is important that the treatment is carried out thoroughly and is repeated daily for three consecutive days. It is necessary to check that the treatment has been effective by further sampling for the organism three or more weeks after treatment or by limited use on susceptible cows or heifers. These test females are then examined for the presence of organisms or vaginal immune response.

Although there is no natural immune response in the bull, one successful form of treatment depends on vaccination of the bull (Clark & Dufty, 1982). The vaccine is licensed for use in a number of countries but not in the UK though on occasion licences have been issued.

Treatment of cows with local or systemic antibiotics is unreliable and because cows develop resistance to the infection it is usually best to wait for this to develop. Whatever course is followed an infected cow should be regarded as potentially infective for at least two gestations after infection. Even after this time a few cows may remain infected. As it takes only one cow to infect a bull when natural service is practised, it is clear that it is hazardous to allow natural service of any cows that have ever been infected unless the bull has been vaccinated. Vaccination of cows (where permitted) is widely and fairly effectively practised in range conditions.

On a herd basis, when campylobacteriosis is diagnosed the best advice is that natural service should stop and all services should be by AI using semen from non-infected bulls. Recently infected cows will continue to return to service for some time.

There is an alternative, which is extremely difficult to carry out successfully over a long period and should be advocated only under special circumstances. This is to use the infected bull(s) on infected cows; and AI or non-infected bulls on non-infected cows and heifers.

Stage of failure unknown. Non-specific endometritis will be dealt with here. There are few areas where the gap between the theory of therapy and its practice as applied in the field is so great!

The two most common therapeutic approaches are (i) promotion of the cow's normal resistance to infection, and (ii) the use of antibiotics. There is a tendency for spontaneous elimination of the infectious agents from the uterus, most likely due to the cow going through successive periods of oestrus. The current practical approach to treatment is discussed by Pepper & Dobson (1987).

1 *Promotion of uterine resistance to infection.* This is brought about in cases where there is a corpus luteum present by the induction of oestrus using prostaglandin $F_{2\alpha}$ or an analogue.

In the absence of a corpus luteum, an oestrogen, such as oestradiol benzoate, may be administered systemically and this may give an effect analogous to natural oestrus. When there is no corpus luteum present, some clinicians treat with prostaglandin $F_{2\alpha}$ or an analogue, possibly inducing uterine contractions.

The intra-uterine infusion of dilute Lugol's iodine (for example a 1 per cent solution in 0.9 per cent saline) is another form of treatment that has been applied widely over the years. It was originally used because of the antiseptic effect but it has been shown that it can cause luteolysis if given early in the oestrous cycle, which may have contributed to its efficacy.

2 *Antibiotic therapy.* Treatment of metritis with antibiotics calls for careful consideration, but unfortunately the published information on field trials is limited. For a useful discussion see Gustafsson (1984). Table 33.19 shows factors that have a significant effect on the outcome of the case.

Choice of antibiotic is best based on sensitivity tests of both aerobic and anaerobic causative organisms. The

Table 33.19 Factors to be considered in antibiotic treatment of metritis

Choice of antibiotic
Dose
Frequency of administration
Type and quantity of the medium
Route of administration

choice of route of administration is between systemic and intra-uterine. When antibiotic is introduced into the uterus it tends to become concentrated in the lumen and in the superficial layers of the mucous membrane and also absorbed into the circulation. A considerable quantity is ejected via the vagina and lost, particularly at oestrus. Some preparations cause necrosis of the endometrium, though whether this is beneficial or not is not known. The presence of pus in the uterus may adversely affect the antibiotic's action.

Systemically administered antibiotic is transferred into all parts of the reproductive tract and ovaries, the concentrations varying with different antibiotics and different vehicles. Dose and frequency of administration should be adequate to achieve and maintain a therapeutic concentration at the site of infection for a long enough period of time. This is possible by repeated systemic administration and for intra-uterine treatment either daily treatment or the use of an in-dwelling uterine catheter would be needed.

If treatment results in adequate levels of antibiotic at the site of infection then antibiotic in the milk will almost certainly be at a level that requires withholding the milk from sale.

It must be rare for these criteria to be met under field conditions. The most common form of treatment is one intra-uterine infusion of either a proprietary product or an antibiotic solution or mixture made up by the clinician.

For the treatment of metritis caused by *Ureaplasma*, Doig *et al.* (1979) advocate intra-uterine infusion of 1 g of tetracycline suspension 24 hours after insemination.

Prognosis

From the client's point of view successful treatment means that the cow becomes pregnant, a two-stage process. Firstly, the cow has to return to normal reproductive function and secondly she has to conceive. While the first stage is mainly the responsibility of the veterinarian, the second stage often depends on the farmer and farm staff. Where poor husbandry (i.e. feeding, housing or breeding management) is thought to be causing return to service, prognosis must be guarded because it is often a difficult and slow task for the veterinarian to effect a marked improvement.

Table 33.20 Response of apparently normal repeat breeders served without treatment

Number of cows	Treatment	Per cent pregnant at first AI after examination	Reference
191	None	59.7	De Kruif (1975)
141	None	60.0	Refsdal (1979)

Results of treatment reported by different workers are rarely comparable because different criteria for selection of cases and assessment of success may have been applied. In many cases self-cure is a phenomenon and because controlled studies are rare, interpretation of results is problematic. Accordingly it is suggested that, as well as reading published reports, clinicians analyse their own practice records of diagnosis, treatment and outcome.

The most common situation is the cow presented after a few unsuccessful inseminations (or services), which on examination appears to be normal. These *apparently normal repeat breeders* have an expected pregnancy rate at the first service after examination that is about the same as the first service pregnancy rate in the herd, as indicated in Table 33.20.

This is not to say that the factors influencing fertility in first service and repeat breeder cows are the same. In the first service cows, fertility may be affected by closeness to calving and the stress of peak yield. The population returning to service will have overcome these problems but will include a higher proportion of cows that will never become pregnant. Unfortunately before their ultimate disposal, cows in the last group will have had two or three different treatments and several examinations at routine visits. In most cases there is no reliable way of identifying these problem cows.

In animals that are hospitalized the owner should be given a definite prognosis as soon as possible to minimize the cost involved in keeping and treating cows over several weeks. Much of this cost is due to the fact that once an animal has been served there is little positive that can be done except monitoring changes until pregnancy or non-pregnancy is confirmed. With modern diagnostic methods it is now possible to reduce the waiting time from service to diagnosis of non-pregnancy to a minimum. If the prognosis is favourable, costs are reduced if the cow is returned to the owner's farm where she can be treated by the local veterinarian.

Accurate prognosis with long-term repeat breeder cows is also difficult. However, the outlook must always be regarded as poor but particularly so in cases with blocked oviducts, persisting metritis and anomalous steroid hormone production from the ovaries. For example, of 33 chronic repeat breeders treated by Boyd *et al.* (1984) only eight became pregnant. Even the use of embryo transfer techniques is not particularly successful. Reported results from these sort of cases are quite variable.

The two most commonly diagnosed specific pathological causes of return to service are cystic ovarian disease and purulent metritis.

Cystic ovarian disease. In data collected from a number of veterinary practices Bartlett *et al.* (1986a) recorded that culling rate for cows that had cystic ovarian disease was 26.6 per cent compared with 21.6 per cent for other cows. Cows with cystic ovarian disease that conceived had an interval from calving to conception 33.5 days longer than cows without cystic ovarian disease.

In general, three factors affect the outcome.

1 The time that has elapsed since calving. Cases of cystic ovaries that occur up to six weeks after calving have a good chance of spontaneous recovery. Cases that are first seen six months after calving have a very poor prognosis.

2 The accuracy of diagnosis. If the type of cyst is misdiagnosed, selection of inappropriate treatment will give poor results.

3 The aetiology of the condition affects the outcome. If the cyst is caused by a temporary environmental influence then prognosis is good even without treatment. At the other extreme, if it is one of the minority of cases caused by deficiency of LH and FSH receptors in the ovary, the prognosis is very poor.

The question of the desirability of treating a condition that may have a hereditary component is discussed under Prevention.

The results presented in Table 33.21 (Ax *et al.*, 1986; Booth, 1988; Nanda *et al.*, 1988), in most of which diagnosis and outcome were checked by progesterone assays, are typical of earlier published field trials. Stolla *et al.* (1980) in a critical field trial noted that 24 per cent of cows with cystic ovarian disease that were 'treated' with normal saline became pregnant to the first service after non-treatment.

Although PRIDs are widely used to treat cases of follicular cysts, there is little published information on success rates. In one trial (van Giessen, 1981) 33 cows that had failed to respond to GnRH treatment were treated with PRIDs. Of these 24 eventually became pregnant; pregnancy rate to first service after treatment was 27 per cent. Better results would be expected when PRIDs are used as the primary treatment.

Guenzler & Schallenberger (1980) treated 66 cows in which luteal cysts had been diagnosed by rectal palpation. After treatment with an analogue of prostaglandin $F_{2\alpha}$ complete luteolysis occurred in the 35 cows with mid-cycle levels of progesterone and all but three of these started normal cycles. The first service pregnancy rate for these cows was 40 per cent. The two groups of cows with lower levels of progesterone cycled erratically after treatment and had first service pregnancy rates of 20 and 24 per cent. Nanda *et al.* (1988) treated 77 luteal cyst cases with an analogue of prostaglandin $F_{2\alpha}$ and 65 per cent of these exhibited initial recovery, i.e. the cyst regressed and a corpus luteum formed; not all became pregnant and in 18 per cent the cyst recurred.

Purulent metritis. Ott & Gustafsson (1981) reviewed reports on over 600 cases and showed that in 85 per cent the uterus was emptied within a few days of treatment with prostaglandin $F_{2\alpha}$ or an analogue. In most reports the authors stated that pregnancy rate

Table 33.21 The treatment of follicular cystic ovarian disease with GnRH

Number of cows	Type of cyst	Confirmed by progesterone assay	Treatment	Successful result: progesterone rose within 14 days	Reference
104	Follicular	Yes	GnRH	73 (70%)	Nakao *et al.* (1983b)
30	Follicular	Yes	GnRH	25 (83%)	Ax *et al.* (1986)
12	Follicular	Yes	None	3 (25%)	Ax *et al.* (1986)
116	Follicular	No	GnRH	61 (53%)	Nanda *et al.* (1988)
55	Follicular	Yes	GnRH	40 (73%)	Booth (1988)
44	Follicular	Yes	HCG + progesterone	32 (73%)	Booth (1988)

after successful treatment was lower than in normal cows. Time from treatment to conception was about 75 days. Arthur *et al.* (1989) also summarized a number of reports on the use of prostaglandin $F_{2\alpha}$ or an analogue and concluded that the results as far as pregnancy was concerned were good.

Factors that affect prognosis have been quantified by Anderson (1985) who modified a system proposed by Studer & Morrow (1978), which was based on a careful analysis of clinical and laboratory observations. Anderson took into account (i) the time since calving, (ii) whether oestrus had occurred since calving, (iii) the amount of pus, (iv) the size of the cervix, and (v) the diameter of the larger affected horn.

By giving points for these factors a cumulative score was calculated that gave a useful prediction about the eventual outcome of the case. Cows that had been in oestrus had a poor prognosis, presumably because they had not responded to the normal defence mechanism.

Pepper & Dobson (1987) found that the relative amount of pus in the discharge gave a (non-significant) indication of the pregnancy rate after treatment and that time from calving to treatment was significantly related to pregnancy rate after treatment. Cows treated with prostaglandin $F_{2\alpha}$ or oestrogen within 40 days of calving had a pregnancy rate of about 55 per cent compared with a significantly poorer result for cows treated later. From Anderson's (1985) data it appeared that in successfully treated cows there was a high incidence of periparturient problems at the resultant calving and a very high culling rate in this group of animals in the year after treatment, observations that warrant further study.

As regards the outlook for *herds* with a return-to-service problem prognosis varies and obviously is related to the diagnosis. Some episodes of herd infertility are of short duration and normal fertility returns spontaneously.

In cases where a definite infectious cause is identified, such as campylobacteriosis the outcome can be completely satisfactory with the elimination of the infection and the return to normal herd pregnancy rate. This depends on treatment being carried out carefully and the subsequent control of breeding management.

Where the problem is related to poor husbandry caution should be expressed until clear signs of improved management are noted.

Prevention

Improvement in pregnancy rates is achieved by encouraging good husbandry and avoiding factors that have an adverse effect on fertility. While it is possible to achieve a very high fertilization rate (up to 100 per cent), some embryonic death is inevitable, which is why it is rare for a herd to achieve a pregnancy rate of greater than 70 per cent.

There are a number of items, listed below, which contribute to good fertility but deficiency in any one of these is likely to produce poor pregnancy rates.

1 Avoidance of dystokia and postpartum abnormalities; and timely veterinary intervention where indicated. This should reduce the incidence of delayed involution, non-specific metritis, blocked oviducts and cystic ovarian disease.

2 Proper nutrition and maintenance of suitable body condition before and after calving.

3 Accurate heat detection.

4 The proper use of records can help to achieve good pregnancy rate and to avoid long interservice intervals. This is done by:

(a) not serving cows too soon after calving (not before 42 days);

(b) being aware of the expected return-to-service date (for example, by using a three-week calendar);

(c) ensuring early pregnancy diagnosis;

(d) checking the fertility of the bulls;

(e) checking the efficiency of the inseminators;

(f) understanding the causes of fertility variations in a specific herd.

5 Avoidance of service contact outside the herd and ensuring veterinary examination of bought-in breeding stock will reduce the risk of introducing venereal diseases.

6 Good housing environment and cattle handling will help to avoid stress, lameness, discomfort and fear in the herd.

7 Consideration should be given to reproductive dysfunction with a hereditary component, e.g. cystic ovarian disease.

8 Avoid interventions that may cause embryonic death, such as drastic changes in feeding and environment, herd medication and IBR vaccination in the weeks after service.

9 Drug therapy, using either antibiotics or hormones, in the postpartum phase has been advocated as a way of improving pregnancy rates. The doubtful value of this is discussed below.

Where drug therapy is applied selectively in cows identified as likely to have poor fertility this is obviously a suitable approach. However, it has been proposed that routine treatments should be applied to all cows, normal and abnormal, and this is much more questionable. There are, of course, special circumstances when treatment of normal cows is acceptable, for example the use of a PRID to promote early breeding in a cow

Table 33.22 The effect of routine treatment of normal cows on first service pregnancy rate (per cent)

$PGF_{2\alpha}$	GnRH	Both	None	Reference
–	57	–	52	Langley & O'Farrell (1979)
–	39/39	–	44	Nash *et al.* (1980)
–	64/71	–	46	Nash *et al.* (1980)
–	–	34	46	Richardson *et al.* (1983)
42	40	38	29	Benmrad & Stevenson (1986)
68	–	–	43	Young & Anderson (1986)

$PGF_{2\alpha}$, prostaglandin $F_{2\alpha}$.

that has calved late in a restricted calving season.

In previous decades the routine use of antibiotics in both normal and abnormal cows after calving or at the time of insemination has been tried. Results have shown no benefit to normal cows.

More recently it has been proposed that the routine administration of either prostaglandin $F_{2\alpha}$, or GnRH or both in the early postpartum period improves pregnancy rate. Table 33.22 shows results obtained in several field trials and no consistent pattern of improved fertility emerges. The numbers of cows in the groups ranged from 29 to 79.

Great attention must be paid to cows that are treated to allow synchronization of insemination because of the size of the potential loss. The technique is best suited for beef suckler herds. For best results the farmer, the veterinary surgeon and a member of the insemination organization should discuss the whole operation well beforehand. Only reproductively normal cows at least six weeks after calving (preferably longer) should be included. First calvers tend to give poor results and should be excluded. Results with dairy cows also tend to be unsatisfactory. Avoid stress and any change in management and diet during preparation and for three to four weeks after insemination. As far as possible all drug therapy should be avoided during the same period. It is essential that preparation is made to deal with the cows that return to the synchronized insemination.

References

Anderson, D.B. (1985) *A clinical study of chronic endometritis in dairy cows.* MVM thesis, Glasgow University.

Andersson, L. & Emanuelson, U. (1985) An epidemiological study of hyperketonaemia in Swedish dairy cows; determinants and the relation to fertility. *Preventive Veterinary Medicine*, **3**, 449–62.

Andriamanga, S., Steffan, J. & Thibier, M. (1984) Metritis in dairy herds: an epidemiological approach with special reference to ovarian cyclicity. *Annales de Recherches Veterinaires (Paris)*, **15**, 503–8.

Arthur, G.H., Noakes, D.E. & Pearson, H. (1989) *Veterinary Reproduction and Obstetrics (Thieriogenology)*, 6th edn., pp. 1–64, Baillière Tindall, London.

Ax, R.L., Bellin, M.E., Scheinder, D.K. & Haase-Hardie, J.A. (1986) Reproductive performance of dairy cows with cystic ovaries following administration of Procystin TM1. *Journal of Dairy Science*, **69**, 542–5.

Bane, A. (1964) Fertility and reproductive disorders in Swedish cattle. *British Veterinary Journal*, **120**, 430–41.

Bartlett, P.C., Ngategize, P.K., Kaneene, J.B., Kirk, J.H., Anderson, S.M. & Mather, E.C. (1986a) Cystic follicular disease in Michigan Holstein–Friesian cattle: incidence, descriptive epidemiology and estimated economic impact. *Preventive Veterinary Medicine*, **4**, 15–33.

Bartlett, P.C., Kirk, J.H., Wilke, M.A., Kaneene, J.B. & Mather, E.C. (1986b) Metritis complex in Michigan Holstein–Friesian cattle: incidence, descriptive epidemiology and estimated economic impact. *Preventive Veterinary Medicine*, **4**, 235–48.

Beghelli, V., Boiti, C., Parmigiani, E. & Barbacini, S. (1986) Pregnancy diagnosis and embryonic mortality in the cow. In *Embryonic Mortality in Farm Animals* (ed. by J.M. Sreenan & M.G. Diskin), pp. 159–67. Nijhoff, Dordrecht/Boston/Lancaster.

Benmrad, M. & Stevenson, J.S. (1986) Gonadotrophin-releasing hormone and prostaglandin $F_{2\alpha}$ for postpartum dairy cows: estrous, ovulation and fertility traits. *Journal of Dairy Science*, **69**, 800–11.

Bishop, M.W.H. (1964) Paternal contribution to embryonic death. *Journal of Reproduction and Fertility*, **7**, 383–96.

Bloomfield, G.A., Morant, S.V. & Ducker, M.J. (1986) A survey of reproductive performance in dairy herds. Characteristics of the patterns of progesterone concentrations in milk. *Animal Production*, **42**, 1–10.

Booth, J.M. (1988) The milk progesterone test as an aid to the diagnosis of cystic ovaries in dairy cows. *Veterinary Record*, **123**, 437–9.

Boyd, H. & Reed, H.C.B. (1961a) Investigations into the incidence and causes of infertility in dairy cattle — Fertility variations. *British Veterinary Journal*, **117**, 18–35.

Boyd, H. & Reed, H.C.B. (1961b) Investigations into the incidence and causes of infertility in dairy cattle — influence of some management factors affecting the semen and insemination conditions. *British Veterinary Journal*, **117**, 74–86.

Boyd, H., Renton, J., Munro, C., Harvey, M., Isbister, J. & Kelly, E. (1984) Clinical studies of a series of long (term) repeat breeder cows and heifers. *Vlaams Diergeneeskundig Tijdschrift*, **53**, 165–9.

Clark, B.L. & Dufty, J.H. (1982) The duration of protection against infection with *Campylobacter fetus* subsp. *venerealis* in immunised bulls. *Australian Veterinary Journal*, **58**, 220.

Clark, B.L., Dufty, J.H. & Parsonson, I.M. (1986) The frequency of infertility and abortion in cows infected with *Trichomonas foetus* var. *brisbane. Australian Veterinary Journal*, **63**, 31–2.

Claus, R., Karg, H., Zwiauer, D., von Butler, I., Pirchner, F. & Rattenberger, E. (1983) Analysis of factors influencing reproductive performance of the dairy cow by progesterone assay in milk fat. *British Veterinary Journal*, **139**, 29–37.

Coleman, D.A., Thayne, W.V. & Dailey, R.A. (1985) Factors affecting reproductive performance of dairy cows. *Journal of Dairy Science*, **68**, 1793–1803.

Curtis, C.R., Erb, H.N., Sniffen, C.J., Smith, R.D. & Kronfield, D.S. (1985) Path analysis of dry period nutrition, postpartum metabolic and reproductive disorders, and mastitis in Holstein cows. *Journal of Dairy Science*, **68**, 2347–60.

Dohoo, I.R. & Martin, S.W. (1984a) Disease, production and culling in Holstein–Friesian cows. III. Disease and production as determinates of disease. *Preventive Veterinary Medicine*, **2**, 671–90.

Dohoo, I.R. & Martin, S.W. (1984b) Disease, production and culling in Holstein–Friesian cows. IV. Effects of disease on production. *Preventive Veterinary Medicine*, **2**, 755–70.

Dohoo, I.R., Martin, S.W., McMillan, I. & Kennedy, B.W. (1984) Disease, production and culling in Holstein–Friesian cows. II. Age, season and sire effects. *Preventive Veterinary Medicine*, **2**, 655–70.

Doig, P.A., Ruhnke, H.L., Mackay, A.L. & Palmer, N.C. (1979) Bovine granular vulvitis associated with *Ureaplasma* infection. *Canadian Veterinary Journal*, **20**, 89–94.

Etherington, W.G., Bosu, W.T.K., Martin, S.W., Cote, J.F., Doig, P.A. & Leslie, K.E. (1984) Reproductive performance in dairy cows following postpartum treatment with gonadotrophin releasing hormone and/or prostaglandin: a field trial. *Canadian Journal of Comparative Medicine*, **48**, 245–50.

Fathalla, M.A., Geissinger, H.D. & Liptrap, R.M. (1978) Effect of endometrial damage and prostaglandin $F_{2\alpha}$ on experimental cystic ovarian follicles in the cow. *Research in Veterinary Science*, **25**, 269–79.

Franco, O.J., Drost, M., Thatcher, M.J., Shille, V.M. & Thatcher, W.W. (1987) Fetal survival in the cow after pregnancy diagnosis by palpation per rectum. *Theriogenology*, **27**, 631–43.

Fredriksson, G. (1984) Some reproductive and clinical aspects of endotoxins in cows with special emphasis on the role of prostaglandins. *Acta Veterinaria Scandinavica*, **25**, 365–77

Fulkerson, W.J. (1984) Reproduction in dairy cattle: effect of age, cow condition, production level, calving to first interval and the 'male'. *Animal Reproduction Science*, **7**, 305–14.

Giessen, R.C. van (1981) Intravaginale behandeling van cysteuze ovariele follikels bij het rund met progesteron (PRID), waarbij een behandeling met GnRH niet tot resultaat leidde. *Tijdschrift voor Diergeneeskunde*, **106**, 881–3.

Grahn, T.C., Fahning, M.L. & Zemjanis, R. (1984) Nature of early reproductive failure caused by bovine viral diarrhea virus. *Journal of the American Veterinary Medical Association*, **185**, 429–32.

Guenzler, O. & Schallenberger, E. (1980) The treatment of ovarian cysts in cattle with prostaglandins — possibilities and limitations. *Acta Veterinaria Scandinavica*, Suppl. 77, 327–41.

Gustafsson, B.K. (1984) Therapeutic strategies involving antimicrobial treatment of the uterus in large animals. *Journal of the American Veterinary Medical Association*, **185**, 1194–8.

Hancock, J.L. (1948) The clinical analysis of reproductive failure in cattle. *Veterinary Record*, **60**, 513–17.

Hare, W.C.D. (1986) Status of disease transmission studies and their relationship to the International Movement of Bovine Medicine. *Canadian Veterinary Journal*, **27**, 37–55.

Henricson, B. (1957) Genetical and statistical investigations into so-called cystic ovaries in cattle. *Acta Agriculturae Scandinavica*, **7**, 3–93.

Hermas, S.A., Young, C.W. & Rust, J.W. (1987) Genetic relationships and additive genetic variation of productive and reproductive traits in Guernsey dairy cattle. *Journal of Dairy Science*, **70**, 1252–7.

Jackson, P.S., Johnson, C.T., Bulman, D.C. & Holdsworth, R.J. (1979) A study of cloprostenol-induced oestrus and spontaneous oestrus by means of the milk progesterone assay. *British Veterinary Journal*, **135**, 578–90.

Jasko, D.J., Erb, H.N., White, M.E. & Smith, R.D. (1984) Prostaglandin treatment and subsequent cystic ovarian disease in Holstein cows. *Journal of the American Veterinary Medical Association*, **185**, 212–13.

Kesler, D.J. & Gaverick, H.A. (1982) Ovarian cysts in dairy cattle: a review. *Journal of Dairy Science*, **55**, 1147–59.

Kruif A. de (1975) *Fertiliteit en subfertiliteit bij het vrouwelijk rund*. Thesis, Utrecht.

Laitinen, E.R., Tenhunen, M., Haenninen, O. & Alanko, M. (1985) Milk progesterone in Finnish dairy cows: a field study on the control of artificial insemination and early pregnancy. *British Veterinary Journal*, **141**, 297–307.

Langley, O.H. & O'Farrell, K.J. (1979) The use of Gn-RH to stimulate early resumption of oestrous cycles in dairy cows. *Irish Journal of Agricultural Research*, **18**, 157–65.

Leslie, K.E. & Bosu, W.T.K. (1983) Plasma progesterone concentrations in dairy cows with cystic ovaries and clinical responses following treatment with Fenprostalene. *Canadian Veterinary Journal*, **24**, 352–6.

Melrose, D.R., Morgan, B., Stewart, W.J. & Thomson, D.M. (1957) The treatment of *Vibrio fetus* infected bulls. *Veterinary Record*, **69**, 691–2.

Morrow, D.A. (1986) *Current Therapy in Thieriogenology 2. Diagnosis, Treatment and Prevention of Reproductive Diseases in Small and Large Animals*, pp. 1–143. W.B. Saunders and Company, Philadelphia.

Nakao, T., Sugihashi, A., Saga, N., Tsunoda, N. & Kawata, K. (1983) Use of milk progesterone enzyme immuno-assay for differential diagnosis of follicular cyst, luteal cyst and corpus luteum in cows. *American Journal of Veterinary Research*, **44**, 888–90.

Nakao, T., Shirakawa, J., Tsurubayashi, M., Oboshi, K., Abe, T., Sawamukai, Y., Sago, N., Tsunoda, N. & Kawata, K. (1984) A preliminary report on the treatment of ovulation failure in cows with gonadotrophin-releasing hormone analog or human chorionic gonadotrophin combined with insemination. *Animal Reproduction Science*, **7**, 489–95.

Nanda, A.S., Ward, W.R., Williams, P.C.W. & Dobson, H. (1988) Retrospective analysis of the efficacy of different hormone treatments of cystic ovarian disease in cattle. *Veterinary Record*, **122**, 155–8.

Nash, J.G., Ball, L. & Olson, J.D. (1980) Effects on reproductive performance of administration of GnRH to early postpartum dairy cows. *Journal of Animal Science*, **50**, 1017–21.

Noakes, D.E., Till, D. & Smith, G.R. (1989) Bovine uterine flora post partum: A comparison of swabbing and biopsy. *Veterinary Record*, **124**, 563–4.

Okuda, K., Kito, S., Sumi, N. & Sato, K. (1988) A study of the central cavity in the bovine corpus luteum. *Veterinary Record*, **123**, 180–3.

Oltner, R. & Edqvist, L.E. (1981) Progesterone in defatted milk: its relation to insemination and pregnancy in normal cows as compared with cows on problem farms and individual problem animals. *British Veterinary Journal*, **137**, 78–87.

Ott, R.S. & Gustaffson, B.K. (1981) Therapeutic application of prostaglandins for post partum infections. *Acta Veterinaria Scandinavica*, Suppl. 77, 363–9.

Pepper, R.T. & Dobson, H. (1987) Preliminary results of treatment and endocrinology of chronic endometritis in the dairy cow. *Veterinary Record*, **120**, 53–6.

Refsdal, A.O. (1979) *Undersoekelse av kviger og kyr utsjaltet paa grunn av ufruktbarhet.* Thesis, Oslo.

Refsdal, A.O. (1982) Ovariecyster hos melkekyr. *Norsk Veterinaertidsskrift*, **94**, 789–96.

Reid, I.M., Roberts, C.J. & Manston, R. (1979) Fatty liver and infertility in high-yielding dairy cows. *Veterinary Record*, **104**, 75–6.

Richardson, G.F., Archbald, L.F., Galton, D.M. & Godke, R.A. (1983) Effect of gonadotrophin-releasing hormone and prostaglandin $F_{2\alpha}$ on reproduction in postpartum dairy cows. *Theriogenology*, **19**, 763–70.

Rowlands, G.J., Lucey, S. & Russell, A.M. (1986) Susceptibility to disease in the dairy cow and its relationship with occurrences of other diseases in the current or preceding lactation. *Preventive Veterinary Medicine*, **4**, 223–34.

Saloniemi, H., Groehn, Y. & Syvaejaervi, J. (1986) An epidemiological and genetic study on registered diseases in Finnish Ayrshire cattle. II. Reproductive disorders. *Acta Veterinaria Scandinavica*, **27**, 196–208.

Schermerhorn, E.C., Foote, R.H., Newman, S.K. & Smith R.D. (1986) Reproductive practices and results in dairies using owner or professional inseminators. *Journal of Dairy Science*, **69**, 1673–85.

Sreenan, J.M. (1988) Embryo transfer: Its use and recent developments. *Veterinary Record*, **122**, 624–9.

Singh, E.L. (1987) The disease control potential of embryos. *Theriogenology*, **27**, 9–20.

Sreenan, J.M. & Diskin, M.G. (1986) The extent and timing of embryonic mortality in cattle. In *Embryonic Mortality in Farm Animals* (ed. by J.M. Sreenan & M.G. Diskin), pp. Nijhoff, Dordrecht/Boston/Lancaster.

Stephens, I.R., Slee, K.J., Poulton, P., Larcombe, M. & Kosior, E. (1986) Investigation of purulent vaginal discharge in cows, with particular reference to *Haemophilus somnus*. *Australian Veterinary Journal*, **63**, 182–5.

Stolla, R., Bostedt, H., Wendt, V. & Leidl, W. (1980) Zur Ovarialzyste des Rindes. III. Vergleichende Wertung von Therapieverfahren. *Berliner und Muenchner Tieraerztliche Wochenschrift*, **93**, 4–10.

Studer, E. & Morrow, D.A. (1978) Postpartum evaluation of bovine reproductive potential: comparison of findings from genital tract examination per rectum, uterine culture and endometrial biopsy. *Journal of the American Veterinary Medical Association*, **172**, 489–94.

Thatcher, W.W. & Collier, R.J. (1986) Effects of climate on bovine reproduction. In *Current Therapy in Theriogenology 2. Diagnosis, Treatment and Prevention of Reproductive Diseases in Small and Large Animals.* (ed. by D.A. Morrow), W.B. Saunders and Company, Philadelphia.

Trimberger, G.W. (1948) Breeding efficiency in dairy cattle from artificial insemination at various intervals before and after ovulation. University of Nebraska College of Agriculture, Agricultural Experimental Station, Research Bulletin 153.

Wagner, W.C. & Li, P.S. (1982) Influence of adrenal corticosteroids on postpartum pituitary and ovarian function. In *Factors Influencing Fertility in the Postpartum Cow* (ed. by H. Karg & E. Schallenberger), pp. 197–219. Nijhoff, The Hague.

Warren, M.E. (1984) Biological targets for fertility and their effects on herd economics. In *Dairy Cow Fertility* (ed. by R.G. Eddy & M.J. Ducker), pp. 1–14. British Veterinary Association, London.

Watson, E.D. & MacDonald, B.J. (1984) Failure of conception in dairy cattle: progesterone and oestradiol-17β concentrations and the presence of ovarian follicles in relation to the timing of artificial insemination. *British Veterinary Journal*, **140**, 398–406.

Watson, E.D. & Munro, C.D. (1984) Adrenal progesterone production in the cow. *British Veterinary Journal*, **140**, 300–6.

Watson, E.D., Jones, P.C. & Saunders, R.W. (1987) Effect of factors associated with insemination on calving rate in dairy cows. *Veterinary Record*, **121**, 256–8.

Young, I.M. (1989) Dinoprost 14-day oestrus synchronisation schedule for dairy cow. *Veterinary Record*, **124**, 587–8.

Young, I.M. & Anderson, D.B. (1986) First service conception rate in dairy cows treated with dinoprost tromethamine early post partum. *Veterinary Record*, **118**, 212–13.

Chapter 34: Fetal Loss and Abnormalities of Pregnancy

by H. BOYD AND D. GRAY

Introduction

This chapter deals with problems that arise from day 42 of pregnancy to term, but mainly during the last three months of gestation. The incidence of loss in this period is low but each individual case is serious. For example, abortion of a seven-month-old fetus results in a very long loss of production time, loss of the calf and in many cases culling of the affected animal.

Fetal loss and abnormalities during pregnancy that are dealt with here are listed in Table 34.1.

Abortion

Manifestation

Individual. The stage of gestation at which fetal death and expulsion occur will influence the detection rate of individual aborting cows. In many cases the manifestation is obvious with the farmer finding a large aborted foetus. However, the expulsion of a small fetus, particularly where animals are housed in accommodation with slatted floors or deep straw bedding, may well go unnoticed. In these situations, the aborted cow may be seen to have parts of the fetal membranes hanging from the vulva or to have an abnormal vulval discharge or signs of a recent calving, such as mammary gland changes. Under extensive beef cattle management systems or where in-calf dairy heifers and dry cows are grazed away from close supervision, the only signs of abortion are that the cow comes into oestrus and is found to be empty on rectal palpation or fails to calve when expected.

Herd. The majority of abortions occurring in a herd will be sporadic in as much as they will be caused by unrelated factors. The incidence of fetal death has been reported to be 3–4 per cent of pregnancies in 'normal' herds (Miller, 1986). Recognition of a true herd abortion problem may be difficult against this background, particularly where a seasonal calving pattern is being aimed at. In this situation abortions will necessarily be seen during a specific time period possibly leading to the false conclusion that an abortion 'storm' is occurring in the herd. Deas (1981) suggested that a 5 per cent or greater abortion rate in a herd should be considered as indicating herds with a true abortion problem.

Aetiology

Death of the fetus, which is the starting point for many abortions, can be caused by a wide variety of factors, including infections, endotoxins, exotoxins, trauma and physical disturbance to the fetal blood supply. Sometimes the cause precedes the manifestation by many weeks.

The aetiology of abortion is complex and one classification of different causes is presented in Table 34.2.

Infectious causes of abortion. The majority of cases of abortion in which the cause is diagnosed are due to infectious agents. Reports of the incidence of different agents that have been published, for example by Kirk-

Table 34.1 Fetal losses and abnormalities during pregnancy

Abortion (including live premature calves)
Fetal mummification
Fetal maceration
Hydrops allantois
Hydrops amnion

Table 34.2 Classification of causes of abortion

Infectious
Non-specific
Specific
Miscellaneous
Drug induced
Insemination/intra-uterine infusion
Hypothyroidism
Trauma/stress
High fever and endotoxins
Exotoxins
Nutritional
Twin pregnancy
Genetic

bride (1985) and Jerrett *et al.* (1984). The incidence reported by state laboratories vary quite considerably from country to country, within countries and seasonally. This is partly due to the variety of environments and husbandry practices to which cattle are exposed. As laboratory techniques change the apparent importance of some conditions, such as leptospirosis, increases. Veterinarians will find it useful to keep informed about changes in their own areas by reading the reports of the state laboratories, which are published in the local veterinary press. For example, in the UK reports from the local state veterinary laboratories are regularly reported in the *Veterinary Record*.

Non-specific infections can cause abortion: cows that suffer from an acute infectious illness may abort without any infectious involvement of the uterus and contents. There are several possible reasons for this. For example, in salmonellosis, bacterial toxins may cause localized placental necrosis, which interferes with placental hormone production and results in abortion (Hinton, 1986). It has been suggested that increased corticosteroid production may be the abortifacient mechanism. Fredriksson (1984) has shown that endotoxins from Gram-negative organisms can cause luteolysis, which could affect the maintenance of pregnancy. In other infections, such as tick-borne fever (see p. 742), the febrile response itself is thought to cause fetal loss.

In *specific infections* systemic infection is followed by localization of the organisms in the placenta and usually also in the fetus, with a wide range of pathological effects.

Table 34.3 lists some of the infectious agents reported as having been associated with bovine abortion. Many of these agents cause sporadic abortions as a result of opportunistic invasion of the gravid uterus following bacteraemia or septicaemia. Impaired immunity associated with pregnancy often allows low-grade pathogens or even commensals to overcome host defences and invade the placenta and fetus. These sporadic infectious abortions are important in the individual affected cow but are not conducive to practical control measures.

Certain pathogens are recognized as being of major importance in abortion, either because they can result in a high incidence of abortion in a herd or because they are zoonotic infections transmissible to humans as a result of contact with infected cattle or the consumption of contaminated cattle products. In some cases both criteria apply and these are often the diseases chosen for national control or eradication programmes (e.g. brucellosis, leptospirosis, salmonellosis). An understanding of the epizootiology and pathogenesis of these infections is necessary to allow relevant control

Table 34.3 The agents causing infectious abortion

Bacteria
Actinomyces pyogenes
Bacillus licheniformis
Brucella abortus
Campylobacter fetus subsp. *venerealis*
C. fetus subsp. *fetus*
C. jejuni
Erysipelothrix rhusiopathiae
Escherichia coli
Haemophilus/Histophilus group
Klebsiella pneumoniae
Listeria monocytogenes
Pasteurella haemolytica, *P. multocida*
Pseudomonas aeruginosa, *Ps. pseudomallei*
Salmonella spp.: *S. dublin*, *S. typhimurium*, *S. montevideo*, etc.
Spirochaetes
Borrelia coriaceae
Leptospira interrogans: serovars *hardjo*, *pomona*, *canicola*, *grippotyphosa*, *icterohaemorrhagiae*
Staphylococcus aureus
Streptococcus spp.
Yersinia pseudotuberculosis
Mycoplasma/Ureaplasma
Mycoplasma bovis
Ureaplasma diversum

Table 34.3 (Cont.)

Fungi/yeasts
Absidia spp. (*A. corymbifera*, *A. ramosa*)
Aspergillus flavus, *A. niger*, *A. fumigatus*, *A. terreus*, *A. nidulans*
Candida parapsilosis, *C. tropicalis*, *C. pseudotropicalis*, *C. albicans*, *C. krusei*
Mortierella wolfii
Mucor spp.
Rhizopus spp.
Torulopsis candida
Trichosporon cutaneum
Zygomycetes
Rickettsia/Chlamydia
Tick-borne fever (*Cytoecetes phagocytophila*)
Heartwater (*Cowdria ruminantium*)
Q fever (Coxiella burnetii)
Chlamydia psittaci
Protozoa
Babesia bovis
Sarcocystis spp.
Toxoplasma gondii
Trichomonas foetus
Trypanosoma congolense
Virus
Adenovirus
Akabane
BHV-1 (IBR/IPV)
BHV-4
Bluetongue
BVD MD
Louping ill
Orbivirus
Parvovirus
PI_3

measures to be applied. Detailed descriptions for each agent are outwith the scope of this text, but an outline of the important factors for the more common groups follows.

1 *Salmonellosis* (Hinton, 1986). *Salmonella dublin* causes septicaemia, dysentery and abortion and is the commonest cause of salmonella abortion. The pathogenesis of abortion is complex because there are various different pathways. In the acute stage of the disease abortion may be due to non-specific factors that have been described previously. Abortion also occurs two to four weeks after the acute phase, caused by infection of the placenta and the fetus but many also occur in symptomless latent carriers. Salmonella abortions are most common from June to November and more frequent in the south west of the UK where they account for about 1 per cent of all abortions investigated. Other *Salmonella* species causing abortion include *S. typhimurium*, *S. montevideo*, *S. hadar* and *S. agama* (see also Chapter 13).

2 *Listeriosis* (Gitter, 1979). Listeriosis in cattle is associated with feeding contaminated silage, particularly of poor quality. The route of infection is oral as well as possibly via upper respiratory tract or eyes. Bacteraemia results in placentitis and widespread infection of the fetus leading to late abortions (sixth to eighth month), which are sporadic, tend to occur in the winter and recur year after year. A high incidence of retained fetal membranes and resulting metritis has been reported. Intra-uterine death of the fetus results in moderate to severe autolysis at the time of abortion but fetal liver shows numerous minute necrotic foci in a majority of cases. The organism is very widespread and occurs in many species including man (see p. 703).

3 *Brucellosis* (Morgan & Mackinnon, 1979). *Brucella abortus* is the cause of infectious bovine abortion (Bang's disease) world-wide. Infection is by ingestion or through the conjunctiva. The organisms have a predilection for the pregnant uterus and cause varying degrees of placentitis, their growth being stimulated by the presence of the saccharide alcohol erythritol in the placenta. During non-pregnancy and early pregnancy the bacteria are found in the udder and lymph glands. Infection may lead to abortion from about seven months gestation onwards or to the delivery of a live full-term calf. Cattle often become chronically infected and although cows usually only abort once, subsequent apparently normal calvings may be associated with the spread of organisms in discharges.

4 *Campylobacteriosis* (Garcia *et al.*, 1983). There are various subspecies of *Campylobacter fetus* and sporadic abortion may follow either venereal infection (*C. fetus* subsp. *venerealis*) or infection following ingestion (*C. fetus* subsp. *fetus*). In both cases there is placental and fetal infection. Abortion may result from this direct infection or possibly as a result of endotoxin production. Abortions are most common about the fifth or sixth month.

5 *Leptospirosis* (Ellis, 1983, 1985). There are several serogroups, each containing a number of serovars and their importance varies geographically and seasonally. In the UK *Leptospira hardjo* of the Sejroe group is important whereas in the USA, Canada, Australia and New Zealand *L. pomona* is a serious cause of abortion. In temperate climates the organisms survive best outside in warm damp conditions and infection is commonest in the late summer and autumn with abortions showing a seasonal increase in prevalence during autumn and early winter. Leptospiraemia after pen-

etration of mucous membranes leads to infection of the kidneys and placenta with subsequent fetal infection. Fetal death and abortion occurs from four to twelve weeks after infection and is most common during the last four months of gestation. Abortion is frequently followed by retention of fetal membranes, excretion of the organism in discharges and persistence in the uterus and oviducts.

Leptospira hardjo also causes a milk drop syndrome with fever, fall in milk yield, flaccid udder and later abortion, though abortion may occur with no other clinical signs. It is a cattle-associated serovar and introduction to a herd is associated with the purchase of infected male or female animals, although contaminated water sources and incidental hosts such as sheep, goats or deer may be important (see p. 569).

6 *Fungal abortion* (Pepin, 1983; Foley & Schlafer, 1987). Fungi are the cause of sporadic abortions and small outbreaks of abortion. The source of infection is most commonly contaminated foodstuffs, typically mouldy hay and straw. Cattle that are tied in cow sheds are most often infected (Williams *et al.*, 1977). The routes of infection are oral and respiratory but it is not known whether spores or fragments of mycelium are transported to the uterus. A placentitis results in transcotyledonal spread to the fetus, which may show skin lesions and fungal invasion of the rumen and abomasal walls. Most abortions occur between the fifth and seventh months of gestation.

Yeasts (*Candida* spp.) also produce a necrotizing placentitis with secondary fetal infection of many organs.

Mortierella wolfii abortion in Australia has been associated with poor-quality grass silage (McCausland *et al.*, 1987).

7 *Bovine virus diarrhoea/mucosal disease virus (BVD/MD)* (Brownlie, 1985; Duffell & Harkness, 1987). The epidemiology of infection with this virus is extremely complex. The effect of BVD infection in susceptible pregnant cattle depends on the stage of gestation. Early in pregnancy there will be embryonic death and return to service. Infection later in pregnancy may result in inhibition of fetal growth with abortions, stillbirths and weak live calves resulting. Abortion in early to mid-pregnancy produces a fetus that may have antibody to the virus but from which virus cannot be isolated because of autolysis. Abortion in late pregnancy usually produces a fresh fetus from which virus can be isolated. Owing to central nervous system involvement, ataxia and eye lesions may be noted. The development of mucosal disease in later life may depend on *in utero* infection before day 125 with noncytopathic BVD virus followed by subsequent infection with cytopathic BVD virus during the first two years of life. Infection is introduced into a herd by animal contact, usually a purchase (see p. 660).

8 *Infectious bovine rhinotracheitis/infectious pustular vulvovaginitis virus (IBR/IPV)* (McKercher, 1964; Kendrick, 1973; Kahrs, 1986). This very widely distributed herpesvirus infection is spread by the respiratory or ocular route or venereally. Abortion occurs from a few days up to about three months after infection in a pregnant cow, and may or may not be associated with clinical signs of IBR or IPV before or after aborting. Up to 25 per cent of exposed pregnant cattle may abort after exposure (see also p. 256).

9 *Trichomoniasis* (Skirrow & BonDurant, 1988). This venereal disease occasionally causes abortion but the more typical signs are return to service and pyometra. *Trichomonas fetus* is confined to the reproductive tract of bulls and cows and infection of the cow occurs during natural service. Infection of the uterus results in an endometritis with subsequent infection and death of the embryo or fetus.

Miscellaneous causes of abortion

1 *Drug induced.* Great care is required when treating pregnant cows for non-reproductive disease; similarly, the use of drugs for reproductive system therapy should be undertaken only after making sure the cow is not pregnant. The main concern is with prostaglandin $F_{2\alpha}$ or an analogue used on a cow that is thought to be not pregnant. By around gestation day 200 the cow is producing progesterone from the placenta and therefore prostaglandin $F_{2\alpha}$ or an analogue is less likely to cause abortion after gestation day 150 than earlier.

Fetal corticosteroids act as the trigger to initiate physiological birth and there is a serious risk that their administration will cause abortion if given in the second half of pregnancy. Abortion after vaccination against foot-and-mouth disease has been recorded (Ahlers *et al.*, 1985).

It is unlikely that other approved drugs will cause abortion unless administered into the uterus, but the reader is advised to check the data sheets supplied by the manufacturers. Deliberate induction of abortion or parturition by the use of drugs may be carried out for a variety of therapeutic reasons (Chauhan *et al.*, 1984).

2 *Insemination/intra-uterine infusion.* A small percentage of pregnant cows come into oestrus and if they are inseminated they are liable to abort. The same outcome will follow intra-uterine treatment of a pregnant cow, hopefully a rare event.

3 *Hypothyroidism*. The association of goitre with late abortion, premature delivery and stillbirth can be related to areas deficient in iodine. It is also a danger where large quantities of brassicas containing goitrogenic substances are fed and has higher incidence in severely cold climates, where the metabolic requirements for maintaining body temperature are high leading to an increased demand for thyroid hormone.

4 *Trauma/stress*. It is difficult to assess the role played by trauma or stress in any particular case of abortion. The pregnant cow appears to be able to withstand quite considerable trauma to the abdomen without abortion resulting. As farmers may be intending to sue the perpetrator of the trauma or stress the veterinarian should be cautious in expressing an opinion in individual cases. In most cases it is impossible to be categorical about the cause and the veterinarian must ensure that there is a thorough investigation of the case. It is then possible for a certificate to be written which states that no other cause of abortion has been discovered. The same applies where the farmer attributes abortion to fright, for example caused by low-flying aircraft. The suspicions of the client should be made clear to the laboratory when any samples are submitted. Noise stress causing abortion has been reported (Zoldag *et al.*, 1983) and Jerrett *et al.* (1984) suggested that high cortisol levels in 17 per cent of aborted cows in which no diagnosis had been made might indicate a role for acute stress in the aetiology.

5 *Exotoxins*. Many toxic plants, mycotoxins and toxic chemicals have been recorded as causing abortion. Specific examples are narrowleaf sumpweed in the USA, ergot in the UK, aflatoxicosis and zearalenone oestrogenic toxin produced by *Fusarium* species moulds. Nitrate/nitrite poisoning resulting from increased use of nitrogenous fertilizer is becoming recognized as a significant cause of abortions in the USA and several European countries.

6 *High fever and endotoxins*. Abortions associated with these factors have been discussed under non-specific infectious causes of abortion.

7 *Nutritional*. Severe malnutrition or starvation may lead to fetal death at any stage of gestation but should be uncommon where normal husbandry practices are followed. Specific nutritional deficiencies or imbalances resulting in abortion or stillbirth include vitamin A deficiency (p. 220) and goitre (p. 221), which has been discussed previously. Maternal deficiencies of selenium or vitamin E have been associated with the birth of dead, weak or premature calves and a high incidence of retained placenta.

8 *Twin pregnancy*. Jerrett *et al.* (1984) reported that in all cases of aborted twins in their study no specific diagnosis was reached. This implies that some cows have difficulty in maintaining twin gestations.

9 *Genetic*. Genetic defects in the embryo that render it non-viable usually result in early embryonic loss rather than later abortion. However, fetal death and consequent abortion may occur with chromosomal abnormalities which normally result in congenital malformations. Hare (1980) suggests that fetal death may result from placental development lagging behind fetal development or asynchronous cellular development in fetal organs.

Diagnosis

Diagnosis of the specific cause of individual abortions is usually dependent on laboratory investigation. However, the clinician has an important role in ensuring that the appropriate samples reach the laboratory in good condition. A knowledge of the pathogenesis and epizootiology of the different sorts of abortion is essential for sample selection as well as for dealing with an outbreak.

It is desirable to investigate all abortions. Although this is expensive it is the best way to establish the disease status of a herd and provides the basis for formulation of management policies to reduce the incidence of abortion. In many countries there are statutory regulations which require that all abortions are reported and samples taken for screening for infectious causes such as brucellosis. This has the advantage that all abortions are (or should be) seen by the clinician and it also means that samples go to an approved laboratory so that some of the cost of a more complete examination may be covered.

Only about one-quarter to one-third of abortion investigations yield a diagnosis, which does mean, however, that after investigation of five consecutive abortions from one herd there is a reasonable chance of arriving at a diagnosis, assuming that all cases have the same cause. The difficulty of laboratory diagnosis is one reason why a careful examination of the cow and the products of abortion may be valuable. If, for example, only one of a series of abortions is diagnosed in the laboratory, it will be important to know if the signs presented in the other cases and the physical lesions are typical of the disease that has been diagnosed.

Two series of articles dealing with bovine abortions in the USA cover diagnosis (Canant, 1985) and managing abortion, including diagnosis (Kirkbride, 1985).

A *systematic examination* should be carried out under the headings shown in Table 34.4.

Table 34.4 Systematic examination of abortion

History
General examination of the cow
Examination of the fetus and placenta
Collection of samples for the laboratory
Interpretation of results

The history will give the gestational age, evidence of illness in the dam or herd generally before the abortion, and if there have been many abortions in the herd. As some causes of abortion also affect other stages of reproduction, it is useful to discover if there is an infertility problem in the herd, and if stillbirths and weak calves are common. Any increase in incidence of retained fetal membranes or endometritis should be recorded. Details of vaccination can be gathered but as Kirkbride (1985) points out, vaccination does not equal immunization and the farmer's memory or records about vaccination may be unreliable.

Details of the dates of entry of purchased animals into the herd and the sources of such purchased animals, including bulls, may be valuable in determining sources of specific infection.

Where several abortions have occurred, the age distribution and management group distribution of affected cows should be noted. This may disclose possible common risk factors associated with management practices or changes. In particular where heifer replacement stock are managed separately from the milking herd until after their first calving, these animals will often be susceptible to infections endemic in the adult cows. Abortions in cows carrying their second calf may be especially common under these circumstances. Information on the breeding history of aborting cows should include whether pregnancy resulted from artificial insemination or natural service. Particularly in the latter case, the identity of the specific bull or bulls should be recorded to determine if a genetic or venereally transmitted factor may be involved.

The nutritional history of the group of affected cows should be taken. This may disclose long-term deficiencies in nutrition or changes in nutrition at vital stages of fetal development that can be related to the gestational age of the aborted fetus. An assessment of the quality of concentrates and forage being fed should be made including any gross evidence of fungal contamination of hay, straw, silage or cereals.

Chemical analysis of silage is often carried out for ration formulation purposes and a copy of such an analysis will give an indication of the efficiency of fermentation, which could influence the numbers of potential pathogens such as *Listeria monocytogenes*, *Bacillus licheniformis* and *Mortierella wolfii*.

Any evidence for seasonal incidence of abortion may be helpful since specific agents may show specific seasonal incidence related to management factors.

General examination of the cow may give an indication of possible causes of abortion but is unlikely to lead to a specific diagnosis. It should be carried out in case the cow is ill and requires treatment.

Examination of the fetus and placenta. Examine the fetus for crown–rump length, i.e. a straight line from crown to rump, estimated age, freshness and weight. A formula to estimate the fetal developmental age from the crown–rump measurement is $x = 2.5(y + 21)$, where y is the crown–rump length in centimetres and x is the gestational age in days.

Post-mortem examination of the fetus and placenta may be carried out by the clinician at the same time as samples are collected or it may be part of the laboratory examination. While findings rarely give a specific diagnosis, certain observations can give a strong indication of particular causes as shown in Table 34.5.

Collection of samples for laboratory investigation. In many cases, the clinician will have to rely on a specialist laboratory for diagnostic procedures. In an ideal situation, the entire aborted calf with associated fetal membranes and appropriate samples from the dam should be delivered as soon as possible to the laboratory. Where transport difficulties or other delays preclude this, the field veterinarian should collect appropriate samples while carrying out a post-mortem examination of the aborted fetus. Selection, collection and transport of samples should be discussed with the laboratory personnel. The particular range of tests carried out will vary depending on the causes of abortion that occur in an area and the diagnostic facilities available to the laboratory. A suggested approach is shown in Table 34.6, which indicates specific tests related to specific aetiological agents. As can be seen the emphasis is on demonstrating specific infectious agents or antibodies to them. Many non-infectious cases of abortion will remain undiagnosed and an attempt at diagnosis of these cases will involve close scrutiny of other evidence including history and fetal pathology.

Serological and immunological tests have not been specified since they vary between laboratories and are subject to constant development.

Table 34.5 Indications of cause of abortion from post-mortem findings

Post-mortem observation	Possible causes
Autolytic fetus	
Advanced	*Salmonella* spp. *Leptospira* spp. *Trichomonas foetus* *Actinomyces pyogenes*
Variable	*Campylobacter* spp. *Brucella abortus* *Listeria spp.* BVD/MD, IBR
Fresh or living fetus	*Aspergillus* spp. *Bacillus* spp. *Campylobacter* spp. BVD/MD Nitrate toxicity *Brucella abortus*
Liver lesions	IBR: focal necrosis *Listeria* spp.: shrunken, soft, grey, focal abscesses
Skin lesions	Mycosis
Placental lesions	Mycosis *Campylobacter* spp. *Bacillus licheniformis* *Brucella abortus* *Actinomyces pyogenes* IBR
Enlarged thyroid (>0.03% body weight)	Hypothyroidism (goitre)
Brain lesions, e.g. cerebellar hypoplasia, hydrocephalus	BVD/MD
Meconium staining of skin or lungs	Fetal hypoxia (secondary to placentitis)
Perirenal oedema or haemorrhage	IBR

Interpretation of results. Interpretation of antibody levels to specific pathogens in maternal serum can be very difficult. Ideally, a significant rise in titre (seroconversion) between a sample taken at the time of abortion and one taken three to four weeks later is good evidence of recent active infection. In many cases, however, abortion may have occurred several weeks after exposure of the dam and in the post-abortion period maternal antibody levels may have peaked or even be declining. This is particularly so in leptospirosis where antibody levels at the time of abortion may be very low (Ellis, 1983). It may be helpful in such situations to examine blood samples from cohorts in

Table 34.6 Suggested approach for laboratory testing with different materials

Material required	Appropriate tests	Aetiological agent
Fresh tissues		
Fetal Lung Liver Spleen Kidney Stomach contents Placenta	Microbiological culture methods (transport media may be needed)	Range of bacterial and fungal pathogens Viral pathogens: BVD/MD, IBR
Maternal milk, faeces, vaginal swab		*Leptospira* spp.
Fixed smears		
Vaginal swab	Microscopy	
Cotyledon	Modified Ziel–Neilsen	*Chlamydia*, *Brucella* spp., Q fever
Stomach contents	Dilute carbol fuchsin	*Campylobacter* spp.
Liver	Gram stain	*Listeria* spp.
Skin, stomach contents	Lactophenol cotton blue	Fungi
Lung, kidney	Fluorescent antibody test	*Leptospira* spp.
Fixed tissues		
Brain	Histopathology	BVD/MD, *Sarcocystis* spp.
Thyroid		Goitre
Placenta		Fungi
Liver		IBR, *Listeria* spp.
Other tissues		Non-specific changes
Blood/fluids		
Fetal fluid	Serological methods	BVD/MD, IBR, PI_3
Fetal serum		*Leptospira* spp., Q fever
Maternal serum (paired: acute/convalescent)		*Brucella* spp., *Chlamydia*, etc.
Vaginal mucus (dam)	Agglutination test	*Campylobacter* spp. *Trichomonas foetus*
Preputial washings (sire)	Culture/microscopy	*Trichomonas foetus*
	Fluorescent antibody test	*Campylobacter* spp.

the herd to determine the prevalence of antibodies to the agent. In the case of active infection within the group, some individuals are likely to have high titres whereas in an endemic situation most animals will have low titres. A particularly difficult situation arises with an infection that is widespread in the cattle population such as BVD. As an example of this difficulty consider the criteria listed by Kirkbride (1985) to be fulfilled before abortions in a herd can be attributed to BVD.

1 Virus in several aborted calves.
2 BVD in the herd (clinical episodes of scouring).
3 Precolostral antibodies in the calf.
4 Lesions of the central nervous system in the calf.

The presence of specific antibody in fetal fluids or serum should be good evidence of *in utero* infection with an infectious agent. However, even this has its pitfalls. On the one hand, absence of antibody may reflect infection of the fetus prior to development of immunocompetence or very recent infection that has not allowed time for antibody production. On the other hand, Miller (1986) states that many agents pass through the fetal placental unit without disturbing pregnancy but stimulating fetal antibody production. In addition, Poitras *et al.* (1986) demonstrated antibody transfer from dam to fetus in sheep associated with placental lesions resulting in functional confluence of maternal and fetal circulations. Infectious placentitis in cattle could presumably result in a similar transfer of antibodies.

In all cases a final diagnosis should be made taking into consideration the history of the case and relating any pathogens isolated or serological evidence to specific fetal or placental lesions and to the known epizootiology of the infection.

Treatment

In most cases, abortion has occurred before the veterinarian sees the cow and therefore treatment must deal with any effects on the animal's general health and specific reproductive problems such as retained fetal membranes and metritis. These have been discussed elsewhere (p. 429).

Avoidance of spread of infectious causes of abortion to other cattle is dealt with under Prevention.

Vandeplasche & Bouters (1985) recommend that if abortion is threatened because of severe illness or surgery, it may be prevented by the use of tocolytics (drugs that cause the uterus to relax), progesterone, progestagens or antiprostaglandins, such as indomethacin or aspirin.

Prognosis

For the individual cow the prognosis is usually favourable as long as she is supervised in the immediate period after abortion to detect and treat any signs of systemic illness arising from uterine infection or the systemic condition that caused the abortion is dealt with. After abortion, cows start cycling at least as quickly as after calving and, in general, subsequent pregnancy rates are satisfactory.

Prognosis for the rest of the pregnant animals in the herd is a more serious consideration and varies with the diagnosed cause of abortion and will be discussed below.

Prevention

After one, and particularly after several abortions an owner wants to take steps to avoid more occurring. These are often either not possible or unreliable, which may be difficult for the client to accept. For example, there may be a period of three months between infection with IBR and abortion, which means that whatever measures are taken abortions will continue. In general, prevention is a long-term process.

There are numerous difficulties when considering prevention of abortions. Because abortions are nearly always sporadic or occur in short series, it is hard to assess how effective control measures are. Also, expensive intervention is hard to justify if only a few more animals were likely to have aborted anyway. Control measures for non-infectious abortion require common sense and involve avoidance of further exposure to the cause.

Interim measures for control of infectious abortion. Prevention of spread from aborted to other cows depends on isolation of the cow, destruction of all contaminated bedding and the products of abortion not required for diagnostic purposes, followed by thorough cleaning and disinfection of infected premises. When abortion occurs among grazing cows in summer or in loose housing in winter these ideals cannot be met.

Specific measures for control of infectious abortion (Kirkbride, 1985)

1 *Brucellosis* (Elliott & Christiansen, 1977). Spread of infection from an infected cow to other animals in the herd takes place at the time of abortion or calving and for several weeks after. Immediate isolation of aborted cows and hygienic measures to reduce spread to and exposure of other bovines is necessary. In non-immune

herds there is a grave risk of an abortion storm resulting from exposure of other pregnant cows. In herds where the infection has become endemic, abortions tend to be sporadic or mainly confined to younger age groups. In both cases an increase in herd immunity by the use of an appropriate vaccination programme is the most effective method of preventing future losses (p. 812). Live avirulent vaccines such as Strain 19 are usually used in young female stock before they are bred. Dead vaccines such as Strain 45/20 can be used in adult females. In general, vaccination leads to a reduction in the incidence of abortion but does not by itself result in elimination of infection from the herd.

Attempts of eliminate *Br. abortus* infection from individual cows by the use of antibiotics are usually ineffective because of the intracellular nature of the organism. Milward *et al.* (1984) studied the efficacy of various treatment regimens in eliminating infection from known infected cows. The most successful regimen was a combination of long-acting oxytetracycline and streptomycin. This study showed that serological tests were not good indicators of the efficacy of treatment and it may not be possible to prove elimination of infection in live animals.

In many countries national control or eradication campaigns have been put into effect. These may take several forms but usually include some incentive for owners to vaccinate their stock, notify abortions and provide for serological testing of herds, including bulls, with slaughter of reactors. Antibody titres resulting from vaccination have caused diagnostic difficulties in many countries. Attempts to overcome these problems have included the development of special serological tests, restriction of vaccination with live vaccine to heifer calves under six months and reduced dose vaccination by various routes of administration. National campaigns are dependent for their success on the active support of cattle owners, usually engendered by effective communication of aims and benefits and supported by financial compensation or support.

2 *Campylobacteriosis* (Garcia *et al.*, 1983). Control of abortions due to *C. fetus venerealis* involves those measures that are also used to control herd infertility caused by this organism. These include the use of antibiotics to treat infected bulls and cows as well as semen that is to be used for artificial insemination. In addition, the use of artificial insemination rather than natural service in a herd will allow cows that have been exposed to infection to develop immunity and clear the organism from their genital tracts. In several countries vaccination of bulls and breeding females is available to assist control and eradication of the disease.

Sporadic abortions due to other *Campylobacter* species may be more difficult to control since the infections are usually enteric rather than genital and spread is not usually venereal. Multivalent vaccines have been developed that include *C. fetus fetus* antigen and will confer immunity to that subspecies. Although several antibiotics inhibit *C. fetus fetus* and *C. jejuni* (particularly erythromycin), the sporadic nature of abortions makes the use of antibiotics for prevention impractical.

3 *Leptospirosis* (Ellis, 1983). Control of leptospiral abortion depends on hygienic measures to reduce the spread of infection, both from aborting cows and leptospiruric animals and on increasing herd immunity by vaccination or controlled natural exposure.

Antibiotic treatment of animals affected by milk drop syndrome due to *L. hardjo* may reduce the number of subsequent abortions. However, antibiotic therapy during a *L. hardjo* abortion storm has been found to be of no appreciable value. Although treatment with dihydrostreptomycin has been shown to eliminate leptospires from the kidneys of carrier animals, blanket herd treatment is unlikely to be economically justifiable. Attempts to identify and eliminate carrier animals are at present impractical.

Combined vaccination (p. 812) and antibiotic treatment resulted in cessation of abortions due to *L. pomona* in one herd (Kingscote & Wilson, 1986). Blanket vaccination of pregnant animals in the face of abortions due to *L. hardjo* has the added advantage that vaccinated animals are less likely to become infected and shed leptospires in their urine. This is important from the point of view of reducing risks to humans of acquiring infection. Normally, herd vaccination is carried out before the period of maximum transmission and includes young female stock before they are bred for the first time. Once vaccination is started in a herd, it is usually necessary to continue annual booster vaccination of all adult stock.

4 *Other sporadic infectious causes*. These may be divided into two groups from the point of view of control. In the first group are agents that are related to specific feeding practices and in which prevention of access to the source of infection may result in reduction of the incidence of abortion. In this category, *Listeria monocytogenes*, *Bacillus licheniformis* and *Mortierella wolfii* have all been associated with feeding poor-quality or soil-contaminated silage. Similarly, fungal or yeast-induced abortions are often related to gross contamination of hay or straw. Ideally, any fodder or bedding material that is visibly affected by fungi or moulds should not be used for pregnant cows.

The practicalities of such advice will vary with individual farm situations and the availability of alternative materials. Routine chemical analysis of silage will give information on the efficiency of fermentation and the degree of soil contamination. Poorer quality silage may be fed to non-pregnant cattle. Even where it is practicable to remove the source of infection, occasional abortions may continue in cows that are already infected.

The second group of agents includes organisms that are opportunistic pathogens or obligate pathogens. The source of infection in these cases is usually other cattle. In general, attempts to control abortions by blanket antibiotic therapy or vaccination are not cost-effective since the incidence of abortion is low and significant numbers of further abortions are unlikely even without the application of control measures. In the view of Hinton (1986) this is true even for abortion due to *Salmonella* spp. However, the normal hygienic measures to prevent spread must be carried out to safeguard both animal and human health. One possible exception to the above would be epizootic outbreaks of abortion that occasionally occur due to *Chlamydia psittaci*. Blanket treatment with oxytetracycline could be expected to control such an outbreak. Similarly, where silage known to be heavily contaminated with *Listeria* must be fed, therapeutic antibiotics given continuously for 14 days may prevent abortions.

5 *Bovine virus diarrhoea/mucosal disease*. The complex epizootiology of this infection is reflected in measures to control abortion caused by it. Persistently infected cattle (those that were infected *in utero* before fetal immune competence developed) are the main source of infection in a herd. Persistently infected dams usually give birth to persistently infected calves and such calves are efficient excretors of virus. Control measures are aimed at reducing *in utero* infections and raising the immune status of the herd. The first aspect involves the identification of persistently infected animals. These animals are viraemic but do not have neutralizing antibody in their serum. Once identified they should not be bred from and should be kept away from pregnant animals. The second aspect may involve controlled exposure of susceptible heifers before breeding by allowing contact with known persistently infected animals. Effective dead vaccines are not yet available and the use of live vaccine may precipitate mucosal disease in persistently infected cattle.

6 *Infectious bovine rhinotracheitis* (Kahrs, 1986). Episodes of epizootic abortion due to infection with IBR/IPV virus can occur in susceptible herds. Vaccination in the face of such an episode will not be very successful since the infection can have an incubation period of up to three months and abortions may continue for many weeks after vaccination. Prevention in susceptible herds is based on annual or biannual vaccination of breeding females with modified live intranasal or intramuscular vaccine. The latter vaccine should never be given to pregnant cows.

7 *Trichomoniasis* (Skirrow & BonDurant, 1988). Reducing abortions due to *T. foetus* involves the same control measures as those used to control infectious infertility caused by this organism. Three areas of control have been suggested: (i) stop transmission of the disease by using controlled artificial insemination; (ii) eliminate infection by treating infected bulls preferably with divided doses of ipronidazole and culling aborted cows and non-pregnant cows following pregnancy testing; and (iii) prevent re-introduction of the disease by testing replacement bulls.

Mummified fetus

By the fifth month of gestation the fetus has acquired the main bones and an impervious integument. If it then dies and is retained *in utero* in a bacteria-free environment it will undergo mummification. The fluids in the amniotic and allantoic sacs and in the fetus are absorbed. The fetus becomes a dried-out bag of bones and the uterus clamps tightly around it. There is no adverse effect on the dam's health and pregnancy appears to continue as normal. The cow may deliver the mummified fetus, usually well after the expected date of parturition. Alternatively, the first sign may be oestrus either before or after the expected date of delivery; in some of these cows the mummified remains will have been expelled from the uterus but retained in the vagina.

In the Channel Islands breeds there is an inherited form of haematic mummification in which there is a rubbery layer of modified blood between the fetal membranes and the endometrium.

Aetiology

Factors that cause death of the fetus after about five months of gestation but do not involve pyogenic infection include torsion of the uterus, torsion of the umbilical cord, viral infections and poisons. The genetic involvement in Channel Island cattle has been mentioned above.

Diagnosis

Diagnosis is straightforward. The history is that a pregnant cow does not show signs of preparing to calve, goes over the expected calving date, or comes into oestrus. Rectal examination reveals a thin-walled uterus clamped down on a bony, fetus-shaped structure or the presence of a similar body in the vagina, which can be confirmed by vaginal examination.

Treatment

Treatment rarely presents serious problems. If the mummified fetus is still in the uterus prostaglandin $F_{2\alpha}$ or an analogue systemically is usually effective in inducing delivery. If the mummified fetus is in the vagina it is usually possible to remove it manually using ample lubrication.

Corticosteroids are not effective in inducing delivery of a mummified fetus, presumably because of the lack of functional fetal membranes.

Occasionally, there may be difficulty in removing the fetus because the cervix does not open up sufficiently or the vagina or vulva are too tight. These cases are very difficult to deal with as surgical extraction presents problems of access.

Prognosis

Prognosis is good. The general health is not adversely affected, the response in terms of expulsion of the mummified fetus is good and the return to normal cyclicity is rapid. In fact, return to cyclicity is sometimes one of the presenting signs of the condition.

Apart from the haematic mummification cases in Channel Island cattle, there is no suggestion that the cause is inherited so that the cow can be used for breeding with little risk of repetition of the condition or of handing on any predisposition to the next generation.

There is no way of *preventing* mummification.

Macerated fetus

A fetus that dies, is not aborted and is then exposed to pyogenic infection becomes macerated.

The condition is recognized by the farmer because of a purulent discharge from the vulva, which may contain small bits of bone. The effect on the cow's general health varies: in some cases there is no noticeable effect, in others there is loss of weight and condition.

Aetiology

Maceration results when death of the fetus is followed by infection that causes degeneration of the fetus. Often an abortion starts but the cervix does not open enough to allow passage of the fetus. The attempts by the cow to deliver the aborting fetus cease because of uterine inertia and the uterus is invaded by bacteria from the vagina. In some cases infection may be haematogenous.

Diagnosis

Diagnosis presents few problems. A cow that was thought to be pregnant produces a purulent discharge that may include small bits of bone. Vaginal examination reveals that this is coming through the cervix and on rectal palpation it is clear that the uterus contains a lot of bony material, which is felt through a thickened uterine wall.

Treatment

There is no effective treatment of this condition. Removal of fetal remnants via laparotomy is contraindicated because the uterus is contracted round the macerated fetus and is far from the abdominal wall. Removal of all the bones through the cervix is practically impossible. Administration of drugs that cause uterine contraction will not succeed in getting rid of the degenerating bones; they increase the pre-existing risk that the bones may penetrate the uterine wall.

Prognosis

The prognosis is extremely poor and these cows should be culled. There is no way to *prevent* this condition.

Hydrops allantois and amnion

In the last third of gestation the farmer suddenly notices that the affected cow has gross abdominal enlargement, which affects both right and left flanks and the floor of the abdomen. The 'suddenness' of the discovery is often due to lack of observation in the early stages. As the case develops the effect of the pressure on the thoracic organs and the great blood vessels in the abdomen is exhibited by distress in breathing, inability to get up and loss of appetite with resultant severe loss of body condition and not infrequently death. In many cases the calf exhibits abnormalities such as ankylosis.

Aetiology

Little is known about the aetiology of hydrops and it is even unclear whether the two conditions, hydrops amnion and hydrops allantois, are related. For a recent review see Wintour *et al.* (1986).

Diagnosis

Diagnosis is usually easy but there are some possible sources of error. The history is of a cow in the last trimester of gestation that has rapidly developed gross abdominal enlargement.

The location of the swelling is in both flanks and ventrally, which helps to differentiate from bloat (p. 637), with the swelling on the left side, and ascites, with swelling more ventrally. Percussion on the sublumbar fossa on one side causes a fluid thrill that can be felt on the other side. On rectal palpation an extremely taut uterus is felt, which in extreme cases is as tense as a drum. The uterus is pushed upwards and backwards so that it can be difficult to introduce the arm far into the rectum. Because of the tenseness of the uterine wall it is impossible to feel anything inside the uterus. While this picture is characteristic for hydrops it can also apply to the rare situation in which an extremely large tumour in the abdominal cavity displaces the pregnant uterus upwards and backwards, causing increased intra-uterine pressure and gross enlargement of the abdomen.

The great size of these animals tends to mask their very poor condition and it is important to make a careful general examination of the animal. This is necessary as a guide to prognosis and it draws the client's attention to the poor condition of the animal.

On clinical examination it is not possible to differentiate between hydrops amnion and hydrops allantois, which is by far the more common.

Treatment

A few of these cases go to term and start spontaneous delivery; they require assistance because of uterine inertia and sometimes because the calf has ankylosed joints. Generally, when the excess fetal fluids are discharged at spontaneous birth, the cow does not collapse.

It might therefore be thought that the ideal solution was to leave these cases until they go into spontaneous parturition. Unfortunately, during the waiting period sudden deterioration, collapse and death due to respiratory and circulatory failure may supervene.

On the other hand, removal of all the fluid by drainage via the cervix or flank is contraindicated because it is usually followed by collapse and death. This is why previous treatment was a two-stage surgical operation involving controlled drainage for 24 hours followed by caesarean section.

The treatment of choice today is prostaglandin $F_{2\alpha}$ or an analogue administered systemically to induce parturition. Treatment with corticosteroids is also recommended and oxytocin can be used to hasten uterine contraction after parturition.

Cows with hydrops allantois or hydrops amnion that are slaughtered will most likely be condemned as unfit for human consumption because of the poor condition of the carcass and failure to set.

Prognosis

Prognosis is these cases must be extremely guarded; those that survive are likely to produce abnormal calves and they may take a long time to regain body condition. Once body condition is back to normal, cyclicity and pregnancy rate are not adversely affected. The chance of the condition recurring is small and so this is not a reason for culling. If the condition occurs in the spring and there is ample grazing then the cow is worth keeping till the autumn for breeding.

There is no way to prevent hydrops allantois or hydrops amnion.

References

Ahlers, D., Grunert, E. & Mehrkens, L. (1985) Investigation of abortion in cows associated with vaccination against foot and mouth disease. *Deutsche Tieraerztliche Wochenschrift*, **92**, 423–8.

Brownlie, J. (1985) Clinical aspects of the bovine virus diarrhoea/mucosal disease complex in cattle. *In Practice*, **7**, 195–202.

Canant, J.C. (1985) Diagnosis of the causes of bovine abortion. *Modern Veterinary Practice*, **65**, 929–31; **66**, 47–50, 107–9, 155–8, 271–4, 331–3.

Chauhan, F.S., Mgongo, F.O.K. & Kessy, B.M. (1984) Recent advances in hormonal therapy of bovine reproductive disorders: a review. *Veterinary Bulletin*, **54**, 995.

Deas, W. (1981) Non-brucella abortion in cattle. *In Practice*, **3**, 14–19.

Duffell, S.J. & Harkness, J.W. (1987) The bovine virus diarrhoea–mucosal disease complex. *Veterinary Annual*, **27**, 91–7.

Elliot, R.E.W. & Christiansen, K.H. (eds) (1977) *Brucellosis: A Veterinarian's Guide to the Literature*. Animal Health Division, Ministry of Agriculture and Fisheries, Wellington, New Zealand.

Ellis, W.A. (1983) Recent developments in bovine leptospirosis. *Veterinary Annual*, **23**, 91–5.

Ellis, W.A. (1985) Bovine leptospirosis: some clinical features of serovar *hardjo* infection. *Veterinary Record*, **117**, 101–4.

Foley, G.L. & Schlafer, D.H. (1987) *Candida* abortion in cattle. *Veterinary Pathology*, **24**, 532–6.

Fredriksson, G. (1984) Some reproductive and clinical aspects of endotoxins in cows with special emphasis on the role of prostaglandins. *Acta Veterinaria Scandinavica*, **25**, 365–77.

Garcia, M.M., Eaglesome, M.D. & Rigby, C. (1983) Campylobacters important in veterinary medicine. *Veterinary Bulletin*, **53**, 793–818.

Gitter, M. (1979) *Listeria monocytogenes* infection in bovine abortion. In *Proceedings of the 7th International Symposium on Problems of Listeriosis, Varna, Bulgaria,* 1977 (ed. by I. Ivanov) National Agroindustrial Union, Centre for Scientific information, p. 193.

Hare, W.C.D. (1980) Cytogenetics. In *Current Therapy in Theriogenology* (ed. by D.A. Morrow), pp. 119–55. W.B. Saunders, London.

Hinton, M. (1986) Salmonella abortion in cattle. *Veterinary Annual*, **26**, 81–9.

Jerrett, I.V., McOrist, S., Waddington, J., Browning, J.W., Malecki, J.C. & McCausland, I.P. (1984) Diagnostic studies of the fetus, placenta and maternal blood from 265 bovine abortions. *Cornell Veterinarian*, **74**, 8–20.

Kahrs, R.F. (1986) Effects of infectious bovine rhinotracheitis on reproduction. In *Current Therapy in Theriogenology* (ed. by D.A. Morrow), pp. 250–4. W.B. Saunders, London.

Kendrick, J.W. (1973) Effects of the infectious bovine rhinotracheitis virus on the fetus. *Journal of the American Veterinary Medical Association*, **163**, 852–4.

Kingscote, B.F. & Wilson, D. (1986) *Leptospira pomona* abortion storm in a cattle herd in Saskatchewan. *Canadian Veterinary Journal*, **27**, 440–2.

Kirkbride, C.A. (1985) Managing an outbreak of livestock abortion — 2: Diagnosis and control of bovine abortion. *Veterinary Medicine*, **80**, 70–9.

McCausland, I.P., Slee, K.J. & Hirst, F.S. (1987) Mycotic abortion in cattle. *Australian Veterinary Journal*, **64**, 129–32.

McKercher, D.G. (1964) The virus of infectious bovine rhinotracheitis as a cause of abortion in cattle. *Journal of the American Veterinary Medical Association*, **144**, 136–42.

Miller, R.B. (1986) Bovine abortion. In *Current Therapy in Theriogenology* (ed. by D.A. Morrow), pp. 291–300. W.B. Saunders, London.

Milward, F.W., Nicoletti, P. & Hoffmann, E. (1984) Effectiveness of various therapeutic regimens for bovine brucellosis. *American Journal of Veterinary Research*, **45**, 1825–8.

Morgan, W.J.B. & Mackinnon, D.J. (1979) *Brucellosis in Fertility and Infertility in Domestic Animals* (ed. by J.A. Laing). Bailliere Tindall, London.

Morrow, D.A. (1986) Current Therapy in Theriogenology 2. pp. 1–1143. W.B. Saunders, London.

Pepin, G.A. (1983) Bovine mycotic abortion. *Veterinary Annual*, **23**, 79–90.

Poitras, B.J., Miller, R.B., Wilkie, B.N. & Bosu, W.T.K. (1986) The maternal to fetal transfer to immunoglobulins associated with placental lesions in sheep. *Canadian Journal of Veterinary Research*, **50**, 68–73.

Skirrow, S.Z. & BonDurant, R.H. (1988) Bovine trichomoniasis. *Veterinary Bulletin*, **58**, 591–603.

Vandeplasche, M. & Bouters, R. (1985) The impact of gynaecological and obstetrical problems resulting out of pregnancy and parturition. In *Factors Influencing Fertility in the Postpartum Cow* (ed. by H. Karg & E. Schallenberger), pp. 30–44. Nijhoff, The Hague.

Williams, B.M., Shreeve, B.J., Hebert, C.N. & Swire, P.W. (1977) Bovine mycotic abortion: some epidemiological aspects. *Veterinary Record*, **100**, 382–5.

Wintour, E.M., Laurence, B.M. & Lingwood, B.E. (1986) Anatomy, physiology and pathology of the amniotic and allantoic compartments in the sheep and cow. *Australian Veterinary Journal*, **63**, 216–21.

Zoldag, L., Heuwieser, W., Grunert, E. & Stephan, E. (1983) Steroid hormone profile in pregnant cows after exposure to noise stress, with particular reference to corticosteroids. *Zentralblatt für Veterinarmedizin A*, **30**, 737–48.

Chapter 35: Bull Infertility

by D. LOGUE AND J. ISBISTER

Introduction

Since the domestication of cattle it has been a farmer's dream to breed or buy the best bull in the region. This still applies! However, the outstanding bull is very rare and the purchase of a young bull in the hope of achieving fame and fortune is a considerable gamble. The genuine need for young bulls plus this dream means that there will always be a demand for them.

When all breeding was by natural service the potential for genetic improvement by a good bull was very limited. Furthermore, sharing and hiring animals resulted in the spread of venereal disease with some disastrous results for those affected farms.

Artificial insemination (AI) was introduced to the UK just before the end of the Second World War. It fulfilled two objectives: firstly, the more widespread use of good bulls, and secondly the limitation of venereal disease. Unfortunately, the expression of oestrus in the cow varies in time of occurrence, duration and intensity and many farmers find accurate, and more particularly, efficient oestrous detection difficult and time consuming (see p. 436). This is the major obstacle to the full development of AI and ensures that many farmers continue to use natural service even though, due to the genetic improvement from AI, they could afford to have a longer calving interval and yet still expect to have the same financial returns (Hillers *et al.*, 1982).

The problem is illustrated by a study of UK national cattle population statistics where only approximately half the cows are bred by AI (see Table 35.1). In the USA the proportion bred by AI is probably a little higher (70 per cent) (Doak, pers. comm., 1988). In addition, there have been a number of factors that have counteracted the undoubted improvements in the efficiency of AI.

1 Intensification of dairy production and changes in beef husbandry have resulted in fewer people working on the farm with less time available for oestrous detection. Furthermore, the continuing financial pressure from the banks and other lenders has also made many dairy farmers economize by changing from paying for a technician AI service to inseminating their own cows (DIYAI).

While some farmers use the technician AI service plus a sweeper bull in their herds, a greater proportion of the DIYAI farmers keep a bull(s) as a precaution against poor fertility arising from a doubtful insemination technique.

Unfortunately, no figures are produced for the number of cows inseminated in the DIYAI sector in the UK but an estimate can be made using the average herd size for each UK. However, census area, the number of DIYAI licences issued by areas and the assumption that 75 per cent of the cows in each herd are inseminated (Table 35.2).

2 There has been a gradual increase in herd size and thus the added costs of keeping one or even several bulls are relatively lower. For example, in the UK, dairy herd size has increased dramatically over the last 20 years (see Table 35.3), while in the EC it has increased by over 100 per cent in the last 10 years (Anon., 1988). Similar trends have been apparent in the USA (Niedermeier *et al.*, 1983).

3 A further effect of the larger number of cows per

Table 35.1 Number of cattle and number of first inseminations in UK ($\times 10^6$) using technician service. Source: Federation of the UK MMB

	1975	1988
Number of cows	5.0	4.4
Number of first inseminations	2.8	2.2

Table 35.2 Number of cows in DIYAI herds

	England and Wales	Northern Ireland	Scotland	Total
DIY licences	3300	1000	700	5000
Average herd size	69	37	89	–
Number of cows	227700	37000	54300	319000
Cows inseminated (assuming 75%) by DIY service	170775	27750	40725	239250

Table 35.3 UK cattle statistics. Source: the UK Federation of the UK MMB

Year	Cow numbers $\times 10^6$	Herd size
1960	4.01	20
1965	4.21	25
1970	4.55	31
1975	5.14	43
1980	4.69	55
1985	4.47	64
1988	4.27	65

herd has led to a more predictable production of heifer replacements, i.e. statistical variation of males to females is nearer to the expected 50:50 as the numbers increase. This has meant that a definite block of cattle can be released for service with either a beef sire or one of less genetic superiority for milk.

4 In many beef and dairy herds, calvings, and thus breeding periods, are concentrated into relatively short periods of time for production reasons. This leads to a requirement for high oestrous detection rates and high fertility, both of which are best achieved by using a combination of AI and natural service.

5 Finally, in the past an important reason for using AI has been to reduce the introduction of disease. With the increasing improvement in the health status of the national herd in many countries there is less pressure for AI use for this reason alone.

The role of the veterinarian and bull use

The role of the veterinarian in the control and monitoring of bull fertility is fourfold (see Table 35.4).

It is worthwhile defining the various types of herd breeding policy since this will influence the management of the bull and may give a guide to the needs of the unit with regard to disease control.

Four basic types of policy can be recognized.

1 Beef suckler herd. The principal demand is to produce calves for fattening. The cows are mated while suckling and to ensure that this system operates at highest efficiency a short breeding period would appear to be a prerequisite in most geographical locations (Kilkenny, 1978).

2 Dairy heifers. A considerable proportion of dairy herds use natural service when breeding heifers. This is mainly to avoid oestrous detection and the need to gather the individual heifer for AI. The use of synchronization and fixed-time AI with batches of maiden heifers using an easy-calving dairy sire has to some degree circumvented this. However, most of these heifers which return are served by a sweeper bull.

3 Sweeper bull. This term usually refers to the running of a bull after a fixed period of 'AI-only' breeding. Generally, in dairy cattle, the bull run is a beef breed and thus any calves born are easily distinguished from pure-bred dairy calves.

The timing of the introduction of the sweeper is paramount since mating pressure will obviously depend on the number of non-pregnant cows left after the AI breeding period. Clearly a drop in the pregnancy rates achieved with AI can result in an increase of mating pressure upon the bull run subsequently.

4 Modified sweeper. The 'sweeper bull' is utilized for mating selected cows throughout the breeding season, for example cows of low genetic potential, repeat breeders, cows not exhibiting firm signs of oestrus and cows with a history of being difficult to get in calf. Subsequently, the bull is used as a 'true' sweeper.

Table 35.4 Role of the veterinarian in bull fertility

Advice on disease control
Advice on the selection of bulls and their subsequent examination for breeding soundness either before or after purchase
Advice on bull management and examination of bulls prior to the breeding season
Monitoring herd fertility

Bull infertility

Manifestations and aetiology

Bull fertility is presented as one, or a combination of the four manifestations, namely:
1 failure to mount;
2 failure to achieve intromission;
3 failure to thrust and ejaculate;
4 poor pregnancy rate.
Consequently, the aetiological factors are varied and numerous.

FAILURE TO MOUNT

Failure to mount is either due to lack of libido or physical inability. The following factors have an influence on the ability to mount.
1 Age.
2 Genetic background.
3 Season.
4 Social factors.
5 Overwork.
6 Nutrition.
7 Orthopaedic abnormalities.
8 Housing conditions.

Age

The age at which a bull is capable of mounting, protruding the penis fully, and ejaculating semen (puberty) varies with the bull and breed (see p. 405). However, one would normally expect a bull of a high production dairy breed to be capable of serving a cow at 12 months of age, although usually semen production would have commenced some two months earlier. Indeed mounting behaviour would be normal in the prepubertal state. Continental beef breeds tend to mature at a later age than most dairy breeds and so more care is needed with such animals when attempting to use them at a young age, for example less than 18 months. From a behavioural point of view young bulls often display naivety and awkwardness in their approach to an oestrous cow. There is evidence that this can be affected by how young males are reared, so that young bulls raised with female calves are less likely to exhibit sexual naivety than those kept in the presence of their dams until weaning (Kilgour, 1984).

In extreme cases young bulls may go through a pronounced phase of showing no sexual interest even when presented with a cow in oestrus. This 'sexual inhibition' may be heightened by the presence of another bull. While the condition often indicates an inherently poor libido, the problem may correct itself with time. Similarly, despite being clinically normal, bulls can show a considerable lowering of their sexual drive beyond eight to ten years old (Chenoweth, 1983).

Genetic factors

There is evidence from work with identical twins that many aspects of mating behaviour, in particular sexual drive and mode of approach to service, are inherited (Bane, 1954).

Furthermore, despite the wide variation between individuals there is plenty of evidence that some types and breeds of bulls display better libido than others. For example, dairy breeds tend to show a stronger sexual drive than beef breeds and there is now evidence of a quite high heritability for libido (Chenoweth, 1983).

However, there is little evidence that variation in libido is due to differences in circulating hormone concentrations (Bane, 1954). This was demonstrated dramatically in an endocrinologically abnormal bull with a 60, XXY chromosome complement, in which the mating behaviour was normal (Logue *et al.*, 1979).

There is little firm evidence of any relationship between poor libido in the bull and poor oestrous expression in female offspring, but there is some evidence of a relationship in sheep. Thus libido is a factor that should not be ignored in any selection programme (Chenoweth, 1983).

Season

There is conflicting evidence about the effect of season of the year largely because of the environmental conditions in which the bulls were kept. A sluggish sexual drive has been related to periods of extreme heat, cold and light reduction (Vincent, 1972; Foote *et al.*, 1976; Gwazdauskas, 1985).

Social factors

Age, genetics and season all interact in the herd situation where the bull is running with a group of cows either as the only male or along with several other bulls as a mating team. Thus generally the oldest and largest bulls are dominant and spend most of their time in the presence of the sexually active oestrous females (Chenoweth, 1983). Subordinate bulls spend considerably less time with that group and in some cases their attempts to serve will be totally disrupted by the dominant bull.

Overwork

Bulls do become satiated. This state varies with the individual and the herd structure and in temperate climates seems more likely to present during the winter than longer daylight periods. In simple terms, introduction of a young totally inexperienced 18-month to two-year-old bull to 20 cycling cows is considered to be risking overwork, while introduction to as many as 40 is foolhardy! Finally, poor female fertility can compound the problem because of returns to service.

Nutrition

High planes of nutrition result in puberty and maturity being reached at an earlier age (Salisbury & Van Demark, 1961). There is also some evidence that high energy intakes in early development are detrimental to subsequent libido. This effect has been described in both dairy and beef bulls but without looking closely at whether the regime caused the physical defects in the bulls such as laminitis. There does not appear to be a direct relationship between nutrition and fertility in working bulls. Nevertheless, it is widely believed by farmers that performance testing young working bulls is detrimental to their longevity as working sires.

Orthopaedic abnormalities and housing conditions

Often the bull will show an intent to mount, moving to the cow and standing behind her, but does not mount because of painful or physical limiting orthopaedic abnormalities. Obviously, the extent of this effect is mediated by the level of libido of the bull and on some occasions the frustration becomes so great that the bull will strike the cow.

There is a large number of orthopaedic problems that are liable to interfere with the ability to mount and serve a cow. The most common problem areas are in the foot, the hock, the stifle and the back.

Many of these problems result from injuries to muscles, tendons and joints (see Chapter 29) caused by the bull slipping when attempting to serve on poor underfoot conditions. Thus, adequate housing and service management are prerequisites of good bull fertility. However, some appear to be more specific bull problems, such as spinal changes (Bane & Hansen, 1962) and stifle injuries (Bartels, 1975) and delayed spastic paresis (Fig. 35.1).

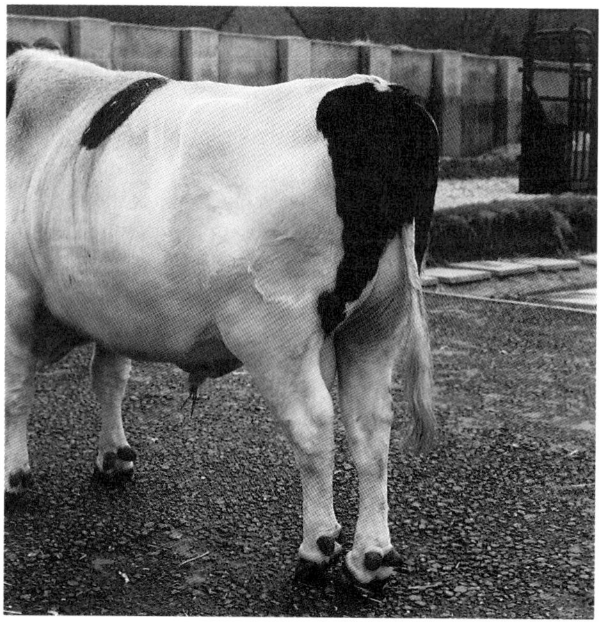

Fig. 35.1 Delayed spastic paresis in the bull.

It should also be remembered that other less specific conditions can cause poor libido simply due to the bull feeling unwell or being in pain. This is particularly relevant if the penis and/or prepuce has been damaged (see below). Finally, other diseases such as bovine spongiform encephalopathy (BSE) and progressive ataxia (see p. 148) of Charolais cattle (Palmer *et al.*, 1972) should be borne in mind.

FAILURE TO ACHIEVE INTROMISSION

The majority of bulls that are presented as being able to mount but then failing to gain intromission suffer from a variety of conditions, which include penile or preputial defects and orthopaedic problems. In order to fully understand penile problems it is necessary to briefly to discuss the anatomy and physiology of erection in the bull.

Intromission can only be achieved if the penis is fully erect. This is a stiffening process brought about by the filling of the corpus cavernosum penis with blood pumped in by the ischiocavernosus penis muscle (Fig. 35.2). Since drainage of the corpus cavernosum penis is very slow in normal bulls, blood pressure in the corpus cavernosum penis builds up well in excess of that in a car tyre (over 200 p.s.i.) (Beckett *et al.*, 1974). This is sufficient to harden and straighten the penis and it is consequently forced out of the sheath. The latter, owing to its elastic nature, envelops the erecting penis up to the start of the free end of the penis. As the penis protrudes and reaches the point of ejaculation, it stiffens still further and spirals in an anticlockwise direction. This 'corkscrew' is caused by the fibrous architecture of the glans, in particular the dorsal apical ligament and spiral distribution of collagen fibres along the tip of the penis, allied to the rise in blood pressure at the corpus cavernosum penis at ejaculation. Further distortion may be caused by the very transitory erection of the erectile tissue at the tip of the penis. It is believed that this may be caused by pressure waves in the corpus spongiosum penis (Ashdown, 1973).

Clinically, there are two major presentations associated with failure to achieve intromission and each can be further subdivided as follows.

1 The penis cannot be protruded sufficiently.
  (a) Balanoposthitis.
  (b) Short penis.
  (c) Rupture of penis.
  (d) Persistent frenulum.
2 Failure to locate vulva.
  (a) Psychogenic.
  (b) Penile problems: fibropapillomata; drainage defects; corkscrew penis; deviations.

THE PENIS CANNOT BE PROTRUDED SUFFICIENTLY

Balanoposthitis. Some cases of inflammation of the epithelium of the penis and prepuce can result in inability to mate because of pain or from physical interference. There are three areas of damage.
1 The region around the preputial orifice.
2 The penile epithelium.
3 The reflected prepuce which, by virtue of its extreme elasticity and mobility, stretches and reflects itself along the extended erect penis.

1 The region around the preputial orifice. Problems in this area may be the result of trauma with subsequent infection (Memon *et al.* 1980–85). An example is where the bull everts his preputial epithelium, which is then damaged and infected (Long & Dubra, 1972). The breeds most commonly affected are the Aberdeen Angus and polled Hereford, which have no retractor preputiae muscle and the *Bos indicus* breeds and crosses (Larsen & Bellenger, 1971). Ubiquitous organisms such as *Actinomyces pyogenes* and *Staphylococcus aureus* can often be isolated from such lesions. The smegma

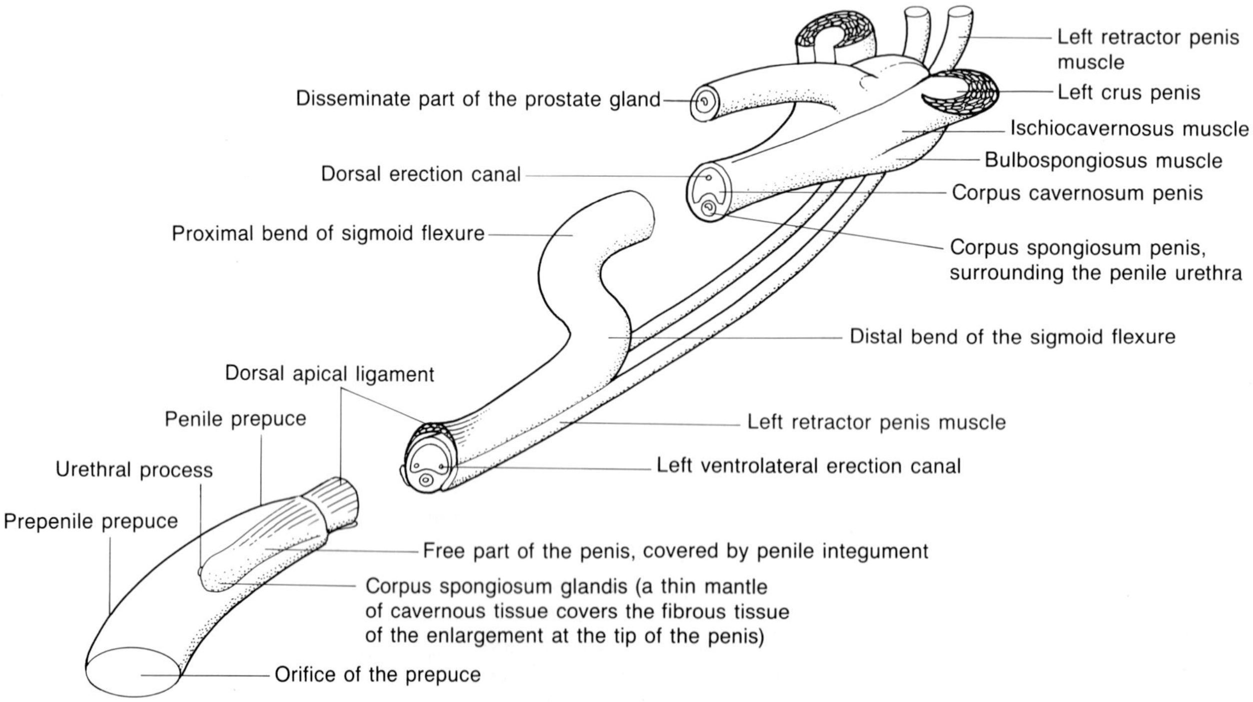

Fig. 35.2 Diagram to show the anatomy of the penis and prepuce of the bull. (Courtesy of Dr R.R. Ashdown.)

produced by the bull is very tacky and the authors know of at least one case where the problem was caused by the firm matting of the hairs over the preputial orifice due to this substance with resultant failure to protrude the penis. Others have described hair rings around the free end of the penis, although this usually produces an annular constriction a few centimetres behind the tip of the penis.

2 The penile epithelium. This can be damaged either traumatically, or by infection, in particular by the infectious bovine rhinotracheitis/infectious pustular vulvovaginitis virus (IBR/IPV). Damage with subsequent scar tissue results in a failure to protrude.

3 The reflected prepuce. This area is extremely important because it must function properly to allow the penis to protrude (Ashdown & Pearson, 1973a). Any traumatic damage with resulting scar tissue formation tends to be self-perpetuating since the scar tissue often limits movement, resulting in further tearing. Furthermore, infection at such sites is common with subsequent abscessation (Fig. 35.3). An extreme example of such damage can occasionally be seen after collection with an artificial vagina and in some of these cases the tear is very large indeed (Fig. 35.4). Usually the bull in question is a young inexperienced animal or one returning to work after a prolonged lay off (Monke, 1980).

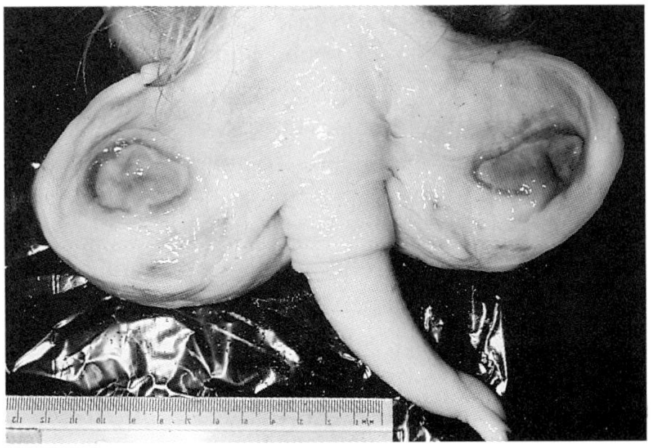

Fig. 35.3 Abcess formation of the preputial epithelium in the bull.

Short penis. As the bull grows so the penis should also develop. In some cases it would appear this does not occur and the bull becomes less and less able to protrude the penis sufficiently to achieve intromission. The exact aetiology of the problem is obscure and may well be due to several different conditions but it does not appear to be a defect of erection since the penis appears to firm up quite normally. Fibrous metaplasia of the retractor penis muscle has been described (Arthur, 1960) and this has been successfully treated by myectomy. However, since the condition appears to be heritable surgery is probably not advisable. At its simplest, a grossly enlarged pendulous abdomen may be a cause of the problem though usually in such cases some of the penis can be protruded. A severe drainage defect problem could also possibly present in this manner (see later).

Rupture of the corpus cavernosum penis. As mentioned earlier the pressures erecting and firming the penis are immense and in some unfortunate cases the tunica albuginea ruptures (Fig. 35.5). It is possible that in some cases the tunica albuginea is unable to sustain integrity because of the pressure alone but it is more likely that it ruptures under additional strains caused

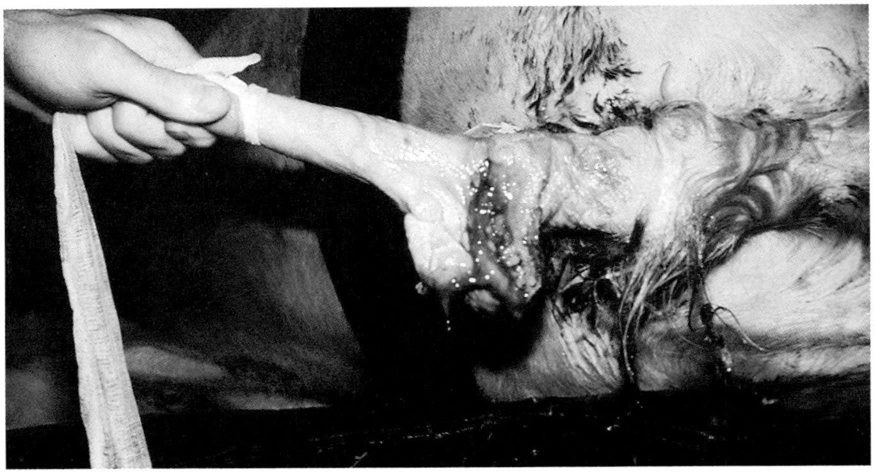

Fig. 35.4 Severe tear of prepuce.

by a sudden penile deflection due to an unexpected movement by the cow while service is taking place, or the bull slipping while the penis is in the vagina. Rupture generally occurs in the region of the sigmoid flexure (see Fig. 35.2). It is most common on the dorsal aspect of the distal bend of the sigmoid flexure but can also occur on the dorsal surface of the penis between the root and proximal bend of the sigmoid flexure. Such rupture results in a haematoma, which subsequently organizes and prevents the full erection and protrusion of the penis. Unfortunately, recurrence is not uncommon (Ashdown & Glossop, 1983).

Persistent frenulum. The penile frenulum, which normally attaches the free end of the penis to the prepuce of the prepubertal bull, is normally 'lost' during early puberty, possibly breaking during play and/or masturbation. Occasionally, this does not occur and its persistence prevents the tip of the penis straightening on erection. It is usually bent ventrally and caudally.

Failure to locate vulva

Psychogenic problems. There would appear to be two distinct problems.
1 Neck or side mounting.

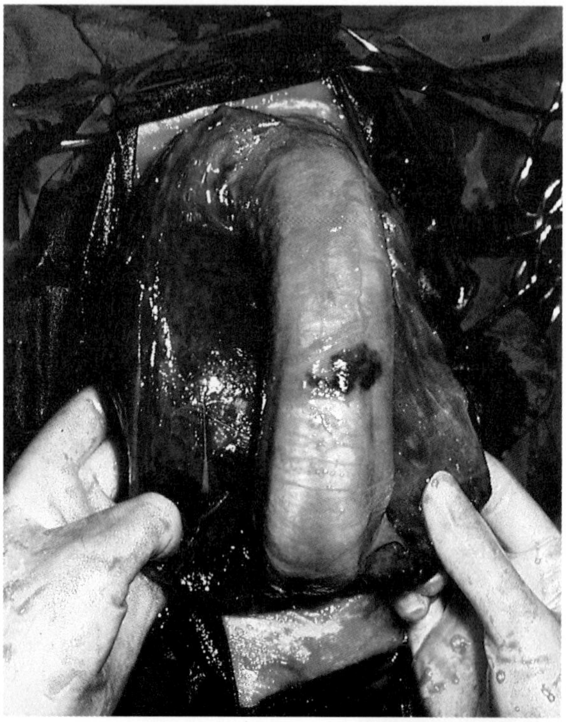

Fig. 35.5 Rupture of the corpus cavernosum penis.

2 Normal mounting, but without success, the bull being incapable of inserting the penis into the vagina despite a good erection and apparently normal seeking movements even to the extent of touching the vulva.

The aetiology for these conditions especially the former is obscure though neck mounting is not uncommon in young inexperienced bulls. However, they usually quickly move round to the rear of the cow. For the latter one could hypothesize either that this could be an early manifestation of a premature partial drainage defect of the corpus cavernosum penis or that there was an inadequate sensitivity of the penile tip resulting in a lack of appreciation of the position of the penis relative to the vulva.

Penile problems. Fibropapillomata. These are generally found on or near the tip of the penis (Fig. 35.6). They are caused by a virus and are thus transmissible. They can occasionally also cause considerable problems in the female (Meischke, 1979). In the bull they usually only affect the penis of young animals less than four years of age and generally regress after a period of two to six months. In some cases however they persist much longer and some become eroded and infected (Walker, 1980).

Drainage defects. Careful anatomical studies of the normal and abnormal penis have revealed a number of arteriovenous shunts, which allow the venous cavities of the penis to drain more quickly than usual. This results in an inability to erect fully or to sustain an erection (Ashdown *et al.*, 1979).

It is now considered possible to distinguish four different venous drainage defects based on history and clinical findings. However, in the last analysis all are associated with inadequate erection in the bull and a diagnosis of venous drainage defect is probably sufficient in most cases (Logue & Greig, 1985).
3 *Corkscrew penis.* Spiral deviation of the penis within the vagina at ejaculation is physiological but in the clinical condition the spiral deviation precedes intromission and so prevents service. This is most commonly seen in beef bulls of around four years of age. (Blockey & Taylor, 1984).

In all cases the spiral is anticlockwise and often it does not occur until the penis makes contact with the vulva of the cow. However, in some cases the condition may be so severe that spiral deviation occurs while the penis is still in the prepuce and it may then prevent protrusion.
4 *Deviations* of the penis, particularly ventral deviations, must be differentiated from drainage defects.

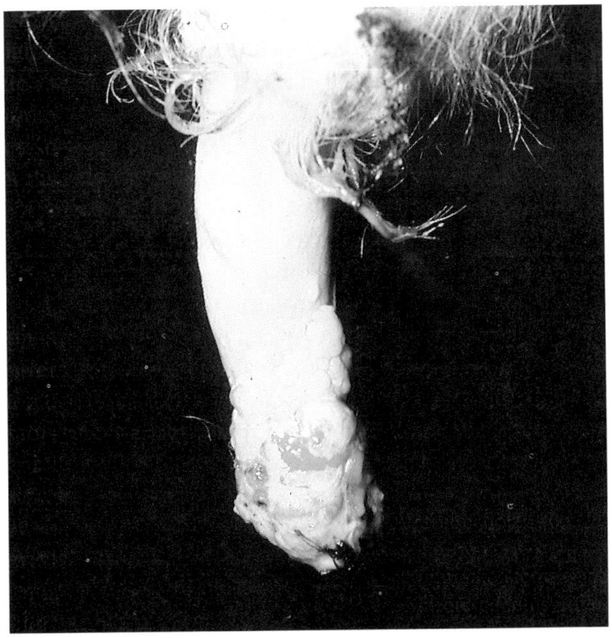

Fig. 35.6 Fibropapilloma on the tip of the penis.

These deviations may be caused by scar formation such as that following acute balanoposthitis or surgery (Walker, 1980).

FAILURE TO THRUST AND EJACULATE AFTER INTROMISSION

Occasionally, one encounters a young bull that is capable of placing the penis in the anterior vagina but then fails to thrust vigorously and ejaculate. In some cases the cause may be orthopaedic, but some may be neural in origin, whether due to local receptor problems causing a lack of sensitivity of the penis or a more general psychosomatic defect. Another possibility is that this problem might be due to a slight defect either in the drainage of the corpus cavernosus penis itself or defect in the corpus spongosum penis or even of the erectile tissue in the tip of the glans. Finally, in some cases it may just be due to inexperience.

NORMAL SERVICE WITH A POOR PREGNANCY RATE

The vast majority of conditions causing this manifestation are related to problems associated with sperm production and transport. An understanding of the complexity of the mechanisms involved in governing and modifying these processes is essential. There are two basic components in the ejaculate, spermatozoa and seminal fluid. The former are produced in the seminiferous tubules of the testes by spermatogenesis and the latter from the testes, epididymes and accessory sex glands.

The clinician should consider the following items when presented with a bull that is serving normal cows satisfactorily but achieving a low pregnancy rate.

1 Age.
2 Overwork.
3 Insult to spermatogenesis.
4 Testicular degeneration.
5 Testicular hypoplasia.
6 Interference with storage and transport of spermatozoa.
7 Abnormalities of accessory sex glands.
8 Influence of fertilization failure and embryonic loss (see Chapter 33).

Age

There is a gradual development towards maximum fertility in the young bull and this is under physiological control. A practical example of these effects can be seen in the increase in scrotal circumference with age (Coulter & Foote, 1978). This parameter is quite valuable as an objective estimate of normal development of the testes and epididymes. Figures from bull examination suggest that while a scrotal circumference of 35–40 cm is desirable in a young bull (approx. 18 months) it is the measurements that are below 30 cm which require the most attention.

One theory for the relatively lower fertility seen in young bulls when compared with adults is related to the development of both testes and epididymis in the young bull, which has roughly half the sperm output of an adult, but less than one-quarter of the storage available in the tail of the epididymis with probably only enough for two to three days' sperm production. Hence it is much easier to deplete the young bull. Furthermore, it will be apparent that relative to the testes the epididymis, particularly the tail, is still enlarging and just how this interacts with sperm maturation in these young bulls is not well understood (Aman & Almquist, 1976; Amann & Schambacher, 1983).

In summary, while the bull may be capable of reproducing quite early in life it is not until after three years of age, or possibly even a little later in the case of late-maturing continental bulls, that one can safely say that the fertility of the bull is unlikely to improve further.

While detailed studies are not really available it does

appear that fertility also diminishes with advancing age (Amann & Schambacher, 1983). In the older bull poor fertility is associated with degeneration of some of the seminiferous tubules and with the development of testicular calcinosis in the seminiferous tubules resulting in non-productive areas of testes. Testicular calcinosis can be quite marked in some older bulls; however, it can also occur in young animals (Turnbull, 1977).

Overwork

Much of the information about semen quality and work rates come from AI centres. However, the demands upon bulls running and mating with a herd of cows are obviously very different from those at an AI centre since young active bulls may serve a cow 10 times or more during oestrus. This sort of pressure (10 ejaculates in 2 hours) results in a diminution of total sperm numbers per ejaculate by a factor of around 10 (Salisbury & Van Demark, 1961) mainly due to a fall in concentration. Concentration in such circumstances falls to as low as 100×10^6 sperm/ml, a level that in a fertility examination would certainly result in the fertility of the bull being questioned. However, theoretically, complete rest of around two weeks should allow a return to normal sperm concentrations in the ejaculate. In practice this is generally the case. In other words the main effect of overuse is to exhaust the epididymal reserves. However, at very high and sustained mating pressures a slower return to normal number of spermatozoa per ejaculate may be found. Furthermore, it has also been noted that as the number of ejaculates increases, sperm motility tends to fall. In addition, the likelihood of an occasional azoospermic ejaculate increases (Salisbury & Van Demark, 1961).

Finally, there is some information indicating that young bulls given a diet below maintenance for energy take considerably longer to replenish their sperm reserves. This is particularly relevant to young post-sale bulls, which are purchased in very good body condition and then put outside with cows in a hard environment thereby losing condition rapidly. By inference such bulls take considerably longer to replenish their sperm reserves (Salisbury & Van Demark, 1961).

Insult to spermatogenesis

Spermatogenesis is a very sensitive process and can be easily upset. Nevertheless, it can also recover, particularly if the insult has been transient. Such insults can be categorized as either local or systemic.

Local

1 *Scrotal sac disruption*. Obviously, severe trauma to the scrotum can have a direct effect upon the testes and epididymes but one of the main functions of the scrotum is temperature control and any disruption of this can interfere with spermatogenesis. The first area of spermatogenesis affected is meiosis, the spermatogonia tend not to be affected and, after removal of the insult, regeneration within six weeks is to be expected providing the Sertoli or nurse cells are not damaged also. These are the most resistant to insult (Kumi-Diaka & Dennis, 1978).

While weather conditions are capable of insult and cause variations in semen quality (Parkinson 1987), it really requires trauma, a severe skin infection, an allergic reaction with scrotal oedema, a scrotal hernia or a deformity of the pampiniform plexus (so-called varicocele) to produce serious infertility.

2 *Orchitis/epididymitis*. Inflammation of the testes is commonly a purely local problem and frequently it only involves one testicle. However, often the infection so interferes with the temperature gradient of the scrotum that the remaining testicle is indirectly affected. A similar effect is seen with epididymitis though in this case there is the further problem of obstruction of spermatozoa and testicular fluid on the affected side. Often orchitis and epididymitis are concurrent.

The causes of orchitis/epididymitis infection are not well documented. In many cases *A. pyogenes* can be isolated from the affected testes but whether this is the original pathogen is uncertain. Other bacteria, such as those of the *Haemophilus/Histophilus* group have been implicated in spermatogenic damage as have viruses.

Systemic

1 *Systemic illness*. Severe illness can disrupt spermatogenesis by one or all of three routes: firstly, by interfering with the temperature gradient of the testes, secondly as a consequence of toxaemic damage to the spermatogenic epithelium and finally by interfering with the complex hormonal secretions which control spermatogenesis and their interactions.

One interesting condition, worthy of mention, is *idiopathic angioneurotic oedema*. This is occasionally seen in young bulls, particularly of continental breeds and generally occurs soon after introduction to grazing. There is often tremendous oedema of all the dependent areas especially the scrotum with consequent azoospermia. The latter is presumably due to a temperature effect. Recovery is usually complete.

2 *Drugs*. Although therapeutic products are subject to

very stringent safety screening there are certain drugs that might affect male fertility.

Anabolic steroids given to young growing bulls have been shown to have an undoubted effect upon spermatogenesis resulting in a reduced testicular size and delayed development of the seminiferous tubules and interstitial cells (O'Lamhna & Roche, 1983; Deschamps *et al.*, 1987a,b). Although it was suggested that these effects were temporary the fact that there was a delay in puberty, that the effect was more severe in younger animals, that there was evidence of interference in the hypothalamic–pituitary axis, and the size and structure of the testes and epididymis, and finally that the studies were relatively short-term makes one very wary of such a claim.

Given the effect of anabolic steroids by inference treatment with *corticosteroids* is also likely to affect semen quality (Li & Wagner, 1983), and indeed some slight changes have been described short term. However, administration to adult Holstein bulls did not appear to cause any practical spermatogenic problems (O'Connor *et al.*, 1985). Nevertheless, there is very recent evidence that some non-steroidal anti-inflammatory drugs such as flunixin could have an effect (Archbald *et al.*, 1990). Field experience has also failed to show any fertility effect associated with the administration of the commonly used antibiotics. However, again the periods of administration were relatively short. Abbitt *et al.* (1984) reported that neither dihydrostreptomycin sulphate nor oxytetracycline hydrochloride had any real effect upon reproductive function even when given in greater than normal therapeutic doses.

Testicular degeneration

In many infertile animals the only apparent histological defect associated with infertility is the absence of dividing spermatogenic cells, the Sertoli cells and interstitial cells still being evident. Evidently, however, histology does not show the defects of function, in particular the delicate interaction between the cells of the testes and their hormonal influences from, and feedback to, other centres.

Studies in the rat have shown firstly that Sertoli cell function was disrupted by a whole variety of noxious stimuli and that one side-effect of such damage was an increase in serum follicle stimulating hormone (FSH) concentrations due to a decreased output of inhibin. Secondly, the Leydig cells were also affected since serum luteinizing hormone (LH) concentrations were higher and testosterone concentrations lower. Finally, there was evidence of a reduced response to human chorionic gonadotrophin (HCG) (de Kretser, 1979).

The inference is that damage to the spermatogenic epithelium interferes with androgen binding protein (ABP) and inhibin release leading to an increased FSH concentration, which in turn alters the balance of testosterone–oestradiol synthesis towards the latter with a subsequent alteration in LH concentrations. Since there is evidence that LH can directly affect the Leydig cell, testosterone release and so ABP release by the Sertoli cell, it can be seen that if events are prolonged or extreme these effects may accumulate and eventually result in a permanent derangement. As mentioned earlier not all derangements are necessarily mediated by hormonal dysfunction. Thus it is believed that chromosomal abnormalities may interrupt the meiotic process to such a degree that infertility or reduced seminiferous tubule output is a result (Chandley, 1979). This does not appear to be as much of a problem in cattle as in man, though there is evidence of reduced fertility in cattle carrying a 1/29 Robertsonian translocation (Gustavsson, 1974; Logue & Harvey, 1979) and bulls with 60, XXY chromosomes are, as might be expected, completely sterile (Logue *et al.*, 1979). However, the nature of the bovine karyotype has meant that identification of reciprocal translocations is not easy and it is likely with improved techniques some will come to light. These abnormalities are more likely to be associated with infertility than the Robertsonian translocations which appear to be quite common within the cattle.

Finally, the roles of bacteria and viruses in the aetiology of this condition are not well understood. For example, a few apparently infertile bulls have been found to be viraemic carriers of bovine virus diarrhoea/mucosal disease virus (BVD/MD) (see p. 660) or to have high titres to *Leptospira hardjo* (see p. 570). However, in some cases the animals have subsequently proved fertile; this even applied to one BVD/MD viraemic animal (Logue *et al.*, unpublished information). Where the derangement of the seminiferous epithelium is permanent then this may result in a gradual diminution in size of the testicle, i.e. testicular atrophy. Unfortunately, unless one had prior knowledge that the affected bull had previously had normal-sized testes this small size could quite easily be considered as testicular hypoplasia.

Testicular hypoplasia

This condition is defined as the congenital presence of either one or two small testes (i.e. bilateral or unilateral)

(Fig. 35.7). It has been closely studied in the Swedish Highland breed of cattle where it has been demonstrated to be a heritable defect caused by a recessive gene with incomplete penetrance. In both unilaterally and bilaterally affected cases sexual behaviour and secondary sexual characteristics are normal (Lagerlöf, 1951).

It is not known whether a similar inheritance pattern applies to other breeds.

It is theoretically possible that toxic or infectious agents affecting the dam at a critical stage of organogenesis of the testes could also cause hypoplasia, either bilateral or unilateral. Mention should also be made of bilateral testicular hypoplasia (Fig. 35.8) that is associated with the abnormal sex chromosome constitution XXY, i.e. an 'extra' X chromosome (Fig. 35.9). As already mentioned other cytogenetic abnormalities are associated with infertility.

Scrotal circumference measurements can be helpful in giving an objective guide to testes size as it is a simple, highly repeatable, measurement. In other species it has been related to spermatozoa production and, intriguingly, ovulation rate in the female offspring (Land, 1978). However, from a practical point of view it is sufficient to note that those males with a below normal scrotal development have a greater likelihood of being infertile.

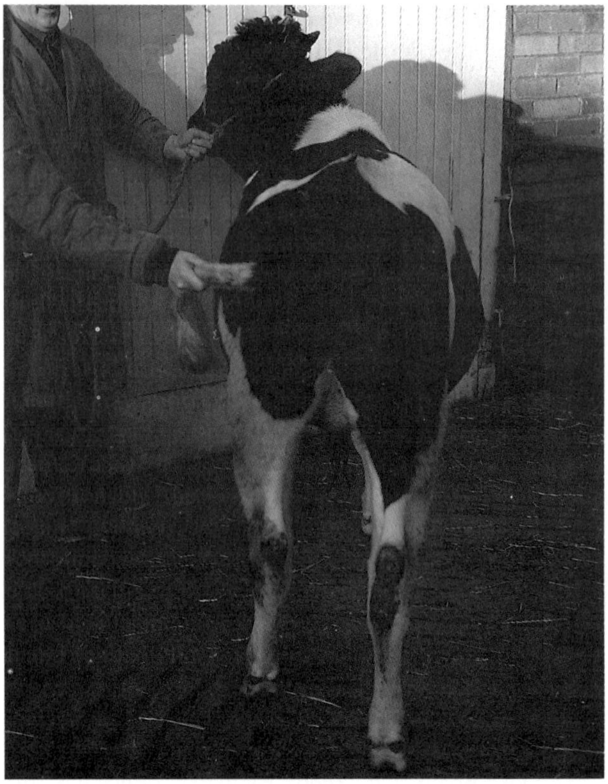

Fig. 35.8 A 61XXY bull with bilateral testicular hypoplasia.

Interference in transport and storage of spermatozoa

It is generally impossible to differentiate clinically which of the local and systemic effects mentioned earlier have an effect solely upon the epididymes, since, as already mentioned, any disruption of testicular function frequently interferes with epididymal function.

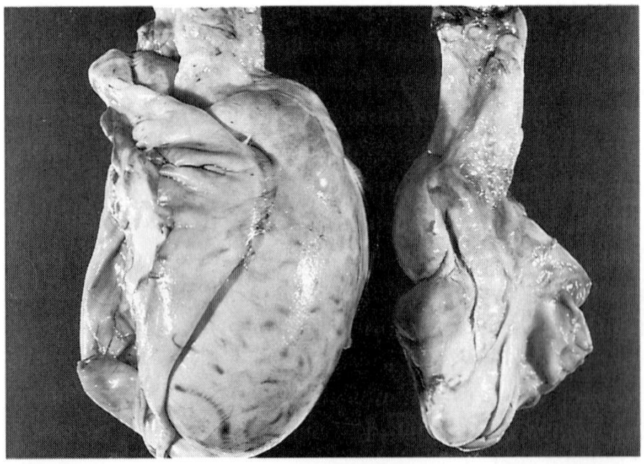

Fig. 35.7 Unilateral testicular hypoplasia in the Ayrshire breed. Note the adhesions on the normal testis caused by needle biopsy.

The epididymis, unlike the testis, develops from the mesonephric (Wolffian) ducts and are prone to several congenital malformations (Blom & Christensen, 1960).

Aplasia of part of the epididymis, ductus deferens and seminal vesicles has been described as a congenital defect in the bull. The aplasia is usually unilateral and can be very specific. It is generally associated with spermatocele formation or so-called sperm granulomas proximal to the aplasia (Blom & Christensen 1960). These are most commonly seen on the head of the epididymis and while they have been described as being a result of segmental aplasia (see above), in some cases spermatoceles arise in this position apparently spontaneously.

Spermatocele formation has been diagnosed in the field following a sudden failure to mount and thus, by inference, it is painful in the acute phase (Logue & Greig, 1986). Since this was the only behavioural demonstration of pain it could be that any discomfort is only appreciated when the bull is sexually aroused. The exact relationship of the spontaneous condition to segmental aplasia is uncertain but one cannot ignore

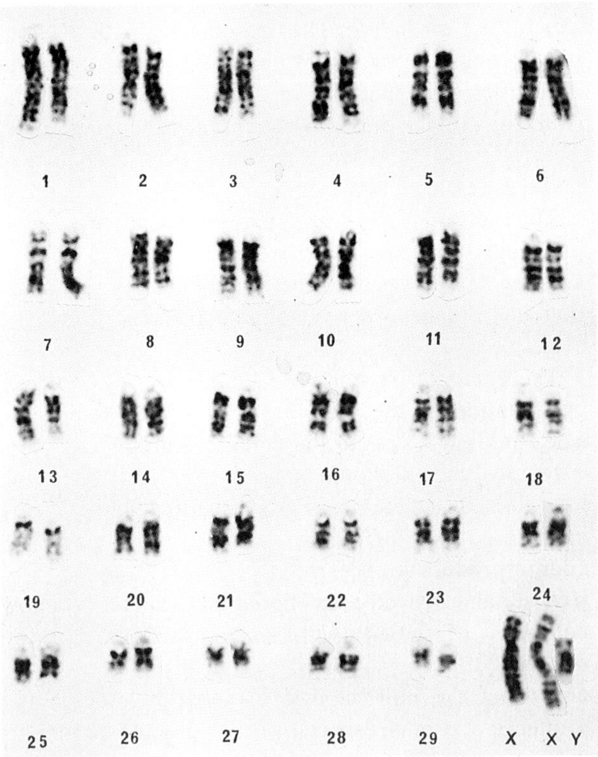

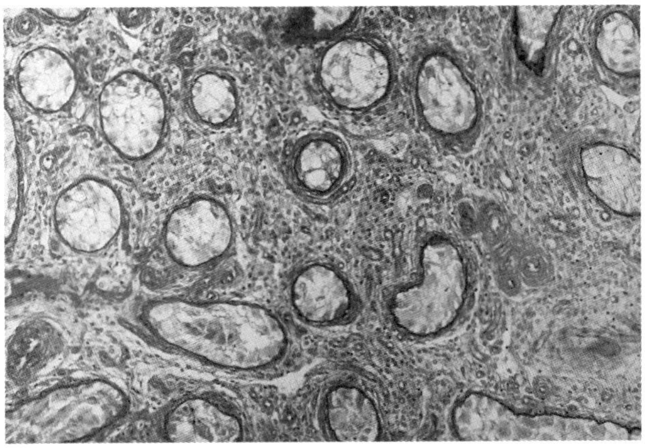

Fig. 35.9 (a) G-band karyotype 61XXY. (b) XXY bull. Tubules lined by Sertoli cells only, Leydig cells moderately increased in proportion. (Masson X195). (Courtesy of the Veterinary Record.)

the possibility of an infectious condition causing an epididymitis and subsequent spermatocele. However, epididymitis resulting from infection by *Brucella* sp. and the *Haemophilus/Histophilus* group appear to occur most frequently in the tail of the epididymes. *Mycoplasma* infections have also been implicated in epididymitis (La Faunce & McEntee, 1982).

Unilateral spermatoceles need not necessarily cause sterility since once the inflammatory reaction has settled the remaining testicle can produce an apparently normal ejaculate. However, it is clearly not advisable to use such an animal with a large number of females and in two cases, known to the authors, where the bulls involved were at an AI centre the concentration of the ejaculate never returned to the level seen before the incident. In one of these bulls the second epididymis also suffered the same problem and had to be destroyed. No significant micro-organism could be found (Logue & Hignett, unpublished information). In some cases small compact masses up to the size of a pea, so-called cysts, can be felt both on the epididymis and on the spermatic cord itself. They are developmental in origin and of no consequence as long as they do not interfere with sperm transport.

Abnormalities of the accessory sex glands

The accessory sex glands consist of the seminal vesicles, ampullae, prostate and bulbourethral glands. Abnormalities of the seminal vesicles are the most commonly diagnosed condition. Segmental aplasia of the seminal vesicle occurs and appears often to be related to a congenital defect (Blom, 1979a,b). Numerous infectious agents have been isolated and implicated in the aetiology of this condition in the bull, such as members of the *Chlamydia* group. *Mycoplasma bovigenitalium* and *Mycoplasma bovis* (La Faunce & McEntee, 1982). However, in severe clinically recognizable cases the most common organism isolated is *A. pyogenes* (Arthur, 1960; McCauley, 1980).

Diagnosis, treatment and prognosis

Diagnosis is based upon a combination of bull and herd history, examination of the bull and the results of the various tests that are undertaken including an examination of a representative ejaculate of semen. Even if the diagnosis is tentative and the aetiology uncertain the findings may indicate a treatment and will probably allow a prognosis.

HISTORY

Usually the client will have given some information about the bull by telephone and ideally will have presented some farm records for perusal prior to the examination of the bull. At the outset, ask and record the answers to the questions in Table 35.5. One is looking for an estimate of the extent of the infertility by comparison to other bulls; when it was first manifest; if it has been continuous or varied and so on (Table 35.5).

In some cases it may be possible to give a firm diagnosis and an accurate prognosis based on the history and visual examination of the bull when presented with a cow in season, i.e. without even collecting and examining a semen sample. However, it is still generally advisable to attempt to collect a semen sample even if only to confirm the history. Insurance companies often insist on a semen examination being carried out.

EXAMINATION OF THE BULL FOR BREEDING SOUNDNESS

The objectives of the visit to the farm are:

1 to see the conditions under which the bull is expected to work;

2 to confirm that the history is reliable and if possible to examine records;

3 to examine the bull;

4 to ascertain the status of the bull as a possible vector of reproductive disease and possibly other diseases of a less specific nature but just as important from an economic point of view.

In order to study semen for abnormal characteristics the operator must use a technique to obtain and prepare semen for examination that will be representative of the ejaculate of the bull in natural service.

For a full clinical examination of a bull and for semen collections it is desirable that a bull be restrained and can be led on halter. The reason for this is obvious but on many farms this is not possible with resultant difficulties particularly in reconciling the safety of the collector with the desire to obtain a good semen sample. The following are some suggestions that may help to make the visit go more smoothly.

1 The bull should be sexually rested for at least one to preferably three weeks prior to the visit.

2 A quiet cow in oestrus, preferably halter-trained and that has not been served at that oestrus, should be available as a teaser.

3 There should be suitable facilities for restraint and examination of the bull, e.g. crush with removable sides to allow access to the penis and prepuce.

4 Ideally, the bull should be used to serving while being restrained by a halter or ringrope. Unfortunately, many are unused to being handled and therefore restraint is counterproductive.

5 A suitable fenced area should be available to allow collection of semen (with an escape route for the collector).

6 Instruct the bull handler or those helping in the sequence of events, especially in relation to bull mounting for collection.

7 Select a small relatively warm area of bench space (which is covered and with an electricity supply) near the collection area where any semen collected may be examined.

8 Any cows that have been running solely with this bull should be nearby — for pregnancy diagnosis or sampling (vaginal mucus or blood) should the occasion demand it. Unfortunately, often these will have been remated by another bull. However, even then examination may allow confirmation of this.

9 If possible, another bull should be available nearby. This can be useful to confirm the teaser cow is in oestrus when the bull under test has failed to mount.

10 Use a check list of equipment and materials (see Table 35.6).

The order of events for the visit involving the collection and examination of semen are as follows.

Table 35.5 Information required to define the problem

Type and breed of bull
Age
Demeanour
Ringed
Type of herd
Role of bull in herd
Extent and duration of problem
More than one bull with a problem
Correlation with introduction of new male
Correlation with introduction of new female
AI figures available
Insurance status

The on-farm laboratory

This should be set up on arrival so that there is time for the oven, solutions, glassware and hot stage to reach the required temperature.

It should contain the following.

1 Microscope with facilities to examine semen by ×50 to ×100 (for initial motility) by ×200 to ×400 (for progressive motility) and ×1000 for morphology.

2 Hot stage (or equivalent). This is a prerequisite for the reliable estimate of motility. Ideally, it should be kept within 1 °C of 37 °C because either a high or low temperature can have dramatic consequences upon sperm motility. Unfortunately, this equipment is quite expensive and therefore many veterinarians use a small prewarmed flat bottle or brass plates as an alternative. If this approach is used then it is best to have two so that they can be alternated and so kept at as steady a temperature as possible.

3 Hot oven. While it is possible to use the farm oven to keep slides, coverslips, pipettes and stains, regulation of a reasonable temperature range (35–40 °C) is often difficult. For this reason it is preferable to have a small portable oven.

4 Stains. It is well worthwhile using more than one stain routinely. The most commonly used are nigrosin–eosin and Indian ink for sperm morphology, methylene blue for examining the semen for extraneous cells, and Giemsa for a combination of the two. Nigrosin–eosin and Indian ink are used directly, i.e. after preheating to 37 °C they are mixed with the semen immediately after its collection and a smear is then made. The second pair of stains are used on a direct smear of the semen, which is air-dried and then fixed before smearing.

Table 35.6 Check list for breeding soundness kit

1	Artificial vaginas, liners, cones, cord
2	Lubricant for artificial vagina
3	Electroejaculator(s)
4	Electric plug adaptors and circuit breakers
5	Cable
6	Semen collection tubes
7	Heated cabinet
8	Transformer packs
9	Microscope and light source plus hot stage
10	Two funnels for collection of electroejaculated semen
11	Wire funnel holder
12	Stains: nigrosin–eosin, Giemsa and methylene blue
13	Slides and coverslips and holder box plus slide labels
14	Paper wipes, cotton wool and swabs
15	Immersion oil
16	50 ml syringe (or flutter valve) with tubing for preputial wash
17	Thermometer
18	Tape measure
19	Pipettes and bulbs
20	Small test tubes for use in staining
21	2.9% sodium citrate
22	0.9% NaCl and phosphate buffered saline
23	Blood tubes, vacutainers, holder and needles and spirit
24	Virus and *Mycoplasma* transport medium
25	Record sheets, markers and pens

5 Solutions for examination of progressive motility. A 'normal' saline solution may suffice although a more physiological solution may be used, such as either phosphate-buffered saline or 2.9 per cent trisodium citrate are preferable. These solutions should also be preheated to as near 37 °C as possible.

6 Artificial vagina. At least two should be assembled and be filled with warm water to a lumen temperature of about 60 °C (they will often have cooled to around 45–48 °C by the time they will be used or if not they should be adjusted to this range when required). In general, inexperienced bulls prefer rough liners and younger bulls a shorter artificial vagina, i.e. about 25 cm long.

Introductory examination of the bull

It is worthwhile giving the bull an initial examination prior to collection, firstly to allow the bull to get used to the personnel involved, particularly the collector of semen, and secondly to allow the collector to judge how potentially dangerous the bull is.

Service behaviour and collection of semen

It is important to interfere as little as possible with the normal service behaviour of the bull to obtain a representative ejaculate.

Artificial vagina and teaser cow. The best technique for the collection of semen is the use of an artificial vagina (Fig. 35.10). The factors for obtaining a representative semen sample are detailed below.

1 *Cow in season.* A cow in oestrus will stand to be mounted. This is essential particularly with an experienced beef bull, which will generally refuse to mount if the cow does not stand steadily when the bull 'tests' her. Furthermore, since many bulls are not used to being handled and therefore have to be allowed to mount free of control it is wise to have something that they are more interested in than the collector! The cow must be physically capable of bearing the weight of the bull and ideally she should be restrained by at least a halter. Unfortunately, many cows have never been haltered so they tend to object to this and thus by struggling put the bull off working. Furthermore, in other cases their stubborn lack of initial movement is itself off-putting to the bull and if nothing is happening it is worthwhile trying to lead the cow in front of the bull.

2 *Good surroundings and surface.* Some bulls can be totally inhibited in the wrong surroundings. Ideally,

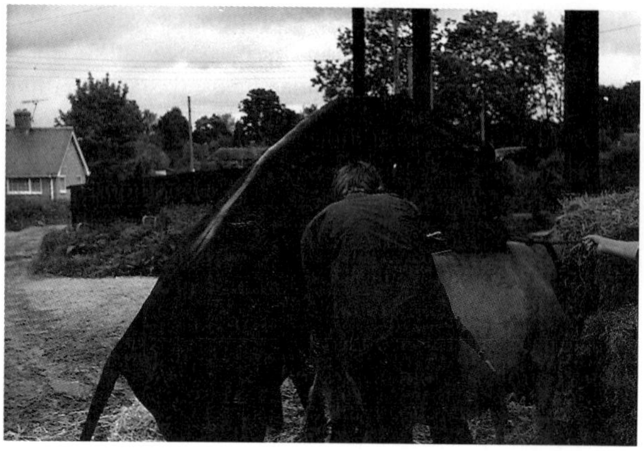

Fig. 35.10 The on-farm collection. The bull has just ejaculated.

one should work in the place where the bull normally serves the cows.

A good surface will encourage a bull to mount, for example a bull with laminitis or an old bull will often work better on a relatively soft surface such as grass rather than on concrete. However, in most circumstances the latter is the preferred surface since most injuries to collectors are caused by the bull falling. It is for this reason that most AI centres use service stocks and obviously if these are available they should be used. However, whatever adaptation or compromise is used, the collector must remember that his safety and that of the others involved is paramount. The main prerequisites are common sense, plenty of room and a safe footing.

3 *Experience of collector*. It is difficult to rationalize just what the collector does to ensure a good collection.

Firstly, there is the judgement as to whether to try and collect when the bull first mounts. Quite often the first mount will be 'premature' with a poor erection of the penis and in most cases it is best just to deflect the penis by using pressure on the sheath and let the bull dismount. However, this carries the risk of putting the bull off mounting again. Nevertheless, time and effort spent in teasing (even to the point of removing the bull or the cow from the scene) is usually rewarding and eliminates any doubts that can arise when a poor sample is obtained, at the very first mount.

Secondly, there is the process of actually allowing the penis to enter the artificial vagina. In some cases, where the bull will not immediately thrust, it may be induced to do so by a short, quick, back and forward movement of the artificial vagina. This should be firm but gentle. Related to this is the decision as to the length of the artificial vagina, the pressure of the water in the liner, the type of liner and temperature. For example, few bulls will thrust well with an artificial-vagina temperature less than 40 °C, but equally there is no need for it to be more than 55 °C. The use of a very warm artificial vagina with a rough liner can leave the penis looking very red. It is vital to remember that the tip of the penis is highly sensitive, and that an ejaculatory thrust is usually induced immediately it enters a properly prepared AV.

Wherever possible more than one collection should be made especially if the first is of poor quality. Moreover, in some cases an even greater number of collections may be required to satisfy the collector that the bull has worked well and that the series of samples obtained is as representative as possible. Only experience allows this judgement.

When the bull is brought out for service the collector should watch only the bull and make the following mental notes:

1 Demeanor. Is he interested in the cow?

2 Gait. Is he lame, if so where?

3 Libido. Is he keen to work? Watch for the pumping of the ischiocavernosus muscle (this will be apparent by a rippling tail–head movement) and the dripping, clear pre-ejaculatory fluid from the prepuce. The penis may also be seen protruding a little from the prepuce: does this appear normal? Usually before mounting an experienced bull will grunt and make a quick movement at the rear of the cow just to test if she will stand. If the cow is not in season she will move, even if restrained, and this may be quite sufficient to stop the bull mounting.

4 Penile erection and ejaculation. The bull should mount, clasp the cow, erect fully and search for the vulval opening with the penis, and, on finding the artificial vagina, thrust and ejaculate in one movement. The search should not take more than 10 seconds and a good thrust takes both hind legs off the ground in a forward direction. The sound of an explosive exhalation indicates ejaculation. Because of the rapidity of service in experienced bulls and the necessity of examining the semen sample as soon as possible after collection it is often difficult to examine the penis fully and collect semen at the same time. However, an appreciation of its firmness is possible as is a quick visual assessment of both penis and the prepuce. Should a more thorough examination be indicated mounting can be repeated later without a collection being made; the penis (that part within the prepuce) being pulled toward the examiner thereby exposing the protruded portion for a more prolonged examination. This posture

can often be held for a few seconds as long as the tip of the penis does not contact the cow. Finally, after a collection of semen it is very worthwhile standing back and observing the bull serving the cow naturally. Obviously, this is only possible with a cow in season and the consent, of the owner who may not wish to have the cow served.

Other techniques of semen collection. Occasionally, the collection of an ejaculate by artificial vagina proves impossible and it is deemed necessary to examine a semen sample. In such circumstances, if the bull will mount and serve an oestrous cow then the removal of semen and vaginal mucus from the vagina of the cow and examination of the spermatozoa in the mucus is a valid technique. It is for this reason that the cow should not be served prior to the visit.

In the last resort, and only if it is felt *absolutely* necessary should one collect semen by electroejaculation. This technique depends on electrical stimulation of the sacral segments of the spinal cord, which are mainly parasympathetic nerves emerging from the pelvic plexus.

This stimulation will often cause a form of erection (possibly incomplete) and ejaculation. The ejaculate often differs from a 'normal' ejaculate by having a considerably greater volume, and a lower sperm concentration (even in the 'sperm-rich' portion). This is due to the excessive contribution of the accessory glands, in particular the seminal vesicles.

Another disadvantage of this technique is that the animal shows tetanic contractions with each series of pulses and these increase in strength with voltage. Initially, he raises his tail, then rocks gently to and fro, then lifts one hind leg, arches the back and eventually, if excessive stimulation is applied, the bull will go down. For this reason it may be advisable in some circumstances to sedate the bull. However, our experience is that the technique can be used without sedation.

Sexual rest before electroejaculation seems to aid obtaining a representative sample. The main value of the technique is to confirm the presence of motile spermatozoa and obtain sufficient to study their morphology.

Examination of ejaculate

While there has been and still is considerable research into the prediction of fertility on the basis of tests upon semen (Linford *et al.*, 1976; Miller & Hunter, 1987), the general form of on-farm semen examination is still largely based on the pioneering work of the early AI industry. In particular, the reader is referred to the study by Bishop *et al.* (1954).

An ejaculate examination generally entails observing and recording the following.

1 Volume.
2 Initial motility of sample.
3 Progressive motility of spermatozoa.
4 Morphology of spermatozoa.
5 Presence of other cells.
6 Concentration of spermatozoa.
7 Final overall assessment.

Volume. Use a graduated collecting tube.

Initial motility. A small drop of semen is dropped on to a warm slide, which is placed on a warm stage (35–37 °C) and examined (×100) as soon as possible after collection. It is scored on a scale of 0–5, ranging from 0 being completely static to 5 being vigorously active. In the bull the major criterion of scoring initial motility is wave motion, which is a function of concentration, proportion of motile sperm and their activity.

This simple test if applied correctly correlates quite well with fertility. Any bull that consistently produces semen with a score of less than 2 should be suspect.

Progressive motility. Although initial motility gives a guide to the percentage of motile spermatozoa, progressive motility is best estimated by diluting the semen (roughly 1 : 50 depending on concentration) in a prewarmed (35–70 °C) physiological solution (see p. 000) and examining this at ×400 magnification.

A figure in excess of 50 per cent is certainly desirable. High percentage motility generally also means rapid progressive movement. Examination at this power (×400) will also allow some initial observation of the morphology of the spermatozoa and the presence of unusual cells in the semen.

Morphology. The morphology of the spermatozoa is closely related to testicular function and appearance of head, midpiece and tail should all be studied. A general morphological examination entails the observation of spermatozoa (and other cells) under high power (×1000) noting any abnormalities and expressing these as the number of abnormal sperm/100 sperm counted. This is best done quietly away from the farm although a cursory look at ×400 will allow *tentative* prognosis for the owner and also satisfies the collector that the smear is acceptable. The use of at least two different staining techniques is recommended one entailing dilution of the semen prior to making the slide and the other using a direct smear which is stained after fixation. These are described more fully below.

1 *Nigrosin–eosin stain*. Freshly collected semen should be mixed with prewarmed stain roughly according to sperm concentration (average 1 : 10) and allowed to incubate at 35–37 °C for one minute. One small drop is then taken and smeared thinly across a prewarmed slide and allowed to dry. This stain will also allow the computation of the live : dead ratio since eosin is a vital dye, staining so-called dead (or immotile) spermatozoa pink but leaving live sperm unstained. The percentage live figure correlates well with percentage progressively motile and not surprisingly gives similar correlation coefficients with fertility.

2 *Indian ink smear* can be prepared in the same way but do not show 'vital staining'.

3 *Giemsa and methylene blue stains*. In this case at least three direct smears of the semen are made on a warm slide and allowed to air dry. One is fixed using 10 per cent formal saline (buffered), one methanol and the third by gentle heat. After washing the first two in water they are stained in a simple buffered 10 per cent Giemsa solution for approximately 3 hours. Depending on its source, ordinary tap water will do. This stain should highlight the acrosome and allow further identification of any abnormalities of this region in particular. If one brings the slides back to the laboratory before fixation the use of the two different fixes can be of particular value, since often one gives a better resolution of the acrosome than the other, presumably due to differences in the relationship or thickness of the smear, time of air drying and the fix. The neat dried slide is stained by methylene blue (see p. 500).

Considerable experience is required before reliable counts of morphological abnormalities can be obtained. Furthermore, the effect upon the fertility of the semen depends upon the type and extent of abnormality (Barth & Oko, 1989); thus head and midpiece abnormalities (including cytoplasmic droplets) are more important than simple reflected tails (Fig. 35.11). Some abnormalities are known to be inherited, for example the knobbed sperm (Fig. 35.12). Results of morphological analysis should be presented in tabular form showing the proportions of the various abnormalities seen (Table 35.7).

Presence of other cells. A variety of cells is normally found in semen and these are best observed either in the direct smear stained by Giemsa and/or a direct smear heat-fixed and stained by methylene blue (Fig. 35.13). The latter demonstrates leucocytes particularly well. Most of the cells are of preputial or urethral epithelial origin and are of little consequence. However, the presence of large numbers of leucocytes, small darkly staining cells that appear to be degenerating spermatids, multinucleate giant cells and so-called 'round' cells are indicative of spermatogenic disruption.

Concentration can be estimated using the criteria in Table 35.8. When a more accurate measurement is needed then resource to a simple haemocytometer, an

Table 35.7 Sperm abnormalities

Head abnormalities
Microhead
Macrohead
Pyriform
Acrosome defect
Neck abnormalities
Detached head
Detached tail
Fractured neck
Other
Midpiece
Double
Swollen
Abaxial
Curved
Other
Tail
Coiled
Tail reflected
Protoplasmic drops
Proximal
Distal

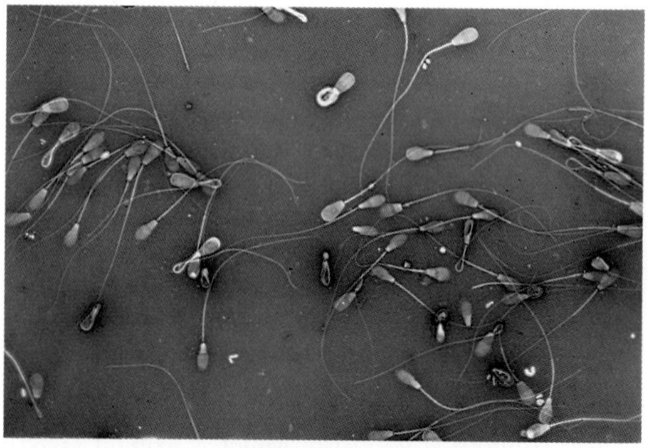

Fig. 35.11 Sperm head, midpiece and tail abnormalities in semen from an infertile bull (nigrosin–eosin) (× 350).

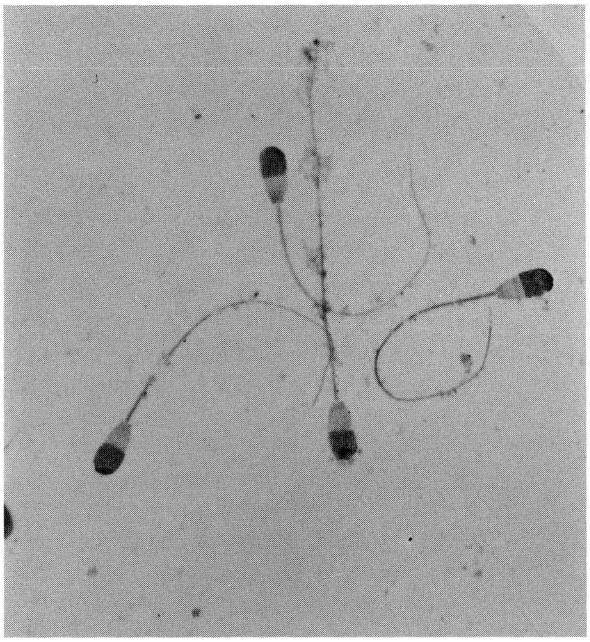

Fig. 35.12 'Knobbed' sperm, an inherited defect of the Friesian breed (Glemsa) (× 700).

opacity measurement using a photometric device or an electronic counter is required.

Physical examination of the bull

During the preliminary examination and during the collection of semen some indication of possible defects may have been highlighted. Whether or not this is the case, a full examination of the reproductive tract is essential to add to the information already available from the history and the preliminary semen findings. In addition examination of several other aspects of the clinical appearance of the bull is worthwhile. Obviously, where lameness or some other defect is apparent during collection the relevant area should be examined.

Table 35.8 Visual criteria for estimating semen concentration ($\times 10^6$ spermatozoa/ml) (from Logue & Greig, 1987).

Thick cream	3000
Cream	2000
Milk/cream	1000
Milk	500
Water/milk	250
Cloudy	100

Mouth. Assess the age of the bull by examining the incisor teeth. This is often very helpful in impressing upon owners how immature their young bulls are. Many bulls of continental breeds have still no adult incisors at two years of age.

Eyes. It is also worthwhile examining the eyes, at the very least to rule out congenital cataracts. Severe cataracts can lead to unpredictable behaviour of the bull and are found in all breeds. A good ophthalmoscope is

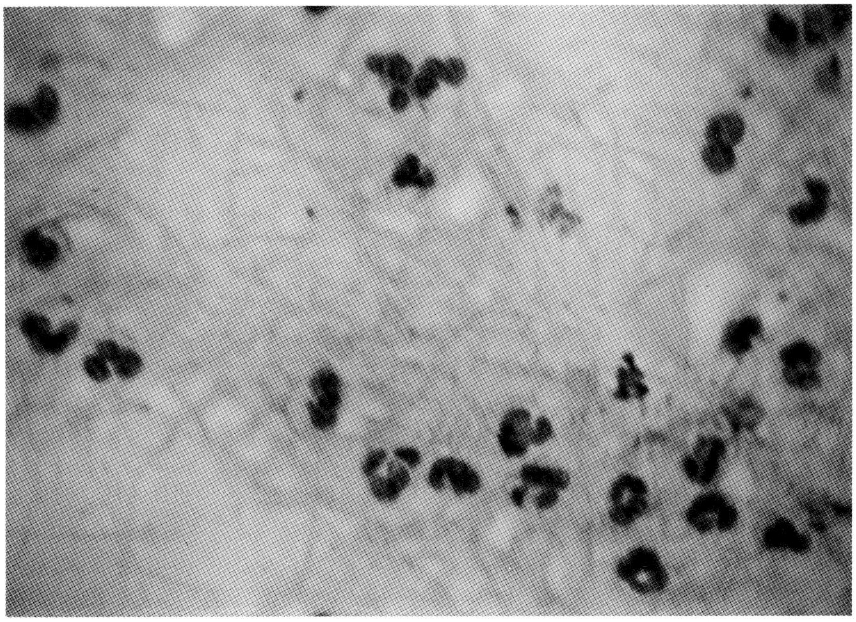

Fig. 35.13 White blood cells in semen (Methylene blue) (× 700).

needed to diagnose less obvious abnormalities such as colobomata of the retina.

Penis and prepuce. Palpate around the orifice of the prepuce, the sheath itself and the penis as it runs back to the scrotum. It is also worthwhile examining the umbilicus for evidence of a hernia.

Scrotum. Palpation of the scrotum allows definition of the following structures:
1 testes,
2 epididymes (head, body and tail),
3 spermatic cords,
4 the scrotal sac itself.

The testes should exhibit freedom of movement within the scrotum and all structures should be of normal size, shape, and free from inconsistency in outline, i.e. bumps and nodules.

A simple subjective measurement of size is the use of scrotal circumference. In the normal adult bull this should be between 33 and 45 cm, depending on breed and mature size.

More recently, the use of real-time ultrasound has been employed as a further diagnostic aid. It remains to be seen precisely how valuable it will be. However, it is now being used by a number of veterinarians including the authors (Figs 35.14 and 35.15).

Pelvis. A rectal examination is needed to examine the accessory sex glands. Some of these are found just under the hand after it has been fully inserted through the anus and the ampullae of vas deferens and seminal vesicles can be identified.

The prostate and bulbourethral glands cannot normally be distinguished. The main part of the former is found at the beginning of the root of penis, while the latter is found just anterior to the ventral bend of the root at the bulbospongiosus muscle.

Again ultrasound has an obvious application, in particular for the examination of seminal vesicles (Fig. 35.16).

Samples for further laboratory investigation. These are influenced in part by the health status of the national herd and that of the herd the bull is being introduced to. The routine employed by the authors in the UK is as follows.

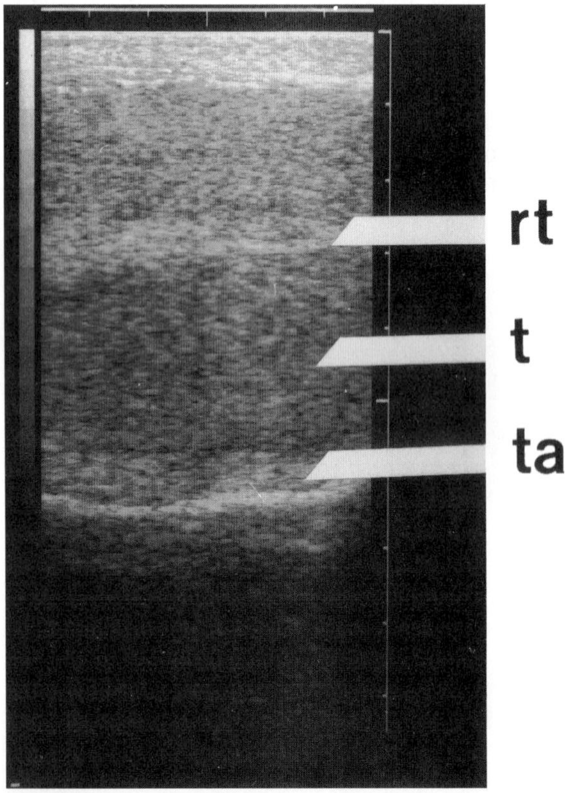

Fig. 35.14 Real-time ultrasound of the testis. rt, rek testis; t, parenchyma of testis; ta, tumia albuginea.

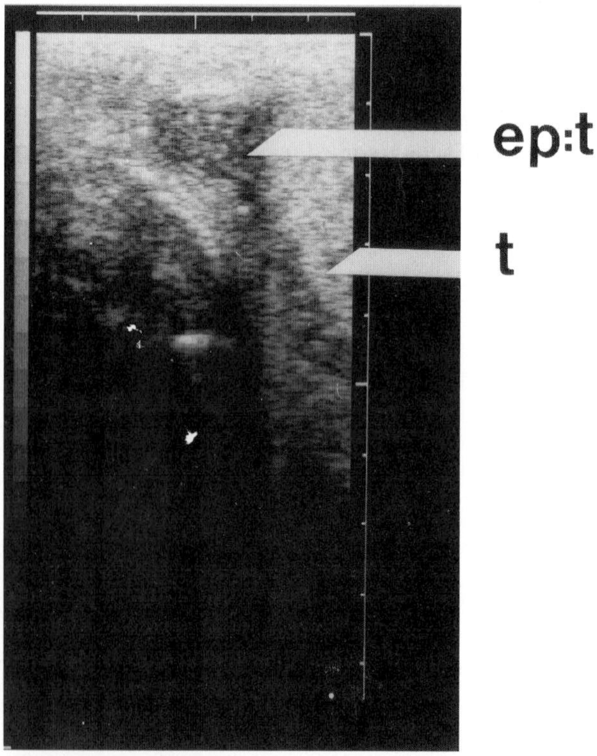

Fig. 35.15 Real-time ultrasound of the tail of the epididymis. ep:t, tail of epididymis; t, testis.

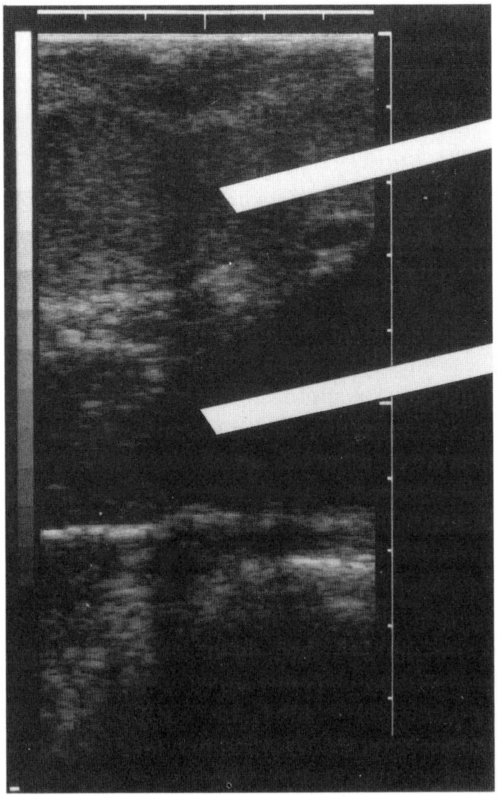

Fig. 35.16 Real-time ultrasound of the seminal vesicle. sv, seminal vesicle; b, bladder.

1 Preputial washing for culture as above and fluorescent antibody test for *Campylobacter fetus* sp.
2 Blood for serology: IBR/IPV, BVD/MD, Leptospires particularly *Leptospira hardjo*
3 Blood for presence of viral antigen: BVD/MD.
4 Semen for culture of bacteria, virus and *Mycoplasma* (if indicated).
5 Blood for routine biochemistry (if indicated), e.g. plasma pepsinogens, routine haematology.
6 Faeces for examination of culture for Johne's disease and *Salmonella* spp. (if indicated) and also examination for fluke and helminth eggs (if indicated).

THE REPORT

Having obtained the history of the bull and examined it fully for breeding soundness (and any cows if necessary) a report should be prepared. This should summarize the history, findings and any laboratory test results. It should then reach a conclusion, which should include a diagnosis, however tentative, and if one is available offer an appropriate treatment and management regime to prevent or control the problem, and finally give a prognosis. A discussion of the aetiology of the problem can also be included. In general the most important aspect of this conclusion is the prognosis. Effectively there are two alternatives: firstly, if the prognosis is hopeless then the bull is best disposed of, and secondly, if there is some hope for recovery then the bull can be kept, treated if necessary and the situation re-evaluated in two to six months depending on the diagnosis.

FAILURE TO MOUNT

Where this is due to a physical problem whether lameness, neck or back ailment, or pain resulting from a penile lesion then the treatment depends upon the type and severity of the problem.

For the major causes of lameness the reader is referred to Chapters 28 and 29 for treatment and prognosis. However, the specific requirements of the bull for service should be borne in mind and thus any prognosis should be guarded. This is because many bulls are prepared to mount before a healing process is complete, thus exacerbating the condition, and also because frequently the bull produces soft dystrophic bone in and around the site of injury resulting in added healing difficulties with subsequent arthritis (Bartels, 1975; Weaver, 1978).

Prevention or at least limitation of the number of physical lesions is possible with good management that centres around an active interest in the bull, his mating behaviour, development and his housing. As already mentioned, it is most important to introduce the bull gradually to an adult workload and to monitor his progress closely at every stage. In particular, the bull should be introduced initially to quiet adult cows which are clearly in season and virtually hand-mated until the bull and his owner are confident that he can work reliably. Table 35.9 gives some general indications of workload.

Attempts to treat low libido by a variety of hormones, either alone or in combination, has rarely proved of value and there is a dearth of recommendations apart from sexual rest in any of the common texts. In fact, matters remain as described by Lagerlöf in 1951!

The prognosis for poor libido of indefinable origin

Table 35.9 Recommended workload of bull with age

<2 years	10 cows
2–3 years	20 cows
3 years	up to 50 cows depending on bull

must be extremely guarded, since, despite any mitigating circumstances, it is likely that this problem is inherent in the make-up of the bull and will recur. In young bulls of around 18 months to two years of age the prognosis is more hopeful but a maximum time-scale of six months in which to show some evidence of overcoming the condition is appropriate.

Where failure to mount is the final outcome of either pain or frustration due to penile or preputial problems then a return to normal behaviour is dependent upon a resolution of the painful condition concerned. The major problems are discussed later but in general there are only two approaches to treatment. The first is conservative symptomatic treatment allied to good husbandry and the second a surgical approach. Unfortunately, in many cases the prognosis is poor and the best course is to cull the bull and obtain the carcass value.

FAILURE TO ACHIEVE INTROMISSION

It is important not to belittle some of the problems of diagnosis, for example an early manifestation of either corkscrew penis or a venous drainage defect could conceivably be masked by the overzealous application of an artificial vagina. However, observation of the natural service behaviour of the bull should avoid this error. As ever prognosis, treatment and prevention depend upon the exact diagnosis.

Balanoposthitis

Treatment of this condition is largely symptomatic; however, in cases with severe scar tissue formation surgery is the only course of action other than salvage (Larsen & Bellenger, 1971; Walker, 1980). Although a guarded prognosis is necessary the chances of recovery will depend on the site, extent and aetiology of the condition. Even in less severe cases sexual rest for at least three months is recommended to ensure adequate healing.

Prevention is best effected by good bull management, regular monitoring of the bull when it is serving a cow and recording of his performance. Should the bull be part of an AI stud then the importance of collection technique must be re-emphasized.

Short penis

Diagnosis is based on the increasing difficulty of the bull to protrude the penis after mounting. The penis should be felt to confirm a firm erection because the condition should be differentiated from either a drainage defect of the corpus cavernosum penis or a long-standing balanoposthitis. The prognosis is hopeless.

Rupture of the corpus cavernosum penis

Diagnosis is based on a sudden onset of an inability to serve coupled with swelling, usually in the inguinal region just above and anterior to the scrotum. Often the bull also presents with a prolapse of the prepuce and because the condition can be painful he may walk stiffly. Where this condition is presented in the acute phase and the surgical approach is adopted, immediate sexual rest followed by surgical removal of the haematoma some five to seven days later, before it can organize (Walker, 1980), is indicated. In more chronic cases and in those acute cases where surgery is not adopted gradual teasing may eventually result in adhesions being broken down sufficiently to allow mating. Progress may also be assisted by frequent gentle massage in the area of the haematoma. Recurrence is quite common and, if possible, identification of the site of rupture is advisable because the prognosis is more hopeful for a rupture at the distal bend of the sigmoid flexure rather than at the proximal bend. This is because the latter is associated with drainage defects of the corpus cavernosum penis (Ashdown & Glossop, 1983). Prevention is clearly difficult but the introduction of young sexually inexperienced bulls to heifers especially at grass should be done with care. Service in slippery surroundings should be avoided if at all possible.

Persistent frenulum

Although this is not a common condition diagnosis is easy as is treatment, which involves simple surgery.

FAILURE TO LOCATE VULVA OR ENTER VAGINA

Psychogenic

A diagnosis of psychogenic depression of libido must be tentative because it is based on a failure to obtain any other. One should always bear in mind that this condition may be the result of penile damage or an early manifestation of a drainage defect of the corpus cavernosum penis, or be of orthopaedic origin.

There is no known treatment apart from initial sexual rest for at least three to four weeks followed by hand-mating after some considerable teasing. Often collection by a small artificial vagina using a rough liner may obtain an ejaculate and start the bull working. The prognosis is very guarded.

Fibropapillomata

Treatment depends on the extent and severity of the tumour. A small single pedunculated tumour is clearly much easier to deal with than a large sessile cauliflower-like lesion. Most authorities advise surgery in severe cases but it is essential to avoid weakening or rupturing the tunica albuginea (Walker, 1980), since this can result in blood escaping at service. Note that possible leakage from the corpus spongiosum penis (CSP) into the terminal part of the urethral lumen has also been described. This could also cause spurting of blood from the penis at service (Ashdown & Majeed, 1978).

Since these lesions are transmissible, segregation of affected cattle, especially heifers, from a young bull is advisable. Contaminated bedding may infect young bulls and sexual play between young bulls may result in superficial abrasion of the penis and thus susceptibility to infection. The use of an older bull on infected females reduces the risk of infection of the bull. Prognosis should be guarded as regards both spontaneous recovery and return to service after surgery.

Drainage defects

Diagnosis is dependent on a careful assessment of the history and a thorough clinical examination of the bull while serving. It is advisable not only to attempt to collect semen by artificial vagina but also to palpate the erect penis as much as possible as the bull attempts to mate and finally, if at all possible, the bull should be allowed to attempt to mate naturally and his lack of ability to mate confirmed. Differentiation between the various categories of corpus cavernosum penis defects is largely academic at present since there is no treatment and the prognosis for all these is hopeless.

Corkscrew penis

This is one of the most dramatic defects and is often diagnosed by the client. It should be remembered that the spiral deviation has been described as occurring normally after entry into the vagina but immediately prior to ejaculation in bulls with apparently normal mating behaviour (Ashdown & Pearson, 1973). The only known treatment is surgical and there are a variety of techniques, all of which depend on either fixing the dorsal apical ligament to the dorsal aspect of the penis or additionally stiffening it by the insertion of fascia lata or carbon fibres. The latter are placed between the ligament and tunica albuginea (Mobini *et al.*, 1982). Postoperative recurrence is quite common after apparent recovery.

Deviations

As with corkscrew penis, deviations are usually obvious, although these conditions can be confused with a drainage defect of the corpus cavernosum penis. The two can be distinguished by the flexibility of the erect penis that is apparent in drainage defects. Some bulls can accommodate deviations surprisingly well and if they are not too pronounced, careful hand-mating may allow these bulls to learn to serve again. Surgical treatment is again a possibility (Walker, 1980) for more severe cases. Guarded prognosis is advisable even for relatively discrete deviations.

NORMAL SERVICE WITH A POOR PREGNANCY RATE

Overwork

This diagnosis will generally be indicated by the history and age of the bull. At worst the semen picture will be of low concentration (200×10^6/ml), marginal initial motility (2/5), but reasonable progressive motility (60 per cent +) and morphology (<20 per cent abnormal). However, often the bull has been removed from the breeding group and rested before examination so the sample appears normal. Treatment as already indicated is sexual rest since it takes nine weeks for development from the spermatogonia stage to ejaculation as a mature spermatozoon. Hence ideally the bull should not serve for at least nine weeks before being re-examined. There is little point in re-examining a bull after less than three weeks' rest. When this diagnosis is made the prognosis is good. However, one must always be aware that such a diagnosis may be complicated by another underlying cause and so it is advisable to be 'guarded but hopeful'.

Insult to spermatogenesis

Local effect

1 *Scrotal sac disruption.* Diagnosis should be determined by a clinical examination. The most obvious problems are varicocele and inguinal herniation. Care needs to be taken when making the latter diagnosis as a pad of fat can lie above the pampiniform plexus and

feel very like a hernia. The treatment and prognosis both depend on the cause.

2 *Orchitis/epididymitis*. These conditions should also be relatively easily diagnosed by a clinical examination. Confirmation of the conditions can be obtained from the semen findings. Generally, there will be low concentration of spermatozoa, poor/marginal motility, poor spermatozoan morphology, especially of the head, and white blood cells and other cells indicative of damage such as large multinucleate cells, so-called 'giant cells'. Culture of semen may allow the identification of a causative micro-organism. However, the findings will to some degree depend on the time-scale. Thus a bull with a spermatocele on the head of the epididymis could have been affected several years previously and the effects of the lesion subsided allowing the semen quality of the bull to return to normal.

The treatment of these conditions by antibiotics is usually ineffective and the main aim should be to prevent testicular degeneration of the sound testis and epididymis. The strategy adopted depends on the severity of infection. Thus assuming the remaining testis is not affected the removal of a grossly infected testis is the treatment of choice. Unfortunately, even then the local, and possibly systemic, damage to the other testis may be sufficient to cause a permanent derangement of semen production. Thus, the prognosis, even in animals that have recovered either after surgery or after conservative treatment, should be guarded. The owner should be reminded that the daily sperm output may be affected in apparently recovered animals and that they should carefully monitor the cows that have been served in the bull's first series of matings to ensure that the proportion of returns to service is acceptable.

Systemic effects

1 *Systemic illness*. Again there is a large number of conditions that can affect sperm production indirectly or directly. Treatment and prognosis are very dependent on the history, the origin of the insult and the age and type of the bull. It should again be remembered that the bull may be presented some time after the incident when recovery is taking place.

2 *Drugs*. It is possible that a bull could suffer from an adverse reaction to one of the common treatments, although such cases are rare. The diagnosis is dependent on the history. Treatment of such adverse reactions is symptomatic while the prognosis depends on the exact form that the adverse reaction takes. The only problem that might arise is with clandestine and improper administration of a drug, such as an anabolic steroid or *B. agonist* with the intent of improving the appearance of the bull or even liveweight performance test results. It is possible to test for residues. The evidence available appears to show that most anabolic steroid effects upon the testis are largely reversible following removal of the drug (Deschamps *et al.*, 1987a, b). Unfortunately, these studies have only involved animals of up to 15 months and may not truly reflect the field situation.

Testicular degeneration

The diagnosis of this condition is dependent upon a history of fertility, followed by infertility with the latter being confirmed by the collection of a semen sample of poor spermatozoan motility, concentration and morphology. In addition there will sometimes also be small darkly staining degenerate spermatids, which in some cases 'raft' together in clumps. In the extreme case the sample may be aspermic. It is of considerable interest to veterinarians in the field that immunization of bulls to gonadotrophin-releasing hormone (GnRH) is generally reversible (Robertson *et al.*, 1982) since this then implies that in many clinical cases where regeneration does not occur the underlying aetiology is more than just a simple hormonal dysfunction. The testes in cases of testicular degeneration may be smaller than normal but often they are within the norm.

While collection of semen is of considerable aid in diagnosis many workers have desired to examine the seminiferous tubules. A number of authors have attempted to use a testicular biopsy as a means of obtaining histological evidence of spermatogenic dysfunction (Galina, 1972). This technique is hazardous even when one uses a modern disposable biopsy needle due to haemorrhage (the testis is very vascular, see Fig. 35.17), spermatogenic disruption and adhesions (see Fig. 35.7). However, with time, good spermatogenic recovery can occur (Galina, 1971; Logue, 1975). The involvement of infectious agents in testicular degeneration is not well understood and so, while BVD and IBR viruses are probably not common causes of the condition, it is nevertheless well worthwhile determining the status of the bull with regard to these viruses, particularly the former.

Testicular hypoplasia

Although testicular atrophy should be dealt with under degeneration from a clinical point of view it is being considered here because unless one has a firm history it can be extremely difficult to differentiate between testicular hypoplasia and testicular atrophy, especially in the bilateral state. Both present as the 'small testes

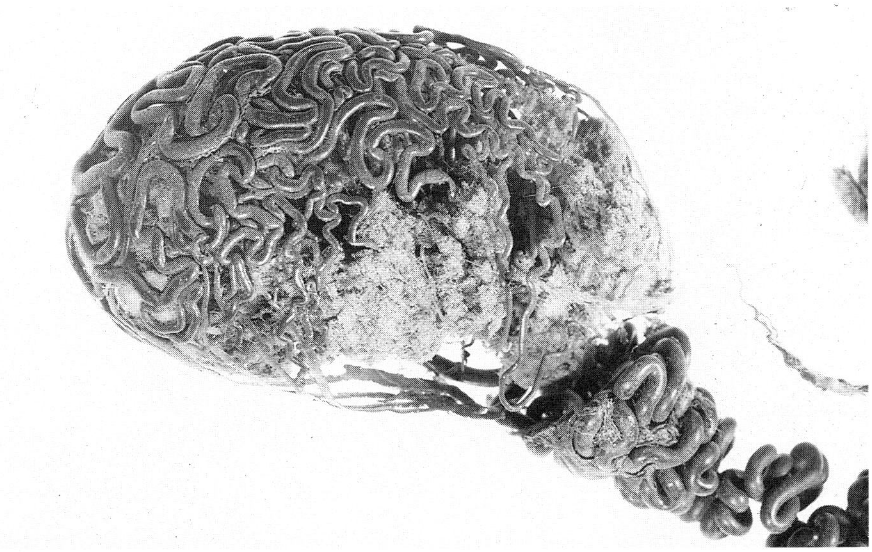

Fig. 35.17 Arterial supply to the testis

syndrome'. Testes that have been affected by atrophy subsequent to a severe infectious condition or trauma may feel small, firm and nodular on palpation while those affected by hypoplasia are usually less firm and more uniform. Frequently, one is left in genuine doubt about the diagnosis.

A diagnostic aid that may prove of value is the determination of the chromosomal constitution of the animal.

Care must also be taken not to jump to conclusions. Surprisingly good quality semen has been collected from bulls with disappointingly small scrotal circumferences. However, such occasions are rare, so that in general the prognosis for the 'small testes syndrome' is poor. As far as the unilateral condition is concerned this is more problematical since often the animal is fertile. Here every attempt to obtain as reliable a history as possible should be made in order to differentiate between hypoplasia and atrophy because of the strong evidence of the heritable nature of hypoplasia. If the diagnosis is hypoplasia the owner should be advised that such stock is only fit for the production of 'slaughter generation' animals, since it is a heritable condition.

Interference with transport and storage of spermatozoa

Abnormalities of the epididymis. Ease of diagnosis depends on the site and the extent of the problem. Should there be a spermatocele then this is generally easily palpated provided one is careful and palpates the entire epididymis. However, some defects can be very small and ultrasound may well prove a very useful diagnostic aid.

Treatment is usually symptomatic and certainly in the early stages antibiotic administration is probably worthwhile. Generally, affected animals are not sterile and thus a prognosis depends upon the other findings.

Abnormalities of the accessory sex glands

Diagnosis of these abnormalities is firstly dependent upon rectal palpation and ultrasonic scanning, and secondly upon laboratory tests, particularly the examination of semen for white blood cells. Hopefully, ultrasound scanning will prove of value in the reliable diagnosis of severe seminal vesiculitis and also segmental aplasia of the seminal vesicle. However, as mentioned before, the application of the technique is still in its infancy (Little & Woods, 1987).

Treatment of an infectious condition obviously requires antibiotic preferably one with a broad spectrum, and given that there is no evidence of severe effects upon the structure of the seminal vesicles prognosis is good. Conditions affecting the other smaller accessory sex glands of the pelvis in the bull have rarely been recognized clinically but this may yet be possible using ultrasound.

Conclusion

The investigation of infertility in the bull is one of the most interesting examinations in farm animal practice. The approach is standard and success is dependent upon attention to detail in all the facets mentioned in this chapter. One of the main advantages the general practitioner has compared with the specialist is an intimate knowledge of the farm, the ability of those involved as stockworkers and also a fair idea of the reliability or otherwise of the history and records. On the other hand the major disadvantages are the small number of cases that the practitioner will see in a year, so limiting the experience that can be built up, the standard of equipment, particularly microscope and other accessories required. Finally the amount of time and flexibility of time that needs to be devoted to such work must be balanced against other possibly more remunerative demands of a busy practice.

References

Abbitt, B., Berndtson, W.E. & Seidel, G.E. (1984) Effect of dehydrostreptomycin or oxytetracycline on reproductive capacity in bulls. *American Journal of Veterinary Research*, **45**, 2243–6.

Amann, R.P. & Almquist, J.O. (1976) Bull management to maximise sperm output. In *Proceedings of the 6th Technical Conference on Artificial Insemination & Reproduction*. National Association of Animal Breeders Inc., pp. 1–10.

Amann, R.P. & Schambacher, B.D. (1983) Physiology of male reproduction. *Journal of Animal Science*, **57**(Suppl. 2), 380–403.

Anon. (1988). *EEC Dairy Facts and Figures*. E&W Milk Marketing Board, Thames Ditton.

Archibald, L., Gronwall, R.R., Pritchard, E.L. & Tran, T. (1990) Acrosome reaction and concentration of prostaglandin E_2 in semen of rams treated with Flunixin meglumine (BANAMINE). *Theriogenology*, **33**, 373–83.

Arthur, G.H. (1960) In *Wrights Veterinary Obstetrics*, 3rd edn, pp. 507–8. Baillière Tindall & Cox, London.

Ashdown, R.R. (1973) Functional anatomy of the penis in ruminants. In *Veterinary Annual* (ed. by C.S.G. Grunsel & F.W.G. Hill), vol. 13, pp. 22–5.

Ashdown, R.R. & Glossop, C.E. (1983) Impotence in the bull: (3) Rupture of the corpus cavernosum penis proximal to the sigmoid flexure. *Veterinary Record*, **113**, 30–7.

Ashdown, R.R. & Majeed, Z.Z. (1978) Haemorrhage from the bovine penis during erection and ejaculation: a possible explanation of some cases. *Veterinary Record*, **103**, 12–13.

Ashdown, R.R. & Pearson, H. (1973) Anatomical and experimental studies on eversion of the sheath and protrusion of the penis in the bull. *Research in Veterinary Science*, **15**, 13–24.

Ashdown, R.R. & Pearson, H. (1973) Studies on 'corkscrew' penis in the bull. *Veterinary Record*, **93**, 30–35.

Ashdown, R.R., Gilanpour, H., David, J.S.E. & Gibbs, C. (1979) Impotence in the bull: (1) Abnormal venous drainage of the corpus cavernosum penis. *Veterinary Record*, **104**, 423–8.

Bane, A. (1954) Sexual function of bulls in relation to heredity rearing intensity and somatic conditions. *Acta Agricultura Scandinavica*, **4**, 95–208.

Bane, A. & Hansen, H-J. (1962) Spinal changes in the bull and their significance in serving ability. *Cornell Veterinarian*, **52**, 363–84.

Bartels, J.E. (1975) Femoral–tibial osteoarthrosis in the bull. Clinical survey and radiologic interpretation. *Journal of the American Veterinary Radiology Society*, **16**, 151–8.

Barth, A.D. & Oko, R.J. (1989) in *Abnormal morphology of bovine spermatozoa*, pp. 1–285. Iowa State University Press, Iowa.

Beckett, S.D., Reynold, T.M., Walker, D.F., Hudson, P.S. & Burphit, R.C. (1974) Experimentally induced rupture of corpus cavernosum penis of bull. *American Journal of Veterinary Research*, **35**, 765–7.

Bishop, M.W.H., Campbell, R.C., Hancock, J.L. & Walton, A. (1954) Semen characteristics and fertility in the bull. *Journal of Agricultural Science*, **44**, 227–48.

Blockey, M.A. de B & Taylor, E.G. (1984) Observations on spiral deviation of the penis in beef bulls. *Australian Veterinary Journal*, **61**, 141–5,

Blom, E. (1979a) Studies on seminal vesiculitis in the bull I. Semen examination methods and post mortem findings. *Nordisk Veterinaermedicin*, **31**, 193–205.

Blom, E. (1979b) Studies on seminal resiculitis in the bull II. Malformation of the genital organs as a possible predisposing factor in the pathogenesis of seminal vesiculitis.

Blom, E. & Christensen, N.O. (1960) The etiology of spermiostasis in the bull. *Nordisk Veterinaermedicin*, **12**, 453–70.

Chandley, A.C. (1979) Chromosomal basis of human infertility. *British Medical Bullettu*, **35**, 181–86.

Chenoweth, P.J. (1983) Sexual behaviour of the bull: a review. *Journal of Dairy Science*, **66**, 173–9.

Coulter, G.H. & Foote, R.H. (1978) Relationship of bodyweight to testicular size and consistency in growing Holstein bulls. *Journal of Animal Science*, **44**, 1076–9.

Deschamps, J.C., Ott, R.S., Weston, P.G., Shanks, R.D., Kesler, D.J., Bolt, D.J. & Hixon, J.E. (1987a) Effects of zeranol on reproduction in beef bulls. Luteinising hormone, follicle-stimulating hormone and testosterone secretion in response to gonadotrophin-releasing hormone and human chorionic gonadotrophin. *American Journal of Veterinary Research*, **48**, 31–6,

Deschamps, J.C., Ott, R.S., McEntee, K., Heath, E.H., Heinricks, R.R., Shanks, R.D. & Hixon, J.E. (1987b) Effects of zeranol on reproduction in beef bulls. Scrotal circumference, serving ability, semen characteristics and pathologic changes of the reproductive organs. *American Journal of Veterinary Research*, **48**, 137–47.

Foote, R.L., Munkenbank, N. & Greene, W.A. (1976) Testosterone and libido in Holstein bulls of various ages. *Journal of Dairy Science*, **59**, 2011–13.

Galina, C.S. (1972) An evaluation of testicular biopsy in farm animals. *Veterinary Record*, **88**, 628–31.

Greenough, P.R., MacCallum, F.J., & Weaver, A.D. (1978) In *Lameness in Cattle*, 2nd edn. pp. 291–321. (ed. weaver, A.D.). *Wright Scientechnica*.

Gustavsson, I. (1974) Appearance and persistance of the 1/29 translocation in cattle. In *Colloque les accidents chromosemiques de la reproduction*. Edit Bové J. et Bové A, pp. 147–53, Institut National de la Santé et de la Recherche Médicale.

Gwazdauskas, F.C. (1985) Effects of climate on reproduction in cattle. *Journal of Dairy Science*, **68**, 1568–78.

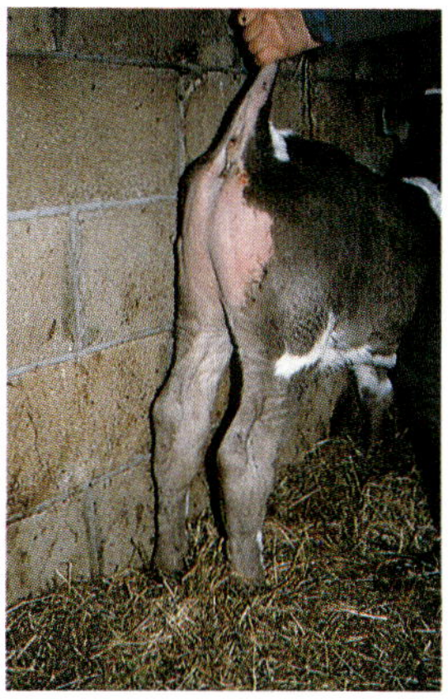

Plate 14.1 Hair loss over legs and perineum associated with steatorrhoea and diarrhoea (from Blowey & Weaver (1990) *A Colour Atlas of Diseases of Cattle*, Wolfe Publications Ltd, London).

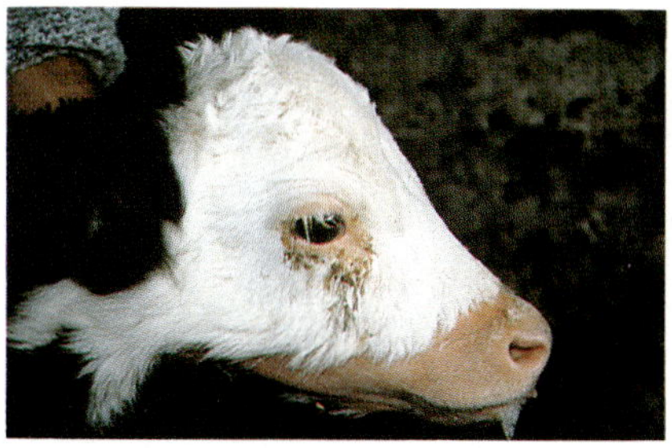

Plate 14.2 Alopecia on muzzle due to adherence of poorly dispersed fats from milk substitute (from Blowey & Weaver (1990) *A Colour Atlas of Diseases of Cattle*, Wolfe Publications Ltd, London).

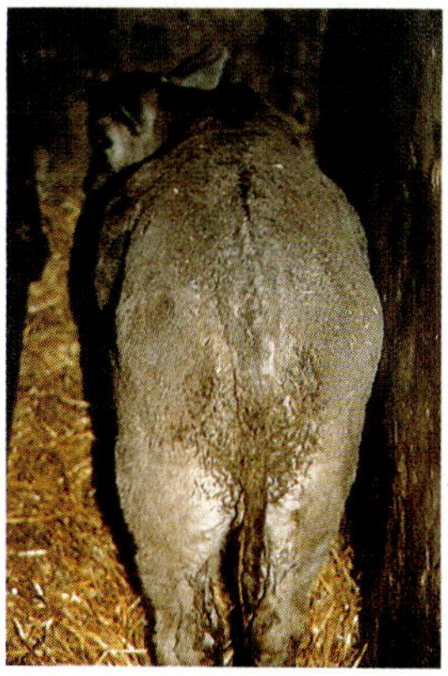

Plate 14.3 Chronic ruminal bloat and scour (from Blowey & Weaver (1990) *A Colour Atlas of Diseases of Cattle*, Wolfe Publications Ltd, London).

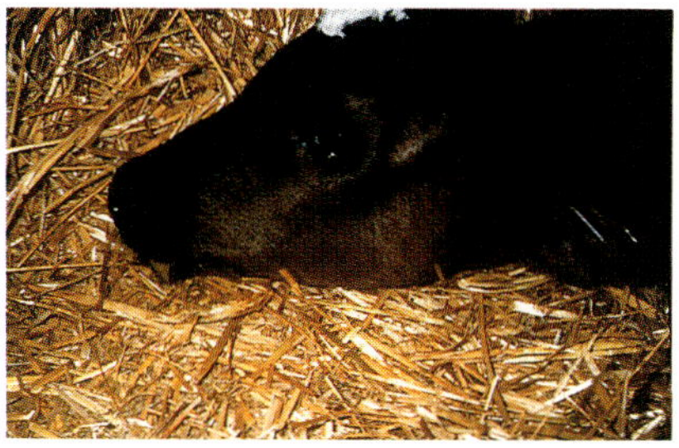

Plate 14.4 Perforated abomasal ulcer: calf *in extremis* (from Blowey & Weaver (1990) *A Colour Atlas of Diseases of Cattle*, Wolfe Publications Ltd, London).

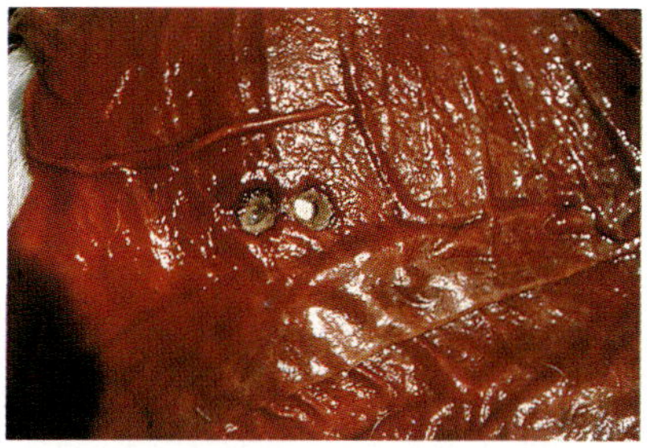

Plate 14.5 Perforated abomasal ulcer: abomasum at post mortem (from Blowey & Weaver (1990) *A Colour Atlas of Diseases of Cattle*, Wolfe Publications Ltd, London).

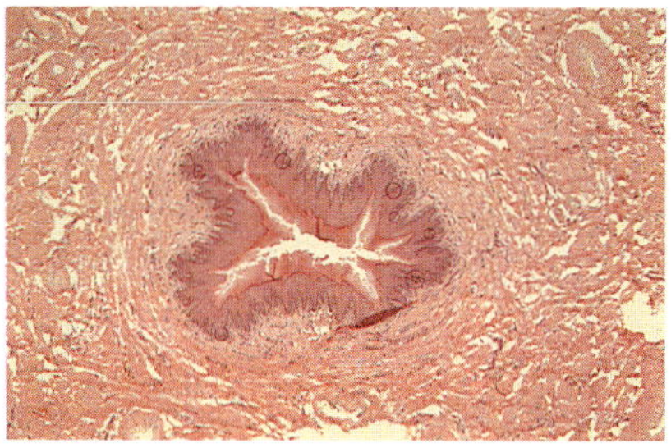

Plate 21.1 Transverse section of teat duct showing lumen and keratinized lining. (×25)

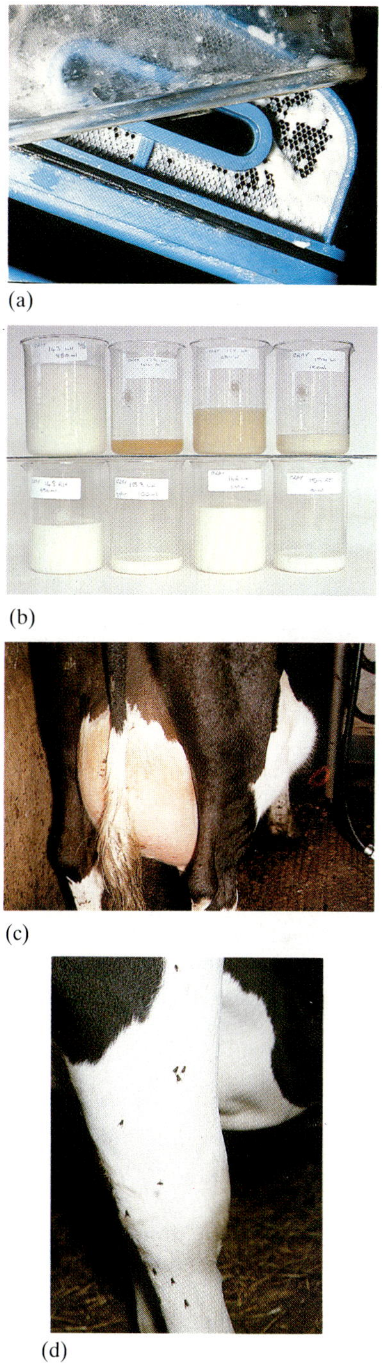

Plate 21.2 Signs of clinical mastitis. (a) Clotting of milk detected on a filter in the long milk tube. (b) Alterations to colour of milk due to mastitis. (c) Swelling and reddening of the rear quarters of a cow with acute coliform mastitis. (d) Oedema of leg of cow suffering summer mastitis. Note biting flies.

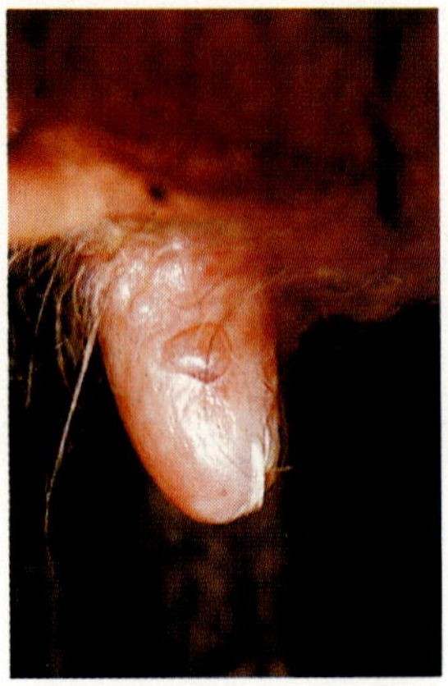

Plate 25.1 Early stage of bovine herpes mammillitis showing unilocular vesicle formation.

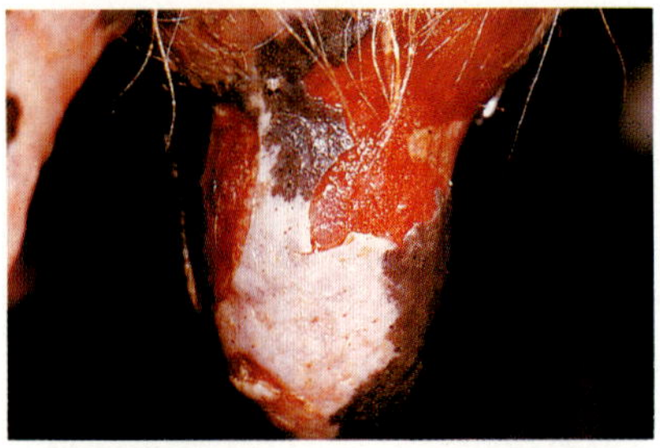

Plate 25.2 Bovine herpes mammillitis (two days). The vesicles have ruptured, producing a serous fluid and exposing a very congested dermis

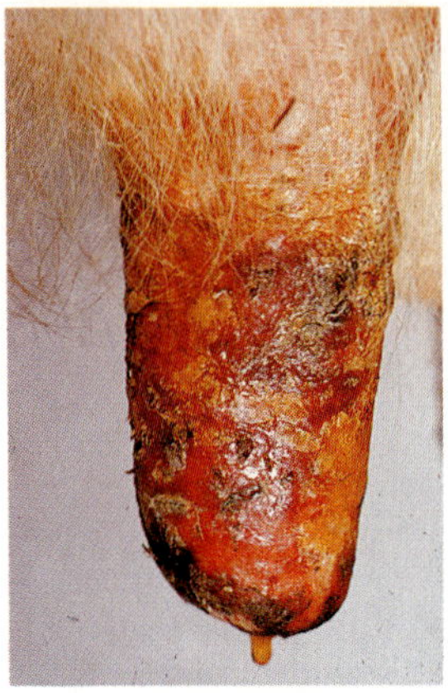

Plate 25.3 Bovine herpes mammillitis (four days). The exudate coagulates on the teat surface producing flat, smooth scabs. These darken to a red–brown colour.

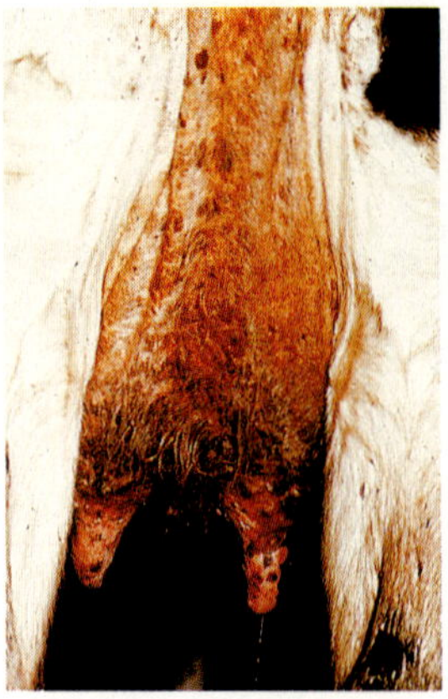

Plate 25.4 Bovine herpes mammillitis. In some cases, particularly in heifers, extensive scab formation can occur over the udder.

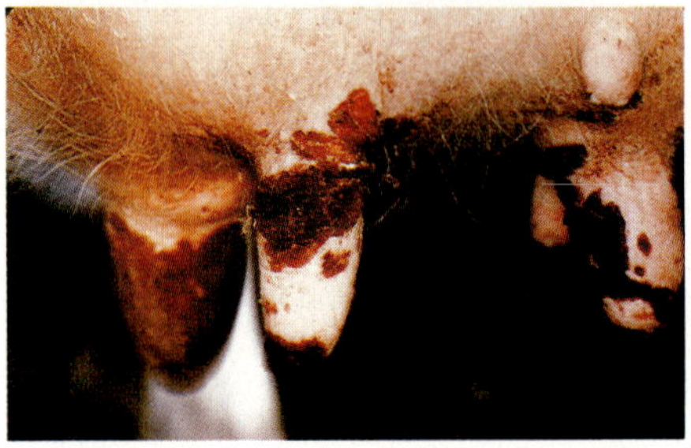

Plate 25.5 Bovine herpes mammillitis (about seven days). The initial oedema subsides and is followed by epithelial necrosis.

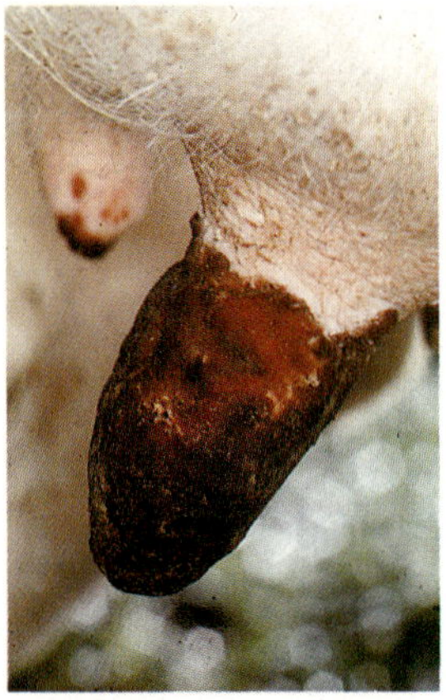

Plate 25.6 Bovine herpes mammillitis (about two weeks). An area of necrosis often involving most of the teat occurs as this is often shed as a whole (see Plate 25.7).

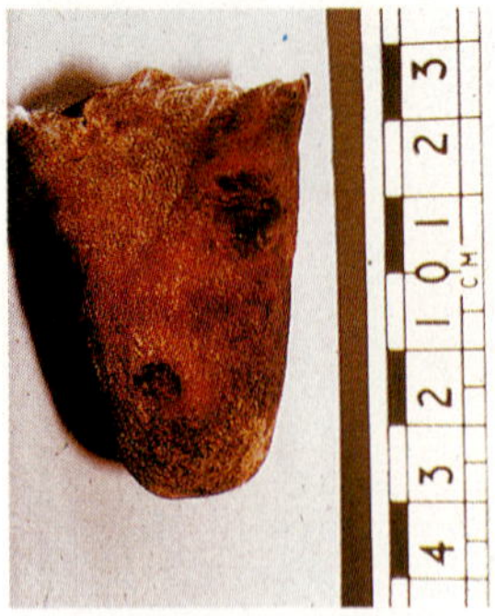

Plate 25.7 Bovine herpes mammillitis (two to three weeks). Necrotic tissue shed from cow.

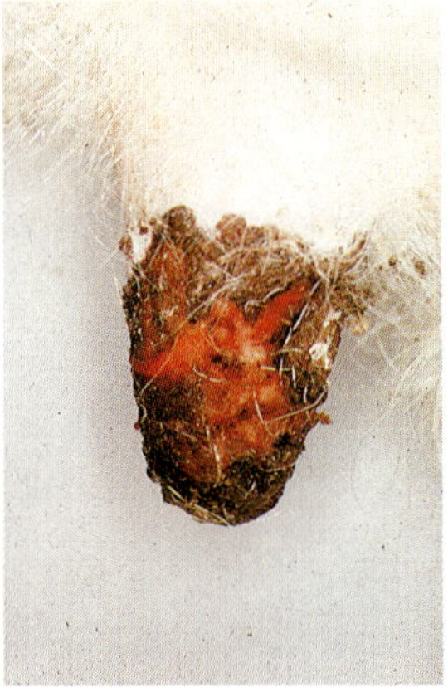

Plate 25.8 Bovine herpes mammillitis. The shedding of the necrotic tissue reveals a raw, granulated area, often becoming secondarily infected with bacteria.

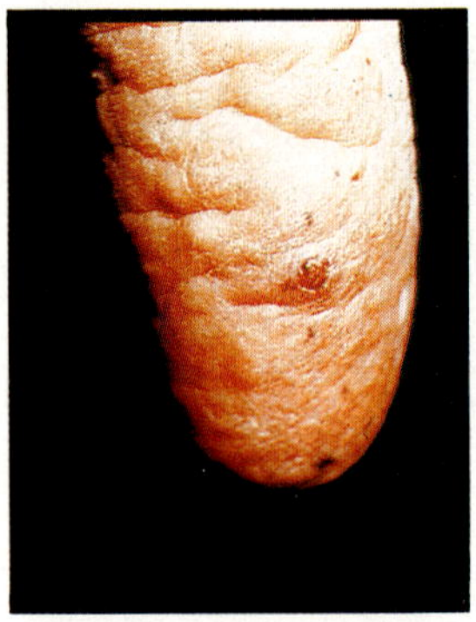

Plate 25.9 Pseudocowpox showing the formation of a small, dark-red elevated scab.

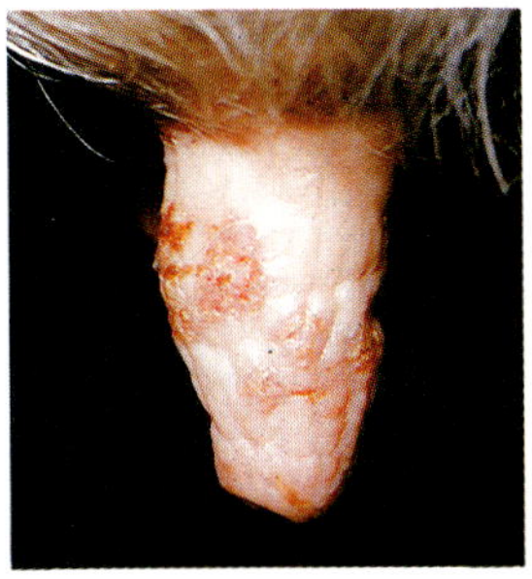

Plate 25.10 Pseudocowpox lesion (seven days), about 1 cm in diameter and somewhat resembling a mild cowpox lesion.

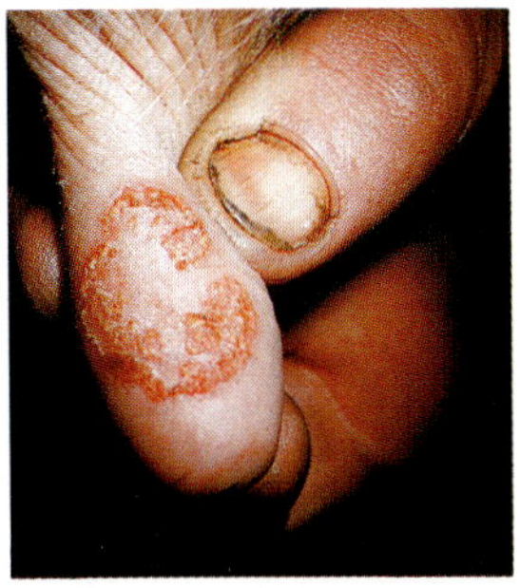

Plate 25.11 Pseudocowpox (10–12 days). A raised scab often known as a 'ring' or 'horse-shoe' scab.

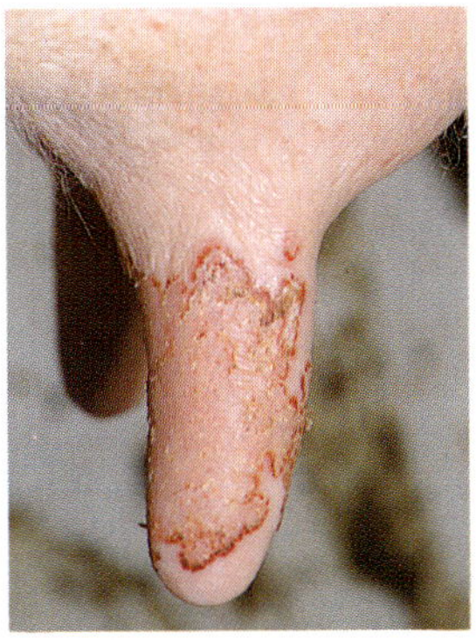

Plate 25.12 Pseudocowpox. Scabs have converged to form a single scab extending the teat length.

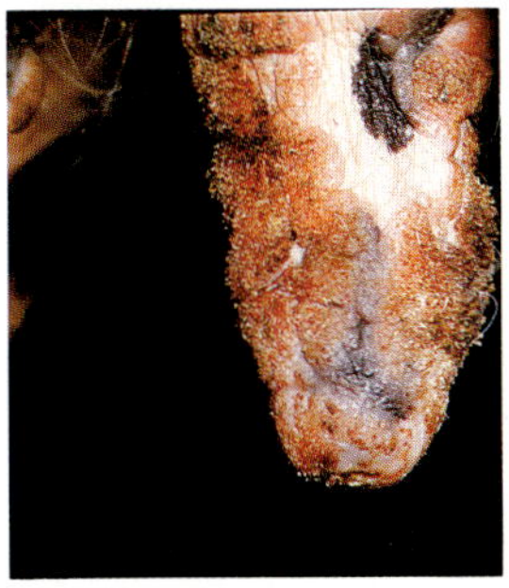

Plate 25.13 An atypical pseudocowpox lesion.

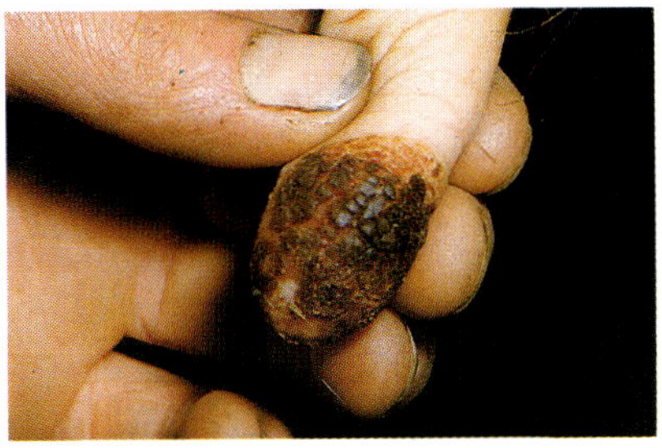

Plate 25.14 An atypical pseudocowpox lesion.

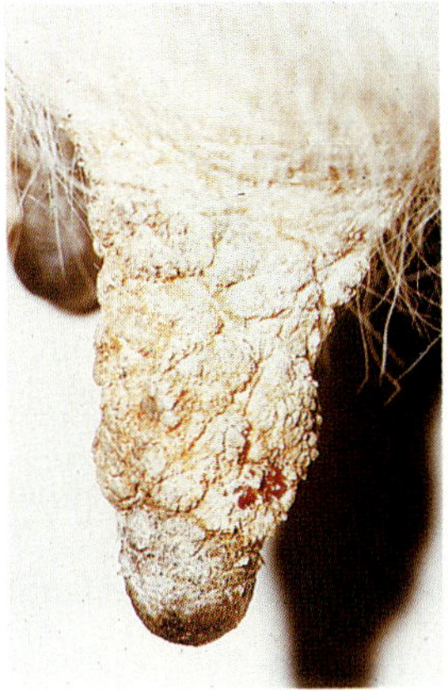

Plate 25.15 An atypical pseudocowpox lesion.

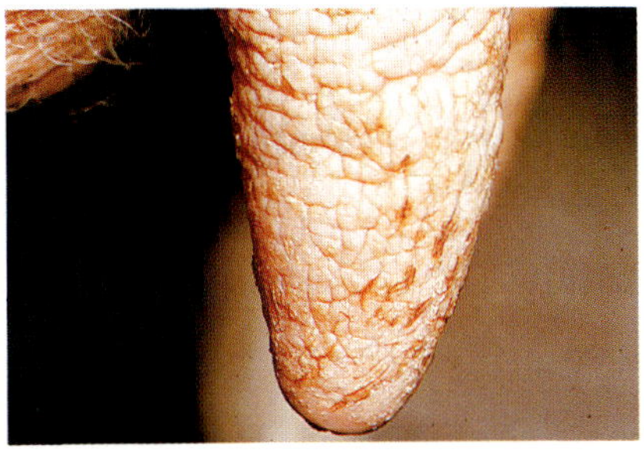

Plate 25.16 An atypical pseudocowpox lesion.

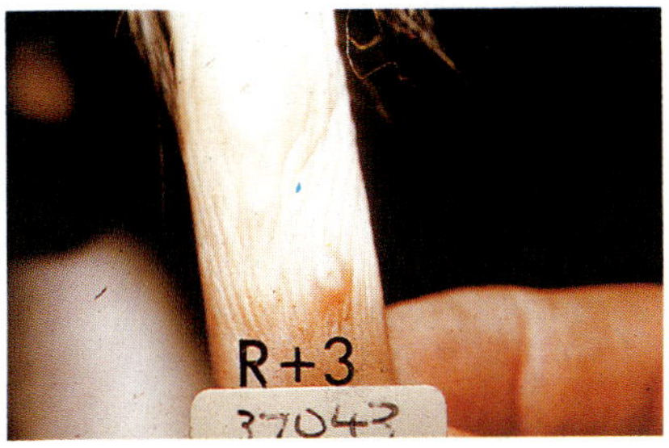

Plate 25.17 Cowpox showing development of a vesicle.

Plate 25.21 (*right*) *Staphylococcus aureus* infection resulting in pustule formation surrounded by erythema (impetigo).

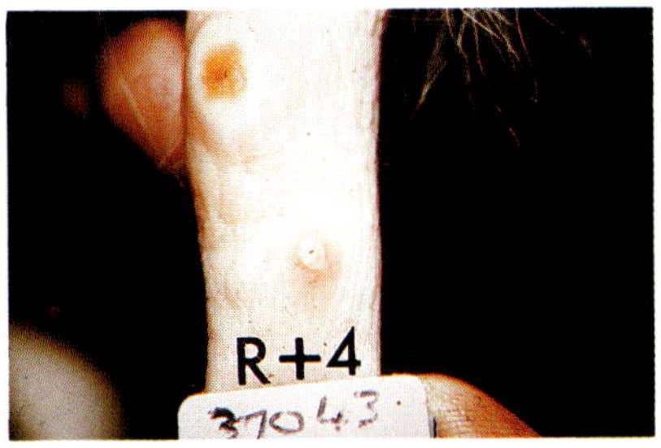

Plate 25.18 Cowpox following rupture of a vesicle.

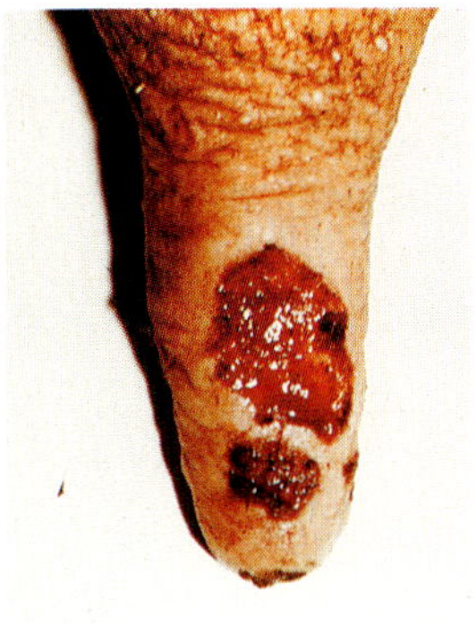

Plate 25.19 Cowpox with scab formation.

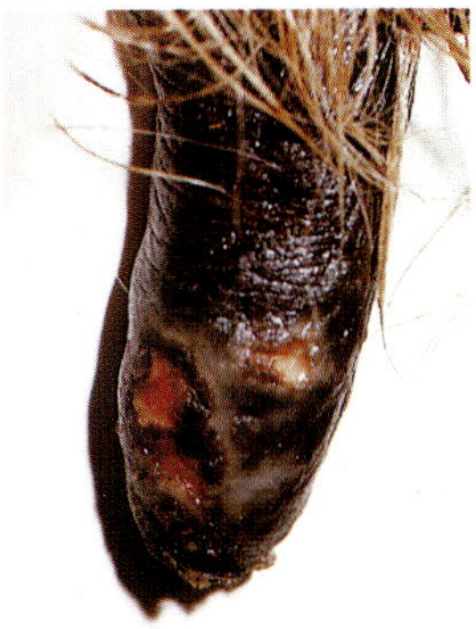

Plate 25.20 A severe cowpox involving most of the teat skin.

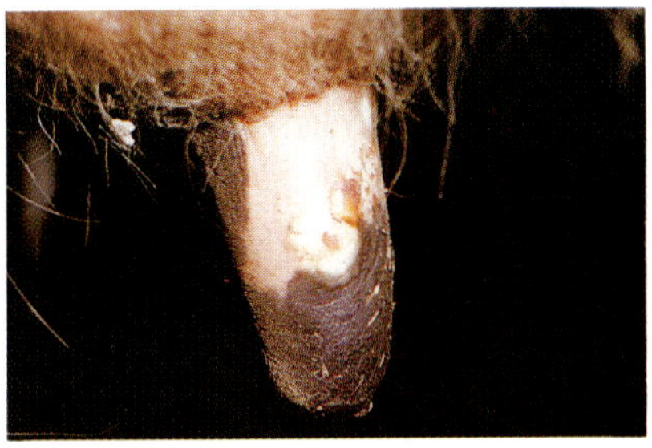

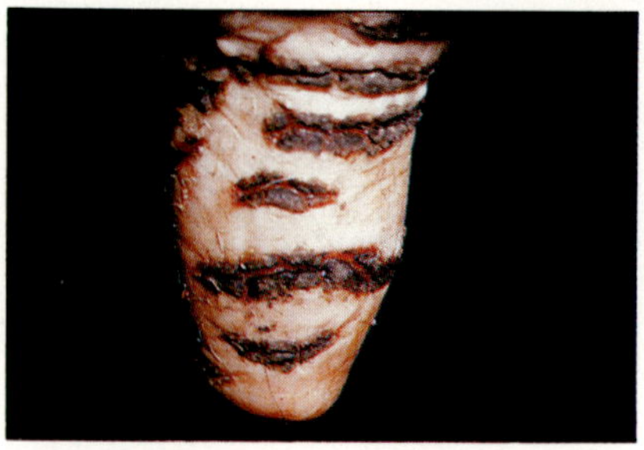

Plate 25.22 Teat chaps.

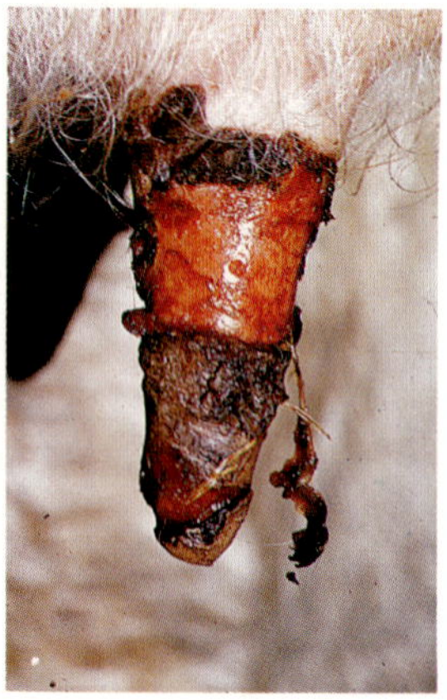

Plate 25.23 A teat with shedding of the skin following photosensitization.

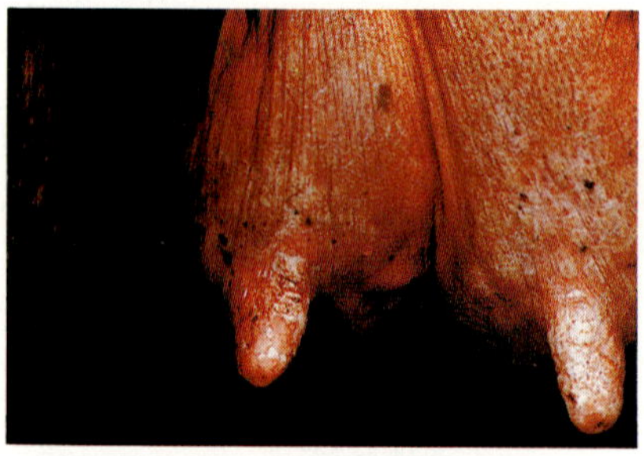

Plate 25.24 Foot and mouth disease. Vesiculation of the teat.

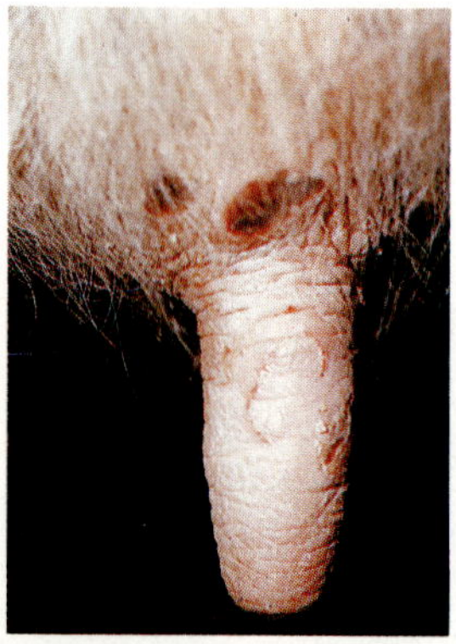

Plate 25.25 Pseudocowpox infection together with cowpox infection.

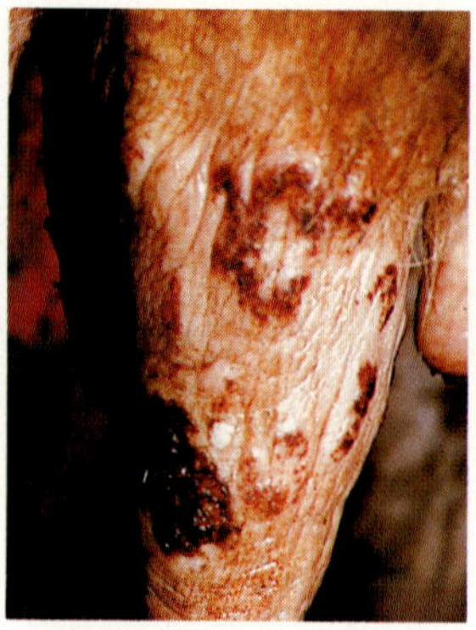

Plate 25.26 Pseudocowpox infection together with bovine herpes mammillitis.

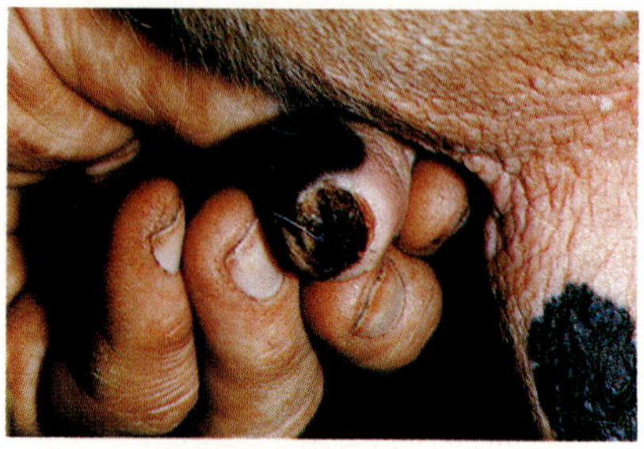

Plate 25.27 Blackspot of a teat orifice.

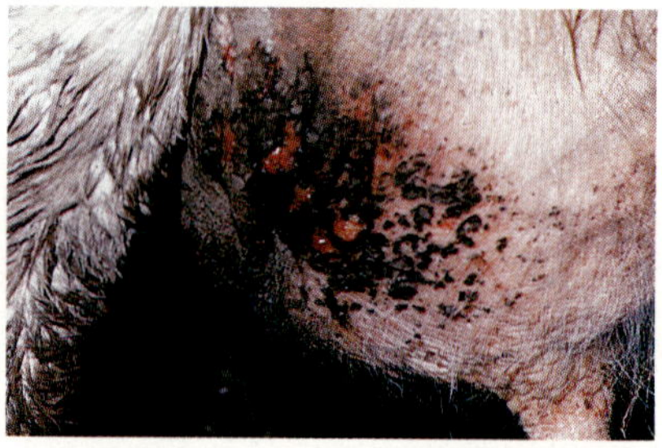

Plate 25.28 Mud abrasion of the lateral surface of the teat.

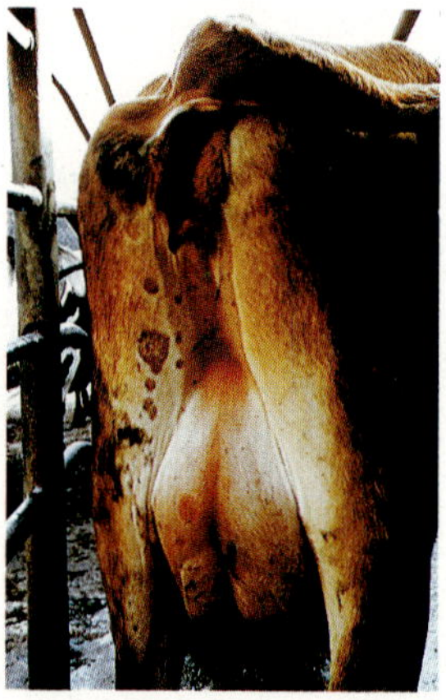

Plate 25.29 Ringworm lesions. Typical *Trichophyton verrucosum* lesions (courtesy of S. Smith, Hoechst Pharmaceuticals).

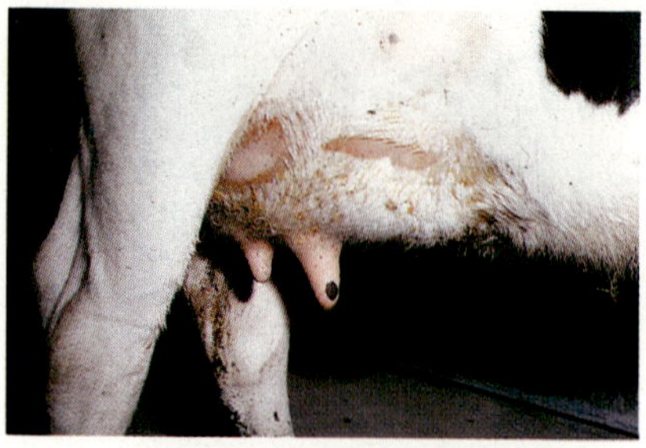

Plate 25.30 Thelitis and serous exudate of the udder skin in peracute mastitis.

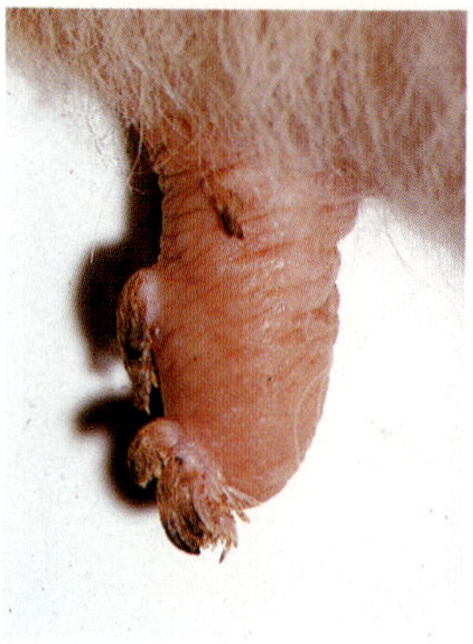

Plate 25.31 Filamentous papillomatosis of the teat.

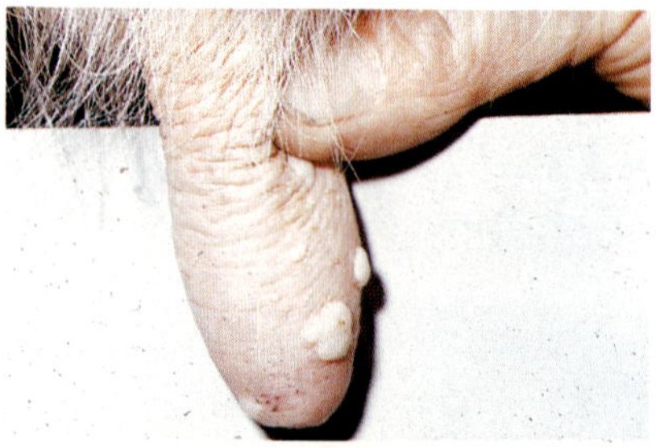

Plate 25.32 Nodular papillomatosis of the teat.

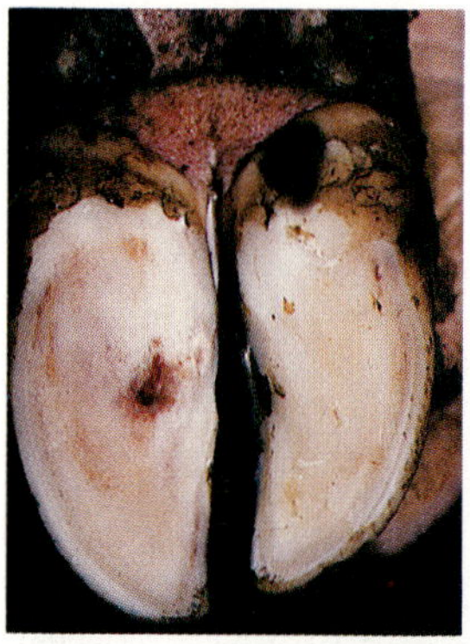

Plate 28.1 The outer hind claw of a cow showing moderately severe haemorrhages. The area involved is characteristic being at the proximal edge of the claw bone and the proximal part of the white line.

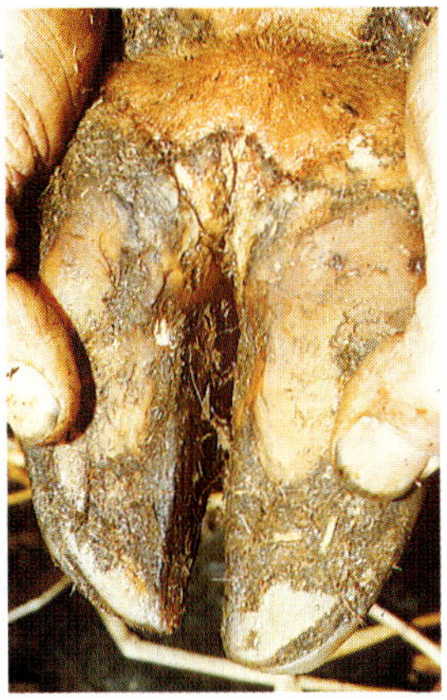

Plate 28.2 Interdigital eczema with the beginnings of underrunning of the heel horn due to interdigital dermatitis.

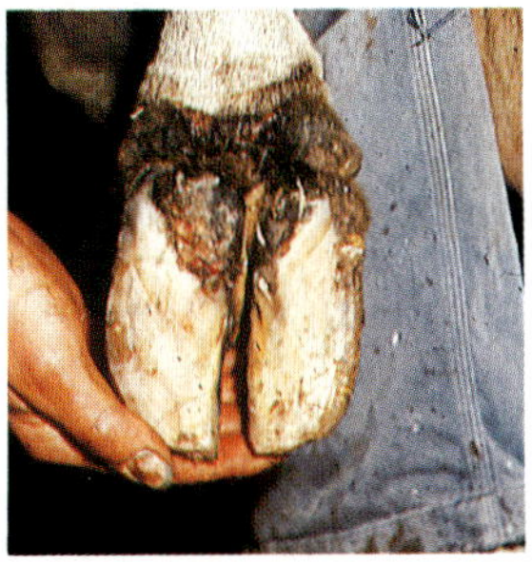

Plate 28.3 Underrunning of the heel horn with an ulcerated pododerm caused by interdigital dermatitis.

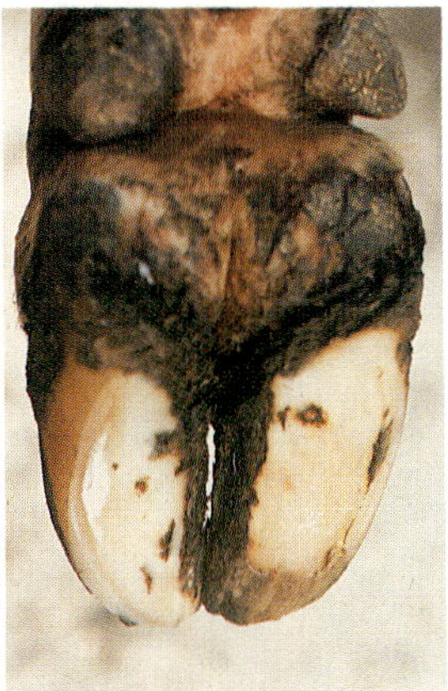

Plate 28.4 Heel horn erosion with underrunning due to interdigital dermatitis. Interdigital eczema is no longer present.

Plate 37b.3 (*right*) Heart. Low power (×80). Neoplastic cells form a dense accumulation in an interfascicular area and a monodiffuse infiltration is seen between the muscle cells (courtesy of Mrs C.K. Dimmock, Animal Research Institute, Yerongpilly, Queensland, Australia).

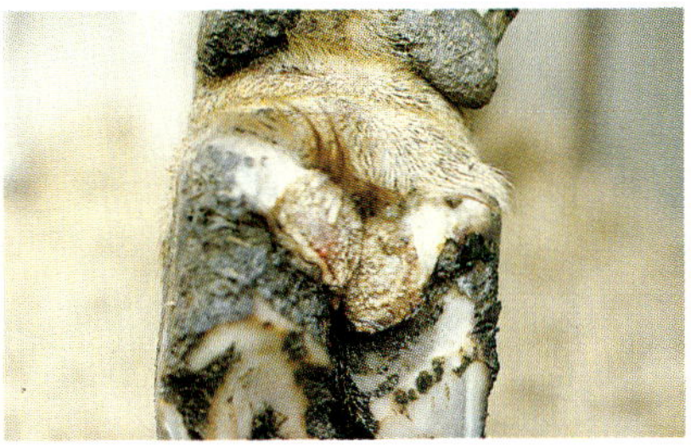

Plate 28.5 Digital dermatitis of long standing. There are long hairs at the edge of the lesion, and the affected area is grey rather than red. The heel horn is deformed and disappearing. The affected areas are probably separated by a band of healthy interdigital skin.

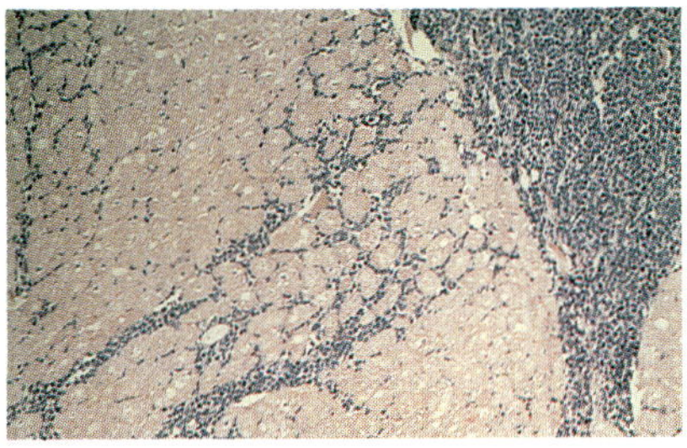

Plate 37b.1 Lymph node. High power (×250) view showing numerous immature lymphoid cells with occasional mitotic figures (courtesy of Mrs C.K. Dimmock, Animal Research Institute, Yerongpilly, Queensland, Australia).

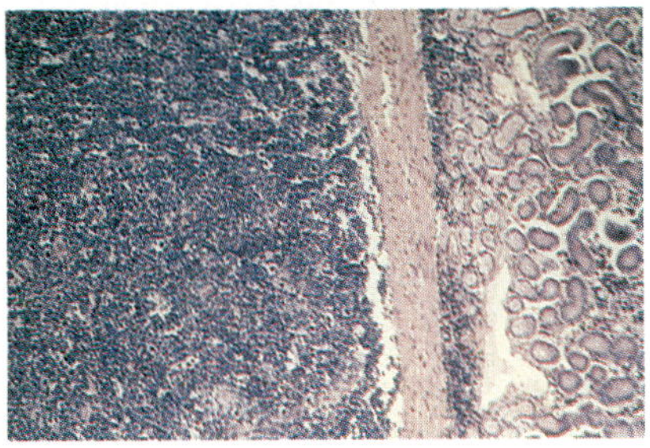

Plate 37b.2 Abomasum. Low power (×50). A mass of neoplastic lymphoid cells occupies the submucosa (right) and small groups of lymphoid cells are present in the lamina propria (left). In this case the muscularis mucosa is spared (courtesy of Mrs C.K. Dimmock, Animal Research Institute, Yerongpilly, Queensland, Australia).

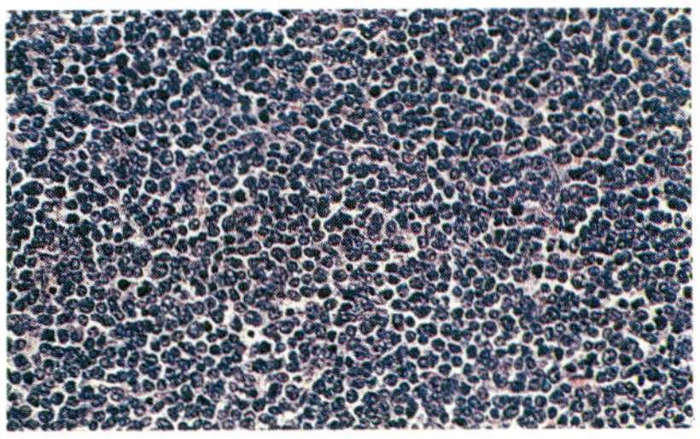

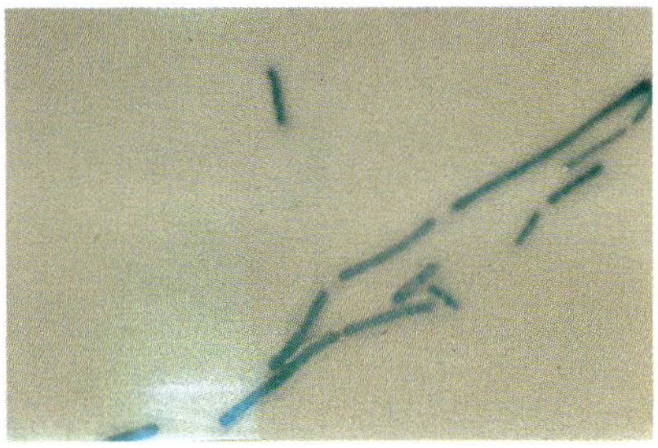

Plate 38.1 *Anthrax bacillium* with typical purple capsules in a smear from blood culture (×850) (courtesy of the Veterinary Investigation Centre, Aberystwyth).

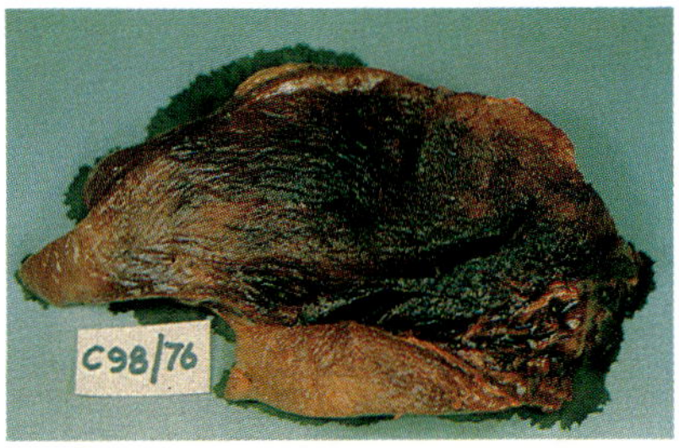

Plate 38.2 Blackleg due to *Clostridium chauveoi* in the thigh muscles of a calf showing the dark, dry and gangrenous lesion (courtesy of the Veterinary Investigation Centre, Carmarthen).

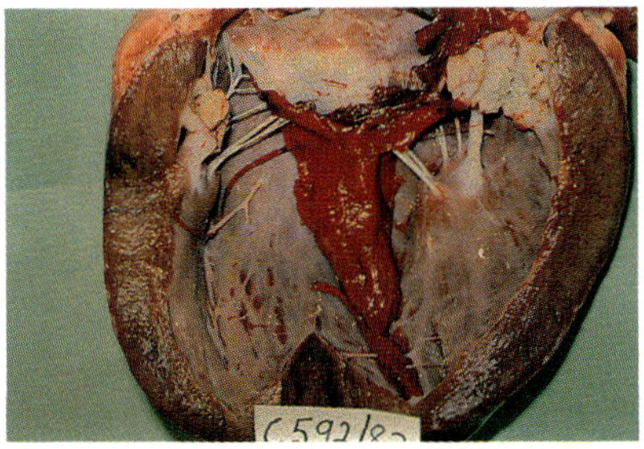

Plate 38.3 Endocarditis. Vegetative growth on the bicuspid valve (courtesy of the Veterinary Investigation Centre, Carmarthen).

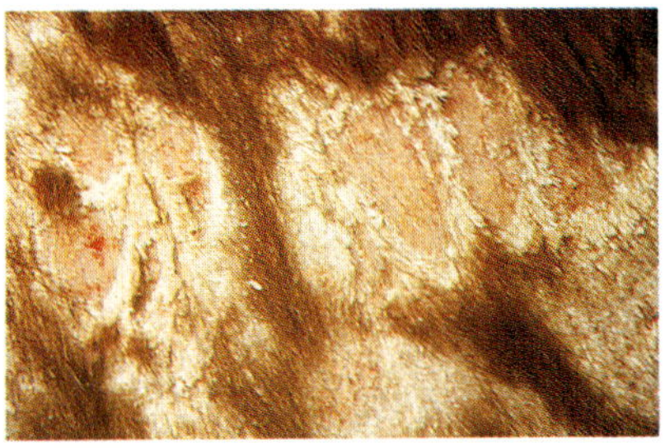

Plate 44.1 Generalized *Trichophyton verrucosum* infection of a beef shorthorn bull.

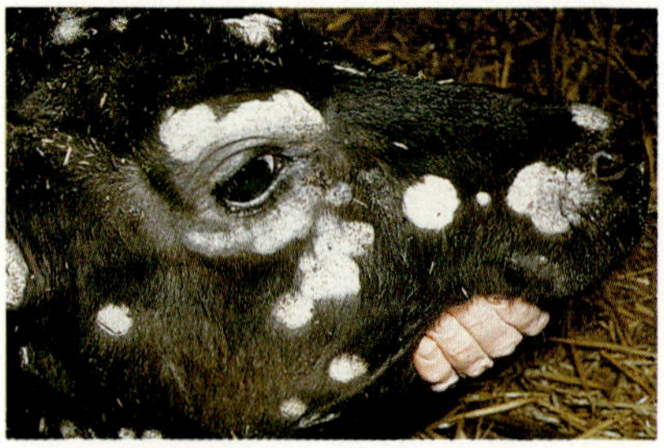

Plate 44.2 *Trichophyton verrucosum* infection of the head of a Friesian calf.

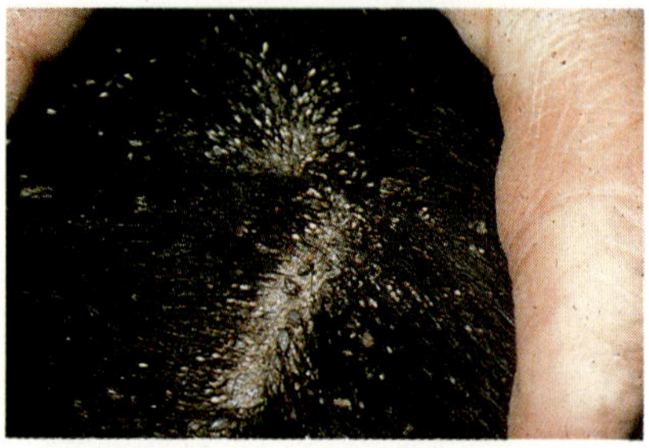

Plate 44.3 *Linognathus vituli* lice and ova (nits) on a calf.

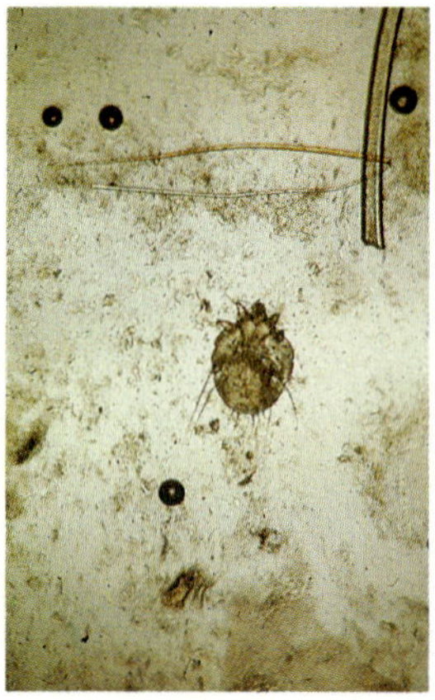

Plate 44.4 Wet preparation in potassium hydroxide solution of *Sarcoptes scabei*. Mite $240\,\mu m \times 200\,\mu m$.

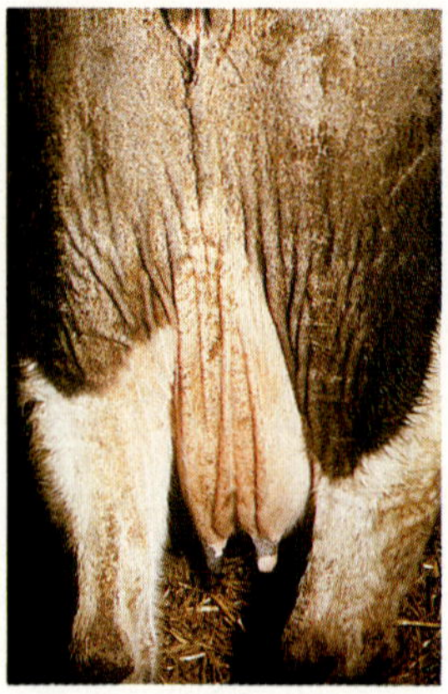

Plate 44.5 Friesian cow with generalized sarcoptic scabies.

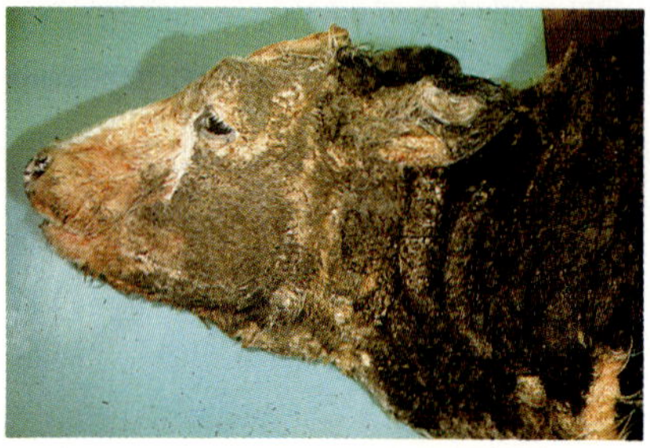

Plate 44.6 Hereford-cross calf with generalized sarcoptic scabies.

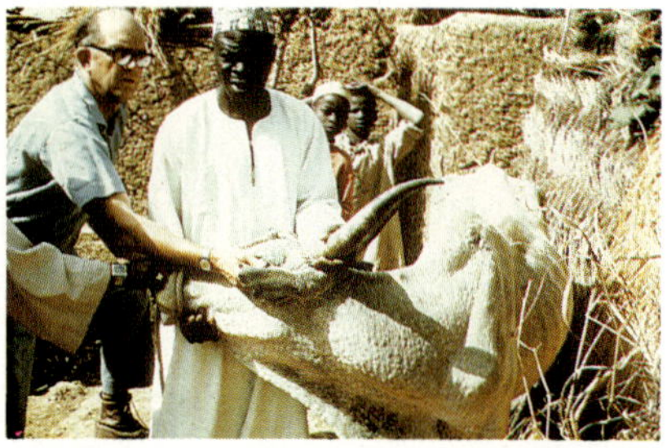

Plate 44.7 Cow with nodular lesions of demodicosis on the neck (northern Nigeria).

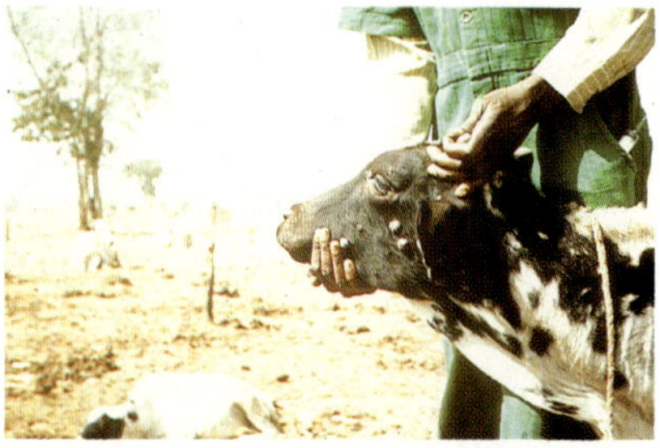

Plate 44.8 Viral papillomatosis. Calf with multiple lesions on the head and neck.

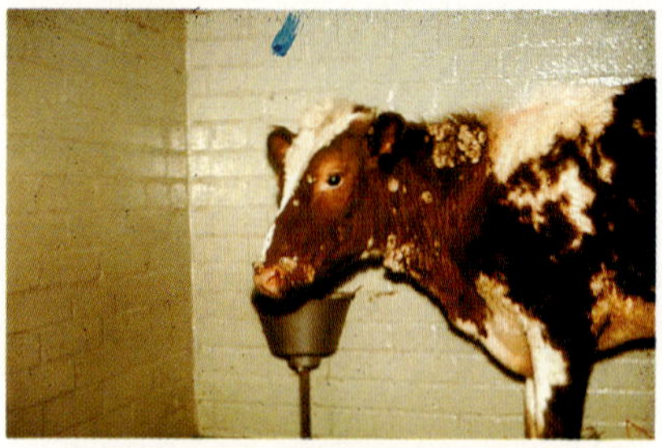

Plate 44.9 Viral papillomatosis. Ayrshire heifer with extensive cauliflower growths on the head and neck.

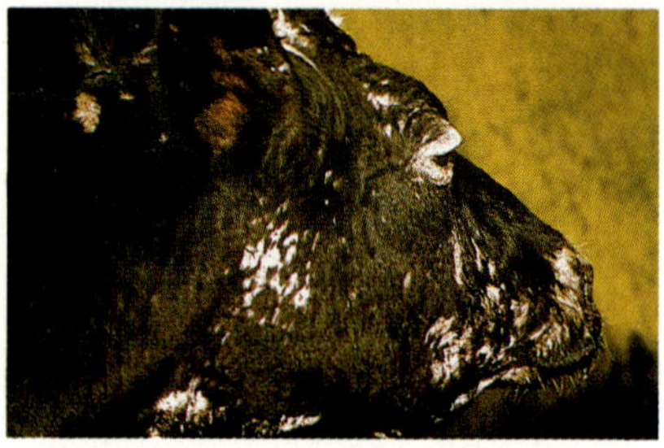

Plate 44.10 Pruritis/pyrexia/haemorrhagic syndrome. Head of a cow showing papule and exudative dermatitis.

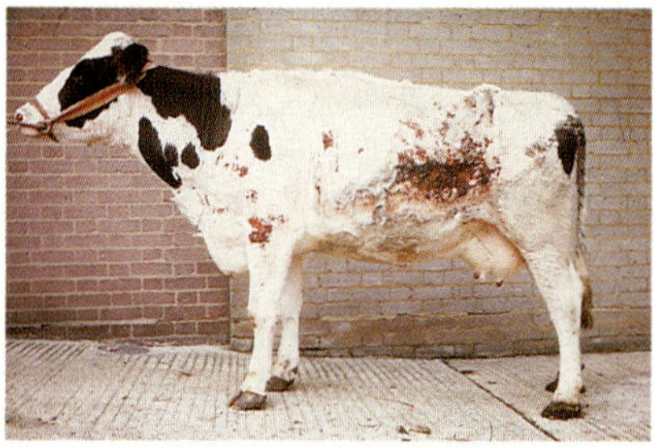

Plate 44.11 Friesian cow with severe photodermatitis.

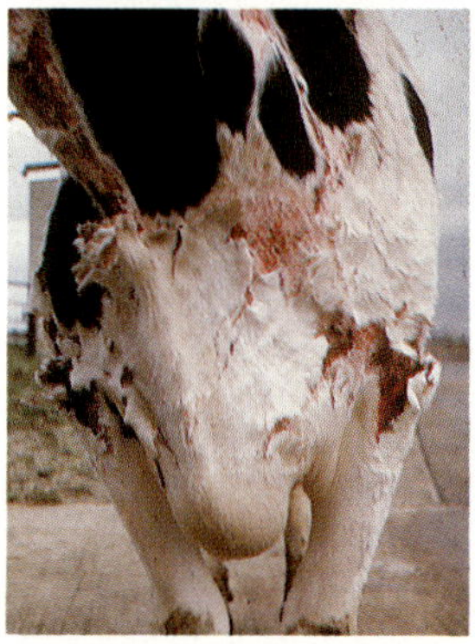

Plate 44.12 Friesian cow with severe photodermatitis. Note the non-affected densely melanotic skin.

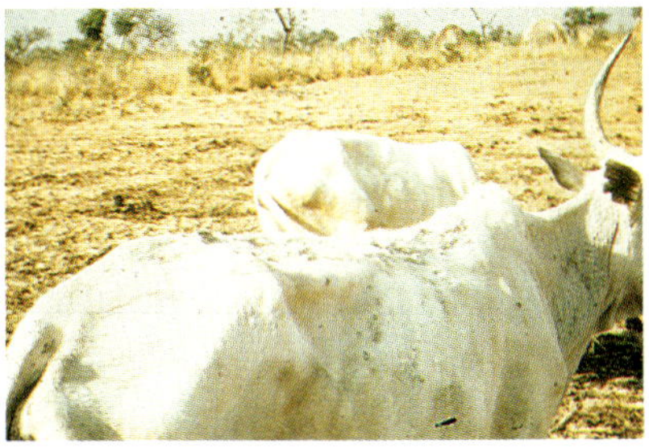

Plate 44.13 Dermatophilosis. Crusted lesions on the dorsum of a cow (northern Nigeria).

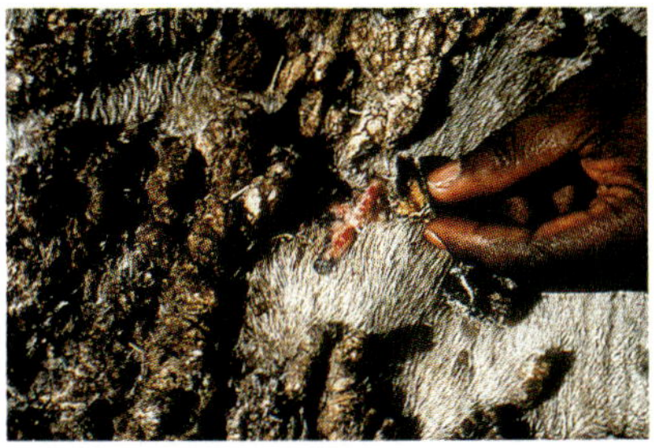

Plate 44.14 Dermatophilosis. Hyperkeratotic scab and crust (northern Nigeria).

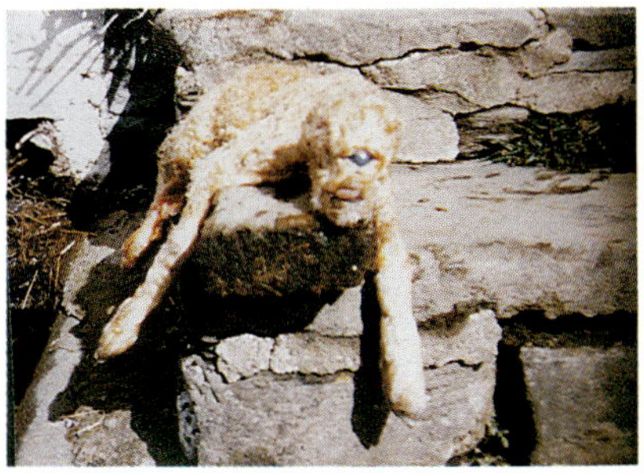

Plate 46.1 Cyclopia in a newly born Jersey calf.

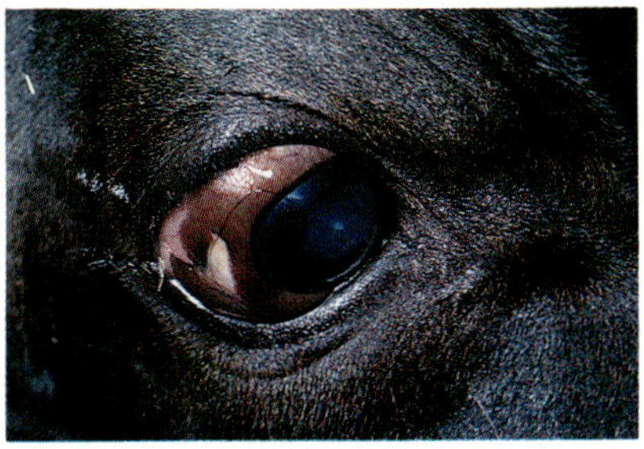

Plate 46.2 (a) Early esotropia (convergent squint) in a three-month-old Friesian calf.

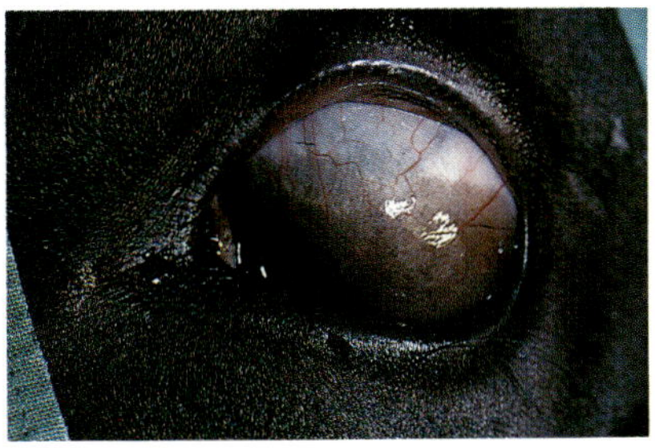

Plate 46.2 (b) Marked esotropia in an eight-month-old Friesian heifer. The globe has rotated medially to such an extent that mainly scleral tissue is visible within the palpebral fissure.

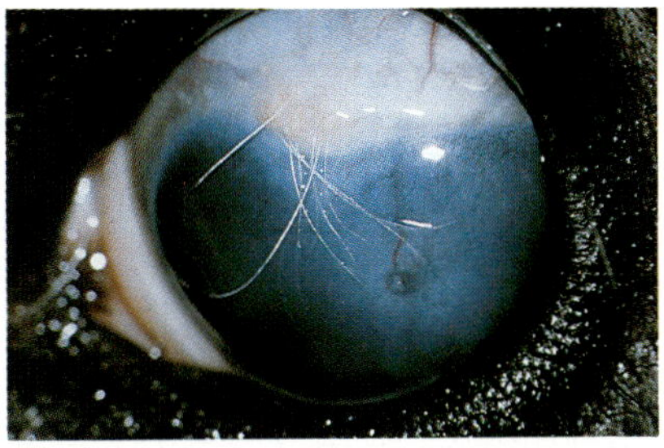

Plate 46.3 Epibulbar dermoid within the dorsal bulbar conjunctiva in a four-month-old Friesian calf; other ocular anomalies were also present (courtesy of S.M. Crispin).

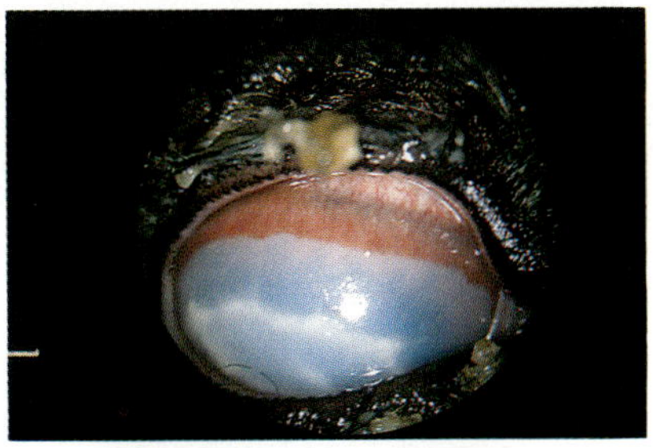

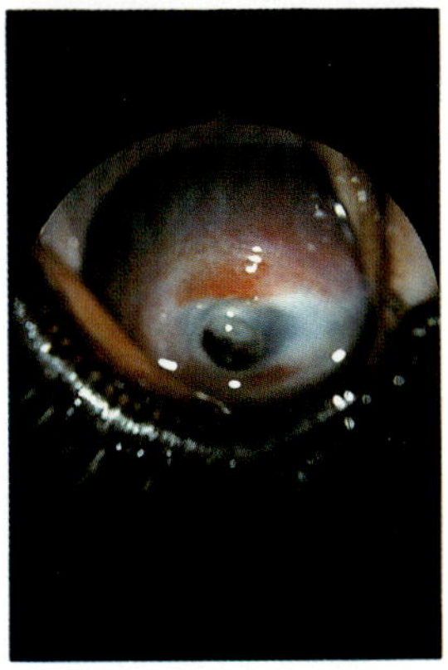

Plate 46.4 (*left*) Infectious bovine keratoconjunctivitis. (a) At eight days corneal vascularization has occurred. (b) Rupture of the cornea and staphyloma formation. Right eye in a six-month-old Friesian.

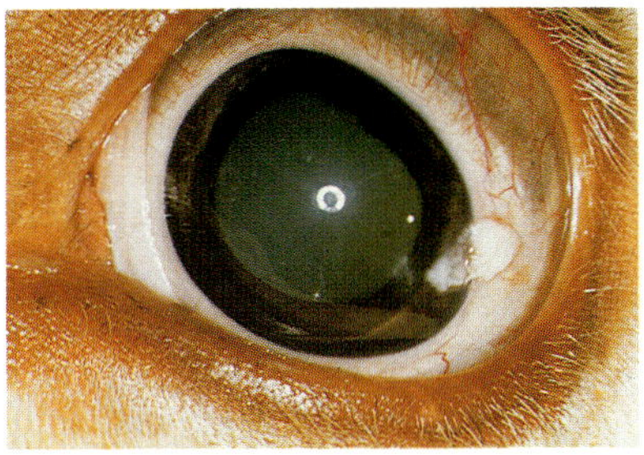

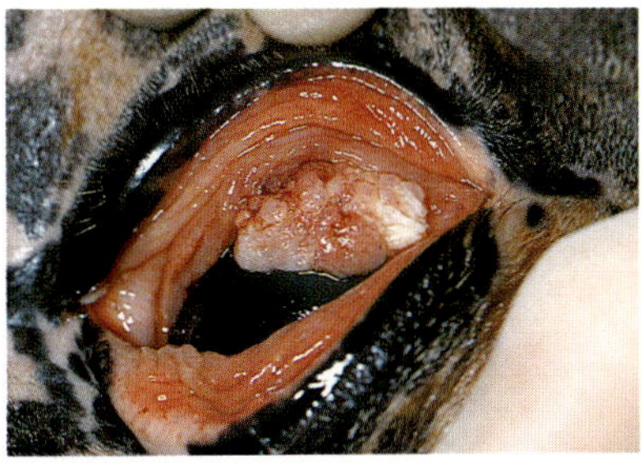

Plate 46.5 Squamous cell carcinoma. (a) Small precursor papilloma at the lateral limbus in a two-year-old Hereford cow, left eye (courtesy of S.M. Crispin). (b) Extensive involvement of the lateral bulbar conjunctiva, right eye.

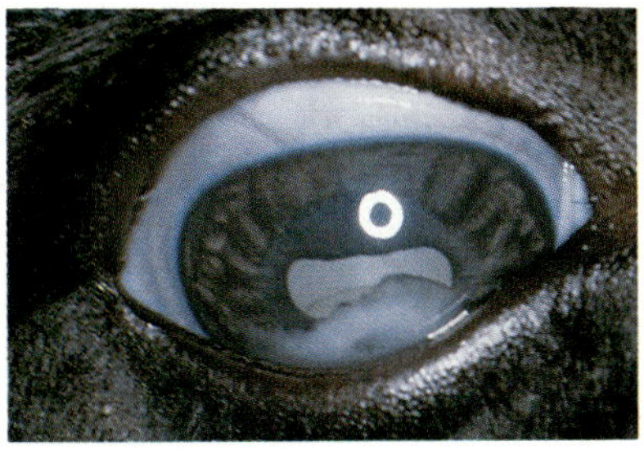

Plate 46.6 Anterior uveitis secondary to a septicaemia of undetermined aetiology. Right eye, two-year-old Friesian (courtesy of S.M. Crispin).

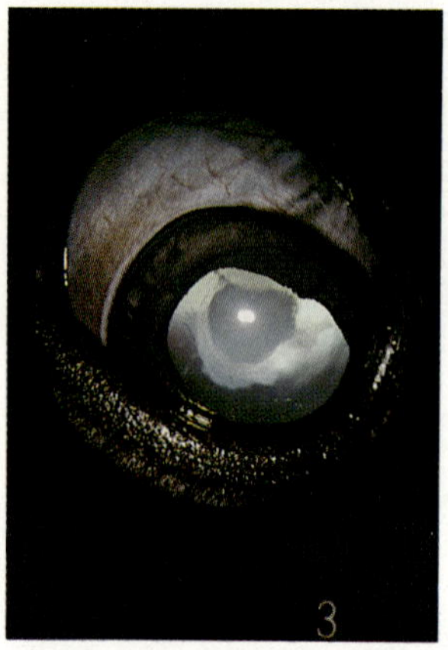

Plate 46.7 Congenital cataract in the right eye of a two-month-old Friesian.

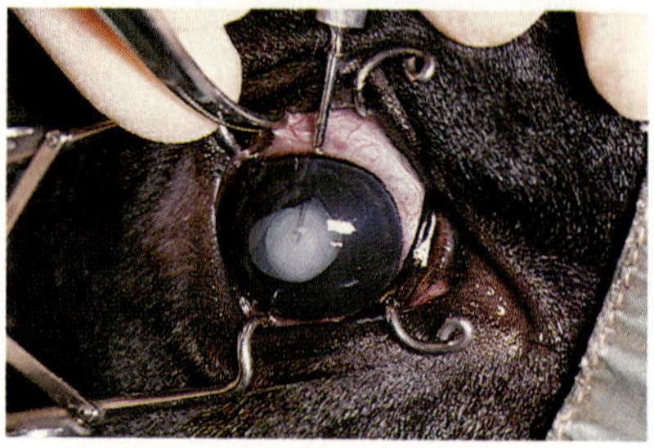

Plate 46.8 Lens discision for the treatment of congenital cataract. The Bowman's discision needle is used to break up the anterior capsule through a dilated pupil, and dislocate the cortical and cataractous lens material into the anterior chamber.

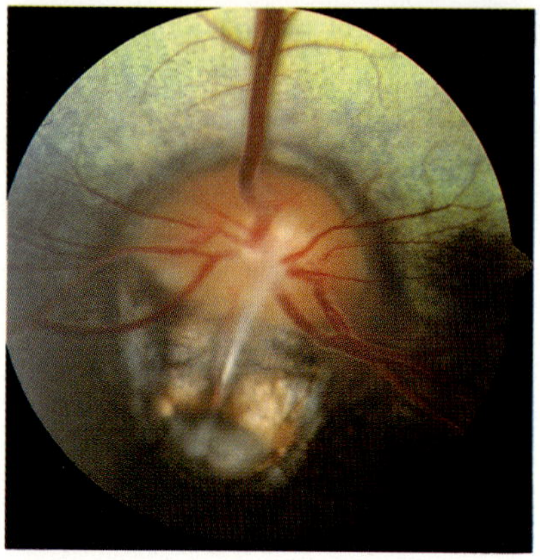

Plate 46.9 Typical papillary coloboma in a 12-month-old Charolais bull (courtesy of K.C. Barnett).

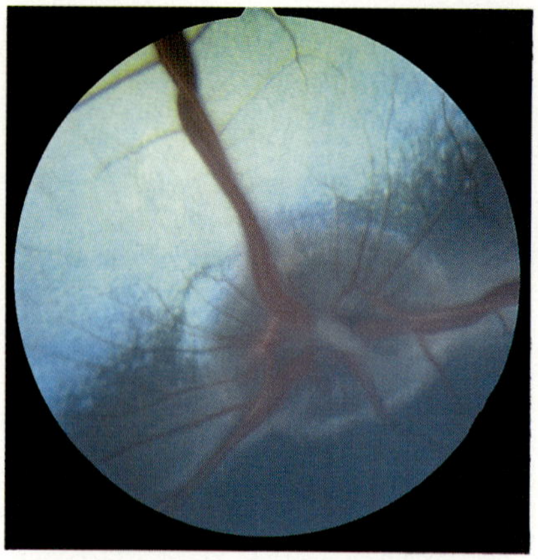

Plate 46.10 Normal bovine fundus with a remnant hyaloid tag over the centre of the optic papilla. Twelve-month-old Friesian.

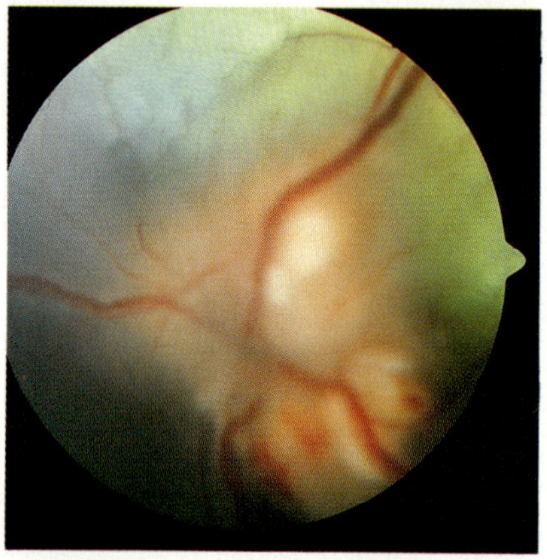

Plate 46.11 Severe papilloedema with disc haemorrhages in a seven-month-old vitamin A deficient calf (courtesy of K.C. Barnett).

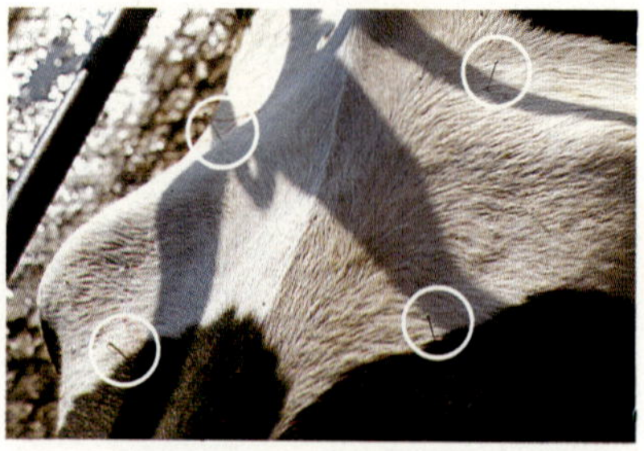

(a)

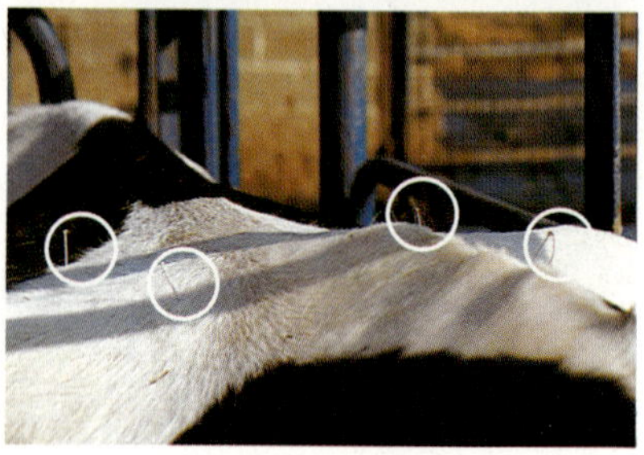

(b)

Plate 59.1 (a & b) Treatment for anoestrus. This comprises needles in Bladder 31 and Bladder 26. Each is bilaterally stimulated. Bladder 26 is antero-lateral to the sacro-iliac joint and Bladder 31 is posterior to this.

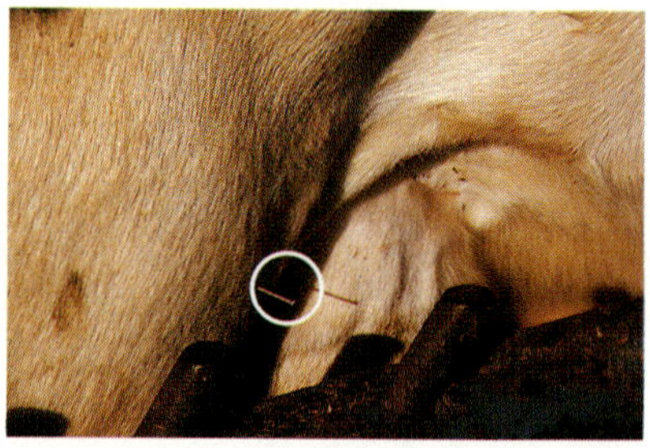

Plate 59.2 Stomach 36. This point is antero-lateral on the proximal end of the tibia in the depression lateral to the tibial crest. This is an important and commonly-used point with a wide variety of actions. This point is called Zusanli and is indicated in the treatment of melancholia, irritability, shyness, posterior paralysis, pain or swelling of the hindquarters, blood pressure defects, malfunction of genital organs and hormonal equilibrium. It is also useful in diseases affecting the skin.

Hillers, J.K., Thonney, S.C. & Gaskins, C.T. (1982) Economic comparison of breeding dairy cows artificially versus naturally. *Journal of Dairy Science*, **65**, 861–5.

Kilgour, R. (1984) Sexual behaviour in male farm animals. In *Male in Farm Animal Reproduction* (ed. by M. Courot), pp. 108–32. Martinus Nijhoff, Dordrecht.

Kilkenny, J.B. (1978) Reproductive performance of beef cows. *World Review of Animal Production*, **14**, 65–74.

Kretser, D.M. de (1979) Endocrinology of male infertility. *British Medical Bulletin*, **35**, 187–92.

Kumi-Diaka, J. & Dennis, S.M. (1978) The Sertoli cell index as a measure of testicular degeneration in the bull. *Veterinary Record*, **103**, 112–14.

La Faunce, N.A. & McEntee, K. (1982) Experimental *Mycoplasma bovis* veniculitis in the bull. *Cornell Veterinarian*, **72**, 150–67.

Lagerlöf, N. (1951) Hereditary forms of sterility in Swedish cattle breeds. *Fertility and Sterility*, **2**, 230–42.

Land, R.B. (1978) Genetic improvement of mammalian fertility: a review of opportunities. *Animal Production Science*, **1**, 109–35.

Larsen, L.H. & Bellenger, C.R. (1971) Surgery of the prolapsed prepuce in the bull: its complications and dangers. *Australian Veterinary Journal*, **47**, 349–57.

Li, P.S. & Wagner, W.C. (1983) *In vivo* and *in vitro* studies on the effect of adrenocorticotrophic hormone or cortisol on the pituitary response to gonadotrophin releasing hormone. *Biology of Reproduction*, **29**, 11–24.

Linford, E., Glover, F.A., Bishop, C. & Stewart, D.L. (1976) The relationship between semen evaluation methods and fertility in the bull. *Journal of Reproduction and Fertility*, **47**, 283–91.

Little, T.V. & Woods, G.L. (1987) Utrasonography of accessory sex glands in the stallion. *Journal of Reproduction and Fertility*, **35**(Suppl.), 87–94.

Logue, D.N. (1975) *A study in bovine cytogenetics*. PhD Thesis, Glasgow.

Logue, D.N. & Greig, A. (1985) Infertility in the bull. 1. Failure to mate. *In Practice*, **7**, 185–91.

Logue, D.N & Greig, A. (1986) Infertility in the bull. 2. Infertility associated with normal service behaviour. *In Practice*, **8**, 118–22.

Logue, D.N. & Greig, A. (1987) Infertility in the bull. 3 Collection and examination in semen. *In Practice*, **9**, 161–70

Logue, D.N. & Harvey, M.J.A. (1978) Meiosis and spermatogenesis in bulls heterozyos for a presumptive V29 Robertsonian translocation. *Journal of Reproduction and Fertility*, **54**, 159–65.

Logue, D.N., Harvey, M.J.A. & Lennox, B. (1979) Hormonal and histological studies in a 61xxy bull. *Veterinary Record*, **104**, 500–3.

Long, S.E. & Dubra, C.R. (1972) Incidence and relative clinical significance of preputial eversion in bulls. *Veterinary Record*, **91**, 165–9.

McCauley, A.D. (1980) Seminal vesiculitis in bulls. In *Current Therapy in Theriogenology: Diagnosis, Treatment and Prevention of Reproduction Diseases in Animals* (ed. by D.A. Morrow), pp. 401–5. W.B. Saunders & Co., Philadelphia, London, Toronto.

Meischke, H.R.C. (1979) A survey of bovine teat papillomatosis. *Veterinary Record*, **104**, 28–31.

Memon, M.A., Dawson, L.J., Vsenik, E.A. & Rice, L.E. (1980–85) Preputial injuries in beef bulls: 172 cases. *Journal of the American Veterinary Medical Association*, **193**, 481–5.

Miller, D.J. & Hunker, A.G. (1987) Individual variation for *in vitro* fertilization success in dairy bulls. *Journal of Dairy Science*, **70**, 2150–53.

Mobini, S., Walker, D.F. & Crawley, R.R. (1982) An experimental evaluation of the response of the bull penis to carbon fibre implants. *Cornell Veterinary Journal*, **72**, 350–60.

Monke, D.R. (1980) Avulsion of the bovine penile epithelium at the fornix. In *Proceedings of the 8th Technical Conference on Artificial Insemination*, pp. 48–65. National Association of Animal Breeders Inc.

Niedermeier, R.P., Crowley, J.W. & Meyer, E.C. (1983) United States dairying changes and challenges. *Journal of Animal Science*, **57** (Suppl. 2), 44–57.

O'Connor, M.L., Gwazdauskas, F.C., McGilliard, M.L. & Saake, R.G. (1985) Effect of adrenocorticotrophic hormone and associated hormonal responses on semen quality and sperm output of bulls. *Journal of Dairy Science*, **68**, 151–7.

O'Lamhna, M. & Roche, J.F. (1983) Effect of repeated implantation with anabolic agents on growth rate, carcass weight, testicular size and behaviour of bulls. *Veterinary Record*, **113**, 531–4.

Palmer, A.C., Blakemore, W.F., Barlow, R.M., Frazer, J.A. & Ogden, A.L. (1972) Progressive ataxia of Charolais cattle associated with a myelin disorder. *Veterinary Record*, **91**, 592–4.

Parkinson, T.J. (1987) Seasonal variation in semen quality in bulls: correlation with environmental temperature. *Veterinary Record*, **120**, 479–82.

Robertson, I.S., Fraser, H.M., Innes, G.M. & Jones, A.S. (1982) *Veterinary Record*, **111**, 529–31.

Salisbury, G.W. & Van Demark, N.L. (1961) *Physiology of Reproduction and Artificial Insemination*, 1st edn. W.H. Freeman & Co., San Francisco, London.

Turnbull, P.A. (1977) An abattoir survey of bull genitalia. *Australian Veterinary Journal*, **53**, 274–9.

Vincent, C.K. (1972) Effects of season and high environmental temperature on fertility in cattle. *Journal of American Association of Veterinary Medicine*, **161**, 1333–8.

Walker. D.F. (1980) Genital surgery of the bull. In *Current Therapy in Theriogenology: Diagnosis, Treatment and Prevention of Reproductive Diseases in Animals* (ed. by D.A. Morrow), pp. 370–401. W.B. Saunders & Co., Philadelphia, London, Toronto.

Chapter 36: Herd Fertility Management

(a) Dairy Herds

by H. BOYD

Introduction

Many veterinarians are familiar with herd fertility control and much written in this chapter is directed at clinicians who already practice fertility control. For those veterinarians who would like to start doing fertility control work, detailed instructions are set out in a section at the end of this chapter, which they are advised to read first (p. 515).

A fertility control programme is a well-established system of preventive medicine in the management of reproduction, successfully practised throughout the world. It is successful because the farmer gains in improved income more than the cost of the programme (Esslemont *et al.*, 1985). For the veterinarian, fertility control represents a profitable outlet for specialist skills. In addition, regular farm visits to carry out fertility control give the veterinarian the chance to promote other aspects of preventive medicine.

It is essentially a simple and practical method of applying knowledge and veterinary skills to an important part of livestock management. Success depends on cooperation between the veterinarian and the farmer. It is based on good husbandry and consistently efficient detailed work by the veterinarian.

Reproduction is particularly suitable for preventive medicine because if treatment is delayed until reproductive failure is recognized by the owner there will be an irretrievable loss of production time.

Because of the effect of husbandry (feeding, housing and breeding management) and general health on reproduction, a fertility control programme should also incorporate other aspects of preventive medicine and encourage the practice of good husbandry.

Table 36.1 The main components of a fertility control programme

Targets and planning
Cow identification and records
Routine veterinary visits
Review of progress

Table 36.1 lists the main components of a fertility control programme.

Components of a fertility control programme

Targets and planning

A fertility control programme requires reproductive targets. These are chosen for economic reasons and are limited by what is physiologically possible. Although the veterinarian guides the farmer in the decision about targets, it is the farmer's responsibility to choose the targets. Only if the farmer really wants to achieve the selected targets are they likely to be achieved.

HEIFERS

Dairy farmers often aim for seasonal calving for the whole herd. To achieve this it is essential that the heifers calve early in the chosen season. If pregnancy rate is 60 per cent and all the heifers are cycling, over 90 per cent should be pregnant nine or ten weeks after the start of the breeding season. Therefore, the minimum target for both the service and calving periods should not be less than 10 weeks.

As age at first calving has a major effect on the proportion of a cow's life that is productive, there is an optimal age for first calving and, for dairy breeds, this is often put at 24 months old. However, farmers have to consider conditions in their own herds before they decide at which age the heifers should calve.

Having chosen the desired season of first calving and the desired age at first calving, various problems arise that have to be thought through. If, for example, the calving season chosen is September, October and the beginning of November and the age at first calving is to be 24 months, what is to be done with heifers that are born in December, January or February? Will they be left until the next calving season when they will be nearly three years old, or will they be made to calve even younger than 24 months old, or will they be allowed to calve in January or February? These are important and difficult decisions.

Once the decision has been made, other consequential targets have to be considered. If a heifer has to calve at 24 months old she must become pregnant at 15 months old. To do this she has to be cycling and well grown. She also has to keep growing to be in a fit condition to calve down with a good-sized calf and to be big enough to thrive in the competitive life in the dairy herd. This means the farmer has to plan the growth rate from birth to meet the targets at these critical times (see p. 444). The veterinarian has an important role in reducing calf diseases to allow planned growth rates.

Other breeding targets have to be established, in particular an acceptable culling rate and the choice of types of sires to use. This again requires careful thought. One aim is to avoid dystokia and this should be considered in choosing the breed of bull and the individual bull to be used for service. If proven artificial insemination (AI) dairy sires are used, there are advantages in breeding replacement heifers out of heifers because each generation should have greater genetic potential than the one before. It may also be a target to use beef sires on some heifers to avoid too many replacement dairy animals. To work out all this is complex and use of previous data from the herd may help.

COWS

The most important targets are a controlled calving interval and season of calving. In addition, consideration of involuntary culling rate is necessary.

In fertility control work, the calving interval is the number of days from the immediately past calving to the next. Farmers are very conscious of the need to have a controlled calving interval, but the ideal target varies from country to country, from farm to farm and indeed from lactation to lactation. In Britain the normal target is a 12-month calving interval.

There are two reasons why calving interval is important.

1 Typically, milk yield reaches a peak about five weeks after calving and starts to decline at about eight or nine weeks after calving. This is why the first part of a lactation is more profitable than latter parts and the dry period. Short calving intervals result in a greater proportion of a cow's productive life being spent in this early, profitable part of lactation.

2 Short intervals produce more calves over a given period of time than long intervals. In a 100-cow herd with a 12-month calving interval there will be (approx-

imately) 100 calves born per year; in a similar herd with a 14-month calving interval the number of calves per year will be about 86.

James & Esslemont (1979) explain the complexities of the 'ideal' calving interval, which are listed in Table 36.2.

It is tempting when marketing fertility control to put a money value on the loss occasioned by every day the calving interval is extended beyond the target. A figure that is used in the UK at present (1991) is £2/day. It should be realized that this (or any other figure) is not necessarily applicable to any individual herd. In the USA a figure of $2.50/day has been suggested (Bartlett *et al.*, 1986).

Table 36.2 Factors influencing the choice of calving interval

Age of the cow
Shape of her lactation curve
Month of the year
Feeding
Cost
Availability
Calving and milking facilities

Once the calving interval has been chosen a series of consequential targets emerge. If the target for calving to calving is 365 days, then the target for calving to conception must be 85 days, which is 365 days minus the gestation length of about 280 days.

Account must be taken of the fact that many cows require more than one service for pregnancy when calculating the target interval from calving to first service. In a specific herd this depends on conception rate, oestrous detection rate and culling rate. In many herds a target for calving to first service of 65 days is satisfactory.

It is clear that cows must be cycling by the target date for first service. A target that is often taken for the start of cyclicity based on the physiology öf the dairy cow is 42 days after calving.

It is quite obvious that a target of first service 65 days after calving has to be modified to become the oestrous cycle that straddles 65 days, often taken as 56–76 days inclusive (eight to eleven weeks) after calving. This modifies the target for calving to conception to the three-week period around 85 days, i.e. up to 96 days after calving.

In a herd with a 55 per cent first service pregnancy rate and reasonable oestrous detection the targets shown in Table 36.3 will achieve a 12-month calving interval given an acceptable degree of culling.

Many farmers have as their prime target the season of calving. Although the calculations involved are in essence the same, the emphasis and methods of calculation tend to be rather different from farmers aiming for a specific calving interval.

The start and end of the service season is controlled by the targeted calving season. It is essential that as many cows as possible are served in the first three weeks (oestrous cycle) of the breeding season. It is particularly important to have all the cows cycling in time and therefore the target for cyclicity is the three weeks before the start of the service period.

VETERINARIAN'S ROLE

The veterinarian's role is to:

1 encourage the farmer to think through his targets, and

2 to ensure that the targets are realistic.

There is no use producing targets that do not take into account bovine reproductive physiology or that are unduly optimistic regarding pregnancy rate, oestrus detection rate or the standard of husbandry on the farm.

Table 36.3 Targets for a 12-month calving interval

Start cycling: by 42 days after calving
Start service: 56 days after calving

Cow identification

A clear reliable cow identification system is needed to run a fertility control scheme. Good identification is needed for accurate records.

Without proper identification there will be no clear system to ensure that cows are served when planned, no way of knowing which animals fail to meet targets and dangerous confusion when animals are presented for veterinary examination. As an example of the latter point consider a cow that has an unrecorded service, is pregnant and is presented to the veterinarian as 'not yet seen in oestrus'. She will have a corpus luteum and the usual treatment with prostaglandin or an analogue would cause abortion. Similarly, if a cow that was presented for pregnancy diagnosis on the basis of a known service date had an unrecorded service at a later date, even the most experienced veterinarian could make an erroneous diagnosis of 'not pregnant'.

The veterinarian should encourage the farmer to choose a system suitable for the conditions in which the herd is kept.

Record systems

A great deal has been written about record systems and the reader is advised to study recent expositions on the subject (Anon., 1984; Esslemont *et al.*, 1985; Morrow, 1986). A simple system for beginners is described at the end of this chapter (p. 515).

WHY ARE RECORDS NEEDED?

1 Records are needed for efficient day-to-day running of the herd, even in herds with no thought-out plans and targets. They tell the stockworker whether a cow that is in oestrus is due for service or should be left till the next oestrus; they indicate when a cow is expected to come in season from the recorded date of last oestrus or service; and they allow the accurate selection of cows for the veterinary visit or for sampling.

2 Records are needed to monitor progress. It is necessary to keep an eye on herd progress as well as individual cow status. Monitoring will indicate how many cows are starting cycling on time after calving, how many cows are being served on time; and it will show the success rate of services and the incidence of long and short interservice intervals.

Monitoring of herd events gives the veterinarian the chance to deal with herd problems at an early stage.

3 Records are useful as an aid to diagnosis. If cows are grouped according to factors that may be related to fertility, it is sometimes possible to pinpoint aetiological factors. Examples include where one bull has a poor pregnancy rate, or the average calving-to-first-service interval is very long in first calvers or if a seasonal effect on fertility is noted.

WHAT ARE RECORDS?

Records consist of the following information written down by a farm worker: a cow number, a date and an event. Errors of two sorts occur: items are written down incorrectly; and events occur and are not recorded. The main events that are recorded in variable detail are listed in Table 36.4.

PROBLEMS IN RECORD ANALYSIS

There are two intrinsic, insurmountable problems in relation to analysis.

1 With very few exceptions the amount of data available, when taking into account the variability of all fertility measurements, is not enough to give statistically valid information. This is particularly the case when the records are subdivided, as suggested above, into age groups, seasonal groups and so on.

2 Information that is up-to-date is practically always incomplete (see below) and as a result may produce incorrect conclusions; complete information is nearly always out-of-date.

Up-to-date, incomplete information will give a more favourable result than is true in the measurement of the time from one reproductive event to another. Consider the important index, the calculation of the herd average and spread of the interval from calving to first service. If the figure is calculated before all the cows in the calculation have been served (or marked as 'not to be served') the result will be biased because it will include all cows served soon after calving and will exclude those problem cows that will eventually be served after a long calving-to-first-service interval.

On the other hand, early calculation of pregnancy rate produces a worse than actual result because the cows that have returned to service will be recorded as failures before the pregnant cows have been confirmed in-calf by rectal palpation.

Incomplete results based on non-return rates or on progesterone assays also distort the real picture.

These errors matter because decisions will be based

Table 36.4 The main events to record

Calving, oestrus, service, result of service, abortion
Veterinary reproductive findings and treatment
Other diseases
Production information
Milk yield
Feeding

on false assumptions. The actual analysis of records is discussed in the section on periodic review.

Routine visits

At each routine visit the owner will have selected animals for examination based on a system agreed between client and veterinarian. The animals presented for examination will vary from herd to herd and between practices. The groups of cows shown in Table 36.5 should be presented at the routine visit. Stage for examination or intervention figures are in parentheses.

Methods of examination, diagnosis and treatment have been discussed in Chapter 32. At each visit the clinician should spend a few minutes looking over the records with the client to pick up any problems at an early stage, to modify targets, to give information to the farm staff and to give them the chance to discuss any veterinary problem that is worrying them.

Table 36.5 Selection of cows for routine visit

Cows with abnormalities at or after calving (21 days after calving) or all cows about 21 days after calving
Cows overdue for oestrus (42 days after calving)
Cows in target service period but not yet served (56–76 days after calving)
Cows overdue for service (77 days after calving)
Cows due for pregnancy diagnosis (42 days after last service)
Cows seen at the previous visit and not served since
Other problem cows Purulent discharge Aberrant sexual behaviour Repeat breeders

RECORD KEPT AT THE VISIT

Apart from the breeding records the veterinarian should keep a simple record sheet that records everything done and advised. An example is shown in Fig. 36.1.

Whatever method is used to transfer the veterinary findings to the records, care should be taken with cows that are found to be non-pregnant to make sure that it is clear to which service 'non-pregnant' applies. Errors arise when the cow is served later and the result 'non-pregnant' may be taken to apply to that subsequent service.

The quality of the work done at the routine visit and the informal discussion of progress and problems is very important. The routine visit supports the advice given at the periodic review.

Periodic review and dealing with problems noted

Detailed description of the many different ways of gathering and analysing breeding records are easily obtained in recent publications (Anon., 1984; Esslemont *et al.*, 1985; Morrow, 1986). Instead of repeating this here, attention is concentrated on what the analysis is trying to achieve and on some of the problems of interpreting records.

While at each visit an eye is kept on the progress of the herd's breeding pattern, periodically it is necessary to look more thoroughly at the fertility of the whole herd. The intervals between periodic reviews will vary with the seasonal calving pattern, with the intensity of the client's interest and with the apparent success rate as noted at each visit.

The basis of the periodic review is an analysis of the herd breeding records and an assessment of the effectiveness of treatment. Cows in the milking herd will be considered separately from heifers.

There are so many ways of recording and analysing herd breeding records that this simple exercise can be unnecessarily confusing. There are two reasons for analysing herd records in these periodic reviews.

1 Assessment of current status to establish whether there is a problem that needs attention or whether things are progressing satisfactorily.

2 Discovery of any particular areas of weakness.

In the analysis of purely reproductive data (not factors which affect reproduction), there are five analyses that can be carried out as listed in Table 36.6. The most important of these are marked with an asterisk.

The first step is to define clearly which cows are to be included in the analysis.

1 The ideal baseline is all cows that calve in a specified period. This period has to end long enough before the day of analysis to allow every cow to have completed her reproductive cycle to the stage of pregnancy diagnosis or to the decision to cull.

2 All cows that are due to be served. It may be necessary when using records kept by an AI centre to take as the starting point all cows that are presented for first insemination. In that case, it should be remembered that some cows will have been culled (or marked to be culled) before they were presented for insemination and so a certain amount of loss is ignored.

Once the group to be analysed has been selected, it is important that the analysis makes it clear what has happened to every cow in the group.

CALVING TO SUBSEQUENT REPRODUCTIVE EVENTS (TO FIRST OESTRUS, TO FIRST SERVICE, TO CONCEPTION)

It is simple to calculate the number of days from calving to first oestrus, to first service and to conception. It is more difficult to express this information in a clear way and to interpret the results correctly.

1 The first thing to note is how many cows actually had a first observed oestrus, had a first service or became pregnant, in relation to the number of animals that started in the group. Culling rates of about 25–30 per cent are common in dairy herds. If the rate is much greater than this, the veterinarian should establish whether something is going wrong in the herd or whether the records are incomplete.

2 The next thing to calculate is the average number of days from calving to oestrus (target: cycling by 42 days); to service (target: 65 days) and to conception (target: 85 days). Targets assume that the object is to have a 12-month calving interval. While averages are not completely satisfactory figures they are worth knowing and comparing with target figures.

The average is of limited value because it may be made up of a wide spread of values. For example, an average calving-to-service interval of 65 days may consist of very short and very long intervals (unsatisfactory), or it may be the result of most intervals being close to the target (satisfactory). If the average is greater than the target, results are certainly not satisfactory and the average does give some idea of the seriousness of the situation.

Farm | Date of visit 30.6.92
minus 42 days* 19.5.92
TSP 56 to 77 days** 14.4.92 to 5.5.92

Pregnancy diagnosis

Date of service	Result	Treatment

Anoestrus etc.

Cow	Calving date	Observation	Treatment

Date of last visit 16.6.92

List of all cows examined at last visit and recommendations (except positive pregnancy diagnosis)

(Check if served or not;
if not served should be in group of cows for the current veterinary examination)

*date for pregnancy diagnosis and oestrus due
**target period for first service

Fig. 36.1 Record of veterinary visit.

Table 36.6 Analysis of reproductive data

Intervals in days between calving and subsequent reproductive events
Calving to first oestrus
Calving to first service*
Calving to conception*
Success rate of services*
Intervals in days from service to service
Involuntary culling rate
Submission rate (in herds with short breeding season)*

* Most important reproductive data.

Table 36.7 Measurement of success rate of service

Percentage: 'successful services' of 'all services'
Ratio: 'all services' to 'successful services'
Visually: as a cusum (Anon., 1984) (can be expressed mathematically)

Consequently, the concept of a 'target period' has been developed. For example, instead of a 65-day target for an average interval from calving to first service, the target changes to getting as many cows as possible served in the oestrous cycle period around 65 days, i.e. from 56 to 76 days (8–11 weeks) after calving. The target for conception is the period around 85 days, i.e. 76–96 days (11–13 weeks) after calving. For first oestrus it is best to aim for as many cows as possible seen in oestrus by 42 days.

Information about the number of animals that fall into the target periods, before the target period and after it can be presented in histogram form. This is very clear, easily understood, and puts the extent of the problem into exact numbers.

SUCCESS RATE OF SERVICES

The success rate of services is again quite simple to work out, but to avoid misinterpretation it is essential to understand the different ways of doing this as shown in Table 36.7. The difficulty arises because of the different ways of defining 'all services' and 'successful services': 'All services' can mean literally that; it can also mean all services up to a certain number of services, say five; or it can mean 'all first services' (first service is defined as the first service after calving or in a heifer's life). 'Successful services' can mean services that result in calving, or that result in positive pregnancy diagnosis by rectal palpation, or positive pregnancy diagnosis by milk progesterone, or by non-return to service at various intervals after calving.

Depending on the definitions used the success rate calculated from the same group of animals can vary enormously.

In most herds that are under veterinary supervision 'success' will be defined as positive pregnancy diagnosis.

There are several points in favour of basing the success rate on first services rather than on all services, especially:

1 the result can be obtained earlier than if one has to wait for the result of the last repeat breeder in the group;

2 each cow contributes the same weight to the calculation.

Therefore, in herds controlled by a veterinarian, success rate is best defined as the first service pregnancy rate = percentage of cows that are pregnant to first service.

Bear in mind that an accurate figure will not be obtained until the result of the last first service is known, which will be about six weeks after that last service if pregnancy diagnosis is by rectal palpation.

Once the first service pregnancy rate has been worked out it is compared with the target rate of between 50 and 60 per cent, the target depending on a variety of factors.

INTERSERVICE INTERVALS

The number of days between services is worked out. The object of doing this is twofold.

1 To assess the efficiency of heat detection. The assumption is made that most cows that do not become pregnant return to service at a normal cycle length of 18–24 days and therefore that returns longer than this represent missed oestrus. While this is not strictly correct the distribution of interservice intervals is quite useful for assessing poor oestrous detection.

2 To observe the incidence of irregular intervals, such as <18 days, between 25 and 36 days, as these can indicate inaccurate heat detection or embryonic death.

The data are presented as one or two normal cycle lengths (18–24 and 36–48 days) or less than one, between one and two, or more than two cycles (<18, 25–35 and >48 days). Alternatively, the figures are set out as a histogram with each day represented separately, which is satisfactory for visual presentation but difficult to describe in a report.

The proportion of cows presented for rectal pregnancy diagnosis that are not pregnant also gives an indication of the number of missed oestrous periods because most non-pregnant cows have been in season once or twice before examination and have not been observed in oestrus.

CULLING RATE

The incidence of culling in relation to the total starting population and the stage at which the decision to cull is taken is presented as a percentage and an actual number. It is desirable to record the reason for culling.

EFFECTIVENESS OF TREATMENT AND ACCURACY OF PREGNANCY DIAGNOSIS

Treatment, including conservative treatment, takes place:

1 at and after calving,
2 in the preservice period, and
3 at and after service.

Accordingly, the targets for treatment vary. Lists should be prepared with appropriate dates, diagnosis, treatment and results of treatment. Laboratory confirmation of the accuracy of diagnosis and of the success of some treatments is possible and will eventually add to the veterinarian's efficiency.

Many veterinarians who have not previously analysed their results will find the effectiveness of treatment disappointing. Better results require more accurate diagnosis, careful selection of cases for treatment and improvement of the client's breeding management, so that practically all cows in oestrus after treatment are inseminated at the right time.

Similarly, a follow-up on accuracy of positive and negative pregnancy diagnosis should be carried out. It is not sufficient to note that a positive diagnosis was followed by a calving; the calving date should be a normal gestation length after the service for which the examination was carried out. If prostaglandin $F_{2\alpha}$ is used routinely to treat cows diagnosed as non-pregnant, there is no point in assessing the accuracy of the diagnosis of non-pregnancy!

Accuracy of pregnancy diagnosis should be very close to 100 per cent.

HEIFERS

Analysis of breeding records for heifers is often restricted because of lack of information, particularly where natural service is employed. Where AI is used analysis is to some extent as for adult cows. The aspects shown in Table 36.8 should be borne in mind.

After the purely reproductive analysis the next stage is to correlate the fertility results with factors that could interfere with reproductive efficiency. Some of these factors have been listed in Table 36.6 on p. 513.

At the periodic review a written report should be presented to the client.

Advice for veterinarians who wish to start herd fertility control

Many veterinarians who are not carrying out fertility control work for any of their clients find it difficult to get started. One problem is lack of confidence as regards skills in rectal palpation. If this is the case it has to be overcome by self-education or by organizing suitable training.

Marketing of the service is best done via practice newsletters and a special client meeting to explain to clients all that is involved in control programmes. Help to arrange a meeting can be obtained from many sources, such as other practitioners who run fertility control schemes, commercial firms or colleagues in veterinary schools.

Beginners often have difficulty in knowing what to do on routine farm visits and particularly how to set up and use a record system.

If client is aiming for a 12-month calving interval

A computer-based system of record keeping is useful, and how to choose a system of this sort is discussed by Esslemont *et al.* (1985). However, a written record system is perfectly adequate. The following simple system, which can be made up in the practice and photocopied, is suggested as a starting point. One sheet of A4 or slightly larger, heavy paper is marked across the top with headings that cover one reproductive cycle for each cow from calving to confirmation of pregnancy or disposal/death. The sheet is lined horizontally and each sheet will take records from about 20 cows (see Fig. 36.2).

This sheet is filled in by the farmer in chronological order of calving. It is usually impossible to get accurate records for more than one or two months prior to starting so that recording should be started at the same time as the rest of the programme. The best recording is likely in herds where there is some other recording system used, such as Milk Records.

Fig. 36.2 Simple herd fertility recording system.

Herd breeding record								Farm				Sheet no.			
Cow	Calving		Lactation no.	Pre-service heat dates		Service dates/bull used						PD	Days from calving to:		
	Date	Normal		1st	2nd	Target	1st	2nd	3rd	4th	5th		1st heat	1st serve	Pregnancy
36	6-3-90	Y	6	8-5-90		1-5-90	25-5-90 GS					P+	63	80	80
20	7-3-90	Dead calf	3			2-5-90	12-5-90 DH	11-7-90 Char				P+	—	66	126
38	9-3-90	Y	6	16-4-90		4-5-90	3-5-90 DH					P+	38	55	55
186	10-3-90	Y	4			5-5-90	1-7-90 DH	×		To be sold		P–	—	114	—
148	8-7-90	CS	1			2-9-90	13-9-90 DH						—	67	
14	11-8-90	Y	1			6-10-90							34		
219	12-8-90	Y	2	15-9-90		7-10-90									

Table 36.8 Analysis of heifer breeding records

Starting population
Per cent cycling when put to bull
First service pregnancy rate
Per cent that become pregnant
Range of calving season
Range of ages at first calving (available from milk records)

Many farmers find that a breeding board is useful to supplement this sheet (Anon., 1984).

Arrange to visit the herd every 14 days and at each visit examine all cows that:
1 are more than 56 days after calving and have not been served;
2 served 42 days or more previously and have not returned to service (if unsure of early pregnancy diagnosis, start later);
3 any problem cows.

Keep a record of everything you do on the farm and find out what has happened to all the cows you saw at the last visit (see Fig. 36.1).

It takes a year before the records are complete enough for sensible analysis. Make an initial analysis after six months bearing in mind the problems discussed on p. 511. After that, analyse the records every six months, or other suitable interval, to show the following.
1 The number of cows that calved.
2 Calving service interval:
  (a) The number that have been served since calving.
  (b) The number not served.
  (c) The average calving-to-service interval.
  (d) A simple, small histogram of distribution of calving-to-service intervals.
3 The same information for calving-to-conception interval.
4 First service conception rate.
5 Culling rate.

With a little imagination all the information can be presented on a single sheet of paper (see Fig. 36.3).

If client is aiming for a tight calving season

Use the same record system. Discuss oestrus detection. Make sure the farmer records all heats in the three-week period before the first day of the service period.

Examine, and treat where needed, all animals that have not been in season at the end of the three-week preservice period. Visit at weekly or fortnightly intervals thereafter to examine all cows not yet seen in oestrus and to follow up treatments.

Carry out pregnancy diagnosis nine weeks after the first day of the service season. Remember this simplified advice covers the first steps to help beginners to get started.

(b) Beef Herds

by A.R. PETERS

Introduction

Beef cattle must be considered as a separate entity from dairy cattle as they are managed under entirely different circumstances. They are usually managed as a herd or group and do not receive the same individual attention as dairy cows. They are, therefore, to some extent less accessible to veterinary involvement. Possibly because they are not exposed to such high levels of production stress, clinical infertility problems do not appear to occur to the same extent. Apart from pedigree herds, it has to be remembered that commercial suckler cows are often kept as a low input and low output enterprise, perhaps of secondary or tertiary importance to other activities. This again militates against extensive veterinary involvement. On the other hand, beef cows may be subjected to other stresses particularly that of marginal nutrition and this can have serious adverse effects on fertility, as will be seen later.

Of course, the same parameters of fertility as used in dairy cows are important in beef cows. For example, the calving interval is one of the most important measures of reproductive performance. In some beef herds cows and bulls are together all year round and there is little attempt to control fertility or the season of calving. In better-managed herds a seasonal calving pattern is adopted and the calving pattern itself becomes an important determinant of reproductive performance.

An excellent review of suckler cow management in the UK has recently been published (Lowman, 1988) and this is strongly recommended if the reader requires further detail after reading this chapter.

Determinants of reproductive performance

In the UK, beef cows traditionally calve either in spring or autumn, although there are trends towards calving in other seasons also. Autumn-calving herds tend to produce a higher gross margin/cow than spring-calving herds under UK conditions (see Table 36.9), due mainly to a greater financial output. However, spring-calving herds tend to be stocked more heavily and thus there is little difference in gross margins expressed on a per hectare basis.

The calf is essentially the sole product of the beef herd; therefore, the rate of calf production is even more critical than it is in the dairy herd. In order to illustrate this a comparison between the average performing and best performing (top one-third in terms of gross margin/cow) suckler herds recorded by the Meat and Livestock Commission (MLC) (1981) is shown in Table 36.10. The top one-third herds showed superior performance in almost all the variables recorded. Whilst there was some variation from year to year the most important factors causing these differences were (i) the calf weight at sale/transfer, (ii) the number of calves reared/100 cows and (iii) the stocking rate. The first two of these, calf weight and the number of calves reared, accounted for a major part of the difference in performance between the average and top one-third herds. Put more simply the most successful herds sold *more*, *heavier* calves than the average.

Table 36.9 Gross margins and performance for upland suckler herds by season of calving (1985) (MLC, 1986)

	Spring calving	Autumn calving
Number of herds	45	47
Gross margin (£)		
Per cow	193	237
Per hectare	345	353
Calf age at sale (days)	242	334
Calf weight at sale (kg)	254	324

Table 36.10 Physical performance of hill herds (1980) (MLC, 1981)

	Average	Top
Cow performance		
Calving interval (days)	386	372
Calving period (weeks)	17	13
Per 100 cows put to bull		
Number barren	6.9	4.4
Number died	2.1	1.2
Number calved	92	95
Live calves	89.9	92.7
Calves born dead	2.6	2.6
Calves dead after 1 week	2.4	2.7
Total dead calves	5.0	5.3
Calves purchased	5.3	4.2
Calves weaned	92.8	94.2
Weight calf/cow/year (kg)	232	262
Calf performance		
Disposal/yarding weight (kg)	261	280
Days to disposal/yarding	272	267
Daily gain (kg)	0.8	0.9
Weaning weight gain (kg)	239	257
Stocking rate (cows/ha)		
Grazing	1.45	1.75
Overall	1.25	1.4

Calf weight and age at sale/transfer are reflections of health and growth rate; obviously, calf weight is further dependent to a major extent on the breed of sire used. The heavy breeds such as Charolais, Simmental and South Devon produce calves with the highest weight. However, this has to be balanced against a higher risk of dystokia and possible calf mortality as illustrated by a recent survey shown in Table 36.11. Also, the gestation period and hence the calving interval can be influenced to a limited extent by the breed of sire (Table 36.11). Average calf weight at weaning and its variation within herds also reflects the length of the calving period (see below).

An important index of reproductive performance in the suckler herd is the length of the calving season or period. A 365-day calving interval is optimal as in the dairy herd but a compact calving season is also desirable because:

1 more cows calve early in the period, therefore the age and weight of calves are higher at the time of weaning and sale;
2 the impact of calf disease and mortality may be reduced if there is only small variation in calf ages;
3 cows are all at a similar stage in the production cycle, therefore feed can be rationed more precisely and the cows managed more conveniently.

The calving season is almost directly dependent on the pregnancy rate to service and the length of the breeding or service period. Obviously, the higher the pregnancy rate, the shorter the service period required to ensure pregnancy of all or the majority of the cows. A theoretical relationship between the conception rate, the service period and the calving period was calculated by ICI and is shown in Table 36.12.

Factors affecting reproductive performance

Infectious disease

In some cases of low herd reproductive performance there may be an underlying infectious cause. However, the main reproductive diseases, e.g. brucellosis,

Table 36.11 Estimated annual suckler cow productivity

Sire breed	Assisted calvings (%)	Calf mortality (%)	Calving interval (days)	Annual production of calf weaning weight/cow (kg)
Charolais	9.0	4.8	374	208
Simmental	8.9	4.2	374	203
South Devon	8.7	4.0	375	203
Devon	6.4	2.6	373	200
Limousin	7.4	3.8	375	199
Lincoln Red	6.7	2.0	373	198
Sussex	4.5	1.5	372	196
Hereford	4.0	1.6	372	189
Angus	2.4	1.3	370	179

Table 36.12 Theoretical relation between conception rate and the calving period in a 100 cow herd (adapted from ICI computer simulation by Allen & Kilkenny, 1980)

Herd conception rate (%)	Service period for 90% cows to be pregnant (days)	Length of calving period (days)	No. of cows calving in first month
30	245	260	12
40	140	155	28
50	100	110	41
60	70	85	54

campylobacteriosis (vibriosis), have almost been eliminated from herds in many countries including the UK following disease eradication programmes and the use of artificial insemination (AI). Notwithstanding, specific disease problems may still exist in individual herds and cause poor reproductive performance. For example, campylobacteriosis is still a problem in some herds where a bull is used. Additionally, some viral diseases may result in poor herd reproductive performance, for example bovine herpes I (BHVI) infection and bovine viral diarrhoea (BVD).

Obviously, it is essential to rectify any infectious problem before attempting to improve herd reproductive performance by other means.

Nutritional management

Nutritional status is of vital importance in the maintenance of a high rate of reproductive performance. The nutrition of cattle is covered more comprehensively in specialized texts and only the basic principles will be described here.

Whilst specific deficiencies of micronutrients are common under particular circumstances and can affect fertility, under normal conditions dietary energy appears to be the main factor limiting reproductive performance. However, other nutritional deficiencies occur but are usually confined to localities or even individual herds. These include problems with phosphorus, manganese and cobalt (p. 261) and some vitamins, particularly A and E. For a fuller account of this problem the reader is referred to Chapters 19 and 39.

The technique of body condition scoring has been developed as a simple semi-objective monitor of cows' energy status. The principle depends on the manual palpation of the thickness of subcutaneous fat cover on various parts of the body (see p. 16).

Methods have been developed for both dairy (Mulvaney, 1978) and beef cows (Lowman *et al.*, 1976) and although the finer details vary slightly the overall principle is the same. The thickness of fat cover over the lumbar and tailhead area is estimated and assigned a score usually from 0 (emaciated) to 5 (very fat) although different scales are sometimes used. Descriptions of the various categories on the 0–5 scale are given on p. 16.

An additional guide to the body condition can be obtained by palpating over the hip bones, ribs and either side of the tailhead. With a little experience an operator can assess the body condition of cows to within one half-unit. Optimum body condition scores for beef cows have been worked out for various stages of the reproductive cycle and these are shown in Table 36.13.

The target body condition score at service is the most critical as this is most closely related to overall reproductive performance. The calving interval has been shown to be negatively correlated with body condition at the time of mating in beef cows although the true relationship is probably curvilinear (see Fig. 36.4). This target score is also most difficult to achieve in autumn-calving cows as they are mated during midwinter when they are lactating and when good quality feed is expensive. In a survey, approximately half of the autumn-calving beef cows failed to reach the target condition score at mating (MLC, 1981). In contrast, the nutritional drain of lactation is offset in spring calvers by the plentiful supply of grazing.

Cows should be fed to calve at a condition score of 2.5–3 and should then lose minimum condition until conception (see Table 36.13). Cows calving in fatter condition may have calving difficulties, which in turn may lead to delayed involution, reproductive tract damage, susceptibility to infection of the tract or a combination of these problems. Also, cows with a score of 4 or more are likely to mobilize their fat reserves excessively during the early postpartum period.

Beef cows calving in a low condition are also likely to undergo prolonged periods before the re-establishment of ovarian cycles, undernutrition being one of the major causes of failure to ovulate after calving. Consequently, pregnancy is likely to be considerably delayed in such cows.

Table 36.13 Recommended target body condition scores of beef cows at various stages of the reproductive cycle (MLC, 1981)

	Mating	Mid-pregnancy	Calving
Autumn-calving suckler cows	2.5	2	3
Spring-calving suckler cows	2.5	3	2.5

As pregnancy progresses the lactational demand for a high level of dietary energy decreases. This enables the cow to replace body energy reserves that were lost during early lactation. Thus the cow can be brought back towards the target body condition for the next mating.

Controlling the length of the calving season

There are a number of ways in which a compact seasonal calving pattern may be established and maintained in a healthy seasonally calving beef herd. These include feeding policy, culling policy and postpartum induction of ovulation.

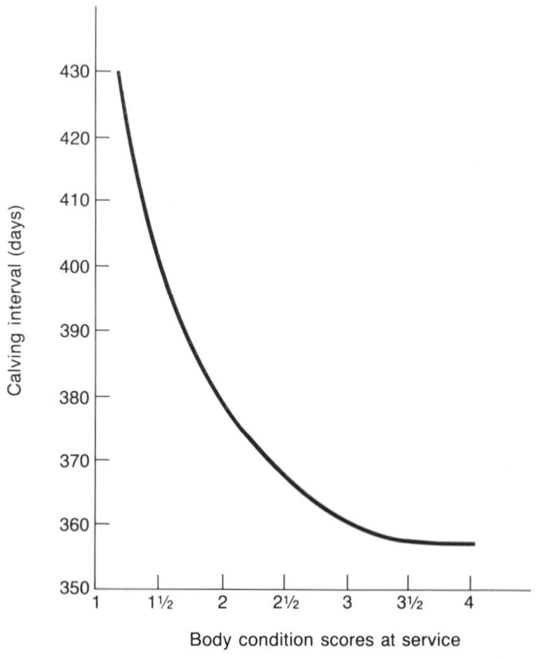

Fig. 36.4 The relationship between calving interval and body condition score at service in beef cows (Kilkenny, 1978).

Feeding policy

It is very difficult to restore compact seasonal calving patterns by nutritional management in herds that have a grossly extended calving season, since this would necessitate the achievement of calving intervals in late-calving cows of well below 365 days. However, it is important to remember that proper nutritional management is vital for the maintenance of a compact seasonal calving pattern.

Culling policy

This is the most extreme but probably the most effective method of modifying a herd's calving pattern. As discussed above, the length of the calving period is highly dependent on the herd pregnancy rate. For example, a five-month calving period is approximately equivalent to a pregnancy rate of 40 per cent. In this situation approximately 70 per cent of cows will calve in the first two months and 30 per cent in the next three months. Therefore, the 30 per cent late calvers should be culled and replaced. Many producers are reluctant to adopt such a high culling rate due to the high cost of purchasing or rearing replacement heifers, particularly during the first year or so. However, such a policy can be of eventual financial advantage due to a decrease in the spread of calving and the consequent management economics as discussed above (see Table 36.14).

Postpartum onset of ovarian cycles

A delay in the onset of ovarian cycles can lead to extended calving intervals and possibly increased variation in calving intervals between cows within a herd. This will result in increases in the length of the calving season.

Factors affecting the postpartum acyclic period

Suckling

Many studies have shown that the onset of ovulation and/or oestrus behaviour are delayed in either dairy or beef-type cows that suckle calves, relative to milked animals, particularly where more than one calf is suckled per cow. In suckling beef cows kept under UK conditions the average time to resumption of ovarian cycles has been reported as 59.9 ± 2.5 days after calving (Peters & Riley, 1982a) but there was considerable variation both within and between herds. Weaning of calves, either temporary or permanent, or at least the prevention of suckling has been reported to shorten the acyclic period.

Table 36.14 Financial effects of a high culling rate (after Allen & Kilkenny, 1980)

	Normal culling policy	High culling rate		
		Year 1	Year 2	Year 3
Number of cows	90	78	86	88
Number of replacements	13	36	20	16
Calving spread (days)	150	100	100	100
Average calf sale weight (kg)	285	285	305	315
Gross margin/ ha (£)	219	174	233	257

Nutrition, body weight and body condition and the postpartum period

Long postpartum acyclic periods in suckling cows may be reduced by the provision of increased dietary energy (e.g. Dunn *et al.*, 1969). Energy intake appears to be more critical than protein intake in the maintenance of reproductive function as positive relationships between energy intake and reproductive performance have been demonstrated in several studies. Low energy intake in prepartum and postpartum cows increases the length of the anoestrous period and in heifers it has been shown to result in fewer ovarian follicles, lower progesterone levels and lower conception rates (Hill *et al.*, 1970).

Nutritional status at and before calving appears to be more important than that during the postpartum period, since Peters & Riley (1982a), using body weight as an index of nutritional status, found a significant negative correlation between body weight at calving and the length of the acyclic period in beef cows, whilst body weight change after calving had no effect. Also, an increase in energy supply to pregnant beef cows has been shown to accelerate the return of ovarian cycles after calving. Target body condition scores are given in Table 36.13.

Season

In the temperate latitudes seasonal variations in conception rates and a longer interval between parturition and first oestrus in the winter and early spring have been reported (e.g. Thibault *et al.*, 1966). Furthermore, spring-calving beef and dairy cows have been reported to undergo longer periods between calving and first ovulation than autumn calvers (Bulman & Lamming, 1978; Peters & Riley, 1982a). Most authors have suggested that such seasonal effects are related purely to nutritional management; however, strong effects of season have been demonstrated after adjusting statistically for the effects of body weight at calving (Peters & Riley, 1982b). Evidence for seasonality in cattle has now been accumulated from Europe, North American, Canada and New Zealand. Thibault *et al.* (1966) have suggested that photoperiod might play some role in seasonality of reproductive activity in the cow and a negative correlation between daily photoperiod during pregnancy and the onset of ovarian cycles after calving has been demonstrated (Peters & Riley, 1982b). It is possible that a vestigial sensitivity to photoperiod may be present in the domestic cow and that in feral cattle this pattern would predispose towards calving during the late spring to early summer, the optimal time for food supply.

In summary, a variety of factors affect the onset of the ovarian cycle in the postpartum beef cow. The order of importance is probably nutrition, season and suckling. However, it is normally impossible in the practical situation to quantify these effects so that the time to first ovulation can be predicted.

Induction of ovulation in beef cows

Most evidence to date suggests that delay in ovulation during the postpartum period is mediated by a low rate of gonadotrophin release; most work has been done on luteinizing hormone (LH) but follicle stimulating hormone (FSH) is probably equally important. Such endocrine changes occur as a result of external factors (some discussed above) acting via the hypothalamus to suppress the release of gonadotrophin-releasing hormone (GnRH).

A reliable hormonal method of inducing ovulation in acyclic cows would obviously be advantageous but it is probably true to say that an ideal treatment has not yet been devised.

Gonadotrophins of non-bovine origin in the form of either pregnant mare's serum gonadotrophin (PMSG) and human chorionic gonadotrophin (hCG) have been extensively used for this purpose in the past but results have been variable; hCG has largely LH-like activity whereas PMSG has mainly FSH-like activity and may result in development of multiple follicles.

The injection of oestrogens in cows results in preovulatory surges of gonadotrophin release (depending on dosage) and oestrous behaviour. However, ovulation may or may not follow such treatment. The response is generally too unpredictable for this to be a useful method of inducing ovulation.

Progestagens have been used extensively to synchronize ovulation in cyclic cows, but may also be used to induce ovulation after calving. Roche *et al.* (1981) reported that 10-day treatment of beef cows with the progesterone-releasing intravaginal device (PRID) resulted in ovulation in about half the cows treated, whereas Bulman & Lamming (1978) reported a 75 per cent success rate with a 12-day PRID treatment in dairy cows. However, in the latter study the conception rate in the responding cows was only 50 per cent and treatment did not affect the mean calving-to-conception interval. Other workers (Ball, 1982; Drew *et al.*, 1982) have reported a reduction in the calving-to-conception interval of up to 14 days following the use of PRID; however, the calving-to-conception interval of PRID-treated beef cows was reduced only if used before day 30 after calving (Peters, 1982).

Mulvehill & Sreenan (1977) have reported the best success in induction of ovulation in beef cows by injecting 750 iu of PMSG at the time of progesterone withdrawal. However, a small number of twin and triple ovulations did occur.

Gonadotrophin-releasing hormone

The injection of GnRH in cattle induces release of both LH and FSH. There have been many attempts to induce ovulation in postpartum cows by single intramuscular injections of 100–500 μg GnRH and these have given variable results. In order to apply these treatments in practice, more consistent responses would be necessary.

At the above dose levels, LH release of preovulatory surge magnitude usually occurs, depending on the responsiveness of the pituitary. However, ovarian follicles appear to require a two to three day period of rising plasma LH concentrations in order to mature fully prior to ovulation. Therefore, a preovulatory LH surge will induce ovulation only if a follicle at the appropriate stage of development is already present. Alternatively, the induced LH release might cause premature luteinization of an unovulated follicle and transient secretion of progesterone sufficient to initiate ovarian cycles.

Two injections of 500 μg GnRH at an interval of 10 days was advocated by Webb *et al.* (1977). However, this treatment regimen has not been particularly successful in larger-scale field trials with beef cattle (Mawhinney *et al.*, 1979). A short-lived rise in progesterone concentrations following GnRH injection has been reported by several authors and may be compared to that occurring naturally in some cows prior to the onset of normal ovarian cycles. There has also been interest in longer-acting administration of GnRH but no product is yet commercially available.

Oestrous synchronization and AI in beef cattle

The full exploitation of genetic progress cannot be made in beef cattle without the use of AI. However, AI is not very widely used in beef cattle, for example fewer than 5 per cent of beef cows in the UK are inseminated artificially. The major reasons for this include the difficulty, trouble and expense of oestrous detection.

It was thought that the advent of techniques for controlling the time of ovulation would overcome the problems of oestrus detection in beef cattle thereby facilitating the use of AI in these herds. Yet these techniques have had little overall impact, possibly because expectations greatly exceeded reality in terms of the capability and efficacy of these products.

Methods

Both prostaglandins and progestagens may be used in beef cows (see Peters, 1986). However, neither would be recommended along with fixed-time insemination. Rather, fertility results will be much better following oestrus observation. In terms of precision of oestrus and ovulation after synchronization treatment the combination of progestagen and prostaglandin is most effective. The progestagen may be either in the form of a synthetic progestagen implant, e.g. norgestomet, or progesterone in the form of PRID. The currently preferred regimen is to give progestagen for seven days and to give the prostaglandin on day 6. This has the effect of synchronizing the decline in progesterone concentrations from endogenous and exogenous sources. Preliminary data on small numbers of animals have shown acceptable fertility results in animals inseminated by appointment (see Table 36.15). There is considerable scope for further investigation of methods to improve the degree of synchronization, possibly by the use of a combination of treatments. For example, the ability of GnRH injections to induce and synchronize the preovulatory gonadotrophin surges has not yet been exploited.

It must also be said that to obtain best results, a very high standard of management and attention is necessary. It has been shown on numerous occasions in the field that these expensive techniques will prove disappointing if management input is not high. Addi-

Table 36.15 Pregnancy rates after various treatments and insemination regimens (after Smith *et al.*, 1984)

Treatment	Timing of AI after last treatment	Per cent pregnant
Control	Observed heat	72
6 day PRID plus PG day 6	Observed heat	82
7 day PRID, PG day 6	Observed heat	73
2 × PG	80 hours	52
7 day PRID, PG day 6	84 hours	66

PRID, progesterone-releasing intravaginal device.
PG, prostaglandin.

tionally, it is important to remember that a sound 'sweeper' bull should be kept to serve those animals not pregnant to the AI.

Management of heifers (see Chapter 5)

Heifers should be bred to calve two to three weeks before the adult herd. Heavy breeds of bull likely to cause dystokia, e.g. Charolais and Simmental, should be avoided. Oestrus synchronization may be used to advantage in heifers along with fixed-time insemination if required, although a bull would still be necessary to serve non-pregnant animals subsequently.

Monitoring reproductive performance in the beef herd

This is very much more difficult in beef cattle than in dairy cows because of the nature of the management systems.

Even in the best-managed units records of reproductive events may be quite rudimentary, possibly including only date of calving. Since bulls are widely used few records of service may be kept. Furthermore, few producers carry out pregnancy diagnosis because of the inconvenience and the lack of perceived benefit. The bull would normally be left with the cows for a length of time that corresponds to the aimed length of the calving season. Whilst it would be advantageous to identify barren cows at the end of the bulling period, in many cases it is not desirable to cull those animals because they are still suckling calves. However, methods of early pregnancy diagnosis would be highly advantageous in the beef herd so that non-pregnant cows could be identified quickly and appropriate action taken. It is unlikely that the milk progesterone test will become popular in beef herds even when a 'cow-side' test is available because of potential difficulties in sample collection. However, the use of real-time ultrasound where embryos/fetuses can be detected by day 30 (White *et al.*, 1985) or earlier offers very exciting possibilities.

It would be desirable for the practitioner to design a 'herd plan' to monitor reproductive performance in beef herds. The following could be used as a guide.

1 Condition-score cows at least two months before the start of the calving season, e.g. at weaning. Those below target (see Table 36.13) should receive supplementary rations to bring them up to target. Any cows above target should have their condition reduced.
2 Condition-score cows at calving: those below target should receive supplementary rations.
3 Special attention should be paid to first and second calvers since these are most likely to be vulnerable to problems, particularly extended periods of anoestrus after calving.
4 The producer should begin to observe and record oestrus three weeks before the bull is introduced.
5 Oestrous periods and services should be recorded throughout the breeding season. Particular attention should be paid to the dates when cows are expected to return to oestrus. The use of chinball markers may assist oestrous observation with cows at grass.
6 Pregnancy diagnosis should be carried out six weeks after the bulls are removed. Barren cows can be culled then. The findings at pregnancy diagnosis in conjunction with the service records will enable the farmer/veterinarian to estimate the likely calving dates and to plan the nutritional management.

Fertility problems arising in beef herds are likely to result from similar causes as in the dairy herd. However, investigation is often hampered by the lack of adequate records. Clinical problems such as retained placenta, cystic ovaries and metabolic disease are much less likely to occur but otherwise the more common problems are similar to those in dairy herds. Similarly, when problems occur they are likely to reflect herd status rather than just involving individual cows.

Analysing herd problems

The following information is likely to be of value in understanding and rectifying problems.

1 Cumulative frequency curve of calvings.
2 The age distribution of cows.
3 The calving dates of first-calving heifers.
4 The culling rate and reasons for culling.
5 An assessment of bull capacity including their ages and clinical histories.
6 Evaluation of the other farm enterprises so that the best calving season can be chosen.

Beef cow stockworkers are capable of achieving rates of heat detection equal to those of dairy stockworkers. If reproductive performance is to be optimized then the stockworker must be prepared to observe and record the herd. For those that do so, techniques such as AI, oestrus synchronization/induction and induction of parturition will be much more successful.

The veterinarian should be able to assess the potential of the farmer and to educate and advise accordingly. This should be on a long-term basis, i.e. five years, by which time optimal targets should have been reached and advisory input can then be reduced to a surveillance role.

References

Dairy herds

Anon. (1984) *Dairy Herd Fertility*, pp. 1–80. Ministry of Agriculture, Fisheries and Food, Reference Book 259. Her Majesty's Stationery Office, London.

Bartlett, P.C., Ngategize, P.K., Kaneene, J.B., Kirk, J.H., Anderson, S.M. & Mather, E.C. (1986) Cystic follicular disease in Michigan Holstein–Friesian cattle: incidence, descriptive epidemiology and estimated economic impact. *Preventive Veterinary Medicine*, **4**, 15–33.

Esslemont, R.J., Bailie, J.H. & Cooper, M.J. (1985) *Fertility Management in Dairy Cattle*, pp. 1–143. Collins, London.

James, A.D. & Esslemont, R.J. (1979) The economics of calving intervals. *Animal Production*, **29**, 157–62.

Morrow, D.A. (1986) *Current Therapy in Theriogenology 2. Diagnosis, Treatment and Prevention of Reproductive Diseases in Small and Large Animals*. W.B. Saunders and Co., Philadelphia.

Beef herds

Allen, D. & Kilkenny, B. (1980) *Planned Beef Production*, p. 183. Granada, London.

Ball, P.J.H. (1982) Milk progesterone profiles in relation to dairy herd fertility. *British Veterinary Journal*, **138**, 546–51.

Bulman, D.C. & Lamming, G.E. (1978) Milk progesterone levels in relation to conception, repeat breeding and factors influencing acyclicity in dairy cows. *Journal of Reproduction and Fertility*, **54**, 477–58.

Drew, S.B., Gould, C.M., Dawson, P.L.L. & Altman, J.F.B. (1982) Effect of progesterone treatment on the calving-to-conception interval of Friesian dairy cows. *Veterinary Record*, **111**, 103–6.

Dunn, T.G., Ingalls, J.E., Zimmerman, D.R. & Wiltbank, J.N. (1969) Reproductive performance of two year old Hereford and Angus heifers as influenced by pre- and post-calving energy intake. *Journal of Animal Science*, **29**, 719–26.

Hill, J.R., Lammond, D.R., Henricks, D.M., Dickey, J.F. & Niswender, G.D. (1970) The effects of undernutrition on ovarian function and fertility in beef heifers. *Biology of Reproduction*, **2**, 78–84.

Kilkenny, J.B. (1978) Reproductive performance of beef cows. *World Review of Animal Production*, **14**, 65–74.

Lowman, B.G. (1988) Suckler cow management. *In Practice*, **10**, 91–100.

Lowman, B.G., Scott, N.A. & Somerville, S.H. (1976) Condition scoring of cattle. East of Scotland College of Agriculture, Bulletin No. 6.

Mawhinney, S., Roche, J.F. & Gosling, J.P. (1979) The effects of oestradiol benzoate (OB) and gonadotrophin releasing hormone (Gn-RH) on reproductive activity in beef cows at different intervals post partum. Annales de Biologic Animale Biochimie et Biophysique, **19**, 1575–87.

Meat and Livestock Commission (1981) *Beef Yearbook*, p. 47.

Meat and Livestock Commission (1986) *Beef Yearbook*, p. 55.

Mulvaney, P. (1978) *Dairy Cow Condition Scoring*. Paper No. 4468, National Institute for Research in Dairying, Reading.

Mulvehill, P. & Sreenan, J.M. (1977) Improvement of fertility in post-partum beef cows by treatment with PMSG and progestagen. *Journal of Reproduction and Fertility*, **50**, 323–5.

Peters, A.R. (1982) Calving intervals of beef cows treated with either gonadotrophin releasing hormone or a progesterone releasing intravaginal device. *Veterinary Record*, **110**, 515–17.

Peters, A.R. (1986) Hormonal control of the bovine oestrous cycle. II. Pharmacological principles. *British Veterinary Journal*, **142**, 20–9.

Peters, A.R. & Riley, G.M. (1982a) Milk progesterone profiles and factors affecting post partum ovarian activities in beef cows. *Animal Production*, **34**, 145–53.

Peters, A.R. & Riley, G.M. (1982b) Is the cow a seasonal breeder? *British Veterinary Journal*, **138**, 533–7.

Roche, J.F., Ireland, J. & Mawhinney, S. (1981) Control and induction of ovulation in cattle. *Journal of Reproduction and Fertility*, Suppl. **30**, 211–22.

Smith, R.D., Pomerantz, A.J., Beal, W.E., McCann, J.P., Pilbeam, T.E. & Hansel, W. (1984) Insemination of Holstein heifers at a preset time after oestrous cycle synchronisation using progesterone and prostaglandin. *Journal of Animal Science*, **58**, 792–800.

Thibault, C., Courot, M., Martinet, L., Mauleon, P., De Mesnil du Buisson, F., Ortovant, R., Pelletier, J. & Signoret, J.P. (1966) Regulation of breeding season and oestrous cycles by light and external stimuli in some mammals. *Journal of Animal Science*, **25** (Suppl.), 119–39.

Webb, R., Lamming, G.E., Haynes, N.B., Hafs, H.D. & Manns, J.G. (1977) Response of cyclic and post-partum suckled cows to injections of synthetic LH-RH. *Journal of Reproduction and Fertility*, **50**, 203–10.

White, I.R., Russel, A.J.F., Wright, I.A. & Whyte, T.K. (1985) Real time ultrasonic scanning in the diagnosis of pregnancy and the estimation of gestational age in cattle. *Veterinary Record*, **117**, 5–8.

Major Infectious Diseases

Chapter 37: Viral Diseases

(a) Bluetongue

by R.P. KITCHING

Bluetongue (BT) is an infectious, non-contagious disease of ruminants characterized by congestion, oedema and haemorrhage. The disease is caused by strains of orbivirus, within the family Reoviridae.

The genus orbivirus, Reoviridae also contains Ibaraki disease virus of cattle, epizootic haemorrhagic disease virus of deer (EHD), African horse sickness virus and Colorado tick fever virus. The outer shell of bluetongue virus (BTV) has a diameter of 65 nm, within which is an inner shell of 32 ring-shaped capsomers. The genome consists of 10 segments of double-stranded RNA, which code for the structural and non-structural viral proteins and which can be separated according to their relative sizes by polyacrylamide or agarose gel electrophoresis. Two of these segments (numbers two and five) code for the outer structural proteins (VP2 and VP5), which determine the serotype of the virus. There are 24 immunologically distinct BTV serotypes that have so far been identified by virus neutralization tests; however, it is probable that more types will be identified in the future. Bluetongue virus is sensitive to low pH, and storage at −20 °C; it is partially resistant to lipid solvents.

Distribution

The distribution of BTV is approximately defined by the latitudes 40° N and 35° S, which includes most of Africa, the Middle and Far East, northern Australia, USA, Central America and South America north from southern Brazil, Paraguay and Bolivia.

Not all the BTV types are found throughout this enzootic region, and the distribution of the different types can vary between years. The BTV types found within a region tend to have greater genome sequence homology, in genome segments other than those which encode the serotype-specific outer capsid proteins, than their designated serotype number would suggest. The type is defined by the outer capsid proteins alone, and while these are found to differ between different serotypes found in a particular region, the remaining genome segments show high levels of sequence homology. The BTV types have therefore been additionally grouped into Australian types and African types, with the North American types being more closely related to the African. The Australian BTV type 1 has more in common with other Australian types than with the African type 1, although sharing with the African type its antigenic determinants. This diversity may explain the marked difference in pathogenicity of the strains of BTV, which does not appear to be related to a specific type designation; it also makes epidemiological studies based on serotype determinations of doubtful significance. Recombination can occur between different strains of BTV, which adds further to the potential for diversity of BTV isolates.

The closely related EHD group of viruses have been isolated in North America, Canada, Nigeria and Australia, whereas Ibaraki disease virus is restricted to South Korea, Japan, Philippines and Indonesia.

History

Bluetongue was first diagnosed in South Africa in sheep at the beginning of this century. It was first seen outside Africa in 1943 in Cyprus, although it had possibly been present in Cyprus as early as 1924. Subsequently, BT was diagnosed in Israel in 1951, in Pakistan in 1959 and in India in 1963. A disease at first identified as sore muzzle of sheep in Texas in 1948 and California in 1952 was the following year diagnosed as BT. Between 1956 and 1960, BTV caused a major epizootic in sheep in Portugal and southern Spain, which reportedly resulted in the loss of 180000 animals, but the virus then disappeared from the region.

Epidemiology and transmission

The distribution of BTV between 40° N and 35° S reflects the distribution of its main biological vectors, certain tropical and subtropical species of *Culicoides* midges, in particular *Culicoides imicola* in Africa and the Middle East, *C. variipennis* in North America and *C. brevitarsis*, *C. fulvus* and *C. wadai* in North Australia.

The adult female *Culicoides* lays her eggs in damp muddy areas containing decaying vegetable material or in cattle dung, two to six days after a blood meal. Depending on the temperature these eggs may hatch in two to three days into larva. The larval stage lasts 12–16 days, followed by pupation and, two to three days later, the emergence of the adult *Culicoides*. In the subsequent 24 hours the adults take a blood meal and mate, and they will continue to take a blood meal every three to four days until the end of their life, which may last for 70 days but probably rarely exceeds 10. Optimum conditions are between 13 and 35 °C. Larvae of temperate species can remain dormant over winter and pupate the following spring. Seven to ten days after taking a BTV-infected blood meal, vector species of *Culicoides* midge are able to transmit virus.

Culicoides usually feed at dusk, during the night or at dawn, and are subject to being transported, sometimes over considerable distances, by strong wind currents. The passive movement of infected *Culicoides* is considered responsible for the introduction of BT into areas usually outside the enzootic region, such as western Turkey and Cyprus. This introduction of BTV into an area may be associated with abnormal wind currents or may be a regular occurrence. The winds of the Intertropical Convergence Zone annually re-introduce BTV-infected *Culicoides* to South Africa from Central Africa. The movement of BTV into Sudan from Central Africa is also associated with a prevailing wind from the South. However, BT may also become enzootic in new regions as climatic changes allow the main vectors to extend their breeding sites or, alternatively, virulent strains of new serotypes of BTV may be introduced into an area already infected with mild or avirulent strains.

Within BT enzootic regions the prevalence of seropositive animals may be very localized around areas particularly suitable for the breeding and survival of *Culicoides*; so-called 'hot spots'. The possibility also exists for new species of *Culicoides* to take on the role of BTV vectors; it has recently been shown that some British species of *Culicoides* can biologically transmit BTV under experimental conditions.

Bulls may shed BTV in their semen intermittently during the viraemia following infection. Bowen *et al.* (1985) classified bulls into three categories: those from which virus could not be isolated from the semen (the majority), those from which only low titres of virus were isolated on less than three occasions, and those which shed virus over a two to three week period. Bluetongue virus could only be isolated from the semen when there was a concurrent viraemia. Six out of nine susceptible heifers inseminated with the BTV-contaminated semen became pregnant, and three of the nine became viraemic. None of the calves born at term showed any clinical abnormality. Considerable importance has been attached to reports of a bull that was persistently infected but seronegative from birth, and intermittently shed virus in semen over an 11-year period (Luedke *et al.*, 1982). Attempts to duplicate the conditions that produce persistently BTV-infected, seronegative calves have been unsuccessful.

Host range

Sheep, goats, cattle, water buffalo, camels and many wild ruminants are susceptible to infection with BTV. However, BT is predominantly a disease of sheep and has only been reported as a disease of cattle in the USA, South Africa, Israel and Portugal.

Pathogenesis

Infection follows the bite of an infected *Culicoides* midge. The virus is carried to the local lymph node where primary replication occurs before dissemination of virus throughout the body. Viral replication then continues in the spleen, lungs, bone marrow and other lymph glands. In sheep, BTV also replicates in the endothelial cells of the blood vessels and, unlike in cattle, has been clearly shown to cross the placenta and can replicate in the developing fetus causing fetal resorption, abortion or developmental abnormalities. The peak viraemia occurs two to three weeks after infection, its duration and severity depending on the strain of BTV.

Clinical signs

Bluetongue in cattle is seen as a transient fever followed by hyperaemia and erosions of the buccal and lingual mucosa and nose and, rarely, the teats. Affected cattle salivate excessively and may walk with a stiff gait. The skin of the nose appears mottled and dark and has been described as 'burnt muzzle', and may completely slough. Fewer than 1 per cent of cattle in the USA infected with BTV show signs, and the lesions may be due to a delayed type hypersensitivity reaction. There is considerable controversy over whether BTV can cross the placenta of the pregnant cow. If the virus is able to cross the placenta it may only do so in association with other placental pathogens, or be restricted to only certain strains of BTV.

Diagnosis

It is not possible to make a diagnosis of BT on solely clinical signs. Cattle infected with BTV develop precipitating antibody detectable on an agar gel precipitation test (AGPT), which is not BTV serotype specific. Type-specific neutralizing antibodies can be titrated in a virus neutralization test using BHK21 cells in a microplate against each of the BTV types present or suspected present in the area. Some cross-reaction is seen on the AGPT with antibodies to EHD virus; however, a group specific competition enzyme-linked immunosorbent assay (ELISA) using monoclonal antibody that does not cross-react with EHD antibody is now available. The viraemia associated with BTV infection can persist up to 120 days, in the presence of neutralizing antibodies. The virus is attached to the red blood cells and appears to be protected from the developing immune response. Intravenous inoculation of sonicated blood into eight to ten-day-old embryonated chicken eggs is a very sensitive laboratory method of isolating virus from blood; whereas the inoculation of suspect material directly into sheep and examining sequential serum samples for evidence of seroconversion is the most sensitive test available. Virus can also be grown in the yolk sac of six-day-old eggs kept between 33.5 and 35 °C, lamb kidney cells, hamster lung cells, BHK21 cells, some mosquito cell lines and following intracerebral inoculation of day-old mice. Chick embryos that die from BTV infection have a characteristic haemorrhagic appearance.

Control

Bluetongue is a non-contagious disease and can only spread by the bite of infected *Culicoides* or the direct transfer of blood or semen from an infected to a susceptible animal. Bluetongue may be controlled by eliminating the vector or vaccinating susceptible animals against the serotypes prevalent in the area. Control of insects has usually been directed towards those insects that carry human disease, and experience gained in these programmes could undoubtedly be of value in BT control. However, there would be little economic justification for attempting to control *Culicoides* solely to prevent BT in cattle.

Cattle can be protected against BTV infection by vaccination with live attenuated vaccine. The practice of mixing together vaccines against each of the prevalent serotypes may result in the failure of one or more of the serotypes present in the vaccine to replicate (Jeggo, 1986). However, vaccination against one serotype, followed one month later with a second serotype can provide protection not only against the two serotypes in the vaccines, but can provide a heterologous protection against a third serotype (Jeggo, 1986). There would still be the difficulty of predicting the probable challenge BTV serotypes. The distribution of the serotypes of BTV tends to be dynamic, with some serotypes being present one year to be replaced the following year by other serotypes.

There is no evidence to indicate that BT can be transmitted during embryo transfer using standard techniques. Bluetongue virus can be transmitted in the semen collected from viraemic bulls, but reports of a persistently infected, seronegative animal (Luedke *et al.*, 1982) have not been confirmed by further research.

Economic significance

The cost of BTV infection in a 1400 dairy cow herd in California, in terms of reduced fertility was $23 000 over a 52-week study period (Osborn *et al.*, 1986). Of particular interest in this study was that the dairyworker responsible for the herd was unaware of the passage of BTV through the herd, and the associated increase in return to service of the affected animals. There is, therefore, the possibility that BT has a greater economic significance in cattle than previously thought, and should not be considered solely in terms of isolated epizootics.

Animals and semen from BTV enzootic areas are subject to movement and export restriction, the cost of which are of greater significance than the direct effects of disease. Many of these restrictions have been formulated on unconfirmed experiments, but they reflect the cautious attitude of the veterinary authorities of importing countries.

(b) Enzootic Bovine Leukosis

by M.H. LUCAS

The disease

Enzootic bovine leukosis (EBL) was first described over 100 years ago in Europe. The disease occurs as multiple cases of lymphosarcoma most frequently seen in animals from three to eight years of age. Tumours may develop in peripheral lymph nodes, in which case the condition is easily recognized, but they may be confined to internal organs resulting in ill-defined signs. In some countries appreciable economic loss occurs through the tumorous form of the disease. Early this century it was recognized that the disease could spread slowly from known foci to adjoining regions. Because lymphosarcoma often occurred in familial aggregations it was interpreted as evidence that the disease was heritable. It is now known that EBL is caused by bovine leukosis virus (BLV). The causative virus was identified first by Miller *et al.* (1969) in the USA since when it has been cultivated *in vitro* and characterized.

The virus

Bovine leukosis virus is an RNA virus belonging to the Retroviridae family. The family includes tumour and non tumour-forming viruses of various species including man. The retrovirus genome is composed of single-stranded RNA, which is converted to DNA by means of the enzyme reverse transcriptase. This enables many retroviruses to become integrated into the DNA of the host cells where they can persist for the life of the animal, bringing about transformation of certain of the cells. Bovine leukosis virus is present in a subpopulation of circulating B lymphocytes where its genetic information is found integrated at a large number of sites in the cellular DNA. Lymphocytes of BLV-induced tumours appear to be of the B cell lineage. Tumour cells are monoclonal or oligoclonal for the site of BLV integration. No evidence has been observed so far for a common integration site for BLV provirus in different tumours.

Several proteins exist in the virion, but as far as diagnosis is concerned two are important, an internal protein antigen with a molecular weight of 24 000 referred to as p24, and a glycoprotein antigen in the envelope with a molecular weight of 51 000 referred to as gp51.

The virus is probably not very stable in situations outside the host. It is destroyed by exposure to ultraviolet light, freezing and thawing, heating at 56 °C for 30 minutes and pasteurization. The virus survives in blood stored at 4 °C for at least two weeks.

Distribution

The virus is distributed world-wide, there being marked regional differences in prevalence. It is relatively common in some parts of Europe and North and South America.

Transmission

Virus is found in the cellular fraction of blood, but not in plasma or serum unless haemolysis has occurred during storage. Virus is also present in colostrum and milk, in tracheal and bronchial secretions, and sometimes in nasal secretions and saliva of infected animals. Virus has not been found in faeces or urine and is probably absent from the semen of most infected bulls.

Very small numbers of blood cells are capable of initiating infection. As little as 0.1 μl of whole blood from an infected cow can be infectious when given intradermally to cattle. Cattle can be infected by the intratracheal route though not as reliably as by the subcutaneous route. Infection can be transmitted by instillation of infected lymphocytes into the nose and by aerosol exposure to cell-free BLV. Calves can be infected orally when newborn but are probably resistant to oral infection by three weeks of age. Adult cattle do not become infected by the oral route. Adult cows can be infected by the instillation of infected lymphocytes into the reproductive tract but semen mixed with the inoculum may have an inhibitory effect on transmission and susceptibility of the genital tract of cows may decrease at the time of oestrus. The virus has been transmitted experimentally to sheep and cattle by rectal inoculation of whole blood from infected cattle.

Sheep can readily be infected experimentally by the parenteral routes but not consistently by the oral route. Between 10^3 and 10^6 lymphocytes from infected cattle, given intravenously, were sufficient to infect sheep. Tumours arise at a higher frequency and after a much shorter time than in cattle. Sheep may die of lymphosarcoma within seven years after inoculation with virus. Tumours develop after 10 months to three years. As in cattle various lymph nodes and visceral organs including heart, abomasum, uterus, kidney and urinary tract are commonly affected. Persistent lymphocytosis is not usual in sheep; once the number of circulating lymphocytes rises it invariably indicates the onset of the tumour stage. Bovine leukosis virus can be transmitted transplacentally to the fetus. In contrast to the situation with cattle, contact transmission does not occur when infected sheep are kept in close contact with susceptible sheep.

Goats inoculated with BLV orally and parenterally become infected and develop antibody but do not usually develop persistent lymphocytosis or lymphosarcoma. The incubation period in sheep and goats varies from about two to sixteen weeks or longer.

Experimental infection with BLV as indicated by persistent antibody production has been reported for chimpanzees, macaques, pigs, domestic rabbits, cats, dogs, deer and rats. No evidence for the production of BLV antibodies followed BLV inoculation in the mouse, chipmunk, ground squirrel, Japanese quail and chicken.

Iatrogenic transmission is probably one of the main reasons for the high prevalence of infection in some herds. Bovine leukosis virus can be transmitted by transfer of infected blood from one animal to another on a hypodermic needle and the use of multidose syringes has been incriminated in virus spread. There is no published evidence to associate tuberculin testing with an increased incidence of enzootic bovine leukosis and experimentally there was no spread when susceptible calves and infected animals were injected alternately by the usual intradermal technique. Protozoal vaccines have been known, or suspected, vehicles for virus spread. Dehorning and ear tattooing have been identified as possible methods of transmission. It has been suggested that the technique of rectal palpation to examine the reproductive tracts of cows could be a means of transmission if separate clean gloves were not used for each animal.

Transmission of virus by contact is one of the most important means of spread of BLV in a herd. The rate of spread of virus is influenced by management and husbandry practices that determine the degree of contact between animals. Because the virus probably does not survive for long in the environment and because infectivity is associated with the cellular fraction of secretions it is therefore assumed that transmission takes place by direct exchange of infected lymphocytes in nasal, saliva and tracheobronchial fluids and possibly vaginal discharges.

The role of milk in transmission under natural conditions does not appear to be very great. The presence of specific antibody in these secretions inhibits virus transmission, and also the susceptibility of the calf to oral infection decreases with age.

Vertical transmission of the virus genome via the gametes does not occur. However, congenital transmission by the transplacental route occurs occasionally. Not all infected cows produce infected fetuses and individual cows may give birth to some infected and some uninfected calves. Fetuses infected *in utero* vary in their serological and virological status, and some may develop neoplastic lesions in the lymphatic tissue.

Transfer of embryos from BLV-infected cows into uninfected cows is not associated with transmission of virus. Virus has nevertheless been found in uterine flush fluid, but this may be due to contamination with blood cells. Virus has not been found in eggs or embryos from infected cattle.

Ova, morulae and blastocysts have been exposed *in vitro* to BLV, but after washing no virus could be detected. Embryos similarly exposed to virus were washed and then transferred to uninfected cows, which did not subsequently develop antibodies to BLV. It was concluded that it was safe to transfer embryos from infected cows providing that the embryos were washed before transfer. Virus transmission to dam or to progeny is not associated with the use of semen from infected bulls for artificial insemination (AI). Transmission by biting insects may be important in tropical and subtropical climates. Statistical evidence of seasonal trends is inconclusive.

Naturally occurring lymphosarcoma in sheep is rare. A retrovirus has been isolated from a diseased sheep and was found to be identical to BLV. Where BLV is found in sheep a cattle origin must be suspected. The virus has also been found in capybaras and water buffaloes. Human beings potentially exposed to BLV do not develop anti-BLV antibodies.

Following infection of an animal with BLV progress of the disease depends on genetic, environmental and unknown factors. Over 60 per cent of infected cattle are asymptomatic. Almost all develop detectable antibodies. Between 30 and 70 per cent of infected animals show persistent lymphocytosis and less than 10 per cent develop lymphosarcoma. Persistent lymphocytosis is seen in 28–85 per cent of tumour cases. In BLV-infected cattle with leukaemia the increase in leucocyte count is due to an increase in B lymphocytes. The percentage of B lymphocytes in the blood can rise to 80 per cent, compared with normal values of 15–20 per cent. In clinically normal BLV-infected cattle without lymphocytosis there can still be an increase in B lymphocytes to 40–50 per cent.

Signs

Clinical signs (Figs 37.1, 37.2) in animals that develop tumours depend on the particular organ or organs involved. One or more superficial lymph nodes may be enlarged and these can be felt as lumps beneath the skin especially in the neck and hind flank areas. However, when the internal lymph nodes are the only ones affected diagnosis may be more difficult. Tumours can occur in the abomasum, right side of the heart, spine, uterus, lymph nodes and the retrobulbar aspect of the orbit. Clinical signs may include depression, indigestion, chronic bloat, displaced abomasum, lameness or paralysis. Abdominal tumours are sometimes detected by rectal palpation during pregnancy examination.

Infection with BLV does not appear to be associated with lower milk production, impaired reproductive capacity in either sex, or with mastitis, lesser longevity or increased susceptibility to other diseases. Bovine leukosis virus does not appear to cause significant immunosuppression in the fetus or adult animal.

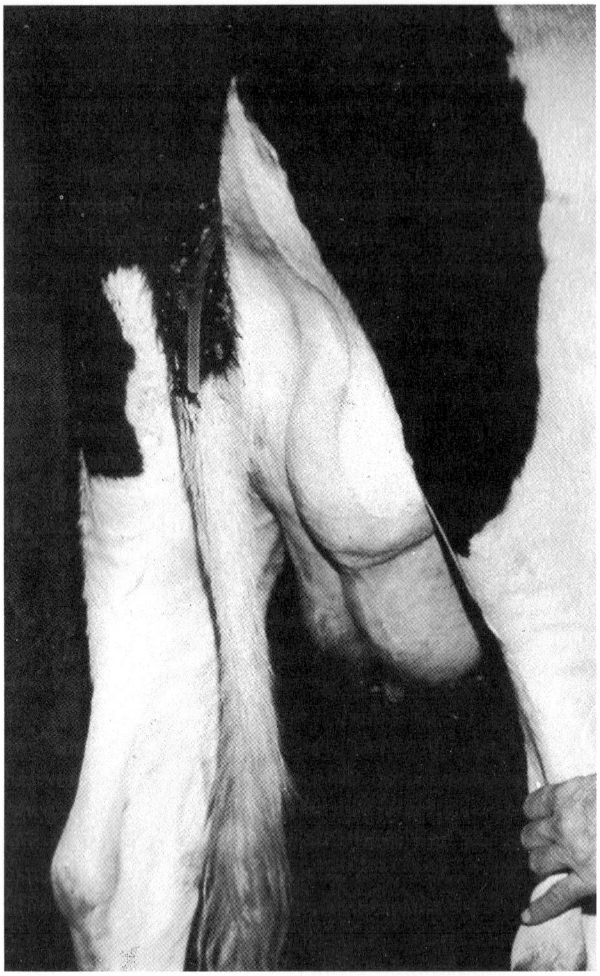

Fig. 37.1 A cow with enzootic bovine leukosis showing enlargement of the mammary lymph nodes. (Courtesy of Dr J. Miller, USDA National Animal Diseases Center, Ames, Iowa, USA and editors and publishers of Modern Veterinary Production.)

Diagnosis

Haematological. Herds with a high incidence of the adult form of lymphosarcoma often contain many clinically normal cattle with persistent lymphocytosis. The development of lymphosarcoma is often preceded by a period in which the animal has persistent lymphocytosis without any clinical signs of disease. Haematological methods were the main diagnostic tools for a number of years and various 'keys' were developed relating lymphocyte counts and age, presenting maximal values above which an animal was declared to have persistent lymphocytosis. The percentage of B lymphocytes in normal cattle varies from 18 to 28 per cent. In BLV-infected cattle with persistent lymphocytosis the percentage of B lymphocytes can increase to as high as 70 per cent. In clinically normal BLV-infected cattle without lymphocytosis the B lymphocytes are increased to 40–50 per cent.

Nuclear pockets are structures that can be seen in lymphocytes using the electron microscope. In normal animals these pockets are seen very rarely, but in BLV-infected animals the number increases.

Serological. The agar gel immunodiffusion test can be used to detect antibody to viral antigens p15, p24 and gp51. The test for gp51 antibody is more sensitive than the p15 and p24 tests or haematology for the detection of infected animals. The test is simple and practical and has been very widely used. The glycoprotein antigen employed in the test is prepared from the supernatant

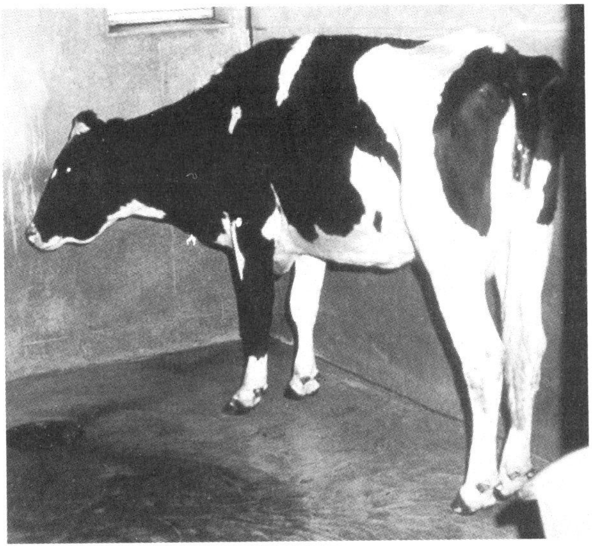

Fig. 37.2 Adult cow with enzootic bovine leukosis showing loss of condition, with wasting of lumbar muscle, brisket and submandibular swelling. (Courtesy of J. Miller, USA.)

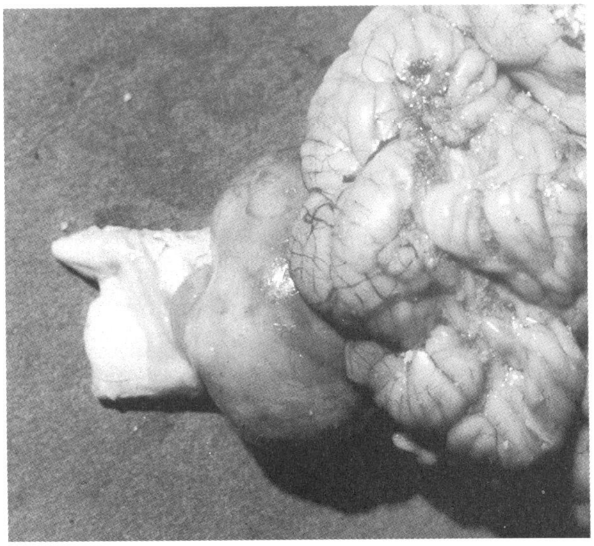

Fig. 37.3 Brain from a cow with neoplasm between cerebellum and medulla. (Courtesy of J. Miller, USA.)

fluid of a cell line persistently infected with BLV. Using cells from BLV-infected monolayer cell cultures, sera can also be tested for specific antibodies by indirect immunofluorescence of immunoperoxidase techniques. Virus neutralization tests have been used that are based on the ability of antibodies to inhibit the effects of BLV in cell cultures. These include a virus neutralization test, a syncytia inhibition or syncytia induction test, early polykaryocytosis test and a pseudotype inhibition test. The last is based on the inhibition of the plaque-forming activity of pseudotypes of vesicular stomatitis virus (or chandipura virus) with envelope antigens of BLV. The complement fixation test using viral antigens from a cell line infected with BLV has been described, but seems to be less sensitive than the agar gel immunodiffusion test for antibodies to the gp antigen. A major disadvantage of the complement fixation test is that many bovine sera are anticomplementary. It is possible to carry out a reverse transcriptase inhibition test based on the fact that serum of some leukaemic cattle inhibits the activity of the reverse transcriptase of BLV. Radioimmunoassay is very sensitive but has the disadvantage that radiolabelled reagents and special equipment are required. Enzyme-linked immunosorbent assay (ELISA) has been adapted in several ways to detect BLV antibodies. The test can be used with milk or tissue fluids as well as serum samples. The test is rapid, sensitive and suited to the testing of large numbers of samples and will probably become more popular as the reagents and test protocols become more standardized.

Isolation and detection of BLV. Virus particles can be seen by electron microscopy in short-term cultures of lymphocytes from BLV-infected animals. Cell culture methods of detection are based on the ability of the virus to induce syncytia in a number of different types of cell monolayers. All the serological tests for the detection of antibodies against BLV can be adapted for the detection of viral antigens. Sheep inoculation is a sensitive method to detect BLV.

Control

Appropriate control measures in any particular situation depend on factors such as prevalence of infection, importance of restrictions on ability to sell cattle, husbandry practices, economic and political considerations, etc. Importers often require animals to be free of virus, which is one reason why many countries are developing control programmes such as eradication or attested herd schemes.

Effective strategies for producing a BLV-free herd include the following.

1 BLV-positive animals are kept physically separated from BLV-negative animals. Check-testing of negative animals is carried out at intervals.

2 Calves born from negative cows are kept apart from infected animals.

3 Calves born from infected cows are reared only on

colostrum and milk from negative cows and are kept isolated. If serologically negative at seven months of age these calves join the negative herd.

4 Introduced animals are tested and found virus free. If they come from an infected herd or from a herd of unknown status they are retested after about 30 days and six months.

5 Embryo transfer and AI are sometimes used as part of a control programme so that new genetic stock can be introduced with minimal risk of introducing BLV.

Vaccination

Preliminary experiments using inactivated BLV, persistently infected cell lines or purified gp51 show that these can produce short-term protection to BLV infection. High antibody titres to gp51 appear to be necessary for protection. Three epitopes that are present on a 15 000 Da peptide fragment of BLV gp51 determine important biological functions of the virus. These epitopes could be the basis of an artificial BLV vaccine. There is some evidence that vaccines prepared from cell lines derived from cases of sporadic bovine leukosis can also produce some short-term immunity to EBL; the mechanism involved is not clear.

Public health

Interest in public health aspects arises for a number of reasons. Virus is present in unpasteurized milk, there is a close occupational contact of humans with cattle, the virus replicates in human cell lines, and virus was apparently transmitted to chimpanzees fed unpasteurized milk from infected cows. Also there is some structural relationship of BLV to the human viruses HTLV-1 and HTLV-2; there is limited evidence so far for a relationship with HIV (LAV/HTLV-3). Some studies have claimed circumstantial evidence for an association between bovine and human leukaemia. There is, however, no incontrovertible evidence that BLV can infect humans.

Sporadic bovine leukosis

Lymphosarcomas are found in young animals in the absence of BLV and these are generally classified as sporadic bovine leukosis. Three forms of sporadic bovine leukosis exist. The *juvenile* form in calves under six months of age involves lymph nodes, liver, spleen and bone marrow (Figs 37.4–37.7). Few signs are seen in this form during the first part of the disease in spite of marked enlargement of the superficial lymph nodes. As the disease progresses internal organs such as the heart and liver become affected (Plates 37b.1 and 37b.2) and this leads to the death of the animal. The *thymic* form is seen in animals 6–30 months old. There is massive tumour formation in the thymus and tumorous changes are also seen in the nodes of the neck and thorax (Fig. 37.8, Plate 37b.3). The condition is fatal. The *cutaneous* form is a rare condition occurring in animals 18 months to three years of age, in which nodular lymphocytic neoplasia is seen in the skin. The first signs are urticaria-like nodules in the skin, especially round the neck, back and thighs (Fig. 37.9). The

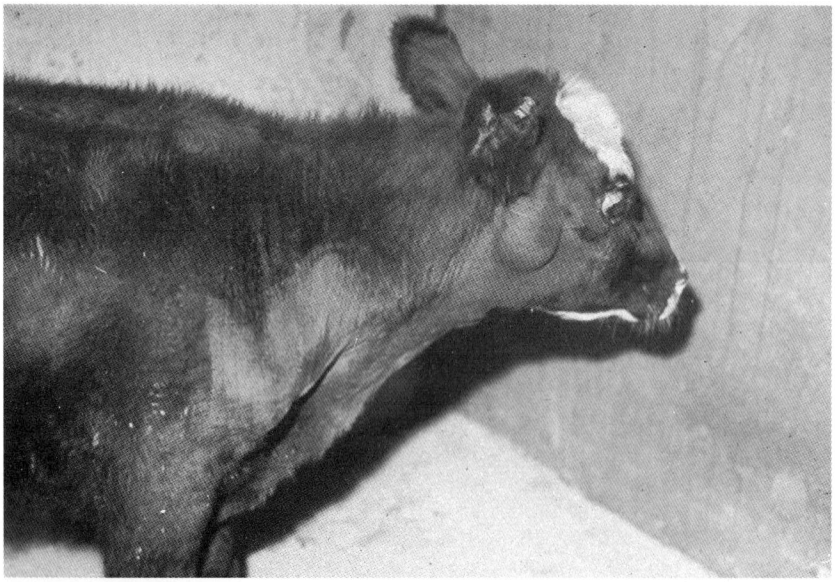

Fig. 37.4 Sporadic bovine leukosis in calf with parotid lymph node enlargement. (Courtesy of J. Miller, USA.)

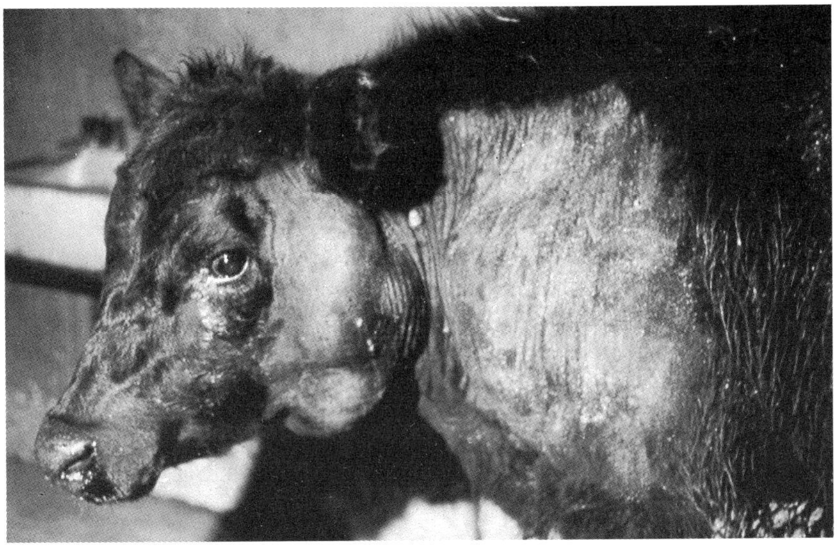

Fig. 37.5 Sporadic bovine leukosis in calf with submandibular, parotid and retropharyngeal lymph nodes on the head and prescapular lymph node enlargement. (Courtesy of J. Miller, USA.)

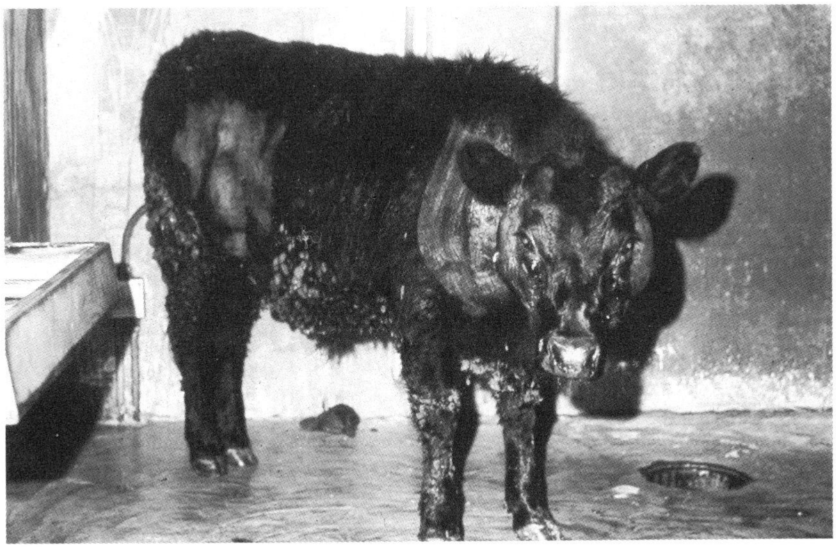

Fig. 37.6 Same calf as in Fig. 37.5 showing gross distension of the head lymph nodes and the prefemoral lymph nodes. (Courtesy of J. Miller, USA.)

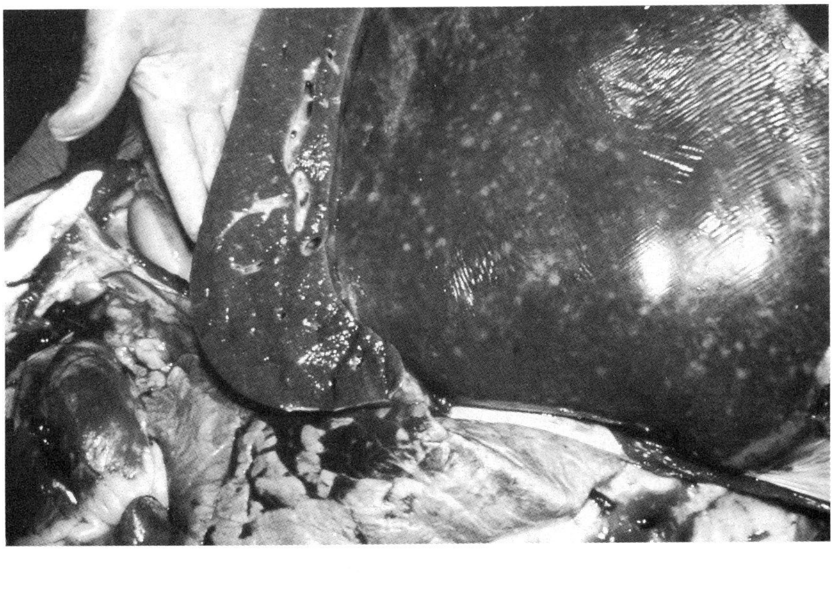

Fig. 37.7 Liver from a calf with sporadic bovine leukosis showing the surface and cut surface with focal neoplastic areas. (Courtesy of J. Miller, USA.)

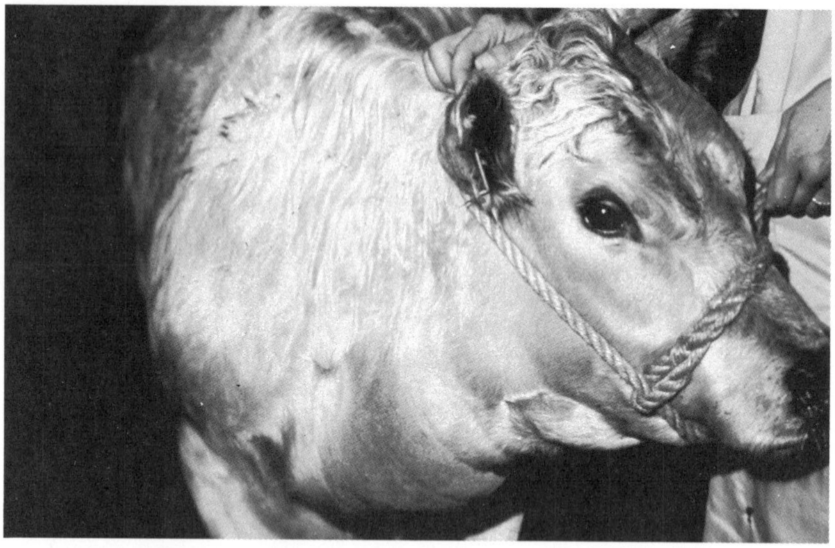

Fig. 37.8 Bullock showing thymic neoplasm. (Courtesy of J. Miller, USA.)

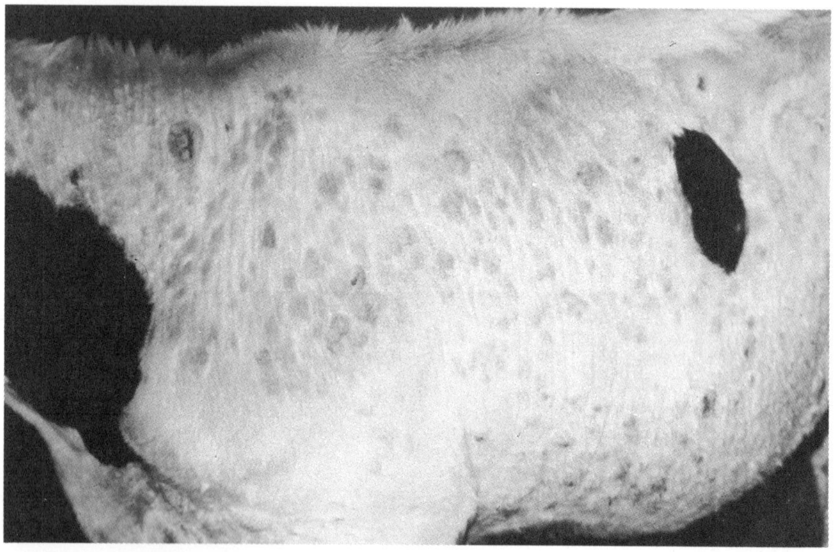

Fig. 37.9 A heifer with acute cutaneous leukosis. (Courtesy of J. Miller, USA.)

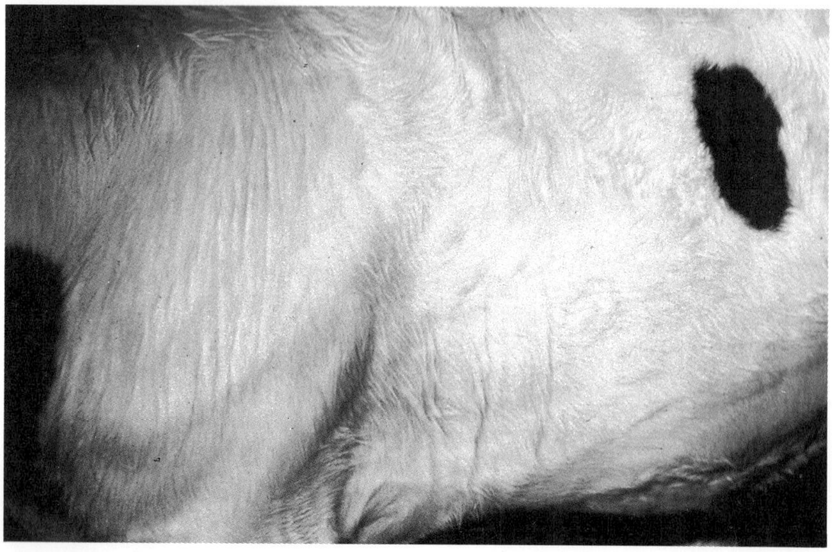

Fig. 37.10 Same heifer as in Fig. 37.9 with cutaneous leukosis lesions subsequently resolving. (Courtesy of J. Miller, USA.)

nodules have a diameter of 1–2 cm. These become encrusted with thick scabs, and alopecia and hyperkeratosis follow. If the animal survives, apparent recovery takes place in several weeks (Fig. 37.10). However, the remission is temporary and lesions develop again but this time with genera lymph node involvement resulting in death. The cause or causes of sporadic bovine leukosis are unknown.

(c) Foot-and-mouth Disease

by R.P. KITCHING

Foot-and-mouth disease (FMD) is a highly contagious disease of domesticated and wild ungulates characterized by vesicles in the mouth and on the feet. Hedgehogs and rarely man may also become infected.

Aetiology

Foot-and-mouth disease is caused by infection with a virus of the genus aphthovirus, in the family Picornaviridae. There are seven antigenically distinct types of FMD virus, identified as types A, O, C, SAT (South African Territories) 1, SAT 2, SAT 3 and Asia 1. Within each of these seven types there are a large number of strains that form an antigenic spectrum, from closely related strains to strains so antigenically different as almost to justify the establishment of additional types. Attempts to classify the strains into subtypes within the types foundered on the ever-increasing number of strains that fulfilled the criteria for creating a new subtype. New isolates of FMD virus are now referred to by the World Reference Laboratory (WRL) for FMD by their type, country of origin, a sequential number relating to the number of isolates received in that year from the same country, and the final two numbers of the year in which they were received, e.g. O India 53/79, Asia 1 India 8/79. Classical subtyping is now only of historical interest.

Aphthovirus has an icosahedral symmetry and a diameter of 24 nm. The outer capsid consists of 32 capsomeres and surrounds a single-stranded molecule of RNA of approximately 8000 bases, and molecular mass 2.8×10^6 Da. This RNA codes for a single large polyprotein that is cleaved into at least six non-structural proteins and the four structural proteins (VP1, VP2, VP3 and VP4), 60 copies of which make up the outer capsid. The RNA base sequence is extremely variable, which is reflected in variations in the amino acid sequence of the proteins for which it codes. The structural characteristics of the outer capsid proteins of the virus stimulates an immune response in the infected host animal. Thus variations in the genome that change the structure of these proteins can reduce the ability of a vaccinated or previously infected animal to resist challenge with a new strain of virus.

Distribution

Foot-and-mouth disease is endemic throughout most of South America, Africa, the Middle and Far East. Canada, Central and North America, Australia, New Zealand, Japan, Scandinavia, Ireland and Great Britain are free of FMD. Most of continental Europe is also free of FMD, but suffers occasional outbreaks of disease in spite of strict quarantine regulations and compulsory cattle vaccination. From 1992 routine vaccination against FMD will cease in all countries of the European Community.

Types O, A and C of FMD virus are the most widespread, especially in South America, the Middle East and Asia; types SAT 1, SAT 2 and SAT 3 are generally restricted to Africa, although they have periodically spread into the Middle East; and Asia 1 occurs in the Far East and India, although it also has spread into the Middle East.

Epidemiology

Foot-and-mouth disease is an extremely contagious disease, with as few as 10 infectious units being able to initiate disease in a bovine by the respiratory route. The virus can survive in dry faecal material for 14 days in summer, in slurry up to six months in winter, in urine for 39 days and on the soil between three days in summer and 28 days in winter. Foot-and-mouth disease virus is, however, very susceptible to inactivation by extremes of pH, i.e. below pH 5.0 and above pH 11.0. It is most stable between pH 7.2 and 7.6. Within this range at 4 °C the virus can survive up to a year but, as the temperature is increased, its survival time is reduced to eight to ten weeks at 22 °C, 10 days at 37 °C and to less than 30 minutes at 56 °C. The survival of airborne virus is optimal when the relative humidity is above 60 per cent. Natural ultraviolet light in sunlight has little direct effect on FMD virus.

Like many diseases, FMD is most commonly spread by the movement of infected animals, and in this respect attention must especially be given to sheep, goats and wild ungulates, because disease in them can be mild, and to pigs because of the amounts of virus they can excrete. An infected pig excretes up to 400 million infectious units/day, 3000 times more than an infected bovine, sheep or goat. In infected cattle, milk products and semen many contain FMD virus up to four days before the appearance of clinical signs and can also be responsible for the spread of disease. Pigs can carry virus for 10 days before disease is manifested. Lorries, fomites and stockworkers may also be contaminated with virus from infected carcasses, although the reduced pH of the carcass following *rigor mortis* is sufficient to inactivate the virus in the meat.

The possibility of wind-borne spread of FMD virus has been given considerable significance, particularly in temperate countries where the climate is conducive to the survival of the virus. There is evidence to indicate that FMD virus has been carried up to 250 km over the sea and up to 60 km over land. The spread of disease by the wind is dependent on the amount of virus generated by infected animals, the weather conditions, the topography over which it is carried, and the susceptibility of the animals contacting the airborne virus. A plume of virus will be subjected to vertical and horizontal dispersion, which is related to wind speed and turbulence, the vertical air temperature gradient and ground topography; the survival of the airborne virus will depend on relative humidity. Cattle have a large respiratory tidal volume compared with other FMD-susceptible stock and can be infected following inhalation of relatively low quantities of virus and thus are most at danger to infection from the airborne virus. Wind-borne spread of FMD virus is believed to have occurred in 1981 when infected pigs in Brittany, France, spread disease to cattle in the Isle of Wight, England, over a distance of 250 km, predominantly over sea. Computer models now exist that can predict the likely wind-borne spread of virus from an infected herd. The maximum daily excretion of virus can be calculated by establishing the number of clinically infected animals and the species infected, and estimating the duration and quantity of airborne virus excreted. The local meteorological office provides information about wind speed and direction, relative humidity and precipitation. When combined with local topographical information and local distribution of livestock holdings, the computer model can give an indication of which herds are most at risk from secondary wind-borne spread of FMD. Manpower resources for surveillance activity can then be concentrated on the herds adjudged to be at greatest risk.

In tracing the movement of FMD between countries, and identifying specific strains of FMD virus, molecular epidemiology has proved very valuable. By precisely characterizing an outbreak strain by the size of its structural proteins and RNA nucleotide sequence, it is possible to show its relationship to strains previously isolated in other countries or in use in vaccines. For instance, in Europe over the last 20 years, there have been a number of FMD outbreaks attributed to the use of improperly inactivated vaccines and escape of virus from establishments producing vaccine. In several instances biochemical analysis of the outbreak strains has shown a clear identity between these and vaccine strains in contemporary use. The techniques currently in use are polyacrylamide gel electrophoresis and isoelectric focusing to identify the viral proteins, and T_1 mapping and RNA nucleotide sequencing to characterize the viral genome (Kitching *et al.*, 1989). However, the variability and rapid mutation rate of FMD virus can sometimes make interpretation of results problematical.

Monoclonal antibodies, which specifically identify some of the individual antigenic determinants on the FMD virus, are also becoming important in FMD virus strain characterization. These determinants may change as the virus mutates through the course of an outbreak, particularly if the outbreak is in a partially immune population.

Cattle recovered from FMD and vaccinated cattle in contact with FMD virus may retain virus in their pharyngeal region for many months. This is the carrier state. Vaccinated cattle that have had contact with disease may also develop a pharyngeal infection without showing any clinical signs. The significance of these carrier animals is not clear but, although it has proven difficult to show transmission from a carrier to a susceptible animal under experimental conditions, circumstantial evidence suggests that they may have initiated outbreaks.

Transmission and pathogenesis

Cattle are most susceptible to FMD by inoculation of the virus intradermally into the tongue and this is commonly used method of challenging cattle during vaccine trials. However, natural infection is most frequently by inhalation of droplets containing FMD virus or by ingestion of FMD virus contaminated material. One infectious unit of FMD virus is sufficient to infect a bovine by intradermolingual inoculation, while between

10 and 100 infectious units can initiate disease in a bovine following inhalation. Many thousand infectious units may be required to infect an adult bovine by ingestion, or a calf by insufflation of infected milk.

The primary site of replication of inhaled virus is in the pharynx and lymphoid tissue of the upper respiratory tract. The virus then enters the bloodstream, is distributed around the body and following secondary replication in other glandular tissues appears in the body fluids such as milk, urine, respiratory secretions and semen, before the appearance of frank clinical signs of FMD. However, it is during the early vesicular stage of the disease that the majority of virus is excreted into the environment. Milk may contain $\log_{10}$ 6.7 infectious doses_{50}/ml, semen $\log_{10}$ 6.2 infectious doses_{50}/ml, urine $\log_{10}$ 4.9 infectious doses_{50}/ml and faeces $\log_{10}$ 5.0 infectious doses_{50}/g.

An infected bovine can excrete up to $\log_{10}$ 5.1 infectious doses_{50}/day by the respiratory route and can provide a potent source of FMD virus to the remaining uninfected cattle in the herd. This may be sufficient to overcome a waning vaccinal immunity.

The incubation period for FMD can be up to 14 days with low infecting doses and with strains of virus of low virulence. However, as the quantity of virus in the environment of an FMD outbreak increases, the incubation period in cattle decreases. For susceptible cattle in contact with an infected animal it is frequently between two and four days.

Clinical signs (Figs 37.11–37.13)

The incubation period is between two and fourteen days, depending on the route of infection, the dose, the strain of virus and the susceptibility of the host. Following an initial pyrexia in the region of 40 °C (104 °F), lasting one or two days, a variable number of vesicles develop on the tongue, hard palate, dental pad, lips, muzzle, coronary band and interdigital space. Vesicles may also be seen on the teats, particularly of lactating cows. Young calves may die before the development of vesicles because of a predilection by the virus to invade and destroy the cells of the developing heart muscle.

The vesicles in the mouth quickly rupture, usually within one to two days of their formation, leaving a shallow ulcer surrounded by shreds of epithelium (Fig. 37.11). The vesicles on the tongue frequently coalesce and a large proportion of the dorsal epithelium of the tongue may be displaced (Fig. 37.12). The vesicles on the feet (Fig. 37.13) may remain for two to three days before rupturing, depending on the terrain or floor surface of the cattle accommodation. Healing of the mouth lesions is usually rapid; the ulcers fill with fibrin and by day 10 after vesicle formation they appear as areas of pink fibrous tissue, still, however, without normal tongue papillae. Healing of the lesions on the feet is more protracted and the ulcers are susceptible to secondary bacterial infection. The horn of the heels may become underrun, both as a consequence of the initial vesicle and secondary bacterial infection.

Acutely infected cattle salivate profusely and develop a nasal discharge, at first mucoid and then mucopurulent, which covers the muzzle. They stamp their feet as they try to relieve the pressure on first one foot and then another. They may prefer to lie down and resist attempts to raise them. Lactating cattle with teat lesions (see p. 327 and Plate 25.24) are difficult to milk and the lesions frequently become infected predisposing to secondary mastitis. Affected cattle quickly lose condition, the drop in milk yield can be dramatic and will not be recovered during the remaining lactation. Some animals fail completely to regain their previous condition, due to the development of lesions in the thyroid gland ('hairy panters').

An outbreak of FMD can be economically devastating in an intensively farmed region. However, in the extensive husbandry systems of South America and Africa where expectations of cattle productivity are low, FMD may seem insignificant compared with the prevalent clostridial, haemoparasite and deficiency diseases. This attitude frustrates programmes completely to control FMD and attempts to introduce intensive farming or a dairy industry.

Pathology

The epithelial cells of the stratum spinosum of the skin undergo ballooning degeneration. As the cells disrupt and oedema fluid accumulates, vesicles develop which coalesce to form the aphthae and bullae that characterize FMD. The cells of the squamous epithelium of the rumen, reticulum and omasum may also become involved. In young animals the virus invades the cells of the myocardium and macroscopic grey lesions may be seen particularly in the wall of the left ventricle, giving it a striped appearance (tiger heart). Cells of the skeletal muscles may also undergo hyaline degeneration.

Diagnosis

Initial diagnosis is usually on the basis of clinical signs, with or without a history of contact between the herd and an infected animal, or reports of FMD in the vicin-

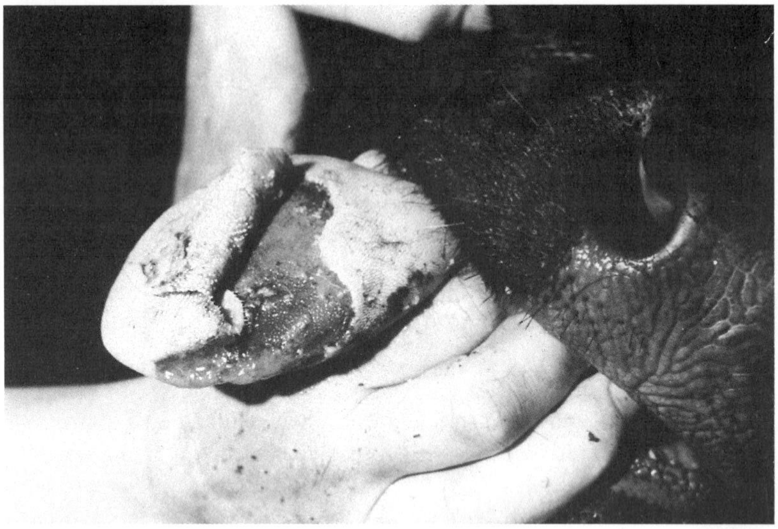

Fig. 37.11 A recently ruptured vesicle in the mouth of a cow with foot-and-mouth disease, showing epithelial separation.

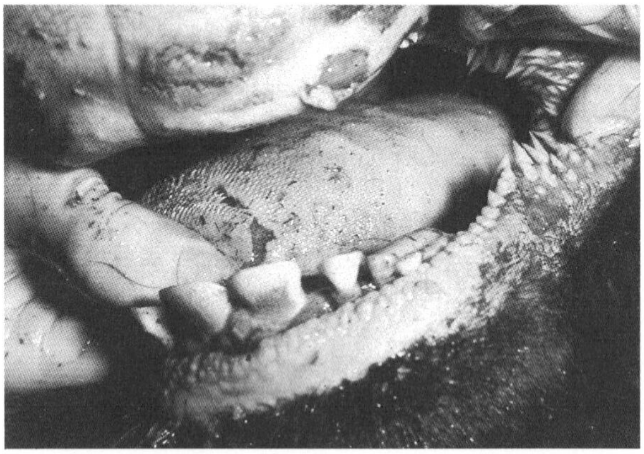

Fig. 37.12 Recently ruptured vesicles on the tongue and dental pad of a cow with foot-and-mouth disease. (Courtesy by A.I. Donaldson.)

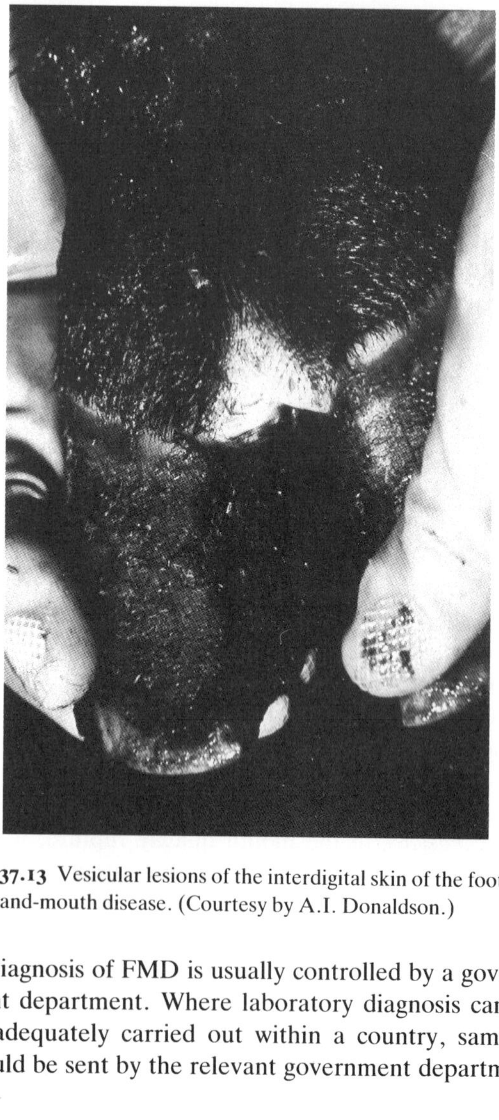

Fig. 37.13 Vesicular lesions of the interdigital skin of the foot in foot-and-mouth disease. (Courtesy by A.I. Donaldson.)

ity. In a fully susceptible herd the clinical signs are frequently severe and pathognomonic. However, in endemic regions in herds that have a partial natural or vaccinal immunity, clinical signs may be mild and may be missed. All vesicular lesions in cattle should be investigated as potential FMD.

The success of the laboratory confirmation of a presumptive diagnosis of vesicular virus infection depends on the submission of adequate material, sent under suitable conditions. A minimum of 2 cm^2 of epithelium from a ruptured vesicle in a 50/50 mixture of glycerine and 0.04 M buffered phosphate (pH 7.4–7.6) should be sent to a laboratory designated for handling FMD virus and equipped with the reagents required to type a positive sample.

Diagnosis of FMD is usually controlled by a government department. Where laboratory diagnosis cannot be adequately carried out within a country, samples should be sent by the relevant government department to the World Reference Laboratory for Foot-and-mouth Disease, Institute for Animal Health, Pirbright Laboratory, Ash Road, Pirbright, Woking, Surrey, GU24 0NF, UK. Even when diagnosis is performed within a country, it is recommended that duplicate samples also be sent to the WRL for confirmation of diagnosis and strain identification. Details of the method of submission of samples are described by Kitching & Donaldson (1987).

Foot-and-mouth disease virus is very sensitive to pH values away from neutrality and is, for example, quickly inactivated below pH 5. Virus can also be isolated from vesicular fluid or from whole blood with heparin collected from the viraemic animal (up to four days after the initial appearance of vesicles). Although high titres of virus can be recovered from milk and internal body organs such as lymph nodes and muscle these specimens should only be sent in addition to, and not instead of, epithelium samples. Negative tests on these tissues could be misleading and cause a false sense of security.

On receipt at the WRL, epithelial samples are prepared as 10 per cent suspensions for the enzyme-linked immunosorbent assay (ELISA). This test identifies virus antigen within the sample and can distinguish between the seven FMD virus types; it has now replaced the classical complement fixation test for FMD diagnosis. Results from this test are available within 3 hours of arrival. At the same time as the ELISA test is being prepared, samples of the epithelial suspension are inoculated onto primary bovine thyroid cells and pig kidney cells (IB-RS-2 cells). If a clear positive is not obtained from the ELISA test, virus growth on either or both of these two cell systems would provide sufficient antigen after 24 or 48 hours for a second ELISA test. In the absence of virus growth on thyroid or pig kidney cells after 48 hours (first passage) the cells are inoculated onto fresh thyroid and pig kidney cells (second passage). Samples are considered negative following negative ELISA and failure of virus growth after 48 hours on second tissue culture passage, i.e. after a minimum of 96 hours following arrival at the WRL.

In countries that use vaccination to control FMD, there is a requirement to relate the outbreak strain to existing vaccine strains. This can be shown using a two-way microneutralization test. Mixtures of field virus and antisera to a vaccine virus, usually prepared in guinea pigs, are incubated at 37 °C for 1 hour and then inoculated with BHK-21 cells into the wells of a microtitre plate. The plates are placed in a 37 °C incubator and examined daily for evidence of a virus-induced cytopathic effect in the cells. The titre of serum that neutralizes 100 Tissue Culture Infective Dose $(TCID)_{50}$ of virus is calculated and compared with the titre of the same serum that neutralizes 100 $TCID_{50}$ of the vaccine virus. The ratio of titre of serum against field virus to titre of serum against vaccine virus is the r_1 value, and gives an indication of the antigenic relationship between the field and vaccine strains and therefore the probable usefulness of that vaccine in controlling the outbreak of FMD.

A similar r_1 value can be derived using the ELISA (Kitching *et al.*, 1988).

The serum antibody titre against FMD virus of cattle vaccinated against FMD can also be measured using the microneutralization test, although this test is now being replaced by an ELISA. Immunity in cattle to FMD can be correlated with the level of serum antibody at 30 days after primary vaccination, although the relationship is not absolute, being dependent on the challenge dose of virus and the closeness of its antigenic relatedness to the vaccine strain. The virus neutralization (VN) and replacement ELISA are FMD virus type specific, so that when used to determine whether an animal has had contact with FMD the VN must be performed separately against each of the FMD serotypes with which the animal may have had contact. In some parts of the world, e.g. Africa, this could be any one of up to six different FMD serotypes. Such testing can be time consuming, expensive and present results difficult to interpret. A non-type-specific screening test has been developed that estimates the presence of antibody to virus infection association (VIA) antigen; VIA antibody is formed in an infected animal in response to RNA polymerase produced by replicating FMD virus. The test may also be used to distinguish between vaccinated animals, in which no virus replication occurs, and animals recovered from infection, although animals that have received multiple vaccinations do also produce some antibody to VIA. Nevertheless, as a screening test the VIA ELISA has many attractions.

Control

The control of FMD depends on prevention of the introduction of virus, prevention of infection of stock and the prevention of spread of virus from infected animals. How this is achieved by individual countries depends on a variety of economic and practical considerations.

Exotic FMD virus may enter an area or country in infected animals and this can include certain zoo animals. Acutely infected animals are usually recognized but sheep and goats frequently only develop very mild clinical signs. Vaccinated cattle can also develop only local lesions of FMD, particularly in the mouth, and may carry infection if imported to FMD-free areas. The importance of cattle and buffalo that are carrying FMD virus in the pharynx is not clear, although there are anecdotal reports of FMD having been introduced with such carrier animals. In order to prevent the introduction of FMD in this manner, some countries refuse entry of any ungulate from FMD-endemic areas, or may insist that any ungulate entering the country has no serum antibody to FMD virus and that oesophageal–pharyngeal scrapings taken by probang are negative for the presence of FMD virus. Any animal vaccinated against FMD is, therefore, prohibited.

Foot-and-mouth disease virus could also enter in the carcass or products of an animal infected before slaughter. In skeletal muscle the virus is inactivated as the pH of the meat falls as the carcass 'sets', but virus in the bone and lymph glands is not subject to this increased acidity and will escape inactivation. Regulations in FMD-free countries require that meat imported from endemic areas has had the bones and lymph glands removed and may also impose additional requirements such as regular vaccination and certification of the absence of FMD from the farm of origin of the meat, the slaughter house and the surrounding areas. If infected meat should still enter in spite of these restrictions an additional safeguard is the prohibition of feeding uncooked meat or other swill to pigs. There are many examples of pigs being the first animals to be infected in an FMD outbreak.

The early detection of an FMD outbreak requires the existence of an efficient veterinary service and a rapid diagnostic capability. The World Reference Laboratorium (WRL), Pirbright, offers a world-wide diagnostic service, although by the time samples are received from abroad an FMD outbreak could be well established. Nevertheless, the service can provide valuable additional support and identify the most suitable vaccine for use to control an outbreak.

Following suspicion of an FMD outbreak the movement of all infected animals must be prevented and local markets and abattoirs closed. The slaughter of all cattle, sheep, goats and pigs on infected premises is practised by all countries that do not routinely vaccinate against FMD, and in many countries that do vaccinate, as this will prevent the establishment of a nucleus of potential carrier animals. Cattle, sheep and goats on surrounding farms that have already been vaccinated should be revaccinated with a vaccine antigenically related to the outbreak strain. Pigs are generally also included in emergency vaccination programmes. All previous movement of animals, animal products and other potentially infected material up to 14 days prior to the estimated appearance of the first clinically infected animals must be investigated. This will not only indicate which other farms may develop secondary outbreaks of FMD but may also identify from where the infection came. Subsequent movement on and off the infected premises must then be kept to a minimum and adequate facilities for cleaning and disinfection provided. Such controllable precautions will identify and considerably reduce the chance of secondary spread. Wind-borne spread of FMD virus prior to the slaughter of the infected animals is, however, uncontrollable. Numerical models developed to predict this wind-borne spread can be used to indicate those farms most at risk and has proved its value in helping to control an outbreak of FMD in the UK.

Vaccination against FMD is an effective method for protecting livestock against infection (p. 813). Only inactivated vaccines are used and they are assessed by their antigen content and the results of potency trials, ideally carried out in fully susceptible cattle. An FMD vaccine is most effective against infection with the homologous strain from which the vaccine was prepared. However, a good vaccine will also protect against closely related strains of FMD virus, although its effectiveness will be reduced the more the antigenic characteristics of the outbreak strain differ from the vaccine strain. It is therefore necessary to identify the types and strains of FMD virus that pose the most significant threat. Nowhere has it been necessary to use more than a quadrivalent vaccine, although there have been occasions when unexpected strains of FMD virus have entered a country. In addition, the characteristic variability of FMD virus has rendered some vaccines no longer effective.

Maternal antibody can interfere with the development of active immunity in young animals. It is therefore recommended that if calves of immune dams are vaccinated in their first three months of life they should be vaccinated twice more at four and five months and possibly again at six months of age. Subsequently, cattle should be vaccinated twice yearly, or even three times yearly in areas where FMD is prevalent.

The method used by different countries to control FMD is dependent on a number of factors. Countries free of FMD and protected on their borders by natural barriers such as desert, sea or mountain ranges can maintain their status by strict import controls and can avoid the recurring cost of vaccination or the possibility of initiating an outbreak through the use of improperly inactivated vaccine or escape of FMD virus from a vaccine production plant. In addition, should FMD virus enter a non-vaccinating country it can usually be immediately identified clinically because of the complete susceptibility of the livestock, whereas FMD virus has been known to circulate in countries that do vaccinate without the knowledge of the veterinary authorities. Finally, countries free of FMD that do not vaccinate have a privileged international trading status. However, should FMD virus enter, there is always the possibility of rapid uncontrollable spread, with severe consequences.

Many countries have no choice but to control FMD by mass vaccination. The movement of nomadic people with their animals, and of wild animals across international borders in Africa, the Middle and Far East, makes disease regulations impossible to enforce. The airborne spread of FMD virus cannot be controlled by legislation. Barrier vaccination can reduce the danger of FMD entering a country or area and has been successful in preventing exotic strains of FMD entering Europe through Turkey and Greece, and in allowing South Africa and Zimbabwe to restrict vaccination to their borders and around game reserves. Countries that do not vaccinate or vaccinate against two or three strains may use emergency vaccination to control an outbreak due to a new strain of FMD by slaughtering affected animals and ring vaccinating around the infected area with a vaccine specifically against the exotic strain.

Economic importance

The economic importance of FMD is hard to quantify accurately. The direct costs of vaccination, slaughter of infected animals, movement restrictions and closure of markets can be measured. The indirect local and national costs, e.g. loss of potential export markets, may be the most significant and yet most uncertain cost.

Assuming that a country wishes to prevent FMD remaining or becoming endemic, two options are available. Either all cattle (and possibly sheep, goats and pigs) are routinely vaccinated or no vaccination is carried out and outbreaks are controlled by slaughter as they occur. Which policy is the most economic can be assessed by critical point analysis or estimating the critical point at which the cost of one policy equals the cost of the other policy. Costs that must be considered are the cost of vaccine and its administration or its storage as a strategic reserve. If it is also assumed that neither policy will eliminate the possibility of FMD outbreaks, the cost of controlling an outbreak must be assessed and multiplied by the estimated total number of outbreaks.

The cost of an FMD outbreak must include the cost of controlling the outbreak, including ring vaccination, the cost of slaughtered animals, the loss of production and the interruption of domestic and international trade. The international trading status of a country that vaccinates already will be considerably less affected than that of a country that does not vaccinate. Similarly, the status of a country that does not use routine FMD vaccine but vaccinates in order to control an FMD outbreak may be affected by very lengthy trade restrictions with other non-vaccinating countries following the cessation of vaccination.

The difficulty in assessing these uncertain costs may be illustrated by an analysis of the cost of annual vaccination (Policy A) and the cost of a stamping-out with ring vaccination (Policy B) carried out in the Federal Republic of Germany (Lorenz, 1987). The average annual cost of Policy A was estimated to be between 52 and 286 million DM, while the average annual cost of Policy B was between 2.5 and 321 or more million DM. The wide range reflected the number of assumed FMD outbreaks that could occur under each regimen. The estimates considered most likely, however, were between 183 and 227 million DM for Policy A and between 47 and 61 million DM for Policy B.

Any scenario for assessing the cost of FMD control must ultimately assume the existence of an efficient veterinary service, capable of diagnosing the disease and with facilities available to control it. Without this infrastructure any, even approximate, estimate of the economic significance of FMD becomes academic.

(d) Rinderpest

by E.C. ANDERSON

The State Veterinary Service in the UK was brought into being specifically to deal with rinderpest or cattle plague. In the eighteenth and nineteenth century devastating outbreaks of rinderpest were responsible for millions of deaths in cattle in Europe. By 1930, with the exception of parts of Turkey, Europe was free of the disease and since that time only small outbreaks of the disease have occurred. The disease has however continued to persist in Asia and the Indian subcontinent and is still present in India, Bangladesh and

Nepal. In 1982–83 it was present throughout the Middle East. Rinderpest was introduced into Africa in the early 1800s and was responsible for a massive pandemic between 1889 and 1897. Africa has not been free of rinderpest since, although it has largely been confined to countries north of the Tropic of Capricorn. In spite of an international vaccination programme carried out between 1962 and 1975, which almost eradicated the disease (Scott, 1985), extensive outbreaks of the disease are again occurring in this region.

Aetiology

The causal agent of rinderpest is a paramyxovirus of the genus morbillivirus. The other members of the morbillivirus genus are measles, canine distemper, phocine distemper (Osterhaus & Vedder 1988; Mahy *et al.*, 1988; Kennedy *et al.*, 1988) and peste des petit ruminants (PPR) to which rinderpest virus is antigenically related. The morbilliviruses are pleomorphic, enveloped, helical particles of between 150–300 nm diameter and contain a non-segmented negative-strand RNA genome. This codes for six structural proteins and possibly one non-structural protein. The virus structural proteins comprise the nucleocapsid protein (N), which surrounds the genomic RNA, a large polymerase protein (L) and a small polymerase-associated protein (P), a matrix protein (M) associated with the virus envelope and two envelope glycoproteins, the haemagglutinin (H) and fusion protein (F). The P gene shows significant homology between members of the morbillivirus group (Barrett & Underwood, 1985).

There is only one serotype of rinderpest virus and rinderpest virus can be distinguished from PPR virus in reciprocal cross-neutralization tests. At present it is not possible to distinguish between the two diseases using the sera of recovered animals. However, the two viruses can be distinguished by comparing the protein patterns in polyacrylamide gels as the N proteins have been shown to have markedly different molecular weights (Diallo *et al.*, 1987). They can also be distinguished by cross-hybridization using specific cDNA probes (Diallo *et al.*, 1989).

The virus is sensitive to lipid solvents, is relatively heat sensitive and is unstable at low pH. It is also labile when exposed to light and survives best at low or high relative humidities but is rapidly destroyed when the relative humidity is between 40–60 per cent. Infectivity is lost when it is suspended in glycerol or water but it is stable in 0.86 per cent sodium chloride at low temperatures with the loss in infectivity rising exponentially with temperature. The use of molar concentrations of magnesium sulphate improves the thermostability of the virus.

Species susceptible

Rinderpest is potentially infective for all members of the order Artiodactyla (Scott, 1964) but in particular infects members of the families Bovidae, Suidae and Cervidae (Plowright, 1968). Of these cattle, water buffalo, Cape buffalo (*Syncerus caffer*) and yak are most susceptible. The disease occurs in sheep and goats in India where it is also seen in pigs. It may be seen in camels. It has been recorded in a large number of wildlife species including eland (*Taurotragus oryx*), lesser kudu (*Tragelaphus imberis*), giraffe (*Giraffa camelopardis*) and warthog (*Phacochoerus aethiopicus*).

Transmission

Rinderpest is spread by direct contact between infected and susceptible animals, by the inhalation of virus-containing aerosols or by ingestion of infected secretions and excretions. On rare occasions it has spread through indirect contact with contaminated fodder and water. Pigs have been infected through eating meat from contaminated carcasses. Different strains of virus vary in their invasiveness and infectivity for different species.

Pathogenesis

Infection is through the upper respiratory tract with primary replication of the virus in the tonsils and local lymph nodes (Plowright, 1968). The virus is disseminated in the blood, where it is closely associated with the mononuclear leucocytes, to all lymphoid tissue and the mucosae of the alimentary and respiratory tracts. The incubation period lasts from two to nine days and viraemia can be detected one to two days before the onset of pyrexia. The prodromal phase usually lasts from two to five days. The virus is shed in all secretions and excretions, the peak of virus production being during the prodromal fever but continuing after the appearance of erosive lesions. Virus levels fall as antibody begins to be produced with viraemia ceasing before the disappearance of the virus from the tissues, about 14 days after the onset of fever. Viraemia lasts on the average about six days but there is considerable variation between strains of virus. Viraemia can occur following exposure to some strains that lasts four to six days without the development of lesions.

Clinical signs

The clinical signs of rinderpest in cattle and other natural hosts are essentially the same but show wide variations in severity depending on the strain involved, and the resistance of the animal, natural or acquired.

The disease may be hyperacute, acute, subacute or chronic (Plowright, 1968). The typical acute disease can be divided into four phases: incubation, prodromal, mucosal and convalescent.

Incubation phase (see above).

Prodromal phase. This is characterized by a sudden onset in fever reaching a peak on the second or third day after onset. It is accompanied by depression or restlessness, loss in appetite and a fall in milk yield in cows. The visible mucous membranes are congested, the muzzle is dry and there may be the beginning of a serous discharge from the eyes and nostrils. There is tachycardia and accelerated respirations, ruminal stasis and constipation. This phase lasts about three days with lesions appearing between two to five days following the onset of pyrexia.

Mucosal phase. The first lesions comprise small foci of necrosis, superficial erosion and capillary haemorrhage in the mucosae of the mouth cavity, which are particularly noticeable on the lower gum and tips of the buccal papillae. They extend to involve the lips, upper gum, hard palate and ventral surface of the tongue. Similar lesions occur in the nasal, vulval and preputial mucosae where they may occur earlier than in the oral cavity. The lesions extend and fuse to produce extensive areas of necrotic erosion with a characteristic fetid smell. There may be excessive salivation and at this stage the lacrimal and nasal secretions become profuse and purulent.

Animals at this stage of the disease are very depressed and respirations are laboured, but pneumonia is rare. Diarrhoea appears usually between four and seven days of pyrexia and one to two days after the appearance of lesions. It is at first watery but later dysentery develops and it may contain pieces of intestinal mucosa. Dehydration is rapid resulting in weakness, prostration and death between six and twelve days after the onset of pyrexia. The mortality rate is over 90 per cent when susceptible animals are infected with virulent strains.

Mild forms of the disease in partially immune animals or following infection with less virulent strains give rise to reduced general signs and less extensive mucosal lesions. However, these may be completely absent with the only sign a transient diarrhoea. Even this may be absent, and some strains of virus result in a complete spectrum of signs from the classical acute febrile disease with extensive lesions and eventual death to a form in which there is fever but no lesions although antigen can be detected in lacrimal secretions (Anderson *et al.*, 1990).

Convalescent phase. Visible mouth lesions may heal within as little as two to three days beginning from the third to the fifth day after their appearance. Diarrhoea may persist for longer. Complete recovery from the acute form takes about four weeks depending on the environment and plane of nutrition.

Pathology

The gross pathology has been described by Maurer *et al.* (1956). The mucosae of the upper alimentary and respiratory tract are eroded and necrotic often being coated with a mucopurulent exudate. Erosions, ulcers and oedema occur in the abomasum, which may also be congested. Peyer's patches in the small intestine are haemorrhagic, oedematous and necrotic. The mucosal surface of the caecum, colon and rectum frequently has characteristic haemorrhagic stripes due to the congestion of the capillaries. Erosion and ulcers also occur in the urogenital tract. The virus has a predilection for lymphoid tissues in which there is extensive necrosis of the lymphocytes of the germinal centres, and the appearance of multinucleated giant cells about eight days after infection. The appearance of cytoplasmic and intranuclear inclusions has been described (Plowright, 1968). The stratified squamous epithelium, particularly of the upper part of the alimentary tract shows syncytium formation and degenerative changes, which are followed by necrosis and detachment to form erosions and ulcers.

Diagnosis

Laboratory confirmation of rinderpest is based on the detection of specific antigens and the isolation of the virus. Retrospective diagnosis is obtained by the detection of specific antibody (Scott *et al.*, 1986).

Antigen detection. Virus is present in the secretions and excretions within two days of the onset of fever. Specific antigen can be detected from this time particularly in the lacrimal secretions but also later in swabs or material from lesions in the mouth, vagina or prepuce. Lymph node biopsies may also be taken.

Rapid diagnosis is desirable and where the disease is suspected specific antigen is readily detected by immunodiffusion or counterimmunoelectrophoresis (CIEOP) in lacrimal secretions in field laboratories. It may also be detected using indicator systems such as red blood cells or latex beads to which specific antibody has been attached in passive haemagglutination or latex agglutination tests. The enzyme-linked immunosorbent assay (ELISA) is a very sensitive test used in suitably equipped laboratories and is often preferred to the complement fixation test. Histochemical methods using fluorescein or enzyme-conjugated antiserum may be used on smears, biopsy material or tissue sections (Scott *et al.*, 1986).

Virus isolation. Virus may be isolated in tissue cultures of primary or secondary calf or sheep kidney cells or Vero cells. It may be isolated from swabs of lesions or secretions, from the leucocyte fraction of blood collected in EDTA or from lymphoid tissue collected at post mortem. Specimens should be transported on ice but glycerol should not be used as a transport medium, as it inactivates the virus.

Antibody detection. The detection of a rising antibody titre in paired serum samples or in disease surveys may be done using the virus neutralization test. This is suitable for small numbers of diagnostic samples but for disease surveillance requiring the screening of large numbers of samples the ELISA is the test of choice. Other tests that are used include indirect immunodiffusion and CIEOP.

Differential diagnosis

In cattle the one disease that cannot be distinguished from rinderpest without laboratory tests is bovine virus diarrhoea. In sheep and goats peste des petits ruminants is identical to rinderpest. Otherwise there are few conditions that should be confused with the acute form of rinderpest. The mild forms in particular, where diarrhoea is the only clinical sign, are indistinguishable from other enteric conditions.

Control

Rinderpest spreads slowly in endemic countries where it affects mainly immature animals. In these countries control is by vaccination annually of all immatures. In such countries attempting eradication, vaccination of the entire cattle population, as well as sheep and goats in those countries where the disease occurs in these species, for three to five years is practised.

In high risk countries adjacent to endemic regions or those importing livestock from endemic countries quarantine and vaccination are combined (see p. 811).

All rinderpest vaccines in use are live attenuated vaccines. Most countries use a tissue culture vaccine (Plowright, 1968) but goat adapted vaccine and lapinized vaccine are still used in some countries.

(e) Vesicular Stomatitis

by R.P. KITCHING

Vesicular stomatitis (VS) is a vesicular disease of cattle, horses and pigs that can also infect a large range of wild animal species. The virus belongs to the genus vesiculovirus, within the family Rhabdoviridae.

There are two serologically distinct types of VS virus (VSV); New Jersey (NJ) and Indiana (IND). The IND type can be further subdivided into Indiana 1 (Indiana strain), Indiana 2 (Cocal and Argentina strains) and Indiana 3 (Alagoas and Brazil strains). In common with all other rhabdoviruses VSV is a single-stranded RNA virus, the RNA being arranged in an enveloped helical nucleocapsid. The intact virus is bullet shaped, measuring 180 nm by 75 nm, and is covered with 10 nm spikes.

Vesicular stomatitis virus will grow in a wide range of primary cells and continuous cell lines, and laboratory animals such as mice, rats, ferrets, guinea pigs, hamsters and chick embryos. Humans are susceptible to VS, the disease being characterized by fever, myalgia, nausea, vomiting, headaches, and occasionally vesicles on the mucosa of the mouth and throat. No deaths have been reported, and the disease rarely lasts more than a week.

Epidemiology

The behaviour of VS in the field has been well documented but in spite of detailed observations there are many aspects of the epidemiology of VS that are still unclear. Enzootic VS has a limited geographical location, within which the appearance of disease is cyclical, apparently related to season or rainfall. The majority of infections are inapparent, and can occur in animals isolated in cages or otherwise separated from other susceptible species. Epizootic spread of VS is associated with simultaneous outbreaks over a wide area, although some herds within this area may remain unaffected. Of the domesticated species, cattle are the most commonly affected, followed by horses and then pigs; sheep and goats never show clinical signs of VS. Few cases are reported in young cattle, most cases appearing in milking cows. Mouth lesions are most frequently reported although in some outbreaks only teat lesions are seen. Insects have been strongly implicated in the transmission of VS, but this has not yet been conclusively demonstrated. The cyclical appearance of VS suggests the existence of interepizootic reservoir hosts, but these have also resisted identification.

A number of theories have been put forward to explain these observations. It has been suggested that VSV circulates in feral pigs, elk, mule deer and antelope and possibly also in water birds and rodents such as wood rats and deer mice. In support of this theory antibody against VSV has been found in all these species and, in some areas, prior to the onset of a VS epizootic in domesticated animals. It has also been suggested without much supporting evidence that VSV could persist in the soil and be circulated by arthropods or even that VSV is primarily a plant virus.

Recent studies using T_1 oligonucleotide mapping of VSV-NJ have helped to identify the origin of recent VS epizootics in the USA (Nicol, 1987). By precisely characterizing the outbreak strains it has been shown that a VS epizootic is not caused by the simultaneous eruption of many strains of VSV within the USA but the rapid spread of a single strain north from the enzootic region of Mexico. A correlation has been shown between outbreaks of VS in North America and wind direction from VS-infected areas, indicating a possible involvement of insect vectors carried by the prevailing wind.

VSV-IND appears to have different epidemiological characteristics from VSV-NJ, and its spread is less associated with clinical disease and has consequently attracted less attention. It is also apparent that the behaviour of VSV need not remain consistent; its mode of transmission for instance can vary even during epizootics.

Distribution

Vesicular stomatitis virus is restricted to North, Central and South America and the Caribbean islands. The disease was transported with horses from America to South Africa in 1884 and 1887, and to France in 1915, but did not persist in either country. The first report of VS in North America was in horses in 1882 during the American Civil War, and there were further reports in 1889, 1904 and 1907. In South America VS was first diagnosed in Argentina in 1939, in Venezuela in 1941 and in Colombia in 1943.

Indiana 1 and New Jersey strains of VSV are enzootic in Mexico and Central America, but a characteristic of both is their periodic movement out of the enzootic areas to cause epizootics in the southern USA and northern South America; VSV-IND has spread as far north as the USA–Canada border. These seasonal epizootics occur typically at the end of the summer, or in the tropics at the end of the rainy season, and usually finish in the temperate regions at the onset of the frosts. The 1982 VSV-NJ epizootic did not, however, follow this cycle and persisted through the winter. Epizootics that spread into the mid-western and western states of North America tend to occur at intervals of approximately five to ten years, while major epizootics have been occurring every 30 years. The predominant serotype causing vesicular disease in the USA is VSV-NJ. Vesicular stomatitis has not been reported in the New England area, eastern Canada or Alaska.

Transmission

The epidemiological characteristics of VS suggest that the disease is predominantly spread by insects. *Culex* and *Aedes* species of mosquitoes, *Phlebotomus* sandflies, *Culicoides*, *Simulium* blackflies, *Musca* species, *Hippelates* eye gnats and Anthromyidae have all been implicated in the transmission of VS. Transovarial transmission of VSV has been shown in the sandfly *Lutzomyia trapidoi*. However, the very low viraemia associated with VS is considered too low to make vector transmission sufficiently efficient to maintain the virus. The vesicular lesions of clinical VS are rich in virus and could provide a potent source for insect infection, but this fails to explain the transmission of VS between subclinically infected animals. Nevertheless, the climatic conditions that predispose to the spread of VS, and the more frequent appearance of VS in animals at pasture, strongly implicates the involvement of insects. In addition, the characteristic termination of a VS epizootic with the onset of subzero night-time temperatures is typical of many vector-borne diseases. The virus does not appear to be totally dependent on insect transmission, as evidenced by the continuation of the North American 1982–83 epizootic through the winter.

Transmission of VS can also occur by direct contact between infected and susceptible cattle, this being frequently associated with subclinical infections. An association has been made between the feeding of abrasive feeds, which compromise the integrity of the buccal mucous membranes, and the spread of VS.

Clinical signs

Vesicular stomatitis in cattle may be an inapparent, mild or severe disease, animals over nine months of age being most commonly affected. Following an incubation period of two to three days, a usually mild fever develops accompanied by depression, lameness and excessive salivation. The fever reduces as vesicles develop on the coronary bands of the feet, or in the mouth or on the teats; rarely are vesicles seen on more than one of these sites. In severe cases, over 50 per cent of the tongue epithelium may be affected, and the resultant difficulty in eating can cause dramatic weight loss. Milk yield is depressed. True vesicles may fail to develop, lesions appearing as crusts or ulcers. Recovery is usually rapid, although milk yield frequently fails to recover during the remaining lactation, and secondary mastitis may be a problem. Some animals fail to recover fully and remain in poor condition. The lesions produced by vesicular stomatitis virus in cattle are clinically indistinguishable from lesions of foot-and-mouth disease (FMD).

Pathogenesis

Vesicular stomatitis virus enters the animal through a skin or mucosal abrasion or possibly is inoculated by an infected insect bite. Aerosol infection has been reported in humans and may also occur in cattle. A low-titre viraemia has been detected in some experimentally infected animals between 11 and 56 hours after infection. Replication of virus occurs at the site of infection in the prickle cells of the Malpighian layer but there is no information on subsequent sites of virus replication. As the cells degenerate, and transudate from the bloodstream accumulates, vesicles develop and the animal becomes febrile. It is not clear why lesions are rarely generalized, but are usually restricted to the teats, mouth or feet. Immunosuppressed or overcrowded animals are more likely to develop lesions. The virus does not cross the placenta, and there are no reports of calves from infected dams being viraemic or having precolostral antibodies to VSV. However, VSV-NJ has once been recovered from an aborted fetus.

Diagnosis

Diagnosis of VS is by clinical examination of affected animals and the demonstration of the presence of VSV, or of a rising antibody titre to VSV. Laboratory confirmation of VS is essential in order to distinguish the disease from FMD.

Vesicular stomatitis virus has a characteristic appearance under the electron microscope. The virus will also grow on a wide range of primary and continuous cell lines, on the chorioallantoic membrane or in the allantoic cavity of fertile eggs and in many laboratory mammals. The Vero-M (green monkey) cell line is used extensively for the growth of VSV for assay of VS antibodies in the virus neutralization test. The complement fixation test and fluorescent antibody test are also used in the diagnosis of VS. Details given for the submission of samples for FMD diagnosis (see p. 542) apply also to the submission of samples for VS diagnosis, although VSV is much less susceptible to pH outside the range of 7.2–8.0. As a differential diagnosis is usually required between FMD and VS, the more stringent requirements of FMD virus should be followed.

Virus neutralization antibodies may be detected 96 hours after experimental inoculation, and they reach a peak by day 12. These antibodies persist for many years and are valuable in showing evidence of previous infection. Their persistence has led to the suggestion that the virus itself may persist in an animal long after recovery from disease, although possibly it remains in a defective, non-infectious form. Complement-fixing antibodies recede in three to six months after infection. A fourfold or greater increase in VSV neutralizing antibodies between early infection and convalescent serum is diagnostic of infection. The presence of neutralizing antibodies does not appear always to prevent reinfection or the development of clinical signs.

Prior to the establishment of suitable laboratory tests, VS was diagnosed by scarifying infective material into the snout of swine and the tongues of cattle and horses, and by intramuscular inoculation of cattle. Vesicular stomatitis virus produced lesions on pigs, cattle and horses, but not in cattle when given by intramuscular injection. Foot-and-mouth disease virus produced disease in swine and cattle, but not horses, and vesicular exanthema virus affected only swine, although occasionally lesions were also produced on the tongues of horses.

Control

Measures designed to control VS reflect the poor understanding of the epidemiology of VS, notably the possibility that animals can remain carriers of VSV. It has been observed that recovered cattle have appeared to spread VSV to susceptible animals, and that some of these recovered cattle have again developed vesicles, usually, but not invariably, on a site different from the original area of infection. These recurrent lesions have usually occurred within 48 hours of moving the recovered cattle, and has led to the suggestion that the recrudescence of clinical disease was brought on by stress. Although it has not been possible to isolate virus from clinically normal animals recovered from VS, the persistence of high levels of neutralizing antibodies in these animals does suggest the presence of a continuous antigenic stimulation.

An additional problem is the high proportion of subclinical cases during epizootics and the possibility that VS could circulate in an area unobserved.

Within the USA animals infected with VSV are quarantined for at least 30 days after all signs of VS have disappeared. Countries free of VS are usually considerably more stringent and will not import any animal with virus neutralizing antibodies to VS. This precaution is intended to exclude the possibility of importing a persistently infected animal.

Living and formalin-inactivated vaccines have been prepared against VSV-NJ. The dead vaccine reduces the incidence of overt disease, while the live vaccine, given by intramuscular inoculation, gives a better protection and does not spread to in-contact susceptible animals. A recombinant vaccine has also been developed by inserting the gene for the VSV glycoprotein into the genome of vaccinia virus. This vector vaccine against VS is reported to be highly effective.

Economic importance

It is difficult to assess the full economic importance of VS because of the effect the presence of disease has on export markets. Direct losses due to disease can be severe, particularly in high-yielding dairy herds, and were calculated to have been between $97 and $253 per clinical case during the 1982 epizootic in the USA (quoted by Monath *et al.*, 1986). Losses due to reduced growth rates in beef cattle in South America are also reported to be significant. Consequent movement restrictions and the closure of local markets can also cause considerable loss. Nevertheless, it is the exclusion of animals in VS enzootic or previous epizootic areas from countries free of VS that causes the most significant economic losses.

References and further reading

Bluetongue

Bowen, R.A., Howard, T.H. & Pickett, B.W. (1985) Seminal shedding of bluetongue virus in experimentally infected bulls. In *Bluetongue and Related Orbiviruses* (ed. by T.L. Barber & M.M. Jochim), Progress in Clinical and Biological Research, Vol. 178, pp. 91–6. Alan. R Liss Inc, New York.

Gorman, B.M., Taylor, J. & Walker, P.J. (1983) Orbiviruses. In *The Reoviridae* (ed. by W.K. Joklik). Plenum, New York, pp. 287–357.

Jeggo, M.H. (1986) A review of the immune response to bluetongue virus. *Revue Scientifique Technologique Office Internationale des Epizooties*. **5**, 357–62.

Luedke, A.J., Jochim, M.M. & Barber, T.L. (1982) Serologic and virologic responses of a Hereford bull persistently infected with bluetongue virus for eleven years. In *American Association of Veterinary Laboratory Diagnosis, 25th Annual Proceeding*, pp. 115–34.

Mertens, P.P.C., Burroughs, J.N. & Anderson, J. (1987) Purification and properties of virus particles, infectious subviral particles, and cores of bluetongue virus serotypes 1 and 4. *Virology*, **157**, 375–86.

Osborn, B.I., Huffman, E.M., Sawyer, I.N. & Hird, D. (1986) Economics of bluetongue in the United States. In *Arbovirus Research in Australia, Proceedings 4th Symposium*, pp. 245–7.

Verwoerd, D.W., Els, H.J., DeVilliers, E.M. & Huismans, H. (1972) The structure of the bluetongue virus capsid. *Journal of Virology*, **10**, 783–94.

Enzootic Bovine Leukosis

Burny, A., Bruck, C., Chantrenne, H., Cleuter, Y., Dekegel, D., Ghysdael, J., Kettman, R., Leclercq, M., Leunen, J., Mammerickx, M. & Portetelle, D. (1980) Bovine leukemia virus. In *Molecular Biology and Epidemiology in Viral Oncology* (ed. by G. Klein), pp. 231–89. Raven Press, New York.

Burny, A., Bruck, C., Cleuter, Y., Couez, D., Deschamps, J., Ghysdael, J., Gregoire, D., Kettmann, R., Mammerickx, M., Marbaix, G. & Portetelle, D. (1985) Bovine leukaemia virus: a tantalizing story. In *Viruses and Cancer* (ed. by P.W.J. Rigby & N.M. Wilkie), pp. 197–216. Cambridge University Press, Cambridge.

Burny, A., Bruck, C., Cleuter, Y., Couez, D., Deschamps, J., Gregoire, D., Ghysdael, J., Kettman, R., Mammerickx, M., Marbaix, G. & Portetelle, D. (1985) Bovine leukaemia virus and enzootic bovine leukosis. *Onderstepoort Journal of Veterinary Research*, **52**, 133–44.

Burny, A., Bruck, C., Cleuter, Y., Couez, D., Gregoire, D., Kettmann, R., Mammerickx, M., Marbaix, G., Portetelle, D. & Willems, L. (1986) Bovine leukemia virus as an inducer of bovine leukemia. In *Animal Models of Retrovirus Infection and their Relationship to AIDS* (ed. by L.A. Salzman), pp. 107–19. Academic Press, New York.

Evermann, J.F. (1983) Bovine leukemia virus infection. *Modern Veterinary Practice*, **64**, 103–5.

Ferrer, J.F. (1980) *Bovine Lymphosarcoma*. Advances in Veterinary Science and Comparative Medicine, Vol. 24. Academic Press, New York.

Ghysdael, J., Bruck, C., Kettman, R. & Burny, A. (1984) Bovine leukemia virus. In *Current Topics in Microbiology and Immunology* (ed. by M. Cooper *et al.*), Vol. 112, pp. 1–19.

Miller, J.M., Miller, L.D., Olson, C. and Gillette, K.G. (1969) Virus-like particles in phytohaemagglutinin-stimulated lymphocyte cultures with reference to bovine lymphosarcoma. *Journal of the National Cancer Institute*, **43**, 1297–1305.

Parodi, A.L. (1986) Enzootic bovine leukosis. Its aetiology, epidemiology and principles of control. *Pro Veterinario*, **1**, 1–4.

Schultz, R.D., Manning, T.O., Rhyan, J.C., Buxton, B.A., Panangala, V.S., Bause, I.M. & Yang, W.C. (1986) Immunologic and virologic studies on bovine leukosis. In *Animal Models of Retrovirus Infection and their Relationship to AIDS* (ed. by L.A. Salzman), pp. 301–23. Academic Press, New York.

Foot-and-mouth disease

Kitching, R.P. & Donaldson, A.I. (1987) Collection and transportation of specimens for vesicular virus investigation. *Revue Scientifique Technologique Officiale Internationale Epizootique*, **6**, 263–72.

Kitching, R.P., Rendel, R. & Ferris, N.P. (1988) Rapid correlation between field isolates and vaccine strains of foot-and-mouth disease virus. *Vaccine*, **6**, 403–8.

Kitching, R.P., Knowles, N.J., Samuel, A.R. & Donaldson, A.I. (1989) Development of foot-and-mouth disease virus strain characterisation — a review. *Tropical Animal Health and Production*, **21**, 153–66.

Lorenz, R.J. (1987) Report of the 27th Session of the European Commission for the Control of FMD, Rome, 21–24 April 1987.

Rinderpest

Anderson, E.C., Hassan, A., Burrett, T. & Anderson, J. (1990) Observations on the pathogenicity for sheep and goats and the transmissibility of the strains of virus isolated during the rinderpest outbreak in Sri Lanka in 1987. Veterinary Microbiology, **21**, 309–18.

Barrett, T. & Underwood, B. (1985) Comparison of messenger RNAs induced in cells infected with each member of the Morbillivirus group. *Virology*, **145**, 195–9.

Diallo, A., Barrett, T., Lefevre, P.C. & Taylor, W.P. (1987) Comparison of proteins induced in cells infected with rinderpest and peste des petits ruminants viruses. *Journal of General Virology*, **68**, 2033–38.

Diallo; A., Barrett, T., Barbron, M., Subbarao, S.M. & Taylor, W.D. (1989) Differentiation of rinderpest and peste de petits ruminants viruses using specific cDNA clones. *Journal of Virologiue Methods*, **23**, 127–436.

Kennedy, S., Smyth, J.A., McCullough, S.J., Allan, G.M., McNeilly, F. & McQuaid, S. (1988) Confirmation of cause of recent seal deaths, **335**, 404.

Mahy, B.W.J., Barrett, T., Evans, S., Anderson, E.C. & Bostock, C.J. (1988) Characterization of a seal morbillivirus. *Nature*, **336**, 115.

Maurer, F.D., Jones, T.C., Easterday, B. & Detray, D.E. (1956) Pathology of rinderpest. *Journal of the American Veterinary Medical Association*, **127**, 512–14.

Osterhaus, A.D.M.E. & Vedder, E.J. (1988) Identification of virus causing recent seal deaths. *Nature*, **335**, 20.

Plowright, W. (1968) *Rinderpest Virus*, Virology Monographs No. 3. Springer-Verlag, Berlin.

Scott, G.R. (1964) Rinderpest. *Advances in Veterinary Science*, **9**, 113–224.

Scott, G.R. (1985) Rinderpest in the 1980s. *Progress in Veterinary Microbiology and Immunology*, **1**, 145–74.

Scott, G.R., Taylor, W.P. & Rossiter, P.B. (1986) *Manual on the Diagnosis of Rinderpest*. Food and Agriculture Organization of the United Nations, Rome.

Vesicular stomatitis

Monath, T.P., Webb, P.A., Francy, O.B. & Walton, T.E. (1986) The epidemiology of vesicular stomatitis — new data, old puzzles. In *Proceedings of 4th Symposium on Arbovirus Research in Australia* (eds. T.D. St. George, B.H. Kay & J. Blok), CISRO, pp. 193–8. Brisbane, Australia.

Nicol, S.T. (1987) Molecular epizootiology and evolution of vesicular stomatitis. *Journal of Virology*, **61**, 1029–36.

Chapter 38: Bacterial Conditions

by B.M. WILLIAMS AND A.H. ANDREWS

Anthrax

Bacillus anthracis infection in cattle causes a peracute or acute disease, which is characterized by a septicaemia and sudden or rapid death. The disease is a zoonosis and is subject to official control measures in a number of countries.

Aetiology

Bacillus anthracis is a Gram-positive capsulated bacillus and its morphology, together with the staining reaction of the capsula, is of diagnostic importance. When stained by Giemsa's, Wright's or similar stains, the capsule stains an intense reddish mauve colour, is square ended and its outline is rather ragged or 'shaggy' (Plate 38.1). A similar reaction is produced by methylene blue, but because of the variability in the content of its oxidized products, azur A and B, which have an affinity for the capsule, the staining reaction is less consistent and the staining of the capsule is a less intense mauve colour. The organism produces a lethal toxin that causes death through shock and acute renal failure.

The organism is a spore-forming bacillus, but mature spores are not formed in the animal before death. The vegetative bacilli are not very resistant to environmental conditions or to physical and chemical agents, and are rapidly destroyed by putrefactive processes in unopened carcasses (Sterne, 1959). However, sporulation occurs when carcasses are opened or when discharges containing bacilli are exposed to air. Mature spores are extremely resistant to environmental conditions and certain disinfectants, and in soil they remain viable for many years.

Anthrax has been reported from most if not all cattle rearing countries of the world, but the incidence of disease is dependent on a number of factors, including climate, soil, animal husbandry and disease control methods. Serious outbreaks of disease are more commonly encountered in tropical and subtropical countries. In such areas, infection persists in the soil and is a major source of infection. The disposal of animal carcasses also presents a serious problem, so that cattle and other animals readily come into contact with the tissues, particularly bones, of animals that die from anthrax. This method of infection is very important in phosphorus deficient areas where cattle develop pica and chew bones in an attempt to remedy the deficiency.

In temperate countries sporadic outbreaks occur involving single or a small number of animals, arising from the ingestion of contaminated feedingstuffs. Campbell (1969) reported that the vast majority of anthrax outbreaks in cattle in England and Wales were associated with compound feedingstuffs containing meat and bone meal derived from imported materials from Asia and South America, but he also emphasized that often vegetable protein became contaminated with anthrax organisms in the holds of ships that were being or had been used for the transport of meat and bone meal. Hugh-Jones & Hussaini (1975) confirmed that in Great Britain, contaminated feedingstuffs were the major source of infection, although infection was sometimes derived from tannery effluent and soil at sites where the carcasses of animals had been buried some years previously.

Infection is acquired through the ingestion of soil or effluent-contaminated fodder or contaminated compound feedingstuffs. Schlingham *et al.* (1956) have demonstrated that clinical disease in cattle can be regularly produced by the oral administration of organisms in feed pellets. The spores penetrate the intact mucosa, or through small abrasions in the mucosa of the mouth and pharynx, and are then transported to the local lymph nodes where germination and multiplication occurs, followed by passage via the lymphatics into the bloodstream, leading to a septicaemia with an explosive invasion of all body tissues.

Signs

All ages of cattle are susceptible to infection. The incubation period is thought to be one to two weeks, although in some incidents it would appear to be three to five days.

At the beginning of an outbreak, the peracute form of the disease is more common, animals usually being found dead within a few hours of being seen in normal health. On the rare occasions that animals are seen ailing, fever, muscle tremors, dyspnoea, collapse and terminal convulsions are the predominant signs, with death occurring in 1–4 hours. In the acute form, which runs a course of 24–48 hours, fever, depression, rapid and laboured respirations, diarrhoea or dysentery, haemorrhagic congestion of the visible mucous membranes and in dairy cattle a sudden drop in milk yield are the main signs. Pregnant animals may abort.

Atypical signs have been recorded in calves receiving prophylactic levels of oxytetracycline or chlortetracycline for the control of salmonellosis. In such animals, a mild fever, bleeding from the nose and eyes and melaena were the only signs observed before death, which occurred 48–72 hours after onset (B.M. Williams, unpublished data).

Pathology

Because of the peracute/acute nature of the disease in cattle, there is little opportunity for ante-mortem laboratory examinations. It may be possible to detect organisms in appropriately stained smears of peripheral blood, but sufficient numbers of organisms are only likely to be present during the later stages of the disease. A haematological examination may reveal a leucocytosis and a shift to the left, but because of the relatively short course of the disease, these changes are not marked.

Before a necropsy is carried out on an animal that has died suddenly or after a very short illness, it is essential that anthrax be eliminated, to prevent contamination of the environment and ensure proper disposal of the carcass. Thus a careful evaluation of the circumstances and a thorough preliminary examination of the carcass must be carried out. If anthrax cannot be eliminated, then a blood sample should be taken from a superficial blood vessel and a stained smear examined microscopically. It is more difficult to identify anthrax bacilli if animals have been treated with antibiotics. The procedures for dealing with suspected anthrax cases vary from country to country and those currently in force in Great Britain are discussed below.

Rapid decomposition of the carcass sets in soon after death and in most instances rigor mortis is absent and dark tarry blood exudes from all the body orifices. There is bloodstained fluid in all body cavities and there are widespread haemorrhages throughout the carcass, particularly on the parietal pleura and peritoneum. Unclotted or poorly clotted blood oozes from the cut blood vessels and there is an intense inflammation of the mucosa of the abomasum and both small and large intestine. The spleen is almost invariably greatly enlarged with sometimes a rupture of the capsule, and a dark semifluid pulp. The lesions in animals that have been treated with antibiotics before death are similar but much less spectacular.

Diagnosis

The diagnosis of anthrax is based on the demonstration of capsulated bacilli in peripheral blood and subsequent confirmation by laboratory isolation and identification. In Great Britain, anthrax is a notifiable disease and the State Veterinary Service is responsible for confirmation.

There are numerous causes of sudden death in cattle, including clostridial infections, hypomagnesaemia, lead poisoning and lightning strike, all of which can be confirmed by a post-mortem examination and appropriate laboratory examinations. As emphasized earlier, such procedures should not be undertaken until anthrax has been eliminated.

Treatment and prevention

Bacillus anthracis is sensitive to a number of antibiotics and treatment of animals during the early stages of the disease is likely to be successful, although severely ailing animals are unlikely to recover. Greenough (1965) successfully treated animals with 5 megaunits of penicillin alone or with streptomycin. The recommended dosage of penicillin is 10 000 units/kg body weight administered twice daily for at least three to five days. Streptomycin, in 4–5 g doses, should also be administered twice daily for the same period. Lincoln *et al.* (1964) consider that septicaemic anthrax is best treated with a combination of large doses of penicillin and streptomycin twice daily, although oxytetracycline and chlortetracycline are the next antibiotics of choice. Bailey (1953) also recommends tetracycline for the treatment of anthrax. Anthrax antiserum administered intravenously is effective but the high cost and large volumes required makes its routine use impractical.

When anthrax has been confirmed in a herd, all animals should be carefully observed at frequent intervals and any that are showing signs of ill health isolated, their temperatures taken and, if elevated, immediately treated with antibiotic.

In Great Britain and elsewhere, anthrax is a notifiable disease under the provisions of the Anthrax Order of 1938 for the protection of both animal and human health. An owner or veterinary surgeon must report any suspicion of disease to a police constable, who informs the Local Authority, which then immediately impose restrictions on the movement of animals onto and off the premises. The carcass(es) of the suspected animal(s) must be detained and the skin must not be incised other than for the removal of a blood sample for diagnostic purposes by the owner's veterinary surgeon or a veterinary officer appointed by the Minister, usually the Divisional Veterinary Officer or a veterinarian acting on his behalf.

The State Veterinary service is responsible for the disease investigation and a stained smear is made from a superficial blood vessel and examined microscopically. If the Veterinary Inspector is satisfied that disease does not exist, the Local Authority is informed and the movement restrictions are withdrawn. If the inspector is not satisfied, an unfixed blood smear and a sample of blood is submitted to the Central Veterinary Laboratory for cultural and biological examination and the Local Authority informed accordingly. On receipt of this information the Local Authority are responsible for disposal of the carcass, usually by burning, and carrying out disinfection of the premises as prescribed in the Order. The disinfectants of choice are 5 per cent lysol, 5 per cent formalin or 5–10 per cent caustic soda. When these procedures have been completed, movement restrictions are withdrawn.

Confirmation of the disease is dependent on the results of the examinations at the Central Veterinary Laboratory, which may take seven or more days. On rare occasions disease is not confirmed; even so the existing procedures are considered effective in view of the serious nature of the disease and the human health implications.

Where enzootic disease exists, then an avirulent spore vaccine is available, and all cattle should be vaccinated on an annual basis. Vaccination is seldom necessary in Great Britain (see p. 806).

The number of confirmed incidents in Great Britain is now very low. This is largely due to the efforts of feedingstuffs compounders, who only use sterilized meat and bone meal or minerals in their finished feeds.

Bacillary haemoglobinuria

Bacillary haemoglobinuria or infectious ictero-haemoglobinuria of cattle was described by Roberts (1959) as a rapidly fatal infectious disease, manifested clinically by a high fever and haemoglobinuria, and pathologically by the presence of an infarct in the liver.

Aetiology

The causal organism is *Clostridium novyi* type D, previously designated *Cl. haemolyticum*. Like other clostridia it is a soil-borne anaerobe, the spores of which are resistant to environmental factors and may survive in soil for weeks if not months. The disease is considered to be one essentially of poorly irrigated or wet swampy land, which favours survival of the organism and is likely to harbour *Lymnaea* spp., the host snail of the liver fluke. The principal toxin produced by the organism is beta, which is haemolytic, necrotizing and lethal.

After ingestion the organism is transported from the alimentary tract to various organs. Smith (1957) recovered the organism from the liver, kidneys and bone marrow of normal cattle, where it remains as a latent infection. It is thought that, as in infectious necrotic hepatitis, the latent spore infection is activated by liver damage, especially by migrating immature liver fluke. The disease has been produced experimentally by infecting calves orally with the spores of *Cl. novyi* type D and carrying out a liver biopsy, and by implanting the organism in the liver suspended in calcium chloride solution (Blood *et al.*, 1983). It has also been postulated that telangiectasis may also be a precipitating factor.

When conditions are favourable for the activation of the latent infection, the damaged liver tissue provides a focus for initial multiplication of the bacteria. An organized thrombus develops in a subterminal branch of the portal vein resulting in a large anaemic infarct in which further rapid bacterial multiplication and toxin production occurs. The toxin produces a haemolytic anaemia, and later a bacteraemia develops. The duration of illness may vary from about 18 hours to four days. Bacillary haemoglobinuria has been observed in North and South America, Australia and New Zealand. Few incidents have been reported in Great Britain.

Signs

Cattle at pasture that are inspected at infrequent intervals may be found dead. The onset of disease is usually sudden, with cessation of feeding, rumination and defecation. Cows in lactation suffer a sudden and dramatic drop in milk yield. Animals are disinclined to move and the temperature is elevated to 39–41 °C (102–106 °F). The mucous membranes are jaundiced and there may be oedema of the brisket, submaxillary region and conjunctiva. Small amounts of bloodstained faeces may be passed in the early stages, but later there may be a frank dysentery. Not all these signs may be seen in individual cases and the variation may be due, in part, to different strains of organisms.

Pathology

One of the obvious features of the disease is the profound anaemia that develops before death. Blood samples from ailing animals show a depressed erythrocyte count, which may be as low as $10^6/mm^3$ and haemoglobin values are in the range of 40–80 g/l. Leucocyte counts are normally elevated to around $20\,000/mm^3$. The organism may be recovered from blood cultures taken during the acute phase. There is a very obvious haemoglobinuria in a proportion of cases, but there are no free red cells in the urine.

In the typical case, the necropsy picture is considered to be pathognomonic, the main features being generalized jaundice often with anaemia; subcutaneous oedema especially over the brisket; accumulation of slightly bloodstained fluid in the pericardial sac, pleural and peritoneal cavities; widespread haemorrhages in the subcutaneous tissues, over the pleural and peritoneal serosa, and endocardium; haemorrhagic abomasitis and enteritis. The liver is usually mahogany coloured with a characteristic yellow infarct, up to 20 cm (8 inches) in diameter, surrounded by a zone of hyperaemia (Fig. 38.1). The kidney cortex is petechiated and deep-red coloured urine may be present in the kidney pelvis and bladder. Evidence of liver fluke damage is not a constant feature.

Diagnosis

Bacillary haemoglobinuria must be differentiated from other conditions in which haemoglobinuria is one of the clinical signs. Acute leptospirosis, due to *Leptospira interrogans* serovar *pomona* (p. 569), is one of these and to confirm a diagnosis in the live animal serological tests and cultural examination of the urine is necessary, although there should be little difficulty in differentiating the two diseases at necropsy. Babesiasis (p. 726) and anaplasmosis (p. 737) can be differentiated by the demonstration of the organisms in blood smears. Post-parturient haemoglobinuria is accompanied by a hypophosphataemia (see p. 588), whilst blood and liver copper levels are elevated in chronic copper poisoning (p. 613). Both these conditions and haemoglobinuria due to the consumption of cruciferous plants (p. 613), such as rape and kale, are afebrile.

Confirmation of a diagnosis of bacillary haemoglobinuria is based on the clinical signs, necropsy findings and demonstration of the causal organism in the liver lesion and other sites by fluorescent antibody techniques. It may also be possible to culture the organism from tissue and demonstrate toxins in the liver infarct, but both procedures are time-consuming and laborious.

Treatment and prevention

Bacillary haemoglobinuria can be successfully treated by the administration of wide-spectrum antibiotics in the early stages (Smith & Holdeman, 1968). Early treatment with large doses of penicillin is also effective (Williams, 1964). Supportive treatment by the administration of electrolyte solutions orally and parenterally and the provision of mineral supplements containing iron, copper and cobalt is also necessary, as well as careful nursing.

The disease can be successfully prevented by vaccination with an aluminium hydroxide adsorbed, formalinized whole culture and it is also claimed that infectious necrotic hepatitis vaccines also confer immunity. Annual vaccination is necessary in enzootic areas (see p. 807).

Botulism

Botulism may be defined as a lethal type of food poisoning in man and several species of animals, caused by the ingestion of *Clostridium botulinum* toxins, which

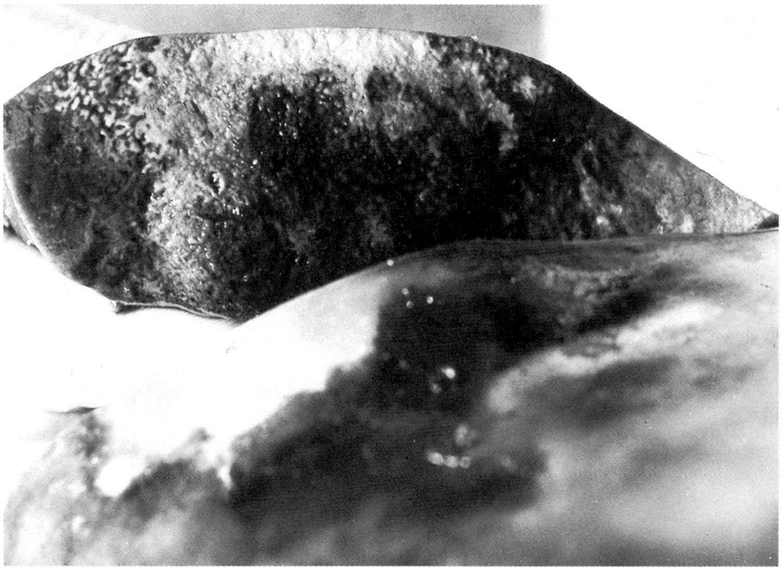

Fig. 38.1 Bacillary haemoglobinuria: a large infarct in the bovine liver caused by *Cl. novyi* type D.

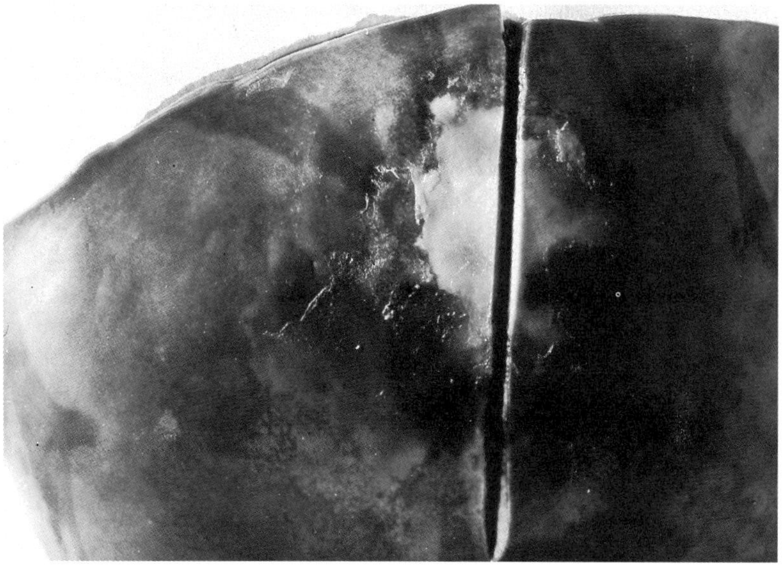

Fig. 38.2 A typical black disease lesion in the vertical lobe of a bovine liver. Note the central necrotic area surrounded by a zone of congestion.

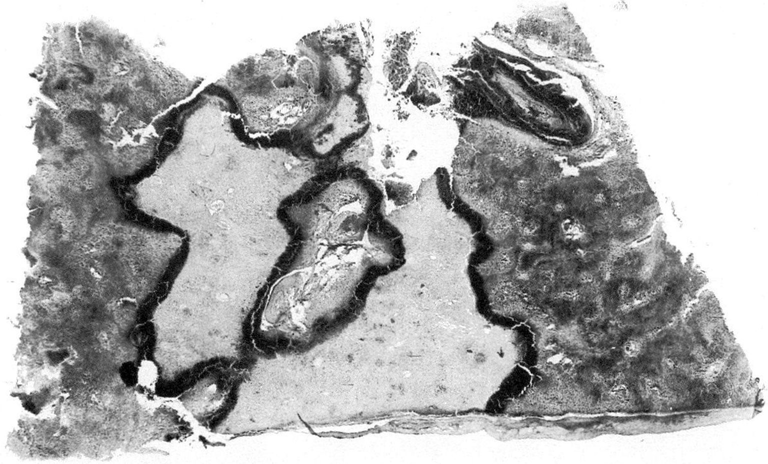

Fig. 38.3 A section through a black disease lesion demonstrating the central necrotic area and the clearly stained leucocyte barrier. (Haematoxylin and eosin, ×5.)

have been produced by the organism in decaying plant or animal tissue.

Aetiology

Smith (1977) defines *Cl. botulinum* 'not as a single species, but as a conglomerate of several distinct culture groups, alike in that they are clostridia and produce toxins with a similar pharmacological action'. There are a number of distinct serological types (A, B, C, D, E, F and G) and although the toxins are similarly designated, the serological specificity of the toxin produced by any strain may not be entirely related to its serological classification.

Like other clostridia, *Cl. botulinum* is a spore-forming organism, which under certain conditions thrives in putrefying animal tissue or decaying plant material. The organism has a world-wide occurrence and is found in the intestinal tracts of herbivores and in soil. It would appear that different soil types favour different types of the organism. Smith (1977) reported that in the USA, type A strains were prevalent in the alkaline soils of the south-west, types B and E in the damp soils of most areas, type C in the acid soils of the Gulf Coast and type D in the alkaline soils of the west.

The toxins of *Cl. botulinum* are neurotoxins, causing motor paralysis without the development of any gross or histological lesions in the nervous system. Although the mode of action is still debated, it appears that the site of action of the toxins is at the synapses of efferent parasympathetic and somatic motor nerves, by interference with the secretion of acetylcholine, which is the chemical mediator of nerve impulse transmission.

Two forms or types of botulism are recognized in cattle. The first is the form that develops after the consumption of, or contact with, carcasses or skeletons of dead animals containing botulinum toxins. The second form of the disease follows the consumption of conserved fodder that is contaminated by the toxins.

The first type of botulism has been widely reported in South Africa (lamsiekte), Australia (bulbar paralysis) and in the USA (loin disease). In these countries it has been associated with low phosphorus levels in soil, poor pastures and drought. Under such circumstances animals including the local fauna, which carry *Cl. botulinum* in their intestines, die and the organisms invade the carcass tissues and produce large amounts of toxin. Muller (1961) has demonstrated that the levels of toxin may reach 10^5-10^6 mouse lethal units/g of tissue. Animals that consume tissue from such carcasses, because of a phosphorus deficiency and a subsequent pica, or feed shortage, ingest both toxin and *Cl. botulinum* spores and will subsequently become a source of toxin and spores for other animals. In Europe, similar circumstances may arise after the spreading of litter from poultry houses on to cattle pastures. Investigations into such outbreaks reveal the presence of poultry carcasses in the litter, which are the source of the toxins (Appleyard & Mollison, 1985; Clegg *et al.*, 1985).

The second type of botulism, forage poisoning, occurs in those countries where conserved forage, especially baled hay and silage, is fed to cattle. The source of toxin has usually been identified as the carcasses of small animals (mice, rats, rabbits and birds) accidentally killed and subsequently baled in the hay or ensiled with the grass or cereal crop. Prevot & Sillioc (1955) recorded that more than half of the cattle botulism in France was associated with the presence of cat carcasses in the feed. Fjolstad & Kluna (1969) also reported an outbreak in which the source of toxin was a cat carcass and demonstrated 500 000 mouse lethal doses/g of the carcass. A hedgehog, discovered in a hay rack, was the source of toxin in an outbreak in cattle with 20 000 mouse lethal doses in its subcutaneous tissue (Ektvedt & Hanssen, 1974). Recently, however, it has been demonstrated that proteolytic strains of *Cl. botulinum* may produce toxin in silage under certain conditions and without the presence of animal tissue (Notermans *et al.*, 1979a, b). It would appear that a low pH prevents toxin formation in silage. The incorporation of poultry manure and poultry waste in cattle feed can also lead to outbreaks of botulism (Egyed *et al.*, 1978) and brewers grains contaminated with *Cl. botulinum* has also been incriminated (Breuknik *et al.*, 1978).

Botulism in any species of animal tends to be associated with certain types of the organism. Ruminants are susceptible to types C and D, although in The Netherlands disease has been associated with type B (Haagsma & Laak, 1977).

Signs

Clinical signs usually appear within two to fourteen days of ingestion of the toxin, although in peracute cases the incubation period may be only a few hours. Illness is afebrile.

In peracute cases the onset of disease is sudden, characterized by a rapid paralysis and death within 12–18 hours. In less acute cases the onset is more gradual, affected animals showing a progressive muscular paralysis of the head, neck and limbs, leading to recumbency, often with the head and neck outstretched or deviated towards the flank.

The majority of cases, however, appear to be of the subacute type. The first signs are periodic periods of restlessness, incoordination especially of the hindlimbs, and an apparent difficulty in chewing and swallowing. These signs progress to ataxia, difficulty or inability to rise, recumbency and an obvious paralysis of the tongue, which protrudes from the mouth. Animals may survive for up to seven days after becoming recumbent, but during the terminal stages respiration becomes laboured and of the abdominal type due to paralysis of the thoracic muscles.

Some animals may recover after showing relatively mild clinical signs over a period of three to four weeks (Clegg & Evans, 1974; Davies *et al.*, 1974). Clegg & Evans reported that surviving animals developed a pronounced respiratory roaring sound, which persisted for three months after recovery.

Pathology

A number of authors have reported on the value of certain biochemical tests on blood and urine from affected animals as aids to diagnosis, but in cattle such tests are of little help in the live animal. However, it is possible in some cases to demonstrate circulating toxins in the serum of clinically affected animals by mouse inoculation tests (Clegg *et al.*, 1985), but such cases are of the peracute or acute type.

As already indicated, the toxins of *Cl. botulinum* do not produce any specific or detectable lesions in the central nervous system, nor do they produce specific changes in the carcass. Those changes that are observed are non-specific and include haemorrhages on the endocardium and epicardium and congestion of the parenchymatous organs and intestinal mucosa. However, it may be possible to demonstrate toxin in the intestinal contents or liver by mouse inoculation tests. Whilst the presence of the organism in the intestine is of little diagnostic value, its isolation from the liver is of significance.

Diagnosis

It must be emphasized that it is not always possible to confirm all suspected cases of botulism by detection of toxin either in the sera of affected animals or in the intestinal contents or liver at necropsy. As *Cl. botulinum* is not normally found in the liver of cattle, isolation from the liver is regarded as significant.

Attempts may be made to demonstrate toxin in suspected feed, but such an approach has its limitations. Suspected feed may be fed to experimental animals of the same species, or an infusion of the feed may be administered to experimental animals. However, toxins in feedingstuffs are not distributed evenly, rather in pockets, and samples of feed for testing must therefore be carefully selected, e.g. from near carcasses or areas of contamination. It is also possible that all the botulinum-contaminated feed will have been consumed before the onset of clinical signs.

Postparturient paresis/hypocalcaemia (p. 577) can be differentiated from the disease by the examination of blood samples and the response to calcium therapy. In some cases of listeriosis (p. 703) there is a paralysis of the tongue, but it is accompanied by fever and other clinical signs such as unilateral facial paralysis and panophthalmia. Bovine spongiform encephalopathy (p. 708) in its later stages might be confused but there is no paralysis and the animal will still eat.

Treatment and prevention

There is little value in the administration of antitoxin, even in the early stages, and there are conflicting views on the merits of purgatives to remove the toxins from the intestine. However, Breuknik *et al.* (1978) reported that symptomatic treatment for dehydration and acidosis seemed to assist recovery. As a general rule, treatment of subacute cases only should be undertaken, as these are the ones most likely to recover.

Vaccination with toxoid is only necessary in enzootic areas and should be given every two years. Where botulism is associated with the disposal of poultry litter on to pasture, every effort should be made to remove any poultry carcasses in it before application.

All poultry waste should ideally be heat treated before incorporation into compound feeds for direct feeding to livestock.

Clostridial myositis: blackleg and malignant oedema

Two forms of clostridial myositis are recognized in cattle: blackleg, which is caused by *Clostridium chauveoi*, and malignant oedema, which is caused by a number of clostridial species and is nearly always associated with wound infection. It is often difficult or impossible to differentiate between the two conditions at a clinical or post-mortem examination (Williams, 1977).

Blackleg

Blackleg or blackquarter is defined as a gangrenous myositis caused by the activation of a latent *Cl. chauveoi* spore infection (Jubb *et al.*, 1983). These authors also refer to a 'false or pseudo blackleg' caused by the activation of *Cl. novyi* and *Cl. septicum* spore infection, but this condition is more appropriately designated malignant oedema.

Aetiology

Clostridium chauveoi is a Gram-positive, spore-bearing anaerobic bacillus, the spores of which are highly resistant to environmental conditions and therefore remain viable for many years. It is, like other clostridia, regarded as a soil organism and following ingestion by cattle, sheep and other animals, the spores localize in the spleen, liver and muscles (Kerry, 1964). The vegetative form of the organism produces a number of toxins, which are capable of inducing local muscle necrosis and toxaemia. The trigger mechanisms responsible for the activation of the endogenous latent spore infection are unknown, but it is assumed that a lowered oxygen tension and a degree of muscle damage are necessary. After activation, rapid bacterial multiplication and toxin formation produce the typical muscle gangrenous lesion and systemic toxaemia.

Most cases occur in animals between 10 months and two years of age at pasture, although incidents may occur in housed animals.

Signs

Often when stock are infrequently inspected animals may be found dead without signs of illness having been observed. The clinical signs that are seen in ailing animals are related to the site of lesion. Limb involvement is manifested as a lameness with a swelling of the upper part which, at first, is hot and painful, but later becomes cold and emphysematous. A lesion of the tongue results in a tongue and throat swelling, with the tongue protruding from the mouth and marked respiratory distress. Stiffness and a reluctance to move is apparent when the sublumbar muscles are involved. In addition to these clinical signs, there is a marked depression, anorexia, rapid pulse rate and high temperature, usually in excess of 40 °C (104 °F). Death occurs in 12–24 hours.

Pathology

The disease usually runs an acute course so that there is little opportunity for collecting specimens for laboratory examination before death. After death the carcass becomes bloated and putrefaction occurs rapidly. Bloodstained froth exudes from the body orifices. It may be possible to palpate the lesion, if it is in a superficial muscle group, but this is usually difficult because of the rapid onset of putrefaction.

Animals dying from blackleg are in good body condition. The body cavities contain bloodstained fluid and the parenchymatous organs show evidence of degeneration and post-mortem decomposition. All the skeletal muscles must be carefully examined by palpation and incision for lesions, which may not be extensive. The lesion produced by *Cl. chauveoi* has a characteristic appearance (Williams, 1977) (Plate 38.2). The muscle is blackened, dry and crepitant with a spongy appearance and a rancid odour. Pale yellow serous fluid surrounds the affected muscle, but this becomes progressively more bloodstained as post-mortem decomposition proceeds.

Diagnosis

A diagnosis can be reached on the basis of clinical signs and necropsy findings, but it is essential that when no clinical signs have been observed, anthrax (p. 551) is eliminated before a necropsy is carried out. *Clostridium chauveoi* can be identified by the staining of lesion impression smears by the specific fluorescent antiglobulins that are now commercially available. Cultural examination is likely to be unrewarding unless fresh tissue is available and special techniques used.

Blackleg may be confused with other conditions especially when death is sudden. Lead (p. 617) and other chemical poisonings (p. 613) require laboratory examination for confirmation, but the typical lesions of blackleg are absent. Black disease (p. 564) and bacillary haemoglobinuria (p. 553) may also have to be considered in a differential diagnosis, but the characteristic liver infarcts are a diagnostic feature of these two diseases.

Treatment and prevention

Antibiotic treatment of affected animals is likely to be effective only if commenced early. Large doses of penicillin (10 000 units/kg body weight) should be administered intravenously, followed by longer acting preparations, some of which should be given into the affected tissue (Blood *et al.*, 1983). However, because of the extensive tissue involvement, even if the infection is eliminated, the subsequent muscle loss is so great that recovered animals are of little economic value. Treatment of animals with tongue infection should not be attempted, because even if successful the whole tongue or most of it will be subsequently lost and early slaughter on humane grounds should be considered.

Blackleg can be successfully prevented by the use of commercially available *Cl. chauveoi* vaccines and all animals over six months of age should be vaccinated prior to being turned out in the spring. There are, however, considerable advantages in the use of multivalent vaccines containing the antigens of *Cl. chauveoi*, *Cl. novyi* and *Cl. septicum*, which offer maximum protection to cattle against blackleg, malignant oedema and black disease (p. 807).

Malignant oedema

Malignant oedema is considered to be an acute wound infection caused by organisms of the genus *Clostridium* (Blood *et al.*, 1983). However, if blackleg is restricted to cover endogenous *Cl. chauveoi* infection then malignant oedema must also include those incidents, albeit relatively few in number, arising from activation of latent *Cl. novyi* and *Cl. septicum*, which undoubtedly occur.

Aetiology

Clostridium chauveoi, Cl. novyi, Cl. perfringens, Cl. septicum, Cl. sordelli and other clostridia have been isolated from, or demonstrated in lesions of clostridial myositis in cattle. Williams (1977) in a survey of 173 cases in Wales demonstrated *Cl. chauveoi* in 75 (43 per cent), *Cl. chauveoi* and *Cl. septicum* in 22 (13 per cent), *Cl. novyi* in 53 (31 per cent), *Cl. novyi* and *Cl. septicum* in nine (5 per cent), *Cl. septicum* in 11 (6 per cent) and *Cl. sordelli* in three (1.7 per cent). In this series *Cl. perfringens* was isolated from about 50 per cent of the lesions, but its presence was not considered to be of significance. There is still some uncertainty about the role of *Cl. septicum* in bovine malignant oedema.

Deep puncture wounds, accidentally inflicted, provide ideal conditions for the multiplication of anaerobes and development of malignant oedema. It may also develop after surgical operations, intramuscular administration of anthelmintic and vitamin preparations, vaccination and parturition. The clostridia are soil organisms that persist in the animal environment and therefore readily gain entry to wounds. The tissue damage and low oxygen tension allow rapid multiplication and toxin production so that clinical signs usually develop within 48 hours. Occasionally, malignant oedema may affect a group of animals that had previously been housed or penned for a short period of time and the absence of any form of wound suggests that some factor, perhaps trauma from bruising, may have activated a latent spore infection.

Signs

The disease is usually sporadic involving single or small numbers of animals. All ages of cattle are affected and clinical signs appear within 48 hours of infection. The clinical signs will vary with the site of infection, but in all cases, anorexia, depression and fever are very marked. A local lesion develops at the site of infection consisting of a swelling, which becomes tense and depending on the type of infection may become emphysematous. Lameness, stiffness and muscle tremors may be evident. Animals usually die within 48 hours.

When infection is associated with parturition, the vulva and perineum swell and there is a bloodstained discharge from the vulva. Death is rapid, usually within 24–36 hours after the onset of symptoms.

Pathology

In malignant oedema there is little opportunity for the laboratory examination of specimens taken from affected animals. As in blackleg, it is necessary for a post-mortem examination to be carried out as soon after death as possible, because of the bacterial invasion of the carcass and rapid onset of putrefactive changes.

The site of infection is surrounded by an extensive oedema of the subcutaneous tissues and intramuscular fascia. It may be possible to identify the initial wound, but tissue damage is usually so extensive that the only trace is a small wound in the skin. The oedema fluid may be clear and gelatinous in *Cl. novyi* infections with very little muscle damage. Infection with *Cl. septicum* produces an extensive bloodstained frothy oedema, with the underlying muscle a dark red colour permeated with gas. *Clostridium sordelli* produces changes similar to those produced by *Cl. novyi* except that the oedema is more bloodstained and has a foul odour. The lesion produced by *Cl. chauveoi* is similar to that described under blackleg.

All body cavities contain bloodstained fluid and the parenchymatous organs show degenerative changes and post-mortem decomposition. If the infection involves the reproductive tract, the uterus will contain a large volume of foul-smelling bloodstained fluid and the uterine and vaginal walls will be greatly thickened, permeated with bloodstained fluid and gas.

Diagnosis

The clinical signs and necropsy findings are so characteristic that diagnosis can be readily reached. It will, however, be necessary to resort to laboratory examination of lesions for the identification of the organisms by fluorescent antibody tests or culture.

Treatment and prevention

Affected animals should be treated with high doses of antibiotics, preferably parenteral penicillin or broad spectrum. In addition, wounds should be drained and irrigated with antiseptic solutions, and packed with a suitable antibiotic preparation.

Trivalent vaccines, containing the antigens of *Cl. chauveoi*, *Cl. novyi* and *Cl. septicum* are available and are effective in preventing malignant oedema (p. 807).

Harwood (1984) highlights the dangers from intramuscular injections administered to cattle, particularly if infection is introduced and if large volumes are used, and under such circumstances routine vaccination is recommended.

Contagious bovine pyelonephritis

This disease is a specific infection of the urinary tract of cattle, which results in a chronic purulent inflammation of the kidneys, ureters and bladder.

Aetiology

Corynebacterium renale is considered to be the specific causal agent, although other organisms, especially streptococci, staphylococci, *Actinomyces (Corynebacterium) pyogenes* and *Escherichia coli*, as well as *C. renale* are present in the urine of some animals with pyelonephritis and may also be implicated. *Corynebacterium renale* is an obligate parasite of cattle and occasionally sheep, and can be readily cultured from the urine of affected and carrier animals.

Goudswaard & Budhai (1975) identified four serotypes, of which type I is the most pathogenic.

It has been demonstrated that the pathogenicity of *C. renale* is dependent to a large extent on the presence of pili on the organism, which assist its adhesion to the urinary epithelium. This process is pH dependent and Takai *et al.* (1980) showed that the proportion of piliated organism adhering to bladder cells is high at a pH above 7.6, but significantly lower at a pH below 6.8, a factor that is important in the pathogenesis of pyelonephritis.

The disease is considered to be the result of an ascending infection, involving successively the bladder, ureters and kidneys. Hiramune *et al.* (1972) established infection in cattle after the introduction of organisms into the bladder and the characteristic lesions developed. Females are far more susceptible than males to infection and the short length of the urethra in the female is thought to be a major factor in the establishment of infection. Stasis of urine is an important predisposing factor in the pathogenesis of pyelonephritis and cystitis and such circumstances may occur when a permanent or temporary obstruction of the urinary tract occurs through the presence of calculi or pressure exerted by a gravid uterus.

The disease is widely recognized in Europe and North America, but the prevalence of infection is largely unknown. Morse (1950) found that *C. renale* could be recovered from the urine of 22.7 per cent of cattle in herds in which pyelonephritis had been confirmed, whereas only 10.7 per cent of cattle in other herds were infected. Clinically infected or carrier cows are the principal source of infection, the disease being mainly transmitted by direct contact, although Morse (1950) reported that infection was transmitted by indirect contact from affected and carrier cows tethered in stalls to those in adjacent stalls. In some herds there is circumstantial evidence to support the existence of venereal spread and the organism has been readily isolated from the prepuce of normal bulls (Hiramune *et al.*, 1975).

Signs

In affected herds, clinical cases appear sporadically with animals under three years of age rarely affected. Most cases occur in dairy herds with the peak incidence usually in winter.

There is considerable variation in the clinical signs observed from case to case, particularly during the early stages. Bloodstained urine may be passed intermittently by an apparently healthy animal over a period of weeks, before other signs appear. In other animals, one, two or more attacks of acute colic lasting up to 6 hours or more may be the first sign. More frequently, however, the onset is insidious. The most common signs are a gradual loss of condition, a slowly declining milk yield, fluctuating or capricious appetite, intermittent fever, and the intermittent passage of bloodstained urine. As the disease progresses, urination becomes more frequent and painful with the passage of small volumes of urine containing blood and tissue debris. During the later stages it may be possible to detect, by rectal examination, enlargement of one or both kidneys, a thickened bladder and enlargement of one or both ureters, particularly the terminal portions where they cross the neck of the bladder. Frequently, palpation of the kidneys induces a pain response. The course of the disease may run from a period of weeks to two or more months, death resulting from a combination of kidney failure and blood loss with an extensive loss of condition.

Pathology

The urine of clinically affected animals is turbid and in

the early stages intermittently bloodstained, but in the later stages the urine is almost constantly bloodstained. Microscopic examination of the centrifuged deposit of the urine reveals the presence of erythrocytes, leucocytes and epithelial tissue debris. *Corynebacterium renale* can be readily demonstrated in Gram-stained smears and Ado & Cook (1979) have reported on the value of fluorescent antibody tests for the identification of the organism. It can be readily isolated on blood agar and other media in common use. The clinical signs are so characteristic that haematological examination and blood chemistry estimations are seldom considered necessary. In any case, such examinations are unlikely to reveal any abnormalities until the disease is well developed when anaemia and uraemia are the most prominent findings.

Animals dying from pyelonephritis are usually in poor condition and the carcass pale and anaemic. Specific lesions are confined to the urinary tract. One or both kidneys are enlarged with less well marked lobulation than normal and a markedly thickened capsule. The surface is mottled by greyish white necrotic areas. On section the renal pelvis is greatly dilated and contains varying amounts of blood, pus and mucoid fluid. Greyish white streaks of necrotic tissue radiate from the pelvis towards the cortex and there may be numerous abscesses in the cortex and medulla of each lobule. The ureters are grossly enlarged and distended by blood, pus and mucus. The bladder wall and the urethra are thickened and the mucosa oedematous, haemorrhagic and necrotic.

Diagnosis

The diagnosis of pyelonephritis is based on the clinical signs, the changes in the urine and the presence of *C. renale* in the urine together with the detectable abnormalities in the urinary tract. Enzootic haematuria (p. 620) has some clinical features in common with pyelonephritis, but it is afebrile, lesions are confined to the bladder and the urine from such cases is sterile or negative for *C. renale*. Similarly, non-specific cystitis may also resemble pyelonephritis, but the bladder only is affected and the urine is sterile or negative for *C. renale*.

Treatment and prevention

Corynebacterium renale is sensitive to a range of antibiotics but penicillin remains the antibiotic of choice for the treatment of pyelonephritis in the bovine. A complete recovery can be achieved if treatment is commenced during the early stages, when little tissue damage has occurred. In advanced cases, however, when there is considerable tissue destruction, only a temporary recovery can be achieved through antibiotic therapy, although this may enable an animal to be fattened and subsequently sent for slaughter. Large doses of procaine penicillin G should be administered, e.g. 10000–15000 iu/kg daily for at least 10 days. The acidification of the urine by the administration of monobasic sodium phosphate is still considered by some as useful supportive therapy and 100 g daily for a period of five days during antibiotic treatment is recommended.

There are no specific control measures other than isolation of affected animals and thorough cleansing and disinfection of the contaminated environment. In affected herds where natural breeding is practised, the introduction of artificial insemination may achieve a reduction in the number of clinical cases.

Endocarditis

Endocarditis may be defined as inflammation of the endothelial lining of the heart. The inflammatory processes usually result in valvular insufficiency or stenosis that interfere with the flow of blood into and out of the heart, leading to congestive heart failure.

Aetiology

Most cases of bovine endocarditis appear to be caused by bacterial infection. Several species of bacteria have been incriminated, but streptococci especially enterococci of Lancefield's group D, *A. pyogenes*, staphylococci and *Pasteurella* species are the commonest (Evans, 1957; Larsen, 1963).

It would appear that a persistent bacteraemia is necessary for the development of endocardial lesions and it is significant that in most, if not all, confirmed cases, a primary focus of infection in the form of mastitis, metritis, reticulitis, limb abscesses, etc. can be identified at post-mortem examination (Evans, 1957; Andersen, 1963; Larsen, 1963).

Although it is generally accepted that the causal organisms are transported to the heart via the bloodstream, the method by which they reach the endocardial lesion is still uncertain. It is possible that some bacteria may be able to adhere to the intact endothelium. However, it is more likely that they adhere to damaged endothelium and it is assumed that trauma and debility are the main factors in producing sufficient damage for the bacteria to localize in the endothelium. This hypothesis is based on the fact that the usual sites of the lesions are on the free edges of the valves exposed to the blood flow and that are in apposition to others. The heart valves of the bovine have their own blood supply and it is thus possible for the bacteria to produce emboli in the capillaries, which form a focus of infection.

The early lesions of endocarditis are seldom seen except in experimental infections. Initially, the leaflet of the valve becomes swollen and an irregular ulcer develops on its surface, in which the bacteria localize. From this ulcerated area the characteristic vegetative structures develop. These have a similar composition to thrombi, except that they contain few platelets. Several layers of thrombus-like material are deposited on the affected valve in response to the bacterial activity, so that vegetations assume a cauliflower or wart-like appearance and the valves become distorted and shrunken and functionally incompetent. Fragments of the vegetation may become detached to form emboli, which lodge in other organs.

Signs

All ages of cattle are affected although Larsen (1963) found that nearly half of the 53 bovine cases he encountered were in animals between two and three years of age. Both Evans (1957) and Biering-Sørensen (1963) found that 3.9 per cent of cattle examined in abbatoir surveys had either died from, or been slaughtered because of, endocarditis.

The published descriptions of the clinical signs of bovine endocarditis are varied and reflect the stage to which the endocarditis had progressed and also the extent to which the clinical signs were attributable to the primary focus of infection (Evans, 1957; Power & Rebhun, 1983). Thus the initial signs may not indicate heart involvement and the onset of the clinical signs of endocarditis may be insidious.

A recurrent or persistent fever of 40–41 °C (104–106 °F), anorexia, depression and a reluctance to move are the usual early signs. Pinching of the withers and ballottement of the sternum ventral to the heart elicit a pain response. The heart rate is accelerated to 100–120 beats/minute and in due course the jugular vein becomes engorged, which is followed by oedema of the brisket and submandibular areas. The detection of a heart murmur on auscultation is an important clinical feature, but this is not easily detected when the right atrioventricular valves are involved. Lacuta *et al.* (1980) have reported on the value of electrocardiography and echocardiography in the diagnosis of endocarditis. Whilst echocardiography is of value in that it will demonstrate reflected echoes from the vegetative lesions and detect abnormal valve movements, electrocardiography is less so because the abnormalities shown are not diagnostic of endocarditis.

As the disease progresses, secondary involvement of other organs and systems occurs, leading to pneumonia, nephritis, arthritis, etc. Progressive weight loss, anaemia and weakness inevitably is followed by recumbency and death. The course of the disease may extend from one or two weeks to two or three months.

Pathology

Blood samples from affected animals show a leucocytosis and a shift to the left, although in the more chronic cases these changes are less well marked. Plasma fibrinogen levels are elevated (Wuijckhuise-Sjouke, 1984) but this is a feature of inflammation of serous membranes as well as endocarditis. The causal organism can be isolated on blood culture during periods of fever but at least 20 ml of blood are necessary and the cultures may have to be repeated on a number of occasions.

The heart lesions found at necropsy are fairly constant (Plate 38.3). The pericardial sac is distended with varying amounts of oedematous fluid and the heart is enlarged and distorted, due to hypertrophy of the myocardium and dilatation of one or more chambers, because of the incompetence/stenosis of the affected atrioventricular valves. In the majority of cases the right atrioventricular valves are affected. The affected valves are shrunken and thickened, particularly in the later stages, and attached to them there are wart-like or cauliflower vegetations.

The parenchymatous organs may show pathological changes. The lungs are passively congested with frequently a number of embolic infarcts, and the liver is usually enlarged due to passive venous congestion and may show evidence of cirrhosis. Numerous small haemorrhagic foci are scattered over the surface of the kidneys and within the cortex and there may be a number of infarcts or abscesses in the cortex.

Diagnosis

The clinical diagnosis of endocarditis is dependent upon the detection of heart murmurs, which may be extremely difficult when the lesions involve the right atrioventricular valves. Thus it may be difficult or impossible to differentiate between endocarditis and pericarditis (p. 566) (John, 1947) or other causes of congestive heart failure. Cardiac lesions of enzootic bovine leukosis (EBL) (p. 530) may also produce signs of congestive heart failure, but affected animals show a persistent lymphocytosis and are positive to the agar gel immunodiffusion test for EBL.

Treatment

The organisms associated with bovine endocarditis are sensitive to a range of antibiotics. However, the nature of the heart lesions is such that therapeutic concentrations of antibiotic may not penetrate through to the bacteria. Furthermore, the permanent damage inflicted on the heart valves and the embolic lesions in other organs cannot be effectively repaired. Thus treatment of ailing animals is unlikely to lead to complete recovery. Although temporary improvement may occur after intensive antibiotic treatment for seven to ten days, a relapse within seven days is the usual outcome. However, Power & Rebhun (1983) reported that nine cows, in which an early diagnosis had been made, responded to long-term penicillin therapy.

Haemorrhagic septicaemia

Haemorrhagic septicaemia, or more appropriately septicaemic pasteurellosis of cattle, is a peracute disease, which is characterized by a septicaemia and a very high mortality rate.

Aetiology

Carter & Bain (1960) and Carter (1982) highlighted the confusion and conflict in the terminology of diseases attributed to *Pasteurella* infection in bovines. Thus it is difficult to assess the accuracy of many of the early reports on haemorrhagic septicaemia. It is now considered to be a primary pasteurellosis caused by *Pasteurella multocida* capsular serotypes B and E, which appears now to be confined largely to the tropical countries of Asia. Shirlaw (1938) reported on the occurrence of septicaemic pasteurellosis in the Northumbrian area of Great Britain in 1926. The lesions in the affected animals were those of a bronchopneumonia and although *Pasteurella* was isolated from the lungs it was not fully typed but likely to have been type B. Since then there have been no further reports of haemorrhagic septicaemia in Great Britain. In the USA only four outbreaks, three in bison and one in cattle, have been confirmed and Carter (1982) speculated on its disappearance from that country.

Pasteurella multocida is not a very resistant organism and it is unlikely to survive for long periods outside the animal body. In soil and mud, for example, where competition for other organisms is strong it does not survive for more than 24 hours (Bain, 1963). Toxins have been demonstrated in culture filtrates, but all the evidence suggests that the most significant of these are endotoxins, which are important in producing the clinical disease and rapid death.

The main source of infection is the carrier animal, the organism localizing in the nasopharyngeal mucosa and tonsils. In herds that experienced haemorrhagic septicaemia 44.4 per cent of healthy cattle were carriers, whereas the carrier rates in three herds in which the disease had not been confirmed were 3.89 per cent, 5.5 per cent and nil (Mustafa *et al.*, 1978). Furthermore, the carrier rate was higher in cattle under two years of age than in adult cattle. It is estimated that approximately 10 per cent of carrier animals become immune.

Spread of infection is through the ingestion of feed contaminated by carrier or clinically affected animals. The role of biting and blood-sucking ectoparasites in the spread of infection is still unclear, although Macadam (1962) suggested on the basis of experimental work in rabbits that ticks could transmit the disease.

It is generally accepted that environmental stress is an important factor in precipitating outbreaks of disease. Outbreaks occur when animals are exposed to cold and wet weather, housed under poor conditions or exhausted by prolonged periods of work. Under such circumstances the immunity of carrier animals wanes, allowing a rapid multiplication of the organism and spread within the carrier animal and its subsequent dissemination to susceptible contact animals.

Signs

The disease may be peracute with death frequently occurring so rapidly that few, if any, clinical signs are observed. In the acute form, there is a sudden onset of fever (41–42 °C, 106–108 °F), severe depression, oedema of the throat, profuse salivation and rapid death, usually in less than 24 hours. The oedematous form of the disease is also acute with the development of hot painful swellings of the head, throat, brisket, perineum and limb(s). Severe oedema of the head and throat may result in dyspnoea and eventually death through asphyxiation rather than death from a septicaemia.

Pathology

Large numbers of *Pasteurella* organisms can be demonstrated in the nasal discharges and saliva of clinically affected animals. The course of the disease is usually less than 24 hours, which limits the opportunities for carrying out laboratory examination on specimens from ailing animals.

On post-mortem examination the most prominent features are widespread petechial haemorrhages on the serous membranes and in various organs, especially the lungs and muscles, and a subcutaneous oedema of the throat region. The lungs are oedematous, may also show an early interstitial pneumonia and often there is a haemorrhagic gastroenteritis. In the oedematous form of the disease, there is widespread oedema of the head, tongue, brisket and/or one or more limbs as well as widespread petechiation. The spleen is not greatly enlarged.

Diagnosis

The regional occurrence of the disease is of some aid in diagnosis, but the clinical signs, rapid course and necropsy findings are similar to those of other diseases, e.g. anthrax (p. 551), clostridial myositis (p. 557), acute leptospirosis, so that confirmation can only be achieved by isolation and identification of the causal organism. *Pasteurella multocida* can be readily isolated from heart blood, spleen, liver and other sites, but identification of the specific serotypes may require submission to specialist laboratories.

Treatment and prevention

Pasteurella multocida is sensitive *in vitro* to a range of antimicrobial substances, including oxytetracycline, chloramphenicol and penicillin/dihydrostreptomycin and, in theory, therefore treatment of clinically affected animals should be feasible. However, the sudden onset and rapid course of the disease are such that treatment during the very early stages only is likely to be successful. Even if all the organisms are eliminated, death from *Pasteurella* endotoxaemia may still occur (Jubb *et al.*, 1985).

The only effective method of control is vaccination of all herds at risk. A dead vaccine in an adjuvant base containing paraffin and lanolin has proved highly effective when used prophylactically and is also of value in reducing losses if used during an outbreak, immunity persisting for at least 12 months. Persistent subcutaneous swellings may develop in some animals and after the administration of some batches of vaccine, anaphylactic shock has occasionally been recorded. A live streptomycin-dependent mutant of *P. multocida* vaccine has been developed (Wei & Carter, 1978) and successfully tested in field trials (De Alwis & Carter, 1980), but does not appear to be commercially available as yet.

The observations of Sawada *et al.* (1985) on naturally acquired immunity to *P. multocida*, capsular types B and E, are of considerable interest. They found, on the basis of serological and passive immunity tests in mice, that 81 per cent of feeder calves were immune to type B and 91 per cent to type E. The immunity appeared to develop in the absence of either of these serotypes in the microbial flora of the calves.

Infectious necrotic hepatitis (black disease)

Infectious necrotic hepatitis is a highly fatal acute or peracute infectious disease of sheep and cattle, characterized by the presence of one or more necrotic areas in the liver, in which *Cl. novyi* type B has multiplied and produced lethal toxins.

Aetiology

The causal organism is *Cl. novyi*, which like other clostridia is a Gram-positive spore-bearing bacillus, widely distributed in the environment, particularly in soil. The more pathogenic types, however, are more prevalent in those areas where infectious necrotic hepatitis occurs. After ingestion, spores are transported to the liver and other locations, where they remain as a latent infection. On the basis of toxin production a number of types are recognized, but infectious necrotic hepatitis in cattle is caused by type B, which produces large amounts of the lethal alpha toxin.

The disease occurs in cattle and sheep in those areas where liver fluke infection also occurs (p. 238), and it has been demonstrated experimentally in sheep that migrating immature liver fluke produce liver damage and through this an environment suitable for the activation of the latent infection. It is assumed that the same sequence of events occurs in cattle, although Williams (1964) noted the absence of liver fluke damage in some confirmed cases. It has been demonstrated that the survival of *Cl. novyi* and *Fasciola hepatica* is favoured by the same type of soil environment (Bagadi & Sewell, 1973). Other migrating parasites, e.g. the intermediate stages of certain canine cestodes, may also activate latent *Cl. novyi* infection.

The organism multiplies rapidly in the damaged liver and large amounts of the lethal and necrotizing toxin are formed, which leads to the production of the characteristic lesion. The toxin is rapidly absorbed, leading to a systemic toxaemic and it is only rarely that the organism can be recovered from other organs in the fresh carcass.

The disease has been confirmed in most countries

where fascioliasis occurs. Cattle of all ages may be affected; Williams (1964) found that in a series of 46 cases, one was in a six-month-old calf, two were in cows over seven years old and the remainder in bullocks and heifers between one and two years old. There is little information on morbidity rates in cattle, but experience in the UK indicates that single animals succumb in most herds. It is likely, however, that the disease is becoming more common in some areas.

Signs

Most cattle with infectious necrotic hepatitis are found dead but, in some, illness may last for one to two days (Herbert & Hughes, 1956). Affected animals develop severe depression, are disinclined to move, with a normal or slightly elevated temperature. Signs of discomfort are exhibited on palpation of the liver region.

Pathology

Because of the acute nature of the disease it is not possible to carry out ante-mortem laboratory examinations.

Animals dying from the disease are usually in good condition. The subcutaneous vessels are engorged and clear gelatinous fluid in variable amounts is present in the axillary and inguinal regions, and over the brisket. Fluid, sometimes bloodstained and containing fibrin strands, is present in the pleural and peritoneal cavities and in the pericardial sac. Haemorrhages are scattered over the endocardium and sometimes over the epicardium, parietal pleura and peritoneum. The mucosa of the abomasum is usually congested and often the abomasal wall is distended by a gelatinous oedema. The duodenum and jejunum may show a patchy mucosal congestion.

The pathological changes in the liver are characteristic. The organ is a dark brown colour due to venous congestion and the gall-bladder is usually distended. One, two or more sharply demarcated yellowish necrotic areas up to 8 cm (3 inches) (Fig. 38.2) or more in diameter may be identified, most frequently on the surface but also in the depths of the parenchyma, where they may be missed unless the liver is carefully palpated and sectioned with a knife. The necrotic area is surrounded by an obvious zone of deep congestion. Lesions may be found anywhere in the liver, but the majority tend to be located in the ventral lobe. Evidence of liver fluke migration in the form of subcapsular haemorrhages and greenish yellow scars (accumulations of eosinophils) may be evident near the lesion.

Microscopical examination of sections prepared from the liver lesions show a central core of necrotic tissue demarcated from the congested parenchyma by a leucocytic barrier (Fig. 38.3). Within the barrier and at the periphery of the necrotic tissue, large numbers of vegetative clostridia are evident. The hepatic cells immediately adjacent to the leucocytic barrier show degenerative changes.

Diagnosis

The post-mortem findings of the characteristic lesions provide a firm basis for arriving at a diagnosis. Fluorescent antibody techniques can be used for the rapid identification of *Cl. novyi* in impression smears made from the periphery of the liver lesion as described by Batty *et al.* (1964). Toxins may also be demonstrated in the liver lesions and peritoneal fluid (Williams, 1964), although the laboratory tests for these are laborious and time-consuming. If the post-mortem findings are inconclusive and the carcass shows evidence of decomposition then the fluorescent antibody and toxin tests cannot be reliably used, since *Cl. novyi* may have multiplied in the liver and other locations after death (Bagadi & Sewell, 1974), and some of the strains found in livers are of low pathogenicity (Williams, 1964) but are detected by fluorescent antibody techniques.

Other cases of sudden or rapid death have to be considered in differential diagnosis and these include anthrax (p. 551), other clostridial infections such as clostridial myositis (p. 557), lead poisoning (p. 617) and metabolic disorders (Chapter 39). It is vital that blood smears for anthrax diagnosis be examined before post-mortem examination is carried out and thereby prevent environmental contamination with anthrax spores.

Treatment and prevention

There is little opportunity for effective treatment, although in those cattle that are ailing for one to two days, the administration of wide-spectrum antibiotics or penicillin and *Cl. novyi* antiserum may be of value.

Effective vaccines have been developed and in areas where liver fluke occurs their use should be advocated. Two doses of vaccine at an interval of not less than one month are required to produce a satisfactory immunity (p. 807). Because of the association with liver fluke infection, control measures should also be adopted for this parasite (see p. 241).

Pericarditis

Infection of the pericardial sac by micro-organisms results in a purulent or non-purulent pericarditis with the accumulation of varying amounts of fluid and consequential masking or muffling of heart sounds, and may lead to congestive heart failure.

Aetiology

A wide range of micro-organisms are associated with bovine pericarditis and they include *A. pyogenes*, *Haemophilus somnus*, *Mycobacterium bovis*, *Pasteurella* species, staphylococci, streptococci and *Mycoplasma* species.

Infection with pyogenic bacteria is nearly always primary and frequently associated with traumatic reticulitis. The organisms are introduced during penetration of the pericardial sac by a foreign body originating from the reticulum, or infection may be the result of direct spread from a traumatic mediastinitis. In some instances a purulent infection may be superimposed on an original non-purulent fibrinous pericarditis. Infection of the pericardial sac also occurs through the localization of a blood-borne infection or through the direct extension of a myocarditis or pleurisy.

During the early stages of a purulent pericarditis there is a marked hyperaemia and deposition of a fibrinous exudate on the epicardium. Varying amounts of fluid accumulate within the pericardial sac and, as the volume significantly increases, both atria and the right ventricle are compressed to such an extent that their function is impaired and congestive heart failure results. A severe toxaemia may also develop. In some instances, however, the volume of exudate is small and adhesions develop between the epicardium and pericardium, which become organized, resulting in complete attachment of the epicardium and pericardium, impaired cardiac function and congestive heart failure.

In non-purulent or fibrinous pericarditis, there is seldom a significant exudation of fluid and therefore no marked distension of the pericardial sac. The epicardium is hyperaemic and fibrinous deposits appear at the base of the heart, which subsequently spread over the whole of the epicardium and internal surface of the pericardium. Adhesions develop between the epicardium and pericardium, but these are not sufficiently dense or strong to impair cardiac movement.

Signs

The early clinical signs of pericarditis are often difficult to identify because they are obscured or dominated by those of the primary disease, e.g. pleurisy, traumatic reticulitis, and the onset of pericarditis may therefore be insidious. Arching of the back, reluctance to move, shallow and rapid abdominal respirations and elevation of body temperature to 40–41 °C (104–106 °F) are the initial signs. The pulse rate is increased, and percussion and palpation over the cardiac area of the thoracic wall elicits a pain response. It may be possible to detect a rough pericardial function sound by auscultation during the early stages, but this is by no means easy and may be missed.

As the condition progresses, fluid accumulates in the percardial sac and the heart sounds become muffled, although sometimes a splashing sound may be detected. The signs of congestive heart failure, engorged jugular veins, a jugular pulse and subcutaneous oedema of the submandibular space, brisket and inguinal region, develop and most animals die within one or two weeks.

Some animals survive the acute phase with antibiotic treatment, and the signs of congestive heart failure abate slowly. However, complete recovery seldom if ever occurs and recovered animals should be sent for slaughter at the earliest opportunity.

Pathology

Blood samples from animals affected with a purulent pericarditis, especially traumatic pericarditis, show a marked leucocytosis and a shift to the left. However, the overall haematological picture depends to some extent on the causal agent and other lesions that may be present, so that the total white cell count may vary from only marginally above the normal range to more than 30 000/μl.

The cardiac lesions found at post-mortem examination depend on the type of infection and the duration of illness. In acute purulent pericarditis the pericardium and epicardium are thickened and covered by a fibrinous deposit, and the pericardial sac distended with fluid, which varies from a dirty grey to a yellowish green colour with a foul odour. The atria and the right ventricle are compressed. When the condition is associated with traumatic injury it may be possible to identify a foreign body, but should this be wire it may have disintegrated. Occasionally, a rupture of one of the coronary vessels, an atrium, or ventricle may occur in traumatic pericarditis and under such circumstances the pericardial sac contains a mixture of blood and purulent fluid. In more chronic cases, the grossly thickened pericardium and epicardium are closely adherent except for loculi containing inspissated or thick creamy pus giving a 'bread and butter' appearance. Signs indicative of congestive heart failure are also identifiable and these include congested liver and lungs, engorged jugular veins and subcutaneous oedema of the submandibular space, brisket and inguinal region. If the pericarditis is associated with other conditions, e.g. traumatic reticulitis, pneumonia or pleurisy, then lesions attributable to them will also be present.

Evidence of a non-purulent or fibrinous pericarditis is sometimes seen in apparently healthy animals dying from other causes. In such animals there is a patchy or diffuse thickening of the pericardium with patchy or diffuse adhesions to the epicardium, which can be easily broken down. There is no evidence of interference with the cardiac function and the lesions are of no pathological significance.

Diagnosis

The clinical diagnosis of pericarditis is not easy because the signs may be dominated or obscured by those of the primary disease and it may be difficult to recognize the pericardial sounds. The characteristic friction sounds in the early stages may be confused with those of pleurisy, although the latter is synchronized with the respiratory movements. Similarly, the pericardial sounds may resemble the murmurs (p. 362) produced by valvular lesions, but unlike the murmurs, they persist for the whole of the cardiac cycle. The heart sounds may also be muffled by effusion associated with pleurisy but under such circumstances there are signs of respiratory involvement.

Treatment

Although long-term therapy with antimicrobial agents is indicated, it seldom results in complete recovery, especially when the pericarditis is traumatic in origin. Thus Blood & Hutchins (1955) report that only about 50 per cent of cattle with traumatic pericarditis treated with sulphamezathine and/or penicillin responded and were sufficiently recovered for salvage. Surgical drainage of the pericardial sac either by pericardiocentesis or pericardiotomy as described by Horney (1960) may also have to be considered. However, it must be emphasized that pericardiocentesis offers only temporary relief of less than 24 hours duration in most cases. There are a number of reports on the successful treatment of fibrinous and traumatic pericarditis by pericardiotomy (Jennings & McIntyre, 1957; Krishnamurthy *et al.*, 1979; Mason, 1979).

Tetanus

Tetanus has long been recognized as a highly fatal disease of all species of farm livestock. The disease is produced by the toxin of *Clostridium tetani* and is characterized by hyperaesthesia, tetany and convulsions.

Aetiology

Clostridium tetani is a spore-bearing organism and is considered to be one of the least fastidious clostridia as far as growth requirements are concerned. The spores are extremely resistant to environmental conditions. The organism has two main habitats, namely the soil and gastrointestinal tracts of animals and humans. It has been suggested that the main reservoir of infection for animals is soil. The organism produces a number of toxins, but the neurotoxin is the one of principal importance.

The portal of entry is usually through a deep puncture, although in cattle introduction into the genital tract at the time of parturition is also important. The organism may also gain entry into surgical wounds, e.g. after castration, and may be introduced into muscle during vaccination and other injections. There are however outbreaks of disease in cattle in which the organism has not localized in any tissue site but remained within the gastrointestinal tract, and such outbreaks are designated as idiopathic tetanus (Wallis, 1963).

After gaining entry into the tissue, the organism remains localized. Multiplication will only occur if optimal conditions develop at the site of infection. If at the time of initial injury there is sufficient tissue damage and a lowered oxygen tension, immediate growth and toxin production will occur. However, such conditions may only be attained after healing at the surface has occurred, so that multiplication and toxin production may be delayed. Thus the incubation period may vary from a few days to four weeks or more. In idiopathic tetanus it would appear that the neurotoxin is produced in the rumen (Smith & Holdeman, 1968).

From the site of production the neurotoxin reaches the central nervous system via the peripheral nerve trunks. The exact mechanisms of transport are not known, nor are the means by which the toxin exerts its influence on the nervous system. Smith & Holdeman (1968) state that the neurotoxin can also reach the central nervous system via lymph and blood.

Individual or small numbers of animals are usually affected in a herd, but in outbreaks of idiopathic tetanus many animals may be affected.

Signs

As the incubation period may vary quite considerably

it is not always possible to relate the onset of clinical disease to specific incidents of injury or surgical interference. The first signs are those of apparent stiffness and reluctance to move, accompanied by muscle tremors that become more pronounced. Another early sign is prolapse of the third eyelid, which becomes more prominent with handling of the head. These signs are progressively followed by the appearance of a slight but persistent ruminal tympany, elevation of the tail, unsteady gait of the hindlimbs, especially when turning, and trismus with saliva drooling from the mouth. Because of inability to adopt the normal urinating posture, urine is retained. Further progression leads to generalized muscular tetany with the adoption of a 'rocking horse'-like posture. Attempts at walking lead to lateral recumbency and an inability to rise. Tetanic convulsions and opisthotonus soon develop. Initially, the convulsions are triggered by external stimuli, but later these occur spontaneously. The duration of fatal disease in young cattle is four to five days, but older cattle may survive for up to 10 days. Non-fatal cases do occur, but generally these do not progress to the convulsive stage and recovery is slow over a period of weeks or sometimes months.

Pathology

There are no tests available for the diagnosis of tetanus in the live animal and any tests undertaken would be for the purpose of eliminating those conditions that produce similar clinical signs. Nor are there any gross or microscopic pathological findings that would confirm tetanus, although attempts should be made to identify the site of infection and culture the organism.

Diagnosis

Because of the distinctive clinical signs, classical tetanus is seldom confused with other diseases. Clinical hypomagnesaemia (p. 219) in calves and cattle (p. 583) is accompanied by tetany and convulsions, but there is no prolapse of the third eyelid or ruminal tympany, and low blood calcium and magnesium levels are diagnostic. Cerebrocortical necrosis (CCN) (polioencephalomalacia) (pp. 225, 701) may produce a similar clinical picture, except that again there is no prolapse of the third eyelid and no ruminal tympany. Also, in CCN the erythrocyte transketolase activity is decreased and blood pyruvate and lactate levels are increased, and classical lesions are obvious at necropsy. Some cases of lead poisoning (p. 617) may also show similar clinical signs, but elevated blood and kidney/liver lead values are diagnostic. Strychnine poisoning is extremely rare in cattle in Great Britain and is usually associated with the ingestion of earthworms treated with strychnine. Strychnine is used for the destruction of moles, and can be identified in the abomasal contents. Bovine spongiform encephalopathy (p. 708) may also need to be differentiated but the signs usually develop over a longer period than tetanus.

Treatment and prevention

Cattle appear to respond better to treatment than horses and sheep, although it is unlikely that fully developed tetanus will respond and therefore under such circumstances euthanasia should be considered.

When treatment is undertaken it should have three objectives: elimination of *Cl. tetani*, neutralization of unfixed neurotoxin and the induction and maintenance of muscle relaxation until all the neurotoxin has been destroyed or eliminated.

Large doses of penicillin administered parenterally is the recommended treatment for *Cl. tetani* infection and this should be supplemented by treatment of the infected site (if located) by irrigation and topical application of antibiotics. Thus treatment should continue for at least seven days.

The administration of antitoxin for the neutralization of unfixed neurotoxin is considered to be of little value unless administered during the very early stages of the disease. If the site of infection has been identified then local injection of the antitoxin may be of value.

A number of drugs have been used to relieve muscle tetany, but because of the need for long-term relaxation some are not suitable because their activity is of short duration. The recommended drugs (Blood *et al.*, 1983) are chlorpromazine (0.4 mg/kg body weight intravenously, 1.0 mg/kg body weight intramuscularly) and acetyl promazine (0.05 mg/kg body weight), administered twice daily for eight to ten days or until the severe clinical signs have disappeared.

Animals that are treated should be kept in dark quiet surroundings with ample bedding and sufficient space to avoid injuring themselves if convulsions occur.

On farms where tetanus is a problem, vaccinations should be routinely undertaken (see p. 807).

Leptospirosis (other than *Leptospira interrogans* var. *hardjo*)

Aetiology

There are many different serotypes of *Leptospira interrogans* present in cattle.

Aetiology

Many serotypes do occur but probably the most important are *L. interrogans* serovar *icterohaemorrhagiae* and serovar *canicola*. *Leptospira interrogans* serovar *pomona* has been found in many countries to be the commonest infection of farm animals. It has only recently been found in Britain and the strain appears to be different from the one causing abortion in pigs. In many cases there are carrier animals and often these are rodents. The leptospires survive in the environment if conditions are wet. However, they are inhibited at a pH less than 6 or greater than 8. Temperatures below 7–10°C (44.5–50°F) or above 34–36°C (93–96°F) are detrimental. The organisms can survive over four months under wet conditions but only 30 minutes when the soil is dried. It often survives in the environment in average conditions for about one and a half months.

Most infection is spread via contaminated feed or water. It must be remembered that most serovarieties are able to infect many species including man.

Mortality rate is usually low at about 5 per cent.

Signs

Acute. The cow is often ill with a pyrexia of 40–41 °C (104–106°F) with dullness and anorexia. The milk yield drops and often there are haemorrhages under the mucous membranes, and there is often jaundice and haemoglobinuria. In some cases there is synovitis or a necrotic dermatitis. Occasionally, meningitis has been recorded.

Subacute. In this form the signs are milder with a temperature of 39–40°C (102–104°F). The animal has a reduced milk yield and is dull. Jaundice occurs in some cases and there is usually some haemoglobinuria. In some cases abortion occurs about a month later.

Chronic. This is not common and results in abortion.

Necropsy

Acute. There are often submucosal and subserosal haemorrhages, jaundice, anaemia and haemoglobinuria. In some animals there is ulceration of the abomasal mucosa and emphysema. Histological examination often shows an interstitial nephritis as well as centrilobular hepatic necrosis.

Subacute or chronic cases are more likely to show a progressive interstitial nephritis with white foci on the surface of the renal cortex.

Diagnosis

This depends on finding the organism. Otherwise, paired serum samples can be examined for a rise in *Leptospira* titres.

Differential diagnosis

Any form of haemoglobinuria will need to be eliminated, including babesiasis (p. 726), which is usually seen in the summer in tick areas. Kale poisoning (p. 613) and postparturient haemoglobinuria (p. 589) should be partly diagnosed by the history and the low plasma phosphorus levels in the latter. Bacillary haemoglobinuria (p. 553) will be differentiated by the presence of clostridia.

Treatment

The main therapy is usually antibiotics such as dihydrostreptomycin or the tetracyclines. Treatment should be given as soon as signs develop. Blood transfusion often helps. The farmer should be warned of possible human infection.

Control

Separate the infected cow. If it is partly due to rodent build-up, control the rodents. Ensure removal of brackish water and provide good drainage. Vaccination could be used, as with *L. interrogans* serovar *canicola* or *icterohaemorrhagiae*, but as cases are usually sporadic this does not tend to be used.

Leptospira hardjo infection ('flabby bag')

Aetiology

Infection with *Leptospira interrogans* serotype *hardjo*, a spiral organism.

Aetiology

This is a common cause of abortion in Britain, although it is one that has only recently been readily diagnosed. Up to 50–60 per cent of British farms may be infected. In Northern Ireland 41.6 per cent of randomly selected aborted fetuses were infected (Ellis *et al.*, 1982) and the level rose to 68.9 per cent of fetuses from farms with abortion problems. A very common problem in New Zealand, most cases are in the dairy herd rather than beef cattle. Humans can be infected but they must be exposed to concentrated infection, i.e. contact via urine while milking. Although infection is present in the milk, it quickly dies off once taken from the udder. Meat does not carry infection. Spread occurs more rapidly in wet seasons in low-lying areas. Colostrum-derived protection normally lasts about three months. Serological rises in *L. hardjo* titres following infection tend to be short-lived, i.e. a few months to a year or so. It was originally considered to be a winter disease. However, carriers often stop or reduce excretion on silage. Most infection now occurs in the summer, often with abortion in the summer or early autumn. Serology in individual animals is difficult because the bacteria are in the lumen of the kidney or uterus.

The spread of infection takes place cow to cow via urine, fetuses and uterine discharge, and from bull to cow by infected semen. The source of infection is via carrier cows or infected calves, which may be chronically infected, but it may possibly be spread by contaminated water or sheep on the farm.

Signs

There are two main syndromes, the udder form and abortion.

Severe udder form. In a cow or heifer the udder signs will not be apparent until the animal has calved. This form occurs soon after the infection enters a herd. There is a sudden drop in milk yield affecting all four quarters, with pyrexia usually between 40 and 41.5 °C (104–107 °F). The udder secretion becomes thickened and clotted, occasionally it is bloody or it can be yellow and colostrum-like. The udder itself is not swollen or inflamed but tends to be flaccid. In a six to eight-week period, 30–50 per cent of the herd may be infected. The condition usually resolves over seven to ten days (see p. 298).

Mild udder form. Many cows are infected and show only a slight drop in milk yield.

Abortion. This usually occurs six to twelve weeks after the dam is infected. Abortion can occur on its own or be preceded by the milk drop syndrome. Most cases of abortion occur in the second half of pregnancy. If infection occurs late in pregnancy then an infected calf may be born. There may be some apparent infertility in the herd (see p. 471).

Necropsy

Abortion. There are usually no useful macroscopic features in the aborted fetus.

Diagnosis

Udder form. History helps in diagnosis, in particular the sudden onset of the problem. The signs, sudden loss of milk, flaccid udder, are useful. The Californian Milk Test is positive and there is a high milk white cell count. Identification and culture of the organisms from urine (it can occasionally be isolated from milk and blood in the acute stages) is a definitive diagnosis. Paired serum samples can be used for the complement fixation test, microscopic agglutination test and plate agglutination test. High titres over 1/300 indicate recent exposure to infection.

Abortion. Identification of the bacterium in the fetus, especially in the lungs, kidneys or adrenal glands, by fluorescent antibody studies, is the main method of diagnosis. Culture of the bacteria can be undertaken. Fetal serology can also be used. Serology of the dam can help but often antibody titres may be static or falling. It is very difficult to detect carrier animals, as up to 25 per cent are serologically negative.

Differential diagnosis

Other leptospiral infections (p. 569), salmonellosis (Chapter 13), foot-and-mouth disease (p. 537), and mastitis (Chapter 21) must all be considered in the udder form. In abortion, (p. 469) salmonellosis, mucosal disease, brucellosis and infectious bovine rhinotracheitis are some common causes to be differentiated.

Treatment

Large doses of dihydrostreptomycin (25 mg/kg body weight) may help remove the organism and prevent kidney and liver damage. All cattle due to calve should be vaccinated.

Control

Vaccination is possible with a killed strain (p. 812). It involves two initial doses at least four weeks apart. If cattle are young when vaccination commences then two doses are required after five months of age. An annual booster is recommended but two vaccinations a year may be required in herds that calve in the autumn. It does not affect animals that already have milk drop syndrome. Vaccination does help prevent abortion but infected cows may still excrete bacteria. It is therefore advisable to treat all adult cattle with dihydrostreptomycin before commencing a vaccination programme.

Haemophilus somnus Infection

Aetiology

A Gram-negative small rod-shaped organism. Most strains of the organism are antigenically similar.

Epidemiology

It is seen in North America and Europe. Inapparent infection occurs more frequently than clinical disease. Problems occur more frequently in younger animals. The portal of entry of infections is often via the respiratory tract although it is also found in the reproductive and urinary tracts. Disease is probably a septicaemia with localization. Single or several cases may occur.

Signs

The peracute form often causes sudden death. The acute form is often seen as the sleeper syndrome or thromboembolic meningoencephalitis (TEME) in growing cattle. The animal is depressed, with closed eyes, and recumbent. Usually there is pyrexia (40–42°C, 104–108°F). Nervous signs can be of muscle tremors and hyperaesthesia. The animal may be blind with retinal haemorrhage. Other syndromes include synovitis with initial lameness. Pneumonia is a common finding, particularly in calves, and often associated with pleurisy. Abortion can occur and so can chronic bloat.

Pathology

There may be focal or diffuse cerebral meningitis with characteristic haemorrhagic infarcts in the brain. Haemorrhages can occur in other organs. In the joint form the synovial membranes are oedematous with petechial haemorrhages. There is often inflammation of the pericardium, peritoneum and pleura which may be serofibrinous or fibrinous. Histologically there is often a vasculitis and thrombosis, often with infarcts and accumulation of neutrophils.

Prognosis

Recumbent cattle often do not recover and usually if there is no response after three days' treatment the condition is irreversible.

Treatment and control

High doses of intravenous tetracycline for at least three days can be useful. Otherwise ampicillin, amoxycillin, chloramphenicol, novobiocin, sulphonamides or potentiated sulphonamides can be administered. Once disease is diagnosed, extra observation must be undertaken of in-contact animals. Control is difficult, although in North America an aluminium hydroxide adjuvenated vaccine is now used.

Pyaemia

Pyaemia is defined as a clinical or pathological state characterized by the formation of multiple secondary abscesses in a number of organs and/or tissues.

The primary pyogenic infection may occur in a number of sites and the formation of metastatic lesions in other organs and tissues follows the entry of organisms into the circulation. Small numbers of organisms may intermittently gain entry via the lymphatic drainage of the primary lesion, to produce a bacteraemia, followed by localization and the formation of secondary abscesses. More frequently, however, a septic thrombus is formed within the primary lesion and portions of this become detached to form emboli, which are then arrested in the capillary bed of an organ or tissues to form the metastatic lesions. The most frequent sites for secondary abscess formation are the valvular endocardium, myocardium, lungs and joints, although the liver and kidneys may sometimes be involved.

In cattle, pyaemia is often associated with septic metritis and mastitis, and *A. pyogenes* is the organism most frequently incriminated. Staphylococcal mastitis may also lead, in some cases, to pyaemia. On occasions, hepatic abscesses and foul in the foot caused by *Fusobacterium necrophorum* may also result in pyaemia.

Because pyaemia is a form of generalization of a primary infection, the clinical signs, diagnosis and treatment must be considered in relation to the primary infections referred to above and which are discussed in the appropriate sections of the text.

References

Anthrax

Balley, W.W. (1953) Anthrax: response by terramycin therapy. *Journal of the American Veterinary Medical Association*, **122**, 305–6.

Campbell, A.D. (1969) Anthrax: A problem of the livestock industry. *Veterinary Record*, **85**, 89–90.

Greenough, P.R. (1965) Anthrax and antibiotics. *Veterinary Record*, **77**, 784–5.

Hugh-Jones, M.E. & Hussaini, S.N. (1975) Anthrax in England and Wales 1963–1972. *Veterinary Record*, **97**, 256–61.

Lincoln, R.E., Walker, J.S., Klein, F. & Haines, B.W. (1964) Anthrax. *Advances in Veterinary Science*, **9**, 327–68. Academic Press, London.

Schlingham, A.S., Devlin, H.B., Wright, G.G., Maine, R.J. & Manning, M.C. (1956) Immunising activity of alum precipitated antigen of *B. anthracis* in cattle, sheep and swine. *America Journal of Veterinary Research*, **17**, 256–61.

Sterne, M. (1959) In *Infectious Diseases of Animals*, 1st edn (ed. by A.W. Stableforth & I.A. Galloway), Vol. 1, pp. 16–52. Butterworth Scientific Publications, London.

Bacillary haemoglobinuria

Blood, D.C., Radostits, O.M. & Henderson, J.A. (1983) *Veterinary Medicine*, 6th edn, p. 548. Baillière Tindall, London.

Roberts, R.S. (1959) In *Infectious Diseases of Animals*, 1st edn (ed. by A.W. Stableforth & I.A. Galloway), Vol. 1, p. 200. Butterworth Scientific Publications, London.

Smith, L.D. (1957) Clostridial diseases of animals. *Advances in Veterinary Science*, **3**, 463–524.

Smith, L.D. & Holdeman, (1968) *The Pathogenic Anaerobic Bacteria*, pp. 339–48. Charles C. Thomas, Springfield, Illinois.

Williams, B.M. (1964) *Clostridium* oedematous infections (black disease and bacillary haemoglobinuria) of cattle in mid Wales. *Veterinary Record*, **76**, 591–6.

Botulism

Appleyard, W.T. & Mollison, A. (1985) Suspected bovine botulism associated with broiler litter waste. *Veterinary Record*, **116**, 535.

Breuknik, H.I., Wagenaar, G., Wensing, T., Notermans, S. & Poulos, P.W. (1978) Food poisoning in cattle caused by the ingestion of brewers grains contaminated by *Clostridium botulinum* type B. *Tijdschrift voor Diergeneeskunde*, **103**, 303–11.

Clegg, F.G. & Evans, R.K. (1974) Suspected case of botulism in calves. *Veterinary Record*, **95**, 540.

Clegg, F.G., Jones, T.O., Smart, J.L. & McMurty, M.J. (1985) Bovine botulism associated with broiler litter waste. *Veterinary Record*, **117**, 22.

Davies, A.B., Roberts, T.A. & Bradshaw, P.R. (1974) Probable botulism in calves. *Veterinary Record*, **94**, 412–14.

Egyed, M.N., Shlosberg, A., Klopper, V., Nobel, T.A. & Mayer, E. (1978) Mass outbreaks of botulism in ruminants associated with ingestion of feed containing poultry waste: Clinical findings. *Reufah.Vet.*, **35**, 93–9.

Ektvedt, R. & Hanssen, I. (1974) Outbreak of botulism in cattle. *Norske Veterinaertidsskrift*, **86**, 286–96.

Fjolstad, M. & Kluna, T. (1969) An outbreak of botulism among ruminants in connection with ensilage feeding. *Nordisk Veterinarmedicin*, **21**, 609–13.

Haagsma, J. & Laak, E.A. (1977) Type B botulism in cattle fed grass silage. Report of an outbreak. *Tijdschrift voor Diergeneeskunde*, **102**, 330.

Muller, J. (1961) Type C botulism in man and animals — incidence in cattle and horses. *Medlemsblad for den danske Dyrlaegeforening*, **44**, 547–57.

Notermans, S., Kozaki, S., Dufrenne, J. & Scothorst, M. van (1979a) Studies on the persistence of *Clostridium botulinum* on a cattle farm. *Tijdschrift voor Diergeneeskunde*, **104**, 707–12.

Notermans, S., Kozaki, S. & Scothorst, M. van (1979b) Toxin production by *Clostridium botulinum* in grass. *Applied and Environmental Microbiology*, **39**, 767–76.

Prevot, A.R. & Sillioc, R. (1955) A biological enigma: resistance of cats to *Clostridium botulinum* toxin. *Annales de l'Institut Pasteur*, **89**, 354–7.

Smith, L.D. (1977) *Botulism, the Organisms, its Toxins, the Disease*, pp. 15, 91–6. Charles C. Thomas, Springfield, Illinois.

Clostridial myositis

Blood, D.C., Radostits, O.M. & Henderson, J.A. (1983) *Veterinary Medicine* pp. 541–5. Baillière Tindall, London.

Harwood, D.G. (1984) Apparent iatrogenic clostridial myositis in cattle. *Veterinary Record*, **115**, 412.

Jubb, K.V.F., Kennedy P.C. & Palmer, A. (1983) *Pathology of Domestic Animals*, pp. 180–4. Academic Press, London.

Kerry, J.B. (1964) A note on the occurrence of *Clostridium chauveoi* in the spleens and livers of normal cattle. *Veterinary Record*, **76**, 396.

Williams, B.M. (1977) Clostridial myositis in cattle: bacteriology and gross pathology. *Veterinary Record*, **100**, 90–1.

Contagious bovine pyelonephritis

Ado, P.B. & Cook J.E. (1979) Specific immunofluorescence of *Corynebacterium renale. British Veterinary Journal*, **135**, 50–4.

Goudswaard, J. & Budhai, S. (1975) Some aspects of the immunological response in cattle with *Corynebacterium renale*. Identification of a new serotype, type IV. *Zentralblatt fur Veterinarmedizin*, **22B**, 473–9.

Hiramune, T., Invi, S., Murase, N. & Yanagawa, R. (1972) Antibody response in cows infected with *Corynebacterium renale. Research in Veterinary Science*, **13**, 82–6.

Hiramune, T., Narita, M., Tomonari, I., Murase, N. & Yanagawa, R. (1975) Distribution of *Corynebacterium renale* among healthy bulls, with special reference to inhabitation of type III in the prepuce. *National Institute of Animal Health Quarterly, Tokyo*, **15**, 116–21.

Morse, E.V. (1950) An ecological study of *Corynebacterium renale. Cornell Veterinarian*, **40**, 178–87.

Takai, S., Yanagawa, R. & Kitamura, Y. (1980) pH dependent adhesion of piliated *Corynebacterium renale* to bovine bladder cells. *Infection and Immunity*, **28**, 669–74.

Endocarditis

Andersen, H.K. (1963) Investigations on pathogenesis, the aetiology and topography of endocarditis in cattle. *Nordisk Veterinarmedicin*, **15**, 668–90.

Biering-Sørensen, V. (1963) Incidence of endocarditis in cattle and its seasonal variation. *Nordisk Veterinarmedicin*, **15**, 691–5.

Evans, E.T.R. (1957) Bacterial endocarditis in cattle. *Veterinary Record*, **69**, 1196–1202.

John, F.V. (1947) Verrucose endocarditis. *Veterinary Record*, **59**, 214.

Lacuta, A.Q., Yamada, H., Nakamura, Y. & Hirose, T. (1980) Electrographic and echocardiographic findings in four cases of bovine endocarditis. *Journal of the American Veterinary Medical Association*, **176**, 1353–65.
Larsen, H.R. (1963) Clinical observations on endocarditis in cattle. *Nordisk Veterinarmedicin*, **15**, 645–67.
Power, H.T. & Rebhun, W.C. (1983) Bacterial endocarditis in cattle. *Journal of the American Veterinary Medical Association*, **182**, 806–8.
Wuijckhuise-Sjouke, L.A. van (1984) Plasma fibrinogen concentration as an indicator of the presence and severity of inflammatory disease in horses and cattle. *Tijdschrift voor Diergeneeskunde*, **109**, 869–72.

Haemorrhagic septicaemia

Bain, R.V.S. (1963) Haemorrhagic septicaemia, Agricultural Studies No. 62. Food and Agricultural Organization, Rome.
Carter, G.R. (1982) Whatever happened to haemorrhagic septicaemia. *Journal of the American Veterinary Medical Association*, **180**, 1176–7.
Carter, G.R. & Bain, R.V.S. (1960) Pasteurellosis (*Pasteurella multocida*). A review stressing recent developments. *Veterinary Review Annotations*, **6**, 105–28.
De Alwis, M.C.L. & Carter, G.R. (1980) Preliminary field trials with streptomycin dependent vaccine against haemorrhagic septicaemia. *Veterinary Record*, **68**, 223–4.
Jubb, K.V.F., Kennedy, P.C. & Palmer, N. (1985) *Pathology of Domestic Animals*, 3rd edn, Vol. 2, pp. 488–9. Academic Press, London.
Macadam, I. (1962) Tick transmission of bovine pasteurellosis. *Veterinary Record*, **74**, 689–90.
Mustafa, A.A., Ghalib, H.W. & Shigidi, M.J. (1978) Carrier rate of *Past. multocida* in cattle herds associated with an outbreak of haemorrhagic septicaemia in Sudan. *British Veterinary Journal*, **134**, 375–8.
Sawada, T., Rimler, R.B. & Rhoades, K.R. (1985) Haemorrhagic septicaemia: naturally acquired antibodies against *Past. multocida* types B and E in calves in the United States. *American Journal of Veterinary Research*, **46**, 1247–50.
Shirlaw, J.F. (1938) Haemorrhagic septicaemia: A criticism of the present position with an account of investigations into the problem in the Northumbrian area. *Veterinary Record*, **50**, 1005–9.
Wei, B.D. & Carter, G.R. (1978) Live streptomycin dependent *Past. multocida* vaccine for the prevention of haemorrhagic septicaemia. *American Journal of Veterinary Research*, **39**, 1534–7.

Infectious necrotic hepatitis

Bagadi, H.O. & Sewell, M.M.H. (1973) An epidemiological survey of infectious necrotic hepatitis of sheep (black disease) in Scotland. *Research in Veterinary Science*, **15**, 49–53.
Bagadi, H.O. & Sewell, M.M.H. (1974) Influence of post mortem autolysis on the diagnosis of infectious necrotic hepatitis (black disease). *Research in Veterinary Science*, **17**, 320–7.
Batty, I., Buntain, D. & Walker, P.D. (1964) *Clostridium oedematiens*, a cause of sudden death in sheep, cattle and pigs. *Veterinary Record*, **76**, 115–17.
Herbert, T.G.G. & Hughes, L.E. (1956) Black disease (infectious necrotic hepatitis) in a heifer. *Veterinary Record*, **68**, 223–4.
Williams, B.M. (1964) *Clostridium oedematiens* infections (black disease and bacillary haemoglobinuria) of cattle in mid-Wales. *Veterinary Record*, **76**, 591–6.
Williams, B.M. (1976) Infectious necrotic hepatitis of sheep: An epidemiological survey on Welsh farms. *British Veterinary Journal*, **132**, 221–5.

Pericarditis

Blood, D.C. & Hutchins, D.R. (1955) Traumatic pericarditis of cattle. *Australian Veterinary Journal*, **31**, 229–32.
Horney, F.D. (1960) Surgical drainage of the bovine pericardial sac. *Canadian Veterinary Journal*, **1**, 363–5.
Jennings, S. & McIntyre, W.M. (1957) Pericardiectomy in a cow. *Veterinary Record*, **69**, 928.
Krishnamurthy, D., Nigam, J.M., Peshin, P.K. & Kharole, M.U. (1979) Thorapericardiotomy and pericardiotomy in cattle. *Journal of the American Veterinary Medical Association*, **175**, 714–18.
Mason, T.A. (1979) Suppurative pericarditis treated by pericardiotomy in a cow. *Veterinary Record*, **105**, 305–1.

Tetanus

Blood, D.C., Radostits, O.M. & Henderson, J.A. (1983) *Veterinary Medicine* p. 538. Baillière Tindall, London.
Smith, L.D. & Holdeman, L.V. (1968) *The Pathogenic Anaerobic Bacteria*, pp. 256–81. Charles C. Thomas, Springfield, Illinois.
Wallis, A.S. (1963) Some observations on the epidemiology of tetanus in cattle, *Veterinary Record*, **75**, 188–91.

Leptospira hardjo infection

Ellis, W.A., O'Brien, J.J., Neill, S.D., Ferguson, M.W. & Hanna, J. (1982) Bovine leptospirosis: Microbial and serological findings in aborted fetuses. *Veterinary Record*, **110**, 147–50.

Metabolic Problems

Chapter 39: Major Metabolic Disorders

by R.G. EDDY

Milk fever (parturient paresis, hypocalcaemia, eclampsia)

Milk fever or hypocalcaemia is probably the most common metabolic disorder affecting cattle. It is normally associated with parturition occurring just before, during or immediately after calving although it has been reported in dry cows and, occasionally, during mid-lactation. The incidence of milk fever is higher in dairy cows than beef cows and increases with age and yield. Milk fever has undoubtedly increased in incidence over recent years due primarily to breeding selection for high yield. The true incidence of milk fever is difficult to determine, although levels of 9 per cent have been reported. However, as the majority of milk fever is treated by farmers' surveys of veterinary practice treatments will be a gross underestimate. Computerized herd health recording schemes such as DAISY (Dairy Information System) operated by Reading University and some veterinary practices in the UK would suggest that the incidence is in the order of 15–20 per cent of all cows calving for the third lactation or above. The incidence does vary considerably between seasons as well as between farms. In some years the incidence in September and October in the UK can be as high as 60 per cent on some farms, whereas during the winter months when dry cows are housed 0–6 per cent would be frequently reported. The disease does appear to be more common when dry cows are fed grass rather than conserved fodder. Milk fever is a common cause of death and is probably the most common cause of apparent sudden death in dairy cows. It is also a common cause of dystokia and hence stillborn calves

Predisposing factors

There are several important predisposing factors that influence the occurrence of milk fever and these account for the wide variation of incidence observed in the UK and other countries world-wide.

Breed. The Jersey and, to a lesser extent, the Guernsey are particularly susceptible to milk fever. This would indicate a genetic predilection for this disease and is probably related to the relatively high production level for a small breed.

Age. It is rare for milk fever to occur at the first calving and relatively uncommon at the second. The incidence does appear to increase with age and incidence levels of 20 per cent or more are common at the sixth calving and beyond. The reason is thought to be that the requirement for calcium at parturition increases as milk yield rises with each lactation and the ability to mobilize calcium quickly from the body reserves, i.e. bone, decreases with age.

Seasonal factors. The incidence in the UK is highest in the autumn months of September and October and at its lowest in the winter months of December, January and February. However, this is more likely to be a result of differing feeding regimens of dry cows than a seasonal effect. In countries where there is little change in dry-cow nutrition during the year, e.g. Israel, there appears to be no seasonal differences in the occurrence of milk fever.

Nutritional factors. The wide range of incidence of milk fever observed between seasons, within a season and between farms in the UK is due to the variation of nutritional input given to dry cows. Dry cows that are fed a diet of hay or silage only, which is now commonplace in the UK, will have a low incidence of milk fever at calving. However, if feeds containing high calcium levels are included in the diet, e.g. sugar-beet pulp or high calcium minerals, the incidence will increase.

The incidence of milk fever in cows at grass varies considerably with the season. In dry weather the incidence is low, but during long wet spells the level is high. A diet of grass with a low dry matter (DM) whether in the spring or autumn can predispose to high incidences of milk fever. There is more than one reason for this. One is that such a diet leads to diarrhoea, which probably reduces the calcium available for absorption. The calcium level of wet grass, particularly in the autumn, can be excessively high, often as high as 1 per cent of DM. More recently, it has been discovered that low magnesium levels in the diet restrict the cow's ability to absorb calcium (Sansom *et al.*, 1983) and the high levels of milk fever found in the spring and autumn in the UK are often due to low magnesium levels in the grass.

Aetiology

Some degree of hypocalcaemia occurs in all cows at parturition but only when this becomes severe do clinical signs develop. Frequently, the hypocalcaemia is accompanied by hypophosphataemia and hypermagnesaemia, although when milk fever is due to low magnesium intake the blood levels of magnesium will also be depressed. The normal concentration of calcium in plasma lies within the range 2.2–2.6 mmol/l (8.8–10.4 mg/100 ml) but will fall to 1.5 mmol/l (6.0 mg/100 ml) in most cows at parturition without milk fever signs occurring. Usually, when milk fever is present the plasma level will be in the range 0.75–1.5 mmol/l (3.0–6.0 mg/100 ml).

The predisposing factor in the aetiology of hypocalcaemia at parturition is the sudden increase in the requirement of calcium for the production of colostrum. The daily calcium requirement of a 600 kg cow in late pregnancy is approximately 28–30 g; this comprises 13–15 g required for endogenous loss in faeces and urine and 15 g to maintain the growing fetus. At the onset of lactation, approximately 1–1.5 g of calcium is required for each litre of colostrum produced so the requirement is increased two or three-fold in a very short period. In order to meet this enlarged demand and to avoid hypocalcaemia, calcium absorption from the gut is increased and further calcium is available from mobilization of the calcium reserves in bone. This explains why mild hypocalcaemia occurs in all cows at parturition. If the cow does not respond quickly to the sudden increase in calcium requirement the hypocalcaemia deepens and signs of milk fever become apparent.

In the normal cow this adaptation process at parturition is under the hormonal control of the parathyroid hormone (PTH). Hypocalcaemia stimulates the secretion of PTH, which in turn stimulates the production of a hydroxylase enzyme in the kidney that is able to synthesize 1,25-dihydroxycholecalciferol ($1,25(OH)_2D_3$), which is produced from vitamin D_3. The $1,25(OH)_2D_3$ stimulates increased gut absorption of calcium and probably the mobilization of calcium from bone (Fig. 39.1).

There are several factors that affect the speed of response to this adaptation process.

1 Age of the cow, as already mentioned. Older cows are less able to mobilize calcium from the skeleton.
2 Oestrogens also inhibit calcium mobilization and as oestrogen levels rise at parturition this will have a negative effect on the adaptation process to maintain calcium levels. Milk fever does occasionally occur during lactation and sometimes in association with oestrus. This again would be due to the inhibitory effect of oestrogens.
3 Food intake is often depressed at or around parturition so the total available calcium in the diet will be reduced. This is particularly the case if diets low in calcium, e.g. straw or cereal-based diets, are fed over the parturition period.
4 The calcium intake during the dry period. If high levels of calcium are present in the diet the reduced PTH output that occurs reduces the rate of absorption from the gut so that when the demand for calcium suddenly increases and the cow's appetite is generally reduced absorption does not satisfy the body requirement.
5 A low magnesium intake in the diet reduces by various mechanisms the ability of the gut to allow calcium absorption. Therefore, diets that are deficient in magnesium will predispose to hypocalcaemia by reducing calcium absorption. Hypomagnesaemia also inhibits mobilization of calcium from bone.
6 Problems associated with digestion, e.g. acidosis and profuse diarrhoea, will reduce the amount of calcium in the gut available for absorption. This could also explain cases of hypocalcaemia that occur at times other than parturition.

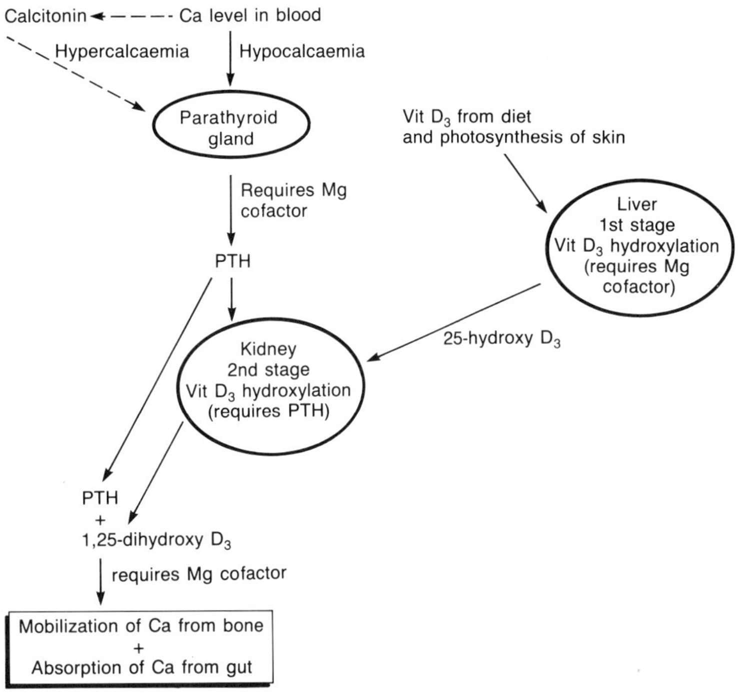

Fig. 39.1 System for mobilizing calcium in cattle. P, parathyroid hormone (Kelly, 1988).

Signs

The clinical signs of milk fever are progressive. In the first stage there is a loss of appetite, lethargy and the rectal temperature is reduced by 0.5 °C (1 °F). This progresses to a stage where the cow stands with the hocks straight and sways laterally, particularly when moving. Constipation is normally seen at this stage. Muscle tremors may be present about the head and limbs. Hyperaesthesia is also often evident at this stage and the cow becomes apprehensive. The lateral swaying develops into incoordination and ataxia and the cow will fall over sideways and rise with increasing difficulty until she becomes permanently recumbent.

The recumbent stage is the one most commonly seen by veterinarians in practice. The cow will be sitting in sternal recumbency often with a noticeable S bend in the neck, progressing to the stage where the head will be resting on her shoulder. The heart rate will be slightly raised but rarely exceeds 90/minute. The pupils will be dilated and the pupillary light reflex will be reduced or even absent. The gut stasis that characterizes this stage of the disease further reduces the availability of calcium for absorption and the disease will progress to the comatose stage. The rumen ceases to function and often becomes tympanic and the cow appears severely depressed. The comatosed stage is characterized by lateral recumbency, increased rumen tympany, total absence of the pupillary light reflex until the cow dies. Death can be due to paralysis of the respiratory muscles but more often death occurs from bloat. Many cows with milk fever are found in ditches or streams, having fallen in during the incoordination phase of the disease. In these situations death can be due to drowning.

The length of time for the disease to progress from first signs of inappetance to death varies from 10 to 24 hours. Many cows are found dead or near to death by the stockworker at the time of morning milking, having been quite normal the previous evening at 7.00 p.m.

If hypocalcaemia occurs at the onset of calving the parturition process will cease due to lack of myometrial contractions. A considerable number of cases of dystokia due to uterine inertia are the result of hypocalcaemia and, if not treated, will result in a stillborn calf or even death of the cow before the calf is born. It is common for the stockworker to find a cow in lateral recumbency in the early morning with the calf presented in the birth canal or even with the head present at the vulva. Frequently, the calf will be dead and occasionally even partially eaten by foxes or other wildlife.

Clinical pathology

The concentration of calcium in plasma is usually below 1.5 mmol/l (6 mg/100 ml) in cows with clinical hypocalcaemia and will fall to as low as 0.25 mmol/l (1.0 mg/100 ml). Phosphorus levels also fall to 1.0 mmol/l from the normal range of 1.4–2.5 mmol/l (4.3–7.8 mg/100 ml). Magnesium levels usually increase to around 1.25 mmol/l (3.0 mg/100 ml) except where the cause of milk fever is related to low magnesium diets when hypomagnesaemia may be present. Hyperglycaemia is also usual during milk fever, but this is frequently seen in normal cows at parturition.

In fatal cases of milk fever there are no gross or histological lesions characteristic of the disease. Bruising of subcutaneous tissue and muscles due to localized trauma may be apparent. The liver is occasionally distended and infiltrated with fat resulting in a yellow discoloration. Cows with this fatty liver are thought to be more prone to milk fever but fatty liver is not pathognomonic of milk fever.

Diagnosis

The diagnosis of milk fever is made on the signs described above and the history of recent or imminent calving. Although blood biochemistry may be considered useful, in practical situations there is not the time available to get a result. A cowside test for calcium is now available in some countries but its value is probably limited to differential diagnosis of the downer cow syndrome or cows failing to respond to treatment for milk fever. The most valuable diagnostic aid available is, once the differential diagnoses have been eliminated, the response to treatment. Intravenous treatment with calcium borogluconate will produce a clinical response within minutes. The cow will become more alert, defaecate and eructate often before the full dose of calcium has been administered.

Differential diagnosis

Although milk fever is an extremely common disease it is essential that a full clinical examination is made for every case. It is common for the new veterinary graduate to diagnose and treat a recumbent cow for milk fever when the cause of the recumbency is toxic mastitis. The clinical examination must therefore include examination of milk from all four teats, the heart rate and the mucus membranes. Misdiagnosis is now more common as farmers treat their own cases of milk fever and frequently confuse the disease with other causes of recumbency.

The differential diagnoses of milk fever are:

1 acute toxic mastitis (Chapter 21);
2 calving paralysis (p. 366);
3 physical injury (p. 374);
4 hypomagnesaemia (p. 583);
5 downer cow syndrome (pp. 368, 594);
6 inanition and other disease;
7 pregnancy toxaemia (p. 593);
8 acidosis (p. 364);
9 hypothermia;
10 bovine spongiform encephalopathy (BSE) (p. 708).

Acute toxic mastitis. In acute toxic mastitis from whatever cause the temperature may be raised but is sometimes subnormal, the pulse may be in excess of 120/minute, the eyes are often sunken, the mucous membranes injected and, in acute colifor mastitis, they are frequently a purple colour. Abnormal milk secretion will be found in one or more teats although in acute coliform mastitis this change in milk character may be less than obvious.

Calving paralysis. The history of dystokia due to fetal oversize and recumbency since calving help in the differential diagnosis but many cases are not clear-cut. Intravenous calcium and the response noted is probably the best aid to differential diagnosis.

Other physical injury. This can occur at any time of lactation or the dry period and can include fractured limbs, pelvic damage and severe muscle damage. These can be the result of excess riding behaviour during oestrus, slipping on ice or slippery concrete or even a collision with a vehicle such as a tractor.

Hypomagnesaemia. This can occur at any time of lactation during the spring or autumn but sometimes is present as a complication of milk fever, particularly during the two seasonal risk periods of spring and autumn. Hyperaesthesia is the main differentiating sign of hypomagnesaemia.

Downer cow syndrome. Initially, this may be difficult to differentiate from milk fever but response to therapy and clinical biochemistry will be helpful. This will be discussed in full later in the chapter (see p. 594).

Inanition. Any condition producing severe weight loss will result in recumbency, particularly in pregnant cows, the most common of which is probably starvation. In seasons where insufficient conserved food is available recumbency due to starvation is extremely common. Body condition is the obvious differentiating feature. However, any disease that causes considerable weight loss will have the same effect, e.g. liver fluke (p. 238).

In seasons when liver fluke prevalence is high, this disease can result in extreme weight loss and anaemia and recumbency prior to parturition is common. Weight loss, red cell count and presence of fluke ova in faeces would be the differentiating features.

Pregnancy toxaemia, particularly in beef cows, can occur in the last two or three months of pregnancy. The sweet smell of acetone on the breath, poor condition or excessively fat and a history of unavailability of food should distinguish this problem. The rumen will also be functioning in the early stages of this condition.

Acidosis. Acute acidosis as a result of the sudden ingestion of large amounts of carbohydrate material, usually cereal-based concentrates, will result in recumbency although hypocalcaemia is often a feature of acidosis. Here the history will help and usually acidosis is accompanied by diarrhoea.

Hypothermia. Mild hypothermia (reduction of 0.5 °C or 1 °F) is a normal feature of milk fever. However, severe hypothermia (reduction of 3–4 °C or 5–7 °F) occurs in cows that have been recumbent all night in winter out of doors. Although these cows have some other primary disease, e.g. milk fever or mastitis, treatment will be unsuccessful unless steps are taken to raise body temperature as rapidly as possible.

In summary, there are many diseases and conditions that result in recumbency of the cow. However, careful history taking and a thorough clinical examination will eliminate most differential diagnoses and if one is still not sure of the diagnosis response to intravenous calcium will always be a useful indicator.

Treatment

The treatment for milk fever is the slow intravenous infusion of 8–12 g of calcium as soon as possible after the onset of clinical signs.

There are a number of licensed preparations available for the treatment of milk fever and most are based on calcium borogluconate (CBG) at 20 per cent, 30 per cent or 40 per cent strength (see Table 39.1). It has been shown that 400 ml of 30 per cent CBG is adequate to treat milk fever in average size cattle and will provide 9 g of calcium, although the most commonly used product in the UK is 400 ml of 40 per cent CBG, which will provide 12 g of calcium. During cold weather the CBG solution should be warmed to body temperature. Approximately 85 per cent of cases will respond to one treatment. In many cases cows recumbent from milk fever will rise within 10 minutes of treatment and others will get up 2–4 hours later.

Table 39.1 Licensed products available for the treatment of milk fever in the UK

Product	Pack size (ml)	Available calcium (g)	Dose required for 600 kg cow (ml)
CBG 20%	400	6	600–800
CBG 30%	400	9	400
CBG 40%	400	12	400
Calcitad 50*	100	4.5	200

* A 100 ml injection of calcium gluconate 3.1 g, calcium borogluconate 42.9 g, calcium hydroxide 1.32 g, magnesium chloride 6.5 g, phosphoryl ethanolamine 0.6 g, methylhydroxybenzoate 0.1 g.

Following the intravenous infusion, which itself should take 5 minutes, it is essential to sit the cow in a sternal recumbency position and turn her so that she is lying on the side opposite to the one on which she was found. Many cases will eructate and defaecate during the treatment. If the cow does not rise immediately she should be turned to lie on the opposite side every 2 hours. Following intravenous treatment milk fever cows should be able to sit comfortably in the sternal recumbent position without the aid of support such as bales of straw. If the cow keeps returning to lateral recumbency following treatment the diagnosis should be re-assessed as it is unlikely to be milk fever.

The use of intravenous treatment cannot be overemphasized as it is essential that the blood calcium levels return to normal as quickly as possible to avoid the complications resulting in the downer cow syndrome. Subcutaneous treatment with CBG is commonly used by farmers treating their own cases of milk fever. This is undoubtedly a factor that has increased the incidence of the downer cow syndrome in recent years. Following intravenous therapy plasma calcium levels rise rapidly and fall to around 2 mmol/l (8 mg/100 ml) 5–6 hours after treatment. Following subcutaneous therapy, the plasma calcium levels may take 3–4 hours to reach 2 mmol/l (8 mg/100 ml). Furthermore, in severe cases of milk fever the peripheral blood circulation will be impaired, which will inhibit the absorption of any fluid material administered subcutaneously. In practice one is often called to attend cases of milk fever that have not responded to subcutaneous treatment administered by the farmer several hours before and the whole of the treatment solution is still present at the injection site.

As already stated approximately 85 per cent of cows will respond to one treatment. If response is not evident by 5–6 hours, then the cow should be re-examined, the diagnosis re-assessed and if necessary a further intravenous infusion of 8–12 g of calcium administered. Some practitioners advocate 400 ml of CBG intravenously plus 400 ml subcutaneously to prevent relapses. Relapse of milk fever occurs in 25 per cent of cases treated and this figure is not affected by additional subcutaneous administration. Blood levels of calcium 6 hours after intravenous or subcutaneous infusions are similar and by 12 hours after administration all the calcium administered, whether by the i.v. or s.c. route, has been eliminated from the body.

Treatment of milk fever should also be accompanied by removal of the calf and advice to the farmer not to milk the cow for 24 hours except to check for the presence of mastitis. As already stated, relapses occur in 25 per cent of cases treated and the likelihood of relapse will be reduced if milk is not drawn from the udder during this 24-hour period. The 8–12 g of calcium given is only a small proportion of the daily calcium requirement, so the treatment is only a holding operation until the normal adaptation process is in full operation. Cases of relapse usually occur at 18–24 hour intervals and should be treated in the same way, i.e. by the intravenous infusion of 8–12 g of calcium. Occasionally cows, particularly Jerseys, have been known to relapse on up to seven occasions.

There is a tendency amongst farmers to give two bottles of 40 per cent CBG, which would amount to 24 g of calcium. Such a procedure is probably counterproductive as there is some evidence to suggest that too high levels of calcium administration will slow up the adaptation process and actually increase the number of cows that relapse.

Some proprietary CBG preparations also contain magnesium (1.0 g) and phosphorus (2.6 g) in addition to calcium. If hypomagnesaemia is a complicating factor of milk fever then the addition of the magnesium may be helpful. However, in cases of clinical hypomagnesaemia more than 1.0 g of magnesium will be required. The presence of the phosphorus has no doubt been added because of the finding that the blood levels of phosphorus in cases of milk fever are also depressed. However, clinical evidence would suggest that the addition of phosphorus has no effect on the percentage of cases that recover or relapse. In fact, it has been shown that plasma phosphorus levels return to normal within a few hours after successful treatment with CBG without the addition of phosphorus.

Historically, the treatment of milk fever was by udder insufflation. This has the effect of slowing down milk production. Plasma calcium levels do rise following udder insufflation and will reach 2.5 mmol/l (10.0 mg/100 ml) by 4–5 hours after treatment. However, the efficacy of CBG intravenously and the dangers of mastitis following insufflation has now rendered this mode of treatment almost extinct except that some clinicians have been known to use the technique in cows that persistently relapse.

Prevention

Much milk fever can and should be prevented (see Table 39.2). If an outbreak occurs in any season where more than 10 per cent of cows are needing milk fever treatment the first action the clinician should consider is to blood test a group of six or seven dry cows to measure the concentration of calcium and magnesium. If the magnesium levels are low, i.e. below 0.85 mmol/l (1.8 mg/100 ml), this should be seriously considered as interfering with calcium absorption, in which case supplemental magnesium should be administered to all dry cows within three weeks of calving. Approximately 10–12 g of magnesium administered daily to dry cows will be sufficient to produce normal plasma levels of magnesium and to allow normal calcium absorption. However, this is often difficult to achieve because of the problem of giving supplemental feeds to grazing cows. A supplement of 25 g daily of calcined magnesite mixed with cereal (1 kg/cow) or silage will produce the desired effect but many farmers are reluctant to give supplemental feeds to dry cows. Recent experience in the UK has shown that the addition of magnesium acetate or magnesium chloride to the drinking water is a practical and effective way to supply magnesium to cows; 50 g daily of magnesium chloride crystals can be added to drinking water if large enough troughs are available. Trough size should be 25 l × the number of cows in the field. If trough size is limited, magnesium acetate can be added to the water supply using a water proportioner plumbed into the water supply pipe.

If the plasma levels of the dry cows are normal then diets restricting calcium intake may be considered, particularly if the plasma calcium levels are at the high end of the normal range. To be certain to prevent milk fever, dry-cow diets should contain less than 30 g/day of calcium. However, in practice, diets producing less than 50 g/day calcium will prevent most cases of milk fever. Autumn grass in the UK often contains 8–10 g/kg DM calcium. Thus with daily intakes of 12–14 kg DM, 90–140 g/day of calcium will be available in the diet. It is impossible appreciably to reduce this level

Table 39.2 Approximate requirements of 600 kg cows for dietary calcium, phosphorus and magnesium (g/day). Source: ARC (1980)

	Ca	P	Mg
Maintenance (non-pregnant)	15	13	9
Maintenance + late pregnancy	28	22	12
Lactation (g/kg milk)	1.65	1.55	0.74

Table 39.3 Approximate calcium, phosphorus and magnesium contents (g/kg DM) of some common feedstuffs

	Ca	P	Mg
Barley	0.6	3.8	1.4
Wheat	0.5	3.5	0.6
Maize	0.2	2.7	1.0
Sugar-beet pulp	10.4	0.9	1.4
Brewers grains	5.0	6.0	1.8
Maize silage	3.7	3.2	3.0
Grass and grass silage (range)	3.0–10.0	1.5–4.5	1.0–3.0
Grass and grass silage (average)	5.9	3.9	1.5

of intake without removing the cows from grass and substituting a diet based on grass silage, maize silage, hay or straw. However, some farmers are prepared to do this to reduce the risk of milk fever, and incidence levels of 5 per cent or less are possible. It should be appreciated that if low calcium diets are advocated for dry-cow use, just before parturition a diet containing more calcium should be administered to ensure adequate calcium being available over the risk period. This can be achieved by feeding cattle concentrate or feeds that are high in calcium, e.g. sugar-beet pulp (see Table 39.3).

Other methods of milk fever prevention involve dealing with individual cows. Maintenance of appetite is essential and, in the past, appetite stimulation by the use of anabolic steroids has been suggested but the use of these products is now illegal in Europe. Maintaining adequate calcium intake by drenching cows daily with 150 g/day of calcium chloride on the day before calving and for four days thereafter has had some success in preventing milk fever and might be considered in cows with a known history of milk fever.

The use of vitamin D_3 and its metabolites given by injection have been advocated in preventing milk fever. The administration of 10 million iv of vitamin D_3 given eight to two days before calving will considerably reduce the incidence of milk fever but the practical problem remains of accurately predicting the time of calving, which in practice has proven more difficult than expected. More recently, the analogue of the vitamin D_3 metabolite 1α-hydroxycholecalciferol ($1\alpha(OH)D_3$) has been used in trials to prevent milk fever. Doses of 350 μg given at least 24 hours and not more than five days before calving do reduce the incidence of milk fever but once again the problem remains of accurately predicting the time of calving. Recently, workers in Israel (Sachs, 1988) have suggested that a single dose of 700 μg of $1\alpha(OH)D_3$ given eight to seven days before expected calving is more effective and that the accuracy of calving date prediction is less important.

Vitamin D_3 or $1\alpha(OH)D_3$ will not be effective if the diet is deficient in magnesium. Before recommending their use the magnesium status of the herd should be assessed by blood testing six or seven dry cows.

Hypomagnesaemia (grass tetany, grass staggers, lactation tetany, Hereford disease)

Hypomagnesaemia is a common feature of a group of syndromes dominated by hyperaesthesia, incoordination, tetany and convulsions that can occur in all ruminants of all ages. Grass tetany or grass staggers is the name given to the syndrome affecting lactating cattle (beef or dairy cows) when grazing grass in the spring or autumn. Subclinical hypomagnesaemia can occur in lactating or dry cows in the spring or autumn and is usually not accompanied by clinical signs. It usually affects the whole herd. Lactating cows will suffer a slight reduction in milk yield and may have a slight nervous disposition, e.g. reluctance to enter the milking parlour. Dry cows will be more prone to milk fever at parturition. If the herd is affected with subclinical hypomagnesaemia some individuals will develop grass staggers, particularly if stressed. Milk tetany occurs in calves fed predominantly milk, particularly calves suckling cows that are subclinically hypomagnesaemic (see p. 219). The incidence of hypomagnesaemia varies considerably from region to region. Some areas of the UK are particularly high in the incidence of the disease in both beef and dairy cows.

The clinical disease is most common around peak lactation, presumably reflecting the secretion of magnesium in the milk. It is also a common cause of sudden death. In 1984 in the UK it was estimated that 0.8 per cent of the dairy cow population died from the disease (Whitaker *et al.*, 1984). This was following the introduction of milk quotas in Europe and a dramatic reduction in the use of concentrate feeds for dairy cows, particularly during the summer months.

Aetiology

As there are no readily available body stores for magnesium, the main factors involved in the aetiology of hypomagnesaemia are the reduction of the amount of magnesium available in the food, and hence available for absorption from the gut, accompanied by a high physiological demand for magnesium. Magnesium is lost from the body in milk, urine and faeces. The endogenous loss in faeces has been calculated to be approximately 1.8 g/day (ARC, 1980). Milk contains 0.12 g/l magnesium so a cow producing 30 kg of milk would lose 3.6 g daily in the milk. Any excess magnesium absorbed will be excreted via the urine, this being the mechanism for stabilizing plasma magnesium levels. If the plasma magnesium levels rise much above 0.8 mmol/l (2.0 mg/100 ml) the excess will be excreted. If magnesium intake levels are excessive, up to 5.0 g/day may be excreted in the urine. However, if magnesium intake falls to the level to maintain homeostasis or below there will no magnesium identifiable in the urine.

To maintain magnesium homeostasis the absorption of magnesium must be continuous so a constant supply is necessary in the diet. Feeds vary considerably in both the content and the availability of magnesium so the choice of pasture is important. Clovers have a higher magnesium content than grasses and grasses themselves vary. Fast-growing Italian ryegrasses have lower levels than perennial grasses. Many broad-leaf plants, such as buttercups (*Ranunculus* spp.), plantains and nettles, have considerably higher magnesium levels than grasses, which probably account to some extent for the increasing incidence of hypomagnesaemia seen in recent years in the UK as old permanent pastures have been replaced with ryegrass leys.

Some soils are known to be deficient in magnesium but also the uptake of magnesium by plants may be influenced by cations such as calcium and potassium in the soil. It has been shown that fertilizers containing potassium applied to grazing areas in late winter or early spring will reduce the absorption of magnesium by plants, and soils containing high levels of potassium are particularly prone to producing hypomagnesaemia in grazing ruminants.

Although this disease has been predominantly a disease of spring grass, in recent years it is becoming increasingly common in cows grazing autumn grass in the UK. The occurrence during winter has also increased in the UK; this can be attributed to the increasing use of grass silage made from young leafy grass low in magnesium during May.

Another important factor in the aetiology of the disease is the energy intake of the animals. This is particularly the case in beef suckler cows grazing inadequate pastures, particularly during times of inclement weather. Experiments have shown that reduced energy intake will interfere with the magnesium available for absorption. The availability of magnesium for absorption from the gut is thought to range from 4 to 35 per cent. Calcium, potassium and ammonium (nitrogen) ions are all thought to interfere with body uptake of magnesium.

It is possible to find animals with low plasma magnesium levels but yet be clinically normal. It would appear that the critical factor influencing the onset of clinical disease is the level of magnesium in the cerebrospinal fluid (CSF). The speed at which magnesium levels fall also influences the onset of clinical signs. In the spring, magnesium levels fall rapidly and clinical disease may become apparent at blood levels at which in the autumn, when the fall is more gradual, the cows remain clinically normal.

The role of calcium in the onset of clinical hypomagnesaemia is also unclear. Approximately 80 per cent of cows with grass staggers have low plasma calcium levels. It has been shown that cows will develop clinical disease within 24 hours after a fall in plasma calcium levels although they have been hypomagnesaemic for several days.

Milk tetany occurs in calves two to four months old reared on whole milk diets without the addition of magnesium supplementation. In young calves absorption of magnesium is good. However, as the calf grows older the ability to absorb magnesium declines. Thus, if the two to four-month-old calf is denied feed supplementation other than cows milk, magnesium absorption will decline to less than requirements and clinical signs will appear. This is seen in suckler calves or veal calves reared on milk or milk substitute that has not been supplemented with magnesium.

Signs

The signs of grass staggers may be classified as subacute, acute or peracute. In the subacute form cows will be apprehensive, and hyperaesthetic. The head will be held high and tremors may be seen around the head (particularly the eyelids), over the shoulder and on the flank. These tremors will be exaggerated if the animal is touched or the skin pinched. The legs may become stiff and a staggering gait may be evident. Cows can remain in the subacute phase for several hours or progress to the acute or peracute form, particularly in response to noise or some other stimulus such as attempting to herd them. The peracute cases will stagger for a few steps and fall over with tetanic spasms of the head, neck and legs followed by clonic convulsions. The legs will paddle furiously, the eyes roll, and there is frothing at the mouth. The heart will pound fast and furious and death can occur at any time. Cows have been known to be grazing one minute and in response to noise from a vehicle or other stimulus to stagger, fall over in convulsions and die in two or three minutes.

The signs in the acute case will be similar but may last for up to an hour or more. In these cases a period of convulsions will be followed by a quiescent period in which the cow may attempt to rise, only to walk a few steps and fall over again followed by convulsions. The rectal temperature, if taken, will be elevated by 1 or 2 °C (2–4 °F). Cows are often found dead with obvious signs that the limbs had been paddling prior to death, thus disturbing the soil around the feet.

In the subclinical form the majority of the herd are usually affected even if acute cases have not been diagnosed. If acute cases are present it can be assumed that the majority of the herd will be affected subclinically. The cows may be slightly nervous, reluctant to enter the milking parlour or be unwilling to be herded. The milk yield will be depressed slightly.

The signs of milk tetany in calves are much the same as for cows with subacute, acute and peracute cases occurring. Often in peracute cases the animals are found dead.

Clinical pathology

Healthy normal cows should possess plasma magnesium levels over 0.85 mmol/l (2.0 mg/100 ml). Any levels below this must be considered at risk and indicative of subclinical hypomagnesaemia, although in acute cases the plasma levels will generally be below 0.4 mmol/l (1.0 mg/100 ml). Magnesium levels in the CSF in acute tetany will generally be below 0.6 mmol/l (1.4 mg/100 ml). Hypocalcaemia is present in at least 80 per cent of acute tetany cases and hyperkalaemia is common. Following tetany or in recovered cases aspartate aminotransferase (AST) and creatine kinase (CK) levels will rise to relatively high levels but return to normal quite soon after recovery.

At post mortem there are no pathognomonic signs. Haemorrhages may be present on the heart muscle and occasionally along the aorta. Regurgitation and aspiration of rumen contents may sometimes be seen. The CSF levels of magnesium will be low and magnesium will be absent from the urine, although the bladder is nearly always empty at post mortem.

Diagnosis

The diagnosis of grass staggers is made on the signs described above. The time of year and type of grazing may help in forming a diagnosis. As there is little or no time in acute cases to conduct blood biochemistry, response to treatment will also confirm a diagnosis. It may be useful for the clinician to take a blood sample before treatment so that analysis can be performed at a later stage should this prove necessary. If animals are found dead then diagnosis must be differentiated from other causes of death. Diagnosis at post mortem is difficult because of the absence of obvious lesions. If quantities of soil have been gouged out of the ground by each of the four feet during the paddling phase this is strongly indicative of acute grass staggers. Absence of magnesium from urine would be a useful indicator but the bladder is generally empty. Blood or tissues are of no value at post mortem because magnesium levels rise rapidly after death. Levels in CSF may be helpful and recently it has been suggested that magnesium levels in vitreous humour taken after death will be depressed in cows that have died from grass staggers. If a cow is found dead and grass staggers suspected from the history and absence of other lesions at post mortem, the wise clinician will blood sample six to seven cows in the group and test for magnesium levels. It is important to make a diagnosis to be able to offer preventive advice for the remainder of the herd.

Diagnosis of death due to milk tetany in calves is possible by measuring the calcium and magnesium levels in bone. A rib or coccygeal bone is usually used for this purpose. A calcium/magnesium ratio in bone of 70 : 1 is considered normal and 90 : 1 considered an indication of severe magnesium depletion.

To diagnose subclinical hypomagnesaemia blood sampling seven cows each from a lactating and a dry-cow group and testing for magnesium is the most useful indicator. Testing urine for magnesium levels has been advocated, absence of magnesium indicating the subclinical state. Urine test strips are available in some countries. However, there are real practical problems in getting a number of cows to micturate on demand.

Differential diagnosis

Acute lead poisoning. In lead poisoning (see p. 617) there may be excitement and occasional convulsions

Hyperaesthesia, as measured by observing muscle tremors in response to pinching the skin, will be absent and blindness is usually a feature of lead poisoning.

Milk fever (p. 577). Some cows in the early stage of milk fever may exhibit hyperaesthetic signs. The history of being close to parturition is the most helpful aid to this differential diagnosis. Many cows are hypocalcaemic as well as hypomagnesaemic and so treatment involves calcium administration; thus being able accurately to differentially diagnose the two conditions is not important in practice.

Acetonaemia (p. 590). Some cows with acute acetonaemia will have hyperaesthetic signs and appear nervous and apprehensive. However, the depraved actions of these cows, such as licking the walls and floor or biting at gates, will usually distinguish this disease from hypomagnesaemia as will a Rothera's test on a sample of milk.

Listeriosis (p. 703). Acute listeriosis may be confused with acute grass staggers but the high rectal temperature and absence of true hyperaesthesia in listeriosis cases should be enough to distinguish this disease.

Bovine spongiform encephalopathy (p. 708). The emergence of BSE in the UK in 1986 has sometimes made the differential diagnosis of the subacute form of hypomagnesaemia more difficult. The ataxia, apprehension and mild hyperaesthesia found in BSE are similar to that found in subacute hypomagnesaemia. Diagnosis is usually confirmed by response to treatment and blood biochemistry, a sample being taken before treatment. It would be wise in all cases of suspected BSE to take a blood sample to eliminate subacute hypomagnesaemia before notifying the suspicion to the authorities.

Others. Lightning strike (p. 762) as a cause of sudden death, some plant poisonings, and in particular Paspalum staggers (*Claviceps paspali* poisoning), are differential diagnoses but can usually be distinguished on grounds of history alone. Rabies (p. 706) may cause problems in countries where it occurs but such animals usually are hyperactive, bellowing and riding other cattle.

Suboptimal production. If production is below expectations, particularly in seasons associated with hypomagnesaemia then subclinical hypomagnesaemia could be present. Blood biochemistry in the form of a metabolic profile that includes magnesium should be considered.

Treatment

Acute cases of grass staggers must be treated promptly. During the course of treatment the operators should be as quiet and gentle as possible as any sudden stimulus will initiate a bout of convulsions. Hence, actually restraining a staggering acute case will often be difficult and when attempting to place a rope or halter on the animal it will sometimes collapse into a fit of convulsions and may even die before treatment has been administered. The success of treatment is also related to the length of time signs have been present in the recumbent acute case. The longer the cow has been showing convulsions the less likely it will be to recover.

Intravenous infusions of magnesium salts, e.g. magnesium sulphate, are sometimes recommended for treatment but this procedure is not without its dangers. Intravenous magnesium sulphate may cause cardiac embarrassment or even respiratory failure. If magnesium sulphate is administered intravenously the concentration should be no more than 6 per cent and must be administered very slowly with the heart being auscultated. However, it is also essential to administer calcium in the form of CBG because most cases of grass staggers are also hypocalcaemic.

The treatment protocol favoured by the author is to discard 100 ml of fluid from a 400 ml bottle of 40 per cent CBG, which also contains magnesium 0.2 per cent and phosphorus 0.5 per cent, and replace this with 100 ml of 25 per cent magnesium sulphate solution. The mixture, which then contains 9 g of calcium and approximately 6 g of magnesium, is infused intravenously very slowly taking 8–10 minutes. The remaining 300 ml of the original 400 ml 25 per cent magnesium sulphate is injected subcutaneously. If during the infusion, or immediately after, the convulsions get worse 10 ml of pentobarbitone sodium 200 mg/ml (euthanasia solution) can be administered intravenously and this will often reduce or even eliminate the convulsions. Following this treatment regimen, if the cow is recumbent, it is important to remain quiet for a further 10 minutes as stimulation even immediately after treatment may initiate convulsions. The recumbent cow should then be raised into sternal recumbency and left for a further 30 minutes before attempting to stimulate the animal to rise.

Treatment is successful, if early, in 80 per cent of acute recumbent cases and nearly 100 per cent in acute standing cases. If the recumbent case is not able to rise within 2 hours of treatment the likelihood of success is extremely poor and slaughter should be considered. Subacute grass staggers should be treated in the same way and success is usually near to 100 per cent.

Relapses are considered normal unless preventative measures are taken. Blood magnesium falls to pretreatment levels within 6 hours of intravenous administration although the subcutaneous injection has a more prolonged effect. Daily subcutaneous injections of 200–400 ml of 25 per cent magnesium sulphate for five days following treatment have been recommended or the oral administration of four magnesium bullets, which are composed of an alloy of 86 per cent magnesium, 12 per cent aluminium and 2 per cent copper weighted with iron shot (Rumbul bullets, Agrimin Ltd), immediately following the intravenous and subcutaneous treatment.

An individual cow suffering from grass staggers is one of a herd and many cows in the herd could be at risk or at least suffering from subclinical hypomagnesaemia. It is important therefore that a group of six to seven cows be blood tested to ascertain the herd magnesium status, and if the blood levels are below 0.8 mmol/l (2.0 mg/100 ml) herd supplementation with magnesium must be instituted.

The treatment of milk tetany in calves is generally academic as most cases are found dead. However, very slow intravenous infusion of 100 ml of 20 per cent CBG with the addition of 20 ml of 25 per cent magnesium sulphate followed by 60 ml of 25 per cent magnesium sulphate subcutaneously would be the regimen of choice. Oral supplementation of magnesium must also follow if the calf recovers. Suggested daily doses of magnesium oxide would be 1, 2 and 3 g for calves up to five weeks, five to ten weeks and ten to fifteen weeks old, respectively.

Prevention

The simplest method of prevention of hypomagnesaemia is to add calcined magnesite (magnesium oxide) to cattle concentrate that is being fed to the cows. However, the main risk periods in northern Europe for hypomagnesaemia are times when concentrate food is not being fed, e.g. spring grazing and autumn grazing for dry cows. In Australia, New Zealand and Ireland very little concentrates are fed, and in many beef suckler herds other ingenious methods must be devised. The magnesium bullets mentioned above will give protection for four to six weeks. However, although two bullets are recommended, in severe hypomagnesaemic areas experience has shown that four bullets are required to prevent problems.

Dusting the pastures with magnesium oxide has been attempted using 50 g/cow/day of magnesium oxide or 0.5 kg/week applied in the early morning when the dew is on the grass. This works best when cows are strip grazed and the magnesium oxide is applied every morning. Weekly applications are effective in dry weather but must be re-applied following rain. However, grass staggers is more common in wet than dry weather.

The increasing practice in recent years in the UK of buffer feeding, where a silage supplement is fed to cows during the grazing season, has meant that magnesium oxide at the rate of 50 g/cow/day can be mixed with or sprinkled on top of the silage.

Supplementation of water supplies using magnesium acetate via a water proportioner is effective but expensive. The proportioner has to be adjusted daily to allow for the variation in water intake that occurs under different weather conditions. The expense and management input required has been a disincentive for this method of prevention to become widespread. The addition of magnesium chloride crystals to the drinking water has increased in popularity in the UK in recent years. It is relatively inexpensive but to be effective the trough sizes must be large enough for all cows to drink the medicated water. The addition of 40 g/cow per day of magnesium chloride to the drinking water has been shown to give reasonable protection. Addition of magnesium salts to the drinking water will depress water intake if the concentration is too high. Troughs with a volume of 20 l of water/cow in the field are required for this method of control to work effectively. Mineral licks and powders containing high levels of magnesium are relatively useless in preventing hypomagnesaemia because of the uncertainty of all cows consuming enough material to give them protection when it is required.

When discussing the long-term strategies for controlling hypomagnesaemia fertilizer policy should be included. All potassium-containing fertilizers should be avoided on soils with high potassium levels and on other soils, if potassium-containing fertilizers are used, they should be applied at low levels in the autumn. If necessary, they can be applied later in the grazing season.

Perhaps plant species should also be considered in long-term control strategies. Clover/grass mixtures should be favoured ahead of grass alone but perhaps above all the use of selective weedkillers should be discouraged. A few buttercups and other wild plants growing in the pasture may not only be aesthetically acceptable but may reduce the incidence of hypomagnesaemia in grazing animals.

The prevention of milk tetany in calves can be achieved by ensuring magnesium supplementation. Proprietary milk substitute powders are adequately supplied with magnesium. If whole milk is used magnesium oxide at the rates given above should be added to the daily diet (see p. 587).

Hypophosphataemia

Hypophosphataemia is the result of a primary deficiency of phosphorus in the diet (see also p. 217).

Occurrence

Dietary deficiencies of phosphorus are widespread under natural conditions. There is a distinct geographical distribution where large land masses are identified as being deficient in phosphorus and livestock cannot be supported without phosphorus supplementation. These areas will be deficient because of the underlying rock formation. Large areas of southern Africa and Australia are well identified as being deficient in phosphorus. Such areas, however, are unknown or rare in northern Europe and if they exist at all, will be localized. Although there are areas of Europe where the underlying rock formation contains no phosphorus, continuous application of fertilizers containing phosphorus and cultivation techniques have improved the soil structure and nutritive value. In consequence, primary phosphorus deficiency is probably a rare occurrence in Europe.

Aetiology

Phosphorus deficiency is usually primary although a severe deficiency of vitamin D (p. 217) may exacerbate the problem. It was once considered that excess calcium would also reduce the availability of phosphorus in the diet and cause deficiencies of phosphorus. Although the calcium: phosphorus ratio in the diet is important in monogastric animals it is probably of less significance in cattle. The maintenance requirements for adult and growing cattle would be approximately 15 g of phosphorus daily. The lactating cow requires approximately 0.75 g/kg of milk produced, so a cow yielding 30 kg of milk daily will require 40 g of phosphorus daily. This level of requirement is considerably less than that currently being recommended in the UK by Agricultural Development and Advisory Service but nevertheless is supported by experimental evidence from the Agricultural and Food Research Council (ARC, 1980).

Signs

In young cattle phosphorus deficiency results in slow growth and rickets. In adult cattle the principal signs are reduced milk yield, weight loss and depraved appetite. Osteomalacia will result from prolonged dietary deficiency of phosphorus. The depraved appetite or pica results in cows eating earth, licking rocks and, where bones are available, osteophagia. The osteophagia frequently results in a high incidence of botulism (p. 556) and in some areas of southern Africa and Australia death from botulism is the most important consequence of phosphorus deficiency. Reduced fertility has been considered a feature of severe phosphorus deficiency but experimental work has demonstrated that fertility is independent of either calcium or phosphorus intakes. Reduced fertility is a feature of malnutrition and frequently animals that are deficient in phosphorus are also suffering from malnutrition. Low energy intake in such animals is much more likely to be the cause of reduced fertility than any specific mineral deficiency.

Cows in late pregnancy often become recumbent particularly in drought seasons. This recumbency is probably a result of general malnutrition rather than a specific phosphorus deficiency.

Hypophosphataemia nearly always accompanies hypocalcaemia in cows with milk fever but this is not thought to be of any significance. Phosphorus levels rarely fall to the levels of 0.3 mmol/l (1 mg/100 ml) seen in severe clinical cases and in any case calcium therapy will result in the blood phosphorus levels quickly reverting to normal.

Diagnosis

The presence of rickets or osteomalacia and/or pica will indicate a dietary deficiency of phosphorus, which can be confirmed by analysis of serum and the diet for the presence of phosphorus. The normal blood level is 1.3–1.6 mmol/l (4–5 mg/100 ml). Levels of 0.5–1.1 mmol/l (1.5–3.5 mg/100 ml) falling as low as 0.3 mmol/l (1 mg/100 ml) of serum in severe clinical cases will be found in hypophosphataemic animals.

Most pastures in northern Europe contain 1.5–4.5 g/kg DM of phosphorus and at these levels phosphorus deficiency will not occur. Osteophagia will occur with pasture levels of 0.2 g/kg DM of phosphorus and rickets and osteomalacia at pasture levels of 0.1 g/kg DM.

The only commonly used feedstuffs in the UK that are deficient in phosphorus are sugar-beet pulp at 0.9 g/kg DM, kale and other *Brassica* spp. crops. These are rarely used at a proportion of the diet significantly reduce the phosphorus intake to dangerous levels.

Control

Under range conditions, where phosphorus deficiency is the most common, supplementation of the diet with phosphorus is often impractical. Bone meal, dicalcium phosphate or disodium phosphate may be provided in feed supplements or free access mineral mixtures. The dietary intake of phosphorus should be at least 15 g/day. Top dressing pastures with superphosphate fertilizers will correct any underlying deficiency and have the added advantage of increasing the yield and protein content of the pasture. However, this is often impractical in areas where the problem exists.

In acute cases where phosphorus therapy is urgent, e.g. postparturient haemoglobinuria, the intravenous administration of sodium acid phosphate (30 g in 200 ml distilled water) is advocated (see below).

Postparturient haemoglobinuria

One specific syndrome associated with phosphorus deficiency is postparturient haemoglobinuria. This is a disease of cows one to four weeks after calving. Haemolytic anaemia and hypophosphataemia are consistent features.

Occurrence

Postparturient haemoglobinuria was first described in Scotland in 1853 and has been reported from many countries including Australia, USA and most of Europe. The occurrence is sporadic and when it does arise it usually only affects one or two cows within a herd. In recent years its occurrence in the UK has been extremely rare. In Scotland it has been associated with the feeding of beets and turnips, in Holland with the feeding of lush spring grass and occasionally it has been reported to accompany the feeding of sugar beet byproducts and alfalfa.

Aetiology

Diets low in phosphorus are incriminated in the cause of postparturient haemoglobinuria. However, it is probable that there is some additional factor that precipitates the problem in hypophosphataemic cattle. This is likely to be a haemolytic factor present in sugar-beet leaves, alfalfa, kale and other *Brassica* spp. plants.

Signs

The principal clinical signs are those associated with anaemia. The cow may be weak and staggering, with mucous membranes pale and heart rate raised. Haemoglobinuria will be a consistent feature. The faeces are firm and dry. If left untreated the cow will finally become recumbent and may die within two to five days. Less severely affected cases may recover, albeit slowly, in three or four weeks. Pica is frequently observed during the recovery period.

Clinical pathology

Serum phosphorus levels are low, usually 0.15–1.0 mmol/l (0.5–3.0 mg/100 ml). Low phosphorus levels will be encountered in other cows in the herd. Red cell counts, packed cell volume and haemoglobin are all dramatically reduced. Serum bilirubin will increase in the later stages of the disease.

At post mortem the liver will be swollen and infiltrated with fat. The carcass is jaundiced and anaemic and red or red/brown coloured urine will be found in the bladder.

Diagnosis

Postparturient haemoglobinuria must be suspected in any cow that is weak, anaemic and exhibiting haemoglobinuria within four weeks of parturition. The haemoglobinuria must be distinguished from babesiasis (p. 726) and copper poisoning (p. 613). A history of feeding large quantities of kale, beet tops or alfalfa will also be a helpful aid to diagnosis. The diagnosis should be confirmed by demonstrating hypophosphataemia and haemoglobinuria.

Treatment

Intravenous therapy with 30 g of sodium acid phosphate in 200 ml of distilled water followed by the provision of 100 g/day of bone meal in the diet is the first line of treatment. In extremely anaemic cases blood transfusion with 5–10 l of blood should be considered. Supportive therapy with large doses of vitamin C intravenously and iron dextran injections will aid the recovery.

Prevention

If brassicas have to be fed to cattle in early lactation their intake should be limited to a maximum of 20 kg wet matter/day. This limitation and an adequate phosphorus intake will prevent the occurrence of postparturient haemoglobinuria.

Acetonaemia

Acetonaemia or ketosis is a metabolic disorder of high-yielding lactating cows characterized by reduced milk yield, loss of body weight, inappetance and, occasionally, nervous signs. Ketone bodies, e.g. acetoacetate, β-hydroxybutyrate or acetone, are present in all body fluids. Hypoglycaemia together with increased plasma free fatty acids and liver fat and decreased liver glycogen are also a feature of this disease. These changes are associated with an inadequate supply of the energy that is necessary to sustain high levels of milk production in early lactation. Pregnancy toxaemia, a common disease of pregnant sheep and characterized by hypoglycaemia and hyperketonaemia, can also occasionally affect pregnant cows particularly when carrying twins.

Acetonaemia is more common in the winter when cows are housed and being fed conserved forage, but it can occasionally be seen in cows at pasture. Cows of any age can be affected and Channel Island breeds, particularly the Jersey, appear to be more susceptible than the Friesian or Holstein. Acetonaemia is less common in the UK now than it was 20 to 30 years ago. This is probably due to higher quality feeds being available although the preponderance of the Friesian breed may have some effect on the disease incidence. Outbreaks are usually restricted to one or two cows but varying numbers of cows in the herd may be affected. If the incidence of the disease is high it can become a severe economic problem due to depressed milk production. The disease usually occurs three to six weeks after calving, when the cow is at her peak milk production but her appetite or DM intake has not yet reached its peak. During early lactation the dairy cow is in negative energy balance. The energy intake in feed is insufficient to meet the energy output in milk. This results in the mobilization of fat reserves to meet the energy deficit and a consequent loss in body weight. This should be considered a normal metabolic situation in high-yielding dairy cows. Such cows will have slightly raised blood ketone levels and may even excrete ketones in urine and possibly in milk. The cow in early lactation is therefore in a delicate metabolic balance and any stress that causes a reduction of feed intake can disturb this balance and result in the onset of clinical ketosis. Factors that can influence the occurrence of the disease include excessive feeding of silage that has a high content of butyric acid, a deterioration in forage quality, sudden changes in types of food on offer and excessive fatness at calving. In the UK the butyric acid content of silage is of considerable importance in the aetiology of this disease because wet conditions, so frequently encountered during silage making, predispose to butyric fermentation of the silage. The role of such silage in the aetiology of acetonaemia is probably twofold. Firstly, there is the direct effect of the presence of butyric acid and secondly there is the reduced dietary intake that accompanies such silage. Cows that are too fat at calving have lower DM intakes in early lactation and are therefore more likely to suffer acetonaemia.

Acetonaemia is occasionally diagnosed in grazing cattle particularly if the grass has a high moisture content and the energy intake is insufficient. Cobalt is required for rumen microbial synthesis of vitamin B_{12} and is also essential for adequate utilization of propionic acid. In areas of cobalt deficiency acetonaemia will be commonly diagnosed in grazing cows (p. 261).

Secondary ketosis is common, if not more common, than primary ketosis and can result from any disease that causes a reduction in appetite in early lactation. Displaced abomasum (see p. 645) and traumatic reticulitis (p. 643) are two common problems frequently associated with secondary ketosis.

Aetiology

To understand the aetiology of acetonaemia one must realize the precarious metabolic balance that exists in all cows in early lactation. To satisfy the requirements of milk production the cow can draw on two sources of nutrients, food intake and her body reserves. In the first two months of lactation a cow producing up to 45 kg of milk daily will use up to 2 kg of body fat and up to 350 g of body protein per day. As far as the dietary supply of nutrients is concerned 80 per cent of the ingested carbohydrates are fermented by the rumen microflora into the volatile fatty acids, acetic, propionic and butyric acids, which are themselves absorbed. Acetate may be oxidized by various tissues or incorporated into milk fat by the mammary gland.

Glucose is synthesized in the liver and renal cortex by the gluconeogenic pathway. Approximately half of the cow's glucose requirement is derived from dietary propionic acid, which is incorporated into the tricarboxylic acid (TCA) cycle and converted to glucose by gluconeogenesis. Glucogenic amino acids, lactic acid and glycerol can be converted into glucose by this process. Reduced production of propionic acid in the rumen will result in inadequate glucose production and a consequent hypoglycaemia. Hyopoglycaemia leads to a mobilization of free fatty acids and glycerol from the fat stores. Hormones such as adrenaline, glucagon, adrenocorticotrophic hormone, glucocorticoids and thyroid hormones all influence this mobilization from the body fat stores. Skeletal muscle and heart can utilize fatty acids for energy production when glucose is short. However, the liver has a limited ability to oxidize fatty acids because acetyl-CoA, which is the endproduct of fatty acid oxidation, cannot be adequately incorporated into the TCA cycle as levels of oxaloacetate, the result of active gluconeogenesis, are low. The excess acetyl-CoA is converted into the ketone bodies acetoacetate and β-hydroxybutyrate and, to a small extent, acetone. Ketone bodies can be utilized by tissues other than liver but, if their production exceeds the rate they are used by muscle and other tissues, they accumulate and ketosis is the result. Ketone bodies are excreted in milk and urine.

The reduction of propionic acid production by the rumen is usually a feature of underfeeding or a reduced feed intake caused by inappetance. Cobalt deficiency, as mentioned above, will also have the effect of reducing propionic acid production. Butyrate is a precursor of acetyl-CoA and is therefore ketogenic. An increase in butyrate uptake from the rumen will therefore be ketogenic. This explains why silage high in butyric acid will induce ketosis in apparently normal cows.

Signs

Hypoglycaemia is the major factor involved in the onset and development of the clinical signs of acetonaemia. There will have been a gradual loss of body condition over several days or even weeks. There is also a moderate decline in milk yield over two to four days before the onset of the obvious clinical signs, which are refusal to eat grain and concentrate feeds and a more sudden drop in milk output. At this stage a sweet smell (as in pear drops) of acetone is apparent on the breath and the discerning stockworker will even detect the same acetone smell in the milk. Once appetite is decreased weight loss is accelerated due to utilization of body stores. Rectal temperature, pulse rates and respiratory rates are normal in the early stages of the disease as are ruminal movements. Faeces will usually be firm with a dark 'waxy' appearance.

A small number of cows with acute acetonaemia exhibit nervous signs, which include excessive salivation, abnormal chewing movements and licking walls, gates or metal bars. Incoordination with apparent blindness will also be a feature. Some cows will even show a degree of aggression and will sometimes charge into walls, occasionally injuring themselves. The other signs observed above are also present. The nervous signs often only last for a few hours with the animals showing more normal behaviour in between.

Clinical pathology

Hypoglycaemia, hyperketonaemia and the presence of ketones in the urine and milk are the features of this disease. Cowside diagnosis is obtained by the detection of ketones in milk and urine using the Rothera's test reaction. A drop of milk or urine is added to a small quantity (which consists of sodium nitroprusside 3 g, sodium carbonate 3 g and ammonium sulphate 100 g) Rothera's reagent on a white tile or piece of white card. The presence of ketones is confirmed by a pink to purple coloration of the reagent. Urine normally contains low levels of ketones so a diagnosis is only positive when the milk is also positive.

Blood glucose levels are reduced to below 1.4 mmol/l (25 mg/100 ml). Total blood ketone levels are raised to over 5 mmol/l (30 mg/100 ml). The plasma glycerol and free fatty acid levels are also elevated. Subclinical ketosis has become more important in recent years with the introduction of the laboratory test for β-hydroxybutyrate (βHB). The level of βHB is frequently used on a herd basis as a measure of energy balance in both lactating and dry cows. Herds with subclinical ketosis have been identified using this test. Serum levels of βHB in excess of 1.75 mmol/l (10 mg/100 ml) will indicate an energy deficit in the diet.

Although mortality is not normally a feature of acetonaemia, affected cows do possess fatty infiltration and degeneration of the liver.

Diagnosis

The diagnosis is made on the history of a cow in early lactation with a sudden fall in milk yield, some weight loss, refusing to eat concentrates, with normal temperature, pulse and respiratory rates and normal rumen movements. Many astute stockworkers will recognize the acetone odour on the breath or in the milk and report this to the attending veterinarian. The diagnosis is confirmed by a positive Rothera's reaction on milk and urine and, if this is not conclusive, a blood sample can be analysed for glucose and ketone levels. It is important to differentiate between primary and secondary ketosis so a complete clinical examination must be performed. Many cases presented by the farmer as acetonaemia are in fact suffering from displaced abomasum (p. 645). Some cows with hypocalcaemia (p. 577) may also show acetonaemia.

The differential diagnosis of the nervous form of acetonaemia can be sometimes confusing. The behavioural changes are similar to listeriosis (p. 703) but usually with listeriosis pyrexia will be present. Hypomagnesaemia (p. 583) should be distinguishable by the presence of hyperaesthesia, particularly the tremors of the eyelids and muscle tremors over the shoulders and the presence of tetanic convulsions. Bovine spongiform encephalopathy (p. 708) may also be confused with acetonaemia because of weight loss. However, the apprehension, kicking and progressive nature of BSE should be distinguishing features, besides which blood glucose, magnesium and ketone levels will be normal in BSE. Rabies (p. 706) is characterized by mania, ascending paralysis and is always fatal.

Treatment

There are three main components of successful treatment.

1 To restore blood glucose levels as quickly as possible.
2 To replenish oxaloacetate, an essential intermediate in the TCA cycle in the liver, so that fatty acids mobilized from the fat deposits are completely oxidized. This will reduce the rate of production of ketone bodies.
3 To increase the availability of dietary glucogenic precursors, notably propionic acid.

An intravenous infusion of 500 ml of 40 per cent glucose will cause a transient rise in blood glucose levels that lasts approximately 2 hours. This should be accompanied by oral administration of glucose precursors such as propylene glycol (150 ml, twice daily). Propylene glycol is preferred to propionate or glycerol because propionate is fermented in the rumen and may cause digestive disturbances and glycerol is converted to ketogenic acids as well as propionic acid in the rumen. Cobalt salts are frequently added to the propylene glycol and in cobalt-deficient areas at least 100 mg/day of cobalt should be administered.

Glucocorticoid drugs are the most commonly used therapy for acetonaemia either used alone or in combination with glucose therapy or when followed by oral administration of glucose precursors. Glucocorticoid therapy results in a reduction of ketone body formation due to utilization of the acetyl-CoA derived from fatty acid oxidation and raises blood glucose levels due to a greater availability of glucose precursors in the liver. The commonly used glucocorticoids are dexamethasone, betamethasone and flumethasone and all are effective. Frequently, a single dose is administered but this does often result in relapses two to three days after the treatment, when the injection can be repeated. There is one disadvantage of repeated glucocorticoid therapy and that is that appetite and milk yield are reduced.

For successful treatment in most cases of acetonaemia the following regimen is to be recommended:

1 500 ml of 40 per cent glucose intravenously, followed by;
2 one dose of glucocorticoid, followed by;
3 oral treatment twice daily with 150 g of propylene glycol containing cobalt for three to four days.

Anabolic steroids are also a useful treatment for acetonaemia and were used in Europe before their use was prohibited under the EC hormone ban. They are effective by increasing the levels of the intermediates of the TCA cycle in the liver. They also stimulate appetite, which ensures an increased supply of the glucogenic precursors. They do not directly raise blood glucose levels. It is important that the cow's appetite returns to normal as soon as possible after treatment so access to good quality fodder is a prerequisite to successful treatment. If butyric silage is implicated in the cause of the problem this should be removed from the diet and only well-fermented silage or good quality hay offered.

If acetonaemia is affecting a high proportion of the herd it would be wise to obtain a supply of ground maize as it has been shown that ground maize is readily digested in the small intestine and results in a rapid rise in blood glucose levels.

Prevention

The prevention of acetonaemia starts before calving. Cows should not be too fat at calving, condition score 2.5–3.0 would be optimum and anything higher would be considered too fat. Access to a plentiful supply of long coarse fibre to promote good rumen digestion is also important during the dry period. Concentrates used during lactation should be introduced in small quantities (1–2 kg/day) two weeks before calving to allow adjustments in the rumen microflora. Changes to diet in early lactation should be made gradually.

Forage containing ketogenic substances such as butyric acid should be avoided in early lactation. Roughage should comprise at least 40 per cent of the diet. In cobalt-deficient areas measures should be taken to ensure adequate cobalt intake, e.g. by spreading cobalt sulphate on to pastures. The concentrates used need to be of good quality. This statement may seem obvious but unfortunately some concentrate manufacturers, under pressure from farmers, will produce substandard concentrates at a lower than normal price. By and large the quality of a concentrate food is reflected in its price.

The use of metabolic profiles (Chapter 40) measuring blood glucose and βHB levels in groups of dry cows and cows in early lactation can be useful in the hands of the experienced veterinarian. This will often indicate an energy-deficient diet and one that could predispose to subclinical if not clinical acetonaemia.

As already stated acetonaemia is less common now than in previous years. This is due mainly to improvements in forage conservation techniques and the improved financial situation amongst dairy farmers in the western world. Thus cows are fed better quality feeds and there is increased awareness that optimum output comes as a result of optimum input.

Pregnancy toxaemia

Pregnancy toxaemia, although primarily considered a disease of sheep, does also affect cattle, particularly beef cattle in late pregnancy. The problem is best described as starvation but the aetiology and pathogenesis is similar to acetonaemia in that an energy deficit in the diet leads to massive mobilization of fat reserves resulting in hypoglycaemia and hyperketonaemia. The problem is most common in beef cattle grazing marginal land, but has been seen in dairy cattle in late winter in seasons where there has been a shortage of conserved forage. Cows of all ages are affected but overfat animals and those carrying twins are the most susceptible. Beef cows often have access to good pastures in the summer months and can get overfat. If the same cows do not have access to good quality forage during the winter months, when they are in late pregnancy they will succumb to ketosis because of the deficit in energy intake. In dairy cows the problem can occur at or around calving and is again the result of insufficient energy intake in excessively fat animals.

Signs

The severity of the clinical signs and their speed of onset are associated with the stage of pregnancy and the degree of nutritional stress. Affected cows are usually seven to nine months pregnant and show the same clinical signs as cows with acetonaemia. They become increasingly dull and depressed and the smell of acetone can be detected on the breath. Many cows become recumbent fairly quickly, within a few days of the onset of hyperketonaemia. Often in poorly supervised herds recumbency is the first sign noticed by the stockworker. Recumbent cows are severely depressed, have an increased respiratory rate, and faeces are scanty, hard and covered in mucus. Some cows develop a bloodstained or fetid diarrhoea in the terminal stages. Most cows die three to fourteen days after recumbency having fallen into lateral recumbency. This often occurs two to five days after sternal recumbency. Cows affected close to parturition often die during parturition.

Clinical pathology

Hypoglycaemia, hyperketonaemia and ketonuria are consistent findings. In recumbent cases the blood levels of βHB are much higher than in acetonaemia; levels up to 22 mmol/l (125 mg/100 ml) may be found. Cows affected close to parturition have hypocalcaemia and occasionally hypomagnesaemia. Recumbent cows in the terminal stages have hyperphosphataemia (up to 6.5 mmol/l; 20 mg/100 ml), hyperglycaemia (up to 9.0 mmol/l; 160 mg/100 ml) and raised AST levels. At post mortem the most consistent findings are an enlarged, yellow, fatty liver with fatty changes in the kidney and adrenal cortex.

Diagnosis

Often several cows are affected before veterinary attention is sought. The usual stimulus to seek veterinary help is when one or two cows are dead or close to death. The history, stage of pregnancy and the nutritional status will usually be enough to enable a tentative diagnosis. Raised blood or urine ketone levels and low blood glucose (plus low calcium in cows close to calving) will usually confirm the diagnosis.

Treatment

Treatment as described under acetonaemia (see p. 592) would normally be indicated. However, so severely affected are the majority of these cows that medical treatments almost invariably fail to succeed. Immediate removal of the calf by caesarean section may save a valuable cow. This should be followed by the full course of treatment described under acetonaemia.

Prevention

Although the problem is more common in fat cows it is essentially the result of starvation and is predominant in years when insufficient conserved fodder has been made. To prevent further cases developing and becoming recumbent a supply of good quality forage is essential even if the farmer has to sell a proportion of his herd to obtain fodder for the remainder.

The downer cow

Attending the recumbent cow is one of the more challenging problems encountered by the bovine practitioner (see also p. 368). Often, accurate diagnosis is not possible but prognosis is extremely important and probably more important than accurate diagnosis. It must be remembered that recumbency is the normal course in the terminal stages of any disease so a full clinical examination is essential in every case plus a thorough history and often supported by biochemical examination of blood. Many workers have offered definitions of the downer cow but the most useful in practice and the one to be used here is: a cow that has been recumbent for 24 hours or more, is in sternal recumbency, and is not suffering from hypocalcaemia or hypomagnesaemia, mastitis or any obvious injury to the limbs or spine.

History

It is important that the clinician obtains an accurate history of the case and the following questions must be asked.

1 How long has the cow been recumbent?
2 When did she calve and was calving difficult?
3 Did she rise after calving?
4 Has she been treated for milk fever, and if so how often and how much CBG has been used?
5 Has the cow moved recently, either spontaneously or with help from the farmer?
6 Where did the cow go down, e.g. concrete, ice, in field, in a ditch, and was this likely to affect the pathogenesis?
7 Is there adequate bedding?

Examination

The first superficial examination will be the position of the animal, position of the legs and degree of alertness. Lateral recumbency, if not due to hypocalcaemia, hypomagnesaemia or bloat is indicative of a terminal state and slaughter should be advised as soon as possible. This includes cows which, although they will sit in the sternal recumbency position for short periods with the aid of supports such as hay bales, revert to the lateral recumbent position when they struggle free of the supports.

The position of the legs is a useful aid to prognosis. If the hindlimbs are in the normal position and the cow attempts to rise the prognosis is guarded to hopeful. If the hindlimbs are rigidly extended forwards so the feet are touching the elbows of the front legs this indicates severe sciatic nerve damage, upper hindlimb muscle degeneration or hip problems, e.g. fracture or dislocation, and the prognosis is hopeless. If both the hindlimbs are spread laterally, with lateral flexion at the stifle the cow has probably 'done the splits' and again the prognosis is hopeless. If one hindlimb is in this position then the prognosis is guarded and careful nursing may succeed. If both hindlimbs are extended behind the animal, and when the position is corrected they return to the original position when the cow attempts to move, again the prognosis is hopeless as this indicates severe muscle degeneration.

The full clinical examination will then be conducted (see Fig. 39.2) and may well reveal other diseases present, e.g. mastitis, metritis (vaginal examination is essential), torn vagina, ruptured uterus, pneumonia, septicaemia, hypothermia, or abdominal catastrophe. It is essential that a rectal examination is performed.

Assuming there is no abnormality in rectal temperature, respiratory rate, mucous membranes and the heart rate is below 80/minute, then ischaemic necrosis of the hindlimb muscles or, as it is more commonly referred to, pressure syndrome should be considered.

Pressure syndrome (ischaemic necrosis). Recent experimental work (Cox, 1982) has demonstrated that if a cow is lying in the same position for 6 hours or more there will be damage to the musculature of the leg on which the cow is lying. Cox describes this as ischaemic necrosis as a result of pressure. If the cow is in the same position for 12 hours continuously then the damage to the muscle is irreversible and the prognosis is therefore hopeless. This situation is most common following milk fever, particularly where treatment has been delayed, or ineffective subcutaneous treatment has been given. Many cows first seen with milk fever at morning milking will have been recumbent for 6 hours, and some for almost 12 hours. Many will be suffering some muscle damage, particularly if they have been lying on unbedded concrete. This is why prompt intravenous treatment for milk fever is essential.

Figure 39.3 shows the pathogenesis of ischaemic necrosis.

Calving paralysis. If the cow has not risen since calving and has not responded to milk fever therapy, and is not suffering from any toxic or septicaemic condition

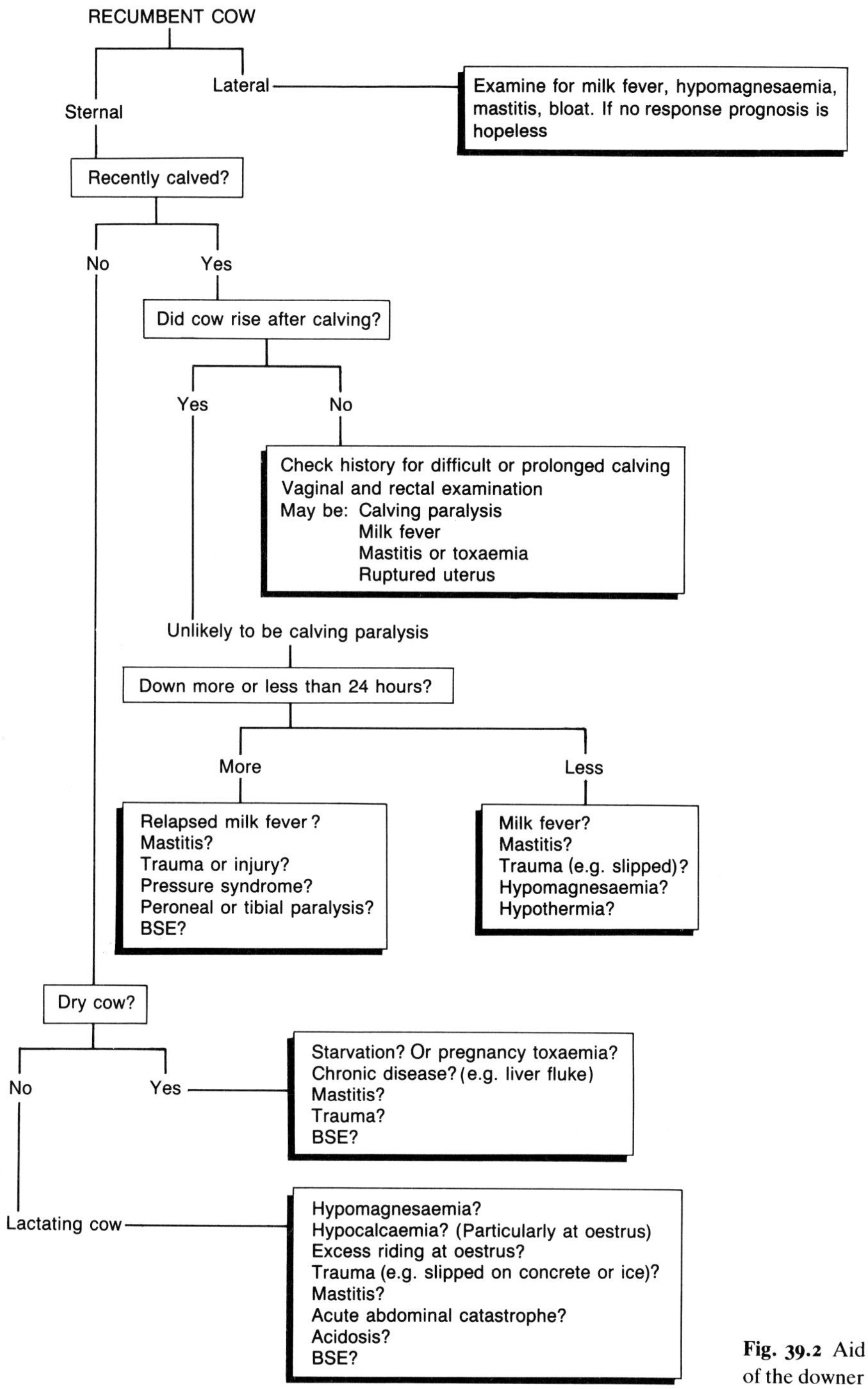

Fig. 39.2 Aid to diagnosis and prognosis of the downer cow.

such as mastitis or metritis, then either pressure syndrome or calving paralysis should be suspected. The history should indicate whether calving has been difficult but occasionally a cow will deliver, with difficulty, a large calf but second stage labour may last 3–6 hours. In such cases, calving paralysis may occur. Calving paralysis as a term is preferable to obturator paralysis, sciatic paralysis, or other defined nerve paralyses. The damage done to the birth canal during prolonged dystokia will result in a variety of lesions in the pelvic cavity. Generally, the bruising and swelling of the soft tissues of the pelvic cavity will damage the sciatic nerve

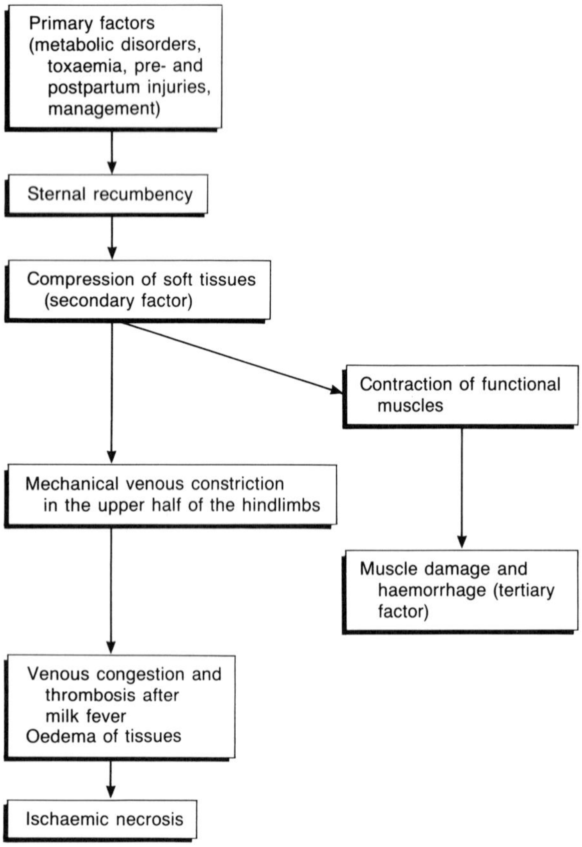

Fig. 39.3 Pathogenesis of ischaemic necrosis (From Andrews, 1986).

and occasionally the obturator nerve. Obturator paralysis (p. 366), on its own, whether it is affecting one or both hindlimbs will not cause recumbency. Such cows can rise, with difficulty, but will show abduction of one or both hindlimbs. Paralysis of the sciatic nerve (p. 367) is more serious and will prevent the cow rising.

Diagnosis and prognosis

Having completed a thorough examination of the recumbent animal that has recently calved and eliminated disease, obvious injury or starvation as a cause of the recumbency, the two most likely problems to be affecting the cow are (i) pressure syndrome (ischaemic necrosis), or (ii) calving paralysis. These cows will be alert, in sternal recumbency, and some will be attempting to rise, or crawling along the ground. Appetite for food and water will be good. At this stage it is essential for the clinician to attempt a more exact diagnosis and offer a prognosis. One of the most important inputs that will aid recovery is tender loving care (TLC). The ability and willingness of the stockworker to nurse and attend these cases will be the most important element in successful treatment. So knowledge of the farm and its staff is essential in forming a prognosis as is the ability to provide soft bedding such as deep litter or a nearby paddock. Diagnosis will be helped if the animal is raised using a Bagshawe hoist and it can be observed if the cow can take weight on one or both hindlimbs and if either or both hindlimbs are abnormal. Abnormalities to observe include the following.

1 Flexion of fetlock and extension of the hock, which will indicate paralysis of the tibial, peroneal or sciatic nerve.

2 Abduction of one or both hindlimbs will indicate obturator nerve paralysis.

3 Swelling of the upper hindlimb musculature of one leg would indicate severe pressure syndrome. If the pressure syndrome is so severe that muscle swelling is obvious and one upper hindlimb is larger than the other, prognosis for that limb is hopeless.

4 Inability to extend or flex the stifle, hock and fetlock joints.

5 The willingness of the cow to take weight on the forelegs. If the cow is so weak she cannot take weight on the forelegs the prognosis is hopeless.

With calving paralysis one can generalize that if both hindlimbs are showing signs of nerve paralysis, e.g. extension of stifle and hocks and flexion of the fetlock, then the prognosis must be hopeless. If only one leg is affected and as long as TLC will be available, the prognosis would be guarded but hopeful. It is surprising how many cows suffering from calving paralysis affecting one hindlimb only will rise seven to ten days after calving.

As an aid to prognosis, several workers have attempted to use blood biochemistry. Serum CK rises to astronomically high levels following muscle damage but its half-life is short and on its own has not proved a reliable indicator of success. Raised serum AST levels will also indicate muscle damage and this parameter is probably more useful than CK levels. As a prognostic indicator in cows that have been recumbent four days or more AST levels can be quite useful. Recently, interest in serum myoglobin levels has been reported from Sweden (Holmgren, 1988) where early work would suggest that in the first three days of recumbency serum myoglobin levels could be a valuable prognostic indicator. Levels below 3 μg/ml would indicate likely recovery.

It is unlikely that any one parameter will be shown to be of value for accurate prognosis. However, a combination of biochemical parameters and clinical signs, particularly attempting to rise, should be useful. Cows recumbent for three days or more must be attempting to rise, as well as bright, alert and eating well, for there to be any likelihood of eventual recovery. The quality of nursing available on the farm must also be considered in making a prognosis. Without good nursing, continual attention to bedding, feed and water, prognosis will be poor. Unfortunately, on many large dairy farms where labour is in short supply, there is often an unwillingness to break from the normal farm routine to provide extra attention to a recumbent cow. This information will be available to the regular attending veterinarian to the farm and will influence the prognosis. On such farms, in the interests of the welfare of affected cows, one will advise immediate slaughter of many cows, which on other farms where TLC is available, they would be likely to recover.

Treatment

All cows where the prognosis is considered hopeless or where it is known that TLC is absent should be slaughtered humanely as soon as possible. In some countries, particularly the UK, such animals can be fit for human consumption if they are not suffering from septicaemia, excessive bruising or any other infectious disease. However, in the interests of welfare, slaughter must take place on the farm. This is perfectly legal in the UK as long as the cow is bled on the farm and transported as soon as possible to the nearest slaughterhouse and the carcass is accompanied by a veterinary certificate that complies with the Slaughterhouse Hygiene Regulations (1977). If the slaughterhouse is EC approved, the carcass must reach it within 30 minutes of being bled.

Treatment will of course depend on the diagnosis, but for the cow that has been recumbent for 24 hours or more a soft bed is essential. A box or barn with an earth floor, or deep litter bedding would be ideal, but if the weather is reasonable the best place for recumbent cows is in a field. Cows can be transported to the field on a gate, on a buck rake or with a cattle net on a fore-end loader. Wherever the cow is moved it must have continuous access to food and water. It is surprising how many stockworkers will forget to provide water to a cow recumbent for 24 hours or more.

If the hindlimbs are continuously abducted either due to bilateral obturator paralysis or injury from slipping on ice or concrete the application of hobbles (Save A Cow, Arnolds Ltd) or a soft rope to tie the hindlimbs approximately 50 cm apart will prevent further muscle damage. This will sometimes result in the cow rising immediately, the only factor causing the recumbency being the persistent hindlimb abduction.

If there is any doubt as to whether the cow may still be suffering from milk fever 8–12 g of calcium should be administered intravenously. This situation could occur where farmers, treating their own cows, have administered subcutaneous CBG on two or more occasions within 24 hours, the calcium has not been absorbed completely, and a state of hypocalcaemia still exists. Some cows with milk fever that recover will relapse so, if in doubt, intravenous calcium should be administered. A blood sample analysed for calcium levels would provide valuable information, if performed quickly, either as a cowside test or in the practice laboratory.

The most important element of treatment, once the cow is on a soft bed or in the field, is frequent turning so that she does not spend more than 3 hours in one position or on one side. Cows that are attempting to rise will frequently change their position and will move from side to side. Cows with an injury, whether it is a nerve paralysis or pressure syndrome, can often be turned to lie on the side opposite to which they are found but at the next attempt to rise they fall back on to the side that is paralysed or injured.

The Bagshawe hoist, which attaches to the pin bones and is lifted using a fore-end loader or pulley blocks, is often advocated for treatment. This equipment will cause muscle damage and its continuous use on the same cow must be questioned on welfare grounds. However, it can be a useful instrument to aid diagnosis. Occasionally, a cow raised by the hoist will take weight on her hindlimbs, remain standing and slowly walk away.

In recent years interest has increased in various inflatable rubber bags (Bovijac, Alfred Cox; Henshaw Airlift, J.M. Henshaw; Downer Cow Cushion, Hamco Products). The reasoning behind the use of these air cushions is to allow improved blood circulation to the affected legs. Unfortunately, with most of the inflatable bags available, once inflated and the cow raised, she frequently struggles and falls off the side of the bag. Cow nets are available and a supportive harness (Downacow Harness, Alfred Murray) can be quite useful.

In Denmark, water flotation is being used. The recumbent cow is hauled into a drop-sided water tank and the tank filled with warm water. The cow will then stand aided by the water, and is left in the same position for up to 7 hours a day. The system is called an Aqua Lift (Rasmussen, 1988).

The use of the Bagshawe hoist (apart from aiding

diagnosis) and the various slings and inflatable bags should be questioned. If a cow cannot stand unaided there is little point in raising her to the standing position. Repeated use of the Bagshawe hoist will cause extensive muscle damage and must be discouraged. Until an inflatable bag has been designed that will prevent a raised cow falling off the side these air bags have only limited use.

The Danish Aqua-lift would appear to be the most practical aid to the recumbent cow but the capital cost of making the lift and providing transport for it may prevent its widespread adoption.

Therapeutic agents frequently used in treating downer cows would include corticosteroids, the analeptic tripelennamine hydrochloride (Vetibenzamine, Ciba Geigy) and phosphorus-containing products (e.g. Foston, Hoechst Ltd) Tripelennamine, whether given on its own or in combination with calcium salts, will change the appearance of the recumbent cow. She will become more alert and appear to be stimulated to the extent that she will often attempt to rise. Intravenous glucose can be useful as supportive therapy.

Prevention

Calving paralysis can, in part, be prevented by selecting bulls with known shorter gestation lengths and ease of calving scores. Feeding of dry cows should also be monitored and frequently rationed, particularly in seasons where grass is plentiful. Overfat cows (condition score 3.5 or over) more frequently develop dystokia due to relative fetal oversize. If a particular bull has been identified as causing dystokia, then all cows remaining that are pregnant to him should be considered for induced parturition using long-acting corticosteroids.

The pressure syndrome is a preventable problem. The majority of cases are a sequel to milk fever where treatment has been delayed or is inadequate. Intravenous therapy with 8–12 g of calcium as soon as possible after the cow becomes recumbent, accompanied by moving the cow into sternal recumbency and turning her so that she is lying on the side opposite to that in which she was found, will prevent pressure syndrome occurring. If the cow is down on concrete she should be moved onto a soft bed or into a field. Many pressure syndrome cases are the result of subcutaneous calcium therapy that fails to be absorbed completely.

Fatty liver syndrome

In the 1970s and early 1980s the syndrome of fatty liver (FLS) or fat cow syndrome (FCS) was widely reported in dairy cows at or around calving. Reports of its occurrence came from many countries, including the UK, USA, France, Hungary and the USSR. The syndrome appears to occur in high-producing dairy cattle where overfeeding in the dry period results in overfat cows at calving. Depressed appetite after calving and the consequent energy deficit result in a rapid weight loss and an accumulation of intracellular fat in the liver. The syndrome is associated with an increased incidence of metabolic, infectious and reproductive disorders such as milk fever (p. 577), ketosis (p. 590), mastitis (Chapter 21) and retained placenta (Chapter 31). Fat cow syndrome as described by Morrow (1976) is clinically the most extreme mainfestation of the syndrome but is probably only the 'tip of the iceberg' and a much larger number of cows were affected by subclinical FLS as described by Reid & Roberts (1982).

Occurrence

The FLS was thought to be widespread in UK dairy cows in the late 1970s and was probably related to gross overfeeding of cows during late pregnancy, particularly with the use of high levels of concentrate foods during the late dry period. However, 'steaming up' with concentrates has recently gone out of favour and is now rarely practised in the UK, which is probably why the incidence of FLS has apparently declined in recent years. However, in seasons where grass is in abundance there is still a danger of cows becoming excessively fat if their diet is not restricted during the dry period and hence FLS can and still does occur. At worst 50–90 per cent of freshly calved cows have been reported to be affected with FLS although on some farms the incidence was very low or even non-existent. Mortality up to 25 per cent has been reported in herds where severe FCS exists.

Pathogenesis

As most dairy cows in early lactation are in negative energy balance they mobilize energy reserves of fat and muscle and consequently lose body weight and condition. The mobilization of body weight reserves involves the release into the blood of free fatty acids from fat depots and glucogenic amino acids from protein stores. The fatty acids are transported via the blood to various organs, e.g. the kidney, liver and muscle, where they are deposited as intracellular droplets of triglyceride. Thus at one to four weeks after calving there is an increased level of fat in the liver. Even before calving there is a rise in liver fat levels occurring two to three weeks before calving. This fat mobilization before calving is probably brought about by the changes in hormonal status as the cow approaches calving. The extent of fat deposition in the liver and other organs after calving is probably determined by a number of factors including high milk yield potential, body fatness or condition at calving and loss of body condition after calving. Excessively fat cows tend to have depressed appetites so the fat mobilization is exacerbated resulting in even higher liver fat levels and increased weight loss.

Signs

The most common indication of the existence of FLS is a high incidence of peri- or postparturient disease, e.g. retained placenta, milk fever, mastitis and ketosis. Cows with FLS will subsequently prove to be less fertile. However, if FLS is suspected it should be noticed that a high proportion of the dry cows are excessively fat (in excess of body condition score 3.5) and many of the cows four weeks after calving are thin (body condition score less than 2).

Clinical pathology

Cows with FLS one week after calving will have significant alterations in their blood constituents. Free fatty acids, bilirubin, AST will all be increased and glucose, cholesterol, albumin, magnesium, insulin and white blood cell count (WBCC) will all be decreased. In cows with severe FCS the WBCC may fall to as low as 3×10^9/l.

Pathology

At post mortem, cows with FCS will have large deposits of fat around the heart, kidney, pelvis and in the omentum. The liver will be enlarged, with rounded edges and a pale yellow colour. Intracellular droplets of triglycerides will be found in liver cells, kidney, adrenal glands, skeletal muscle fibres and cardiac muscle. In the liver the triglyceride globules are deposited within the hepatocytic cytoplasm. The extent of deposition may be as high as 70 per cent of total hepatocyte volume.

It is important to realize that the findings described above may be seen in animals that have been deprived of food 24–48 hours before death. Therefore, post-mortem findings can only assist in the diagnosis of FCS or FLS when used in conjunction with the herd history and clinical pathology.

Diagnosis

The history of increased disease incidence just after calving followed by examination of body condition of dry cows and cows three to four weeks after calving will often give a strong indication of the presence of FLS. Confirmatory evidence is best obtained by liver biopsy of five or six cows immediately after calving. The liver biopsy samples can then be assessed for fat level percentage. The technique of liver biopsy in cattle is relatively easy to perform and should be a technique used by all cattle practitioners. Levels of fat, as assessed by staining sections of liver with toluidine blue or oil red O, in excess of 20 per cent would indicate the presence of FLS. Levels in excess of 50 per cent fat would indicate severe FLS.

Blood biochemistry has been widely explored as a measure of fatty liver and various parameters have been explored, e.g. non-esterified fatty acids (NEFA), glucose, AST and glycerol but these cannot, as yet, be interpreted with great confidence. In the USA another method of estimating liver fat levels is based on the buoyancy of needle biopsy samples in water or copper sulphate solutions.

Treatment

There is no proven treatment for either FCS or FLS. Various empirical treatments have been suggested but there is little evidence that any are of value. The logical approach would be to use the same treatments as are used for acetonaemia. Increasing the glucose supply by the administration of glucose, glycerol or propionate and a glucocorticoid followed by the stimulation of protein synthesis by the administration of an anabolic steroid would appear to be the most logical approach to treatment.

Prevention

Fatty liver is a sign of cows overfat at calving and losing excessive weight in early lactation. The main element of a prevention programme is to restrict the feeding of dry cows so that they calve in a body condition score of 2.5–3.0. The big reduction in the use of concentrates before calving in recent years has almost certainly reduced the number of cows suffering from FLS at calving. Cows in condition score 2.5–3.0 at calving certainly have appetites greater than fat cows and hence lose less weight in early lactation. However, dry cows can become fat on grass diets alone in northern Europe during the spring and early summer, when grass quality is at its best. At such times, therefore, grazing for dry cows should be restricted or supplemented with low quality fibre such as straw or hay. The rules for prevention of FLS are therefore the same as for acetonaemia.

References

Andrews, A.H. (1986) The downer cow. *In Practice*, **8**, 187–9.

ARC (1980) *The Nutrient Requirements of Ruminant Livestock*. A technical review by an ARC Working Party. Commonwealth Agricultural Bureau.

Cox, V.S. (1982) Pathogenesis of the downer cow syndrome. *Veterinary Record*, **111**, 67–9.

Holmgren, N. (1988) Proceedings of XV World Conference on Cattle Diseases, pp. 276–7.

Kelly, J. (1988) Magnesium and milk fever. *In Practice*, **10**, 168–70.

Morrow, D.A. (1976) Fat cow syndrome. *Journal of Dairy Science*, **59**, 1625–9.

Rasmussen, J. (1988) *Proceedings of XV World Conference on Cattle Diseases*, p. 282.

Reid, I.M. & Roberts, C.J. (1982) Fatty liver in dairy cows. *In Practice*, **4**, 164–8.

Sachs, M. (1988) *Proceedings of XVth World Buiatrics Congress*, Palma Mallorca, Spain.

Sansom, B.F., Manston, R. & Vagg, M.J.(1983) Magnesium and milk fever. *Veterinary Record*, **112**, 447–9.

Whitaker, D.A., Kelly, J.M. & Smith, E.J. (1984) Hypomagnesaemia increase. *Veterinary Record*, **116**, 451–2.

Further reading

Hibbitt, K.G. (1979) Bovine ketosis and its prevention. *Veterinary Record*, **105**, 13–15.

Spence, A.B. (1978) Pregnancy toxaemia in beef cows in Orkney. *Veterinary Record*, **102**, 459–61.

Chapter 40: Metabolic Profiles

by R.W. BLOWEY

Introduction

The term 'metabolic profile' was introduced by Payne *et al.* (1970) to describe a system of serological monitoring of dairy herds, as an aid in the assessment of their nutritional, metabolic and health status. In the initial work, cows from 12 herds were sampled and 12 blood parameters, namely glucose, urea, albumin, globulin, packed cell volume (PCV), haemoglobin, calcium, magnesium, phosphorus, sodium, potassium and copper, were measured on each cow. This was later extended to a survey of 75 herds and then to another involving 191 herds, comparing blood levels in summer and winter (Payne, 1978). The combined data were analysed statistically to identify the major sources of variation in blood parameters. These were:

1 the herd from which the cows were selected;
2 level of yield and stage of lactation;
3 season of year.

Variations due to analytical error had been carefully calculated and an allowance made. The findings from a detailed study in Sweden (Hewett, 1974) were similar, namely that the herd of origin produced the greatest variation in blood metabolite level, with stage of lactation and level of yield being the second most important factors. It is the fact that the *herd* is the greatest source of variation that adds validity to the metabolic profile test. There must be a factor(s) relating to nutrition, housing or management, which affects blood chemistry. In the Compton Metabolic Profile test, the effects of level of yield were compensated by looking at results from three groups of animals: (i) seven high-yielding cows, (ii) seven mid-lactation cows, and (iii) seven dry cows.

Although individual variation was such that statistically only five cows were needed for each group, seven animals were sampled to allow for greater randomization, accidental loss of samples, etc. The metabolic profile is a herd or group test, not a test on individual animals. From the initial surveys, *group* mean (or 'normal') values were established and a herd was said to be showing abnormal blood chemistry if the mean value of one of the groups sampled fell outside ± two standard deviations (SD). In the second survey of 75 herds (Payne, 1978), it was found that there was a good correlation between serological abnormalities (i.e. group mean ± 2 SD) and the existence of clinical problems within the herds.

Sampling 21 cows (i.e. three groups of seven animals) and analysing each sample for a range of 12 metabolites was an expensive procedure and as a consequence the system of mini-profiles (Blowey *et al.*, 1973) was introduced. Six cows at between four and eight weeks of lactation were analysed, primarily for energy and protein status, although if required this was extended to include major minerals and some trace elements. This system was found to have considerable practical value in the field.

Basic concepts

The traditional system of assessing the nutritional status of a dairy cow is to calculate the amount of nutrients being supplied (namely the product of quantity times quality) and compare this with the requirements of the animal. This remains the standard procedure and such a system has withstood the test of time. However, it is not without its problems. In practical circumstances it may be difficult to estimate the quantity of food being eaten, for example on self-feed silage or grazing systems. In addition, nutritional interactions, leading to variations in absorption or utilization of nutrients, cannot always be allowed for, or indeed may not even be known. The metabolic profile test is intended to be a measure of the *balance* between 'input' in terms of nutrients absorbed from the gastrointestinal tract and 'output' in terms of the requirements of those nutrients for maintenance, pregnancy and lactation. Therefore, if input is inadequate to match the demands of output then levels of metabolites in the blood may fall. Initially, this fall may be slight and not manifest as a clinical abnormality. As the reduction in metabolite concentration progresses, there comes a stage when it may be seen as clinical disease. A good example of this would be hypomagnesaemia. The metabolic profile test can therefore be used both as an early warning indicator of subclinical disease and as a diagnostic procedure.

The properties of an ideal biochemical parameter for the metabolic profile test are as follows.

1 The metabolite should be stable in the blood sample for a considerable period after collection. To facilitate this preservatives may be used, for example oxalate-fluoride for blood glucose estimation inhibits glycolysis, which would otherwise reduce the glucose content.

2 It must be possible to analyse the metabolite accurately and the amount of laboratory error must be small in proportion to other possible sources of metabolic variation, i.e. the herd, milk yield, etc.

3 The metabolite should be consistently related to nutritional status or some other well-understood metabolic pathway and variations due to diurnal, prandial and other factors should be kept to a minimum.

4 Factors such as age, sex, genotype and environmental stress should have no significant influence on the metabolite.

These factors have been reviewed by Field (1972).

Of course it should be borne in mind that a single blood sample measures the *concentration* of a metabolite at a particular moment of time. For some metabolites, e.g. albumin, it is the total amount of albumin in circulation that gives the best indicator of nutritional status. For other metabolites, e.g. calcium, hormonal and other homeostatic mechanisms maintain a constant blood concentration, irrespective of dietary status. The rate of *throughput* of calcium through the circulation may change and the rates of absorption from bone and gut and of excretion via the kidneys may alter, but plasma concentration is maintained constant. When it does fall, clinical disease (hypocalcaemia) is seen. Calcium is therefore a poor indicator in the metabolic profile test.

For some metabolites, urine may be a better body fluid to analyse. For example, although blood magnesium falls when there is a dietary deficit, at times of dietary excess serum magnesium reaches a maximum level only slightly above normal and the excess is excreted in the urine. Urine concentrations can rise to very high levels therefore and, conversely, in periods of deficit urinary magnesium excretion falls to virtually zero before there is any significant fall in blood magnesium. Urine is therefore a better indicator of magnesium status than blood.

Prandial and diurnal variations in blood metabolites can also cause problems. For example, Payne (1978) considered that the diurnal variation in β-hydroxybutyrate was so great that it produced problems with interpretation and similar considerations have been applied to plasma glucose and plasma non-esterified fatty acids (NEFA) (Parker & Lewis, 1978). Often it is not possible to determine whether diurnal variation is due to a prandial effect, or the time period after milking, when milk secretion reaches a maximum.

Factors relating to sampling

As with many such systems, the value of the metabolic profile is very much related to the quality of the sample taken. The following gives a few guidelines.

When to sample

It is estimated that it takes some two to three weeks for dairy cows to become accustomed to a new ration. This time period is partly to allow the rumen microbes to adjust to the new diet and partly the physical response of the cow in learning new feeding patterns and adjusting to the palatability of a ration. Clearly, the required delay between a feed change and sampling must therefore depend on the nature and degree of the feed change. Under European conditions, suggested sampling times throughout the year would be:

1 autumn, after housing and when the full winter ration is being fed;

2 mid/late winter, as a check on performance;

3 early to mid-grazing season.

If a herd is being sampled on a regular basis, then blood samples should be taken at the same time on each occasion, to try to reduce the effects of prandial and other diurnal variations.

One very important factor is that, if dealing with a 'problem' herd, then unaffected animals should be sampled. For example, if there is a rapid reduction in yield from an early or disappointing peak, then affected cows are *not* the animals that should be sampled. Clearly, cows that have dropped from peak have already reduced their yields to match the food intake being received and as such their blood levels will be returning to normal. It could be said that these animals have already compensated for the poor feeding. The correct animals to sample in this instance would be those cows that have reached and are maintaining a reasonable peak yield, since they are the animals that are most likely to be affected by an imbalance between input and output. It is a failure to appreciate this critical point that has resulted in many people finding little value in the metabolic profile test.

Animals to be sample

The full Compton Metabolic Profile test sampled seven high-yielding cows, seven mid/late lactation and seven dry cows (Payne *et al.*, 1970), whereas others (Blowey, 1975) have used only six early lactation cows. Early lactation animals were chosen because they would be more likely to produce economically beneficial results, for the following reasons.

1 They are approaching the period of service, when nutrition needs to be at an optimum.

2 Peak yield is also reached at this stage and the importance of reaching a satisfactory peak to achieve an overall high lactation production is well known.

3 Cows are sampled before the period of 'equilibration'. If an animal is underfed from calving, she will eventually reduce her yield to match the food intake being received. Blood values may then return to normal. The time needed for 'equilibration' to occur cannot be stated precisely. Clearly, it depends on both the degree and nature of the underfeeding and on the genetic potential of the cow. Cows of high potential may continue milking longer, with abnormal blood chemistry, than those of lower potential. As an approximate guide, however, cows sampled at four to eight weeks after calving should give reasonable results. If sampled at less than three to four weeks, they are unlikely to have settled adequately onto the lactation ration and hence will show underfeeding anyway.

It is clearly important that 'normal' cows for that particular herd are sampled. Any animal that is an exceptionally low or high yielder, has a longstanding health problem, e.g. lameness, is in oestrus, or has any other condition that might affect blood chemistry should not be used.

Although a fairly specific stage of lactation has been suggested, there will be instances when other groups of animals need to be sampled. For example, in a herd with a high incidence of milk fever, late-pregnant cows and, if possible, a few clinically affected animals should be sampled. If fatty liver syndrome (Reid, 1980) is suspected, blood samples taken at seven to fourteen days after calving and analysed for glucose and aspartate aminotransferase (AST) have been found to give the best prediction.

Site of sampling

Bloods may be taken from jugular or coccygeal vessels, although the site of sampling must be stated and the correct normal values used. Although there is a statistically significant variation in blood concentration between the two sites for a wide range of metabolites (Parker & Blowey, 1974), only the difference in blood phosphorus is great enough to affect the interpretation of the metabolic profile. Phosphorus levels in jugular blood are approximately 15–20 per cent lower than in coccygeal blood, due to the drain of phosphate by the salivary gland for its use as a ruminal buffer. Potassium levels are also approximately 5 per cent lower than in coccygeal samples. The mammary vein should not be used as a sampling site, since glucose levels especially tend to be lower and very variable.

Interpretation of results

The most important factor to be borne in mind is that blood analyses are only an *aid* in the assessment of the nutritional and metabolic status of dairy cows. Blood results should not be interpreted in isolation. They need to be considered in conjunction with a whole range of supplementary data, including the following.

1 Details of the individual animals sampled (age, stage of lactation, yield, etc.).

2 A working knowledge of the ration, to enable a diet balance sheet to be calculated. Although some of the data may only be approximate, considerable value can be obtained from this.

3 Cow condition, consistency of faeces and general cow 'contentment'.

4 Total herd milk production and milk quality.

5 The reason for carrying out the metabolic profile. Any clinical signs being shown by the animals sampled, or any other animals, should be noted.

Each one of these items of information, including blood results, will contribute a little towards the assessment of the overall nutritional status of the dairy herd. It is hoped that each item will lead towards the same conclusion. If conflict occurs, then this is where the experience and knowledge of the veterinarian carrying out the interpretation must be applied.

Blood parameters measured

Different authors have used slightly different ranges of blood metabolites. The following provides a few notes on some of the more common parameters measured.

Energy status

Glucose

Glucose is commonly used as an indicator of energy status, although the correlation is by no means precise (Hewett, 1974; Parker & Blowey, 1976; Parker & Lewis, 1978). There are a number of non-nutritional factors, e.g. stress, excitement, severe cold and corticosteroid therapy, that elevate glucose levels and as glucose is subject to fairly precise homeostatic control, large changes in the rate of glucose utilization, i.e. the throughout rate, are initially reflected in only relatively small changes in plasma glucose concentration. Glucose is an essential metabolite for milk production (the rate of availability of glucose to the udder is one of the major determinants of milk yield), for the fetus and for the brain. The quantities required for the brain and for early pregnancy are very small however and hence glucose can only be considered as an indicator of energy status in lactating or late-pregnant animals. It cannot be used in non-pregnant heifers or steers and using such animals Holmes & Lambourne (1970) found that NEFA gave a better indication of energy balance.

Non-esterified fatty acids (free fatty acids, FFA)

In response to underfeeding, an animal mobilizes body reserves by hydrolysing the neutral fat molecule. The long-chain fatty acids (NEFA) thus produced pass to the liver for degradation and subsequent release of energy. In the blood they are transported bound to albumin and their concentration can be measured. A high concentration indicates excessive mobilization of body fat and hence an energy deficit. Although they are a useful indicator of energy status, they are subject to considerable diurnal and prandial variations and also increase rapidly with stress and excitement. It was for these reasons that Russell (1978) discounted their use as an indicator of energy status in late-pregnant sheep, although Lindsay (1978) and Parker & Lewis (1978) considered that they were one of the better indicators of energy status. Animals that have been trained, i.e. have become accustomed to handling and blood sampling, show much less variation with stress and handling (Holmes & Lambourne, 1970).

β-Hydroxybutyrate

β-Hydroxybutyrate (βHB) and other ketone bodies also increase in response to underfeeding and they are not affected by stress. Acetoacetate is present in only low concentrations in plasma and as it is also unstable it is not a satisfactory indicator. Thus βHB is the most commonly used parameter. It is the ketone that is present in greatest amounts in normal well-fed cows, is stable and is not subject to such strict homeostatic control as glucose. Herdt *et al.* (1981) concluded that neither βHB nor glucose could be used as *direct* indicators of energy balance, as even factors such as the level of concentrate being fed affected blood levels of the two metabolites, high concentrate diets leading to an increased plasma glucose and decrease βHB concentrations, irrespective of the overall energy balance of the ration. However, it appeared that βHB might be used to adjust factors in the ration that influenced the rate of glucose availability to the cow, in that there was an inverse correlation between βHB and plasma glucose at all levels of energy balance. The same authors also found that the relationship between βHB and energy balance was stronger on low protein diets. Russell *et al.* (1983) concluded that βHB was closely related to energy status in animals where there is a high metabolic demand for glucose, e.g. during late pregnancy and lactation.

Protein status

Protein digestion in the ruminant is basically a two-step process. Part of the protein entering the rumen (the rumen degradable protein, RDP) is degraded into ammonia by microbial action, the ammonia produced being re-assimilated into microbial protein by a further group of rumen micro-organisms. This is eventually digested by the cow when microbial protein passes into the small intestine. The remainder of the protein (undegradable protein, UDP) passes through the rumen unchanged to undergo primary digestion in the small intestine.

Urea

Urea levels in plasma are primarily derived from rumen ammonia, although a certain amount will also arise from the hepatic deamination of amino acids. Part of the circulating urea is excreted via the kidney, although part is also recycled into the rumen, particularly at low plasma urea levels, via both the saliva and directly across the rumen wall. The metabolism of urea has been reviewed elsewhere (Blowey, 1972) and it was concluded that there was a range of factors that could lead to an increase in urea levels.

1 An increase in protein intake. This has also been shown experimentally in dairy cattle by Treacher (1978).
2 An increased proportion of RDP in the ration, since this would result in a higher proportion of dietary protein being converted to ammonia.
3 A decrease in energy intake, leading to depressed rumen microbial ammonia assimilation and an increased 'leakage' of ammonia from the rumen.
4 An increase in ruminal pH, again allowing a greater 'leakage' of ammonia from the rumen, since free ammonia (NH_3) diffuses across the rumen wall more rapidly than the ionized ammonium (NH_4^+) radicle.
5 Increased body tissue catabolism and/or renal failure. This is unlikely to occur on a herd basis.

Although there is a relationship between dietary protein status and blood urea therefore, the interpretation of abnormal blood urea values in a metabolic profile needs to be carried out with caution.

Albumin

Albumin is a protein synthesized in the liver, and although it in no way acts as a protein store, it is used as an indicator of long-term protein status and of UDP intake. In experiments, Treacher (1978) showed that albumin was related to protein intake, although this was not consistent, possibly due to variations in dietary protein precalving. In addition to a reduced protein intake, other factors that can lead to a depressed serum albumin level include the following.

1 Stage of lactation. Albumin values fall sharply after calving in some cows, but by no means all animals are affected (Little, 1974). A more rapid rate of recovery as lactation proceeds has been correlated with improved fertility and higher milk yield (Rowlands, 1978).
2 A recent increase in protein intake. Urea values will rise within two to three days but albumin may take several weeks to reflect the change.
3 Decreased energy status, depressing the rate of rumen microbial non-protein nitrogen assimilation.
4 Chronic infection, leading to elevated globulins and a compensatory decrease in plasma albumin levels.
5 Any chronic liver damage could depress albumin synthesis. On a herd basis, this could be seen, for example, with fatty liver syndrome (Roberts *et al.*, 1981).
6 Chronic intestinal parasitism (unlikely in adult dairy cattle).

Other blood parameters that have been found to be useful indicators of protein status include PCV, haemoglobin and total protein (Hewett, 1974; Treacher, 1978) all of which may take several weeks to respond to changes in dietary protein intake. Winter anaemia of unknown aetiology occurs in dairy herds on apparently adequate protein status, while high intakes of kale and other brassicas could also result in anaemia. In both instances, PCV and haemoglobin could be depressed, but with an adequate dietary protein intake.

Mineral status

Aspects of mineral metabolism are considered in even less detail than the rather superficial review of energy and protein status, since many of the relevant points will be covered in the specific chapters on minerals and trace elements.

The firm homeostasis for calcium previously referred to is well recognized, making it a poor indicator for the metabolic profile test. Low plasma magnesium indicates dietary deficiency, but at very high intakes blood magnesium rises only to an upper limit and excess is excreted in the urine. Phosphorus levels are also difficult to interpret. Under temperate grazing conditons, pasture alone may supply sufficient phosphorus for maintenance and 20 l only. Low blood phosphorus levels are commonly found in grazing cattle (Parker & Blowey, 1976) and dietary supplementation may be beneficial. In a large field survey, the same authors found a significant relationship between plasma inorganic phosphorus and dietary phosphorus (intake expressed as a percentage of requirements) in four of the 15 herds being monitored. However, in some herds low blood levels were also seen on winter rations, when dietary status was adequate. It is possible that this represents poor absorption, although Underwood (1966) considered that there were significant diurnal and daily fluctuations in plasma phosphorus and that a series of blood samples over a limited period of time would be needed to assess dietary status.

Both copper and selenium status are best assessed by sampling pregnant animals receiving no supplementary concentrates, since such products normally contain quite high levels of trace elements. The standard 'four to eight weeks stage of lactation' of the metabolic profile would not apply therefore. Both trace elements are dealt with in greater detail in Chapter 19. Blood samples can also be analysed for iodine and cobalt status, but interpretation is difficult. Although serum vitamin B_{12} is a reasonable indicator of cobalt status in sheep, the correlation in cattle is poor.

Uses of metabolic profiles

The technique can either be used as a routine monitoring procedure, or in the investigation of health and performance problems. Examples of the latter include a high incidence of ketosis, milk fever, hypomagnesaemia or fatty liver; poor fertility; inadequate cow condition, poor milk production or disappointing milk quality; and in other situations where feeding could be implicated, for example an increased incidence of retained placenta. In all cases it should be remembered that metabolic profiles are only an *aid* in the assessment of nutritional status. Trials have repeatedly shown that there is not a consistent relationship between diet and blood metabolite levels, and as such results should be interpreted in conjunction with the many other aspects of farm data discussed earlier in this chapter. Failure to do so, and failure to select the correct animals for the test, is one of the major reasons why, in many hands, the techniques has been found to be of limited value.

References

Blowey, R.W. (1972) Metabolic profiles — some aspects of their use and interpretation in the field. In *Veterinary Annual*, 13th edn, pp. 21–30. J. Wright Ltd, Bristol.

Blowey, R.W. (1975) A practical application of metabolic profiles. *Veterinary Record*, **97**, 324–7.

Blowey, R.W., Wood, D.W. & Davis, J.R. (1973) A nutritional monitoring scheme for dairy herds based on blood glucose, urea and albumin levels. *Veterinary Record*, **92**, 691–6.

Field, A.C. (1972) An assessment of the value of metabolic profiles (summary of BVA Congress paper). *Veterinary Record* (suppl.), **xix**.

Herdt, T.H., Stevens, J.B., Linn, J. & Larsen, V. (1981) Influence of ration composition and energy balance on blood β-hydroxybutyrate (ketone) and plasma glucose concentrations of dairy cows in early lactation. *American Journal of Veterinary Research*, **42**, 1177–80.

Hewett, C. (1974) On the causes and effects of variations in the blood profile of Swedish dairy cattle. *Acta Veterinaria Scandinavica*, Suppl. No. 50.

Holmes, J.H.G. & Lambourne, L.J. (1970) The relation between plasma free fatty acid concentration and the digestible energy intake of cattle. *Research in Veterinary Science*, **11**, 27–36.

Lindsay, D.B. (1978) The effect of feeding pattern and sampling procedure on blood parameters. In *The Use of Blood Metabolites in Animal Production*, pp. 99–120. Occasional publication of BSAP, No. 1.

Little, W. (1974) An effect of the stage of lactation on the concentration of albumin in the serum of dairy cows. *Research in Veterinary Science*, **17**, 193–9.

Parker, B.J.N. & Blowey, R.W. (1974) A comparison of blood from the jugular vein and coccygeal artery and vein of cows. *Veterinary Record*, **95**, 14–18.

Parker, B.J.N. & Blowey, R.W. (1976) Investigations into the relationship of selected blood components to nutrition and fertility of the dairy cow under commercial farm conditions. *Veterinary Record*, **98**, 394–404.

Parker, B.J.N. & Lewis, G. (1978) The effect of dietary energy level on body condition and some blood components in dairy cattle. In *The Use of Blood Metabolites in Animal Production*, pp. 121–32. Occasional publication of BSAP, No. 1.

Payne, J.M. (1978) The compton metabolic profile test. In *The Use of Blood Metabolites in Animal Production* pp. 3–12. Occasional publication of BSAP, No. 1.

Payne, J.M., Dew, A.W., Manston, R. & Faulks, M. (1970) The use of metabolic profile test in dairy herds. *Veterinary Record*, **87**, 150–8.

Reid, I.M. (1980) Incidence and severity of fatty liver in dairy cows. *Veterinary Record*, **107**, 281–4.

Roberts, C.J., Reid, I.M., Rowlands, G.J. & Patterson, A. (1981) A fat mobilisation syndrome in dairy cows in early lactation. *Veterinary Record*, **108**, 7–9.

Rowlands, G.J. (1978) Change in the concentrations of serum albumin in dairy cows at calving, their possible significance in relation to milk yield and fertility during lactation. In *The Use of Blood Metabolites in Animal Production*, pp. 59–70. Occasional publication of BSAP, No. 1.

Russell, A.F.J. (1978) In *The Use of Blood Metabolites in Animal Production*, p. 31. Occasional publication of BSAP, No. 1.

Russell, A.F.J. & Wright, I.A. (1983) The use of blood metabolites in the determination of energy status in beef cows. *Animal Production*, **37**, 335–43.

Treacher, R.J. (1978) Dietary protein levels and blood composition of dairy cattle. In *The Use of Blood Metabolies in Animal Production*, p. 133. Occasional publication of BSAP, No. 1.

Underwood, E.J. (1966) *The Mineral Nutrition of Livestock*. Food and Agriculture Organization, Commonwealth Agricultural Bureau.

Miscellaneous Conditions

Chapter 41: Major Poisonings

by C.J. GILES

Introduction

The nature of many farming practices such as the widespread and increasing use of agrochemicals and the wide variety of potentially toxic plants, coupled with the innate inquisitiveness of cattle to investigate (often by licking) new or unusual substances, means that many cattle live in a potentially toxic environment. It is perhaps surprising therefore that despite this, incidents of poisoning remain comparatively uncommon in cattle. Most toxic dangers to cattle are well understood and documented. This fact, together with the usually responsible and diligent approach to the handling of toxic chemicals and the correct and proper management of pasture, considerably reduces the risk of cattle gaining access to poisonous substances. Most instances of poisoning arise, therefore, by accident usually as the result of human error, ignorance, neglect or, rarely, malice. Such errors, of course, may not always be under the direct control of the stockworker, for it may be the actions of a third party, often unconnected with livestock that is to blame for a poisoning incident. As an example, the environment and feed of cattle, like all livestock and indeed humans, may be subjected to the effects of industrial pollution. However, incidents where there is gross contamination of the environment or where an accident results in the release of highly toxic substances are very uncommon and for the maintenance of such a state the livestock farmer, like the population in general, must rely on the vigilance and safety standards of industry and the monitoring authorities.

Most instances of poisoning in cattle therefore are not the result of large-scale incidents but arise from accidental access by cattle to toxic substances at the local farm level either by cattle moving from a safe to a toxic environment or by the inadvertent introduction by man of a toxicant into the animals' previously safe environment.

Poisoning in cattle can vary greatly in severity, morbidity and mortality. In the most severe cases, where a large number of cattle have consumed toxic quantities of poison very high morbidity and mortality can result. In contrast, mild episodes occur where the clinical effects are transient and few animals suffer harmful effects. Some of such cases are often so insignificant that they are missed or misdiagnosed.

Diagnosis of poisoning

The diagnosis of poisoning in cattle is not easy, as often it is the last thing a clinician will consider when presented with an outbreak of disease and not infrequently it is a subject about which he knows little. In many cases the evidence of intoxication is merely circumstantial, the materials required to establish a definitive diagnosis have long disappeared and in many cases the clinical signs are vague and confusing. However, poisoning incidents are often serious, potentially litigious and hence must always be handled with care and vigilance.

There are essentially three stages in establishing a diagnosis of poisoning.

1 Recognition that the incident is probably a case of intoxication.

2 Reaching a presumptive diagnosis of the toxicant or class(es) of toxicant.

3 Establishing a definitive diagnosis of the intoxication.

It is not possible in many cases for the three stages to be the accomplished.

RECOGNITION OF APPARENT INTOXICATION

Rarely is an outbreak of disease in cattle immediately attributable to poisoning on clinical or pathological grounds alone. Before the clinician comes to such an opinion he needs to consider fully the history, epidemiology and clinical signs presented and consider carefully the differential diagnosis in order to exclude the more common non-toxic causes of the condition.

Poisoning incidents should be suspected in the following circumstances.

1 The onset of disease is clearly associated with a change in management of the affected animals, for example a change in feed, movement to a new environment or a concurrent agricultural management practice, e.g. spraying or dipping.

2 The epidemiology of the disease is not that expected of an infectious disease, for example the condition may quite obviously arise simultaneously in several animals or groups rather than appear to be the result of spread.

3 The clinical signs as presented are not typical of the more common infectious, parasitic or metabolic diseases with broadly similar clinical pictures.

4 There is circumstantial evidence that animals may have had access to unusual materials.

5 The differential diagnosis of the disease as determined by clinical and post-mortem examination includes poisoning as a possible cause.

PRESUMPTIVE DIAGNOSIS OF THE TOXICANT

Having established the incident may be a case of intoxication the clinician needs to consider what agent or type of agent might be responsible. In some cases this may be straightforward as the history and circumstantial evidence of poisoning may direct the clinician immediately to the probable cause. More frequently, however, it is far from obvious and requires a detailed consideration of the clinical signs, the post-mortem findings (if appropriate) and the circumstantial evidence. The overall aim should be to answer the question: What possibly could the cattle have had access to that could account for the signs and post-mortem picture as observed? This inquiry needs to be wide-ranging. A full history should always be taken; the clinician should examine the animals in the housing or pasture in which they developed the condition but should not merely concentrate on the animals themselves as it is necessary also to inspect the environment for possible sources of toxicants. It is vital, of course, always to inspect the feed but this should not automatically be viewed as the prime suspect source, although a recent change in feed is strong supportive circumstantial evidence that it may be the source of intoxication. In grazing animals the pasture shoud be thoroughly inspected for the presence of known toxic plants.

Any recent use of agrochemicals should elicit questioning of farm staff as to their correct usage and the disposal and storage of concentrate. Anything in the environment of the cattle that would not normally be present should be investigated with suspicion, for example old farm machinery or rubbish left in fields, lead from old batteries and discarded sump oil may be the sources of various toxicants. The water supply must always be critically examined, especially if the supply is provided by means other than a piped mains supply. Could the supply have been contaminated by local dumping of toxic rubbish, or run-off from nitrogenous fertilizers from fields? Only when there is no known indication of local contamination should more distant sources, e.g. industrial sites, be considered.

The clinician's best initial guide to the type of toxicant involved is detailed appraisal of the clinical signs and post-mortem findings, where appropriate, and to correlate these with the known effects of the major types of toxicant (Table 41.1). However, few toxicants produce a clinical picture not shared with other poisons or non-toxic causes and several can produce a wide array of clinical signs.

ESTABLISHING A DEFINITIVE DIAGNOSIS

Having attempted to form an opinion as to the type of toxicant involved, the veterinary clinician is now in a position to attempt to reach a definitive diagnosis. To achieve this, in most cases, especially when chemical rather than plant toxicants are involved, he will require the assistance of a diagnostic laboratory. In some cases a routine thorough gross and histological examination by the laboratory may provide strong supportive evidence of the toxicant as may the botanical examination of rumen contents in cases of plant poisoning but in the majority of instances a definitive diagnosis of poisoning is dependent on the finding, by chemical analysis, of

Table 41.1 Initial linking between clinical abnormality and type of poisoning

System	Abnormality	Suspected class of poison	
		Chemical	Plant
Alimentary	Diarrhoea	Heavy metals, organophosphates, ionophores	Solanine containing, oak, GI* irritants, ragwort
	Colic abdominal pain	Heavy metals, formaldehyde, urea	Oak, GI irritants
	Hypersalivation	Organophosphates, urea	GI irritants
Central nervous system	Depression, coma	Ionophores	Oxalate containing, solanine containing
	Hyperexcitability, hyperaesthesia, convulsions	Heavy metals, nitrofurans, organochlorines	Atropine containing
Eye	Mydriasis	Lead	Atropine containing, Hemlock, *Cicuta* sp.
	Miosis	Organophosphates	
	Blindness	Lead	
Respiratory	Dyspnoea	Nitrate/nitrite	Cyanide containing
Skin	Photosensitization		St John's wort, ragwort
	Gangrene		Ergot
Locomotor	Lameness	Fluoride	Ergot
Urinary	Haematuria		Bracken
	Haemoglobinuria	Copper	*Brassica* spp.
			Allium spp.
All	Wasting		Pyrrolizidine containing
	Sudden death		Cyanide containing, yew, water dropwort

* GI, gastrointestinal.

toxicant in the tissues, ruminal or intestinal contents or food of the poisoned animal. The results of such chemical analyses must always be interpreted carefully and in conjunction with the history, clinical picture and post-mortem findings. The question to be answered is: Would the observed level of chemical (as determined by analysis) in the particular tissue at the time of examination account for the signs and disease picture originally observed? Only when this question can be answered in the affirmative can a definitive diagnosis result. This is not always possible, especially with the economic constraints usually imposed on veterinary laboratory examinations, and the clinician must view attempts at establishing a definitive diagnosis in this light. The required evidence is often not available, for example a suspect batch of feed may have long since disappeared and despite a diligent examination the analyst is unable to determine a chemical cause of the signs observed. The veterinarian at this stage must conclude the case, after referral if necessary, as merely one of *suspected* intoxication.

Relationship between the veterinary clinician and the diagnostic laboratory

If a significant number of investigations are to be concluded beyond the stage of 'suspected intoxication by . . . a working cooperation must develop between the veterinary clinician and the diagnostic laboratory. Once intoxication is suspected the golden rules are to contact the laboratory earlier rather than later and to take too much material for examination rather than too little. When the clinician suspects intoxication and has concluded the initial clinical and environmental assessments contact should be made with a laboratory experienced in diagnostic toxicology. The clinician should inform the laboratory of the following: history, clinical signs, post-mortem findings (if appropriate) and the results of the environmental assessment, indicating an opinion as to possible toxicants. The clinician must then be guided by the laboratory as to what samples to submit, the size of specimens, how they should be packaged or sent and any special instruc-

Table 41.2 Specimens submitted for toxicological examination

Tissue	Amount usually required
Serum (separated from clot, not haemolysed)	up to 10 ml
Urine	50 ml
Liver	100 g
Kidney	100 g
Other tissues	100 g
Rumen contents	500 ml
Feed	minimum 100 g

tions. Accompanying all specimens must be the clinical information as above together with details of any treatments given and the time of death. As a general rule, containers should be glass or plastic, tightly sealed, different organs should be packaged separately and no preservative added. As tests for different toxicants require different samples the need for prior discussion between the clinician and the laboratory is paramount. Detailed discussion is not warranted here. Table 41.2 serves as a guide.

Principal toxicoses

There are a vast array of potentially toxic chemical compounds and toxic plants which can, theoretically at least, cause poisoning in cattle due to the fact that they contain known toxic agents and/or have been proven as toxic by experimental observation. In practice, a few principal toxicoses are commonly observed in a given region or country and the majority are rarely, and a few almost never, encountered.

Local, regional and geographic factors greatly influence the importance of the various toxicoses in different regions and countries, so much so, particularly with toxic plants, that attempting to define the principal toxicoses is fraught with difficulty. Nevertheless, certain types of toxicant are encountered much more frequently than others. These common toxicoses, based generally on the position in the UK, are accorded detailed treatment in the text, whereas for those considered of lesser importance a summary of the principal facts is given in Table 41.3.

Organophosphate and carbamate poisoning

The organophosphate compounds are widely-used agrochemicals in agriculture, horticulture and livestock production and accidental overdosage or overexposure can lead to toxicosis.

Source of toxicant

The principal uses of organophosphates are as insecticides and acaricides, and preparations are made for animal treatment (dusting powders, sprays, washes, dips, pour-on, etc.), sprays for application to plants and granules for application to soil. Carbamates, which have a similar mode of action, are used as molluscicides and herbicides.

Cattle may become poisoned by a variety of methods, principally due to human error, negligence or ignorance. The compounds can be absorbed orally, dermally or by inhalation. Cattle may gain access to stored compounds, they can be mistaken as feed ingredients, and they may also consume treated seed. Containers may be used for feed or water without cleaning. Sprays for pest control in crops may directly contaminate animals or pollute feed or water courses. Inadvertent overdosage can occur with insecticidal sprays, dips or topical pour-on preparations or by a combination of topical and oral therapy or by rapid retreatment.

Signs

The organophosphates and carbamates block the action of cholinesterases (by phosphorylation or carboxylation respectively) at cholinergic nerve endings and myoneural junctions. The continued presence of acetylcholine at these sites produces continued nerve stimulation and accounts for the clinical signs observed. The time of onset of clinical signs varies with the dose and route of absorption from 5 minutes to a few hours. Clinical signs are similar for both organophosphate and carbamate toxicoses and are broadly threefold, namely stimulation of the parasympathetic nervous system (muscarinic effects), stimulation of the skeletal muscles (nicotinic effects) and central nervous effects. The muscarinic effects in general precede the nicotinic. The first effects are excessive, followed by profuse, salivation. This is accompanied by nasal discharge, cough, dyspnoea, colic, diarrhoea, excessive lacrimation, frequent urination and miosis. These are then joined by the nicotinic signs, muscle fasciculations, stiffness, adoption of a 'saw-horse posture', which then progresses to muscle paralysis. Cattle usually show marked central depression although rarely they may show central nervous excitation. As the condition progresses the muscarinic signs become very pronounced with profuse salivation, severe colic, sweating and dyspnoea progressing to collapse and death. Death is the result of hypoxia due to severe bronchoconstriction with respiratory hypersecretion and irregular slowing of the heart.

Table 41.3 Summary of the less commonly observed toxicoses of cattle

Poison	Usual source(s)	Clinical signs	Management guidelines
Aflatoxin	Feeds containing groundnut, cottonseed or maize contaminated with the toxigenic fungi *Aspergillus flavus* and *A. parasiticus*. Growth of toxigenic fungi is only possible when moisture content of stored grain exceeds 15%, feed levels should not exceed 50 p.p.b.	Reduced feed intake, poor weight gain (or decreased milk yield), inappetence, rough hair coat, reduced resistance to infectious disease. Less commonly acute severe signs may be observed especially in calves less than 6 months, including nervous signs, circling, blindness, convulsions, death.	No specific treatment. Remove all suspect feed, submit samples of feed for analysis (permitted levels of dietary aflatoxin controlled).
Arsenicals	Accidental contamination of feed with inorganic arsenicals or organic (herbicides, pesticides). Formerly in dips and weedkillers, industrial chemicals, horticultural sprays.	Often sudden death. Acute — severe colic, salivation, teeth grinding, weakness, incoordination, rapid collapse and death. Subacute — similar with ruminal stasis, diarrhoea, severe thirst, dehydration, collapse and death.	Rarely successful. Adsorbents orally, sulphur compounds, e.g. dimercaprol (4 mg/kg i.m.) or sodium thiosulphate 15–30 g in 100–200 ml water i.v. and up to 60 g orally (adult).
Atropine-containing plants	Deadly nightshade (*Atropa belladonna*), black or stinking henbane (*Hyoscyamus niger*), thorn apple (*Datura stramonum*).	Those of atropinization, dilation of pupils, dryness of mouth progressing to excitement, incoordination, convulsions and death.	Uncommon, often little can be done, pilocarpine can be given by injection but is not widely available and can itself be dangerous.
Brassica	Conversion of S-methyl cysteine sulphoxide in the plants to dimethyl disulphide. Kale (*Brassica deracea*) fed as fodder crop, rape (*B. napus*) and cultivated cabbages. Usually need to eat kale as sole fodder for about three weeks.	Peracute — collapse and death; acute — haemaglobinuria, pallor, weakness, jaundice, tachycardia, diarrhoea, low haematocrit. Heinz–Ehrlich bodies in RBCs. Can be fatal. Within a group usually a high prevalence of subclinical anaemia.	Stop feeding kale, blood transfusion, vitamin injections, iron. Feed good quality hay before and as well as kale.
Copper	Excessive intake of copper from the diet (especially in circumstances where dietary molybdenum is low) and retention in the liver, improper use of copper supplements. Uncommon in cattle.	Acute (rare) — depression, colic, blue–green diarrhoea, collapse, death; chronic — acute haemolytic crisis following prolonged access to excess copper, anorexia, depression, haemolytic jaundice, pallor, haemoglobinuria, death.	Avoid levels of copper in excess of 40 p.p.m. in concentrate feed. Blood test animals for copper levels before using supplements, treatment often of little value but calcium versenate, and oral sodium thiosulphate (1 g) and ammonium molybdate (100–400 mg) may help.
Cyanide	Cyanide release by hydrolysis from cyanogenetic glycosides in plants including cherry laurel (*Prunus laurocerasus*), linseed cake, sudan and sorghum grasses, couch grass, white clover.	Dyspnoea, bright red mucosae, recumbency, convulsions, opisthotonus, rapid death. Often less acute; depression, staggering, muscle tremor, dyspnoea, death within 2 hr, fresh blood is bright red.	Inject sodium nitrite 16 mg/kg i.v. followed by sodium thiosulphate (40 mg/kg i.v.). Repeat only thiosulphate, 30 g doses of sodium thiosulphate orally.
Ergot	Ergots (sclerotia of *Claviceps purpurea*) are found on rye and also on other cereal grains and rye grasses particularly in warm wet seasons.	Acute (convulsive) rare — depression, staggering, blindness, convulsions. Chronic (gangrenous) — lameness, abnormal gait, extremities	Remove from feed source, avoid heavily ergotized pastures or uninspected stored grain following warm wet summers.

Table 41.3 (*Continued*)

Poison	Usual source(s)	Clinical signs	Management guidelines
		swollen, reddened, gangrenous, particularly tail, ear tips, distal limbs.	
Formaldehyde (formalin)	Formalin used for agricultural purposes, e.g. foot baths. Usually associated with a lack of available drinking water.	Mild — salivation, inflammation of buccal mucosae. Severe — dullness abdominal pain, weak pulse, coma, death.	Do not leave cattle unattended near source of diluted formalin. Symptomatic therapy.
Furazolidone	Accidental overdosage following therapeutic or prophylactic use, improper mixing in milk substitute.	Acute — hyperaesthesia, convulsions, death. Chronic — haemorrhages, necrotic lesions in mouth, dysentery.	Stop administration of furazolidone, sedatives to control hyperaesthesia.
Hemlock; spotted hemlock, *Conium maculatum*	Umbelliferous plant common in wasteland and neglected pasture. Characterized by permanganate-coloured spots on stems and mousey odour when crushed, may be eaten when grazing is sparse, palatibility decreases as plant gets woody in late summer.	Dilation of pupils, weakness, staggering, muscle tremor, death from respiratory failure.	Avoid contact with plant and overgrazing especially in early part of the grazing season.
Hemlock; water hemlock, cowbane, *Cicuta virosa*	Plant grows in wet ditches and on edges of ponds and swamps. Contains the very toxic cicutotoxin, the roots being the most dangerous.	Dilated pupils, frothing at the mouth, abdominal pain, violent convulsions, rapid death.	None, awareness of the potential danger.
Mercury	Organic mercury compounds from grain dressed with fungicide, no longer common due to control of seed dressings.	May not appear for three to four weeks after feeding dressed grain, inappetence, blindness, staggering, weakness, nervous signs.	Poisoned animals can be treated with sodium thiosulphate (20 mg/kg i.v. and orally) or dimercaprol (BAL) 2.5–5 mg/kg i.v. 4× daily.
Metaldehyde	Molluscicide for slug/snail control.	Incoordination, hyperaesthesia, salivation, tremor, dyspnoea, fever, ataxia, convulsions, opisthotonus, cyanosis, death.	Sedation or anaesthesia to control hyperaesthesia and convulsions. Consider rumenotomy.
Molybdenum	High soil levels on teart pastures, exacerbated by low copper and high sulphate levels. Induces a relative copper deficiency, high dietary molybdenum and low available copper are interlinked.	Diarrhoea, often green or black with offensive odour, depigmentation, poor condition, stiff gait in young, anaemia, osteoporosis, fractures, poor milk yield.	Test group for low blood copper, careful administration of copper supplements or injections. A perennial problem on known pastures and xerophylactic measures should be introduced.
Ionophores (monensin, salinomycin, lasalocid)	Accidental overdosage or incorrect mixing in cattle diets.	Anorexia, depression, diarrhoea, ataxia, recumbency, dyspnoea, can be fatal. Signs develop in up to two days or longer with lower toxic doses.	History of recent access to changed feed useful in presumptive diagnosis. Feed assays, remove ionophore from feed of affected group, ensure correct levels in feed.
Onion, wild garlic, *Allium* sp.	Large quantities of unwanted onions fed to stock, access to wild garlic in woodlands.	Haemolytic anaemia, haemoglobinuria, pallor, possibly jaundice. Can be fatal.	Remove from source, feed well, multivitamin and iron by injection.
Organochlorine compounds	Accidental access or overexposure to insecticides for animal or agricultural use.	Acute and chronic syndromes occur — abdominal problems and typically salivation,	Give adsorbents orally and/or wash skin contamination with soap and water. Control excitation with

Table 41.3 (*Continued*)

Poison	Usual source(s)	Clinical signs	Management guidelines
		incoordination, muscle tremor, clonic spasms, convulsions, possibly aimless or frenzied movements, clonic–tonic convulsions, collapse, death.	pentobarbitone or sedatives, exposure of food-producing animals to these chemicals may result in high and persistent tissue residues particularly in fat.
Oxalate-containing plants	Unwilted leaves of sugar beet, fodder beet, mangels, also fat hen (*Chenopodium album*), docks and sorrells (*Rumex* sp.). Oxalate is detoxified by ruminal microflora and hence previous sublethal exposure will increase tolerance to oxalate. Large quantities of unwilted leaves need to be consumed over a short period.	Rapid ingestion of soluble oxalates induces hypocalcaemia, paresis, muscle tremor, recumbency, coma, death. Ill-thrift due to chronic renal damage.	Treatment of clinical cases with calcium borogluconate as in milk fever. The response is not as certain and is often unsuccessful. Affected forage should be introduced gradually, is best fed wilted, and not as the sole feed source.
Plants causing gestrointestinal signs	In addition to those described elsewhere there are a large number of hedgerow and wild plants which will induce salivation, colic and diarrhoea, these include: cuckoo pint (*Arum maculatum*), black bryony (*Tamus communis*), Autumn crocus (*Colchium autumnale*), monkshood (*Aconitum napellus*), hellebores (*Helleborus* sp.), buttercup (*Ranunculus* sp.), spindle tree (*Euonymus europaeus*), white bryony (*Bryonia dioica*), dog's mercury (*Mercurialis perennis*), box (*Buxus sempeuirens*), greater celandine (*Chelidonium major*), charlock (*Sinapis arvensis*).	Generally salivation, teeth grinding, abdominal pain, severe diarrhoea, may be accompanied by nervous signs. Fatal in some cases.	Uncommon, symptomatic treatment of colic and diarrhoea, remove from access to suspect plants.
Plants causing photosensitization	St John's Wort (*Hypericum perforatum*) is a common plant in hedgerows and rough grazing and is the most frequently implicated in primary photosensitization. It contains the photodynamic hypericin which is retained when dried. Buckwheat (*Fagopyrum esculentum*) is also photodynamic. Several plants including the ragworts (*Senecio* sp.) and bog asphodel (*Narthecium ossifragium*) cause secondary photosensitization following liver damage.	Photosensitization, erythema, swelling, necrosis of skin in white areas only, pruritus, oedema, later sloughing and self-inflicted injury.	House animals out of direct sunlight, debride raw areas, protect against infection and blowfly strike.
Rhododendron	*Rhododendron ponticum* grows as a cultivated shrub but also extensively in the wild on acid soils where it can form large thickets. Poisoning usually occurs	Salivation, staggering gait, abdominal pain, collapse, death in a few days. Projectile vomiting, green froth around mouth.	Symptomatic treatment, purgatives, ensure adequate fencing of stock.

Table 41.3 (*Continued*)

Poison	Usual source(s)	Clinical signs	Management guidelines
	when hungry cattle break out into woodland or gardens or from hedge clippings dumped in fields.		
Selenium	Toxic levels of selenium may accumulate in certain plants including certain forage plants and grasses growing on high selenium soils. Increased levels may occur accidentally in feeds, the diet should contain under 5 p.p.m.	Acute (rare) — blindness, depression, circling, head-pressing, colic, paralysis, death. Chronic — loss of condition, lameness, emaciation, hair loss from base of tail, hoof damage.	Test forage for selenium levels and withdraw suspect feed (>5 p.p.m. is suspect). Levels in blood >2 p.p.m. indicates excessive exposure.
Solanine-containing plants	Plants of the genus *Solanum*. Green tubers and leaves of the potato (*S. tuberosum*). The woody nightshade (*S. dulcamara*) is common in hedgerows, this plant together with the black nightshade (*S. nigrum*) are common in neglected pasture. All parts of the nightshades are toxic, the berries being the most dangerous.	Salivation, dyspnoea, diarrhoea, depression, prostration, coma. Can be fatal.	Symptomatic treatment, green potatoes should not be fed to livestock but boiling and feeding at less than 25% of diet reduces risk.
Tremorgenic mycotoxins	Certain fungi of the genera *Penicillium* and *Aspergillus* which grow at the base of the grass sward produce tremorgens. Toxicity is most likely to occur in hot, dry summers with cattle grazing at the bottom of the grass plant.	'Ryegrass staggers', usually not observed until animals are disturbed, muscular tremors, stumbling, swaying; when forced to run develop a high-stepping gait, staggering, sternal recumbency, will then recover if left undisturbed.	Recovery is usually uneventful when removed from suspect pasture and given alternative feed.
Urea	Inadequate mixing or diluting of dietary urea, accidental access to concentrated amounts, feeding to unadapted animals, or with high-fibre, low-energy rations. Overconsumption of urea-containing blocks or licks.	Begin within 1 hour, excessive salivation, frothing at mouth, bellowing, bloat, muscle fasciculations particularly of the head, colic, dyspnoea, death.	Drenching with vinegar (4–7 l daily) together with cold water (20–40 l). Ensure adequate mixing of urea, continuous access is preferred, tolerance will build-up in cattle accustomed to urea feeding. But is short-lived on withdrawal.
Water dropwort (*Oenanthe crocata*)	Root tubers from the plant which grows commonly in ditches and marshes. Usually exposed tubers on pasture following ditching or drainage operations.	Often sudden death, salivation, dilated pupils, convulsions, death.	No treatment, awareness of potential danger to grazing animals when ditches are cleared.

Diagnosis

The history and characteristic clinical signs of parasympathetic stimulation are suggestive of poisoning. This will be reinforced if there is circumstantial evidence of exposure to organophosphates or carbamate compounds. Particular attention should be paid to the possibility of inadvertent therapeutic overdosage, for example by combinations of oral and topical exposure. Chemical analysis of blood or tissue for the toxicant is usually of no value due to the fast breakdown of organophosphates; the analysis of contaminated feed or rumen contents is likely to be more successful. However, the preferred method of confirmatory diagnosis is by the determination of the reduction in cholinesterase activity. This test is often performed, for convenience or necessity, on whole blood but examination of brain tissue is better. The test is a specialized laboratory procedure and the testing laboratory should preferably be consulted before the submission of samples.

Principal differential diagnoses

The respiratory signs may resemble fog fever (p. 674) in which the muscle fasciculations are not however usually observed. The syndrome is similar to acute urea poisoning (p. 616), and it may clinically resemble nitrate toxicosis (p. 622) but without the cyanotic mucosae. The nicotinic effects may resemble hypomagnesaemia (p. 577).

Treatment and prevention

Atrophine sulphate is the specific antidote to organophosphate or carbamate toxicosis. It acts by blocking the effects of acetylcholine at nerve endings and will thus only counteract the muscarinic effects. The recommended dose is 0.1 mg/kg body weight by slow intravenous injection followed by 0.4 mg/kg given subcutaneously. The effects are usually observed within minutes. Treatment may need to be repeated during the first 48 hours depending on clinical response. Cattle should be removed from the suspected source and washed with soap and water if exposed via the skin. Intestinal adsorbents such as activated charcoal given by drench or stomach tube are also useful. Prevention is dependent on recognition of the wide diversity of uses of organophosphates and carbamates in the environment and the possibility of accidental exposure or overdosage.

Lead poisoning (see also p. 704)

Poisoning by lead is one of the most common intoxications of cattle, which are more susceptible to this toxicant than other farm species.

Sources of toxicant

There are many potential sources of lead in the environment and accidental access by cattle to a lead-containing product is the usual predisposing cause which, combined with their natural inquisitiveness and a tendency to lick foreign objects, means that a toxic dose is soon ingested. Common sources of lead include old flaking paint, batteries, discarded engine sump oil, grease, putty, plumber's materials, linoleum and mine washings. Grass from verges of heavily used roads can also contain significant amounts of lead from leaded petrol. Lead poisoning is more frequently observed in calves than adults. Poisoning can result from a single ingestion of a toxic amount or from a continued ingestion of lead from the environment with accumulation in the body tissue.

Signs

The onset of disease and, to some extent, the clinical picture that ensues depends on the dose of lead ingested. Both neurological and gastrointestinal signs are seen. Ingestion of large quantities, particularly by calves, tends to lead to an acute syndrome with the neurological signs predominating. Ingestion of lesser amounts results in a subacute pattern. In very acute cases sudden death may be the presenting sign. Acute cases are characterized by sudden onset of muscle fasciculations, particularly of the head and neck, frothing at the mouth, teeth grinding, jaw champing and abnormal movements of the head and eyelids. There is a staggering gait and apparent blindness with pupillary dilation. Colic may be observed. This may progress to collapse, tonic/clonic seizures, hyperaesthesia and death. In adults, abnormal patterns of behaviour, including pushing through fences, charging or mania can be seen.

Subacute cases are dull and anorexic and are apparently blind. There may be aimless wandering, there is muscular tremor and a staggering gait, tooth grinding, signs of colic and a ruminal stasis resulting in constipation followed by diarrhoea. The palpebral eye reflex is absent. Rarely, a more chronic form may be observed with poor growth and anaemia.

Necropsy

In very acute cases there may be no gross lesions but the lead-containing material, such as flaked paint, oil or grease, may be found in the reticulum and rumen. In less acute and subacute cases lesions of the gastrointestinal tract are frequently observed including abomasitis and enteritis. The liver and kidneys may be abnormally pale and show some degeneration. There are frequently epicardial and sometimes endocardial haemorrhages. The brain may be oedematous. Histological changes may be observed in the brain depending on the length of exposure. The hepatic and renal cells may also show degeneration.

Diagnosis

Often the history and circumstantial evidence (suspected lead-containing material in the environment) strongly support a tentative diagnosis of lead poisoning particularly when the neurological signs are observed in calves. This being the case treatment should be instituted immediately, a successful outcome of which is highly supportive of the diagnosis. A confirmatory diagnosis in the live animal rests on a measurement of blood lead levels. A heparinized blood sample should be submitted, and levels in excess of 0.4 p.p.m. are considered diagnostic. From the dead animal, kidney, liver and stomach contents should be submitted. Measurement from the kidney is most reliable and levels in excess of 20 p.p.m. are diagnostic.

Principal differential diagnoses

In the absence of compelling circumstantial evidence of poisoning, lead intoxication can closely resemble several other disorders of calves characterized by neurological signs. These include infections, e.g. listeriosis (p. 703), *Haemophilus somnus* infection, brain abscess, rabies, coccidiosis (p. 243), together with hypomagnesaemia, tetanus, cerebrocortical necrosis (pp. 225, 701), vitamin A deficiency, other poisonings (e.g. mercury) (p. 614) and in older animals nervous acetonaemia (p. 590) and bovine spongiform encephalopathy (BSE) (p. 708).

Treatment and prevention

Treatment is threefold: (i) supportive and symptomatic, (ii) oral salts to precipitate soluble lead and (iii) intravenous administration of lead-chelating agents, which can increase by up to 50 times the rate of lead excretion.

Convulsions and nervous signs can be controlled by the use of tranquillizers and sedatives including acepromazine, xylazine and chloral hydrate. Magnesium sulphate, egg whites and strong tea will precipitate any soluble lead remaining in the gut as insoluble salts of lead. Calcium disodium edetate should be given by slow intravenous injection at a dose of 110–220 mg/kg body weight. This dose should preferably be divided between two or three separate injections per day. Treatment should be given for two to three days, withheld for two days and then repeated, repeating this pattern again if necessary. Good nursing care and oral fluid replacement is required to combat dehydration. Clinical improvement may take two or three days to be apparent and blindness can persist for up to three weeks. Prevention of poisoning by lead is largely a matter of education of those responsible for the care of livestock. A knowledge of the common lead-containing commodities and the need to be vigilant about accidental access should be stressed.

Ragwort poisoning

Poisoning of cattle by the pyrrolizidine alkaloids found in certain genera of plants is a common problem in many parts of the world and can result in severe losses.

Sources of toxicant

The principal genus of plants containing pyrrolizidine alkaloids is *Senecio* of which there are in excess of 1200 species. The quantity and type of alkaloid varies between species, for example the widespread groundsel (*Senecio vulgaris*) is much less harmful than the most important single species the common or tansy ragwort (*S. jacobaea*). In temperate regions the ragwort is widespread in wasteland and neglected pastures and poses a serious potential toxic threat to livestock. Plants of the genera *Crotalaria*, *Heliotropium* and *Amsinckia* also contain the toxic alkaloids.

Circumstances of poisoning

Common ragwort is not attractive to grazing animals and cattle will usually avoid eating the fresh vegetative plant. However, this is not always the case and should never be relied upon. The plant is relatively late in emerging through the sward in the spring and, particularly following widespread seeding from the previous year, small, young plants can become finely distributed within the grasses. This is then non-selectively grazed. In dry conditions and where grass growth is poor, cattle may also be attracted to ragwort. The unattractiveness of the plant is lost, but its toxicity largely retained, when it is dried in hay or ensiled and this represents the single most important cause of intoxication. Cattle will readily consume hay or silage containing ragwort.

Pathogenesis

The pyrrolizidine alkaloids are hepatotoxic, damaging the hepatocytes. The speed at which this cell damage occurs and the consequences thereof are dependent on the dose of alkaloid and the duration of consumption. The liver has a large functional reserve and thus can withstand the functional loss of many hepatocytes before gross dysfunction occurs. An animal would therefore only rarely ever ingest sufficient quantities of alkaloids over a sufficiently short period to result in acute poisoning. Much more commonly cattle will ingest smaller amounts of the toxicant over a period of weeks or even months resulting in a more gradual loss of hepatocyte function, it only being when the functional reserve of the organ has been exceeded that gross hepatic dysfunction and hence clinical disease results.

Signs

The clinical picture can vary, although the principal cause is a subacute to chronic intoxication, acute clinical syndromes may be observed, although more usually a subacute pattern is seen in cattle. Affected cattle will lose weight and usually develop a mild to moderate jaundice, and may show photosensitization. Diarrhoea, colic and straining characteristically occur. Subcutaneous oedema and ascites may be present due to hypoalbuminaemia. Affected cattle are usually dull and depressed. They may show signs of hepatic encephalopathy, resulting from the effects of raised blood ammonia levels on the brain due to the inability of the damaged liver adequately to remove urea arriving via the portal circulation. Signs of encephalopathy include an unawareness of surroundings, staggering gait, aimless wandering, circling and apparent blindness. Head pressing and aggressive syndromes are rare in cattle. Death usually occurs a few days after the commencement of such clinical signs.

Necropsy

The carcass may be jaundiced and in poor condition, and ascites may be present. The liver is characteristically shrunken, fibrosed, slate-grey or mottled. The histological picture of the liver in pyrrolizidine alkaloid toxicosis is characteristic and highly suggestive of the condition but not pathognomonic. The lesions are a fine pericellular cirrhosis, bile duct proliferation and hepatocytomegaly.

Diagnosis

The history and circumstantial evidence are extremely important. It is vital to understand the chronic nature of the intoxication; in most cases animals will often have eaten the plants for several weeks or months prior to the development of clinical signs. Bearing this in mind examination of hay, silage and pasture for the plants is vital, but their absence does not necessarily eliminate pyrrolizidine alkaloid toxicosis unless a history of an unchanged, uncontaminated diet can be positively established. Histological examination of the liver is the method of choice in establishing a diagnosis and, in the live animal, liver biopsy is the most useful diagnostic aid. Serum biochemistry will usually demonstrate an elevation of γ-glutamyl transferase (GGT), and in some cases an elevation in aspartate aminotransferase (AST). Chemical analysis for the alkaloids is not often of value.

Principal differential diagnoses

Particularly where hepatic encephalopathy is marked, ragwort poisoning can resemble rabies, brain abscess/tumour, encephalomyelitis or lead poisoning (p. 617). Where wasting, jaundice and diarrhoea are the dominant clinical signs, intestinal parasitism (p. 231), fascioliasis (p. 238), hepatitis and biliary obstruction should be considered.

Treatment and prevention

Once the clinical picture has developed there is no worthwhile treatment for pyrrolizidine alkaloid toxicosis, but clinically normal cattle in the same group should be immediately switched to a non-contaminated food supply. Prevention relies upon control of the plant and an understanding of the syndrome. Hand pulling and burning of plants before seeding and thëuse of herbicide sprays is to be recommended on affected pastures. Sheep are less susceptible than cattle and can often graze affected pasture or eat hay if not too heavily contaminated. Hay or silage should never be prepared from ragwort-infested grassland.

Bracken poisoning

The bracken fern (*Pteridium*) is widely distributed in the UK, the USA and in many other temperate hilly and forested areas. It can relatively quickly become dominant in a grassland pasture. Where cattle have continued access to bracken-contaminated grazing, toxicosis can result.

Source of toxicant

Cattle are often reluctant to eat bracken and will usually only do so when grassland grazing is sparse. Cattle need to graze bracken as a significant constituent of the diet for several weeks or months before clinical disease may become apparent. The rhizomes, exposed after ploughing of bracken-infested pasture, are more attractive and dangerous as are newly sprouted young fronds. Some of the toxicity remains when bracken becomes dried in hay. Bracken contains a thiaminase but, unlike the situation in herbivorous non-ruminants, cattle are largely unaffected by it. Bracken also contains a variety of other toxic chemicals including a cyanogenetic glycoside (which is only usually present in harmless amounts), toxins that depress bone marrow and a carcinogen (ptaquiloside). These last two can cause disease in cattle.

Signs

Acute poisoning. Acute or subacute toxicosis is the result of bone marrow depression producing leucopenia and thrombocytopenia and occurs following consumption of comparatively large amounts of bracken. Clinical signs may develop for up to several weeks after the exposure to bracken has ended. Signs may be sudden in onset and include anorexia, depression and dysentery, and there may be pyrexia; various signs of capillary fragility and haemorrhage become obvious including petechiae on mucosae, bleeding from nose, vagina and conjunctiva. Trauma may produce haematomata. Heart and respiratory rates are increased. Progressive weakness ensues and death may occur in one to five days. In calves there is often pyrexia, dysentery, frank haemorrhage and petechiation of visible mucosae. Death is often the result of heart failure. There may be laryngeal oedema and marked dyspnoea. Due to the leucopenia, a bacteraemia or other secondary infections are often complications.

Enzootic haematuria. Where cattle have consumed comparatively small quantities of bracken over prolonged periods, neoplastic changes can develop in the transitional cell epithelium of the bladder. Various tumour types may occur including haemangiomas, transitional cell carcinomas, adenocarcinomas and haemangiosarcomas. The resulting clinical picture is termed enzootic haematuria. The condition varies from a mild, persistent haematuria as the only clinical sign to severe cases in which there is pallor of the mucosae, dysuria and tenesmus. The urine in severe cases has visible blood clots in it.

Upper alimentary squamous cell carcinoma (see also p. 632). A third less common clinical syndrome resulting from prolonged exposure to bracken is upper alimentary squamous cell carcinoma, which may accompany changes or tumour formation in the bladder wall. The disease has strong regional incidence, e.g. in western Scotland and Wales, often in suckler cows. Four clinical syndromes are recognized depending on the site of tumour formation. Oropharyngeal tumours produce loss of condition, drooling of saliva, coughing or snoring, halitosis. The nasal discharge may contain ingesta, submandibular lymphadenopathy and diarrhoea. Oesophageal tumours produce diarrhoea, halitosis, coughing, drooling and palpable masses in the oesophagus. Ruminal tympany can result from tumours in the lower oesophagus; there is initially intermittent bloat with loss of condition, then diarrhoea and resistance to the passage of a stomach tube. Tumours in the dorsal rumen produce loss of condition, diarrhoea, distended abdomen and bloat. Oropharyngeal papillomas may often accompany tumours at any site.

Diagnosis

This is based on the clinical signs and an association with bracken feeding or of prolonged exposure to bracken. In acute or subacute cases, bone marrow depression results in thrombocytopenia and leucopenia, prolonged bleeding time and clot formation time.

Necropsy

In acute or subacute cases there are multiple internal haemorrhages of varying size and petechiation. The bone marrow is pale. Tumour changes are evident in the bladder wall and/or carcinomas may be found in the upper alimentary tract.

Principal differential diagnoses

Acute disease can resemble leptospirosis, kale anaemia, or babesiasis. Enzootic haematuria should be differentiated from babesiasis (p. 726) and postparturient haemoglobinuria (p. 589). The syndromes caused by upper alimentary squamous cell carcinoma can resemble Johne's disease (p. 664), copper deficiency (p. 263) and mucosal disease (p. 598).

Treatment and prevention

In acute cases the clinical outcome is probably more influenced by the degree of bone marrow damage than by treatment. Broad-spectrum antibiotics should be administered to counteract bacteraemia and secondary infections. Blood transfusions can be considered. The use of bone marrow stimulants including DL-batyl alcohol has been described. There is no successful therapeutic management of urinary bladder or alimentary neoplasia. Despite its widespread abundance in certain areas the bracken fern should always be viewed as a potentially toxic plant to cattle. Access to bracken-infested pasture should be always limited, especially if grass growth is poor. In particular, cattle should never be allowed access to recently ploughed land with bracken present and where the rhizomes are exposed, especially if they have started to reshoot. Limited areas of bracken infestation can be fenced off, and burning, ploughing and reseeding or herbicide control are all measures that can reduce the level of bracken contamination.

Yew poisoning

Cattle that gain access to yew trees (genus *Taxus*) are frequently fatally poisoned.

Sources of toxicant

The various species of yew (*Taxus baccata*, English yew; *T. lineata*, Irish yew; *T. cuspidata*, Japanese yew) are common ornamental trees or hedgeing plants particularly of old established gardens. The leaves and woody twigs of the yew contain various toxic alkaloids collectively termed taxines. The taxines are also present in the seeds but not the fleshy red outer part of the fruit.

Circumstances of poisoning

Yew is well known as a toxic plant among the agricultural and rural community and poisoning is thus usually the result of neglect, ignorance or (rarely) malice. Cattle will often consume the fresh plant if they are allowed access and will also eat fresh hedge clippings or trimmed branches dumped into their field. The taxines are severe cardiac depressants.

Signs

If moderate amounts of yew have been ingested, sudden death is often the presenting sign. If seen alive, cattle may show dyspnoea, abdominal pain, muscle tremor, weakness and collapse. The pulse later becomes slower before finally disappearing with the heart stopping in diastolic arrest. Recovery is rare and is dependent on ingesting only relatively small amounts of the plant.

Necropsy

Frequently, there are no significant gross findings except the presence of yew leaves and twigs among the ruminal contents or sometimes still in the mouth. The characteristic leaves of the yew when separated by careful washing from the general ruminal contents are thus highly suggestive of poisoning.

Diagnosis

History or circumstantial evidence of access to yew, and presence of leaves and twigs in the rumen contents will usually establish a diagnosis.

Principal differential diagnoses

Yew poisoning should be distinguished from other causes of sudden death, for example lightning strike (p. 762), anthrax (p. 551), blackleg (p. 558), etc.

Treatment and prevention

There is no specific therapy. Symptomatic treatment can be offered to clinically affected animals but the likelihood of recovery or death is principally influenced by the amount of the plant already ingested. Rumenotomy is possible immediately after observing cattle consuming yew. Generally, yew is well known as a toxic plant but the necessity of preventing cattle from gaining access to the plant should be constantly stressed.

Fluoride poisoning (fluorosis)

At normal levels the ingestion of fluorides causes no harm or is even beneficial to cattle. However, at higher levels a chronic (or rarely acute) intoxication results.

Sources of toxicant

Cattle normally gain access to excess fluoride from grazing contaminated pasture. Historically, this commonly arose from industrial effluent, for example from brick manufacture, aluminium smelters, steel works or phosphate production. More recently, other sources of excess fluoride have been recognized including geothermal spring water (when used either as a source of drinking water or for pasture irrigation) and high fluoride-bearing soils. Inorganic rock phosphate is often highly toxic and requires defluorination prior to use as a phosphorus supplement.

Circumstances of poisoning

Rarely will cattle consume sufficient fluoride to result in acute intoxication, but this may result following heavy pasture contamination. More commonly, the grazing of fluoride-contaminated pasture over months or years results in an insidious chronic disease.

Signs

In the acute disease there is anorexia, depression, restlessness, dyspnoea, excessive salivation and muscle tremor leading to convulsions, collapse and death.

Chronic fluorosis. The developing teeth of young cattle are sensitive to excessive fluoride and dental lesions are common in animals exposed before the full adult dentition has developed. The dental abnormalities observed are: increased attrition and liability to fracture, mottling of enamel with white areas, abnormal pigmentation, and yellow or brown discoloration. Teeth may be poorly developed and mineralized.

Bones are also affected by excessive fluoride intake. Although the bones of young cattle are more susceptible, the bones of cattle of any age can be affected by fluoride-induced changes. These are principally periarticular calcification and the formation of exostoses resulting in an intermittent lameness and stiffness of gait, particularly of the hind legs. Palpable exostoses appear on the metacarpals and metatarsals, ribs and mandible and these are painful on pressure. In severe cases fractures of the third phalanx are not uncommon. Affected cattle are unthrifty and have a dull staring coat.

Necropsy

Dental lesions are found, as described above. Bones have a roughened surface and are chalky white, and new bone formation is evident.

Diagnosis

The history, clinical signs and post-mortem findings, together with circumstantial evidence of access to suspect sources of fluoride, are usually suggestive of fluorosis. Radiographic examination of lower limb bones may demonstrate the presence of exostoses. Chemical analysis of urine, blood and bone for fluorine content may be useful. The levels in bone rise with age and elevated levels are indicative of previous exposure to fluoride. Fluorides are chiefly excreted via the urine and do not accumulate in soft tissues.

Attempts should be made to identify the source of fluoride and feed, water and pasture analysed for fluoride content. As a guide the diet should contain less than 50 p.p.m. fluorine on a dry matter basis, and drinking water less than 8 mg/l.

Principal differential diagnoses

The dental and bone lesions are fairly characteristic of fluorosis but in their absence other causes of ill thrift including mineral deficiencies, parasitism and the common forms of lameness must be differentiated.

Treatment and prevention

There is no specific antidote and dental lesions are permanent. After removal from the source of excess fluoride the bones of affected cattle will gradually be remodelled, with normal bone deposition ensuing, but severely affected cattle will never completely recover. Mildly affected cattle should be removed from the source and given a good quality balanced diet. Where ingestion of high or suspect levels of fluoride is unavoidable, aluminium sulphate or calcium carbonate added to the diet may be beneficial in reducing fluoride deposition in teeth and bone.

Nitrate/nitrite poisoning

Under certain circumstances various types of grazing and forage crops may accumulate toxic levels of nitrate within their foliage. In addition, the widespread use of inorganic nitrate fertilizers poses a potential threat of nitrate poisoning in grazing cattle.

Source of toxicant

The *Brassica* plants, green cereals (wheat, barley, rye and maize) as well as the *Sorghum* and Sudan grasses, docks, nightshades and sweet clover may accumulate excess levels of nitrate in their tissues. Nitrate accumulation may occur after excessive use of inorganic nitrate fertilizers or following heavy rain after a period of drought, which leaches accumulated nitrate into the water table. Water run-off from heavily fertilized fields or excess application of nitrogenous fertilizers are the commonest dangers in intensively managed pastures and can lead to problems on grassland pasture or even hay made shortly after exposure of the sward to high nitrate levels. Cattle thus become poisoned by consuming normal amounts of the fresh pasture containing the abnormal nitrate load.

Nitrate ions in the rumen are reduced by the ruminal microflora to nitrite ions, which are subsequently absorbed. The nitrite ion oxidizes the iron in haemoglobin (to its ferric state) producing methaemoglobin, which is unable to bind oxygen. A single intake of nitrate over a short period is more toxic than accumulating the same amount over several days or weeks. A degree of tolerance may also build up in stock receiving sublethal amounts over a prolonged period. High grain diets tend to be somewhat protective against the effects of excess nitrate.

Signs

The condition is usually acute, less commonly subacute. In the acute condition, signs are seen within a few hours of consuming high levels of nitrate. The clinical picture is due to methaemoglobinaemia and the associated anoxia. The visible mucosae become blue and cyanotic, the pulse is weak and rapid, there is drooling of saliva and tachypnoea, exercise is resented and, if forced, may result in severe dyspnoea with mouth breathing. If untreated the condition deteriorates, and there is weakness, ataxia, prostration, coma and death. The rapidity of onset of the clinical signs is dependent on the dose consumed; death can occur in one hour or up to a day following acute intoxication.

Necropsy

High methaemoglobin levels impart a chocolate-brown discoloration to the blood, which is particularly evident in the fresh cadaver. This brown coloration is evident throughout the mucosae, viscera and possibly in the urine.

Diagnosis

The history may be suggestive if a link can be established with known exposure to nitrates. The clinical picture and particularly the post-mortem findings are also highly suggestive. Methaemoglobin can be detected in blood but is not stable and a fresh sample needs to be analysed within 4 hours. Alternatively, a sample of heparanized blood can be preserved, consulting the diagnostic laboratory for the preferred method. Nitrate levels in all sources of feed and water should be analysed but tolerance to nitrate may be apparent in some circumstances as described above. Levels in feed in excess of 1 per cent nitrate on a dry matter basis are highly suggestive of intoxication.

Principal differential diagnoses

Circulatory collapse or severe respiratory conditions can result in tissue anoxia and acute cyanosis, but in few other circumstances does methaemoglobinaemia with its characteristic chocolate-brown blood result. Intoxication with chlorates will also result in methaemoglobinaemia.

Treatment and prevention

The animal should be immediately removed from the suspected source of nitrate. The specific antidote is methylene blue, which restores the iron in haemoglobin to its ferrous state thus again allowing oxygenation of the blood and so reversing the tissue anoxia. Methylene blue should be given by intravenous injection at up to 4 mg/kg body weight in a 2 per cent solution. It can be repeated if necessary. Defining the nitrate source and reducing exposure is the key element in control. Ensiling will usually reduce the nitrate content of forage as will allowing the pasture to age and set seed, since nitrate is found mostly in stems rather than in grain.

Oak poisoning

Poisoning by the various oaks of the genus *Quercus* can be a serious seasonal problem in grazing cattle.

Sources of toxicant

Cattle may be poisoned at any time when they gain access to quantities of oak leaves or acorns, which contain the toxic tannins. Cattle can consume small quantities of acorns or oak leaves without ill effects.

Circumstances of poisoning

In temperate countries the autumn fall of acorns is the principal source. The acorn crop varies considerably from year to year and hence there is wide variation in prevalence. Storms and windy conditions that cause a heavy sudden drop of acorns are also predisposing factors. Cattle may also be poisoned from browsing on new leaves and buds or oak seedlings.

Signs

Although sudden death may be observed, poisoning is usually seen as a subacute condition. Affected cattle become depressed and anorexic. Early on in the disease constipation occurs, often with marked straining perhaps accompanied by groaning and abdominal pain; small, dry faecal pellets may be observed at this stage. Later on this gives way to a dark coloured or tarry diarrhoea often with blood; straining may be persistent and severe. As the condition progresses polyuria and subcutaneous oedema may be observed. Cattle then become progressively weaker and collapse with death supervening in four to seven days from the onset of clinical signs.

Pathogenesis

The tannins are nephrotoxic and damage the renal tubules but the precise mechanism of their action is unclear. There is a necrosis of the renal tubular cells and the consequent renal dysfunction leads initially to oliguria or anuria, later progressing in the subacute to chronic stages of intoxication to polyuria with the production of a very dilute urine.

Necropsy

Gross signs include those of oedema, particularly hydrothorax, ascites and ventral subcutaneous oedema, oedema fluid may contain blood, and there is often perirenal oedema together with swollen pale kidneys. The contents of the rumen are frequently doughy in consistency and often contain large numbers of acorns and/or oak leaves, although this is not invariable in the more chronic cases. There may often be colitis, with tarry, bloodstained faecal contents. Histologically, the acute renal lesions include hyaline cast formation and a coagulative necrosis of the tubular epithelium; later mononuclear cell infiltration and fibrosis are observed.

Diagnosis

The history and circumstantial evidence of poisoning together with the clinical signs usually strongly suggest a diagnosis of oak poisoning. This is usually confirmed by finding large amounts of acorns and/or oak leaves in the rumen at post-mortem examination together with the characteristic gross and histological changes. In live animals there will be an elevation of serum urea and creatinine, and glucose and protein will appear in the urine.

Principal differential diagnoses

The main differential diagnoses include clostridial infections (Chapter 38) and other toxicoses.

Treatment and prevention

There is no specific antidote. Cattle may survive poisoning by oak but are frequently left with chronic renal damage, such that they will often perform poorly. The only treatment that is likely substantially to affect the outcome of clinical cases is expensive and specialized involving full-scale renal supportive therapy including measurements and adjustment of plasma electrolytes, oral and parenteral rehydration and the re-establishment of diuresis. Anticipation of potential outbreaks by the recognition of the seasonal nature of the disease and inspection of pastures (particularly if the meteorological conditions would produce a sudden heavy acorn drop) followed by removing cattle from sources of contact is the key to successful prevention.

Chapter 42: Alimentary Conditions

by R.G. EDDY

The mouth and associated structures

Examination of the mouth, muzzle, mucous membranes, tongue and teeth should form a part of the normal clinical examination. Mouth lesions can be signs of systemic diseases such as foot-and-mouth disease, mucosal disease, bluetongue and various poisonings. Lesions of the muzzle and lips and occasional congestion of the oral mucosa can be a feature of photosensitization. Injuries occasionally occur and there are a number of infections and allergic diseases that produce lesions of the lips, tongue and jaws. Diseases of the gums and teeth are rare in cattle, although chronic fluorosis (see p. 621) where it occurs will cause mottling, discoloration or hypoplasia of the teeth, particularly in growing animals. Even problems associated with excess tooth wear are uncommon, presumably because the majority of cattle are slaughtered well before they reach 'old age'.

The main signs associated with mouth lesions are salivation, excess chewing movements, frequent protrusion of the tongue and licking of the lips and muzzle.

Swellings of either jaw will indicate lesions of the jaw, the most common of which are abscesses, infections of the buccal mucosa, e.g. calf diphtheria, or lumpy jaw (actinomycosis). Submandibular swelling may indicate mouth lesions, e.g. wooden tongue (actinobacillosis), or be a sign of cardiac or liver dysfunction, e.g. liver fluke or severe hepatitis.

Swelling of the submandibular and retropharyngeal lymph nodes may be the result of infections such as tuberculosis or actinobacillosis. Swollen salivary glands do also occasionally occur due to tuberculosis infection or infections resulting from penetrating wounds.

Salivation

Ruminants normally produce large quantities of saliva, which acts as a buffer in the rumen to maintain the normal ruminal pH. Adult cattle normally produce 5–10 ml/100 kg body weight/minute. A 600 kg cow can therefore produce 60 ml/minute of saliva.

Excess salivation occurs as a result of many diseases.

1 Foot-and-mouth disease (p. 537) and infectious bovine rhinotracheitis (p. 256).

2 The various causes of stomatitis, e.g. wooden tongue (p. 627), calf diphtheria (p. 214), and teeth-related problems (p. 629).

3 Pharyngeal paralysis, although rare in cattle, is a sign of rabies (p. 706), Aujeszky's disease (p. 705), botulism (p. 556) and occasionally tetanus (p. 567).

4 Obstruction of the oesophagus, the most common of which is choke (p. 631).

5 Eating plants or chemicals that are themselves irritant and cause inflammation in the mouth.

6 Certain chemicals such as copper, lead, mercury and arsenic also stimulate excess saliva production.

Salivation can be controlled using atropine at a dose of 30 mg for adult cattle and can be used 20 minutes prior to anaesthesia. However, the use of atropine to control excess salivation is not to be recommended or considered necessary. The primary cause of the problem should be diagnosed and corrected.

Simple stomatitis

Inflammation of the oral mucosa is characterized by redness and excess salivation. There are a variety of causes, which include the following.

1 Traumatic injuries from the use of balling and drenching guns, mouth gags and stomach tubes may occasionally be encountered.

2 Foreign bodies, such as sticks and vegetable roots, may damage the roof of the mouth, or be wedged between the teeth and the buccal mucosa.

3 Injuries to the tongue may also occur, for example it may be accidentally amputated by sharp metal.

Stomatitis caused by chemicals is more common. Creosote, discarded engine oil, formalin, acids or caustic soda used for forage preservation, chemical dips or sprays are all found on most livestock farms and if left unprotected from animals the inquisitive cow may well consume small quantities resulting in inflammation to the oral mucosa.

Inflammation or infection of the buccal mucosa is occasionally seen. Also, decaying cud may be found wedged between the mucosa and the teeth; this produces a swelling on the side of the face. Removal of the offending material and treatment with a course of parenteral antibiotics (penicillin and streptomycin) results in recovery, although further accumulation of cud material may occur and this has to be removed daily until the lesion heals.

The treatment of these conditions is generally symptomatic. The foreign bodies are removed, antibiotics may be administered and corticosteroids or non-steroidal anti-inflammatory agents may help to reduce the painful effects of the inflammation. Most conditions recover quickly when removal of the offending material has occurred.

Necrotic stomatitis

Fusobacterium necrophorum will be associated with necrotic lesions of the mouth, tongue and larynx. In calves the condition is extremely common (calf diphtheria, see p. 000) but it does occasionally occur in growing or adult cattle. A frequent site is the buccal mucosa and this may be a cause of decaying cud accumulating between the teeth and buccal mucosa as described above. The lesions are necrotic and often contain caseous material. Necrotic glossitis has been reported in feedlot cattle with the necrotic lesions present on the tongue. The aetiology is unknown but is probably infectious and may be viral. The signs are of excessive salivation, swollen cheeks when the buccal mucosa is affected and a foul smelling breath. Treatment with parenteral antibiotics or sulphonamides is generally very effective if given over a period of three to five days.

Popular stomatitis

Popular stomatitis is a virus condition producing vesicles that rupture and produce ulcerative lesions. It is a common condition in calves (see p. 216) but is of little economic significance. It is however a differential diagnosis of foot-and-mouth disease and lesions caused by mucosal disease but there are not usually any signs of systemic disease and there is no excess salivation.

Mucosal disease

Erosions or shallow ulcerative lesions of the dental pad, the mucosa below the tongue, the roof of the mouth and occasionally the tongue occur as a sign of mucosal disease, which sporadically affects growing cattle around nine to eighteen months of age. The lesions are similar to popular stomatitis, except that they are not preceded by vesicles. Diarrhoea and wasting are also present. Mucosal disease and bovine viral diarrhoea (BVD) are described in detail on p. 660.

Mycotic stomatitis

Mycotic stomatitis caused by *Monilia* spp. is thought to be a specific disease entity and is characterized by yellow necrotic lesions on the buccal mucosa, which erode, coalesce and become covered in a fibrinous necrotic membrane. It is likely that the fungal infection is secondary and it has been suggested that the primary disease may be caused by bluetongue virus (see p. 527). Muzzle lesions similar to mycotic stomatitis also occur occasionally.

Phlegmonous stomatitis

Phlegmonous stomatitis and deep-sited cellulitis occur sporadically in adult cattle. It takes the form of an acute, deep-seated, diffuse, rapidly spreading inflammation of the oral mucosa, pharynx and surrounding structures. It may often follow injury to the mucosa by a foreign body. *Fusobacterium necrophorum*, streptococci and *Escherichia coli* have all been isolated from lesions.

The onset of signs is sudden, commencing with excessive watery salivation and lacrimation. The rectal temperature is raised to 40.5–41.5°C (105–107°F) and the heart rate and respiratory rate are increased. There is marked swelling of the face, mouth, muzzle and the submandibular area. There is a foul or fetid smell to the breath and the oral epithelium frequently peels off. In severe cases death may ensue within 24 hours.

Treatment is successful if commenced early and the condition usually responds to sulphonamides or a course of injections with penicillin and streptomycin.

Wooden tongue (actinobacillosis)

Wooden tongue is a well-defined disease producing stomatitis and glossitis, mainly in adult cattle. The causal agent is *Actinobacillus lignieresii*. The disease is found world-wide but the incidence varies considerably between countries. In the UK the incidence of the disease has declined considerably in recent years; whereas 25 years ago the annual incidence was of the order of 20–30 per 10 000 cattle it has declined to around 5 per 10 000.

Aetiology and pathogenesis

The aerobic, Gram-negative coccobacillus *A. lignieresii* is the causative organism and it produces small abscesses commonly referred to as 'sulphur granules' in soft tissues. The bacteria do not survive outside the animal host for longer than five days but have frequently been isolated from the faeces of normal healthy animals. It is considered to be a normal inhabitant of the upper respiratory and alimentary tracts.

The organism does not normally invade healthy skin or mucosa but trauma to the mucosal surface from sharp objects such as sticks, straw or barley awns will allow entry of the organism. Although wooden tongue is the most common clinical manifestation of *A. lignieresii*, the organism will produce lesions elsewhere, e.g. the oesophageal groove, the rumen wall, and other soft tissues of the head and neck. It is frequently isolated from cervical and pharyngeal lymph nodes. The organism, once it has gained entry into tissues, produces small multiple swellings that develop into small abscesses 2–5 mm in diameter. The surrounding tissues swell as a result of the inflammation and the tongue may increase in size by 50 per cent.

Signs

Wooden tongue has a sudden onset, with excess salivation, difficult mastication and therefore reduced feed intake. There is considerable submandibular swelling and frequently swollen submandibular and retropharyngeal lymph nodes. The tongue will frequently protrude from the mouth. The tongue (particularly the dorsum) will be swollen, hard to the touch and on the surface will be seen round, discrete, yellow lesions 2–5 mm in diameter. These are abscesses situated just below the tongue epithelium. If left untreated the disease progresses so that eating becomes impossible and weight loss follows. Eventually death will occur due to starvation.

Treatment

If initiated early in the course of the disease, treatment is generally successful. However, if treatment is delayed beyond two weeks it is less likely to be so. Traditionally, treatment consisted of intravenous sodium iodide 7 g/100 kg body weight administered as a 10 per cent solution and repeated in 10–14 days. Oral treatment with sodium or potassium iodide is also effective.

Iodine treatment should continue until signs of iodism occur, such as dry scaly skin rather similar to dandruff. Sodium iodide should not be administered to heavily pregnant animals because of the risk of abortion.

Antibiotics are effective. Streptomycin at a dose rate of 10–15 mg/kg daily given intramuscularly for 10 days is effective in most cases. However, penicillin is less satisfactory. Some workers advocate the streptomycin should be injected into the lesion. Besides being extremely painful to the animal this does not appear to be necessary.

Animals that have been affected and untreated for two weeks or more and animals that do not recover within two weeks of treatment should be slaughtered.

Prevention

In most situations the disease of wooden tongue is sporadic. However, herd outbreaks have been known to occur, which may be the result of feeding hay or straw containing thistles, gorse or brambles. In any case affected cattle should be isolated to prevent spread of the infection and feeds such as those described above should not be offered. The reduction in UK incidence in recent years may well be related to a sharp decrease in the use of hay and a corresponding increase in silage as a method of grass conservation.

The jaw

A number of conditions affect the jaw of adult cattle, usually the lower jaw or mandible. Fractures of the symphysis (annual incidence 1 per 100 000) are a result of falling on ice or slippery concrete and hitting the jaw on a hard surface. Fractures of the mandible usually result from accidental collision with a farm vehicle or occasionally a pathological fracture due to lumpy jaw (actinomycosis) or neoplasia. Jaw abscesses are seen in calves and growing cattle. In calves these are the sequel to untreated calf diphtheria but in growing cattle they may be caused by infections being introduced at the time of tooth eruption. Actinomycosis is a well-defined infection of the mandible but only occurs rarely.

Fractures

Fractures of the symphysis are presented as an acute onset problem. Some swelling, occasionally blood-stained, of the lower lip will be noticed and some excess salivation. The animal continues to eat but with obvious difficulty.

Examination of the jaw will reveal bruising of the lower lip and excess mobility of either side of the mandible. The front teeth may or may not be displaced, loose or even lost.

These animals will recover in about three weeks, provided they are isolated from the herd and food is cut and brought to the animal. Grazing or feeding from self-feed silage faces will prove difficult for affected animals. Abnormal positioning of the front teeth may be present after healing has completed.

Trauma-induced fractures of the mandible may be more difficult to manage. If there is no obvious displacement of bone at the fracture site and no dislocation, healing will take place in three weeks providing food is cut and brought to the animal. If there is severe displacement at the fracture site or dislocation is present, casualty slaughter is usually the wisest course of action.

Pathological fractures due to infection will not heal and immediate slaughter should be advised.

Abscesses of the jaw

Jaw abscesses present as round discrete swellings of the cheek and are quite common in calves and growing cattle. Their size varies but frequently they are about the size of a tennis ball (7.5 cm or 3 inch diameter). Diagnosis is usually confirmed by paracentesis. Treatment by incising into the abscess, removing the pus and flushing with clean water should only be attempted if a soft area is apparent on the abscess surface. If palpation of the abscess reveals the external surface to be hard all over, treatment should be delayed until a softening and pitting of one area is noticeable. This is called pointing of the abscess. Abscesses that are opened and drained prematurely have a tendency to recur.

Retropharyngeal abscess

Abscesses of the retropharyngeal lymph nodes occur occasionally. These are presented as discrete round swellings the size of a tennis ball (7.5 cm or 3 inch diameter) behind the vertical ramus of the mandible. The cause may be actinobacillosis or the result of infection entering a pharyngeal wound. The treatment is the same as for jaw abscesses. There are a few differential diagnoses to consider. However, the author once encountered such a round hard swelling the size of a tennis ball in a Friesian cow. As the swelling was hard with no defined softening the farmer was advised to wait three weeks by which time lancing the abscess should be possible. Three weeks later, as no softening had occurred and the cow was experiencing some difficulty with swallowing, the animal was anaesthetized and the pharynx explored where a tennis ball was discovered!

Lumpy jaw (actinomycosis)

Lumpy jaw is a chronic infectious disease characterized by suppurative granulation of the bones of the head, particularly the mandible and maxilla. There is gross swelling, abscesses are present, fistulous tracts and extensive fibrosis all contribute to the granulomatous lesion. Its occurrence is quite rare in the UK (1–2 per 100 000 annual incidence) but is said to be more common in the western and mid-western states of the USA. However, it is found at varying incidence levels world-wide where grazing cattle exist.

Aetiology and pathogenesis

The causative organism is *Actinomyces bovis*, a Gram-positive filamentous anaerobe, which is a normal inhabitant of the mucous membranes of the oral cavity, upper respiratory tract and digestive tract of most animals. The organism gains access to the soft tissues as a result of mucosal damage caused by sharp objects or erupting teeth. It generally affects cattle two to five years old.

The organism causes a low-grade inflammatory reaction. There follows a proliferation of connective tissue, invasion with leucocytes and the resulting formation of a walled tumour-like mass. The granuloma then invades the bones of the mandible or occasionally the maxilla. The hard, immovable, circumscribed lesion that results may reach a considerable size (15–25 cm in diameter) and will eventually interfere with mastication. The development of the lesion takes several weeks. Interconnecting abscesses and fistulae breaking to the exterior and discharging small quantities of pus are a frequent sequel. The pus may contain yellow granules that, on compression and staining, will reveal the Gram-positive filaments of *A. bovis*. The granulomatous lesion will continue to invade the soft tissues of the head and neck and the teeth are frequently displaced or become dislodged and the lower jaw may be displaced laterally. Pathological fracture of the mandible may occur (see p. 628).

Pathology

Rarefying osteitis, osteoporosis interspersed with granulomatous tissue and pockets of thin pus-containing yellow sand-like granules are the main pathological changes found in this condition. The soft tissues of the head, the oesophagus and oesophageal groove may also be involved. The lymph nodes are not involved.

Diagnosis

Diagnosis is straightforward and based on the clinical signs. Confirmation of diagnosis is made by staining the crushed yellow granules found in the pus and demonstrating the Gram-positive filamentous rods.

Treatment

Treatment with iodides as recommended for actinobacillosis is sometimes advocated (see p. 627). Injecting the swelling with penicillin is also occasionally recommended; however, because of the nature of lesions such treatment is unsatisfactory. Intramuscular injection of penicillin may assist but once better casualty slaughter should be advised as lesions are likely to recur.

Teeth

Dental problems are rare in cattle. Fractures of the mandibular teeth occur occasionally and traumatic injuries can result in incisor teeth being displaced or lost. Excessive wear of the incisors indicates advancing age. Discoloration of the teeth may result from prolonged treatments with oxytetracyclines during the teeth development phase. Discoloration and pitted enamel will occur as a sign of fluorosis.

Jaw abscesses may result from infection gaining access during tooth eruption.

Occasionally, heifers will experience problems with feed when teeth are erupting. This will be particularly noticeable if the forage is in the form of self-feed silage and the clamp well compacted.

Foreign bodies do occasionally become lodged between the teeth or between the teeth and the buccal mucosa.

Anatomy

Cattle have both temporary and permanent dentition. The upper front teeth are absent and the premaxilla is attached by a layer of fibrous tissue covered by a thick horny epithelium. There are 20 deciduous teeth with a dental formula of:

$$I\frac{0}{3}\quad C\frac{0}{1}\quad P\frac{3}{3}\quad M\frac{0}{0}\quad \times 2 = 20$$

In the permanent dentition the three pairs of premolars in each jaw are supplemented by three pairs of upper and lower molars:

$$I\frac{0}{3}\quad C\frac{0}{1}\quad P\frac{3}{3}\quad M\frac{3}{3}\quad \times 2 = 32$$

The front teeth, three incisors and one canine are all spatulate and arranged in a broad arch. The fixation of the teeth allows some dorsoventral movement within the alveoli. There is a large gap or diastema separating the front teeth from those of the cheek. The cheek teeth increase in size caudally and the lower premolars and molars are narrower than the upper ones.

The age of tooth eruption varies between *Bos taurus* and *Bos indicus* and also depends on breed, sex and state of nutrition. Examination of the permanent incisors is frequently used to give an indication of age.

The deciduous teeth have little use in age determination. Calves are frequently born with fully erupted incisors and all will be in place by one month of age.

The average age for tooth eruption in European-type cattle is shown in Table 42.1. However, the standard deviation is approximately 10 per cent of the average age. Thus for a given age of development, e.g. 2.5 years, 95 per cent of the population will be 2.5 years ± 0.5 years, i.e. 2–3 years.

Table 42.1 Average age for tooth eruption in European-type cattle (*Bos taurus*)

Tooth	Deciduous	Permanent
1st incisor	Before birth	22 months
2nd incisor	Before birth	27 months
3rd incisor	Before birth to 2 weeks	37 months
Canine	Before birth to 2 weeks	44 months
1st premolar	Birth to 3 weeks	27 months
2nd premolar	Birth to 3 weeks	24 months
3rd premolar	Birth to 3 weeks	33 months
1st molar	—	6 months
2nd molar	—	12 months
3rd molar	—	24 months

The oesophagus

Emesis or vomiting (see p. 111)

Emesis (vomiting) is not a common sign in ruminants. Reverse peristalsis of the oesophagus is a normal physiological process in rumination.

However, vomiting (when rumen contents are ejected from the mouth) does occasionally occur in actinobacillosis of the oesophageal groove or with painful conditions of the mouth caused by teeth erupting. The ejection of rumen contents is also frequently seen in the terminal stages of milk fever, the result of rumen pressure caused by tympany accompanying oesophageal relaxation that occurs with hypocalcaemia, not by reverse peristalsis. Grain overload (rumen acidosis), traumatic reticulitis, diaphragmatic hernia, vagal indigestion and abomasal impaction have all been reported to produce emesis but in the author's experience vomiting is not normally associated with these conditions. Emesis as a herd problem has been reported to occur following the consumption of spoiled maize silage. In the UK poisoning with azalea or rhododendron species (see p. 615) is probably the most common cause of vomiting in cattle, although poisoning by lily of the valley (*Convallania majalis*) and sneezeweed (*Helenium loopesii*) have been reported to cause vomiting in cattle in the USA.

Diseases of the oesophagus

Disorders of the oesophagus are relatively rare. Mucosal disease/BVD does produce shallow ulcerative lesions of the oesophagus (see p. 660). Malignant catarrh also produces characteristic lesions of the oesophagus and occasionally oesophageal lesions may be found in calves suffering from calf diphtheria (see p. 214). Primary conditions of the oesophagus are:

1 traumatic lacerations,
2 stenosis caused by pressure from outside the oesophagus,
3 obstruction or choke,
4 Dilatation (see p. 111).

Oesophageal trauma

The usual cause of lacerations to the oesophagus is the result of careless use of a probang or stomach tube, which can sometimes cause rupture. As the probang is rarely used in cattle practice nowadays this problem is uncommon. If rupture of the oesophagus is suspected, then immediate slaughter should be recommended.

Oesophageal stenosis

Stenosis due to pressure outside the oesophagus can be caused by gross swelling of the mediastinal lymph nodes. This used to be a problem associated with tuberculosis, but more recently it has been reported to be associated with lymphomatosis. Oesophageal stenosis caused by swollen mediastinal lymph nodes resulting in chronic bloat in calves three to six months old is sometimes reported in calves recovering from pneumonia.

Choke

Oesophageal obstruction or choke is a relatively common problem in cattle. As cattle consume food rapidly, incomplete mastication is normal. Regurgitation and remastication of food boluses is relied upon to ensure food is ground into small particles. Apples, potato tubers or portions of root vegetables, such as turnips, fodderbeet or mangolds, will all be swallowed in relatively large pieces, often without any mastication. The occurrence of choke therefore mirrors the fashions in feeding cattle. When potatoes are in excess and inexpensive they are used as cattle feed and when mangolds and turnips were widely used choke was common. The presentation of the root crops also affects the occurrence of choke. If large roots such as fodderbeet or mangolds are fed whole then choke is uncommon but if chopped they will attempt to swallow without mastication pieces of root that are too big to pass down the oesophagus. Strip-grazing root crops, such as stubble turnips, also rarely results in choke. Presumably cattle bite relatively small pieces at a time. This is probably why the most common causes of choke are apples and potatoes, which are the right size to obstruct the oesophagus, are difficult to masticate being round and slippery, and are rarely chopped before being fed. If potatoes are being fed, ample bunker space is essential for all cows to eat simultaneously. If not, cows trying to barge through to reach the feed bunker may cause the cow eating inadvertently to swallow a whole potato it might otherwise chew.

Signs

Profuse salivation, followed by bloat, are the principal signs of choke because the obstructed oesophagus prevents swallowing of saliva and eructation of rumen gas. Affected cows will look distressed, the head is extended forwards and frequent attempts to swallow are often evident. Excess chewing movements are frequently observed and coughing, due to saliva accumulation in the pharynx, may occur.

The extent of the rumen tympany is related to the length of time choke has been present and the nature of the object. A round object such as an apple or potato will completely obstruct the oesophagus and death from bloat may be a sequel. If the offending object is irregularly shaped, such as a root or a portion of a potato, some gas may escape past the obstruction and death from bloat will be avoided.

Diagnosis

Diagnosis is usually made on the basis of the signs of excess salivation, rumen tympany, forward extensions of the head and the history of the availability of offending feeds. The obstruction is usually at one of three sites.

1 Alongside the larynx in the upper oesophagus.
2 At the entrance to the chest.
3 In the thoracic portion of the oesophagus.

The cervical sites are more commonly involved than the thoracic oesophagus and occasionally the obstruction will be between the laryngeal area and the entrance to the chest.

Usually the obstruction can be seen and palpated as a discrete swelling, although if it is present alongside the larynx confusion with the thyroid cartilage may occur. If in doubt or an obstruction in the thoracic oesophagus is suspected the passage of a stomach tube will aid the diagnosis. If the stomach tube reaches the rumen and the tympany relieved, an obstruction, if it existed, will probably have been dislodged. The differential diagnosis should not present problems, although indigestion and tympany may be mistaken for bloat. Bronchitis, because of the cough and protruding tongue, may be, but should not be, confused with choke. Once the obstruction has been located, either by palpation or by stomach tube, diagnosis presents no problems except with rabies (p. 706). Excess salivation is the only sign both rabies and choke have in common so the possibility of rabies must be eliminated by assessing other signs before proceeding along the diagnostic pathway to choke.

Treatment

Before treatment commences, the animal will need to be restrained in a cattle crush or at least tied in a byre stanchion. A bulldog-type nose handler is used by an assistant further to restrain the animal and keep the head from moving. The first element of treatment is to assess the severity of the rumen tympany. If the animal is in distress because of bloat, this is relieved by inserting a cannula into the rumen in the left sublumbar fossa, using a standard bovine trochar and cannula.

If the obstruction is in the cervical oesophagus a spasmolytic such as hyoscine *N*-butylbromide and dipyrone is administered by intravenous injection and 5 minutes allowed to elapse before attempting to move the obstruction. The spasmolytic will relax the smooth muscle of the oesophagus, which is in spasm and contracted firmly around the obstruction. Five minutes after the spasmolytic has been administered the operator, using his fingers in the jugular groove with an assistant holding the head forward, gradually pushes the obstruction up the oesophagus until it reaches the laryngeal area. Frequently, when at this position and the spasmolytic has taken effect, upward pressure with the fingers will cause the object to be ejected into the mouth. If this does not happen then a mouth gag has to be applied to keep the mouth open and a second assistant places his forearm into the mouth and pharynx and, simultaneously with the operator pushing the object upwards, will grasp it and be able to remove it. If the object is large and appears reluctant to move, this latter procedure can be carried out under anaesthesia. It is the author's experience that anaesthesia has not been required since spasmolytics have been available.

If the obstruction is in the thoracic oesophagus this will have been detected by the use of a stomach tube. The application of gentle pressure with the stomach tube will dislodge the obstruction and push it into the rumen. Again spasmolytic administration will enable the obstruction to be more readily moved. On occasions the obstruction will move on into the rumen without pressure following the spasmolytic injection. If the efforts described do not remove a thoracic oesophageal obstruction, a probang may be used. However, care must be exercised when using the probang, as the pressure applied must not be too severe for fear of lacerating the oesophagus. If the probang fails to dislodge the obstruction a rumenotomy may be considered and the object removed from the oesophagus manually via the rumen.

In preference to a rumenotomy and if it is certain that the obstruction is caused by vegetable matter, a rumen trochar may be sutured in place in the left sublumbar fossa to prevent bloat and the obstruction allowed to macerate. This may take two to four days but is usually effective.

Prevention

Choke can be prevented by the shredding or chopping of root vetegables into small pieces that will not cause obstruction. If potatoes are fed, ample feeding space is required and if they are offered at pasture they should be placed in the field before the cows enter. Cows will follow a vehicle that is unloading food and will attempt to eat while on the move. If they attempt to eat potatoes or apples while on the move they are more likely to choke. It is rare for apples to be intentionally fed to cattle. However, when orchards are grazed by cattle, windfall apples should be collected before allowing cattle access. This will not only prevent choke but also rumen acidosis (see p. 634) from overeating apples.

Upper alimentary squamous cell carcinoma

Occurrence

Squamous cell carcinoma of the upper alimentary tract occurs sporadically in cattle grazing bracken areas. The problem usually affects beef cows and has been reported in Scotland and North Wales. It occurs on farms with a high bracken cover but is less common than another bracken-induced disease, enzootic haematuria. Both conditions have been reported in the same animal. The disease generally occurs in animals over six years old. Almost invariably alimentary papillomata, in which papilloma virus can be demonstrated, occur in animals affected with bracken-induced squamous cell carcinoma. It is thought therefore that the disease is caused by a toxic factor present in bracken that activates papillomata in the alimentary tract to develop into squamous cell carcinomas.

Signs

The clinical signs can be divided into four main syndromes that are related to the site of the carcinoma, which can occur in the pharynx, oesophagus or rumen.

Oropharyngeal syndrome. The presence of the carcinoma in the oropharyngeal region will produce a chronic wasting condition of one to six months' duration. A cough may be present in the last two to four weeks of the disease and excess salivation and drooling will often the evident. Snoring may also be a feature and halitosis is frequent. Examination will reveal a tumour in the mouth or pharynx. Papillomas will also be present. The submandibular lymph nodes may be enlarged.

Oesophageal syndrome. If present in the oesophagus the carcinoma will produce signs similar to choke with partial or complete occlusion of the oesophagus. Halitosis, coughing and drooling may be present and gurgling sounds may be heard coming from the oesophagus. The passage of a stomach tube may prove difficult. The history will include a gradual weight loss over a period of one to three months. Papillomata may be present in the mouth or pharynx. A palpable mass in the oesophageal region will be present.

Ruminal tympany syndrome. Carcinoma of the cardia or thoracic oesophagus will produce intermittent ruminal tympany following a period of one to six months of gradual weight loss. The passage of a stomach tube will prove difficult. Papillomata of the mouth and pharynx will usually be present and profuse diarrhoea is a common feature.

Wasting and diarrhoea syndrome. If the carcinoma is present in the dorsal pigmented area of the rumen symptoms of rumen indigestion will be present. The tumours in the rumen can reach 30–50 cm (12–20 inches) in diameter. A slow loss of weight over up to nine months is followed by diarrhoea, which contains much fibrous undigested material. Ruminal tympany is usually present and the abdomen is often pendulous. Papillomata are usually found in the mouth or pharynx.

Diagnosis

The diagnosis may at first be difficult as the signs may resemble choke (p. 631) or rumen indigestion (see p. 633). However, the history of the slow weight loss, the presence of bracken and the occurrence in older beef cows will considerably aid the diagnosis. As papillomata are almost invariably found in the mouth or pharynx of affected animals a thorough examination of the mouth should be made if the other signs are present. Johne's disease (p. 664) may also be confused with this condition but the distinguishing feature is the consistency of the faeces. In Johne's disease the faeces are homogeneous, there being no signs of undigested fibrous material.

Treatment and prevention

There is no treatment and as the condition is invariably fatal affected animals should be slaughtered as soon as possible.

To prevent the condition, cattle should not have access to bracken. Where bracken exists on a farm cows will rarely eat the bracken if adequate food is available.

Diseases of the rumen

There are a number of diseases that affect the rumen, all of which cause inappetance, reduced milk yield and failure to thrive. An essential element in a thorough clinical examination of the bovine is to observe whether the rumen is tympanic by observing distention of the left sublumbar fossa, the animal is chewing its cud, eructating normally and normal rumen contractions are taking place. Rumen contractions can be detected by palpating with slight pressure in the left sublumbar fossa and detecting the rumen movements, which occur approximately every 30 seconds. Eructation will accompany every second rumen contraction.

Indigestion

Simple indigestion is to be suspected if the rumen contractions are weaker than normal, are less frequent and the clinical examination has revealed no other evidence of disease.

Simple indigestion is frequently seen in dairy cows when new feeds are suddenly introduced to the diet. Intakes of large quantities of very wet grass, frosted feeds, sour or spoiled feed, e.g. butyric or soil-contaminated silage, or the sudden introduction of large quantities of concentrate feeds may all predispose to the onset of indigestion. The accidental intake of small quantities of antibiotics, which disturb the rumen flora, will also precipitate indigestion as is seen in feedlot beef cattle when rations containing monensin sodium are first introduced. Dairy cow concentrate rations containing as little as 0.005 mg/kg dry matter (DM) of lincomycin have been incriminated in causing severe indigestion of whole dairy herds with a consequent 50 per cent reduction in the herd milk production. The lincomycin contamination occurred at the compound mill where the milling equipment was used to produce dairy concentrate immediately following the production of a pig feed containing lincomycin.

Relatively minor changes in rumen pH are likely to cause atony of the rumen. The intake of any indigestible, stale or sour feeds will interrupt the process of rumen fermentation, which changes the pH resulting in rumen atony. The sudden introduction of new feeds to which the rumen is unaccustomed will have a similar effect.

The rumen is a versatile fermentation chamber and will accommodate a wide variety of feeds, e.g. 100 per cent cereal diets in feedlot beef production, extremely wet grass in some seasons and highly fibrous foods such as hay or straw. However, if changes to the diet are made the rumen flora have to adapt to the new feed and to prevent indigestion occurring the changes should be gradual. Thus new food should be introduced in small quantities at first with the intake being gradually increased daily.

Signs

The first clinical sign of simple indigestion will be reduced appetite and in dairy cattle a simultaneous milk yield reduction will be apparent. The reduction in feed intake may be as much as 50 per cent with no other obvious signs. The cow may be slightly depressed. Rectal temperature will be normal and heart rate raised slightly to around 80/minute. There may be a mild diarrhoea and a mild rumen tympany may be present. In chronic cases of indigestion undigested fibre may be present in the faeces. Rumen contractions will be reduced in strength and frequency, often to as few as one contraction every 3 or 4 minutes.

Diagnosis

Diagnosis of simple indigestion will be based on the clinical examination and the elimination of any other disease. There is very little in the way of laboratory tests that can be useful. An increase or decrease in rumen pH may be a useful guide but tends not to be used in practice because of its impractibility. The history may be the most useful clinical indicator and may suggest a 'feed problem'. If only one cow in the herd is affected the history may not be helpful and the diagnosis more difficult. However, if the whole herd or a substantial part of the herd is suddenly affected with inappetence it would be quite logical to suspect a 'feed problem'.

Other diseases that may be readily confused with simple indigestion are displaced abomasum, traumatic reticulitis, lesions of the oesphageal groove, early milk fever and acetonaemia. A thorough clinical examination will eliminate these other diseases.

Treatment

Many animals suffering from indigestion will recover spontaneously in two to three days if they are removed from the offending diet and allowed access to good quality hay.

A large number of treatments for indigestion have been employed and are usually administered as drenches (Table 42.2). Mixtures containing nux vomica, gentian, sodium bicarbonate, magnesium carbonate, etc. are frequently used and act by altering the rumen pH and stimulating appetite and even providing vitamins and trace elements essential for rumen microbial synthesis.

Table 42.2 Preparations available for the treatment of indigestion in the UK

Name	Presentation	Manufacturer
Leo Cud	Powder	Leo Laboratories Ltd.
Proviton	Powder	B.K. Veterinary Products Ltd.
Vetrumex	Powder	Willows Francis
Pro-rumen	Powder	Univet Ltd.
Bykodigest	Powder	Intervet U.K. Ltd.
Stomach Powder	Powder	Arnolds Vet. Products Ltd.
Stomach Powder	Powder	Animal Care Ltd.

If the rumen is atonic for more than 24 hours the administration of rumen inoculum obtained either from an abattoir or a healthy cow will aid recovery. Probiotics may also be helpful.

Prevention

The prevention of indigestion is not always straightforward. The avoidance of abrupt changes in feeds, and of indigestible, sour or putrefied feeds is relatively easy. However, cows will break out into pastures where they should not be and will, if given the opportunity, consume foods of dubious quality in large enough quantities to be harmful. The frequency of occurrence of simple indigestion on a farm is likely to be inversely related to the quality of management that exists.

Rumen acidosis (grain overload, overeating syndrome, barley poisoning)

Wherever intensive livestock production is practised acute indigestion as a result of excessive intakes of grain, beans or compound feed is common, either as a result of cattle gaining accidental access to grain stores or by the sudden introduction of unlimited supplies of grain to the diet. There are two distinct syndromes associated with overeating.

The most common is acute acidosis as the result of consuming excess carbohydrate, which rapidly ferments leading to lactic acidosis followed by acute dehydration and depression. Accidental access to compound feed stores by cattle, who will readily consume 15–20 kg of concentrate, is the most common scenario but the problem is also seen in feedlot beef cattle fed *ad libitum* cereal-based diets, particularly when the diet is first introduced. Excess intake of apples by cattle grazing orchards is also a common cause of rumen acidosis.

Alkalosis. A less common syndrome occurs as a result of excessive intake of highly fermentable proteinaceous feeds, e.g. soya bean, which results in excess ammonia production in the rumen leading to alkalosis with excitement and hyperaesthesia.

Pathogenesis

The rumen can be visualized as a continuous culture fermentation vat. The rumen microflora constitute the culture, which grows on the substrate or medium being provided by the feed the animal consumes. The rumen microflora is a balanced colony of bacteria and various protozoa. If the feed content changes the balance of the microflora will need to change, e.g. increase in intakes of highly fermentable carbohydrate will lead to streptococci and lactobacilli organisms predominating. With a normal balanced microflora the fermentation endproducts are the volatile fatty acids (acetic, propionic and butyric acids), which are absorbed from the rumen. Bacterial cell protein for digestion and absorption in the lower intestine and water-soluble vitamins are also products of the fermentation process.

The streptococci and lactobacilli organisms that predominate when excess carbohydrate is ingested produce lactic acid as a fermentation endproduct. Lactic acid production increases the rumen osmotic pressure and fluid is drawn into the rumen from body tissues. The rumen pH also drops and the majority of Gram-negative bacteria and protozoa are destroyed. The pH may drop to 4.5. The lactic acid is converted to sodium lactate, which is absorbed directly from the rumen into the blood or is passed down the intestinal tract and absorbed from the abomasum or small intestine. The presence of sodium lactate in the small intestine produces an osmotic gradient and draws water into the small intestine thus contributing to the diarrhoea. The sodium lactate in the blood reduces blood pH.

Chemical damage to the rumen mucosal epithelium results in bacterial and fungal organisms penetrating the rumen wall and in chronic acidosis will lead to the occurrence of liver abscesses, which are frequently seen in beef cattle raised on 100 per cent cereal diets.

Urine output will be decreased as a result of the dehydration and will also be acidic, containing high levels of lactate. The damage to the rumen epithelium leads to a chronic rumenitis, which in turn causes an increased incidence of bloat. This is often seen in feedlots as a cause of sudden death. Although the main signs of acidosis are the result of lactate absorption an additional component may be the absorption of endotoxins released from the destruction of large numbers of Gram-negative bacteria in the rumen.

Signs

The speed of onset and the severity of clinical signs will depend on the quantity and nature of the food consumed and whether the rumen is adapted to that particular feed. Newly introduced feeds may well prove fatal to animals that are not accustomed to the particular feed in quantities that other animals consume regularly. Also, feedlot animals that are apparently accustomed to cereal diets will sometimes overeat for no apparent reason. Feedlot cattle being fed cereal diets are probably in a continuous state of mild acidosis and a relatively small increase in intake will produce enough lactic acid to destroy the remaining Gram-negative bacteria and produce clinical signs of acidosis. Problems also arise should cattle on *ad libitum* feed run out of cereal and then be immediately introduced to the old level. Water deprivation can also produce a problem.

Clinical signs usually become apparent 12–36 hours after the engorgement. Incoordination and ataxia are the first signs to be noticed with the stockworker reporting the cattle as 'drunk'. The animals will be anorexic, they may appear to be blind and will rapidly become weak and depressed. The rumen will be distended producing abdominal pain, which causes the animal to grunt or grind its teeth and ruminal movements cease.

Dehydration becomes apparent within 24–48 hours and severe diarrhoea will be evident in animals that do not die immediately. The faeces will be a pale 'pasty' colour. Respiratory rate will be raised because of the acidosis, the rectal temperature depressed by 1–2 °C (2–4 °F), the heart rate is in excess of 180/minute and the pulse weak. Severe cases will become recumbent with the head resting on the shoulder, as in milk fever. Death will occur within 24–48 hours in acute cases.

In feedlot cattle that recover some animals fail to thrive even after apparent recovery and this can be due to chronic rumenitis, liver abscesses, or chronic laminitis (p. 360).

Alkalosis. The signs are not completely typical but they do involve muscle tremors, convulsions and slow shallow respiration. In the later stages there may be dyspnoea and hyperpnoea.

Clinical pathology

Affected animals are dehydrated and show haemoconcentration. Blood pH may also be depressed. The pH of rumen contents will be 4 or lower and urine pH around 5.

However, in practice, laboratory tests are rarely performed because of the necessity to institute treatment quickly and the diagnosis is rarely a problem. In order to assess blood pH, bicarbonate and total carbon dioxide levels need also to be measured.

At post mortem of acute cases the rumen will be distended containing excess fluid with evidence of grain particles present. Rumen pH evaluation at post mortem is of no value unless done immediately after death because post-mortem changes will increase the pH. Chronic acidosis as a result of long-term cereal intake may be characterized by rumenitis although to observe this the examination must be performed soon after death. Multiple liver abscesses may also be present in chronic acidosis.

Alkalosis. If the less common syndrome of alkalosis is present due to the ingestion of excess soya beans or similar high-protein feeds, the rumen pH may be alkaline and the urine and blood pH will also be raised.

Diagnosis

Diagnosis is not usually difficult and is frequently made on the history together with signs of incoordination and ataxia. In feedlot beef animals it is usual for several of the group to be affected but with dairy cattle any number may be affected depending on how many cows had accidental access to the grain store, which is the most common scenario. Cows grazing orchards will consume large quantities of apples, particularly after a storm and again the history should be of considerable help in reaching a diagnosis.

Laboratory tests are not normally necessary and unless a result can be available within an hour or so are of no value in the practice situation because to be effective, treatment must be administered as quickly as possible. The prognosis for peracute recumbent cases is very poor, but for the less acute standing cases the prognosis is relatively good provided treatment is not delayed.

Treatment

In peracute recumbent cases the rumen should be emptied by rumenotomy and the dehydration and acidosis corrected using a balanced electrolyte, e.g. McSherry's solution (see Table 42.3), and 5 per cent sodium bicarbonate solution intravenously. Up to 60 l of electrolyte solution will be required for an adult cow over a 24-hour period. Up to 300 ml of 5 per cent sodium bicarbonate solution may also be administered, the quantity required depending on the degree of acidosis present and can be assessed by observing a slowing down of the respiratory rate during its administration, if given slowly. Supportive therapy should include intravenous calcium borogluconate (400 ml of 30 per cent solution) and 400 ml of 40 per cent dextrose solution.

Table 42.3 McSherry's solution

Sodium chloride	4.95 g
Sodium acetate	7.50 g
Potassium chloride	0.75 g
Calcium chloride	0.30 g
Magnesium chloride	0.30 g
Water	1 litre

For less acute cases that are still standing, the oral administration of magnesium hydroxide, magnesium carbonate or aluminium hydroxide at a dose rate of 1 g/kg body weight mixed in 10 l of warm water and administered by stomach tube will help restore rumen pH. The dehydration and acidosis is corrected using an electrolyte solution and sodium bicarbonate intravenously as for peracute cases. Intravenous administration of a vitamin B/vitamin C mixture is widely used in the UK with apparent success. Doses of 30–50 ml intravenously are frequently used and are thought to aid detoxification of lactate in the liver.

Antihistamines are also considered to be of value by some clinicians. Calcium borogluconate and 40 per cent dextrose are also useful as supportive therapy when administered intravenously.

Alkalosis. Treatment of alkalosis resulting from soya bean or high-protein engorgement should consist of an electrolyte mixture containing excess chloride such as Ringer's solution. Volumes of 30–50 l will be required over a 24-hour period but no bicarbonate should be used. All concentrate feeds should be withdrawn from the diet and only hay or silage offered.

Prevention

Bulk storage of concentrates in large bins has reduced the incidence of acidosis in many dairy herds where accidental access of feed stores with concentrate stored in bags was once quite common.

In feedlots where concentrated food is fed *ad libitum*, often to the exclusion of long fibre, introduction to the concentrate must be gradual and the feed bunkers should be of adequate size to allow all animals to feed together. The feeders should not be allowed to empty to avoid excessive intake by hungry animals once the feeders are refilled. Continuous access to the food will allow 'little and often' intakes of food. Ideally, some roughage should always be available even if it only represents 10 per cent of the DM intake. Roughage availability has been shown to reduce the incidence of liver abscesses in cereal produced beef in the UK. It is also advisable that the grains should not be finely ground, which in itself encourages rapid fermentation. The grain should be cracked or rolled and more recently whole grain has been fed without seriously affecting the digestion of the cereal.

Rumen parakeratosis

Parakeratosis of the rumen epithelium is a common sequel to the feeding of 100 per cent concentrate diets to cattle. The disease is characterized by enlargement and hardening of the rumen mucosa papillae and may affect 100 per cent of animals reared on 100 per cent cereal diets. The disease syndrome also includes the associated lesions of liver abscesses and possibly laminitis. Parakeratosis may occur as a secondary stage of acute rumen acidosis.

Pathogenesis

The association between liver abscesses, lesions of the rumen mucosa and the feeding of 100 per cent concentrate diets to ruminants has long been recognized. The lower rumen pH associated with concentrate diets and the consequent increase in lactic acid production produces an inflammatory reaction of the rumen mucosa. This damage to the mucosa allows debris to adhere to the mucosa causing ulceration and infection and resulting in abscess formation in the rumen wall. The rumen papillae become enlarged and thickened and may clump together to form bundles in response to the inflammatory reaction. The papillae may contain excessive layers of keratinized epithelial cells, particles of food and bacteria. A sequel to the damage to the rumen mucosa is the presence of liver abscesses. Some workers also report that laminitis is a later sequel but as laminitis has been found in the absence of rumen and liver lesions the role of acidosis in the aetiology of laminitis is far from clear.

Signs

Rumen parakeratosis does not necessarily produce signs of disease, although it has been reported that the addition of 10 per cent hay or silage to the diet of 100 per cent cereal-fed cattle will improve appetite and weight gain. Some individual animals that are seriously affected with abscesses in the rumen wall and liver may show reduced appetite and reduced growth rate particularly towards the end of the feeding period. Complications such as peritonitis, septicaemia or even endocarditis may occasionally be evident.

Diagnosis

The diagnosis in the live animal is extremely difficult because the reduced growth rate and inappetance are signs of many diseases. As it is a group problem the detection of the rumen wall lesions and liver abscesses at post mortem will be the best diagnostic indicator.

Treatment and prevention

The treatment of individual cases by the time they show inappetance and poor growth rates is unrewarding because of the severity of the damage to the rumen wall and liver. However, if the problem is suspected (by the post-mortem examination of some animals from the same farm at the abattoir) feeding 10–20 per cent of the diet in the form of long roughage will prevent deterioration and allow the animals to reach slaughter weight. Prevention depends on the inclusion of 10 per cent long fibre in the diet, although recent experience has shown that feeding whole grains will reduce if not eliminate the problem of rumen parakeratosis and liver abscesses.

Bloat (rumen tympany)

Bloat or rumen tympany is a disease easily recognized and feared by cattle farmers. Bloat refers to an excessive accumulation of gas in the rumen and, because of a failure to eructate, rumen distension occurs, frequently resulting in death. It is a major cause of death in cattle in all intensive livestock areas of the world.

There are two types of bloat, gaseous bloat or secondary rumen tympany and frothy bloat or primary rumen tympany.

Gaseous bloat (secondary rumen tympany). Any condition that causes an oesophageal obstruction or that interferes with eructation will produce gaseous bloat.

The condition is generally sporadic in occurrence and is less common than frothy bloat. The following conditions will lead to gaseous bloat.

1 Lesions of the oesophageal groove, e.g. vagus indigestion, abscessation or infection with *A. lignieresii* obstruct the groove and prevent eructation.

2 Physical obstruction of the groove with afterbirth has been reported.

3 Physical obstruction of the oesophagus with potatoes or other root vegetables causing choke will prevent eructation.

4 Pressure on the oesophagus by enlarged mediastinal or bronchial lymph nodes prevents gas escaping through the oesophagus. This is a common problem in growing cattle three to six months old, particularly those that have been affected with pneumonia.

5 Inability to eructate is also a feature of tetanus (p. 567) and milk fever (p. 577) and gaseous bloat is a frequent feature of these diseases.

6 Prolonged lateral recumbency as a result of disease or animals that are cast for prolonged surgery will frequently lead to gaseous bloat because of the inability of the rumen gas to escape. Cattle that inadvertently fall in dorsal recumbency into ditches will generally die of bloat if not retrieved in time.

7 Severe damage to the rumen epithelium following acute acidosis may lead to rumen atony and accumulation of gas.

8 Excess cereal ingestion usually results in gaseous bloat.

Frothy bloat (primary rumen tympany). Frothy bloat is much more common than gaseous bloat and usually affects several animals in the group at the same time. Although frothy bloat does occur in feedlot cattle it is more generally associated with pasture feeding. Pastures that are most commonly incriminated in the cause of frothy bloat usually contain high levels of leguminous plants, particularly clover or alfalfa.

Frothy bloat is extremely common in some countries, e.g. New Zealand, due to the high content of clover in the sward. In these situations the problem is well recognized and anticipated so that prevention regimens are universally applied. In the UK, frothy bloat can appear suddenly without warning on lush spring or autumn pastures and up to 25 per cent of the herd may be suddenly affected. Some of these pastures may not contain a high clover content. The onset may be extremely sudden, often 4–6 hours after milking and return to the grazing areas. The only warning that the farmer experiences is the bellowing of several cows in extreme pain, and on reaching the field there may be several cows recumbent or even dead with many others exhibiting rumen tympany to varying degrees of severity.

Pathogenesis

Bloat is the result of the inability to eliminate gas from the rumen by eructation. With gaseous bloat this is secondary to some other condition or disease.

With frothy bloat eructation is prevented by the accumulation of froth, which prevents gas escaping into the oesophagus. The production of froth or foam is a result of the raised viscosity of the rumen fluid and the small bubbles of gas, the natural product of rumen fermentation, cannot coalesce. Under certain conditions some naturally occurring plant substances, e.g. saponins, pectins, hemicellulose, and certain proteins will raise the viscosity of rumen fluid. There also appears to be an individual animal susceptibility. Succulent, high-protein plants, particularly the leguminous plants in the pre-bloom stage, undoubtedly predispose to the occurrence of frothy bloat. Frothy bloat does also occur in feedlot cattle, particularly if fed on finely ground grain. This may be due to the gases being trapped by the fine particles of feed but the rapid fermentation that follows the feeding of finely ground grain is undoubtedly a contributory factor. Adaptation to a particular feed is also important. As the rumen microflora adapts itself to the particular pasture or ration there is a tendency towards reduced susceptibility.

Signs

Rumen tympany, as evidenced by distension of the left sublumbar fossa, is well recognized by most stockworkers and should present no problems. With severe tympany the animal will be exhibiting signs of pain, e.g. kicking its ventral abdomen and bellowing. The bellowing can frequently be heard up to 500 m ($\frac{1}{3}$ mile) away. In acute frothy bloat the disease progresses rapidly and the animal soon becomes recumbent and can die in 30–60 minutes from the onset of tympany.

Pathology

Post-mortem bloat in ruminants that die from other causes can be confusing to the diagnosis of the condition. If the animal is seen soon after death, death from bloat will be obvious because of the gross abdominal distension and at post-mortem examination oedema in the inguinal and ventral perineal region together with congestion and haemorrhage in the anterior parts of the carcass will be evident. The liver will be extremely pale due to compression and the rumen will be grossly distended and contain froth. The quantity of froth present declines after death. Rupture of the diaphragm and the abdominal musculature, particularly in the inguinal regional, may also be apparent. Death from gaseous bloat is less common but the absence of froth and the finding of a primary lesion should differentiate it from frothy bloat.

Diagnosis

The preliminary diagnosis presents no problems and is based on distension of the left sublumbar fossa. If only one animal is affected in the herd the bloat is probably a gaseous bloat but if several animals are affected to varying degrees and they are at pasture the diagnosis will certainly be frothy bloat. However, if there is any doubt the passage of a stomach tube will provide the answer. If the problem is one of gaseous bloat and the stomach tube reaches the rumen and possibly removes an obstruction on the way, the gas will escape through the stomach tube and the rumen will rapidly revert to its normal size. If gaseous bloat is confirmed and the bloat relieved, a full clinical examination should be performed to ascertain the cause of the failure to eructate.

If the bloat is due to froth little or no gas will escape via the stomach tube, which will itself become blocked with froth.

Treatment

The traditional treatment for bloat was the passing of a 5 mm diameter trochar and cannula into the rumen via the left sublumbar fossa. Many farmers possess such a trochar and cannula. However, this instrument is of little use because gaseous bloat can nearly always be relieved by stomach tube and only when this is not possible should a rumen trochar and cannula be used. For frothy bloat the cannula itself becomes blocked with froth and does little to relieve the tympany.

Treatment for all but the peracute cases necessitates the passing of a stomach tube and, if this reveals the bloat to be frothy, antifoaming agents that reduce the viscosity of the rumen contents and disperse the froth can be passed down the stomach tube. Vegetable oils such as linseed, peanut, corn or soya bean oil are all useful antifoaming agents. Traditionally, 500 ml of linseed oil to which is added 50 ml of turpentine was effectively used as a bloat drench but this does tend to taint the milk. Oil mixed with detergent will disperse faster in the rumen ingesta.

Table 42.4 Treatments available for frothy bloat in the UK

Name	Active ingredient	Manufacturer
Birp	Dimethicone	Arnolds
Rumoxane	Organo-poly-siloxane 1%	Willows Francis
Antibloat	Methyl silicone 2.5 g	Bimeda

Proprietary bloat drenches containing silicone or poloxalene are available (Table 42.4) and are equally effective. Within 5 minutes of administration of the antifoaming agent the animal will start to eructate and in most cases the tympany will be relieved within 1 hour. If tympany still exists after 1 hour, a further administration of an antifoaming agent by drench may be given. If tympany still exists 1 hour after the second drench the diagnosis should be re-assessed and a stomach tube passed to ensure there is no oesophageal obstruction. Once the diagnosis of frothy bloat has been established in a group of affected animals the less acute cases can be treated by drenching alone.

In peracute cases where death is imminent and the animal is recumbent, it will be necessary to conduct an emergency rumenotomy. A 10–20 cm vertical incision is made in the midpoint of the sublumbar fossa, using a sharp knife. On incising the rumen there will be an explosive release of rumen contents and marked relief for the cow. Following the release of the frothy rumen contents the wound is cleansed and sutured using the standard surgical closure. Antibiotics are administered postoperatively and recovery is usually uneventful.

Chronic gaseous bloat in calves and feedlot animals is often treated by establishing a 10–15-cm rumen fistula. Under local anaesthesia the skin and musculature of the sublumbar fossa are incised and the rumen exposed. The rumen is then incised and the rumen wall sutured to the skin. Alternatively, a prosthetic device may be sutured into the abdominal wall and the rumen allowing gas to escape. This device may be removed two to three months later and the wound allowed to granulate by which time the primary cause of the bloat will have corrected itself.

Prevention

To prevent further cases of frothy bloat occurring when a sudden acute outbreak is encountered at pasture the cattle should be removed immediately, provided with dry food such as hay or straw and all cows showing any degree of rumen tympany drenched with an antifoaming agent. The pasture should not be used for grazing for at least 10 days.

Where risk pastures exist, e.g. those containing high proportions of legumes, gradual access to the pasture should be practised starting with 10 minutes a day and increasing by 10 minutes each day. Long fibre should be fed before being allowed access to the pasture. Strip-grazing to restrict intake can be practised but is not favoured by stock farmers who currently prefer paddock grazing or set stocking. However, during high-risk periods in problem areas, these methods alone will not be satisfactory. In New Zealand and Australia, where the risk from bloat can be exceedingly high, during the spring, when the pasture is fast growing, the only satisfactory method of control has been the daily administration of antifoaming agents by drench after milking. Oils may be given at doses of up to 240 ml/day in high-risk periods although 60–120 ml/day would be more common. Poloxalene, a non-ionic surfactant, is frequently used at 10–20 g/head/day and up to 40 g/day in high-risk periods.

If strip-grazing is practised, the antifoaming oils can be emulsified with water and sprayed on the grass daily. Addition to the water supply is sometimes used but effectiveness does depend on adequate individual intake.

Poloxalene can be added to grain mixtures or compound feed or even mineral blocks. However, in grass-rich areas, grain is rarely fed to cattle, particularly in the bloat-risk season of fast grass growth, and mineral blocks suffer from variable individual intake. Daily drenching has therefore become the preferred method of bloat prevention. The rumen implantation of a slow-release device containing an antifoaming agent is being developed in New Zealand and Australia.

The ultimate objective in bloat control is to develop pastures that have a low bloat-producing potential yet still possess the characteristics for high levels of production. The direction of development will be to develop strains of leguminous plants that have a low bloat-producing potential. To date little progress has been made in identifying the strains of red clover with the ability to produce less bloat, although it is recognized that sainfoin produces less typanitic problems than clover. At the moment, pastures should not contain more than 50 per cent clover until such strains of clover are developed.

Vagal indigestion

Vagal indigestion is a chronic condition of adult cattle with a slow insidious onset but is still a differential diagnosis of rumen atony, simple indigestion or mild bloat. The incidence of vagal indigestion is now quite rare, the annual incidence being less than 1 in 10 000, having decreased in recent years, probably mirroring the decline in the incidence of traumatic reticulitis.

Aetiology

Vagal indigestion is thought to be caused by interference with the function of the vagus nerve. The condition has been produced experimentally by severing the vagus (Xth cranial) nerve. The clinical syndromes vary slightly depending on the site of the nerve severence. In practice, the most common cause of nerve damage is the adhesions formed around the reticulum in advanced cases of traumatic reticulitis. The vagus nerve passes through the diaphragm in the region of the reticulum and is susceptible to damage in that area from the inflammation and infection that follows traumatic reticulitis. Other lesions that may damage the nerve would include actinobacillosis of the reticulum, infections of the mediastinal lymph nodes, e.g. tuberculosis, ruptured diaphragm or pleurisy. Sometimes cattle that survive surgery for abomasal torsion later develop signs of vagal indigestion. This could be the result of damage to the nerve caused by the torsion.

Because of the loss of function of the vagus nerve, ingesta is not transported from the rumen to the abomasum or from the abomasum through the pylorus, with the consequent result that the rumen and often the abomasum distend with fluid and ingesta producing abdominal distension.

Signs

The clinical signs are variable in that the abomasum is not always directly involved. Depending on the level at which the vagus nerve is damaged various syndromes can develop that are clinically classed as follows.

1 Pyloric obstruction and abomasal impaction.
2 Ruminal distension with atony.
3 Ruminal distension with hypermotility.

In some cases combinations will occur.

Pyloric obstruction and abomasal impaction. If the abomasum is involved there is a pyloric stenosis, which prevents ingesta leaving the abomasum. The ingesta accumulates and the abomasum becomes distended and can be palpated in the abdominal flank. Later the rumen becomes atonic and distends with fluid and ingesta.

Ruminal distension with atony. This is due either to a primary effect of the paralysed vagus nerve on rumen function or it can occur following (1) from a backflow from the distended abomasum. The effect of this is to produce a characteristic shape to the abdomen. The left flank is distended and well rounded as in mild bloat and the right flank is distended in the lower regions of the abdomen, giving the right flank a pear-shape appearance. This shape is characteristic of vagal indigestion. In some cases of vagal indigestion where only the rumen is affected the organ will be grossly distended, containing large quantities of fluid. Rumen contractions are infrequent and no rumen sound will be audible. Faecal output is decreased and the faeces are frequently of a pale pasty consistency. Rectal temperature is normal, the heart rate may be normal but in some cases is markedly decreased to around 40/minute. There is also dehydration, decreased milk yield and a gradual but progressive loss of body condition. Rectal examination will reveal a grossly distended rumen, reaching into the pelvic canal and also the ventral rumen distended well over to the right side of the abdomen. The abomasum is not usually palpated per rectum. The fluid content of the rumen and the abomasum can be assessed by ballottement of the abdominal wall on both flanks.

Ruminal distension with hypermotility. There is slight ruminal tympany, and frequent and forceful rumen contractions. Recent body weight loss will be evident. Faeces are scant and pasty. Rectal palpation will reveal a gross distension of the dorsal sac of the rumen and the ventral sac will possess an 'L'-shaped distension.

Clinical pathology

The experienced clinician will make his diagnosis on the clinical signs described and there are no laboratory tests that can be considered specific for vagal indigestion. The dehydration will increase the packed cell volume. If pyloric stenosis is present a metabolic alkalosis will be present with the effect of reducing serum chloride to 40–50 mmol/l. An elevation of rumen chloride concentration (above 30 mmol/l) indicates abomasal reflux into the rumen.

Diagnosis

Veterinary advice is usually sought by the stockworker because it is noticed that the cow has slowly developed an abdominal distension and it is considered that the animal may be affected with bloat. A thorough clinical examination must be performed to establish the differential diagnosis.

If the animal is passing small quantities of pale pasty faeces, the left flank is rounded and distended, the right flank distended in the lower half only and the distension is due to fluid accumulation in the rumen and abomasum, and if the rectal temperature is normal and heart rate normal or slightly depressed, then a diagnosis of vagal indigestion can be made. However, many cases are brought to the veterinarian's attention before all the signs have fully developed and perhaps the right flank distension is not obvious. The insidious onset will distinguish the condition from bloat as will the fluid-filled rumen. Abomasal impaction must be distinguished by ballottement, which will indicate firm abomasal contents in impaction and fluid contents in pyloric stenosis.

Accumulation of fluid within the peritoneal cavity from ascites, peritonitis (p. 655) or ruptured urinary bladder can be differentiated by paracentesis. Hydrops allantois or amnii (p. 479) will also produce severe abdominal distension but will be differentiated on rectal examination.

Treatment

The prognosis in vagal indigestion is generally poor to hopeless and in most cases immediate slaughter is advised.

If treatment is embarked upon because of the value of the animal the dehydration and any chloride deficit should be corrected. As much as 40–50 l of Ringer's solution may be required over 24 hours and given intravenously. It must be remembered that oral fluid therapy must not be contemplated because of the fluid retention in the rumen.

Following rehydration an exploratory laparotomy and rumenotomy may be performed. Adhesions around the reticulum can be palpated. A rumenotomy partially to empty the rumen is then performed and the reticulum and oesophageal groove examined for tumours or other lesions. The author, on one occasion, found a complete afterbirth wedged in the oesophageal groove in a cow that had not eaten since calving 10 days previously and was showing signs of rumen atony and distension. Removal of the afterbirth led to an uneventful recovery.

Even if tumours, adhesions or oesophageal lesions are discovered the prognosis is still likely to be hopeless so surgery should only be contemplated in valuable animals and a poor prognosis given before surgery commences.

Cold cow syndrome

Another rumen indigestion syndrome that has been reported from different areas of the UK has been named the cold cow syndrome. This syndrome usually occurs in early spring in lactating cows when grazing ryegrass pastures. The onset is sudden but not related to change in pasture use. Both poor and lush pastures have been involved and the occurrence is not related to levels of fertilizer use. The morbidity is high and varies from 8 to 100 per cent of the herd, but mortality is nil. Milk yield may be depressed by up to 50 per cent but recovers within two days. The condition was first recognized in Northern Ireland in the late 1970s and in the south-west of England in 1982 and has been reported in several years since.

Aetiology

The aetiology is unknown but several suggestions have been made. These include unusually high levels of soluble carbohydrate found in grass being grazed by affected herds (Jack, 1985). Other suggestions have been the oestrogenic zearalenone or other metabolites of field microfungi or the presence of high levels of soluble proteins or a protein metabolite. Climatic conditions have been investigated and cases have occurred during periods of frost, cold wet weather and during warm dry springs. Large night/day fluctuations in atmospheric temperature of the order of 17–18 °C (30–32 °F) accompanied one series of outbreaks.

Clinical pathology

Blood samples from affected cows have been examined for a wide range of biochemical parameters but no abnormalities have been detected.

Signs

A sudden onset of ataxia and incoordination, with a few animals being weak and becoming recumbent, followed by a copious non-smelling acute diarrhoea are the principal clinical signs. The cows behave as though they are drunk. The cows are characteristically cold to the touch as though in a state of shock but rectal temperatures are normal. Appetite is much reduced if not absent and the milk yield falls by up to 50 per cent in the herd and in some individuals by up to 100 per cent. The duration of the disease is short as appetite and milk yield return to normal in two to three days. If cows regraze the same pastures later in the season no disease in seen.

Treatment and prevention

Because of the rapid recovery treatment appears unnecessary, except that the herd should be housed on dry food for 24 hours and then moved to new pasture. Symptomatic treatment of recumbent cows may be required.

Until the aetiology of this condition is understood, preventative measures will not be possible.

The oesophageal groove

Lesions of the oesophageal groove will interfere with the normal rumen digestion process. Tumours or granulomatous lesions will occlude the oesophagus and prevent eructation and lead to a gaseous bloat or secondary rumen tympany. The same lesions may interfere with normal rumen contractions and cause signs of simple indigestion. Although not common (annual incidence 1 per 10 000 cattle) actinobacillosis of the oesophageal groove does occasionally occur. Some lesions of the oesophageal groove may be due to upper alimentary squamous cell carcinoma in bracken areas (see p. 632).

Signs

The presenting signs of actinobacillosis of the oesophageal groove will be inappetence, reduced milk yield, and possibly mild tympany evidenced by distension of the left sublumbar fossa. The rumen contraction will be weak and occur at once every 1 or 2 minutes. Rectal temperature and heart rate will be normal. Examination of the faeces will reveal strands of undigested fibre. Although this latter finding is in itself only an indication of indigestion, and several lesions of the rumen or rumen wall or dental problems may lead to undigested fibre appearing in the faeces, the most common cause is likely to be actinobacillosis of the oesophageal groove.

Diagnosis

Only a tentative diagnosis can be made based on the clinical observations described above. Although diagnosis would be confirmed by performing an exploratory laparotomy and a biopsy of any oesophageal groove lesion discovered, this is unlikely to be performed in practice because of economic considerations.

Treatment

Although the prognosis in these cases must be guarded because of the uncertainty of the diagnosis, cows presenting the above described lesions are worthy of treatment. Treatment using antibiotics over a prolonged period of at least 10 days can be successful. The antibiotic of choice is streptomycin and a dose of 5–6 g daily for 10 days is effective in a proportion of cows exhibiting the above described signs.

Traumatic reticulitis (traumatic reticuloperitonitis, hardware disease, wire)

Traumatic reticulitis is a well-described disease affecting mainly adult cattle. Because of the rather undiscerning eating habits of the cow, it is quite common for cattle to ingest metallic objects with their food. Some abattoir surveys have demonstrated over 50 per cent of cattle reticula to contain foreign objects of either metal, wood or stone. If pieces of metal wire or nails 5–10 cm long are ingested these will accumulate in the reticulum and when rumen contractions occur may penetrate the reticulum wall. The incidence of this disease varies considerably around the world. The incidence in the UK has declined in the last 30 years and the present annual incidence is around 5 cases per 10 000 cows. However, in some areas the disease is still extremely common and may reach an annual incidence of 100–200 per 10 000 cows.

This disease is probably related to standards of management that exist on the farm, e.g. rusty, poorly maintained barbed wire fences are a frequent source of the offending wire. It is thought that the incidence has declined since string has replaced wire to secure bales of hay and straw and much barbed wire fencing has been replaced by electric fences. However, cases of this disease will still be encountered on untidy farms where nails, wire and other metallic objects are left lying around in fields and where they can be accidentally picked up by hay or silage making machinery.

Pathogenesis

Metal objects that are ingested invariably lodge in the floor of the reticulum due to their relative mass and the position of the reticulum. It is only short sharp objects that penetrate the reticulum wall and these are usually 5–10 cm long. The penetration occurs as a result of the ruminal and reticular contractions. On entering the wall of reticulum the wire will continue to penetrate until it reaches the peritoneum. Infection from the rumen then follows the wire and a localized peritonitis is produced causing local abscess formation and adhesions. If the direction of the wire is forward the diaphragm and pericardium may be punctured, which produces a localized pleurisy and pericarditis. If the direction of the wire is left or right of the forward direction the diaphragm may not be involved but extensive peritonitis could well develop with adhesions containing a variety of abscesses being produced. If the peritonitis is extensive, adhesions between the reticulum and liver or spleen may be evident. Sequelae to traumatic reticulitis include localized or diffuse peritonitis, liver abscessation, splenitis, pleurisy and pericarditis. These sequelae may take several weeks to develop.

Signs

The condition is generally progressive and the clinical signs changes as the disease progresses from the initial acute phase through a subacute to a chronic phase.

In the initial acute phase the cow is anorexic, and milk production is reduced. The cow may exhibit an arched back and the abdomen is tucked up. A grunt may be heard when the animal walks, although on occasions there will be a reluctance to move and also a reluctance to lie down.

Rectal temperature will be elevated to 39.1–40 °C (102.5–104 °F) and although the frequency of rumen contractions may be reduced they are more often increased to 3 or 4/minute. Respiratory movements will be shallow, increased in rate and mostly thoracic. Frequently, farmers mistakenly diagnose the condition as pneumonia. The heart rate will be raised to around 75–90/minute.

The acute phase may last three to five days and then the rectal temperature will fall to around 39 °C (102 °F) or sometimes to normal. The subacute phase will last several weeks, showing signs of mild indigestion. Rumen contractions will be weak and infrequent, there may be a mild tympany and undigested fibrous material may be evident in the faeces. Sometimes apparent recovery from the acute phase will occur and the animal will return to near normal production but a relapse will occur several weeks later. This relapse is usually associated with the onset of pericarditis. The animal will be reluctant to move, may occasionally grunt but signs of cardiac insufficiency will predominate. A firm pronounced jugular pulse will be noticeable, together with oedema of the brisket and auscultation of the lungs may reveal signs of congestion or even pleurisy. Auscultation of the heart will sometimes be difficult as the heart sounds will be muffled and difficult to hear. However, splashing and tinkling sounds over the heart region will confirm the presence of pericarditis (see p. 566).

Pathology

During the acute phase there will be a measurable increase in circulating neutrophils with white cell counts rising to 30×10^9/l (30 000/μl). Ketone bodies may be present in urine or milk indicating a secondary acetonaemia. During the subacute phase, when peritonitis is developing, the white cell count may be subnormal.

At post mortem, the degree of peritonitis can be dramatic with adhesions between the reticulum, rumen, diaphragm, liver and spleen. Incising through the adhesions may reveal multiple abscesses. Abscesses may also be present in the liver. The pericarditis, when present, will also be dramatic with gross thickening of the pericardium and large quantities of pus present in the pericardial sac, so-called bread and butter heart. Pleurisy, and localized pneumonia and abscessation may also be present.

Diagnosis

The diagnosis of the acute phase is based on the signs described and discovered during the clinical examination. Cows with traumatic reticulitis can often be made to grunt by pressing down firmly on the withers, thus making the animal lower its back. However, this test is only an indication of peritonitis and not specific for traumatic reticulitis. Grunting can also be induced by applying sharp pressure just to the left of the xiphoid process using a clenched fist. This will specifically indicate pain in the region of the reticulum.

The most successful diagnostic test is known as the 'reticular grunt' or Williams test (Williams, 1975). This test uses knowledge of the cycle of reticulo-rumen contractions.

1 Contractions of the reticulum, followed by contraction of the rumen. There is no eructation at this stage.

2 Following relaxation of the reticulum and rumen, an independent contraction of the rumen occurs. This contraction is accompanied by eructation.

3 Relaxation of the reticulum and rumen completes the cycle. The 'reticular grunt' is based on the correlation of pain with contractions of the reticulum. Since the reticular contractions occur in conjunction with rumen contractions, the clinician should observe for signs of pain during or just before the non-eructating rumen contractions. These signs of pain will be a mild grunt, and shuffling of the forelegs. To help detect the grunt, observation of the left costal arch may reveal the animal holding its breath just before it grunts.

This test is specific for traumatic reticulitis but is only effective in the acute phase of the disease.

Diagnosis of the subacute phase may prove extremely difficult, as the signs are often vague and only indicative of a non-specific indigestion. If such cases are encountered and a diagnosis of indigestion made, but a return to normal is not rapidly achieved, subacute traumatic reticulitis/peritonitis must be considered as a differential diagnosis.

The use of metal detectors have been advocated by some workers. However, because metal objects are frequently found in the reticulum a positive metal detector test will often be misleading.

Diagnosis of pericarditis is more straightforward. The jugular pulse and brisket oedema will lead the clinician to auscultate the heart in detail. Muffled heart sounds and splashing, fluid or tinkling sounds around the heart will confirm pericarditis.

Treatment

Various treatment regimens have been advocated for traumatic reticulitis and they can be classified into surgical and conservative.

If a diagnosis is made during the acute or subacute phase and there are no signs of pericarditis, the surgical approach has much to commend it. In many cases the diagnosis is only tentative and the rumenotomy is exploratory to confirm diagnosis or establish another diagnosis. Under paravertebral anaesthesia, an 18-cm vertical incision is made in the sublumbar fossa, the rumen wall exteriorized and a 10–15-cm incision made into which a McLintock ring is fitted, thus temporarily fixing the rumen wall to the exterior and preventing peritoneal contamination with rumen contents. A scrubbed arm is inserted into the rumen and the reticulum located. Each crypt of the reticulum should be explored as the offending wire may have penetrated to the extent that very little is left protruding into the reticulum. Adhesions between the reticulum and diaphragm or abdominal floor can be detected by attempting to lift the reticular wall. Once located, the offending wire should be slowly withdrawn back through the reticular wall and removed from the rumen. The rumen incision is closed using Lembert sutures and the abdominal wall incision closed in the usual way.

Five days of antibiotic treatment should follow the surgery to prevent the spread of the peritonitis initiated by the foreign body. This operation can be very satisfactory to conduct in practice and the majority of cases make an uneventful recovery.

The conservative treatment involves restricting the animal's movement by tying it in a byre stall with the front feet raised 35–40 cm higher than the hind feet for three weeks. Parenteral antibiotics will also be given for five to seven days, and in some countries a magnet will be inserted into the reticulum using a balling gun.

If pericarditis is evident immediate slaughter must be recommended as there is little likelihood of recovery. On no account should a rumenotomy be considered because even if the wire is located removing it may well cause the heart to stop and death during surgery will be the result.

Prevention

The main thrust of prevention must be to avoid leaving wire or nails lying around to be picked up by cattle during feeding. The use of metal detectors on forage harvesting equipment to prevent damage to the equipment have undoubtedly reduced the incidence of metal objects being found in cattle feeds. Some workers have advocated the routine use of magnets. These are inserted into all cattle on the farm. There is no real evidence that these have been successful.

Abomasum

Diseases of the bovine abomasum comprise an interesting group of conditions only really appreciated in comparatively recent years (Pinsent, 1978).

There are three important conditions that probably have a similar aetiology and epidemiology, yet produce widely differing clinical syndromes. These are left displacement of the abomasum (LDA), dilatation and torsion in the right flank (RDA) and ulceration. Impaction of the abomasum has also been reported. The three important conditions (LDA, RDA and ulceration) appear to be the result of intensive management of cattle and have not been recorded in wild ruminants. In fact their occurrence, particularly LDA, is almost entirely restricted to dairy cattle and rarely found in suckler beef cows. Diet undoubtedly has an important role in the aetiology of these diseases, with the use of concentrated cereal-based feeds and low-fibre diets generally being incriminated. In some countries the feeding of root crops that are heavily contaminated with soil, sand and gravel have also been incriminated. In the UK and USA, LDA is much more common than RDA or ulceration. However, reports from Scandinavia would indicate that RDA is much more frequently seen there than in the UK or USA and may be the result of much greater use of root feeds such as fodder beet.

Displacement of the abomasum to the left

Left displacement of the abomasum is by far the most common of the abomasal diseases encountered in cattle in the UK or USA. Its occurrence is almost entirely confined to dairy cattle, although it has very occasionally been seen in bulls, where it is probably secondary to some other condition. The author has, on one occasion only, diagnosed the condition in a Friesian bull and in that case the animal was suffering from severe endocarditis. It was likely that this particular LDA was a secondary condition brought about by the inappetence caused by the endocarditis. The overall incidence varies considerably between years and between seasons. In some years the annual incidence can be as high as 25–30 per 10 000 and in others as low as 4–6 per 10 000.

There appears, in the UK, to be a definite seasonal pattern to the incidence with the majority of cases occurring in late winter–early spring, i.e. January to April, the period of winter housing in the UK. In the USA, LDA is reported to be more common in the winter housing period. However, the problem is encountered in countries where spring calving predominates and the cows are at pasture during the susceptible period, e.g. Ireland, Australia and New Zealand, although the incidence varies considerably between farms. The author has experienced the condition in eight cows in a 110-cow herd in one year, all occurring from January to April; yet there are many farms that have never, knowingly, experienced the condition. Breed susceptibility has been investigated and there has been no authoritative confirmation that there is a genetic predisposition. However, it is thought that the condition generally affects the higher yielding cows, mainly in early lactation, although occasionally during late pregnancy.

Aetiology and pathogenesis

The precise aetiology of LDA is not readily understood but the occurrence of the problem soon after, or occasionally just before, parturition would suggest that the presence of the gravid uterus or the process of parturition predisposes to the condition. Certainly it has been observed that in normal cows in late pregnancy the presence of the gravid uterus displaces the abomasum forwards and to the left, and after calving the organ returns to its normal position. To remain displaced after calving, the abomasum must have developed atony and the subsequent accumulation of gas. Atony of the abomasum is likely to be caused by one of four factors.

1 The feeding of rapidly fermentable concentrate feeds, which have a tendency towards the production of acidosis.

2 The accumulation of sand or gravel in the abomasum, which damages the abomasal mucosa.

3 Stress conditions or metabolic diseases that frequently occur around the time of parturition. Hypocalcaemia will itself cause atony of the abomasum.
4 The occurrence of systemic diseases that produce toxaemia, such as acute metritis.

It is likely therefore that atony of the abomasum and the accumulation of gas within the organ is the prime factor in the pathogenesis of the condition. The mechanical effect of displacement by the gravid uterus may well have some involvement in originally displacing the abomasum, but once displaced to the left and the organ is located between the left abdominal wall and the rumen the atonic nature of the abomasum and the presence of gas will prevent the organ returning to its normal position.

Signs

The clinical signs of LDA can vary considerably, although in general the signs are similar to chronic acetonaemia. Mild cases are encountered that show little more than a slightly depressed appetite, rumination and milk yield. At the other extreme, acute cases can be encountered with complete inappetence, absence of rumination, loss of condition, scanty diarrhoea and grunting with some signs of mild colic. The most common clinical picture is one of refusal to eat concentrates, some reduction in milk yield and scanty soft or pasty faeces. Rectal temperature will be normal but the heart rate may be raised to 80–100/minute. Rumen movements will usually be absent or at least infrequent and in some cases palpation of the rumen in the left sublumbar fossa will be impossible because of the presence of the gas-filled abomasum between the left abdominal wall and the rumen. A Rothera's test on urine or milk will usually be positive and thus in many instances the cow will be presented as a suspected case of acetonaemia. In the more acute cases, which are more common in late pregnancy, distension of the left flank will be evident.

Diagnosis

The diagnosis of LDA is relatively easy, providing the clinician always keeps the condition in mind when making a clinical examination of dairy cows. Confirmation is based on auscultation, percussion and auscultation, or ballottement and auscultation of the left flank. The stethoscope is placed on the last intercostal space in line with the lower limit of the left sublumbar fossa and the penultimate rib is percussed by 'flicking' it with the finger. If a 'ping' or high-pitched resonant sound is heard, this is indicative of a gas-filled organ inside the abdominal wall. Should the first attempt fail to elicit the characteristic 'ping' the stethoscope is moved so that an area representing a 20 cm square forward and below the first stethoscope site is auscultated and the second to last and third last ribs percussed in the same way as described above. If a high-pitched resonant sound is heard over this area, confirmation of the diagnosis should depend on auscultation only and a short series of tinkling sounds reminiscent of raindrops falling on a metal roof will be heard.

The frequency of these tinkling sounds is quite variable and the clinician may have to auscultate for up to 10 minutes in some cases. Ballottement of the lower left flank at the same time as auscultation of the target area described above may frequently elicit the same tinkling sounds. The diagnosis, by auscultation of the tinkling sounds without recourse to ballottement, is to be favoured because ballottement may elicit splashing sounds from the rumen that can be difficult to distinguish from the high-pitched tinkling sounds diagnostic of LDA. However, a negative diagnosis can fairly quickly be achieved by using the percussion and auscultation technique over a 20 cm square area forward of and ventral to the lower limit of the left sublumbar fossa and only when this technique produces a pinging noise should it be necessary to spend time in auscultation alone.

All cows that are presented with inappetence and have a normal rectal temperature, particularly in early lactatiön or late pregnancy, should be subjected to the percussion and auscultation technique to eliminate LDA as part of a normal clinical examination. If this is performed the clinician is unlikely to fail to diagnose LDA.

However, it must be said that a small number of cases are not diagnosed at the first examination and a diagnosis of acetonaemia or, occasionally, indigestion is made and the corresponding treatment administered. Such cases will show a temporary recovery but the signs will relapse two to five days later. It is essential when treating acetonaemia or indigestion that the farmer is instructed to seek further veterinary advice if the condition regresses. Many cases of LDA are diagnosed in cows that have been treated for acetonaemia two to five days previously either by the farmer or a veterinarian.

Following a complete clinical examination the differential diagnosis of LDA is related to whether the high-pitched resonant sounds can be confused with anything else. Once heard, these sounds are never forgotten. However, similar sounds do occur in conditions of the rumen that produce rumen atony, a rumen mildly distended with gas accumulation, as is seen in vagal indigestion, actinobacillosis of the oesophageal groove, localized peritonitis or mild rumen tympany. However, if the tinkling sounds are heard spontaneously and not induced by ballottement, the likelihood of misdiagnosing these other conditions as LDA is slim. The author has on one occasion, having made a diagnosis of abomasal dilatation in the right side of the abdomen by recognizing the tinkling sounds, performed a laparotomy to discover the sounds were produced by a large subperitoneal abscess in the upper right abdomen.

Treatment

The treatment for LDA falls into two categories, conservative or surgical.

Conservative measures include drug therapy and rolling. Drug therapy using calcium borogluconate solution, neostigmine and saline cathartics has been attempted with very little success. The usual conservative treatment is to roll the cow. The cow is cast, using the Reuff's method, on to its right side. The cow is then rolled into dorsal recumbency and kept in this position for 5 minutes. During this time the animal may be rocked to the left and right and the abdomen massaged vigorously to encourage the abomasum to rise into the ventral abdomen. The animal is then rolled over to a left side lateral recumbency and maintained in this position for a further 5 minutes, allowing time for the abomasum to return to its normal position. During this process, splashing and gurgling sounds can be heard coming from the abdomen as the abomasum moves. The animal is then allowed to rise. The left flank is then auscultated to ensure the abomasum is still not present in the LDA position.

One variation of this procedure reported to be successful by one UK practitioner (B. Jeffrey, pers. comm.) is to cast the cow into left-sided lateral recumbency and restrain the animal in this position for 30 minutes. The gas present in the abomasum allows the organ to 'float' back to its normal position.

It is essential if the LDA has been corrected by rolling that the animal is re-examined 48 hours later to ensure that a relapse has not occurred. In the experience of the author, and many others, relapse is to be expected in over 75 per cent of cases of LDA that have been corrected by the rolling technique. Quite frequently if relapse does occur, the signs may not be so severe as those present before the correction and the animal may well complete its lactation albeit with a reduced total milk yield. In such cases, chronic LDA exists and ulceration of the abomasum with adhesions to the abdominal wall may well develop thus shortening the productive lifetime of the animal.

The surgical approach to treatment consists of laparotomy, returning the abomasum to the right side of the abdomen and suture fixation of the organ to the abdominal wall. Many different surgical techniques have been described for this procedure but the one favoured by the author is the right flank approach with the animal standing. The animal is starved of water and food for 24 hours prior to surgery to reduce the size of the rumen. Using paravertebral anaesthesia, a 20-cm incision is made in the abdominal wall, starting at the lower limit of the right sublumbar fossa and extending vertically downwards. The left arm then enters the abdominal cavity and moves carefully down the right side of the abdomen, along the floor and up the left side with the hand always in contact with the peritoneum. The hand can then locate the distended abomasum situated high in the left flank between the rumen and the abdominal wall. The hand is then placed over the top of the abomasum and downward pressure exerted. Several attempts at downward pressure may be required to disperse the gas present in the organ. The organ is then pushed down and below the rumen. It is important that contact by the hand is maintained with the abomasum during this stage of the operation because if it is lost it may be difficult to find the abomasum without causing trauma to the small intestines.

When the organ has been brought across to the right side, the pylorus is located and brought to the abdominal wall incision. Using non-absorbable suture material, e.g. monofilament nylon, and a round-bodied needle a suture is placed in the greater curvature of the abomasum close to the pylorus and this is then sutured to the peritoneum and abdomen wall at the base of the incision. The abdominal wall incision is closed in the normal way and postoperative antibiotics administered. Appetite is stimulated by the administration of rumen-stimulant drenches and the animal allowed immediate access to good quality fodder and water. This technique has been used by the author for over 20 years and on one occasion only has correction not been possible. In this case adhesions were present between the abomasum and the left abdominal wall. A second incision was then made in the left sublumbar fossa, and the adhesions were broken down revealing a perforated ulcer. The ulcer was excised, sutured using a purse string suture and the abomasum returned to the right flank where an assistant located and sutured it as described above. This right-sided approach has been used widely in the UK and is suitable for operating on the farm.

The right paramedian approach is also widely used. The animal is cast into dorsal recumbency and local anaesthesia administered for an incision posterior to the sternum and midway between the midline and the right subcutaneous abdominal vein. The abomasum is located, returned to its normal position and fixed using catgut or monofilament nylon sutures 2–3 cm from the margin of the incision. This technique does return the abomasum to its normal position, whereas in the former the fixation of the pylorus to the abdominal flank wound results in the abomasum being slightly out of position. In the author's opinion the abomasopexy should be performed with non-absorbable suture material as the few cases that have relapsed following abomasopexy were mostly sutured with catgut.

Another technique involves a left flank approach, pushing the abomasum back to the right side and then entering the rumen as in a rumenotomy to transfix the rumen to the floor of the abdomen by using a large needle and a long suture. The suture needle is passed vertically down through the rumen wall and abdominal wall to the exterior. The needle is removed from the suture and the procedure repeated with the other end of the suture material and the suture tied as a mattress suture on the exterior of the ventral abdomen. This produces an adhesion between the ventral rumen and the ventral abdomen that will prevent a recurrence of the LDA.

Prevention

Advice on prevention is difficult because the precise nature of the aetiology is unknown. Furthermore, most cases occur only sporadically and it is rare for farms to experience more than one or two cases in a season. If the incidence is higher on a particular farm, attention to the feeding regimens may prove worthwhile. Dry cows should be fed a diet of long fibre and very little concentrates. Dry-cow diets should always contain less than 30 per cent concentrate on a DM basis. Maize silage, which itself contains up to 50 per cent grain on a DM basis, should be restricted to no more than 15 kg/day during the dry period. The change in diets that occur at calving should be made as gradually as possible. Ideally, 2 kg daily of concentrates for the last two weeks of the dry period will help the rumen microflora adjust to the increased concentrate intake that occurs in early lactation. The approach to prevention of LDA is much the same as the approach to the prevention of acetonaemia.

Right-sided abomasal dilatation and torsion

Occurrence

Right-sided abomasal dilatation and torsion occurs much less frequently than LDA in the UK and USA, although it appears to be more common in Denmark. The annual incidence in the UK is of the order of 2–3 per 10 000. It normally occurs in early lactation and rarely in the dry cow, but although predominantly affecting dairy cows it has been reported in bulls, young animals, beef cows and feedlot cattle.

Pathogenesis

As with LDA, the aetiology of RDA is not fully understood but the pathogenesis is probably similar to that of LDA. Atony of the abomasum followed by the accumulation of feed, fluid and gas produce a grossly distended organ. The presence of gravel and sand in the abomasum has commonly been observed in affected animals, which may account for the higher incidence in Denmark where large quantities of fodder beet are fed that often is contaminated with soil. Torsion is frequently a sequel to the dilatation and this is purely a mechanical effect of the increased weight and size of the dilated organ. The torsion can be in several directions, e.g. the organ may be rotated dorsally 90–180°, or counterclockwise up to 180° as viewed from the rear, or the torsion may incorporate the omasum.

Signs

The onset of dilatation is insidious with inappetence, milk yield reduction and varying degrees of ketosis. Rumination ceases and rumen contractions are weak and infrequent. Faecal quantity is reduced but its consistency is usually diarrhoeic, foul smelling and often contains occult blood. Rectal temperature is normal and heart rate raised to 80–100/minute. Mild colic signs may also be evident and there is often a noticeable distension of the right flank. Once torsion occurs, the signs become peracute. Then there is a subnormal temperature, with a heart rate up to 160 minute, cold extremities and extreme dullness. These signs indicate severe shock and frequently colic may be observed. At this stage the animal is anorexic and the rectum will be empty except for some tar-like mucus.

Diagnosis

Diagnosis should not present any problems if the techniques of percussion and auscultation, ballottement and auscultation and auscultation alone are applied to the right flank in the same way as described for the diagnosis of LDA on the left flank. The same 'ping' and tinkling sounds if heard on the right flank will indicate a RDA. Determination of whether torsion exists will rely on the severity of the signs exhibited, e.g. the presence of a very fast heart rate, subnormal temperature, the signs of shock and the consistency of the rectal contents. Rectal palpation may also reveal the presence of a grossly dilated viscus in the right sublumbar region. Differential diagnosis of RDA plus torsion will include all causes of acute abdominal obstruction, particularly caecal dilatation and torsion, torsion of small intestines, intussusception and perforated abomasal ulcer. However, being able to palpate the organ on rectal palpation and hearing the characteristic high-pitched sounds should not cause problems in diagnosis.

Treatment

If torsion is not present there is often a temptation to try conservative treatments using antacids by mouth and spasmolytics, vitamins or antibiotics by injection. This is not to be recommended. Although some cases of dilatation do recover spontaneously, many do not. Many cases will remain dilated and a chronic state of abomasal dilatation develops where the animal loses weight and milk production, and eventually is culled as a 'poor doer'. Often the dilatation progresses to torsion and surgery to correct abomasal torsion is much less successful than correcting dilatation without torsion. This is because of the severe shock that is induced in the animal by the torsion. The decision on whether to attempt surgery in cases of RDA plus torsion will depend on the degree of shock that exists. In severe cases casualty slaughter should be advised. Recently, successful treatment of dilatation without torsion has been reported using metoclopramide hydrochloride.

However, in valuable animals and less severely affected cows, surgery can be successful. Intravenous drip therapy should be set up immediately using Ringer's solution or isotonic sodium chloride. Cows with RDA plus torsion will be suffering from metabolic alkalosis and will be short of chloride ions. Sodium bicarbonate or sodium lactate should not be used. To restore normal hydration, 40–50 l of electrolyte are likely to be required over a 24-hour period.

Having set up the intravenous drip, surgery should commence immediately. Under paravertebral anaesthesia an incision is made in the right abdominal wall with the animal standing. If the animal cannot stand it is likely her condition is so severe that surgery would not succeed and casualty slaughter should be advised. On entering the abdomen and the abomasum located the first procedure is to deflate the organ using a wide bore (12G) needle and rubber tube. Having deflated the organ the direction of the torsion should be identified and an attempt made to correct the torsion without removing the fluid. If correction of the torsion is not possible than half of the fluid should be siphoned out of the abomasum. This will ease the recognition of the torsion direction and more readily allow repositioning of the abomasum. Abomasopexy is carried out as for LDA correction. The abdomen is closed in the normal way. If RDA exists without torsion the abomasum should be emptied of fluid by siphoning and then the organ opened and all debris, which may include straw or hair balls, stones or gravel, should be removed. The abomasum incision is then closed, returned to its normal position and the abdomen closed in the normal way. Abomasopexy is not normally required in this situation. Fluid therapy is continued until the animal has rehydrated and postoperative antibiotics administered for five days. Following recovery diarrhoea will be present for two or three days.

Recovery rates of 75–80 per cent are reported by some workers in hospital situations and around 50 per cent when the omasum is involved in the torsion. Recovery rates for on-farm surgery are likely to be less and this must be appreciated before embarking on surgery in preference to casualty slaughter. The likelihood of recovery will depend on the length of time that elapses from torsion occurring to operation and the level of shock that exists at the time operation commences.

Prevention

Measures to prevent RDA are the same as for LDA (p. 648) but as the condition is relatively rare, specific measures to prevent RDA are academic. If root vegetables are used in large quantities for fodder they should be washed before feeding to remove the soil contamination.

Abomasal ulceration

Ulceration in the form of small multiple ulcers occurs in the abomasal mucosal surface in a number of systemic diseases but these are rarely diagnosed, their presence being masked by the other signs present of the systemic disease.

However, a syndrome of peptic ulceration in adult cattle does occur sporadically and may result in perforation and peritonitis or haemorrhage, which can be mild and recurrent or acute and be a cause of death. The actual incidence of abomasal ulceration is probably much more common than generally realized as many cases are difficult to diagnose and may produce little harmful effect until perforation or haemorrhage occurs. The aetiology is uncertain but feeding regimens involving a sudden introduction of concentrate feeds are likely to be implicated much the same as in the presumed aetiology of LDA and RDA. The author has experienced three sudden deaths in a herd of 120 dairy cattle that were caused by perforated abomasal ulcers. The abomasum contained large quantities of sand and gravel, which were the result of a depraved appetite. The cows were constantly eating soil, which was later confirmed to be due to hypocuprosis. The aetiology of peptic abomasal ulceration is therefore similar to LDA and RDA and is considered by some workers to be another manifestation of the same syndrome. Certainly, ulcers are found in the abomasum of both LDA and RDA.

The ulcers occur singly or occasionally in twos and threes and vary in size from 2 to 6 cm in diameter. Fungal hyphae are frequently found in the depths of the ulcers, which tend to extend into the submucosal layers until, in some cases, perforation occurs. If the perforation occurs at a point covered by omentum the ulcer may be sealed by omental adhesion. However, if the ulcer perforates at a point lateral to the omental covering, the abomasal contents spill into the peritoneal cavity and death soon follows. Another complication occurs when the ulcer erodes into a blood vessel producing haemorrhage. This may be only temporary and the blood vessel heals but more often the haemorrhage does not stop and the animal dies from blood loss. This can be a cause of sudden death. The annual incidence for abomasal ulcers with haemorrhage would be in the order of 5–10 per 10 000.

Diagnosis

The only occasion where the syndrome can be diagnosed with certainty is when haemorrhage occurs. A cow presented with inappetence, reduced milk yield and passing black tarry faeces, which contain large quantities of occult blood, will almost certainly be suffering from a haemorrhaging abomasal ulcer. Severe cases will be anaemic, the heart rate fast and loud and death can occur within 24 hours. The prognosis in such cases is extremely guarded for, although animals do appear to make a recovery, relapses are common.

The diagnosis of abomasal ulcers with perforation is difficult. The signs are of mild colic and pain in the right ventral abdomen. Confirmation will only come from an exploratory laparotomy. Abomasal ulcers may well be present in many apparently normal cows and undoubtedly many do heal but the sudden onset of signs associated with acute haemorrhage or perforation would indicate that until such dramatic consequences occur the ulcers may not be harmful.

Treatment

Treatment is purely academic. Ulcers without perforation or haemorrhage are unlikely to be diagnosed. The prognosis in haemorrhaging ulcers is so uncertain that casualty slaughter should be advised. Perforated ulcers, if not sealed with omentum, are usually only discovered at post-mortem examination. Ulcers that have perforated and become sealed with omentum are unlikely to be diagnosed except on exploratory laparotomy in a cow showing signs of right-sided anterior abdominal pain and when discovered they are probably best left undisturbed.

Prevention

With the current state of knowledge on aetiology, the best advice on prevention is to follow that for LDA and RDA (p. 648).

Abomasal impaction

Impaction of the abomasum may occur occasionally but is certainly of no great significance in adult cattle. Its annual incidence would be less than 1 per 100 000 and appears to be more common in beef cows than dairy cows as a result of feeding poor quality fibrous material. The impaction occurs with the accumulation of large quantities of fibrous food, sand or gravel close to the pyloric outlet. The onset is insidious, with a gradual loss in milk production and inappetence. Progressively, rumen impaction occurs, rumination ceases and constipation sets in. Rectal temperature is normal but heart rate will exceed 100/minute. At first there is little or no abdominal pain but progressively pain becomes evident in the anterior right ventral abdomen (as distinct from the left anterior abdomen in traumatic reticulitis). Pinching of the withers at this stage may elicit a painful grunt. It is unlikely that a positive diagnosis will be made without recourse to an exploratory laparotomy when an enlarged doughy abomasum will be palpated.

Pinsent (1977) was of the opinion that many cases of abomasal impaction reported in the past may well have been vagus indigestion as workers reported enlargement of the fundus of the abomasum, which contained dry rumen contents and an accumulation of fluid within the rumen.

However, if such a case is encountered at exploratory laparotomy, abomasotomy and removal of the offending contents can be attempted.

Abomasal impaction in calves

Abomasal impaction does appear to be more common in calves than adult cattle. Calves from three weeks to three months can be affected although six to ten weeks is the most common period. Depraved appetite, causing the calves to eat bedding and lick hair, are thought to be the cause. Finely ground grains made into pellets have also been incriminated in the aetiology, presumably the result of rapid fermentation. Coarse ration where the grain ingredients are rolled or cracked is preferred to pellets by many calf rearers because less 'digestive upsets' appear to occur.

Diagnosis

Affected calves usually have a brown, mild diarrhoea and normal rectal temperature. The most striking feature is the result of ballottement of the lower right abdomen, which will reveal loud splashing noises over a large area usually indicating an enlarged abomasum containing excess fluid.

Treatment

Treatment using antacids such as magnesium hydroxide or magnesium carbonate or mild laxatives such as liquid paraffin or linseed oil may be helpful. In early cases surgical interference to empty the abomasum can be effective. It is interesting to note that the abomasum of veal calves slaughtered at 14–16 weeks old and reared solely on liquid milk substitute diets frequently contain one or several hairballs many up to 20 cm in diameter without abomasal ulceration or any abnormal effects being noticed before slaughter.

Colic and acute intestinal obstruction

Colic signs are frequently reported in adult cattle. They may indicate a tympanic intestinal colic or they may signal some more serious problem. This section will discuss the differential diagnosis of colic signs and will describe in detail: tympanic intestinal colic, intussusception, caecal dilatation and torsion, prolapse of small intestine through a ruptured mesentery, and torsion of small intestine around the root of the mesentery.

Occurrence

Colic is a sporadic condition affecting only individual animals, it being extremely rare for more than one animal to be affected at any one time. Signs of colic are reported quite frequently in all ages of cattle and under all types of management, whether extensive or intensive. A thorough clinical examination will be required to differentiate the many problems that produce colic. By far the most common cause of colic is tympanic intestinal colic, which is very similar to the syndrome so frequently seen in the horse. Intussusception, caecal dilatation and prolapse of the small intestine through the mesentery are much less common and in the UK each would have an annual incidence of less than 1 per 10 000.

Signs

The clinical signs of colic in cattle are firstly reduced appetite or even anorexia, reduced milk yield and a noticeable change in behaviour. Kicking at the ventral abdomen, shifting weight from one hind foot to the other, licking at the flank or chest wall, frequently lying down and then standing and generally restless. The intensity of the signs exhibited will vary with the degree of pain. On some occasions the signs are quite mild with only occasional kicking at the ventral abdomen and may be missed by all but the most astute stockworker. The above signs are all indicative of pain but not necessarily abdominal pain. Conditions that will produce similar signs include photosensitization (p. 686), particularly if the teats are affected, strangulated scrotal hernia, uterine torsion, urolithiasis (p. 226) and ureter obstruction.

Diagnosis

The diagnosis of the cause of the signs of colic will include a thorough clinical examination. The rectal temperature may be raised, the pulse will certainly be increased and the more acute the problem the faster and weaker will be the pulse. Abdominal sounds may be present or absent. In intestinal obstruction the sounds will be absent. The mucous membranes will be injected in acute problems and the eyes sunken. Ballottement of the ventral abdomen should always be performed and may reveal splashing fluid sounds. A rectal examination should also be performed. In intestinal obstruction the rectum will be empty and sticky. Enlarged viscera or abnormal positioning of the viscera may be palpated on rectal palpation. A detailed description of the use of rectal palpation in the diagnosis of abdominal disorders has been recorded by Stober & Dirkson (1977).

In many cases of intestinal obstruction diagnosis may only be confirmed on exploratory laparotomy. Exploratory laparotomy as a diagnostic procedure as opposed to its use solely as a surgical treatment is to be recommended (Pinsent, 1978) where the attitude of the farmer and conditions conducive to surgery exist. Many farmers, with their increased education and training, will understand the value of an exploratory laparotomy if the problem is fully explained. Furthermore, exploratory laparotomy may well reveal the cause of acute intestinal obstruction and allow surgical correction and recovery to take place, whereas if surgical intervention is unnecessarily delayed the likelihood of recovery is always reduced. The author has, on two occasions, performed an exploratory laporotomy where an unknown intestinal obstruction was thought to exist to find that on both occasions a thin fibrous strand or adhesion was present in the abdomen and a loop of small intestine had become entwined around the strand, thus causing the obstruction. Severing the strand released the bowel and in both cases the animal made an uneventful recovery.

Tympanic intestinal colic

Tympanic intestinal colic is by far the most common condition to produce colic signs. It can occur at any age and calves are presented with colic signs as frequently as adult animals. The signs are of sudden onset but in lactating cows they are frequently observed at milking time and in calves during or just after feeding.

Diagnosis

As all the usual colic signs are present the clinical examination will reveal normal rectal temperature, raised heart rate (80–90/minute) and normal mucous membranes. Abdominal sounds will be present, sometimes at an increased intensity. Rectal examination will reveal faeces in the rectum and it is unlikely that any abnormality to the viscera will be palpated. It is important to ensure that the differential diagnoses mentioned above are not present. Uterine torsion will only be present in late pregnancy but photosensitization is fairly common (5–10 per 10 000) and must be eliminated from the diagnosis by careful examination and palpation of any white areas of skin.

In the calf, abdominal palpation should be performed as intussusception is relatively common and can sometimes be palpated. The diagnosis will be confirmed by response to treatment or spontaneous recovery within 24 hours.

Treatment

The most effective treatment is the intravenous administration of a spasmolytic such as hyoscine-*N*-butylbromide and dipyrone. Oral treatment with mild purgatives, such as linseed oil or liquid paraffin, have been used in the past but these are unnecessary and not as effective as spasmolytics and may well be contraindicated.

Torsion of intestines (red gut in calves)

Torsion of the intestines around the root of the mesentery is extremely rare in adult cattle (1 per 10 000) but has been reported to occur spontaneously and the cause is unknown. It has also been reported to occur following rolling of cows to correct uterine torsion or left displacement of the abomasum. The entire small intestine twists up to 360° around the root of the mesentery.

In calves, the condition is more common and is known as *red gut* and is associated with the feeding of milk substitutes. It appears to have increased in incidence in recent years and is more commonly seen in loose-housed machine-fed calf rearing systems, where the intake of milk is uncontrolled and can be quite excessive. Although the aetiology is uncertain, the pathogenesis is thought to be the rapid fermentation of lactose in the ileum, which leads to gas production and gross dilatation of the intestine, which then twists at the mesentery root. Affected calves are normally three to six weeks old and are presented showing severe colic signs with death following within 12 hours. It can also be a cause of sudden death. Diagnosis is rare in the live animal, mainly because of the rapid progression of the disease and it is not possible to differentiate it from tympanic intestinal colic.

At post mortem the findings are quite dramatic. The small intestines are grossly dilated with gas, are a bright-red colour and the whole of the intestinal mucosa is bright red. To detect the torsion, the post mortem must be performed with care because if the abdomen is fully opened and the intestine allowed to spill out, the torsion will untwist and therefore not be detectable.

In adult cows the presenting signs of intestinal torsion are those of severe colic Rectal temperature may be raised, the pulse weak and fast, mucous membranes are injected and the eyes sunken. Rectal examination will usually reveal multiple gas-distended loops of small intestine in the right side of the abdomen and these may distend into the pelvic cavity. The site of the mesentery twist will normally be beyond reach but tense strands of mesentery may be palpable.

Treatment

Immediate surgery is indicated. Laparotomy is performed under paravertebral anaesthesia in the right sublumbar fossa. Loops of distended bowel may protrude through the abdominal incision. The root of the mesentery will be located in the region of the left kidney and the direction of the twist should be determined. The torsion is corrected by manipulation of the intestines, some of which will need to be exteriorized to allow room in the abdomen to correct the twist. This surgery is certainly of a heroic nature but nevertheless can succeed if the animal is not too severely shocked when the operation commences. Follow-up treatment with intravenous fluids and antibiotics should always be administered.

Prolapse of intestines through mesentery

This condition is usually only seen in adult cattle and is more common than torsion at the mesentery root. Its annual incidence is still only approximately 1 per 10 000. The acute nature of the signs are identical to torsion at the mesentery root and rectal palpation will reveal gas-distended loops of small intestine, which make it clinically indistinguishable. If untreated, death will occur within 12 hours.

Treatment

Immediate exploratory laparotomy will reveal the grossly gas-distended intestine but it may be difficult to distinguish from torsion of the intestines. Palpation of the root of the mesentery must be performed first to distinguish the condition from torsion. One clue to the problem being one of prolapse of intestine through mesentery will be the presence of normal intestine. Palpation of the gas-distended intestine will reveal that it is protruding through a hole in the mesentery. The hole must first be enlarged and the intestines slowly fed back through the aperture after which the mesenteric rupture is sutured. It must be emphasized that surgery should only be contemplated if the animal is not too severely shocked. As death can occur quickly with this condition, casualty slaughter is commonly advised.

Caecal dilatation and torsion

Caecal dilatation is a distinct clinical entity in adult cattle. Its occurrence is sporadic (approximately 1–2 per 10 000) and usually occurs in early lactation, although the condition has been reported in bulls. The aetiology is thought to be related to high levels of volatile fatty acids in the caecum, which originate from the rumen or from fermentation of undigested starch in the caecum. The fatty acids cause atony of the caecum and the gas accumulates. Mild dilatation probably causes no signs but severe dilatation will produce typical colic signs. However, many cases of caecal dilatation progress to caecal torsion. Strictly speaking this is not a torsion but due to the gross size of the dilated caecum and the large quantity of fluid it contains the distal end falls forward producing a kink in the organ. Occasionally, the weight of the distended caecum produces a torsion at the mesentery root and the colon, caecum and small intestine are involved in a torsion rather similar to the torsion of the small intestines at the mesentary root.

Diagnosis

Diagnosis is based on the presence of the signs of colic, although sometimes the colic signs are quite mild. Ballottement of the right flank will elicit copious splashing and fluid sounds and the right flank may be noticeably distended. Rectal examination will reveal an empty rectum and if a reliable history is available the animal will not have passed any faeces for 24 hours or more.

Usually, the dilated caecum will be palpable at the entrance to the pelvic cavity and many even protrude into the pelvic cavity. If the caecum has 'kinked' rectal exploration of the abdominal cavity will be required to detect the dilated organ.

Treatment

The only treatment is surgical intervention and should always be considered in an animal that is not too shocked and where the condition has not been present for too long.

A right-flank laparotomy is performed and, on exploration, the grossly enlarged caecum can be detected. Palpation of the root of the mesentery should be carried out to try and determine if a torsion exists.

The first stage of the operation is to siphon off the fluid present in the caecum thus reducing its volume to a manageable size. It is possible in some cases to siphon off 30–40 l of dark foul-smelling fluid. When as much fluid and gas as possible has been removed a purse-string suture is used to repair the incision through which the siphon tube was inserted and an attempt is made to relocate the caecum back to its normal position. If the caecum is kinked or twisted, removal of the fluid may well allow the torsion to correct itself. The laparotomy is closed in the normal way. Postoperative treatment is usual with fluid therapy if dehydration is evident and antibiotics to prevent peritonitis developing. This can be a rewarding operation and most animals make an uneventful recovery.

Intussusception

Intussusception or telescoping of the bowel occurs in adult cattle and calves. The annual incidence in adult cattle is around 1 or 2 per 10 000 but may be more common in calves. The condition is caused by strong peristaltic movements of the intestine and either the small intestine telescopes into small intestine or occasionally through the ileo-caecal valve into the caecum. In calves the condition is usually a sequel to profuse diarrhoea but this appears not necessarily to be the case in adult cattle. Some workers have suggested that a tumour or inflammatory growth in the lumen of the affected part may be a causative factor in adult cattle.

Signs

When the intussusception first occurs there will be mild signs of colic. These signs frequently go unnoticed by the stockworker or if they are seen they are discounted because they do not last for long and the animal makes an apparent recovery. Two to three days later the animal's milk production declines, inappetence sets in and the astute stockworker may notice the animal to be constipated. This is the most frequent time veterinary attention is sought.

Examination will reveal a normal rectal temperature, the heart rate raised to 80–120/minute and auscultation will reveal bowel stasis. A rectal examination will reveal an empty rectum or the presence of scanty bloodstained faeces or thickened mucus. On questioning, the stockworker may admit that colic signs were evident two to three days earlier.

Diagnosis

In many cases rectal palpation will reveal a hard, sausage-shaped mass in the right abdomen. The absence of any dilated organ and complete bowel stasis will indicate a strong likelihood that an intussusception is present even if it cannot be palpated, although simple rumen indigestion may be difficult to differentiate. Palpation of the offending intussusception may be made easier if the floor of the abdomen is raised using a pole under the ventral abdomen and lifted by two persons. The course of this disease is not as acute as other causes of intestinal obstructions; thus if the clinician is not certain of the diagnosis, mild purgatives such as liquid paraffin or linseed oil may be administered orally and the case re-assessed 24 hours later. These will do no harm if an intussusception exists and if the problem is one of indigestion faeces will be passed within 24 hours. It is important to instruct the stockworker to isolate the animal in a clean pen for this period so that any faeces voided will be observed. One of many problems with loose-housing systems is that accurate history of whether an animal is eating forage, defecating or urinating is frequently unavailable.

If no faeces have been voided in the 24 hours of isolation an exploratory laparotomy must be contemplated.

Treatment

An exploratory laparotomy in the right sublumbar fossa should be carried out if the farmer is willing. Failing this, casualty slaughter should be carried out. Exploration of the abdominal cavity will reveal the hard mass of the intussusception, although when it is exteriorized it may not be recognizable as such. It may appear more like a bloodstained tumour. Normal gut should be identified entering and leaving the mass, which should then be surgically removed and intestinal anastomosis performed. If the mass is recognizable as an intussusception, as may be the case if diagnosis was prompt, on no account should an attempt be made to unravel the intussusception. Although this may well be possible, the offending length of gut must be considered to be diseased because it will certainly reform as an intussusception within 24 hours of correction. Some workers have suggested that if intussusceptions are not removed surgically, but conservative treatment principles applied, the necrotic tissues of the intussusception will slough out in 10–14 days and the animal will recover. This approach to treatment is not to be recommended because in the author's experience animals that are not treated surgically will die.

The intestinal anastomosis does require some surgical skill but should not be beyond the majority of large animal surgeons. The technique has been performed quite satisfactorily on the farm.

INTUSSUSCEPTION IN CALVES

In calves intussusception is a sequel to acute diarrhoea. Signs of colic will be present in the initial stages of the disease but frequently the animal is presented because it is not defecating or is collapsed. Occasionally, the intussusception can be palpated through the abdominal wall and if the calf is not in an advanced state of shock an exploratory laparotomy may be considered and the offending lesion removed surgically and intestinal anastomosis performed. Unfortunately, in calves the condition is most commonly encountered at post mortem.

Diaphragmatic hernia

Diaphragmatic hernia has occasionally been reported in cattle but the condition is rare and the incidence is probably less than 1 per 100 000 per year. The clinical signs will depend on which abdominal organs are prolapsed through the hernia. The condition may be a sequel to traumatic reticulitis where the diaphragm has been weakened.

The most commonly prolapsed organ seems to be the reticulum and the result is interference with the motility and function of the rumen and reticulum. Colic signs will be noticed at the time of the rupture but they do not persist. Signs similar to vagus indigestion may be apparent, although low-grade pain in the posterior thorax/anterior abdomen region rather like traumatic reticulitis has been noticed. Respiratory signs may be apparent due to reduced thoracic space. A definitive diagnosis is unlikely to be made without recourse to an exploratory laparotomy and then if a diagnosis is made it is unlikely that surgical correction will succeed.

Fat necrosis (lipomatosis, peritoneal fat necrosis)

Lipomatosis or peritoneal fat necrosis occurs sporadically (annual incidence 1–5 per 100 000) in old cows with a suggested predisposition towards Channel Island and Aberdeen Angus breeds. Affected cows may not present any signs and the condition is detected at routine rectal examination. Advance cases of the condition will show signs of weight loss, underperformance and inappetence. The diagnosis will be based on rectal palpation findings when large hard masses can be palpated in the abdominal cavity. Occasionally, fat in the pelvic canal will be affected and the canal will be almost completely occluded, and it is nearly impossible to carry out rectal palpation because of lack of space.

There is no treatment and slaughter should be advised. On post mortem as much as 20–25 kg of hard necrotic fat may be present in the omentum and mesentery.

Peritonitis (see also p. 113)

Peritonitis is a local or general, acute or chronic, inflammation of the peritoneal cavity. Peritonitis usually occurs as an accompanying condition of other specific diseases, e.g. traumatic reticulo-peritonitis (p. 643) or metritis (p. 427). The most common cause of peritonitis is traumatic reticulitis followed by peritonitis as a sequel to metritis, dystokia or retained afterbirth. However, peritonitis may be a sequel to abdominal surgery, a ruptured abomasal or intestinal ulcer, penetration of the intestinal tract by foreign bodies, pancreatic necrosis, rupture of biliary or urinary tracts, an infected umbilicus in calves, rupture of the rectum, uterus or large intestine, tuberculosis, liver abscesses, and chronic right- or left-sided displacement of the abomasum. Peritonitis can also be associated with septicaemic conditions such as anthrax and calf septicaemia.

Signs

The clinical signs include a raised rectal temperature, which is frequently in the range 39–40 °C (102.5–103.5 °F), respiration is frequently shallow and pulse and respiratory rates are increased. The back is moderately arched, there is a reluctance to move and walking sometimes instigates grunting. Appetite and milk production are invariably depressed and rumination ceases.

Diagnosis

The diagnosis of peritonitis can be difficult and is based on the history and clinical findings. However, the condition should be suspected in all cows that are presented with the above clinical signs and a thorough examination may reveal which organ is responsible. Ballottement of the lower right flank may reveal splashing sounds indicating the presence of fluid in the peritoneum and also may cause the animal to grunt. For a more detailed description of the diagnosis of traumatic reticulo-peritonitis see p. 643. The history may also be helpful in arriving at a diagnosis, e.g. recent dystokia or abdominal surgery. If metritis is suspected, a rectal or vaginal examination will aid the diagnosis. Abdominal paracentesis should reveal the presence of peritoneal fluid, which will be foul smelling and contain a large number of white blood cells.

The severity and extent of the peritonitis is usually

reflected in the severity of the clinical signs. If the peritonitis is generalized and acute, the animal groans on expiration. When only a limited area of the peritoneum is involved, as in traumatic reticulo-peritonitis, pain will only be evident when the exact location is percussed.

It is important to attempt to determine the cause of the peritonitis in order to give an accurate prognosis and to determine the line of treatment that should be followed.

Prognosis

Localized peritonitis has a favourable prognosis, providing the offending organ can be identified and corrective action taken. However, in acute generalized peritonitis the prognosis can be poor, particularly if the peritonitis is a sequel to abdominal surgery, dystokia or a ruptured abdominal viscus. The prognosis will be related to the severity of the clinical signs, the degree of depression, the weakness of the pulse and the extent of the signs of toxaemia.

Treatment

Treatment may first be directed to correction of the initial problem. However, the peritonitis itself will be treated with large doses of antibiotics administered intraperitoneally, intravenously and intramuscularly. An initial dose of 5 g of benzylpenicillin and 5 g of dihydrostreptomycin is administered into the peritoneum via the right sublumbar fossa, using a 2-inch 16-gauge needle followed immediately by 5 g of procaine penicillin G and 5 g of dihydrostreptomycin by intramuscular injection and every 12 hours for three to five days. Some workers have reported success using heparin by intramuscular injection at a dose of 50 000 iu twice daily for three days in addition to antibiotic therapy (Breukink, 1980).

Diarrhoea

Diarrhoea in adult cattle is a frequent sign and is present in many diseases. It may occur sporadically, affecting only individual animals or it may be present in a large number if not the whole of the group. If the whole group is affected, one must consider the feed or the possible presence of a virus infection as in winter dysentery. Blood may be present, in which case dysentery is used to describe the sign. The diarrhoea may be very watery or even projectile as in redwater (pipe stem diarrhoea). The colour and odour may be distinctive. Dark, foul-smelling, liquid faeces would indicate the presence of occult blood and haemorrhage in the upper small intestine. Pale, pasty-coloured faeces may indicate rumen acidosis. Diarrhoea with air bubbles is frequently attributed to Johne's disease. Endotoxaemia from a coliform mastitis or metritis will produce dark watery faeces. Infections with agents such as *Campylobacter* spp. or BVD/mucosal disease virus will also produce diarrhoea and *Salmonella* spp. often produce dysentery. Intestinal parasitism will produce diarrhoea of varying intensity depending on the severity of the problem, although this more commonly affects growing cattle than adults.

Non-inflammatory diseases, e.g. cardiac failure, lymphosarcoma and systemic amyloidosis, also produce diarrhoea by increasing intestinal secretion into the bowel lumen.

The clinician is frequently presented with an adult bovine where the only sign is an afebrile diarrhoea. Clinical examination may reveal sluggish rumen movements but no other signs of indigestion or of abomasal disease. Many of these cases will be the result of ingestion of toxic plants if the cattle are grazing or being fed conserved fodder and frequently the cause may be a small batch of soiled or spoiled silage.

Some cows with such acute diarrhoea die rapidly and post-mortem examination reveals a severe enteritis, frequently haemorrhagic but the examination for infections or parasite counts proves unrewarding. One usually assumes that the cause of death is poisoning but frequently the toxic agent is not discovered. When presented with individual cows showing diarrhoea and no systemic disease or other signs present, the cow must be removed from its present food source, isolated and given only dry feed, such as hay, to eat. Treatment with antibiotics such as streptomycin may be instituted, although the efficacy in these situations is not proven. Spasmolytics may help and oral therapy with gut sedatives such as chlorodyne or absorbents such as kaolin are frequently used but again their efficacy is not proven. The addition of glycine/electrolytes to the drinking water has more recently been suggested, but in cases where severe dehydration is present intravenous administration of 20–40 l of balanced electrolytes is indicated.

If the herd or group are all affected, one must remember that lush spring grass will produce diarrhoea as will wet autumn grass in the UK. Wet grass silage will also produce fluid faeces. In some areas of the UK and in other countries molybdenum toxicity is common, e.g. on the so-called teart pastures of Somerset, and this will produce severe diarrhoea in the whole grazing herd but can be corrected by the administration of copper in the form of copper sulphate to the diets.

An infectious cause of a whole group of cattle to be affected with diarrhoea is winter dysentery (see p. 659) but infection with *Salmonella typhimurium* or *S. montevideo* may spread rapidly through a herd but the animals will also be pyrexic.

Thus diarrhoea is a sign of many disease conditions of cattle but frequently enteritis will occur in individual animals and the cause will remain undetermined. There remains a challenge for the bovine practitioner.

Salmonellosis

Infection of adult cattle with a variety of *Salmonella* spp. is frequently encountered in cattle practice (see Chapter 13). In the UK as many as 100–200 herds per 10 000 may suffer the disease each year where it affects a considerable proportion of the herd. The incidence of sporadic salmonellosis, where only one or two animals in the herd are affected, may be as high as 500–1000 per 10 000 herds. These sporadic occurrences are usually abortions due to *S. dublin*. A variety of *Salmonella* spp. have been known to affect cattle but the two most prominent are *S. dublin* and *S. typhimurium*. *Salmonella newport* and *S. montevideo* are less frequently reported and sporadic outbreaks with other species occasionally occur. The most serious problems are associated with enteritis and septicaemia, but sporadic outbreaks of abortion with no concurrent septicaemia or enteritis are frequently encountered due to *S. dublin*. Abortion appears different from the enteritis and septicaemia syndrome and will be dealt with separately (p. 471).

Epidemiology and aetiology

The aetiological agents *S. typhimurium* and *S. dublin* are those most frequently encountered although other species are reported sporadically. The epidemiology of *S. dublin* and *S. typhimurium* appear to differ.

It has been known for some time that to establish *S. dublin* carrier status in the adult cow there needs to be damage to the liver and/or bile ducts. The most frequent cause of liver damage is liver fluke and in areas where liver fluke is endemic, the incidence of *S. dublin* enteritis is more common. The source of infection for *S. dublin* is therefore carrier cows, most of which are suffering liver damage from liver fluke and if liver fluke is endemic in a herd, *S. dublin* may spread rapidly. In areas where *S. dublin* infection is unusually high, the organism can frequently be isolated from rivers, streams and ditches. It is difficult to postulate the role this contamination has on the spread of the infection as one would expect the watercourses to be infected if carrier cows exist in the area.

The carrier status probably also exists with *S. typhimurium* but this is much less common than with *S. dublin*. The majority of *S. typhimurium* outbreaks in adult cattle are of sudden onset and indicate a recent introduction of the infection into the herd. The most common sourse of infection is probably purchased contaminated compound feeds. These feeds often used to contain processed animal protein, which was frequently infected with *Salmonella* spp. Cross-infection to cereals also occurs when common storage bins and mixing equipment are used. Cross-contamination of animal feeds may also be caused by wild birds or rodents that may live in animal feed production premises. A further source of infection for *S. typhimurium* is rivers or streams. In many rural areas public sewerage facilities do not exist and septic tanks or cess pits are used. If these do not function satisfactorily, raw or part-treated sewage finds its way into rivers. Human infection has also been the cause of infection when cattle have grazed fields in which human defecation is known to have occurred or fields that are situated next to lay-bys on busy main roads.

On occasions cows have been shown to be excreting *S. typhimurium* but yet not show signs of disease, i.e. they are carrier cows. The presence of a carrier cow within a herd may go undetected and no problem exists with the rest of the herd. The reason why the infection does not spread in these situations is not clear. It may be that a minimum infective dose is required to establish disease or the immune system of the animals may be depressed with a virus infection spreading within the herd and this allows *Salmonella* infection to develop into disease.

Signs

The principal signs produced by *Salmonella* infections are acute enteritis and septicaemia with a sudden onset of severe diarrhoea or dysentery. Frequently, the mucous membrane lining of the small intestine is passed with the faeces and, occasionally, blood clots are present.

The rectal temperature is 40.5–41.5 °C (105–107 °F) and the cow is severely depressed. The severity of the signs varies considerably. If the disease occurs at or near parturition, septicaemia sets in and mortality may be as high as 20 per cent of affected animals, particularly with *S. dublin* infections. *Salmonella typhimurium* produces morbidity varying from 10 to 70 per cent of the herd but mortality is generally not high except that it will be higher if infection occurs at or around calving.

If infection with *S. typhimurium* or *S. dublin* occurs during late pregnancy, seriously affected animals will frequently abort. This is probably a result of the fever and septicaemia rather than the infection directly affecting the fetus or placenta. *Salmonella dublin* will cause abortion without enteritis and septicaemia being present but the epidemiology and pathogenesis is different. This will be discussed under *Salmonella dublin* abortion (see p. 471). Animals that abort following septicaemia and enteritis frequently develop acute septic metritis and peritonitis and frequently die.

Diagnosis

The diagnosis is confirmed by the isolation of *Salmonella* spp. from faeces of affected animals. The faeces of all cattle presented with acute enteritis accompanied with fever should be sampled and tested for *Salmonella* spp. by bacteriological isolation. Affected animals should be kept in isolation until the result is known.

Treatment

Antibiotics administered parenterally are used for the treatment of salmonellosis. Due to resistance to some antibiotics an *in vitro* antibiotic sensitivity test should be performed as soon as possible. Resistance to penicillin, streptomycin, the tetracyclines and ampicillin is widespread with *S. typhimurium*. The neomycin, framycetin, are frequently effective and resistance to chloramphenicol and gentamycin is rare. The combination of trimethoprim and sulphadiazine is also frequently used. There is always some controversy regarding the use of antibiotics in treating salmonellosis in adult cattle. Septicaemic cases and complications following abortion should always be treated with antibiotics. However, in a herd outbreak, some animals will be less severely affected than others and will recover spontaneously without the use of antibiotics. Antibiotic therapy will need to be administered for three to five days.

Oral rehydration therapy is indicated where dehydration is evident and if the dehydration is severe, intravenous administration of 30 l of balanced electrolyte solution will prove to be a valuable support to antibiotic therapy. Recovery time can be quite variable. Cattle with mild enteritis will recover within two days, whereas severe septicaemic cases may take one to two weeks to recover their previous appetite and will not normally return to previous levels of milk production.

Control

Once the diagnosis has been confirmed in a herd, it is important to limit the spread within the herd. Isolation of affected animals will help but by the time cows are identified with enteritis, *Salmonella* organisms will be isolated from any site on the farm frequented by the cattle. Vaccination of non-affected animals should be considered. In the UK there are two vaccines available, a live vaccine prepared from an avirulent strain of *S. dublin* (Mellavax, Cooper Pitman Moore Ltd) and a dead vaccine prepared from formalin-killed cells of *S. dublin* and *S. typhimurium* (Bovivac, Hoechst UK Ltd) The live vaccine is not licensed for use in adult cattle and although it only contains *S. dublin* antigens, it does produce some cross-protection against *S. typhimurium*. In the face of an outbreak and the need rapidly to limit the spread of infection, the live vaccine is preferred to the dead vaccine, which requires two injections 21 days apart. Although not licensed for use in adult cattle, a number of practitioners in the UK have used the live vaccine in herds of cows when either *S. dublin* or *S. typhimurium* have been spreading through the herd, with apparently favourable results. Following vaccination, new cases of enteritis occur for up to 14 days after injection after which the problem appears to stop.

If *S. dublin* is identified as the causal organism, a representative number of faeces samples (usually six to twelve) should be examined for the presence of liver fluke ova and if positive the herd should receive appropriate anthelmintic therapy.

It is essential when salmonellosis occurs on a farm that the utmost care should be taken regarding personal hygiene. All the staff should be made aware of the zoonotic implications and should not consume milk during the course of an outbreak. In the UK, *Salmonella* isolation must be reported to the relevant departments of agriculture, who monitor the infection nationally although very little action is taken against the farmer unless there is a perceived human health risk, e.g. fresh milk is being used for yoghurt, cream or cottage cheese production, in which case the public health authorities may insist on pasteurization of the milk prior to processing. The question is frequently asked: Should recovered cases be kept and will they become permanent carriers? Practice experience would indicate that in the majority of outbreaks of *S. typhimurium* the problem rarely recurs. It is only very occasionally that a herd may become chronically infected and sporadic cases will continue to occur. More usually the infection is confined to the calves in endemically infected herds. In the case of *S. dublin* enteritis the main thrust in control following vaccination is to control liver fluke in the herd. If this is successfully achieved, enteritis caused by *S. dublin* will be infrequent.

Attempts to identify carrier cows within endemically infected herds are sometimes recommended. This is achieved by faeces sampling the entire herd and culturing the sample for *Salmonella* spp. Unfortunately, *Salmonella* spp. are excreted intermittently in carrier cows and animals need to be sampled on several occasions, probably as many as six or seven, to be reasonably certain all carrier cows are identified. This procedure has proved to be neither practical nor necessary in most outbreaks.

Prevention

To prevent infection with *S. typhimurium* may be difficult because of the frequency in which it is found in animal feeds. Contamination of feed can also be caused by rodents and birds. However, legislation has been implemented in the UK to supervise all protein processing plants and to ensure the protein material is sterilized. It is likely that in the future infections entering the herd via purchased feeds will become less frequent.

Preventing infection spreading from the human population to cattle can be achieved to some extent by the supply of clean wholesome water for cattle to drink. For the effective control of a variety of infections cattle should not be allowed to drink from natural watercourses. Effective fencing of fields may also be required, particularly alongside main roads and lay-bys to prevent humans using grazing fields as a lavatory.

Winter dysentery

As the name implies, winter dysentery occurs during the period of winter housing and affects cattle of all ages. It is obviously an extremely infectious disease because when it enters a herd it rapidly spreads through all animals in the herd. Also, once infected and the animals have recovered, the herd will not usually experience the problem for four or five years thus indicating a herd immunity developing.

Moreover, once one herd in an area becomes infected, it appears to spread rapidly to other herds nearby. Perhaps this is a disease that can be spread by veterinary surgeons! However, it is interesting that there has been very little mention of its occurrence in the UK during the last 15–20 years, whereas during the late 1950s and early 1960s it was frequently encountered. It has been reported to be present in several countries in Europe and the northern States of the USA and Canada have experienced large outbreaks in past years. Although the morbidity is almost 100 per cent, mortality is normally absent. Milk production, however, may be reduced by up to 50 per cent and take up to two weeks to recover and so it is of economic importance.

Aetiology

Campylobacter fetus var. *jejuni* was once thought to be the causative organism. But the speed of spread, the short incubation period of around three days and the inability to reproduce the disease using cultures of *C. jejuni* leads one to suspect the aetiological agent is a virus, which to date has not been identified. However, coronaviruses have been encountered in several outbreaks.

Signs

The main sign is of a severe, watery, dark brown diarrhoea with a foul-smelling odour. The faeces may be tinged with blood. The diarrhoea is sometimes described as explosive or projectile. At first only one or two cows in the herd are affected but within three or four days several cows will show signs and within two weeks all the older cattle on the farm will have become affected. The rectal temperature is usually normal, and appetite is reduced in only a small number of more severely affected animals. However, milk yield may be reduced by up to 50 per cent and such animals may show signs of abdominal pain, e.g. colic, arched back or a 'hunched up' appearance may be apparent. The course of the disease in most cows is two to three days.

Diagnosis

The severity and speed of spread of the disease presents no real problems in diagnosis except with the initial cases, which may be misdiagnosed as a poisoning (Chapter 41) or non-specific enteritis. Once several cows are affected and the disease is occurring during the housed period, diagnosis is based on the clinical signs present.

Bovine virus diarrhoea would involve fewer animals, which would have a pyrexia and characteristic oral lesions. Coccidiosis (see p. 243) normally affects younger animals but this can be differentiated by the presence of tenesmus and the identification of oocysts in the faeces.

Treatment

Most affected cattle recover spontaneously in two to three days and treatments do not speed recovery. However, a proportion of the cases are more severely affected and some may become weak enough to become recumbent. Severely dehydrated animals will require intravenous administration of 20–30 l of balanced electrolytes and electrolytes added to the drinking water should prove advantageous. Oral astringents, such as 50 ml of 5 per cent copper sulphate administered every 12 hours, may prove effective. Morphine and chloroform (chlorodyne) reduce intestinal motility and absorbents such as kaolin or bismuth salts have also been recommended. Oral sulphonamides have been reported to be useful by some practitioners.

Prevention

This is an extremely infectious disease and when it occurs in an area cattle or unnecessary personnel should not enter the farm. Veterinary surgeons should take the utmost care in thoroughly disinfecting their boots and protective clothing before entering and leaving farms when this infection is present locally.

Bovine virus diarrhoea/mucosal disease

Bovine virus diarrhoea and mucosal disease are both diseases caused by bovine virus diarrhoea virus (BVDV), which is similar to the viruses that cause Border disease in sheep and swine fever in pigs. These three viruses are together classified as pestiviruses. The pestiviruses and rubiviruses are at present classified together in the family Togaviridae. It is worth noting that both rubella virus in humans and all three pestiviruses can cross the placenta and damage the fetus.

In 1946, veterinary workers at Cornell demonstrated that a virus was the cause of a transmissible bovine diarrhoea, and thereby named BVDV. The disease has since been identified in Australia, New Zealand, Europe, Canada as well as Great Britain. There would appear to be an increase in reported incidences of the problem in recent years. However, this is most likely the result of improved diagnostic techniques.

Aetiology (Figs 42.1 and 42.2)

Infection with BVD virus is generally a mild or even subclinical event, except on two occasions, i.e. infection of the pregnant animal and in mixed infections, e.g. with other respiratory viruses such as respiratory syncytial virus (RSV), infectious bovine rhinotracheitis virus (IBR) or parainfluenza virus (PI3).

Many isolates of BVDV occur but all appear to cross-react with convalescent BVDV sera. There are two distinct forms of the virus, distinguishable in tissue culture, cytopathic and non-cytopathic. This distinction is important in the pathogenesis and understanding of mucosal disease. Cytopathic virus in tissue culture causes severe damage to the cells and complete destruction within 48–72 hours. The non-cytopathic virus causes no cell damage and is identified by staining with fluorescein-labelled BVDV antisera.

Non-cytopathic virus can exist on its own as an infectious agent, whereas cytopathic virus, isolated from field cases of mucosal disease, is usually superimposed on to a non-cytopathic virus infection. Bovine virus diarrhoea virus is shed in nasopharyngeal secretions and urine and perhaps by aerosol droplets. Faeces is a poor source of virus.

Pathogenesis

Postnatal infection of the young or growing animal with non-cytopathic virus is usually a subclinical event. In most herds where the virus is present there is no disease-related problem. However, infection of the seronegative pregnant cow before 120 days of gestation, before the immune system of the fetus has become fully developed, can result in disease. The fetus becomes infected and may result in abortion, mummification or early fetal death. If the fetus survives until neonatal life, it may have developed a state of immune tolerance and then the virus will persist for life. The fetus at birth will be virus positive but seronegative to the persisting virus. Infection after 120 days will still cause damage to the fetus, but it does not become immunotolerant and viraemic. Such damage would include cerebellar hypoplasia resulting in ataxic calves.

Infertility. Infection of the cow in early pregnancy will cause infertility due to embryo or early fetal death. Evidence of this has been seen in North America, where an infected bull was used on two groups of heifers. One group was seropositive and the other seronegative. The seropositive heifers conceived normally but the seronegative heifers suffered infertility that lasted several weeks. These heifers eventually con-

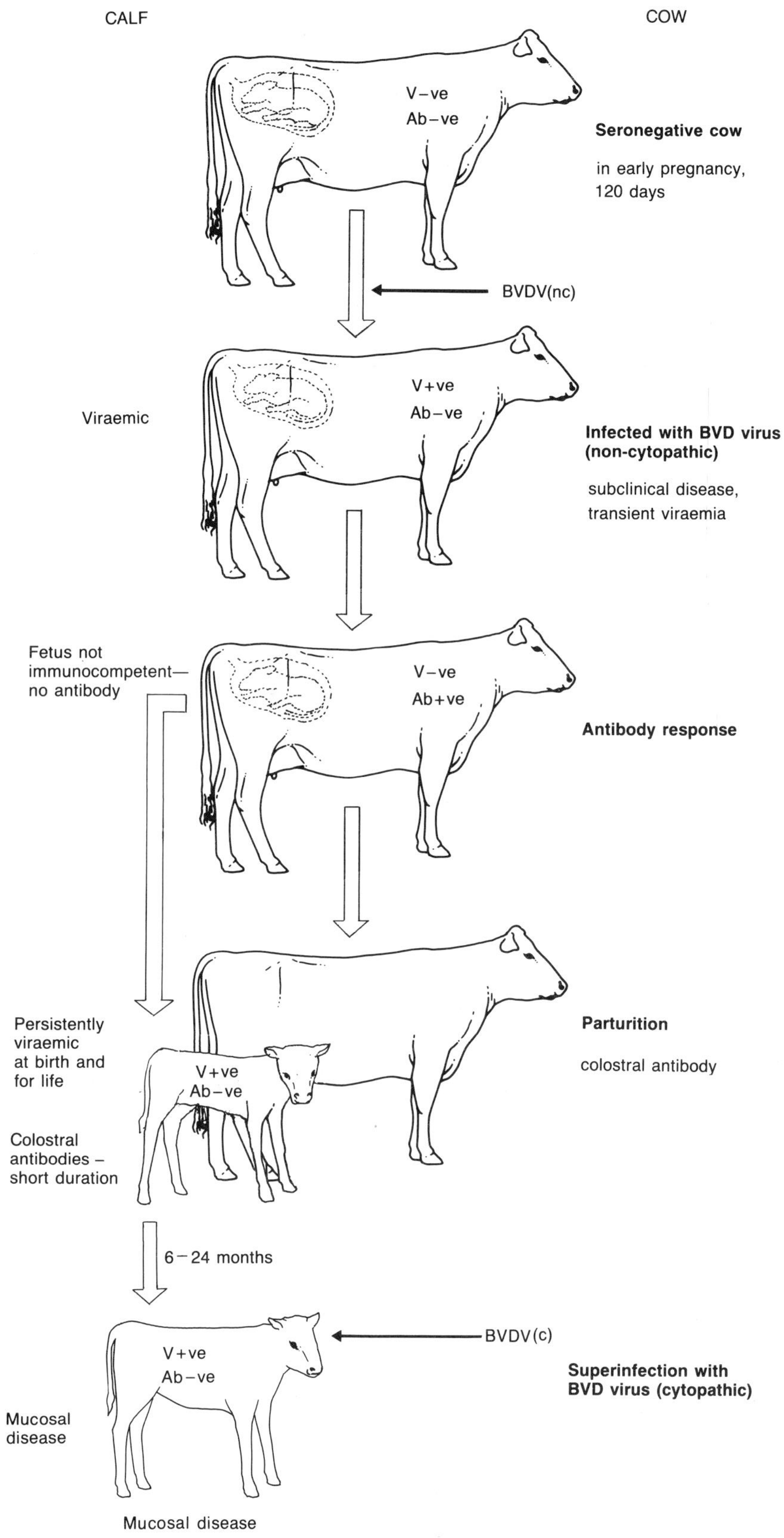

Fig. 42.1 Hypothesis for the aetiology of mucosal disease. V, BVD virus; Ab, antibody to BVD virus; nc, non-cytopathic; c, cytopathic (after Brownlie, 1985).

Category	Animal	Status	Result of exposure to BVD virus	Final antibody status
1	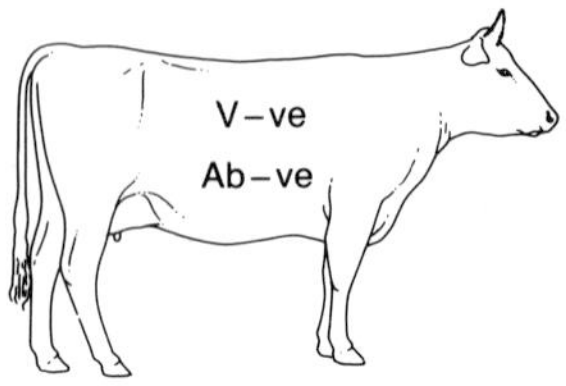 V−ve Ab−ve	No previous exposure to BVD virus	Transient mild infection	+ve
2	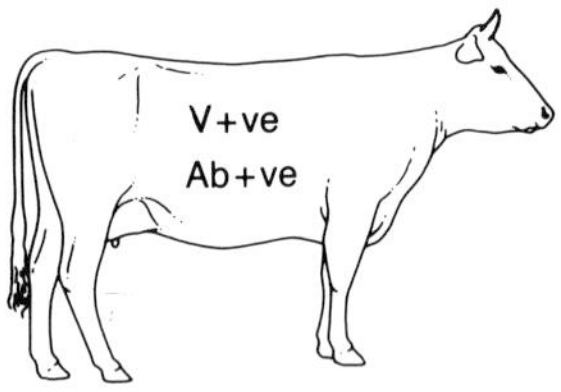 V+ve Ab+ve	Previous exposure to BVD virus from 120 days gestation onwards	Immune	+ve
3	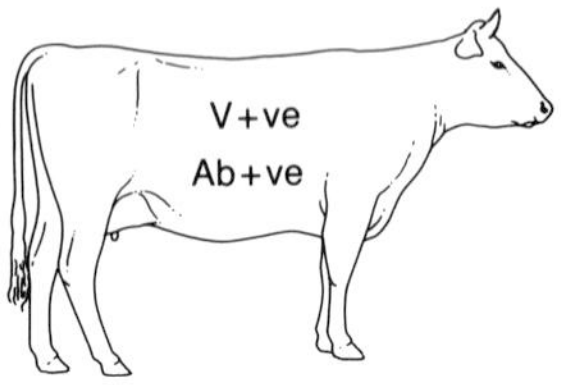 V+ve Ab+ve	(a) Acute viraemia presently sero-converting	Will become immune	+ve
		(b) Persistently viraemic; occasionally these animals may have low levels of antibody	May later succumb to mucosal disease	±ve
4	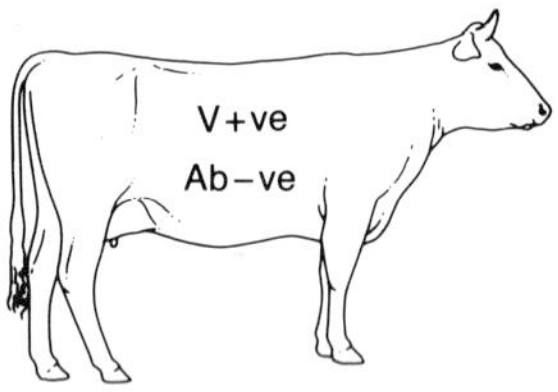 V+ve Ab−ve	(a) Acute viraemia	Will become immune	+ve
		(b) Persistently infected with BVD virus	May later succumb to mucosal disease	−ve

Fig. 42.2 Combinations of BVD virus and antibody in cattle and their significance (after Brownlie, 1985).

ceived when they had seroconverted some six to eight weeks after the initial infection.

Mixed infections. Bovine virus diarrhoea virus is immunosuppressive. Although infection of calves with BVD virus alone is generally subclinical if RSV, IBR or PI3 viruses are also present the pneumonia will be more severe than infection with respiratory viruses alone (see Chapter 15).

Mucosal disease. Mucosal disease occurs as a result of a calf that was born viraemic and seronegative becoming superinfected with cytopathic virus. Mucosal disease is generally sporadic in nature affecting young cattle six to eighteen months old. It is usual to find only one, two or three cases occurring on any one farm at the same time; however, larger outbreaks can occur. The disease is characterized by weight loss, severe diarrhoea and inevitably death. Death from mucosal disease usually occurs two to three weeks after infection with cytopathic virus.

Signs

The first signs to appear are anorexia accompanied by reddening and erosions around the dental pad, along the gingival border and under the tongue. These are followed by reddening and erosion around the muzzle. The erosions are shallow, varying sizes and shapes and frequently coalesce. These are to be distinguished from ulcers following vesicular damage, e.g. in foot-and-mouth disease (p. 537) or vesicular stomatitis (p. 546), which are deeper than mucosal disease erosions. Diarrhoea then follows and sometimes lameness may be apparent due to heat and reddening on the coronary band and erosions present in the interdigital space. Because of the sudden onset, diarrhoea is often the first sign that is noticed although salivation is frequently present. The animals are occasionally pyrexic. Weight loss is rapid and death inevitably occurs five to ten days later. Acute infections in adult cows can lead to diarrhoea and agalactia.

Necropsy

The post-mortem findings are usually strongly suggestive of mucosal disease. Oval erosions or shallow ulceration may be seen in the buccal cavity, oesophagus, abomasum, the small intestine beneath the Peyer's patches and in the colon. Oedema and erythema in the intestinal epithelium may also be a feature. The prime sites are oesophagus, small intestine and abomasum. Care must be exercised in opening the small intestine, which must be opened at the mesenteric attachment in order not to incise through the lesions. Virus can be cultured in tissue culture from all the lesions and also from mesenteric lymph nodes, spleen, thymus and tonsil.

Diagnosis

The diagnosis of mucosal disease will be based on the clinical signs and laboratory tests. Pyrexia, diarrhoea, erosions in the mouth and on the muzzle and recent weight loss in an animal six to eighteen months old should be highly suggestive of mucosal disease. In the live animal, clotted and EDTA blood samples and a nasopharyngeal swab should be taken and must be submitted to the laboratory within 24 hours for both virus isolation and for BVDV antibodies. It is also helpful to submit fresh spleen, mediastinal lymph node, thymus and small intestinal tissue (particularly with Peyer's patch tissue) for virus isolation.

Differential diagnosis

The main features of mucosal disease are mucosal erosions, diarrhoea and death. Foot-and-mouth disease (p. 537), malignant catarrh and rinderpest (p. 543) are the principal differential diagnoses. With foot-and-mouth disease morbidity is 100 per cent and vesicles precede the mucosal ulcerations. With malignant catarrh corneal opacity is a feature; there is also gastroenteritis and enlarged lymph nodes. Lymph node enlargement is not a feature of mucosal disease. Rinderpest has vesicles preceding the erosions, morbidity is high and intestinal oedema and lymph node enlargement is common. *Salmonella* (p. 657) enteritis should not present a problem with differential diagnosis as it generally affects either young calves or adult animals and there are no mouth lesions. Acorn poisoning can look similar on post mortem but biochemistry and histology of the kidney should distinguish it from mucosal disease (see p. 623). Other poisoning events may also be considered as a differential diagnosis but the characteristic oval erosions are generally absent.

Treatment

There is no effective treatment for mucosal disease. If the disease is suspected all efforts should be towards a diagnosis so that effective control measures may be instituted.

Control

When a positive diagnosis has been made, the dam of the affected animal and all the animals in the same group as the affected animal should be blood sampled and the blood cultured for the presence of virus. Persistently viraemic cows invariably give rise to viraemic calves so all dams of viraemic offspring need to be identified. If infection is a recent introduction then several calves in the same age group as the affected one may also be persistently viraemic. Most of these are likely to succumb to mucosal disease at some time in the future.

When testing for BVDV, one should be aware of the possibility of sampling a calf that is only acutely infected and not persistently viraemic. To differentiate this possibility all virus-positive animals should be retested at an interval of six weeks. Persistently viraemic calves should be slaughtered. There is no vaccine available in the UK; however, in the USA vaccines prepared from attenuated cytopathic virus are available, but it is believed that these have occasionally caused disease. An effective killed vaccine is required but as yet is unavailable.

It is important to recall that surveys have suggested that 1 per cent of adult animals in the national herd are persistently viraemic. The retention of viraemic animals in the herd is one strategy used to maintain herd immunity. However, there is always a risk that susceptible cows in early pregnancy can become infected. Therefore, once persistently viraemic animals have been identified they should be slaughtered unless they can, with certainty, be kept away from cows in early pregnancy. All newly introduced animals should be isolated and screened for the presence of antibody and virus before mixing with the herd. Persistently viraemic animals should not be kept.

Johne's disease (paratuberculosis)

Johne's disease is a chronic, infectious enteritis that results in progressive wasting and eventual death. The disease has been reported world-wide wherever ruminants exist and the causal organism is the acid-fast bacterium *Mycobacterium johnei* (*paratuberculosis*). The prevalence of Johne's disease varies between countries and within countries.

There appear to be endemically infected farms on which the incidence can be as high as two or three confirmed cases every year, yet in the same district there will be many farms that do not experience the disease, except occasionally in a purchased animal. In the UK the incidence has declined considerably over the last 30 years, although the incidence in some northern European countries is still rather high.

Pathogenesis

Infection with *M. johneii* occurs in young calves usually from their dams or contact with faeces of carrier cows. There follows a long incubation period of two to six years during which lesions develop in the small intestine and the animals intermittently excrete the organism in the faeces. Not all infected animals progress to the disease state. Where the disease does develop, the organisms multiply and cause extensive lesions in the small intestine that produce overt clinical disease.

Signs

The usual presenting signs are profuse diarrhoea accompanied by gradual weight loss. Frequently, the stress of calving initiates the onset of symptoms and affected cows are presented two to four weeks after calving. Rectal temperature, appetite and ruminal contractions remain normal. Submandibular oedema is sometimes present. In advanced cases the weight loss leads to an emaciation and the diarrhoea remains profuse often with bubbles in the faeces.

Necropsy

The main pathological features are thickening of the lower part of the small intestine, the ileo-caecal valve and sometimes the colon. The mucosal surface has a corrugated appearance. The organism may be present on the mucosal surface or tissue sections of the intestinal wall may reveal both intracellular and extracellular organisms.

Diagnosis

Any debilitating disease that results in emaciation may be confused with Johne's disease. However, the profuse diarrhoea, frequently containing bubbles, will distinguish the condition from weight loss caused by liver fluke (p. 238), liver disease, chronic traumatic reticulo-perito-nitis or malnutrition. Johne's disease should always be considered as a possible diagnosis when a cow, four years old or more, and recently calved is presented with weight loss and chronic diarrhoea. The history of the prevalence of the disease on the farm will also be helpful. Diagnosis is best confirmed by the demonstration of clumps of acid-fast bacteria in smears of faeces stained with Ziehl–Nielsen stain. As excretion can be intermittent, repeat testing is sometimes necessary. The faeces sample is best taken from the rectum using a gloved hand, scraping faeces from the rectal mucosal surface. Failure to detect the organism in faecal smears does not rule out the possibility of Johne's disease. However, the organism can usually be detected at post mortem in stained impression smears of the mucosal surface of the terminal ileum or in histological sections of the same area of ileum.

A complement fixation test for Johne's disease antibodies in blood is available in the UK but this is generally regarded to be of little value as many false positives occur, presumably due to cross-reaction with other non-pathogenic *Mycobacterium* species.

In some countries, Johnin is used as a diagnostic test and can be administered intradermally or intravenously. Injected intradermally, Johnin produces an oedematous swelling at the site of injection in some cattle that are infected with Johne's disease. When injected intravenously Johnin will initiate a rectal temperature rise of at least 0.8 °C (1.5 °F) 4–8 hours after injection. However, as with the complement fixation test the use of Johnin as an accurate diagnostic indicator is not to be regarded as reliable.

If a definite diagnosis is required, the organism can be cultured from faeces, portions of terminal ileum, or mesenteric lymph nodes but positive results will not be available for six to eight weeks.

Treatment

Treatment of Johne's disease is not to be recommended as the clinical signs are only evident in the terminal stages of the disease. Antibiotics effective against Gram-negative bacteria, e.g. streptomycin, have been used but without any long-term success. A short remission of the diarrhoea is sometimes possible following a seven-day course of streptomycin and may be considered if for some reason it is not practical to cull the affected animal immediately. If dehydration is evident rehydration with intravenous fluid therapy may allow the animal to be sent for human consumption.

Control

As infection with the Johne's disease organism occurs in calf-hood the main plank in any control programme is to separate the calves from their dams immediately after birth and rear them completely separate from the adult herd. They should not be allowed access to faeces from adult cows at any time during the growing period and all drinking water should be from uncontaminated sources, namely mains water.

In the UK and elsewhere a live vaccine (p. 811) is available for use in endemically affected herds. The vaccine used is licensed by the Ministry of Agriculture, Fisheries and Food and can only be used on farms where a positive diagnosis has been made from faeces or postmortem material. Calves are separated from their dams at birth and the vaccine administered subcutaneously in the brisket area in the first seven days of life. A fibro-caseous nodule 2–5 cm in diameter is produced at the injection site and this remains for life.

Vaccinated animals will produce positive reactions to both the avian and bovine tuberculin administered during tuberculosis testing. Usually, the avian reaction is greater than the bovine so differentiation from tuberculosis is possible if the comparative intradermal tuberculosis test is used.

Vaccination in endemic herds has met with considerable success in reducing the incidence of disease in them. However, to be successful separation of the calves from the adults and good hygiene is necessary in addition to vaccination.

Tenesmus

Tenesmus or ineffectual straining to defecate is commonly a sign of disorders of the pelvic cavity, the rectum and some diseases of the alimentary canal.

Tenesmus can be produced by profuse watery diarrhoea or dysentery, constipation, parturition, prolapsed vagina or rectum, vaginitis, urethral calculi, cystitis, lipomatosis of the pelvic cavity and coccidiosis. Tenesmus is also an important sign of ragwort poisoning. Manual examination of the rectum or vagina will produce tenesmus, which will be all the more severe if diarrhoea is present. Rectal or vaginal lacerations as the result of sticks or broom handles being inserted into the vagina or rectum by sadistic individuals will also cause tenesmus. In practice, the most commonly encountered reason for tenesmus is a cow that continues to strain after calving. This can be due to a second calf in the pelvic canal, a retained afterbirth or lacerations to the vaginal wall. The most effective treatment in these situations is to remove the calf if one is present or administer a local epidural anaesthetic.

A thorough examination is essential in cattle exhibiting tenesmus. Vaginal examination should be carried out using a vaginascope to prevent further damage, although frequently signs of vaginal damage may be apparent by separating the vulval lips. A rectal examination will normally be necessary, particularly if constipation is suspected, but a gloved well-lubricated arm should be used because this procedure may exacerbate the condition. Every effort must be made to identify the cause of the tenesmus so that corrective therapy can then be applied.

Diseases of the rectum and anus

Rectal prolapse

Rectal prolapse is less common in cattle than in other species. However, it may occur as a result of prolonged tenesmus associated with vaginal lesions, or coccidiosis and it has been associated with laurel poisoning. The condition appears to be more common in the Hereford than other cattle breeds.

Treatment

The rectum, if not excessively swollen, can be replaced under epidural anaesthesia and a pursestring suture using umbilical tape inserted around the anal ring.

In recurrent cases a submucosal resection may be required.

Rectal tears

Rectal lacerations are occasionally produced during rectal examinations. They may also be produced by sticks or poles being inserted into the rectum by sadistic individuals. If the tear is completely through the rectal wall repair via a laparotomy may be possible, although it is not easy to reach the pelvic cavity from a laparotomy incision. Also, to succeed the repair must be effected immediately the laceration occurs, otherwise faecal material will have entered the pelvic and abdominal cavities. The judicious clinician will advise immediate casualty slaughter in such cases.

Recto-vaginal fistula

Recto-vaginal fistulae are invariably the result of severe dystokia, usually in first-calving heifers. Tearing of the vulva can sometimes involve the anus or occasionally a foot of the fetus punctures the roof of the vagina and the floor of the rectum and a fistula results. These normally heal and the animal thereafter defecates via the vagina. Attempts at surgical repair are sometimes recommended because pneumovagina or vaginal contamination with faeces produces infertility. Although conception will not occur in cows so affected if natural service is used, it may be successful using artificial insemination because the semen is deposited in the anterior cervix or the body of the uterus thus bypassing the vaginal damage.

References

Breukink, H.J. (1980) The effect of heparin in the treatment of general peritonitis in cows. In *Proceedings of the XIth International Congress on Diseases of Cattle*, Tel Aviv, pp. 1442–45.

Jack, E.J. (1985) The cold cow syndrome — the Cornish experience. In *Proceedings of British Cattle Veterinary Association Meeting, London, January 1985*, p. 203.

Pinsent, P.J.N. (1977) The diagnosis of the surgical disorders of the bovine abomasum. *Bovine Practitioner*, **12**, 40–57.

Pinsent, P.J.N. (1978) The diagnosis of the surgical disorders of the bovine abomasum. *Bovine Practitioner*, **13**, 45–50.

Stober, M. & Dirkson, G. (1977) The differential diagnosis of abdominal findings (adspection, rectal examination and exploratory laparotomy) in cattle. *Bovine Practitioner*, **12**, 35–9.

Williams, E.I. (1975) The 'reticular grunt' test for traumatic reticulo-peritonitis. *Bovine Practitioner*, **10**, 98.

Further reading

Brownlie, J. (1985) Clinical aspects of bovine virus diarrhoea/mucosal disease complex in cattle. *In Practice*, **7**, 195–202.

Pinsent, P.J.N. (1977) The diagnosis of the surgical disorders of the bovine abdomen. *Bovine Practitioner*, **12**, 40–7.

Chapter 43: Respiratory Conditions

by A.H. ANDREWS

Acute exudative pneumonia

Aetiology

This is thought in many cases to be a primary bacterial condition and usually *Actinomyces* (*Corynebacterium*) *pyogenes* (Gram-positive rods) can be isolated, or in some cases *Pasteurella haemolytica* and *P. multocida* (Gram-negative short rods) (Pirie, 1979).

Epidemiology

This condition is not uncommon and is usually seen as respiratory disease in individual animals. It can be present in cattle of any age, particularly when there has been chronic pneumonia in the housing period. In can be seen in dairy-bred cattle as well as in suckler animals, both indoors and at grass. Individual cases usually occur but outbreaks can follow some form of stress. The condition is one of sudden onset and is mainly differentiated from acute pneumonia by the fact that it affects individual animals.

Signs

The animal shows signs of suddenly going off its feed and is dull. There is an oculo-nasal discharge which may be mucoid or mucopurulent. The temperature is usually 40–41 °C (104–107 °F), respiratory rate is between 20 and 60/minute, usually with hyperpnoea. There is often some coughing but this is not pronounced. On auscultation there are usually squeaks, humming and wheezing often at inspiration, particularly the latter. Cranio-ventrally, there may be moist sounds and there may be pleuritic rub (sandpaper-like) sounds in a few cases.

Necropsy

At post mortem there are dark areas of consolidation in the ventral parts of the apical and cardiac, and in some animals, the thoracic lobes. The areas of pneumonia may be small and scattered, but in more severe cases there are large areas of consolidation and, in some animals, abscess formation. Microscopically, there is exudation and vascular congestion with the bronchioles and alveoli showing infiltration with neutrophils and macrophages (Pirie, 1979).

Diagnosis

Diagnosis depends on the history of usually only a single animal being involved with pyrexia and respiratory signs normally being evident.

Differential diagnoses involve chronic pneumonia but normally the animals are less ill and several are affected. Inhalation pneumonia usually results in a very dull animal and also there is often a history of drenching.

Treatment and control

When treating, the affected animal should be isolated. Antibiotic therapy with oxytetracycline, penicillin and streptomycin, ampicillin, amoxycillin, sulphadimidine, trimethoprim and sulphadiazine for three to five days is usually successful. Most cases respond well to therapy, but a few cases relapse and some ultimately develop chronic suppurative pneumonia.

Prevention is by trying to ensure adequate ventilation when housed and to avoid chilling.

Aspiration pneumonia

Aetiology

This is also known as inhalation pneumonia and although not a common condition, it still occurs too frequently. Obtaining an adequate history is important and often the stockworker may realize what has happened, but will be reluctant to admit it or even that the animal has been drenched. Obstruction or paralysis of the larynx, pharynx or oesophagus may produce the problem, as with parturient paresis, or the rupture of a pharyngeal abscess or the products of laryngeal diphtheria. The signs will depend on the nature of the fluid introduced, the quantity and the bacteria introduced. If a large quantity is administered into the lungs, then instantaneous death may occur. If the substance given is soluble, then absorption into the body is rapid because of the highly vascular nature of the lungs, and few, if any signs will occur. Less soluble products will result in a varying degree of toxaemia and respiratory signs, which are often fatal, after between one and three days.

Signs

In the peracute form death occurs rapidly after drenching. However, in the acute form only one animal is usually affected and there is a history of drenching. Signs develop rapidly and include a varying degree of dullness and inappetence, a cough and tachypnoea. The temperature is usually elevated to about 40 °C (104 °F) and on auscultation there are areas of dullness present, normally in the cranio-ventral parts of the lungs, and moist bubbling and crackles may be heard in the area. There is often also a pleuritic rub sound and some degree of thoracic pain. If the condition progresses, the signs of dullness and anorexia become more pronounced, and there may be a fetid odour to the breath.

In the subacute form there are few signs present except for episodes of coughing and tachypnoea following the introduction of the fluid. Some animals will survive the immediate episode and become chronic cases. These will show ill-thrift and intermittent bouts of respiratory problems.

Necropsy

At post mortem there is often an acute exudative or gangrenous pneumonia of the ventral parts of the apical, cardiac and usually also the diaphragmatic lobes. In some animals there is extensive suppurative necrosis.

Diagnosis

Diagnosis is helped if a true history is obtained and is indicative that the condition is present. Usually only a single animal is affected and the signs are of sudden onset. The respiratory signs are severe and there is usually a leucopenia and neutrophilia present.

Differential diagnoses include septicaemia, which has less respiratory signs, enteritis but then diarrhoea is present, and acute exudative pneumonia, but in this case there is no history of drenching and usually the animal is less dull.

Treatment and control

If there is to be a hope of effective therapy, it must be administered as soon as possible after the drenching incident. The use of antibiotics or a sulphonamide is indicated and it is best to give the first dose intravenously. Thus oxytetracycline, amoxycillin, ampicillin, sulphadimidine, sulphamethoxypyridazine or sulphapyrazole can be used. In exceptional circumstances chloramphenicol might be indicated. Therapy should be continued in most cases for about five days. In addition, fluid therapy may be required. The animal should be encouraged to eat and drink. It should be kept on its own in a well-bedded, airy pen.

Control is by ensuring that all drenching and dosing is undertaken slowly, allowing the animal time to swallow.

Bovine farmer's lung

Aetiology

This is a form of chronic atypical interstitial pneumonia. The condition appears to be a chronic reaction to certain fungi found in badly made hay, such as *Micropolyspora faeni*.

Epidemiology

The problem is quite common during the winter in housed cattle fed poor quality mouldy hay or straw. More cases occur in the wetter western parts of Britain and in other countries with high rainfall. Where much rain falls in the summer months, hay may need to be baled at very high moisture contents. This allows overheating to occur and thermophilic microflora then predominate. Disease is often only seen in adult cattle and in some cases the farmer will also have farmer's lung. In Britain this is defined as an industrial injury and is considered to be due to the inhalation of dust from mouldy hay or other mouldy vegetable produce. It results in a defect in gas exchange due to a reaction in the peripheral parts of the bronchopulmonary system. In cattle the condition is usually a herd problem but occasionally a farmer will consider that there is sudden onset in one animal. In such cases the examination of other animals will show varying lesser degrees of the problem.

Signs

The acute signs follow housing and there is often a sudden onset of dullness, a fall in milk yield and a decreased appetite. The animal shows respiratory signs, normally including some respiratory distress, and coughing. On auscultation there are crackles over the cranio-ventral parts of the lung. Although some cases are pyrexic, most animals will have a normal rectal temperature.

In the chronic form there is progressive weight loss and coughing, often with the production of green mucus, which tends to occur with each winter but resolves during the summer months with outside grazing. Occasionally, such animals will develop a sudden crisis following a stress such as calving, a sudden heavy exposure to the antigen, unaccustomed exercise or due to congestive heart failure. Usually there is obvious tachypnoea and hyperpnoea but no pyrexia or thoracic pain or alteration in the resonance of the thorax. Auscultation may produce harsh crackles over the cranio-ventral aspects of the lung and in some cases there are widespread whistles, squeaks and wheezing. It is uncommon for animals to die of the condition unless there are complications.

Necropsy

At necropsy all lung lobes may be affected and there is often overinflation of the peripheral acini. Small grey–green foci tend to be present in the lobules. Histologically, the alveolar walls show interstitial infiltration with plasma cells, lymphocytes and macrophages. Another change is bronchitis obliterans and also epithelial granulomata can occur.

Diagnosis

Diagnosis depends on a history of occurrence in wet areas and feeding poor quality mouldy hay in winter. The problem improves in the summer. Signs include loss of weight with the respiratory disease. An intradermal skin test with *Micropolyspora faeni* produces a reaction 4–6 hours after injection. On serological examination precipitating antibodies to *Micropolyspora faeni* are found but they may also be seen in unaffected cattle within the same herd.

Treatment and control

The use of long-acting corticosteroids may help reduce signs. Where mouldy hay or straw has to be fed or used for bedding then it must be shaken out outside before being offered to the animals. As human problems can arise, a face mask should be worn.

Control involves improving hay-making, which may mean the use of hay additives to upgrade hay quality. Otherwise, the provision of silage might be useful but this does normally mean investment in new machinery for producing the conserved roughage.

Bovine tuberculosis

Aetiology

This is infection with *Mycobacterium bovis* (Gram-positive, acid-fast rods).

Epidemiology

At one time the condition was very common in many countries. However, following tuberculin testing, pasteurization of milk and adequate meat inspection the disease is uncommon in most countries today, but is still seen periodically mainly in dairy herds. In most cases infection breaks out in the growing heifers or younger cows. The condition is still prevalent in south-west England. In many regions infection has reappeared and is associated with the finding of tuberculosis in the European badger (*Meles meles*). Infection of deer with *M. bovis* can also spread disease and in New Zealand a problem occurs with the brush-tailed possum (*Trichosurus vulpecula*). The organism is killed by sunlight, but is resistant to desiccation and can survive in a wide range of acids and alkalis. It is also able to remain viable for long periods in soil that is moist and warm. In cattle faeces, *M. bovis* can survive for as little as a week or as long as eight weeks. Man can occasionally be infected and the disease can occur in goats and pigs, and very occasionally in horses and sheep.

When infection is by inhalation, a lesion often occurs at the point of entry and the local lymph node. When ingestion is the route of entry, alimentary lesions are rare but lesions may be present in the tonsils, pharyngeal or mesenteric lymph nodes. Lesions may then disseminate from the primary areas to others.

When the badger is involved, most infection is thought to be by ingestion, but a higher infection level is necessary to establish alimentary than respiratory infection. In most cases the lesions are respiratory and are thought to be due to the inhalation of ruminal gases.

The organism can be present in sputum, milk, faeces, urine, vaginal and uterine discharges and any discharging lesions. Entry is usually by inhalation (especially if housed) or ingestion (when outside or badgers are the source of infection). Drinking infected milk can infect the calf. Once in a herd, infection probably spreads from cow to cow by inhalation. However, spread from cows to calves may be via the milk. Occasionally, intrauterine infection has resulted from a coital transfer.

Signs

Various body systems can be infected. Often signs are few and usually are confined to the respiratory tract. There is a soft, productive, chronic cough occurring once or twice at a time. It can be elicited by pressure on the pharynx. If the condition continues there is a marked increase in the depth and rate of respirations as well as dyspnoea. In advanced cases, areas of dullness in the chest are heard on auscultation or percussion. In other cases there are squeaks and whistles. A snoring respiration can occur.

The alimentary form is unusual. There are few signs but occasional diarrhoea occurs. Bloat can arise through enlargement of the mediastinal and bronchial lymph nodes.

Mammary involvement these days tends to be rare but results in udder induration and the supramammary lymph nodes are enlarged. The udder form can be a serious potential source of spread to humans. The uterine form is also uncommon. Swelling of various lymph nodes can occasionally be seen, and abortion may sometimes occur.

A generalized form can occur with signs following calving. There is a progressive loss of condition with a variable appetite. There may be a variable rectal temperature but usually it is only about 39.7 °C (103.7 °F). The animals are more docile than normal but still bright and alert.

Necropsy

A focus of infection occurs within a week of bacteria entering the cow and, after the third week, calcification can occur. Depending on the route of entry, and where the condition becomes generalized, one or several lymph nodes may contain tuberculous granulomas. In the respiratory system it is the mediastinal or bronchial lymph nodes that are involved, possibly with abscesses in the lungs. The pus is thick, cheese-like and yellow or orange in colour. Sometimes the pleura and peritoneum contain nodules.

In practice, an attempt is made to determine whether infection is active and if cases are 'open' and therefore likely to infect other animals. Active infection is designated by lung infection with limited encapsulation and hyperaemia. This categorization is now thought to be erroneous and it is considered that most lesions are potentially infective. Other organs often show small, transparent, shot-like lesions and these may also be present in the lymph nodes. Tuberculous cystitis and metritis tend to be open cases. Closed infection is seen as discrete lesions enclosed within well-developed capsules. The enclosed pus tends to be caseous and yellow or orange in colour.

Diagnosis

Diagnosis depends on the history of an area where tuberculosis occurs in cattle, badgers or other wildlife. The signs often result in chronic respiratory lesions with loss of condition and a soft, productive, single cough. The comparative tuberculin test is useful. It uses avian (0.5 mg/ml) and bovine tuberculin purified protein derivative (1.0 mg/ml) injected into the neck skin. There is a greater skin thickness increase in bovine than avian tuberculin. Interpretation depends on whether there is no history of reactions, one or more reactions without confirmation at post-mortem examination or a herd with a recent history of reactions confirmed post mortem.

Johne's disease (p. 664), skin tuberculosis or avian tuberculosis can result in false positive bovine tuberculin reactions but usually the avian reaction arises more than the bovine. False negatives occur following protracted infection, desensitization following tuberculin testing, early cases of infection, old cows and those animals recently calved.

The single intradermal test is used in many countries. Its main disadvantage is that it will give reactions to avian tuberculosis, skin tuberculosis or Johne's disease. A short thermal test can be used by injecting tuberculin subcutaneously and measuring the animal's temperature every 2 hours. A rise in temperature of 1 °C (1.8 °F) is considered significant. Intravenous tuberculin also results in a temperature rise. The Stormont test is often used to detect disease in infected cattle. A single intradermal test is used, followed by a second at the same site after a week. If the area then swells it is considered to be positive. Various serological tests have been used and recently the enzyme-linked immunosorbent assay (ELISA) test has shown promise.

Differential diagnosis

Differential diagnosis includes enzootic bovine leukosis (Chapter 37b) but this can be detected by serology. Chronic lung abscesses can cause problems in diagnosis. Traumatic reticulitis (p. 643) may produce similar signs but there is usually a history of an acute attack. Chronic pericarditis (p. 566) can present problems but will result in a jugular pulse and muffled heart sounds and endocarditis (p. 561) cases usually produce a murmur. Contagious bovine pleuropneumonia (p. 672) can cause problems but can be differentiated by a complement fixation test. Lymph node enlargement due to actinobacillosis (p. 627) may be difficult to detect but can be done with a tuberculin test.

Treatment and control

Treatment is not usually undertaken because of the chronic nature of the disease and its potential zoonotic effects. Control in many countries, including North America and Europe, is by tuberculin testing and slaughter of reactors. Hygiene standards need to be upgraded and efficient meat inspection and tracing back to the farm of origin is useful.

Chronic suppurative pneumonia

Aetiology

Various initial causes may result in one or more pathological conditions such as bronchopneumonia, bronchiectasis and pulmonary abscesses. These are often encompassed by the term chronic suppurative pneumonia.

Epidemiology

Most cases occur in adult cattle rather than those still growing. It is, however, a very common cause of respiratory signs in the individual animal. Often there has been an outbreak of acute pneumonia in the history. Although most cases seem to progress slowly over a period of weeks or months, the odd case will appear to be of sudden onset, due to a rapid exacerbation of a suppurative area in the chest.

Signs

Severe signs of disease include a sudden marked loss of condition with dullness, obvious thoracic pain, pyrexia (40.5 °C; 105 °F). In some animals there is halitosis due to a necrotizing bronchopneumonia and pleurisy. Death in these animals often occurs within a few days.

More usually the animal becomes progressively duller and thinner, with a fall in milk yield and intermittent pyrexia, up to 40 °C (104 °F). A cough is usually present with the production of mucus and there is a variable degree of tachypnoea. Thoracic pain may be obvious by an abduction of the elbows and reluctance to move, but in other cases it is only discernible on ballottement. On auscultation there are usually whistles, squeaks and wheezing sounds in the cranio-ventral part of the chest and there are often areas of dullness.

Necropsy

If the main lesion at post mortem is a bronchopneumonia, there is usually marked consolidation of the cranio-ventral parts of the lung, with exudate filling the bronchi and bronchioles. On histological examination, inflammatory cells pass the alveoli and bronchi. When the main problem is a bronchiectasis, often bronchi in the cranial and middle lobes, with dilated air passageways, contain mucus and fibrous tissue. In severe cases the histological sections show complete destruction of the alveolar tissue. When lung abscesses are the main feature, these are usually found in the ventral lung border. Necrotic tissues and pus-containing structures are found within a fibrous capsular wall.

Diagnosis

Diagnosis is based on a history of a chronic loss of condition with respiratory disease in a single animal with signs such as pyrexia, thoracic pain and cough.

Differential diagnosis needs to include acute pneumonia (p. 667), which may be in a single animal or several animals; salmonellosis (p. 657), but at this age there is usually diarrhoea; infectious bovine rhinotracheitis (IBR) (p. 256) infection, but this usually results in a marked conjunctivitis. Inhalation pneumonia (p. 668) on the other hand has a specific history and tuberculosis (p. 669) will probably have a history of herd infection, whereas malignant catarrhal fever will involve ocular lesions and enlarged lymph nodes, etc.

Treatment and control

Often therapy is of limited use. Any treatment may need to be prolonged for 10 days to two weeks or more. Antibiotic therapy with amoxycillin, ampicillin, oxytetracycline, penicillin and streptomycin, sulphadimidine, or trimethoprim and sulphadiazine may be helpful. Most cases that respond are likely to break down again and so infected animals should be slaughtered when convenient.

Control involves culling animals that have had previous bouts of respiratory disease and ensuring all cases are treated early and thoroughly.

Contagious bovine pleuropneumonia

Aetiology

This is the result of infection with *Mycoplasma mycoides* var. *mycoides*.

Epidemiology

The condition is not seen in Great Britian, the last cases being in 1898. Eradication has also been achieved in other countries such as the USA in 1892 and Australia as recently as 1972. The condition is, however, seen throughout much of Eastern Europe, Asia, Africa and the Iberian Peninsula (Blood *et al.*, 1983). It is still one of the major farm animal plagues in certain parts of the world.

Infection tends to spread more quickly in housed animals than those at grass. Once outside the animals, the organism soon dies. On hay it lives for up to six days. On products of animal origin such as urine it can remain longer. The disease results in thrombosis of the pulmonary vessels. Death is from anoxia and possibly toxaemia.

The source of infection is from carrier or infected animals and the source of infection for a herd is the introduction of carrier animals. The main route of entry of infection is via infected droplets. The incubation period is variable but is usually three to six weeks, although it may be extended to six months.

Morbidity in totally susceptible herds is about 90 per cent with a mortality of around 50 per cent. Of the surviving infected animals about 25 per cent become carriers and 25 per cent make a complete recovery.

Signs

Signs are of a sudden onset of pyrexia (40.5 °C; 105 °F) with a loss of milk, anorexia, cessation of rumination and depression. The affected animals trail behind the rest of the herd and a cough is heard, at first only with exercise. As the condition progresses there is obvious pain with abduction of the elbows, an arched back and an expiratory grunt. The respirations become increased and shallow and the head starts to be extended. On auscultation there is a pleuritic rub and then there are areas of dullness and gurgling sounds present. Percussion produces dull areas, which in recovered animals are often inactive sequestra. In carrier cattle these sequestra may break down again under stress, producing disease with toxaemia, loss of weight and mild respiratory signs. Occasionally, oedema develops in the submandibular and brisket areas.

Necropsy

On necropsy there are only lesions in the thoracic cavity and the pleura tends to be thickended with deposits of fibrin and clear, serous fluid. One or both lungs have areas of consolidation with red or grey hepatization. The interlobular septa are distened with exudate producing the classical 'marbling' effect. In the carrier animal areas of necrosis become enclosed in a thick, fibrous capsuled-sequestra. The organism can be isolated from the pleural fluid or lung. In some cases there is oedema of the brisket area, as well as the thoracic lymph nodes and the tonsils.

Diagnosis

Diagnosis depends on the history — an imported animal or entry of infected animals to the herd. The signs are helpful with sudden onset of pyrexia and respiratory distress with pain. Serological examination using the complement fixation test (CFT) is useful but tends to be negative early in the disease or when the condition has been resolved. Carrier animals are often easily detected by the CFT. A plate CFT has been introduced and is more accurate than the standard CFT. Other tests have been used but most are less accurate.

A single intradermal test for contagious bovine pleuropneumonia is of use on a herd basis and in chronic cases. However, it does not always detect acute infection.

At post-mortem examination there is a thickened pleura and marbled lung from which the organism can be detected in the effusion fluid and it can be cultured from lung or pleural fluid.

Differential diagnoses include pasteurellosis (p. 253) but bacteriology differentiates this. Parasitic bronchitis (p. 236) could cause problems but usually there is less pyrexia and the faecal larval count will differentiate. Fog fever (p. 674) could be suspected but the history helps. Chronic suppurative pneumonia (p. 671) could also confuse but usually only one animal is infected and there are intermittent periods of pyrexia.

Treatment and control

Treatment would not be undertaken if the disease occurred in countries where it has been eradicated. In countries where the condition is enzootic, tylosin is used at a dose of 10 mg/kg (5 mg/1b) every 12 hours for three days. Other drugs such as erythromycin or spiramycin may be useful and chloramphenicol and oxytetracycline have some value.

The disease is notifiable in many countries including Britain, most of Europe, North America and Australasia and affected herds would be slaughtered. In other countries vaccination is undertaken with live vaccine. Pleural exudate from natural cases has been used but can produce a severe reaction. Vaccines produced from *Mp. mycoides* growth in broth culture give a short immunity and require annual booster vaccination. A T1 strain broth culture is used in many African countries as it produces a two-year duration of immunity. Recently, the development of avianized vaccines has lengthened the duration of immunity to three to four years, as well as being of limited virulence. Other vaccines have been developed and work is still being undertaken to produce a dried vaccine. Products presently available only last for a few hours after reconstitution (p. 812).

Diffuse fibrosing alveolitis

Aetiology

The cause is unknown but many cases occur in animals with chronic bovine farmer's lung and have precipitating antibodies to *Micropolyspora faeni*. However, it is probable that there are other precipitating causes as some cattle do not possess antibodies to this organism.

Epidemiology

The condition affects individual animals and is uncommon although more frequently seen in herds with a history of bovine farmer's lung. Both dairy and suckler cows are affected and cases can occur indoors or outside, particularly in animals older than six years. The condition is usually a progressive problem and may actually start following a stress such as calving. The condition has normally been present for weeks or months before advice is sought and the animal will have lost condition with coughing or respiratory signs when subjected to mild exercise. Congestive heart failure occurs in about 12 per cent of cases.

Signs

Affected cattle are bright and do not have a raised temperature or pulse rate. The appetite is good but there is a progressive loss of condition. The respiratory signs tend to be quite severe, with a persistent cough always present as well as tachypnoea and hyperpnoea present even in the resting animal. On auscultation of the chest, rhonchi (whistles, squeaks, wheezing) are heard over both lungs and crackling sounds in the cranio-ventral chest. There is no thoracic pain.

Depression and inappetence only occur in the late stages of the condition with congestive heart failure resulting in subcutaneous oedema and an increased heart and respiratory rate. The liver may be palpably enlarged and there may be diarrhoea.

Necropsy

At necropsy alveolar changes predominate but there may be bronchitis with excessive thick mucus in the bronchi. There is thickening and fibrosis of the alveolar walls. Histologically, large numbers of mononuclear cells are seen in the alveolar air spaces. There may be hyperplasia of type 2 pneumocytes or metaplasia of the alveolar epithelium so that it contains ciliated and mucus-secreting cells. Pulmonary hypertension can occur and this results in right-sided heart failure.

Diagnosis

Diagnosis depends on the history, i.e. a single animal, with gradual loss of condition with respiratory signs present at rest, coughing, no thoracic pain or fever and a bright animal.

Treatment

As the cause is unknown, little can be done to alleviate the problem. However, corticosteroids can reduce the cellular changes in the lung. Casualty slaughter of the animal should be undertaken before the loss of condition is too severe.

Dusty feed rhinotracheitis

Aetiology

Particles of different sizes meet varying fates in the respiratory system following inspiration (see Table 43.1). Most of the particles will be in the nasal passages or the trachea, bronchi and bronchioles. The condition results from the introduction of dry, fine-particled feed, or very dusty bedding.

The introduction of a dusty dry feed to animals indoors causes the problem. The signs occur most frequently in the hour or two following feeding. Removal of the feed causes recovery in a few days. The condition occurs most commonly when the relative humidity is low.

Signs

Following feeding or bedding, there is the sudden onset of coughing. The cough tends to be dry and can be single or paroxysmal. Several cattle are normally affected. The animals are otherwise bright and alert; they eat well and there are no abnormal lower respiratory sounds. Respirations are normal in rate and extent, and temperature is normal. There is conjunctivitis and usually a copious ocular and nasal discharge, which is mucoid but sometimes slightly purulent.

Treatment and control

Treatment involves replacing the feed or bedding used. Otherwise dampen down the feed before giving it, or molasses can be added to it. In the case of bedding, new bales should be opened up outside before the cattle are bedded.

Control is by not feeding dusty hay. If the feed is found to be dusty then 5 per cent molasses should be added to it. Dusty bedding should not be used. As the particles affecting the animals can affect humans, it is advisable for workers to wear face masks.

Table 43.1 The fate of various-sized particles entering the respiratory system

Particle size (μm)	Fate
>10	Removed in nasal passages
2–10	Deposited at varying levels in respiratory tract, but above alveoli. The smaller the particle, the further down the respiratory airways it is deposited. Removed by mucociliary action
1–2	Deposited in alveoli
0.5–1	Exhaled with air
<0.5	Deposited in alveoli due to diffusion forces

Fog fever

Aetiology

This is a form of atypical interstitial pneumonia. Although not fully authenticated, the condition is considered to be a toxicosis following the ingestion of large quantities of L-tryptophan.

Epidemiology

The condition is seen in cattle over two years old, particularly those in suckler herds, and affects several cattle to a varying degree at the same time. Often the cattle have been receiving little nutrition and are put onto a more lush pasture in the autumn (September to November). The field may have been top-dressed with a nitrogenous fertilizer. The condition is normally seen within two weeks of entry to the new pasture. The Hereford and Hereford-cross breeds seem to be particularly susceptible.

It is thought that L-tryptophan in the grass is ingested and metabolized in the rumen to indole acetic acid (IAA), which is decarboxylated by *Lactobacillus* spp. to produce 3-methyl indole (3MI). This metabolite can enter the blood and is usually acted upon by the mixed function oxidase system to produce indoles and other metabolites in the urine. 3-Methyl indole can cause the destruction of pulmonary cells such as type 1 pneumocytes and monociliated bronchiolar secretory cells, resulting in various pathological changes. Mortality in severely affected animals can be high (up to 75 per cent) but usually only a small number (5 per cent) are so involved.

Signs

Several animals will show signs but the degree will vary widely and often the farmer only notices one to be ill at the start. The cattle tend to be much quieter and more approachable than normal and to have a sleepy or tranquil expression. The respiratory signs are usually of distress but vary in degree. Coughing is normally little heard.

In the severe form there is the sudden onset of dyspnoea with a loud respiratory grunt, mouth breathing, and often the animal froths at the mouth. Auscultation reveals little considering the severity of the illness, but it may produce soft, moist sounds and a few crackles. Death can occur as the result of excitement. Less severely affected animals show tachypnoea (rate 50–80/minute) with hyperpnoea and usually there is no dyspnoea. The rectal temperature tends to be normal and the animal is again quiet and tranquil. Coughing is only heard occasionally and in some recovering animals a subcutaneous emphysema may develop. Auscultation may reveal harsh sounds.

Necropsy

Dead animals have haemorrhages in the larynx, tracheal and bronchial mucosae. The lungs tend to be swollen, heavy and dark red in colour. The cut surface glistens, is smooth and has a red appearance. Emphysema may be present in the interlobular septa and pleura. Histological examination reveals severe congestion and oedema of the pulmonary tissue, hyaline membrane formation, severe interstitial emphysema and moderate epithelial hyperplasia of type 2 pneumocytes.

Cattle slaughtered in the later stages do not usually show haemorrhages of the respiratory mucosa. There is an overall pale pink colour with variable amounts of interstitial emphysema.

Diagnosis

Diagnosis involves the history of a group condition, mainly in suckler animals moved to a lush pasture in autumn. The signs help, particularly the acute respiratory signs with little to hear on auscultation, no cough and the animals being more tranquil than usual. Postmortem findings indicate the condition, with pulmonary oedema and emphysema.

Differential diagnoses include husk (p. 236), but a cough is present and there would be a history of no vaccination. Pneumonic pasteurellosis (p. 253) would produce pyrexia and a mucopurulent discharge. Nitrate poisoning (p. 622) would produce some signs but the blood would tend to be brownish and the urine contain methaemoglobin. Infectious bovine rhinotracheitis (p. 256) would usually involve pyrexia and a loud explosive cough. Thrombosis of the caudal vena cava would usually involve a single animal and eventually haemoptysis would occur. *Brassica* spp. (p. 613) poisoning would have a different history of feeding and would usually be later in the autumn.

Treatment and control

Treatment is to remove the cattle from the incriminated pasture. Most other treatment tends to be empirical. Interference with a severely distressed animal may result in its death. Atropine at 1 g/450 kg (990 lb) body weight intravenously acts as a bronchodilator and corticosteroids may be useful. Flunixin meglumine has been beneficial in experimentally produced acute bovine pulmonary emphysema.

Control means that if animals are hungry when they enter a new pasture in the autumn, restrict their feed by only allowing grazing for short periods during the first two weeks. This should be for about 2 hours on the first day, increasing by an hour a day so that the cattle can be left out for the whole day after about 12 days. Otherwise the area can be strip-grazed or initially grazed with a less susceptible species such as sheep. If monensin sodium is given at the rate of 200 mg/head per day before entering the pasture, this can stop problems.

Thrombosis of the caudal vena cava

Aetiology

The cause is a septic focus, usually in the liver, resulting in a septic thrombus in the caudal vena cava, from which there is the haematogenous spread of infection to the lungs.

Epidemiology

This is an uncommon condition affecting single animals over one year old, although many cases occur in the growing animal. A few cases of thrombosis of the cranial vena cava have been recorded with similar signs. Most cases result from a liver abscess. This causes a localized phlebitis, usually in the area of the vena cava, adjacent to the liver. Septic emboli pass to the lungs where they can produce chronic suppurative pneumonia and multiple lung abscesses, or they can cause pulmonary arterial lesions. Endarteritis, arteritis and thromboembolism occur, resulting in aneurysms of the pulmonary artery, which then rupture causing haemorrhage in the bronchi and alveoli. Usually, there is a history of sudden onset of respiratory disease, although in some cases there is a history of chronic loss of weight and coughing. A few cases show obstruction of the hepatic venous return with chronic venous congestion of the liver, its enlargement and no access to the collateral venous drainage. Bacteriological examination often reveals little because of previous therapy. However, some cases reveal staphylococci, *A. pyogenes* and *Fusobacterium necrophorum* spp.

Signs

Peracute signs result in an animal dying suddenly with no premonitory signs but usually there is a pool of blood in front of it. In the acute case, cattle with the condition show respiratory disease for a few days or some months, with tachypnoea and shallow breathing. The animal develops haemoptysis and frothy blood can be found in the nasal passages and mouth. There are often blood stains around the animal and in many cases there is melaena. There is a variable amount of thoracic pain with abduction of the elbows. On auscultation there is a widespread whistle, with wheezing sounds.

The chronic form involves animals developing congestive cardiac failure and ascites with an enlarged liver, which may be palpated on the right sublumbar fossa. This often occurs some time before haemoptysis is present.

Once animals start to show haemoptysis then death will ensue, usually within a week or two but occasionally it may take up to 40 days.

Necropsy

Following death, often one or more abscesses are found in the liver, and usually the caudal vena cava thrombosis is in the area of the liver. Multiple septic emboli are normally present within the pulmonary artery. In the lung itself there is usually embolic suppurative pneumonia, intrapulmonary haemorrhage, often concentric and globular in shape, and multiple red areas where blood has been aspirated. When there is obstruction of the hepatic veins then there is marked hepatomegaly and ascites.

Diagnosis

Diagnosis involves the history of loss of condition and respiratory signs in a single animal. The signs help, particularly haemoptysis with thoracic pain, and are almost pathognomonic. Post-mortem findings are relatively diagnostic with thrombosis of the vena cava, emboli in the pulmonary artery and intrapulmonary haemorrhage. Haematological examination shows the packed cell volume is often low (11.0–22.5 per cent).

Differential diagnosis includes an accident, but signs would be highly unlikely unless there is an immediate history of trauma. Tuberculosis (p. 669) could also give rise to some of the signs but is usually much slower and the tuberculin test would reveal this.

Treatment and control

There is no effective therapy. Cattle can be casualty slaughtered if necessary after a course of four or five days' antibiotic therapy using a broad-spectrum compound and then leaving the required withdrawal time.

Control is not possible, but any septic focus should be treated adequately as soon as it occurs. Make sure that all changes in feeding are undertaken slowly so as to avoid the possibility of acidosis.

References

Blood, D.C., Radostits, O.M. & Henderson, J.A. (1983) *Veterinary Medicine*, 6th edn, pp. 692–6. Baillière Tindall, London.

Pirie, H.M. (ed.) (1979) *Respiratory Diseases of Animals. Notes for a Postgraduate Course*, Glasgow University, Glasgow, pp. 41–2.

Chapter 44: Skin Conditions

by L.R. THOMSETT

The skin of the ox shows general conformity with the anatomical characteristics of the large domestic animals (Fig. 44.1). Approximately 7 mm in thickness, it consists of epidermis and dermis and their adnexa. The hair follicles are simple and carry a single hair, the colour of which, depending on body site and breed, may be black, white or a wide variety of variants of brown or grey. Single hairs leave the skin surface at an angle, each follicle having an erector pili muscle allowing the hair to be raised to a more upright position.

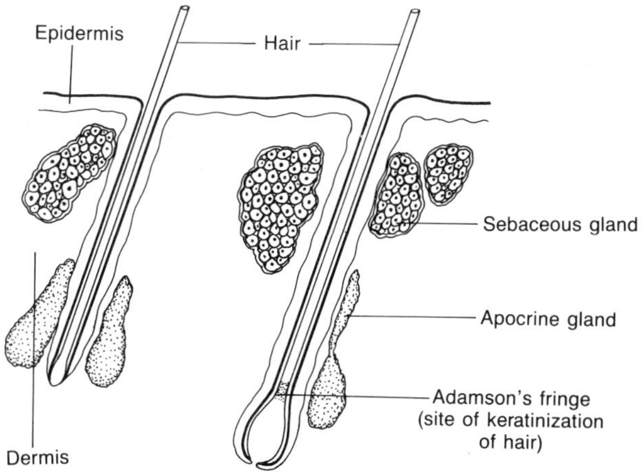

Fig. 44.1 Diagrammatic representation of bovine skin.

Hair growth and replacement is a cyclic process of active growth (anagen) when the hair follicle is producing a new hair, and a period of rest (telogen) when the mature hair, which now has a constricted bulb and is referred to as a 'club' hair, is held in the hair follicle before being shed.

Sweat and sebaceous glands are distributed over the body surface and show specialization in certain areas, e.g. the mammary gland, naso-labial glands of the muzzle. At the extremities of the limbs and on the head of horned breeds the skin is specially modified to form the hooves and horns.

SKIN DISEASES OF CATTLE

Primary disease of the skin of cattle is more commonly attributable to parasite infestation or fungal infection. Bacteria and viruses play a minor role except when skin signs are associated with systemic infection by these organisms. Allergic disorders are also uncommon and genetic diseases rare.

THE EFFECT OF SKIN DISEASE ON THE LIVESTOCK INDUSTRY

Where animals are reared to provide food and other byproducts, skin disease, although clinically not in itself serious and rarely life-threatening, may cause significant losses to the agricultural industry through the following effects.

1 The debilitating effect of pruritus on the affected animals. Heavy louse infestations or infestation by sarcoptic mites causes irritation, restlessness and weight loss.
2 Damage to hides from self-trauma or the migration of parasitic larvae.
3 Damage to tissue from bacterial infection or larval migration resulting in condemnation or trimming of meat at slaughter.
4 Limitation of sale value or show potential of infected animals and their danger as vectors of disease to other stock.

Warble fly

This is also known as warbles, cattle grubs, gad fly or *Hypoderma* infestation and is due to the migrating stages of a parasitic insect (see p. 249). Two species of warble fly are recognized in many countries of the northern Hemisphere, namely *Hypoderma lineatum* and *Hypoderma bovis* and they differ little in their territorial distribution. These parasites are not found in the southern Hemisphere as they have not become established, despite importation of infected cattle.

Cattle, particularly young stock at pasture, are the definitive host for the parasitic stages of the life cycle although other species are recorded as occasionally being infested, such as horses, deer, goats and even man. In species other than cattle the life cycle is rarely, if ever, completed.

Life cycle (see Figs 44.2 and 44.3)

Warble flies become active in the spring and on warm days in the summer months adult females (up to 15 mm long) home in on grazing cattle and alight on the hairs of the lower limbs, on which they lay their eggs. *Hypoderma bovis* lays its eggs singly while *H. lineatum* lays a row of six or more on a hair. The egg-laying behaviour of the flies causes irritation and restlessness to cattle and attempts are made to avoid the flies by running away. Characteristically, this is seen as initial apprehension among a group or an individual animal, followed by suddenly taking flight at a gallop, tail in the air, suddenly turning and repeating the movement in an effort to shake off the pursuing flies. This is known as 'gadding'.

Once ova are attached to the hairs they hatch in four days and larvae crawl to the skin surface, through which they penetrate to the connective tissue and wander for four to five months. Migratory patterns within the host differ: *H. lineatum* moves to the submucosal connective tissue of the oesophageal wall while *H. bovis* goes to the region of the spinal canal and epidural fat. At these sites they remain for the autumn and winter. As second-stage larvae they migrate towards the back of the host where further maturation takes place.

Large domed nodules are formed under the skin within 30–45 cm (12–18 inches) on either side of the spine, in which the now third-stage larva produces a ventral breathing pore. Grubs within the nodules progressively increase in size to 25–28 mm in length, depending on species. In the spring the larva emerges from its cyst, falls to the ground and pupates. After a period of four to six weeks the adult fly emerges.

Effect of Hypoderma *larvae on the host*

Fly attacks. Considerable 'worry' is caused to cattle when approached by these flies; this results in restlessness that interferes with grazing and may result in poor weight gain. Milking cattle show a fall in milk yield.

Damage by larvae
1 Carcasses. The presence of grubs may necessitate trimming of meat at slaughter or, in some cases, condemnation. Trimming makes the carcass less aesthetically acceptable and so it can disproportionately reduce the price when meat is plentiful.
2 Hides. Maturation of warble fly grubs to the stage where they make breathing pores causes serious damage to the dermis and results in downgrading of affected hides.
3 Rupture of larvae. This occasionally precipitates an immunological reaction.

When migrating in the earlier stage of the life cycle, *H. lineatum* larvae may cause an oesophagitis when they reach the oesophageal wall; *H. bovis* larvae can result in posterior paralysis.

Treatment and control

Treatment of lesions associated with the maturation of the migrating larvae has now been superseded by preventive measures.

Since the range of activity of *Hypoderma* flies is limited to 5–14 km (3–9 miles), control of infestation by eradication is feasible provided neighbouring stockkeepers treat their animals.

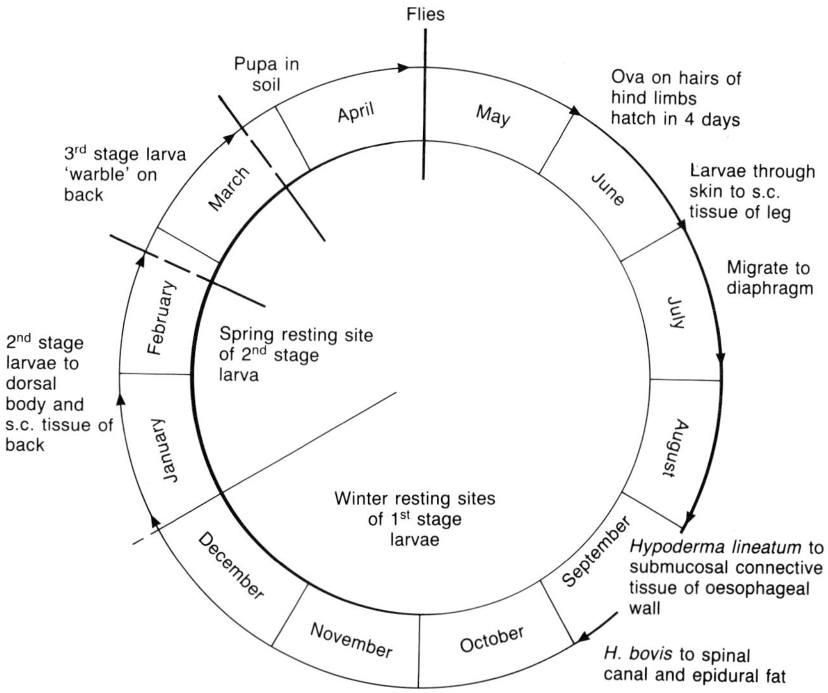

Fig. 44.2 *Hypoderma* spp. life cycle.

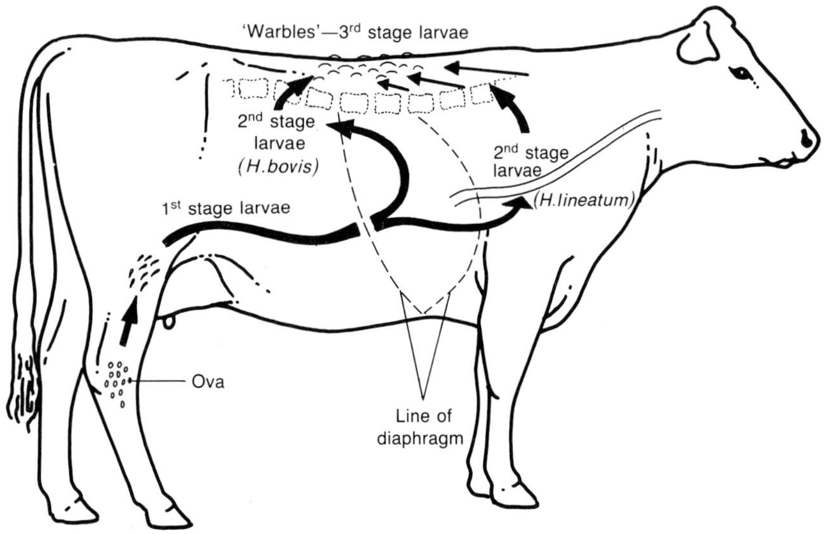

Fig. 44.3 Migration of warble fly larvae within cattle.

Organophosphorus preparations. Organophosphate systemic insecticides have been found to be the most effective agents for the eradication of *Hypoderma* larvae, the aim being to destroy them early in the infestation before they reach resting sites near the neural canal or are themselves very large.

Preparations used include Phosmet, trichlorfon, Ronnel, coumaphos and fenthion. All are cholinesterase inhibitors and knowledge of their actions, in particular their toxic effects and antidotes, is essential before using them for warble treatment (see p. 612).

Organophosphorus preparations have been employed by dip, spray and wash. The most satisfactory method of application has been shown to be the 'pour-on' procedure. An example of pour-on treatment, using Phosmet 13.3 per cent w/v solution, is shown in Table 44.1.

Cattle should be treated in autumn (15 September to

Table 44.1 Dose rate for pour-on treatment using Phosmet 13 per cent w/v

Weight of animal (kg)	Dose (ml)
Up to 130	20
131–200	30
201–260	40
261–330	50
Over 330	60

30 November) or in the spring (15 March to 31 June). Best results are obtained by autumn treatment and prevent skin nodule formation by the third-stage larvae in the spring. No treatment should be given between 1 December and the following 14 March because of possible reactions at the winter resting sites due to the death of the warbles.

Animals being treated on the above regimen should not be given organophosphorus anthelmintics, levamisole or diethylcarbamazine citrate at the same time.

Special precautions regarding the use and handling of organophosphorus preparations, particularly with regard to wearing protective clothing, are applicable and reference to the manufacturer's data sheet is essential before their use.

In Great Britain warble fly infestation is a notifiable disease.

Ivermectin. The systemic parasiticides based on ivermectin are also effective in their ability to destroy warble grubs. A 1 per cent ivermectin injection should be used according to the manufacturer's instructions.

Dermatophytosis (ringworm)

The infection of hair and skin keratin with the dermatophytes *Trichophyton verrucosum*, and less commonly *T. mentagrophytes*, causes lesions commonly referred to as ringworm. This disease has a world-wide distribution, the incidence of which is considered to be high although an accurate figure for its occurrence is not known. It is particularly common in young stock between two and seven months of age and during the autumn and winter months of the year. Adult cattle are also quite frequently affected.

Animals kept in close contact with one another, e.g. under intensive management systems, are particularly at risk. Other species may also be infected, including horses, sheep and also man in whom it may cause serious skin lesions. Although not giving rise to serious systemic debilitating symptoms, the effect of ringworm is on the value of the animal or its hide.

Show animals with the disease may not be shown or sold, infected stock carry a depreciated market value when offered for sale and the hides of animals slaughtered show defects that render them less valuable for top-quality leather manufacture.

Epidemiology

The spores of ringworm fungi survive for many months and in some cases years in the farm environment. They may be transmitted either by fomites or by asymptomatic carrier animals to susceptible hosts.

The *incubation period* of the disease is generally considered to be approximately one week although four weeks has been suggested as the period in some outbreaks. Once in contact with the skin surface of a susceptible animal, the fungus invades the anagen hairs (telogen hairs are not affected) by enzymatic destruction of keratin. Hyphal growth extends only as far as the point at which keratinization of the hair takes place (Adamson's fringe).

The hair, so weakened, breaks off, leading to the partial alopecia seen on clinical lesions of dermatophytosis. A generally mild inflammatory reaction accompanies the infection; only occasionally is this severe in cattle, leading to excess production of skin scale, folliculitis or furunculosis.

Signs

The disease is usually non-pruritic in cattle. Lesions are characteristically greyish-white and have an ash-like surface. Their outline is circular and they are slightly raised due to the accumulation of many layers of scale and the swelling of tissues beneath due to a moderate inflammatory reaction. Some lesions may show areas of mild exudation and yellow crust formation where the skin reaction is more severe. Removal of hair tufts or some of the accumulated crust will often leave a raw bleeding surface. Broken hairs remain as hair stubble encased in scale and crust (Plate 44.1).

The size of lesions varies, 3–5 cm (1–2 inches) diameter being common; in the more severely affected animals lesions become confluent to form extensive areas of infection (Plate 44.2).

The distribution of lesions in calves commonly involves the periorbital skin, ears and back, while in adult cattle the thorax and limbs are the more favoured sites. In show cattle subjected to grooming, multiple small lesions develop over the whole of the body and limbs following the spread of infective spores by contaminated grooming brushes. Very occasionally the udder can be affected (Plate 25.29).

Duration of the disease

Ringworm infection is generally considered to be self-limiting and the course of the disease to be one to four months, although in some cases a period as long as nine months has been necessary for resolution to take place. These periods may be shortened by implementing the appropriate therapeutic measures.

Diagnosis

Diagnosis is made on the clinical signs of classic lesions of dermatophytosis confirmed by the laboratory examination of hair and crust samples.

Collection of samples

1 By forceps epilation of hair from areas of active infection.

2 Scrapings of crust, hair and scale using a scalpel blade.

Using either of these procedures the material obtained is collected in a paper envelope (ensuring that the quantity of sample is adequate for the diagnostic procedures to be carried out), sealed and labelled for transmission to the laboratory.

If culture is contemplated, swabbing the area with 70 per cent alcohol prior to collection of material may reduce contaminants in the specimen.

Laboratory diagnosis. Arthrosporic hyphae on hairs can be demonstrated using the microscope.

1 Wet preparation of suspect material on a microscope slide with coverglass mounted in 20 per cent potassium hydroxide solution and gently warmed.

2 Wet preparation in lactophenol cotton blue on a microscope slide under a coverglass.

3 Wet preparation on a microscope slide under a coverglass mounted in potassium hydroxide/Super Quink solution.

In all procedures using the microscope for the examination of wet preparations care is necessary in adjusting the microscope illumination in order to visualize arthrosporic hyphae. This is equally applicable to the examination of portions of cultured material.

Definitive diagnosis of the species of fungus may be obtained by culture techniques using Sabouraud's agar, mycobiotic agar, or dermatophyte test medium (DTM), and observing the characteristics of the organism, i.e. colonial morphology and that of the hyphal growth. In order to arrive at a conclusive answer culture time may need to be extended, i.e. for as long as three weeks.

Using Sabouraud's agar, rapid identification of *T. verrucosum* may be achieved by culture at 30–37 °C (34 °C), when the colony shows long chains of chlamydospores characteristic of the organism.

The DTM may be used to suggest a positive diagnosis of a pathogen by observation of the indicator colour change.

Definitive diagnosis is only by identification of cultural characteristics.

Treatment

Owing to the difficulty in eliminating the organism from the environment in which many cattle are kept, and the number of animals involved, the reward for treating the disease with such preparations as are suitable (these may only succeed in moderately reducing the duration of the disease) has brought the therapy of ringworm in cattle into question. Scott (1988) refers to 'a sea of antifungals' for the treatment of animal ringworm, many of which are of questionable efficacy.

Systemic treatment

1 *Griseofulvin.* An oral feed supplement given at a dose of 10 mg/kg body weight for seven to fourteen days. In the USA an alternative routine of 15–35 mg/kg body weight for 18–30 days is considered more effective. Pregnant animals should not be treated with this preparation.

2 *Sodium iodide.* A dose of 1 g/14 kg body weight as a 10–20 per cent aqueous solution is given by intravenous injection, followed by a repeat injection seven days later. Pregnant cattle should not be treated with iodide therapy.

Topicals

1 *Imidazoles.* Applications ot sprays, ointments and creams, e.g. miconazole, 5 per cent thiabendazole.

2 *Other preparations* include copper naphthenate and cod liver oil spray, and sodium benzuldazate wash.

Prophylaxis

Griseofulvin at a dose of 7.5–60 mg/kg per day for five weeks has been suggested as a prophylactic against dermatophyte infection. Pregnant animals should not be treated. However, animals so treated will not be immune to disease and so may become infected at a later date.

Immunity

There is still scant knowledge of immunity to dermatophyte infection. Re-infection after natural infection with a dermatophyte is, however, uncommon.

Vaccination

Immunization of cattle against *T. verrucosum* has been carried out in the USSR and Norway. Two doses of a live vaccine made from a non-pathogenic strain of *T. verrucosum* are given, the initial dose followed by a second 10–14 days later. Adverse reactions to this procedure have been recorded. However, apparently vaccination is effective in preventing clinical disease.

Disinfection

Viable spores of ringworm fungi may remain in buildings and particularly on porous surfaces, e.g. wood, brick, for months or years, making disinfection difficult.

Cleansing with high pressure water jets, scrubbing down with hot detergent solutions or disinfectants (e.g. benzalkonium chloride) or alternatively, disinfection with 2 per cent formaldehyde solution after prior scrubbing can remove infection.

Parasitic skin disease

Lice (pediculosis) (Plate 44.3)

Lice are somewhat dorso-ventrally flattened insects up to 6 mm in length that are host-specific parasites.

The distribution of lice is world-wide. The species infecting cattle are the biting louse *Bovicola* (*Damalinia*) *bovis*, and the sucking lice *Haematopinus eurysternus, Linognathus vituli*, and *Solenopotes capillatus*. The biting lice feed on tissue debris while the sucking species suck blood and tissue fluid (see p. 250).

Life cycle

The entire life cycle of approximately three to six weeks' duration is spent on the host. Adult females lay their eggs and attach them singly to hairs. These appear as pearly or opalescent bodies (nits) 1–2 mm long. From the egg immature nymphs emerge, and pass through several moults before becoming adult. Survival off the host is short, usually less than one week. However, under certain conditions lice have been recorded to survive for periods up to three weeks.

On the host, populations of lice vary seasonally, being highest in colder seasons when the coat is long and transmission by contact from animal to animal readily occurs. Lower populations in the warmer seasons are due to the higher environmental temperature of the skin and coat in which lice cannot survive.

In spite of these factors, small populations may survive in protected areas, i.e. the ears, axillae, jowl, tail, ready to multiply when environmental conditions become beneficial.

Distribution of infestation on the host

Biting lice occur mainly on the neck, withers and tail head. Sucking lice are commonly found as a more generalized infestation, occurring on the head, neck, withers, down the brisket, tail, axillae and groin.

Signs

The cardinal sign is pruritus, the resulting restlessness leading to poor feeding and poor weight gain. The coat is poor in condition, often with alopecia and excoriation due to self-trauma, with loss of coat lustre and excess dandruff as well as hide damage. Animals in milk may show lowered production. Infestations with sucking lice may give rise to anaemia and consequent increased susceptibility to concurrent disease.

Diagnosis

This depends on the demonstration of lice and eggs within the coat. Because of pruritis, the only major disease to be differentiated is mange.

Treatment

Louse infestations of cattle may be controlled by the application of antiparasitic sprays, powders, washes, 'pour-ons' and certain injectable preparations. The use of these should be complemented by attention to management and husbandry aimed at eliminating reservoirs of infection and improving nutrition.

Antiparasitics for louse control, of which there are many, are based mainly on organochlorine, organophosphorus and synthetic pyrethroid active principles, e.g. Gamma BHC powder (0.625 per cent), Coumaphos powder (1 per cent), Diazinon wash (2 per cent), Phosmet 'pour-on' (13.3 per cent) and Permethrin 'pour-on' (4 per cent).

Ivermectin 200–300 µg/kg subcutaneously is effective against sucking lice but of variable efficacy against the biting species. Before use reference should be made to the manufacturer's data sheet for details of special precautions to be observed, e.g. milk withholding times of dairy cattle, permissible intervals between treatment and slaughter of meat animals.

Mite infestations: mange, scabies

Infestation of the skin of cattle with parasitic mites may be by any of four species: *Sarcoptes scabiei, Psoroptes communis, Chorioptes bovis or Demodex*. The incidence of disease due to these shows variation in different parts of the world in respect of the species of mite and pathogenicity (p. 251).

SARCOPTIC MANGE, SARCOPTIC SCABIES

Sarcoptes scabiei (bovis) (Plate 44.4) has a life cycle of 10–17 days and may infest cattle of any age, breed or sex. Infection takes place by direct contact with infected cattle or with environmental fomites, although survival of the mites in the environment is limited to a few days.

Signs

Sarcoptes scabiei causes an intensely pruritic papular dermatitis due to the burrowing activities of the female mites within the superficial epidermis and a concurrent hypersensitivity reaction. This results in a non-follicular papular response, exudation and crusting with self-trauma in an attempt to relieve the itching. This produces excoriation, alopecia and thickening of the skin (Plate 44.5).

Lesions commonly commence about the head and spread to become generalized with gross thickening of skin folds. In some animals these lesions may be accompanied by secondary infection with bacteria (Plate 44.6).

The persistent intense pruritus causes debility, loss of condition, poor food conversion, hide and skin damage and in dairy cattle a reduction in milk yield. Workers in close contact with affected animals may show papular skin lesions.

Diagnosis

Physical examination, history, possible human involvement, demonstration of *S. scabiei* in skin scraping material examined microscopically all help the diagnosis. In exceptional cases skin biopsy may be helpful.

The main differential diagnosis is with psoroptic/chorioptic mange.

Treatment and chontrol

1 Organophosphorus, organochlorine washes, dips, sprays.
2 Gamma BHC 7.5 per cent (not milking cows) 5–25 ml in 6 l water.
3 Diazinon 2 per cent wash, 28 ml in 4.5 l water.
4 Phosmet 20 per cent pour-on.
5 Ivermectin 200–300 μg/kg by subcutaneous injection.

These are examples of preparations available. Application routines may vary and response to treatment will determine how many applications may be required. Reference to the appropriate data sheet is essential for information on special precautions and withdrawal times to be observed (see p. 682, louse control).

PSOROPTIC MANGE, PSOROPTIC SCABIES

Psoroptes mites are non-burrowing and have a two-week life cycle. Survival off the host may be as long as three weeks. Transmission of infection is by direct or indirect contact.

Signs

Infection commences over the withers and spreads to the rest of the body. Lesions are papules accompanied by severe pruritus leading to extensive serous exudation and crusting with alopecia and lichenification. Irritability and consequent debility may result in unthriftiness, poor weight gain, hide damage and reduced milk yield in lactating animals.

Diagnosis

The diagnosis is by demonstration of mites by microscopic examination of wet preparations of skin scrapings. Differential diagnosis is with sarcoptic scabies, and chorioptic scabies.

Treatment

Treatment is the same as for sarcoptic scabies, although care is needed to ensure that infection has been eradicated. Resistance to treatment has been recorded.

CHORIOPTIC MANGE, CHORIOPTIC SCABIES

Chorioptes bovis is a superficial, non-invasive inhabitant of cattle skin. Living on epidermal debris, it has a life cycle on the host of two to three weeks. It survives only a few days off the host under natural environmental conditions although under experimental conditions it may live as long as 10 weeks.

Transmission of infestation is usually by contact. Outbreaks among housed dairy cattle are higher in the winter time when mite populations are greatest.

Signs

Non-follicular pruritic papules result in self-trauma accompanied by erythema, excoriation, exudation, alopecia and the formation of crusts. These mostly involve the limbs, particularly the hindlimbs, the udder, scrotum, perineum and tail. The neck and flanks may also be involved.

Diagnosis

Diagnosis is by the microscopical demonstration of causal mites in wet preparation of skin scrapings. The differential diagnosis is with infestations with lice (p. 682) and other parasitic mites.

Treatment

Treatment is the same as for sarcoptic scabies. Apparent spontaneous regression may occur in the summer months when infestation appears to be confined to the distal limbs.

DEMODICOSIS

Demodectic mites are considered to be normal residents of the skin of many species of wild and domestic animals. They are apparently host specific and live mainly within the hair follicles and sebaceous glands. Three species of *Demodex* mites have been identified in cattle, the life cycle of which, as in other hosts, is obscure. Transmission of infection occurs from dam to calf by contact during suckling. No age or sex predilection has been established, nor is it clear why an organism living as a commensal should suddenly become a pathogen by its rapid unpredicted multiplication; immunodeficiency has been suggested as one cause.

Signs (Plate 44.7)

Multiple nodules, sometimes secondarily infected, result in folliculitis and furunculosis of the face, neck and shoulders, occasionally becoming generalized. The disease is usually non-pruritic but nevertheless results in severe hide damage and consequent economic loss.

Diagnosis

With skin scrapings, wet preparations of expressed nodule contents examined microscopically show caseous sebaceous masses and large numbers of mites.

Histology of skin biopsy shows distended hair follicles packed with mites. Secondarily infected lesions show folliculitis, furunculosis and dermal granuloma formation.

Differential diagnosis is with dermatophytosis (p. 680) and dermatophilosis (p. 688).

Treatment

Demodicosis is often difficult to treat and prognosis is always guarded. Organophosphorus 'pour ons' have in some cases been found to be beneficial.

Warts (viral papillomatosis)

Bovine papillomatosis is commonly thought of as an infectious disease of the skin of mainly young cattle, usually self-limiting, widely distributed about the world, posing little difficulty in diagnosis, prognosis or treatment. The causal agent of the condition is a virus.

This is not, however, the whole story of bovine infection with DNA papovaviruses of which the bovine papilloma virus has certainly five, if not more, strains. Cross-reactivity between strains does not occur.

Papilloma virus appears to be host specific and transmission of bovine warts to humans handling infected cattle and cattle products has not been proven.

Of the strains of virus isolated, it appears that each has an anatomically determined predilection site of infection.

1 BPV type I causes frond-like lesions on the nose, teats or penis: fibropapillomas in young cattle (Plate 25.31).
2 BPV type II causes papillomatosis of the skin of the face, head, neck and dewlap, eyelids and occasionally legs of young cattle.
3 BPV type III causes atypical warts, small smooth white sessile lesions on the udder and teats (Plate 25.32).
4 BPV type IV causes alimentary tract and urinary bladder papillomas and ocular lesions possibly progressing to squamous cell carcinoma.
5 BPV type V causes non-regressing rice-grain warts on the teats.

Interdigital fibropapillomatosis, although wart-like in character, has no proven viral aetiology.

Epidemiology

Infection may be spread either by direct contact with infected animals or indirectly by fomites, e.g. from fences by trauma through minor abrasions or by direct or indirect effects of ectoparasitism. Following infection lesions appear after a two to six-month incubation period.

Signs

Viral papillomatosis is commonly seen in young cattle and once established lesions will resolve in a period of one to twelve months. Commencing as small, smooth, hairless, firm, button-like elevations projecting slightly above the skin surface, they may be from 1 mm to several centimetres in diameter (Plate 44.8). They may develop to become coarse and cauliflower-like (Plate 44.9), sessile or pedunculated and single or multiple in number. Lesions are commonly sited on the head, neck and brisket and extensive generalization may occur.

Diagnosis

On clinical grounds the lesions are characteristic as is their distribution pattern on the skin and also the age group affected.

Histological examination shows epithelial proliferation with or without connective tissue proliferation: BPV I and II produce epithelial and fibrous proliferation; BPV III, IV and V produce epithelial proliferation.

Prognosis

In infection with BPV I and II, spontaneous regression within one to twelve months is the rule, while in the case of BPV III, IV and V and 'interdigital papillomatosis', lesions tend to be persistent.

Treatment and control

With uncomplicated cases little treatment is required since spontaneous regression in young animals is the rule. Occasional cases of generalization may be encountered and are likely to be due to a failure in cell-mediated immunity.

Autogenous vaccines (p. 814) for the treatment of bovine papillomatosis are of doubtful value. Where large, persistent growths are present, e.g. on the neck, removal by cryosurgery or cold steel surgery may be attempted.

For the prevention of infection with BPV I and II, commercial and autogenous vaccines are claimed to be effective. The use of lithium antimony thiomalate 6 per cent w/v solution by deep intramuscular injection, 15 ml on each of four to six occasions at 48-hour intervals is claimed to aid enucleation and necrosis of pedunculated warts.

Disinfection

While control of infection by disinfection is not commonly undertaken, where recurrent outbreaks of disease have occurred in housed cattle attempts at disinfection may be justified. Solutions of formaldehyde or caustic soda in appropriate dilution may be used, hosing down all treated surfaces well with water after these solutions have been allowed to act and prior to restocking.

Urticaria

The physical manifestation of urticaria in the form of oedematous skin plaques or of angioneurotic oedema may be caused by a wide variety of factors. These may be immunologic, as in Coombs type I and II reactions, or non-immunologic associated with injected irritants or non-immunologic histamine release.

Some non-immunologic factors that may precipitate urticarial responses or intensify an already established reaction are pressure, sunlight, heat, exercise, drugs, chemicals, even psychological stress. Certain genetic disorders have also been implicated in the aetiology of urticarial reactions.

Urticaria is usually seen as an acute onset disorder having no age, breed or sex predilection, which runs an acute or chronic course. It mostly affects a single individual or, on occasion, a small group.

Signs

In cattle, urticarial reactions are associated with insect and arthropod bites and stings, infection, the administration of antibiotics, vaccines or other biological products, some feedingstuffs as well as stinging plants.

Lesions of urticaria may vary in size, often being plaque-like wheals, localized or generalized over the neck, body and upper limbs in particular. They are usually cold to touch and may pit on pressure. Pruritus is variable as is the tendency for serum leakage onto the skin surface or for there to be haemorrhage. Urticarial lesions commonly show a well-defined shape or pattern, e.g. being ovular, serpiginous or arciform, or in the case of angioneurotic oedema involve certain structures with extensive oedematous swellings.

Acute onset angio-oedema has been seen in the UK on turning out housed cattle onto spring pasture, manifest as oedematous swelling of the periorbital skin, muzzle, perianal and perivulval tissue and occasionally the udder and teats. The condition is usually transient and apparently causes little distress. More severely affected animals may show evidence of respiratory distress.

In the USA a form of auto-allergic urticaria has been described in Jersey and Guernsey cattle. Affected individuals are believed to have a genetic predisposition to an allergic response when there is unusual engorgement of the udder or undue retention of milk. Clinical signs are of allergic urticarial skin rash and, in some individuals, respiratory distress.

Diagnosis

Diagnosis is mainly on history and lesions of rapid onset. Urticarial-like plaques with superficial exudation and crusting closely resemble the discrete active lesions of dermatophytosis (p. 680).

Treatment

Treatment is with subcutaneous or intramuscular injection of 3–5 ml of 1/100 adrenaline solution. Cattle with milk allergy should be milked out. In urticaria spontaneous resolution is often rapid and may have commenced or taken place by the time a visiting veterinarian arrives to attend the case.

Pruritus/pyrexia/haemorrhagic syndrome (PPH)

A disease of cattle, the pathophysiology of which is unclear, was first reported in cattle in the UK and in The Netherlands in the late 1970s. In The Netherlands the outbreaks were associated with the feeding of concentrates containing a urea compound, diureidoisobutane. In the UK this compound was not implicated and the causal factor has not been identified. Most cases were on self-fed silage, often after the introduction of a different silage additive to the farm. All cases were in cows, with a morbidity of 10.9 per cent and up to 25 per cent mortality, although almost all cases are culled due to loss of condition.

Signs

The systemic response is of a high fever (40–41 °C; 104–106 °F) with petechiation of the conjunctiva and visible mucous membranes, with general dullness. An extensive papular to exudative dermatitis with pruritus of variable intensity develops over the head, neck, perineum, udder, back and tail-head (Plate 44.10). These signs are accompanied by self-trauma (rubbing, kicking and licking), which leads to excoriation with bleeding and hair loss over a period of days to several weeks. Although the dermatitis may subside, the febrile response may persist for four to seven weeks.

Seriously affected animals may die, while those less so are unthrifty and ultimately have to be destroyed.

Diagnosis

The blood picture shows leucopenia followed by leucocytosis. Skin biopsy shows superficial and deep perivascular dermatitis with eosinophils and mononuclear cells predominating.

The post-mortem generalized petechiation particularly subserosal, with some cases showing free blood at external orifices.

The differential diagnosis is with other acutely febrile diseases of dairy cattle, such as anthrax (p. 552), and exudative dermatitis with severe pruritus of parasitic origin.

Treatment

This is non-specific and usually there is little response. A few cases have improved following prolonged use of injectable corticosteroids.

Photosensitization

Aetiology

This biophysical phenomenon occurs when skin becomes sensitized to certain wavelengths of sunlight, particularly within the ultraviolet range of the spectrum, in the presence within skin cells of specific photodynamic agents (see also pp. 326, 615).

Photodynamic agent in circulation → skin → irradiation by sunlight → cell death → necrosis → sloughing

Substances giving rise to these reactions in cattle may be porphyrins originating from defective haemoglobin metabolism, e.g. congenital porphyria, bovine protoporphyria, or they may be substances of plant origin, e.g. hypericin, which is found in the plant St John's wort (*Hypericum perforatum*). This process of photosensitivity is often referred to as *primary* or *direct* light sensitization.

Alternatively, another set of circumstances can lead to photosensitization, referred to as *secondary* or *hepatogenous* light sensitization. Although the final outcome, skin necrosis and sloughing, is the same as in the primary form, the process by which this is brought about differs.

Where liver damage (of diverse aetiology) interferes with the metabolism of the chlorophyll metabolite, phylloerythrin, this latter substance enters the circulation. As with other porphyrins, it initiates a light sensitivity response when present in the skin.

Both of these manifestations of photosensitivity are

systemic in origin. A third, localized, form of skin reaction to sunlight may on rare occasions be induced by contact with the sap of certain plants containing psoralens. Localized lesions are more likely to be found on the distal limbs, muzzle or ventrum.

In order for photodynamic cell destruction to take place, the following circumstances are necessary.

1 The photodynamic agent must be present in the skin at the time of exposure to sunlight.
2 The exposed skin will be non-pigmented (the greater the density of melanin pigmentation, the greater is the protection against ultraviolet solar radiation).
3 The density of hair cover should be such that sunlight can penetrate to the skin surface.

Photosensitization leading to photodermatitis is essentially a physical process. The activation of porphyrins within skin cells by ultraviolet irradiation releases energy that causes cell death, the clinical signs of which are erythema, oedema and necrosis of exposed non-pigmented areas of skin. In some animals vesication is present prior to necrosis, sloughing and ulceration of affected areas. Pruritus and pain may also be shown.

Sites most likely to be involved in cattle are those most exposed to direct sunlight, e.g. the head, neck, back and lateral aspects of the body, udder and teats (more extensively when the photosensitive animal is lying down) (Plates 25.23, 44.11 and 44.12).

Diagnosis

The dramatic lesions of skin necrosis and sloughing should not present diagnostic difficulty in the established case. The presence or absence of systemic signs of illness, e.g. jaundice, positive blood screens for hepatic disease, should determine whether the condition is primary or secondary.

Very localized lesions on distal limbs, ventrum or muzzle would suggest a topical plant contact aetiology.

Prognosis

In the primary form of the disease, provided the underlying cause is not genetic, then removal to housed, well-ventilated, shaded and cool conditions should be adequate to allow resolution of the lesions. Where severe liver damage is confirmed, prognosis is poor and may well be terminal.

Treatment

Cool, shaded, fly-free housing to avoid myiasis is necessary. Where necrosis and sloughing has taken place then lesion hygiene is essential to prevent fly strike and the application of powder dressing to that end is beneficial. Resolution in severely affected animals is often a long process. Antibiotics to limit secondary infection may be justified, as may the short-term administration of corticosteroids in certain cases. In secondary photodermatitis, the justification of therapy will be determined by the acuteness or chronicity of the underlying disease.

Bovine farcy

A chronic nodular and ulcerative disease of the skin of cattle, the causal organisms of which may be either *Nocardia farcinica* or *Mycobacterium farcinogenes*. The disease is only found in Africa, Asia and South America.

Aetiology

Nocardia farcinica is a soil saprophyte that becomes inoculated into wounds by contamination or enters the skin by inoculation via tick vectors, which themselves carry the organism for long periods of time.

Signs

Once inoculated, slowly developing painless nodules appear more commonly over the head, neck, shoulders, limbs, perineum and groin. Infection may give rise to mastitis and whilst following the lymphatics cause cording of these vessels as well as lymphadenopathy. Ulceration of lesions occurs with the discharge of thick, grey/yellow material.

Infection may be protracted and confined to the skin but generalization, particularly to the lungs and viscera, can occur with a progressive loss of condition leading to death.

Diagnosis

Diagnosis is dependent on the clinical signs. The organism may be demonstrated in smears of exudate (acid-fast filaments, which are beaded). Culture of *Nocardia farcinica* is also possible.

Histopathology shows the presence of pyogranulomatous dermatitis.

The differential diagnosis is with so-called skin tuberculosis due to acid-fast bacilli, particularly nodules found on the lower limbs or cording of lymphatics of forelimbs.

Treatment

Inorganic iodides have been used but the advice given is usually to have the affected animals destroyed.

Dermatophilosis (bovine streptothricosis)

This is a chronic or acute exudative dermatitis that may affect many species of animals and is of world-wide distribution. It also occurs in humans.

The disease in cattle is of particular importance in Africa, where it is thought to have been known since the nineteenth century, in America, the Middle East and Mediterranean Europe.

In cattle the disease is of importance for its role in causing economic loss through down-grading of hides and skins, reduced milk yield, marked debility in severely affected animals with dehydration and death.

Aetiology

The agent responsible for infection is the actinomycete, *Dermatophilus congolensis*, a Gram-positive filamentous bacterium. Infection with *D. congolensis* is confined to the epidermis where the motile zoospore stage of the organism, activated under suitable conditions of climate and skin damage, grows to form a filamentous mycelium within the epidermis. In dry conditions the spore stage of the bacterium may remain dormant in dry crust, scab and hyperkeratotic skin debris for many months.

A number of factors influence the incidence of the disease, of which high temperature and humidity play an important role. Similarly, breed susceptibility is of importance, indigenous cattle being more resistant to infection than imported exotic breeds.

The initiation of lesions requires skin damage, albeit superficial, by abrasion, e.g. thorn scratches, insect bites (biting flies or ticks may themselves carry the infective organism).

The incubation period may be as short as two weeks.

Signs

Bovine cutaneous streptothricosis commences as a circumscribed moist patch, often with raised or matted hairs, giving a characteristic 'paint brush' appearance. Discrete lesions occur in the initial stages which coalesce to form large areas of hyperkeratotic scab and crust (Plates 44.13 and 44.14). In severe infections as much as half the skin surface may be involved. Scab may be of variable thickness and on removal show a concave underside coated in thick, yellowish exudate, leaving a raw, bleeding epidermis.

Diagnosis

Impression smears of the exudate, fixed and stained by Gram's method or methylene blue, reveal numerous rows of cocci formed into branching filaments. Organisms may not be readily demonstrable in material taken from old lesions or those affected by secondary infection. *Dermatophilus congolensis* may be cultured on blood agar under microaerophilic conditions.

Differential diagnosis is with dermatophytosis (p. 680) and sarcoptic scabies (p. 683).

Treatment

Antibiotic therapy using penicillin and streptomycin as a single dose regimen (70 000 iu penicillin and 70 mg/kg body weight streptomycin intramuscularly) will prevent epidermal invasion by zoospores as well as re-infection. Alternatively, five daily doses of 5000 iu penicillin and 5 mg/kg body weight streptomycin may be given (Lloyd, 1981). Long-acting oxytetracycline by deep intramuscular injection at 20 mg/kg body weight has also been found to be effective (Lloyd *et al.*, 1990). Topical application of solutions of cresols and copper salts in appropriate dilution may have a preventive effect.

Prevention

Since predisposition to the disease is due to skin trauma from vegetation, ectoparasite infestation with poor husbandry resulting in malnutrition and/or the presence of concurrent disease, many of these factors are difficult to control. Efforts directed towards the establishment of herds of breeds resistant to *D. congolensis* may be of long-term benefit.

The quest for an effective vaccine continues but is still in the experimental stage of development (Lloyd, 1984). A combination of improved husbandry with vaccine therapy may eventually be the effective means of control.

Horn cancer

This disease, which results in neoplasia of the horn core, is usually an extension of squamous cell carcinoma that arises from the mucosa of the frontal sinus. Involvement of the horn core causes loosening of the horn, which drops off leaving the tumour exposed. While metastases occur in such conditions as squamous cell carcinoma of the eye, they do not occur in horn core lesions.

Diagnosis

This is by biopsy and clinical examination.

Treatment

Treatment has been found to have variable degrees of success and recurrence is common following surgery. Cryotherapy, surgical excision, radiodiathermy and immunotherapy have all been tried.

Lumpy skin disease and pseudo-lumpy skin disease (see also p. 748)

Two forms of lumpy skin disease are recognized.

1 True 'lumpy skin' disease, the causal agent of which is the Neethling pox virus, infection with which gives rise to acute or subacute disease among cattle in parts of Africa.

2 Pseudo-lumpy skin disease due to infection with Allerton virus, bovine herpes virus type 2, which has a world-wide distribution amongst all types of cattle.

Lumpy skin disease

A seasonal disease that occurs particularly at times of high insect population and can affect cattle of any age, breed or type.

The mode of transmission of infection has not been fully determined although the association with periods of high insect population and proof that *Stomoxys calcitrans* can carry the virus suggests that the organism is insect-borne. The incubation period is one to four weeks.

Lumpy skin disease causes high economic loss through decreased milk production, abortion, loss of condition and hide damage.

Signs

The initial viraemia is associated with a febrile response, nasal discharge, excess salivation and possibly lameness. After a period of one week the first signs of skin lesions may be seen as papules/nodules with enlargement of the superficial lymph nodes.

Skin lesions can be localized or generalized, circumscribed firm and flattened intradermal nodules up to 5 cm in diameter. While lesions can be confined to the skin of the chest, neck, back, limbs, perineum, udder and scrotum, more severely affected animals may show involvement of the nasal and turbinate bones. Oedema of the ventral chest and abdomen, also the limbs, may occur.

Skin lesions may well ulcerate and be slow to resolve, persisting for months to years in some cases. In most instances the skin lesions necrose, passing through phases of ulceration and scarring before resolution in a period of one to three months.

Morbidity is usually around 50 per cent but may be as high as 90 per cent with mortality in the region of 10 per cent.

Prognosis

This is always guarded. Those animals that progress to respiratory tract involvement may well die.

Diagnosis

History, clinical examination, skin biopsy and virus isolation are all helpful. Apart from other histopathological changes present, eosinophilic intracytoplasmic inclusion bodies may be found in keratinocytes, and glandular and ductal epithelium of the skin glands.

Treatment

None is effective. Antibiotics may be given to combat secondary infection. Measures to minimize the possibility of fly strike and subsequent myiasis should also be taken.

Prevention

Some protection is gained by vaccination with modified Neethling virus vaccine. Vaccination with sheep pox virus has also conferred some protection.

Pseudo-lumpy skin disease

A much milder condition than 'true' Neethling virus lumpy skin disease and due to infection with bovine herpes virus type 2. The organism is also responsible for outbreaks of herpes mammillitis (p. 321).

Signs

There is absence of a systemic response or superficial lymphadenopathy with a clinical course similar to herpes mammillitis, resolution occurring in two to three weeks. In exceptional cases lesions may persist for considerably longer.

Skin lesions have a similar distribution and appearance to those of lumpy skin disease, with limbs, body, neck, back, udder, perineum and scrotum showing superficial raised plaques having a central depression and superficial necrosis.

Diagnosis

History, physical examination, virus isolation and skin biopsy are helpful. Skin biopsy shows, among other changes, eosinophilic intranuclear inclusion bodies in keratinocytes of the stratum spinosum.

References and further reading

General

Scott, D.W. (1988) Structure and function of the skin. In *Large Animal Dermatology*, pp. 2–28. W.B. Saunders & Co., London.

Warble fly

Fadok, V.A. (1984) Parasitic diseases of large animals. *Veterinary Clinics of North America: Large Animal Practice*, **6**, 3–26.

Scott, D.W. (1988) Parasitic diseases. In *Large Animal Dermatology*, pp. 245–8. W.B. Saunders & Co., Philadelphia.

Soulsby, E.J.L. (1982) *Helminths, Arthropods and Protozoa of Domestic Animals*, 7th edn, pp. 432–7. Baillière Tindall, London.

Dermatophytosis

Scott, D.W. (1988) *Large Animal Dermatology*, pp. 179–82. W.B. Saunders & Co., Philadelphia.

Parasitic skin diseases

Blood, D.C., Radostits, O.M. & Henderson, J.A. (1983) *Veterinary Medicine*, 6th edn, p. 964. Baillière Tindall, London.

Fadok, V.A. (1984) Parasitic skin diseases of large animals. *Veterinary Clinics of North America, Large Animal Practice*, **6**, 3–26.

Linklater, K.A. & Gillespie, I.D. (1984) Outbreak of psoroptic mange in cattle. *Veterinary Record*, **115**, 211–12.

Scott, D.W. (1988) Parasitic diseases. In *Large Animal Dermatology*, pp. 207–30. W.B. Saunders & Co., Philadelphia.

Warts

Gibbs, E.P.J. (1984) Viral diseases of the skin of the bovine teat and udder. *Veterinary Clinics of North America: Large Animal Practice*, **6**, 187–202.

Hunt, E. (1984) Infectious skin diseases of cattle. *Veterinary Clinics of North America: Large Animal Practice*, **6**, 155–74.

Scott, D.W. (1988) Epithelial neoplasms. In *Large Animal Dermatology*, p. 420. W.B. Saunders & Co., Philadelphia.

Pruritis/pyrexia/haemorrhagic syndrome

References to outbreaks are all prior to 1980, since which time there have been no reports in the scientific literature. However, a few outbreaks still occur each year.

Blood, D.C. & Radostits, O.M. (1989) *Veterinary Medicine*, 7th edn, p. 1300. Baillière Tindall, London.

Photosensitization

Manning, T.O. (1984) Non-infectious skin diseases of cattle. *Veterinary Clinics of North America: Large Animal Practice*, **6**, 176–9.

Scott, D.W. (1988) In *Large Animal Dermatology*, pp. 76–83. W.B. Saunders & Co., Philadelphia.

Bovine farcy

Lloyd, D.H. (1981) Bovine farcy. In *Current Veterinary Therapy, Food Animal Practice* (ed. by J.L. Howard), p. 1136. W.B. Saunders & Co., Philadelphia.

Dermatophilosis

Lloyd, D.H. (1981) Streptothricosis. In *Current Veterinary Therapy, Food Animal Practice* (ed. by J.L. Howard), pp. 1134–5. W.B. Saunders & Co., Philadelphia.

Lloyd, D.H. (1984) Immunology of dermatophilosis: recent developments and prospects for control. *Preventive Medicine*, **2**, 93–102.

Lloyd D.H. & Sellers, K.C. (1976) *Dermatophilus* infection in animals and man. Symposium Proceedings, Ibadan. Academic Press.

Lloyd, D.H., Hawkins, J.P. & Pragnell, J. (1990) Efficacy of long-acting oxytetracycline in the treatment and control of bovine dermatophilosis. *Veterinary Dermatology*, **1**, 78–82.

Horn cancer

Bastianello, S.S. (1982) A survey of neoplasia in domestic species over a 40-year period from 1935 to 1974 in the Republic of South Africa. I. Tumours occurring in cattle. *Ondersterpoort Journal of Veterinary Research*, **49**, 195–204.

Pachauri, S.P. & Pathak, R.C. (1969) Bovine horn cancer. Therapeutic experiments with autogenous vaccine. *American Journal of Veterinary Research*, **30**, 475–7.

Lumpy skin disease and pseudo-lumpy skin disease

Martin, W.B. (1986) Bovine mamillitis. In *Current Veterinary Therapy: Food Animal Practice II* (ed. by J.L. Howard), pp. 472–3. W.B. Saunders & Co., Philadelphia.

Njoku, C.O. (1986) Lumpy skin disease. In *Current Veterinary Therapy: Food Animal Practice II* (ed. by J.L. Howard), pp. 481–2. W.B. Saunders & Co., Philadelphia.

Scott, D.W. (1988) *Large Animal Dermatology*, p. 108. W.B. Saunders & Co., London.

St George, T.D. *et al.* (1980) A generalised infection of cattle with bovine herpes virus 2. *Australian Veterinary Journal*, **56**, 42.

Chapter 45: Neurological Disorders

by R.M. BARLOW

Introduction

The central nervous systems (CNS) of all mammals are vulnerable to developmental aberrations, attack by micro-organisms, toxic insults and metabolic disturbances.

Though in some respects the bovine nervous system may appear to be more robust than those of some other domestic ruminants, a growing number and variety of conditions that involve neural dysfunction are being recognized in cattle. In some, the nervous system is the primary target, whereas in other conditions the nervous system is involved concomitantly with, or as a consequence of, disease in other systems.

In this chapter an attempt is made to present in a readily assimilable form some of the more clinically relevant aspects of development, structure and function and the ways in which the various components of the nervous system respond to injury. In this way it is hoped to provide the reader with a basic appreciation of the varied pathogenetic mechanisms that may operate in neurological disorders. Such an appreciation should be helpful in diagnosis, prognosis and the assessment of benefits, if any, of therapeutic measures.

Development, structure and function of the nervous system

Development

Of all body systems the nervous system is perhaps pre-eminent in the importance that proper development of structure and function have on the well-being of the individual.

Development of the nervous system of mammals takes place as a sequence of intensely active events that occur from early embryogenesis and continue in cattle into postnatal life. During these phases cells undergoing rapid division and differentiation are uniquely susceptible to a wide variety of noxious influences, which include physical, chemical and infectious agents.

The physical factors include extremes of temperature, especially maternal hyperthermia, exposure to ionizing radiations and direct or indirect trauma. Chemical factors include organic, inorganic and plant poisons, nutritional imbalances and toxic products of microbial activity in the maternal or external environment. The direct invasion of the fetus by micro-organisms presents a further hazard and, of course, inherited defects or spontaneous errors in nucleic acid templating may produce effects at all stages of development. At certain stages immunological phenomena of the graft–host rejection type are also possible.

Fertilization of the ovum occurs in the fallopian tube

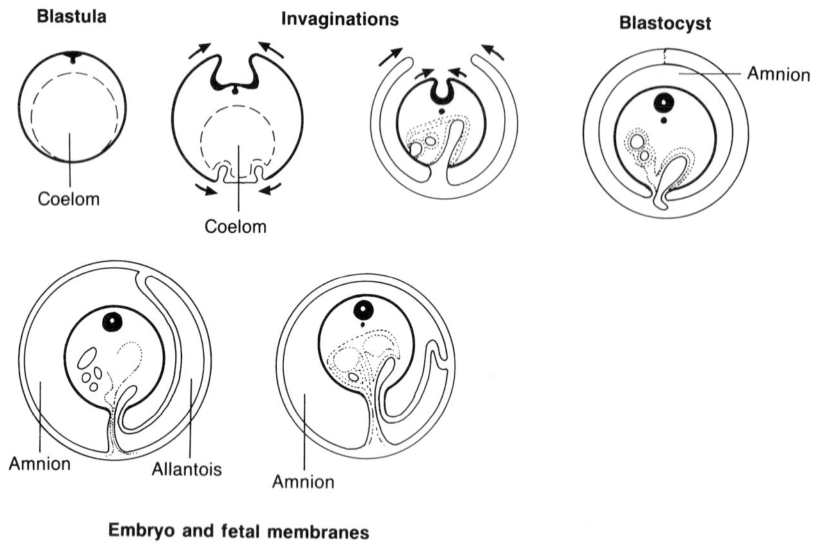

Fig. 45.1 Diagram of embryogenesis showing formation of embryonic and fetal membranes.

and the dividing zygote within its zona pellucida reaches the uterine horn three to four days later at the 16-cell stage. By the eighth day the morula has become a blastocyst in which embryonal and placental elements have differentiated and the zona pellucida has been lost. The blastocyst elongates and a part of it thickens and differentiates into three fundamental layers, ectoderm, mesoderm and entoderm. This thickened portion elongates to establish the long axis of the embryo and by a sequence of invaginations of the cyst wall the embryonic portion becomes enclosed by the extra-embryonic ectoderm, which forms the amniotic cavity and chorion (Fig. 45.1). The origins of the nervous system (the neural tube) and the gut are formed by similar invaginations and within the mesoderm differentiation of the cardiovascular system and liver commences.

By the 18th day the chorionic portion of the blastocyst (also called the trophoblast) has grown to fill the uterine horn and make firm contact with the uterine caruncles. These are gradually eroded and invaded by the rapidly vascularizing trophoblastic epithelium to establish the cotyledonary placenta.

During the preimplantation phases of embryogenesis and organogenesis (Fig. 45.2) the neural tube closes to form the cavity of the ventricular system. Dilatations at the cranial extremity, the prosencephalic vesicles, form the precursors of the cerebral hemispheres and the inner cell layer of the lining of the neural tube differentiates into ependymal cells, from the basal surface of each of which a fibre radiates to the margins of the CNS. The subependymal cells proliferate and migrate along these fine fibres whilst differentiating into neuroblasts and glioblasts.

Though the preimplantation embryo is insulated from many exogenous hazards by virtue of floating in an avascular fluid-filled sac, some 30 per cent of embryos are lost during the first three to six weeks of gestation. It is during this period also that many gross malformations, e.g. midline defects such as cyclopia (Plate 46.1), or spina bifida, have their origins.

Implantation in cattle is a gradual process that extends from about 25–30 days of gestation until the end of the third month, whereafter the placenta continues to grow and mature for about another month. This is the period of placental primacy, during which growth of placenta exceeds that of the fetus. Within the fetus the genesis and maturation of organs proceeds apace and the increasing vascularity of the placenta to meet the growing demands for nutrients and oxygen also exposes the fetus to a greater range of hazards than before implantation. Migration of neuroblasts and maturation of nerve cells with outgrowth of axons occurs and is followed by maturation of glioblasts into oligodendroglia, Schwann cells and astrocytes. Schwann cells and oligodendroglia commence the process of myelination, first in peripheral nerves then spinal cord and brain stem, cerebellum and forebrain.

The final phase of intra-uterine life is concerned mainly with growth and maturation of fetal organs and the onset of function. During this period the fetus is not only vulnerable to concomitant insults, but also to deficiencies of nutrients and oxygen arising from earlier insults that have caused stunting of the placenta during the period of placental primacy.

Birth is initiated by events intimately involving the fetal nervous system. Stimulation of the fetal hypothalamus, possibly by hypoxia, causes the pituitary to

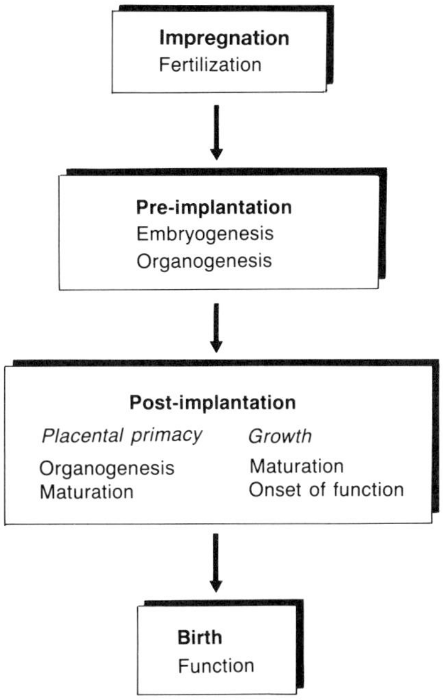

Fig. 45.2 Sequence of developmental events during pregnancy.

release adrenocorticotrophic hormone (ACTH), which in turn stimulates the fetal adrenal, the glucocorticoid hormones of which regulate the production of progesterone, oestrogens and prostaglandins at uterine level to induce myometrial contractions. Difficult or prolonged labour may result in hypoxic or traumatic damage or haemorrhage within the CNS, or avulsions of peripheral nerves, e.g. femoral.

In cattle, neural development is almost complete at birth. The cerebellum, however, continues to mature for some weeks and growth of spinal cord and peripheral nerves may continue for some months.

Structure and function

Structurally, the nervous system of higher vertebrates is at the same time both simple and exceedingly complex. It is simple in that the functional units are essentially only of two types, neurones and neuroglia. The neurones form the conducting system for neural impulses, receiving stimuli via their dendrites and transmitting them via the axon, these being extensions of the nerve cell body. The neuroglia are also of two types. The first are the oligodendroglia, which are responsible for the formation and maintenance of the myelin sheaths of the axons and also act as satellites subserving nerve cells. The second glial cell type are the astrocytes, which provide the supporting scaffold of the CNS and through their intermeshing processes provide nutrient pathways and also contribute to the blood–brain barrier, which prevents access of some molecules, e.g. immunoglobulins to nervous tissue. In the peripheral nervous system the Schwann cell is the homologue of the oligodendrocyte.

Complexity derives from the interactive and intricate nature of neuronal circuits, some of which are excitatory and others inhibitory. The complexity and diversity of structure and function are greatest in regions of highest neuronal density and are not yet fully understood. In general terms, however, the cerebral hemispheres are concerned with cognitive functions, receiving impulses from organs of special sense, together with tactile positional and other sensory information, all of which are integrated and formulated into conscious responses. The cerebellum, whose output is inhibitory, serves to modulate and control these responses. The brain stem serves many of the same functions as the cerebrum at a subconscious level and acts as a relay station for impulses passing to and from the cerebrum, cerebellum and spinal cord. The spinal cord and peripheral nerves are concerned with reflex activity and the transmission of impulses to and from the higher centres. The spinal cord and brain stem also contain the central connections of the autonomic or vegetative nervous system, which controls and maintains homeostatic mechanisms over a wide range of environmental situations.

To sustain functional activity the nervous system is heavily dependent upon glucose and oxygen; consequently there is a rich capillary network, especially in regions of high neuronal density. Even brief interference with the blood supply will rapidly cause hypoxia, interfere with membrane function and with accumulation of toxic metabolites such as lipid peroxides, resulting in swelling or cell death. When a nerve cell is lost it cannot be replaced and the circuit containing it is diminished. If substantial numbers of nerve cells are lost, functional deficits will result.

Infectious agents, toxic incidents and traumatic events may damage not only the neurone but also the glial components of the nervous system. Astrocytes are particularly reactive. Following injury they can proliferate to produce an astroglial scar, which itself may distort the tissue and further interfere with neural function. Oligodendroglia can also be regenerated from stem cells but in the mature CNS the ability to replace myelin is to a large extent dependent upon the viability of the neurone.

Reactions of nervous tissue to injury

Essentially, there are three ways in which cells may respond to injurious influences. These are destruction, depression and stimulation.

Destruction or cell death is followed by mineralization of the necrotic cell debris by calcium or iron, or its removal by lysis or active phagocytosis. *Depression* may reduce the purposive activities of the cell or if more severe, may compromise its vital functions leading to accumulation of metabolic products within the cytosol or organelles and ultimately to necrosis.

Stimulation is the response to the mildest forms of insult and is arguably an attempt by the cell to dilute the effects. This may be accomplished by hypertrophy or by cell division in tissues capable of mitotic activity. In nervous tissue neuroblasts lose this capability as they migrate and nature into nerve cells. Thus the full range of responses to noxious influences affecting the nervous system can occur only during the embryonic and early fetal stages.

Susceptibility of developing nervous tissue to injury is influenced not only by the nature and intensity of the insult but also by factors such as the rate of cell division taking place at the time of the injury in the particular region of the nervous system, and the degree of differentiation which the target cells have achieved. Since development is a finely integrated sequence of processes, local disruption of the sequence may affect the subsequent development of other tissues, directly or due to competition for substrates.

Injury to the blastocyst may be lethal or it may be fully overcome. Injury at a slightly later stage of development may result in gross malformations such as deletion or reduplication of a primordial structure, or by midline defects such as spina bifida or encephalocele, which are not incompatible with continued existence. The later in fetal life that cellular injury is sustained the more selective and subtle the primary pathology is likely to be, though the primary lesion may be overshadowed by the effects it has on organs and tissues quite remote from it.

By comparison with the responses of the developing nervous system to injury the reactions of the mature nervous system are relatively simple in themselves. Complexity arises from the anatomical distribution of the lesions and their functional significance.

Cytotoxins, or anoxia lasting a matter of minutes, can cause irreversible damage to nerve cells resulting in necrosis. A number of special terms have been used to describe subtle differences in the appearance of nerve cells undergoing necrosis (Sullivan 1985), but these can be resolved into two basic types. In the acute process the cytoplasm swells becoming pink and homogeneous whilst the nucleus swells and then shrinks. When the necrotizing process is less severe and more enduring the Nissl substance disappears from the margins of the cell, the cell body and nucleus shrink and the nucleolus becomes eosinophilic. This latter type of change may be difficult to distinguish from post-mortem change.

Less severe, potentially reversible damage to neurones may occur following damage, such as rupture of the axon, is accompanied by swelling of the cell body with margination of the Nissl granules (central chromatolysis). The nucleus at first swells then also moves to the cell margin. If the damage becomes irreversible the nucleus becomes shrunken and pyknotic, the cell body meanwhile developing a glassy or hyaline appearance, which may persist for some time before lysis or phagocytosis occurs.

Sublethal damage to neurones may also lead to the formation of localized axonal swellings variously described as spheroids or as axonal torpedoes. When such swellings occur at the proximal stump of a severed axon they are known as retraction bulbs.

Astrocytes respond to injury by swelling and hyperplasia, or if the damage is lethal, by retraction and fragmentation of processes and necrosis of the cell body. Unlike neurones, however, astrocytes can be regenerated from residual stem cells or the division of persisting cells at the margins of the lesion. Astrocytes resemble connective tissue cells in other organs in that, following deletion of parenchymal elements, they will proliferate to form a glial scar. Such a scar can result in kinks and twists in adjacent nerve fibres. In such situations it is thought that astrocytes may become involved in the transmission of nerve impulses and by spreading them to other nerve fibres in the vicinity they may contribute to the enhancement of neuronal firing. In this way glial scars could contribute to the development of postencephalitic forms of epilepsy.

The reactions of oligodendrocytes to injury resemble those of astrocytes and are most readily appreciated in the satellite cells that support the nerve cell body. Acutely injured oligodendrocytes show swelling and vacuolation of cytoplasm whereas in chronic neuronal injury they proliferate around the damaged neurone in what is termed neuronal satellitosis.

The myelin-forming and sustaining oligodendrocytes respond to injury in like manner. The normal myelin sheath forms from a spade-like oligodendroglial process wrapped spirally around an axon. As successive spirals are laid down the cytosol and contained organelles are squeezed out except at the inner, outer and end 'loops' of the process so that the plasma membranes of each spiral lie in contact. Sublethal damage to the oligodendrocyte resulting in cell swelling leads to separation of contacting plasma membranes and distension of the inner, outer and end loops, often referred to as periaxonal or intramyelinic oedema. Lethal damage to an oligodendroglial cell results in primary demyelination of that segment of the axon. Remyelination will occur if the insult is overcome and residual oligodendrocytes or undifferentiated stem cells are available.

The close functional relationship between neurones and oligodendroglia is also evident in the process of Wallerian degeneration. If an axon is sectioned, the portion distal to the section, separated from its cell of origin dies, and the myelin sheath surrounding it first collapses and is formed into digestion vacuoles in which phagocytosis by macrophages occurs. In short, the myelin-forming and sustaining activities of oligodendrocytes are in some way dependent on the presence of an intact axon.

The nature and causes of signs of neurological disorder

Endogenous biochemical causes

This group of conditions includes those metabolic diseases that are associated with the stresses of production and systems of management, and also the so-called 'inborn errors of metabolism'. The former include milk fever, transit tetany associated with hypocalcaemia (p. 577), hypomagnesaemic tetany (p. 583) and acetonaemia (p. 590). These disorders produce no specific pathological changes in the CNS and the clinical condition in most instances can be readily reversed by rapid correction of the specific deficiency. These conditions mainly affect high-yielding adult dairy cattle and are related to the stresses associated with calving, lactation or transport. Hypomagnesaemic tetany, however, may also be a cause of rapid death in weaned calves grazing on heavily fertilized lush young leys. The magnesium content is often low, and the high protein and potassium content of such diets reduces the absorption of magnesium from the gut (Field & Suttle, 1979). Though some individuals or families appear to be particularly susceptible to hypocalcaemia and other such metabolic disorders, the degree of heritability is insignificant.

On the other hand, the inborn errors of metabolism presently recognized in cattle are usually considered to be heritable, mainly with an autosomal recessive mode. A gene may control a specific enzyme or enzyme system and a defect therein will block the normal metabolic pathway. In some cases, however, there may be alternative pathways to modulate or minimize the consequences and these may influence the time of onset and rate of progress of clinical disease.

In inherited congenital myoclonus in the polled Hereford (Harper *et al.*, 1986), affected calves, though bright and alert, are unable to stand from birth and show stimulus-responsive myoclonic spasms (p. 149). Pathological changes are confined to the coxo-femoral joints which, in the majority of cases, show eburnation and fracture of the articular cartilages and contusions of the joint capsule and surrounding tissues. These findings suggest that severe myoclonic spasms may have been occurring during intra-uterine life. The cause of these spasms has as yet not been fully established, though recent evidence suggesting a loss of glycine receptors in the spinal cord has been supported by the finding of reduced [^{3}H]-strychnine binding to membranes (Grundlach *et al.*, 1988).

A second genetically mediated disorder that may be confused with inherited congenital myoclonus is neuraxial oedema. This also occurs in Herefords, polled Herefords and possibly other breeds. Affected calves appear normal at birth but within a day or two they become dull and recumbent with opisthotonus. The urine contains elevated ketone concentrations and has an aroma of burnt sugar (Healy *et al.*, 1986). The significant pathology is in the CNS and consists of vacuolation at all levels of the neuraxis. The vacuoles are about 40 μm diameter and are present throughout the white matter and deeper laminae of the cerebral cortex. In many instances there is evidence of defective myelination. Axonal swellings may be present on Purkinje cell axons in the cerebellar cortex and mineralized (Ca^{2+} and Fe^{2+}) bodies may be encountered in the deep granular layer and adjacent white matter of the arbor vitae. These findings together with raised ketones and burnt-sugar aroma of urine are consistent with a diagnosis of 'maple syrup urine disease' resulting from defective amino acid metabolism (p. 149).

There are several inborn errors of metabolism in which the abnormal metabolites cannot be readily discharged and therefore accumulate in the tissues. Nervous tissue is particularly liable to accumulate such metabolites, especially compounds of high molecular weight. This is because cell turnover is low in most cell types and absent in nerve cells. Thus neurones tend to accumulate such compounds preferentially.

Lysosomes normally contain large numbers of hydrolytic enzymes, active at pH 5 or less, which can degrade proteins, glycolipids and carbohydrates into simpler monomeric compounds. If the normal enzymatic processes are overloaded or defective, lysosomes will store the materials they normally degrade. In an important group of genetically mediated diseases, the lysosomal storage diseases, the products of faulty degradation accumulate in lysosomes and the cell bodies swell. The type of storage product can be determined by histochemical and biochemical methods and the specific enzyme defect pinpointed. Since these are autosomal recessive (or sometimes sex-linked) phenomena, they are gene-dose dependent. That is to say the cells of the heterozygote contain approximately half the normal concentration of enzyme, but the animal itself appears normal, whilst the diseased animal is homozygous for the defect and the enzyme is absent. Heterozygote recognition by appropriate enzymic assay therefore offers a means of controlling the disease within a population.

Examples of lysosomal storage diseases that occur in cattle are the lipidosis GM_1 gangliosidosis in the Friesian, the glycoproteinosis mannosidosis in the Angus, Murray Grey and Galloway and the ceroid lipofuscinosis, which has been described in Beefmaster cattle.

GM_1 gangliosidosis is a consequence of reduction in the enzyme β-galactosidase. The clinical signs are reluctance to feed, dullness, progressive ataxia and ill-thrift, and appear one to three months after birth. The glycolipid storage product causes ballooning of neurones throughout the neuraxis.

Mannosidosis (pseudolipidosis) is the result of deficiency of the enzyme α-mannosidase (p. 148). Clinically, the disease presents as wasting, altered behaviour with aggression and progressive ataxia. Superficial lymph nodes may be palpably enlarged. Weakly periodic acid–Schiff (PAS)-positive storage products (oligosaccharides) distend the cytoplasm of neurones, particularly those in the brain stem, cerebellum and spinal cord. Storage products are also found in fixed macrophages in lymphoreticular organs, in the renal tubular epithelium and in the cells of the exocrine pancreas.

Lysosomal α-mannosidase is also inhibited by swainsonine, an alkaloid present in the Australian plant, the Darling pea (*Swainsonia*) and American loco weeds of the genera *Oxytropis* and *Astragalus*. Intoxication of grazing ruminants by these plants mimics the genetic disorder but there may be slow regression of clinical signs when animals are prevented having further access to the plant.

Exogenous biochemical causes

The range of exogenous biochemical causes of neurological disorder is wide. It includes organic and inorganic compounds, phytotoxins and mycotoxins, snake venoms and overdosage with prophylactic and therapeutic substances. Some compounds, e.g. organophosphorus compounds and carbamates, are specific neurotoxins whose mode of action is known. However, a great many toxicants whose primary targets appear to be gut, liver or cardiovascular system also cause neurological disturbances. In the early phases these usually take the form of excitement, muscle fasciculations, tachycardia and hyperpnoea, whilst convulsions and coma frequently characterize the terminal phases. The mechanisms of this toxic stimulation and depression of the nervous system are poorly understood. A partial explanation may be that acute intoxications often produce fulminating clinical disease within minutes and death within a few hours thus giving little time for morphological changes in the CNS to develop. It seems probable, however, that interference with the functions of respiratory enzymes or mediators of synaptic transmission could be a crucial factor.

Though the gut is the most common route of entry, toxicants may also gain access through the skin, the respiratory tract or by injection. The liver is the organ principally concerned with the metabolism and detoxification of poisonous substances though paradoxically some biologically inert substances are transformed into toxic compounds in the liver. For example, parathion becomes metabolized to paraoxon, which is a powerful inhibitor of cholinesterase.

The metabolism of many poisonous substances involves firstly oxidative reactions to produce more polar molecules, which can then be conjugated with substances such as glucuronic acid and excreted by the kidney. Other routes of excretion include expired air (e.g. coniine, selenium) and milk (e.g. lead, pyrolizidine alkaloids).

Toxic substances may have a particular affinity for certain organs and tissues, e.g. iodine for the thyroid gland, or selenium for heart muscle, whilst lipid-soluble compounds are liable to accumulate in nervous tissue. Neural function may also be affected indirectly as a result of toxic dysfunction of the cardiovascular system, liver, or kidneys. As a major organ of storage and detoxification of substances, the liver itself is liable to chronic damage from compounds such as carbon tetrachloride, pyrrolizidine alkaloids, aflatoxins or excess dietary copper, all of which may compromise its ability to handle nitrogenous compounds. Oligodendrocytes appear to be the CNS cells most affected by the hyperammonaemia that may result. They undergo hydropic change resulting in the formation of vacuoles 30–60 μm in diameter in the white matter, notably in cerebellum, brain stem and spinal cord. These vacuoles are attributable to periaxonal and intramyelinic oedema and the condition is termed hepatic encephalopathy.

In cattle, intoxication by chemical compounds is not uncommon for reasons that include their innate curiosity, considerable appetite and non-selective habits of grazing and licking. The most common intoxicants of cattle in the UK in decreasing order of importance have been listed as lead, fluoride, bracken (*Pteridium aquilinum*), nitrates, ragwort (*Senecio jacoboea*), copper, arsenic, organophosphorus compounds, metaldehyde, urea, paraquat, furazolidone, sodium chloride, kale (*Brassica oleracea*), thiabendazole and monensin (Humphreys, 1988). Of these only lead, the organophosphorus compounds, ragwort, copper, urea and sodium chloride are known to cause neuropathological changes. Lead is by far the most important and is considered in detail later (p. 704).

Organophosphorus compounds used as insecticides, herbicides, flame retardants and lubricating agents are variably potent inhibitors of cholinesterase. The clinical signs of acute intoxication, miosis, salivation, polyuria, muscle fasciculations, apprehension and ataxia are the consequences of cholinergic overstimulation, but produce no characteristic neuropathology. Prolonged cholinesterase inhibition, which is most commonly associated with the triaryl phosphates, e.g. tri-orthocresyl phosphate, induces a neuropathy characterized by 'die back' of long myelinated fibres in the peripheral nerves and spinal cord, leading to disturbances of proprioception, and ataxia, locomotor weakness and paralysis (p. 162).

Ingestion of ragwort (p. 618) or excess copper (p. 613) over long periods of time will lead to cirrhosis, which may result in hyperammonaemia and hepatic encephalopathy. Subclinical cirrhosis may predispose to hepatic encephalopathy in cattle on diets containing only a moderate excess of urea. The clinical signs of hepatic encephalopathy may be intermittent and slowly progressive, or acutely fatal depending upon the severity and duration of hepatic overload by nitrogenous compounds. There are behavioural changes, with compulsive walking, circling, twitching of ears and eyelids, apparent blindness, and in severe cases recumbency with opisthotonus and extensor spasms or paddling movements.

Salt poisoning is liable to occur following several days of high salt but restricted water intake followed by free access to fresh water. In its pathogenesis it is comparable to water intoxication. It is thought that rapid reduction of the plasma salt concentration produces an osmotic gradient towards the tissues (which contain high concentrations of electrolyte). This will cause the tissues to swell, increasing intracranial pressure and restricting blood flow in the capillaries in the terminal territories of the major cerebral arteries. Tissue anoxia leads to necrosis of neurones and malacia of some cortical laminae. High-yielding dairy cows in early lactation are said to be especially susceptible because their electrolyte balance is less stable.

Acute poisoning may be suspected in a herd when there is the sudden appearance of neurological or systemic disturbance affecting several members of a group over a short period of time. As the clinical signs are similar for many poisons a detailed history and a careful search of the environment may help to narrow the range of possibilities. Liver, kidney, ruminal and abomasal contents should be collected for chemical confirmation of the diagnosis. In cases of suspected organophosphorus poisoning depression of cholinesterase in a fresh anticoagulated blood sample may be of value, though there can be difficulties in the interpretation of assays.

Control of exogenous biochemical causes of neurological disease is clearly and fundamentally a matter of good management.

Genetic causes

According to Mendelian theory, transmission of a particular familial trait to subsequent generations may occur in either the dominant or the recessive mode. This means that a trait transmitted by a dominant of full penetrance will exhibit the phenotype in at least 75 per cent of offspring, whilst expression of a recessive trait is dependent on gene dose and may vary from 0 to 100 per cent depending on the genotype of both parents. In practice, matters are more complicated because some genes may not be fully penetrant or expression of the trait polygenic. Furthermore, genetic mutation may occur fortuitously or as a result of environmental influences acting during gametogenesis or during recombination of DNA at fertilization. As well as resulting in defective enzymes, as for example in the inborn errors of metabolism (see p. 695), anomalous coding of the genome can result in structural aberrations. The fundamental biochemical mechanisms of such anomalies are obscure and may be complex. The literature contains many references to congenital hydrocephalus in cattle with a putatively genetic basis (p. 147). However, in ascribing a genetic aetiology to a given disease it should be remembered that transmission of disease in a Mendelian pattern does not exclude the possibility of predominant environmental influences, nor does the demonstration of a transmissible agent necessarily mean that expression of disease is not genetically determined. For example, the occurrence of

Table 45.1 Inherited neurological diseases of cattle

Disease	Mode R/D	Breed(s)	Age at onset	Clinical features	Pathology	Reference
Cerebellar abiotrophy	R	Holstein	3–8 months	Progressive spastic ataxia, dysmetria. Loss of menace response	Degeneration of cerebellar neurones sparing the vermis	White *et al.* (1975)
Hereditary congenital ataxia 'jittery'	R	Jersey	Birth to 3 months	Ataxia and intention tremor	Hypomyelination and oedema of cerebellar white matter	Saunders *et al.* (1952)
Cerebellar ataxia	R?	Shorthorn Hereford	1–3 days	Rapidly progressive ataxia with recumbency	Spongy transformation of cerebellar white matter, shrinkage and loss of neurones	Hulland (1957)
Familial cerebellar hypoplasia and degeneration	R	Hereford	Birth	Recumbent, stuporose, intermittent rigidity	Narrow disorganized cerebellar folia. Paucity of cerebellar cortical neurones	Innes *et al.* (1940)
Familial convulsions and ataxia	D	Aberdeen Angus	Birth to 6 months	Recurrent seizures with gradual development of spastic ataxia and hypermetria	Swelling and vacuolation of Purkinje cells and Purkinje cell axons	Barlow (1980)
Doddler	R	Hereford	Birth	Muscular spasms and convulsions, nystagmus, respiratory difficulties	Calcification of cerebellar and medullary neurones	High *et al.* (1958)
GM_1 gangliosidosis	R	Friesian	1 month	Reluctance to feed, dullness and progressive ataxia	Cerebrospinal lipidosis with ballooning of neurones by accumulations of glycolipid	Donnelly *et al.* (1973)
Mannosidosis	R	Angus, Murray Grey, Galloway	Birth onwards	Wasting, aggression and progressive ataxia, lymphadenopathy	Vacuolation of neurones and fixed macrophages, renal epithelial cells and exocrine pancreas	Hocking *et al.* (1972)
Neuraxial oedema: maple syrup urine disease	R	Hereford and polled Hereford	1–3 days	Dullness, recumbency and opisthotonus: nystagmus. Urine smells of burnt sugar	Raised urine ketones. Vacuolation throughout neuraxis especially white matter	Healy *et al.* (1986)
Inherited congenital myoclonus	R	Polled Hereford	Birth	Stimulus-responsive myoclonic spasms	Contusions of coxofemoral joint with fractures/ deformity of articular cartilage	Harper *et al.* (1986)

Table 45.1 Cont.

Disease	Mode R/D	Breed(s)	Age at onset	Clinical features	Pathology	Reference
Bovine generalized glycogenosis	R	Shorthorn	12 months	Muscular weakness, incoordination, deficiency of α-1,4-glucosidase or acid maltase	Accumulation of PAS-positive and Bests carmine plus granules in neurones of midbrain, medullary and cerebellar roof nuclei	Richards *et al.*(1977)
Chediak–Higashi syndrome	R	Hereford, Brown Swiss	Young adults	Partial albinism (ghost pattern colouring). Susceptibility to infection. Premature ageing	Yellow pigmented PAS, LFB and Sudan black B-positive inclusions in nerve cells of brain, cord, myenteric plexuses. Similar to lipofuscin granules	Padgett (1968)
'Weaver syndrome': progressive degenerative myeloencephalopathy	R	Brown Swiss	8–12 months	Motor dysfunction with swinging gait progressing to loss of movement and inability to stand	Axonal degeneration predominantly in spinal white matter, axons in some brain stem nuclei and Purkinje cells of cerebellar cortex. Paramembranous densities at synaptic junctions	Stuart & Leipold (1985)
Neuronal lipodystrophy	R	Beefmaster	12 months	Blindness, circling, recumbency and coma	Neuronal multilamellar and curvilinear inclusions. Similar structures may be found in fixed macrophages in spleen and lymph nodes.	Read & Bridges (1969)
Progressive ataxia of Charolais	R?	Charolais	8–24 months	Progressive weakness and ataxia terminating in recumbency	Segmental demyelination of CNS with retraction of internodes, formation of eosinophilic plaques formed from oligodendroglial processes	Palmer *et al.* (1972)
Recumbent calf syndrome	R?	Red Danish milk breed	6 weeks	Progressive ataxia, paresis and immobility	Degeneration of neurones in ventral horns of spinal cord	Hansen *et al.* (1988)

R, recessive; D, dominant; PAS, periodic acid shift

hydrocephalus and cerebellar hypoplasia in a familial pattern may be a consequence of persistent infection and vertical transmission of bovine virus diarrhoea virus (p. 660).

Another example is spastic paresis (p. 149). This is a condition characterized by contraction of the gastrocnemius muscle, straightening of the tarsus with the calcaneus pulled forward towards the tibia. It occurs with a familial tendency in growing calves of several breeds. Engel (1970) in a study of 100 cases considered that environmental factors associated with conception during winter influenced the prevalence of the clinical disorder and other extended studies have suggested that spastic paresis is not inherited as a simple recessive (Stolzenberg & Schonmuth, 1971; Baird *et al.*, 1974).

There is a substantial number of putatively genetic disorders of the bovine nervous system, the biochemical mechanisms of which are unknown and whose expression may be modulated by factors in the environment (Table 45.1). The plurality of genetic neurological disorders in cattle is possibly a reflection of intensive selection for particular production traits from within small populations of superior animals and is facilitated by artificial breeding techniques.

Control of genetic disease is difficult and probably feasible only in populations with a high incidence of disease in which is implicated either a dominant of full penetrance (a rare event) or a recessive in which the heterozygote carrier animal can be identified.

Micro-organisms

Neurological disorders in cattle can result from the activities of all types of infective agents. Some invade the nervous system usually causing inflammation of the brain (encephalitis), spinal cord (myelitis) or the membranous coverings (meningitis). Others that may be present in the alimentary tract or external environment produce neurotoxins or antimetabolites, which cause degenerative encephalopathies and myelopathies. Calves and young adults are usually the susceptible groups though with some micro-organisms it is the fetus that is most at risk.

Viruses

Viruses of several families, together form an important group of neural pathogens. The oronasal route is the most common portal of entry, but some viruses gain access via the conjunctiva or percutaneously by the bite of an insect vector or infected animal. Initial replication at the site of infection and in local lymphoid tissues is typically followed by viraemia with fever during which the virus penetrates the blood–brain barrier and invades the neural parenchyma. In some viral infections viraemia is insignificant or absent, the virus reaching the neuroparenchyma by centripetal intra-axonal transport. Continued viral replication in the neuroparenchyma causes pathological changes in neurones, sometimes associated with the formation of inclusion bodies, and also in glial cells, which may result in demyelination. Typical inflammatory responses are focal and diffuse proliferations of microglial cells and perivascular and meningeal infiltrations of lymphocytes. As the CNS is normally relatively impermeable to circulating immunoglobulins, synthesis of antibody by B cells in the perivascular cuffs may play an important role in the recovery of the individual.

Other virus infections, e.g. Akabane disease (p. 753) (Inaba *et al.*, 1975) and bovine virus diarrhoea/mucosal disease (Trautwein *et al.*, 1987), generally cause mild or inapparent disease in the adult but cause severe transplacental infections of the fetus. Fetal meningoencephalitis or gross intracranial malformations from destruction of the granuloprival elements of the developing fetal brain may be the result depending upon the stage of fetal development at infection.

Bacteria

Bacteria, with possibly *Listeria monocytogenes* (see p. 703) as the sole exception, do not invade the neuroparenchyma as a primary event. Infection of the neuraxis usually arises from a bacteraemia causing meningitis, which may be purulent or non-purulent depending on the organism involved. Infection of the meninges may also arise directly following local trauma. Subsequent invasion of the neuroparenchyma, however, depends upon damage to the blood–brain barrier, such as may occur following rupture of a meningeal abscess, devitalization of the tissue by toxic products or infarction due to infective emboli as in thromboembolic meningo-encephalitis (Ames, 1987). This condition is caused by *Haemophilus somnus*, a not infrequent inhabitant of the respiratory tract of cattle (p. 571). Under conditions of stress or intercurrent disease a fulminating *Haemophilus* bacteraemia may occur with disseminated intravascular coagulation. Thromboemboli may lodge in meninges, brain, muscles and joints causing depression, blindness and recumbency with muscular weakness. Retinal haemorrhages may be found.

Other manifestations of bacterial involvement in neurological disease include those caused by the exotoxins of clostridial infections occurring elsewhere in the body, e.g. focal symmetrical encephalomalacia (Buxton *et al.*, 1981) and tetanus, which is discussed elsewhere. Also in this category are the thiaminolytic organisms that proliferate in rumen contents and are implicated in cerebrocortical necrosis (see below).

Bacterial toxins produced in the environment have also been implicated in bovine neurological disturbance. In Australia a soil bacterium, *Corynebacterium rathayi*, is carried to the developing seed head of annual ryegrass, *Lolium rigidum*, by a small nematode (*Anguina* spp.). The worm forms a gall within which the bacterium multiplies and elaborates the toxin, which when ingested by cattle causes increased permeability of cerebral blood vessels with leakage of plasma or frank haemorrhage (Berry *et al.*, 1980).

Diseases due to *Chlamydia* and *Rickettsia* are considered elsewhere (see pp. 706, 707).

Protozoa

Protozoan infections with *Toxoplasma gondii* and *Sarcocystis* species have been implicated in neonatal necrotizing non-suppurative encephalomyelitis in calves (O'Toole & Jeffrey, 1987). Severe coccidiosis in calves is not uncommonly associated with neurological disorder. This may vary from mild muscular spasms to tetanic convulsions. This 'neural coccidiosis' appears to be associated with a labile neurotoxin present in the serum of affected calves (Isler *et al.*, 1987).

Fungi

The occurrence of neurotropic mycotoxicoses in Britain has not been firmly established. In New Zealand, however, a condition characterized by trembling ataxia and tetanic convulsions occurs in cattle grazing the stubbles of perennial ryegrass infected with an endophytic *Penicillium* fungus. The tremorgenic neurotoxins lolitrem A and lolitrem B have been demonstrated in this material and produce axonal torpedoes on Purkinje cell axons (Fletcher & Harvey, 1981; Gallagher *et al.*, 1981).

Nematodes

The intermediate stage of the dog tapeworm *Multiceps multiceps* is not confined to sheep but may also occur in cattle and other species including man.

Insects

On rare occasions the larval stages of the warble fly *Hypoderma bovis* and *H. lineatum* may enter the vertebral canal during migration, damage the spinal cord to cause local neural dysfunction before leaving to continue their migration to the subcutis (p. 678).

Specific diseases

Cerebrocortical necrosis (CCN)

This is a sporadic, acute, frequently fatal condition that affects most ruminant species. It is characterized clinically by dullness, blindness, opisthotonus, recumbency and paddling movements and pathologically by patchy cerebral poliomalacia.

Aetiology

Polioencephalomalacia and CCN are pathological descriptions that in themselves have no aetiological significance. In most cases, however, the clinical disorder is responsive to the administration of thiamine. Though the aetiology of this disease is incompletely understood, biochemical observations support the concept that thiamine or vitamin B_1 deficiency at cell level is crucially involved.

Vitamin B_1 is synthesized by higher plants, bacteria, algae and some fungi and most animals are dependent on dietary sources for their requirements. However, healthy ruminants obtain their requirements from thiamine synthesized by the rumen flora. Free thiamine is readily absorbed and is actively phosphorylated to thiamine pyrophosphate (TPP) by an adenosine triphosphate (ATP)-dependent enzyme. Thiamine pyrophosphate is less diffusible than thiamine and is stored mainly in heart, liver and kidneys. The TPP formed within the cell unites with protein moieties to form the holoenzymes of intermediary metabolism.

The brain is critically dependent on carbohydrate for energy and TPP has a coenzyme role in decarboxylation of α-ketoacids, e.g. pyruvate to acetyl-CoA for entry into the tricarboxylic acid cycle and also in the oxidation of α-ketoglutarate to succinyl-CoA. Thiamine pyrophosphate is also a coenzyme in the transketolase reaction of the hexose monophosphate shunt and the alternative, glycolytic, pentose phosphate pathway. Much of the energy produced is used to sustain membrane potentials via the Na^+, K^+-ATPase ionic pump. Impaired efficiency of this pump upsets water and electrolyte balance with several neuropathological consequences, which include varicose dilatations of blood vessels with haemorrhage; hypertrophy and degeneration of synapses and nerve endings (dieback); swelling of perivascular astrocyte foot processes and cell bodies; splitting of the myelin sheath at the intraperiod line and neuronal degeneration. Biochemically, TPP and transketolase activity are reduced and pyruvate and lactate accumulate in the tissues (Edwin, 1970).

Pathology

Subserosal petechiation of the wall of the intestine may be evident, but usually macroscopic changes are confined to the brain. It usually appears pale and swollen with flattened gyri, which in the frontal, dorso-medial and parietal regions often shows a patchy, bilaterally symmetrical, yellow discoloration. There is swelling of the cingulate and parahippocampal gyri, which may herniate beneath the tentorium cerebelli. The posterior vermis may have herniated through the foramen magnum and appear necrotic. The cut surface of the cerebrum reveals that the necrotic cortical tissues have a laminar configuration and may have separated from the underlying white matter. When viewed in ultraviolet light (wavelength 365 nm) affected regions of cortex have a bright white autofluorescence, which has been attributed to ceroid lipofuscin (Little, 1978).

Histologically, there is increased prominence of capillary endothelium (neovascularization), and dilatation of perivascular spaces with occasional small perivascular haemorrhages. Astrocytes and neurones show hydropic changes and nuclear pyknosis, which proceeds in time to a laminar necrosis that faithfully follows the contours of the gyri but spares the depths of the sulci. Necrosis is most severe in the most superficial and also the deeper cortical laminae and may extend into the subjacent, oedematous, gyral white matter. In well-established cases there is a massive influx of macrophages into the necrotic areas and adjacent leptomeninges. In cattle that survive there may be total ablation of the affected areas of cortex with formation of cystic cavities or glial scars.

Symmetrical lesions of the same basic type, but which rarely become necrotic may be found in the basal ganglia and brain stem. The caudal vermis may also contain a necrotic focus attributable to pressure.

Ultrastructural studies of the disease in sheep (Morgan, 1973) have indicated that the earliest changes are cytopathic swelling and accumulation of glycogen granules in the cytoplasm of astrocytes and satellite oligodendroglia. It is considered that the resultant generalized brain swelling may reduce cerebral circulation to the point at which the terminal territories of the cerebral arteries are susceptible to ischaemic necrosis.

Signs and diagnosis

This is a disease principally affecting weaned calves and young feedlot cattle. It is frequently associated with diets low in fibre though cases have occurred in animals grazing lush aftermath. Under these circumstances, changes occur in the rumen flora that permit multiplication of micro-organisms such as *Bacillus thiaminolyticus* and *Clostridium sporogenes*, both of which synthesize thiaminase type I. This enzyme not only destroys thiamine but participates in a base exchange reaction leading to the production of pyrimidinyl nicotinic acid, which acts as a competitive antagonist of thiamine.

Some external dietary sources of thiaminase type I have been implicated in CCN. These include bracken rhizomes (*Pteridium aquilinum*) and Mexican fireweed (*Kochia scoparia*). In Cuba a condition known as molasses drunkenness or molasses toxicity, indistinguishable from CCN, has been described in cattle fed large amounts of immature molasses in a low fibre diet (Geerken & Figueroa, 1971).

In the prodromal phase of CCN there is frequently a brief period of diarrhoea before nervous signs appear. Then there is dullness, cortical blindness with inappetence and a tendency to head pressing. As the disease progresses twitching, muscular tremors and intermittent opisthotonus are evident, followed by salivation, bruxism (teeth grinding), recumbency and clonic convulsions with intermittent periods of spasticity and terminal flaccidity.

Diagnosis of CCN is based primarily on the history, clinical signs and the response to parenteral thiamine administration. Assays of blood thiamine, ruminal and faecal thiaminase may identify other members of the herd at risk of developing the disease. Perhaps the most useful biochemical laboratory procedure is the measurement of the 'TPP effect', i.e. the increase in blood transketolase activity following the addition of excess thiamine diphosphate to the sample.

Treatment and prevention

Given early in the disease the response to large doses (10–15 mg/kg) of thiamine hydrochloride or multi-B vitamin preparations given intravenously is usually evident in 3–6 hours. If thiamine is used the dose should be repeated at least every 4 hours for 24 hours, by which time there should be full clinical recovery. In more advanced cases the prognosis is not as good and more aggressive therapy may be indicated. In established disease daily administration of dexamethasone intramuscularly and mannitol by intravenous drip for three days may facilitate recovery.

For treatment or prophylaxis by the oral route the less water-soluble thiamine derivatives such as thiamine propyldisulphide or tetrafurfuryldisulphide have the advantage that they are not destroyed by thiaminase type 1 and yet are readily absorbed from the gut. Control of CCN may be through the prophylactic use of such drugs, but prevention is by the maintenance of normal rumen fermentation with adequate production of volatile fatty acids, which curtail the growth of thiaminase-producing organisms.

Listerial encephalitis (see also p. 471)

Listerial encephalitis is the result of infection of the brain substance with *Listeria monocytogenes*.

Aetiology

Listeria monocytogenes is a micro-aerophilic Gram-positive, flagellated coccobacillus in which five serotypes and several subtypes have been identified. The organism is present in a wide range of moist environments and may cause disease in man and a variety of domestic species. Many cases are associated with poorly fermented silage. Alimentary and mammary infections may be clinically silent and disease usually takes the form of septicaemia, abortion or encephalitis. Encephalitis is most commonly associated with serotypes 1/2a and 4b.

Pathology

The pathogenesis of listerial encephalitis is probably unique in that available evidence suggests that infection of the brain is by centripetal passage of the organism along branches of the trigeminal nerve from minor breaches in the buccal mucosa, facial skin or conjunctivae. Intracranial pathology initially consists of a small focus of necrosis in the lateral part of the pons, which is associated with activation of microglial cells and astrocytes followed by an influx of inflammatory cells. These are mainly monocytes but a few neutrophils may be found at the centre of the lesions. The initial focus may be unilateral but thereafter (intraneural) spread results in micro–abscesses forming bilaterally in the midbrain and lower medulla. Longer-established lesions are associated with more widespread, predominantly lymphocytic infiltrations of the meninges and perivascular spaces. Listerial encephalitis is thus a unique example of a true bacterial encephalitis.

Signs and diagnosis

Early signs include extreme dullness, difficulty in prehension and mastication, accumulation of cud in the cheek, salivation and deviation without head tilt. There may be ptosis and drooping of the ear on the deviant side and circling in the direction of the deviation. The tongue may also protrude toward the deviant side and be incapable of retraction. Some affected cattle develop panophthalmitis. The animal is febrile and in the later stages there may be persistent bellowing, and frenzy followed by coma and death. The course in cattle lasts 10–14 days.

Listeriosis is frequently associated with the feeding of silage and may be suspected on the basis of the clinical signs and supported by finding a monocytic pleocytosis in the CSF. Rabies (p. 706), bovine spongiform encephalopathy (p. 708) and nervous acetonaemia (p. 590) should be considered in the differential diagnosis. Confirmation of diagnosis is a post-mortem procedure. Isolation of the causal organism from the brain may require extended periods of 'cold enrichment' but the neurohistopathology is usually sufficiently characteristic to permit firm diagnosis.

Treatment and prevention

Chloramphenicol is one of the few antibiotics that will pass the blood–brain barrier and is probably the treatment of choice in the early stages of disease. In established cases where the blood–brain barrier has been breached, penicillin and streptomycin have been found effective when high doses are used over several days. Though progress of the disease may be halted it is unlikely that severe neurological deficits will resolve.

Prevention of listerial encephalitis by vaccination is not an established procedure. Control measures should include attention to the making and management of silage to ensure minimum soil contamination and good fermentation and the withdrawal of poor quality or spoiled ensilage. Cases of listerial encephalitis are usually sporadic but, in the face of a severe outbreak, consideration should be given to prophylactic administration of suitable antibiotics.

Louping-ill

Louping-ill is a tick-borne viral encephalitis which, though primarily a disease of sheep, has also been reported in cattle, goats, horses, pigs, deer and grouse. Humans are also susceptible.

Aetiology

Louping-ill virus is a flavivirus of the Togaviridae that is closely related to that causing Russian spring–summer encephalitis (p. 750). It is transmitted by the tick *Ixodes ricinus*, which is endemic in the upland regions of northern and western Britain. Larval and nymphal stages of the tick acquire the infection during a blood meal on a viraemic host and will transmit to a susceptible host during the blood meal at their next developmental stage. Transovarial spread of infection in the tick does not appear to occur.

Pathogenesis and pathology

Following inoculation of a susceptible host the virus replicates in local lymphoid tissue. Three to five days later viraemia accompanied by fever results in widespread dissemination of virus. A second febrile phase may develop as the virus enters nervous tissue and establishes infection.

The lesions of louping-ill are microscopic and confined to the CNS. In all species they consist of necrosis of neurones, focal and diffuse microglial accumulations in the neuropil and perivascular cuffing by lymphocytes. Inclusion bodies are not found. In cattle and deer, in which the disease tends to be mild with a longer clinical course than in sheep, there may be evidence of neuronophagia. The lesions have a characteristic distribution affecting mainly the medulla, the cervical spinal cord and, to a lesser extent, also the cerebellum (Doherty & Reid, 1971). However, it has recently been shown (Reid *et al.*, 1984) that virus present in the milk of viraemic goats induced more generalized meningoencephalitis in their progeny. It was uncertain whether the route of entry was olfactory or alimentary.

Signs and diagnosis

Evidence of recent or active infestation by *I. ricinus* in a febrile animal raises the possibility of louping-ill virus infection. Neurological signs initially include dullness, fine tremor of muscle groups and congested conjunctivae, progressing to weakness and incoordination, especially of the hindlimbs, followed by prostration, coma and death. In cattle, the neurological disturbance is usually mild and recovery is common. Recovered animals are solidly immune.

Virus is quickly eliminated from extraneural tissues by a rapid and effective immune response. Thus examination of serum for specific IgM antibody by haemagglutination inhibition is preferable to blood culture for *in vivo* diagnosis of louping-ill. Post-mortem diagnosis depends upon virus isolation from brain tissue, histopathology of CNS and the presence of antibody in cerebrospinal fluid.

Treatment and prevention

There is no specific treatment for louping-ill encephalitis. Affected animals should be isolated in quiet darkened surroundings and carefully nursed. Hand feeding, deep bedding and regular turning may be required in some cases. An effective tissue culture vaccine is available (p. 814) and should be used on all young stock and introduced animals in louping-ill endemic areas, in which vaccination titres can be sustained by repeated exposure to infection. Vaccinated and acclimatized cows secrete colostral antibody sufficient to protect their progeny during the first months of life. Control of ticks by dipping or spraying whilst useful in itself is generally insufficient to prevent louping-ill as sometimes ticks will remain. It would be prudent to destroy the milk of infected dairy cattle.

Lead poisoning (see also p. 617)

Cattle through their innate curiosity, indiscriminate feeding habits and relative susceptibility to lead are the species most commonly poisoned by lead compounds.

Aetiology

The most frequent source of lead is from electric storage batteries that have been discarded or used to secure the covers of silage clamps. Other sources include flaking old lead-based paint, boiled linseed oil, putty, asphalt roofing materials, used motor engine oil, linoleum, and atmospheric fallout onto pastures from nearby smelters. Intoxication may result from a single large dose of lead or from ingestion of smaller amounts over a long period of time. In both forms the neurological signs are acute in onset and similar in type.

Pathology

The severity of neuropathological change in lead poisoning correlates more closely with survival time than with the concentration of lead in the tissues, being most severe in cases that survive longest.

Grossly, the brain appears pale and slightly swollen

with flattened gyri but without herniation of the hippocampal gyrus beneath the tentorium or cerebellar coning (cf. CCN). Some gyri, most commonly those in the occipital region, show a yellow discoloration. The cut surface may show separation of these yellow zones of cortical tissue from the underlying white matter at the tips of the gyri with actual cavitation in the deeper cortical laminae. In cases of longer survival these changes may extend to the tips of almost all gyri and extend down the sides of the convolutions (Christian & Tryphonas, 1971).

Histologically, the earliest changes in affected gyri comprise swelling and prominence of capillary endothelial cells, which is sometimes referred to as neovascularization. Swelling of astrocytes, and fine microvacuolation of the neuropil, also occurs at an early stage, advancing to spongy transformation with necrosis of neurones, malacia, and infiltration by macrophages. In cattle with long survival periods these cortical lesions may be extensive, and similar lesions may be present also in the thalamus and hypothalamus, medulla and spinal cord. Acid-fast intranuclear inclusion bodies may be present in the epithelial cells of the proximal convoluted tubules of the kidney and occasionally also in hepatocytes.

Signs and diagnosis

Irrespective of the rate of uptake of lead the clinical signs of intoxication are sudden in onset and characterized by behavioural changes. Cattle become frenzied, bellow, staggering and crashing into obstacles probably as a result of developing central blindness. Death may follow rapidly, or the animal may suffer repeated convulsive episodes with muscle twitching, especially of the palpebral muscles. In some cases there may be dullness, depression, ataxia or circling, head pressing and evidence of abdominal pain.

The diagnosis of lead poisoning is suspected on the basis of clinical signs and the presence of a source of lead. Confirmation depends upon the histopathological findings and the chemical determination of the concentration of lead in tissues. In kidney and liver concentrations >4 p.p.m. wet weight and blood values in excess of 0.2 p.p.m. are considered diagnostic.

Treatment and prevention

Cattle with severe neurological signs of some duration probably have extensive neuropathological changes and are unlikely to respond to treatment. However, if a source can be identified, in-contact animals at risk from a single large dose may be drenched orally with magnesium sulphate (500–1000 g) to precipitate and remove lead from the alimentary tract and injected with calcium disodium edetate at 110 mg/kg by intravenous drip on alternate days for three treatments. The similarity of the pathological changes with those of CCN has encouraged the use of thiamine (10–15 mg/kg intravenously) along with EDTA therapy and is reportedly beneficial. Barbiturate or chloral hydrate sedation may be necessary to control convulsive episodes.

Prevention is a matter of good management, not allowing access by cattle to sources of lead.

Aujeszky's disease

Aujeszky's disease is a herpesvirus infection principally of pigs, which can be transmitted to most other mammalian species.

Aetiology

In common with many other herpesviruses, that of Aujeszky's disease or pseudorabies causes latent infections in the natural porcine host. The introduction of a carrier animal to a 'clean' piggery results in rapid spread of infection and high mortality in sucking piglets. Nasal discharges from infected swine contaminate the environment with virus particles, which can remain infective for several weeks. Infections in cattle are generally sporadic and result from contact with infected pigs, foodstuffs or other materials contaminated with virus. The disease in cattle is usually fatal.

Pathogenesis and pathology

Infection in cattle is generally by the oro-nasal route, although infections arising from cutaneous abrasions, or subcutaneous injections with virus-contaminated needles have been recorded. Following inoculation, virus replicates locally and travels to the CNS in the axoplasm of the olfactory or other cranial or peripheral nerves (McCracken & Dow, 1973). In cattle a low-grade viraemia may occur but is not thought to be important in the pathogenesis or epidemiology of Aujeszky's disease. Virus is not present in bovine secretions or excretions. Centripetal intra-axonal transport of virus causes first a severe ganglioneuritis followed by meningo-encephalitis or myelitis. Following infection by the olfactory route, lesions are most severe in the olfactory lobe, hippocampus and cerebellum, whereas infection of a spinal peripheral nerve results initially in a segmental myelitis. Grey matter is principally affected with degenerative changes in nerve cells and astrocytes in which multiple, small, granular, eosinophilic, intranuclear inclusion bodies may be found. The inflammatory response is essentially non-suppurative and characterized by lymphocytic perivascular cuffing and focal microgliosis.

Signs and diagnosis

The clinical course is short, rarely extending beyond 48 hours in adult cattle, whilst calves may die without obvious prior signs of illness. Usually, however, there is a brief period of excitement with high fever, bellowing, and aggressive behaviour accompanied by trembling, hyperpnoea, salivation and compulsive licking of the nostrils. Intense pruritus of the neck, trunk or hind legs is accompanied by frantic efforts to relieve the itch. Affected animals may become bloated and there is incoordination and terminally, recumbency, convulsions and coma.

Except in calves, the clinical signs are usually distinctive enough for a provisional diagnosis of Aujeszky's disease to be reached. Confirmation is dependent upon demonstration of the characteristic neuropathology or virus isolation from nervous tissue.

Treatment and prevention

There is no effective treatment and prevention of disease in cattle is dependent upon control of disease in the pig population. Attenuated and inactivated vaccines are available and are effective in preventing disease in pigs. However, they will not protect pigs from infection with field virus, which will replicate and be shed for some time after infection. Thus control in pigs must be through the establishment and maintenance of clean closed herds by serological testing and slaughter. This has been undertaken as a successful national campaign in Britain.

Sporadic bovine encephalomyelitis (SBE, Buss disease)

Sporadic bovine encephalomyelitis is a generalized inflammatory disorder of serous membranes, synoviae and vascular endothelium. It has no specific neurotropism, the neurological signs being a consequence of inflammation of the mesodermal elements in the CNS.

Aetiology

Sporadic bovine encephalomyelitis is a specific disease of cattle and buffalo caused by a strain of *Chlamydia psittaci* containing an antigen similar to one found in sheep in polyarthritis strains, but not in abortion strains. The disease has been observed in the USA, Eastern Europe and the Middle East, Japan, Australia and South Africa. Infection is probably world-wide.

Pathology and pathogenesis

The disease is usually fatal within four to five days. The gross post-mortem findings include a serofibrinous peritonitis, pleurisy and pericarditis. A serofibrinous exudate is also found over the surface of the brain, especially the cerebellum and medulla. Histological examination of the brain reveals a predominantly histiocytic and plasma cell infiltration of the meninges, whilst within the neuroparenchyma there is a vasculitis with swelling of the endothelium, which may lead to local ischaemic necrosis. Chlamydial elementary bodies can be demonstrated in brain lesions and lymph nodes. Chronic cases may also develop a lobar pneumonia (Menges *et al.*, 1953a, b).

Signs and diagnosis

The disease rarely affects calves more than six months old in which it tends to be mild with recovery after a few days of diarrhoea. Younger, more severely affected animals also develop a staggering, stiff gait with circling and stumbling. Affected calves are dull and depressed and may exhibit muscle tremors. About 70 per cent of infected animals recover slowly and are solidly immune to re-infection. Clinical diagnosis of sporadic bovine encephalomyelitis may be confirmed by rising titres of group-specific chlamydial antibody in complement fixation or enzyme-linked immunosorbent assay (ELISA) tests in the live animal, or by isolation of the organism from brain and lymph nodes, on McCoy cell tissue cultures or on fertile eggs.

Treatment and prevention

Though *in vitro* the organism is sensitive to tetracycline, successful therapy depends upon treatment very early in the course of the disease using high sustained dosages (50 mg/kg per day).

Rabies

Rabies is a neurotropic viral disease that can affect all warm-blooded animals. The virus is excreted in saliva and transmitted by the bite of an infected animal. It is manifested by irritability, mania and paralysis. It is usually fatal, although recoveries have been documented.

Aetiology

The causal agent is a delicate rhabdovirus readily destroyed by disinfectants and desiccation. It causes pathological changes only in nervous tissue and though most isolates are antigenically similar (Crick & Brown, 1976) pathogenicity is variable. Rabies occurs worldwide except in certain island territories (Australia and New Zealand) and a few countries from which it has been eradicated, such as the British Isles and Scandinavia. In the western hemisphere the infection is endemic in dogs, foxes, wolves, skunks, raccoons and bats of several species. In Europe the fox is the main vector although in recent years insectivorous and fructivorous bats have also been implicated. Infection is transmitted with the bite of a rabid animal.

Pathology and pathogenesis

Cattle are very susceptible to rabies and become infected, usually on the hindquarters or limbs from the bite of a rabid fox, dog or bat. Following local replication, virus travels centripetally in the axoplasm of a peripheral nerve to reach the spinal cord and thence to the brain. *En route* it replicates in neurones to produce acidophil intracytoplasmic inclusion bodies, Negri bodies, which vary in size, number and shape depending upon the pathogenicity of the strain of virus and the morphology of the particular cell. Inclusions may be present in all regions of the nervous system in nerve cells of all types, but they are found most readily in the pyramidal cells of the hippocampus (Ammon's horn) and the large cerebellar Purkinje cells. From the brain, in the later stages of the incubation period, the virus passes centrifugally along nerves to the salivary and lacrimal glands and is excreted in their secretions. Rabies virus is highly neurotropic, and viraemia is minimal or absent. Consequently, the perivascular lymphocytic cuffs that characterize the majority of viral encephalitides are relatively mild. Apart from Negri bodies, characteristic features of the neuropathology include astrocytic swelling leading to the formation of pericapillary and perineuronal spaces, which give the tissue a spongy appearance, and also the presence of small clusters of microglial cells, which develop in both grey and white matter and are known as Babes nodules. It is thought that strains of low pathogenicity produce fewer smaller Negri bodies and more severe inflammatory responses than do more pathogenic strains.

Signs and diagnosis

The incubation period of rabies in cattle varies from about two to three weeks to several months. Clinical signs classically occur in two distinct forms, the mild paralytic or dumb form and the furious form, depending upon the pathogenicity of the strain of virus. In paralytic rabies there may be partial loss of sensation in the hind legs, knuckling of the fetlocks, locomotor weakness and paralysis of the tail. Flaccid dilatation of the anus may be accompanied by straining and passage of air in and out of the rectum. Drooling of saliva and yawning are common features. The entire clinical course lasts about one week and is terminated by recumbency, generalized paralysis with death probably due to respiratory failure.

In the furious form the animal is hyperaesthetic and sexually excited. It bellows hoarsely and becomes violently aggressive towards people, other animals and inanimate objects. Purposeful attacks, however, are frustrated by rapidly progressive incoordination and ataxia. Death occurs quickly following recumbency and paralysis.

Cattle are normally 'end hosts' with respect to rabies, though human infection may follow manual examination of the oral cavity in which virus in saliva is inoculated into scratches caused by teeth.

Clinical diagnosis of rabies is difficult, especially in those countries in which it rarely occurs. The possibility of rabies should be borne in mind in the differential diagnosis of nervous acetonaemia (p. 590), listerial encephalitis (p. 703) and bovine spongiform encephalopathy (p. 708). Rabid cattle invariably die and fluorescent antibody staining of impression smears from appropriate parts of the CNS will establish the diagnosis rapidly.

Treatment and prevention

No treatment of clinical cases should be attempted, nor should they be euthanased prematurely as this may prejudice the post-mortem diagnosis. Postexposure vaccination is a routine procedure in man, but in cattle clinical disease and death would probably occur before an effective immunity had time to develop.

Heartwater (see also p. 744)

This is a disease of reticulo-endothelial cells caused by a tick-borne intracellular organism that affects both domestic and wild ruminants. It is endemic in sub-Saharan Africa and its associated islands and in the Caribbean (Haig, 1955). The neurological manifestations of heartwater are a consequence of damage to the intracranial vasculature and form a variable component of the clinical disorder.

Aetiology

The causative agent of heartwater is a pleomorphic organism *Cowdria ruminantium*. It is transmitted by ticks of the species *Amblyomma*, the bont tick, in which it may be passed through the stages of development but not transovarially. It is this feature that distinguishes *Cowdria* from the *Rickettsia* proper. In the latter transovarian passage in the tick may occur.

Pathology and pathogenesis

Cowdria ruminantium is a tiny rod-shaped or diplococcoid organism that can be demonstrated by May–Gruenwald/Giemsa staining of reticuloendothelial cells. Initially, the organisms are taken up by macrophages, but later they invade endothelial cells in which they rapidly divide to form colonies in the cytoplasm resulting in intimal swelling and increased vascular permeability, capillary occlusion and thrombosis. In severe acute infections there is hydrothorax, hydropericardium, oedema of the lungs and widespread petechial and ecchymotic haemorrhages. Neurological disturbance is referable to oedema, haemorrhages and ischaemic lesions within the brain substance and meninges, especially of the cerebellum and brain stem.

Signs and diagnosis

The incubation period varies from one to four weeks and culminates in peracute, acute, subacute or inapparent disease. Neurological disturbance is associated with the more acute forms with high fever. It usually takes the form of hypermetria, and circling, followed by depression and head pressing, and later by prostration, convulsions and death. In some peracute cases high fever and convulsions may be the first signs of disease and impending death.

Diagnosis is based upon the history and clinical signs. For confirmation in live animals lymph node aspirates may be examined. By light microscopy organisms may be found in the vacuoles of vacuolated reticulum cells. In electron microscope preparations the organisms vary from 0.5 to 3.0 μm diameter and occur as filamentous, horseshoe-shaped, coccoid or polygonal bodies enclosed in a double membrane containing electron-dense granular cytoplasm and less dense fibrillar nucleoid material (Pienaar, 1970). Post-mortem diagnosis is based on the presence of pericardial and pleural effusions and confirmed by finding organisms in films of cells scraped from the endothelium of a large vein, such as the jugular, or in crush preparations of brain tissue.

Treatment and prevention

Tetracyclines administered 12-hourly through the period of fever are effective therapy if begun early in the course of the disease. The convalescent animal, however, remains a carrier for several weeks. A degree of resistance is developed but re-infection can occur. Calves may also be vaccinated by the intravenous injection of 5 ml of infected blood and the signs similarly controlled by tetracycline injections. As there is no passive transfer of resistance there is probably not a significant humoral immune response. Control of ticks by regular dipping can help to reduce the incidence of the disease.

Bovine spongiform encephalopathy (BSE)

This is a recently recognized progressive neurological disorder affecting adult cattle, mainly dairy cattle, in mainland Britain, Orkney, the Channel Islands and Northern Ireland, Saudi Arabia, France and Switzerland. It is characterized clinically by behavioural changes and pathologically by vacuolation of the neuropil and some nuclei of the brain stem. The pathological changes resemble those of certain other neurological disorders of animals and humans collectively known as the transmissible spongiform encephalopathies and classified among the 'slow virus diseases' (Tyrrell, 1979).

Aetiology

As with the other spongiform encephalopathies such as scrapie in sheep, transmissible mink encephalopathy, chronic wasting disease of mule deer, kuru and Creutzfeld–Jakob disease in man, the nature of the aetiological agent has not been firmly established. However, all the conditions mentioned, including BSE (H. Fraser, pers. comm., 1988) have been transmitted to experimental animals by inoculation of brain tissue from affected individuals. There is good evidence to suggest that the infective particle, at least in scrapie, is small as it is associated with membrane fragments present in the microsome fraction of a homogenate. It is also remarkably resistant to physical or chemical disinfection procedures such as boiling, exposure to formalin or ultraviolet radiation. Extended autoclaving at 221 kPa and exposure to 5 per cent solution of hypochlorite (household bleach) will destroy infectivity. All the evidence presently available for BSE indicates a close similarity with scrapie and it is presumed that the causal agents will also prove to be similar.

There have been several theories concerning the nature of the transmissible agent in scrapie. For example, it has been likened to a viroid or naked DNA molecule similar to that which causes potato spindle tuber disease. It has also been suggested that it is a novel kind of infectious protein or 'prion'. The most plausible current hypothesis, however, is that it is a virino or very small scrapie-specific nucleic acid embedded within a tightly packed host-derived protein that is essential for transfection (Kimberlin, 1982).

Pathology and pathogenesis

All the epidemiological evidence presently available strongly suggests that the geographically widespread incidents of BSE are not the result of cow-to-cow transmission but conform to the concept of a single source epidemic with concentrate feedstuffs containing animal protein as the probable source. Since several animals on a single property will have consumed the same batch of concentrate, yet most 'outbreaks' have involved only one or very few animals it follows that either the transmissible agent is very unevenly distributed in the feed, or as in the case of sheep scrapie, host genotype has a profound effect upon susceptibility or the length of the incubation period. It also follows that the alimentary tract is the probable portal of entry. By analogy with scrapie, early replication probably occurs in the gut-associated lymphoid tissue and the lymphoreticular organs before invasion of the CNS (Hadlow *et al.*, 1982).

The pathological changes that result from infection are microscopic and confined to the brain. They consist of bilaterally symmetrical degenerative changes affecting the neuropil and neurones of certain brain stem nuclei (Wells *et al.*, 1987). There is fine vacuolation of the ground substance whilst neurones and neurites develop one or more well-defined intracytoplasmic vacuoles, which may distend the cell body and processes. The nuclei principally involved are the dorsal nucleus of the vagus, the nucleus of the solitary tract, the reticular formation, the vestibular and spinal trigeminal nuclei and in the midbrain the red and oculomotor nuclei. However, specificity of vacuolation in the midbrain nuclei must be discounted as it is an incidental finding in older cattle (Sullivan, 1985). The characteristic lesions of BSE show a mild diffuse reactive astrogliosis, but this is not a feature associated with the non-specific neuronal vacuolation of midbrain nuclei (I. McGill, pers. comm., 1988).

An additional pathological characteristic of the transmissible spongiform encephalopathies is the presence in extracts of brain prepared for electron microscopy of fibrils 100–500 nm in length that are known as scrapie associated fibrils (SAF). These fibrils are composed of either two or four beaded filaments 4–6 nm in width arranged in a helical configuration (Merz *et al.*, 1981).

Signs and diagnosis

Bovine spongiform encephalopathy affects cattle three to six years of age with peak prevalence in the four to five year age group. The disease is rare in beef suckler herds, and in dairy cattle the incidence within breeds appears to be a reflection of population size, a majority of cases occurring in Friesian/Holstein cattle.

The behavioural and locomotor changes are insidious in onset and are relentlessly progressive, though the rate of progression is extremely variable. The initial signs are subtle and include hyperaesthesia, fine fasciculations of the muscles of the neck, shoulder or flank, persistent grinding of teeth, or repetitive agitated purposeless movements of the head or limbs. Affected cattle become increasingly apprehensive when approached and are often reluctant to enter the byre or milking parlour and they can become aggressive when coerced. Locomotor signs include knuckling of fetlocks, ataxia and loss of coordinated movement. At rest, within a group of cows, affected animals appear to be excessively aware and often adopt a roach-backed stance. A sudden loud noise may result in the animal collapsing in a tetanic spasm. Most affected animals are euthanased at this stage because of reduced yield and unmanageable behaviour. The clinical course varies between two to three weeks and several months and there is an indication that disease first appearing around calving time tends to progress rapidly.

A presumptive diagnosis can be made on the clinical signs, although in the early stages of disease, the nervous form of acetonaemia (p. 590), hypomagnesaemia (p. 583), listerial encephalitis (p. 703) and CCN (p. 701) must be considered especially in animals in which the disease has a very acute course. Confirmation of diagnosis depends upon a neuropathological examination for which it is preferable if the animal has been euthanased with intravenous barbiturate overdose. If captive bolt stunning is unavoidable the animal should not be pithed but immediately decapitated.

Treatment and prevention

There is no effective treatment, but temporary sedation may be obtained from diazepam given in the food. In the light of present knowledge prevention depends upon control of possible sources of infection, and notification and elimination of affected animals. Compared with scrapie in sheep, present knowledge indicates that significant vertical/maternal transmission of BSE is unlikely, but it is considered essential clearly to identify and mark permanently progeny of affected animals that are retained.

References

Ames, T.R. (1987) Neurologic disease caused by *Haemophilus somnus*. *Veterinary Clinics of North America*, **3**, 61–73.

Baird, J.D., Johnston, K.G. & Hartley, W.J. (1974) Spastic paresis in Friesian cattle. *Australian Veterinary Journal*, **50**, 239–49.

Barlow, R.M. (1980) Genetic cerebellar disorders in cattle. In *Animal Models of Neurological Disease* (ed. by R. Clifford & P. O'Behan), pp. 294–305. Pitman Medical Series, Tunbridge Wells, Kent, UK.

Berry, P.H., Howell, J. McC., Cook, R.D., Richards, R.B. & Peet, R.L. (1980) Central nervous system changes in sheep and cattle affected with natural or experimental annual ryegrass toxicity. *Australian Veterinary Journal*, **56**, 402–3.

Buxton, D., Macleod, N.S.M. & Nicolson, T.B. (1981) Focal symmetrical encephalomalacia in young cattle. *Veterinary Record*, **108**, 459.

Christian, R.G. & Tryphonas, L. (1971) Lead poisoning in cattle; brain lesions and haematologic changes. *American Journal of Veterinary Research*, **32**, 203–16.

Crick, J. & Brown, F. (1976) Rabies vaccines for animals and man. *Veterinary Record*, **99**, 162–7.

Doherty, P.C. & Reid, H.W. (1971) Louping ill encephalitis in the sheep. II. Distribution of virus and lesions in nervous tissue. *Journal of Comparative Pathology*, **81**, 531–6.

Donnelly, W.J.C., Sheahan, B.J. & Rogers, T.A. (1973) GM_1 gangliosidosis in Friesian calves. *Journal of Pathology and Bacteriology*, **111**, 173–9.

Edwin, E.E. (1970) Plasma enzyme and metabolite concentrations in cerebrocortical necrosis. *Veterinary Record*, **87**, 396–8.

Engel, D. (1970) *Populationsgenetische Untersuchungen zur Aetiologie der spastischen Parese beim Schwartzbunten Rind in Kurhessen*. Dissentation, Giessen.

Field, A.C. & Suttle, N.F. (1979) Effect of high potassium and low magnesium intakes on the mineral metabolism of monozygotic twin cows. *Journal of Comparative Pathology*, **89**, 431–9.

Fletcher, L.R. & Harvey, I.C. (1981) An association of a *Lolium* endophyte with ryegrass staggers. *New Zealand Veterinary Journal*, **29**, 185–6.

Gallagher, R.T., White, E.P. & Mortimer, P.H. (1981) Ryegrass staggers: isolation of potent neurotoxins lolitrem A and lolitrem B from staggers producing pastures. *New Zealand Veterinary Journal*, **29**, 189–90.

Geerken, C.M. & Figueroa, V. (1971) Cerebrocortical necrosis (molasses toxicity) in beef cattle: some preliminary biochemical parameters. *Rev. Revista Cubana de Cienca Agricala (Eng. edn)*, **5**, 205.

Grundlach, A.L., Dodd, P.R., Grabara, C.S.G., Watson, W.E.J., Johnston, G.A.R., Harper, P.A.W., Dennis, J.A. & Healy, P.J. (1988) Deficit of spinal cord glycine/strychnine receptor in inherited myoclonus of Poll Hereford calves. *Science*, **241**, 1807–10.

Hadlow, W.J., Kennedy, R.C. & Race, R.E. (1982) Natural infection of Suffolk sheep with scrapie virus. *Journal of Infectious Diseases*, **146**, 657–64.

Haig, D.A. (1955) Tick-borne rickettsioses in South Africa. *Advances in Veterinary Science*, **2**, 307–25.

Hansen, K.M., Krogh, H.V., Møller, J.E. & Elleby, F. (1988) The recumbent calf syndrome in the Red Danish milk breed — a new hereditary disease. *Dansk Veterinaertidsskrift*, **71**, 128–32.

Harper, P.A.W., Healy, P.J. & Dennis, J.A. (1986) Inherited congenital myoclonus of polled Hereford calves (so-called neuraxial oedema): a clinical, pathological and biochemical study. *Veterinary Record*, **119**, 59–62.

Healy, P.J., Harper, P.A.W. & Dennis, J.A. (1986) Diagnosis of neuraxial oedema. *Australian Veterinary Journal*, **63**, 95.

High, J.W., Kincaid, C.M. & Smith, J.H. (1958) Doddler calves: an inherited disorder of Hereford cattle. *Journal of Heredity*, **49**, 250–2.

Hocking, J.D., Jolly, R.D. & Batt, R.D. (1972) Deficiency of α-mannosidase in Angus cattle: an inherited lysosomal storage disease. *Biochemical Journal*, **128**, 69–75.

Hulland, T.J. (1957) Cerebellar ataxia in calves. *Canadian Journal of Comparative Medicine*, **21**, 72–6.

Humphreys, D.J. (1988) *Veterinary Toxicology*, 3rd edn, p. 8. Baillière Tindall, London.

Inaba, Y., Kurogi, H. & Omori, T. (1975) Akabane disease: epizootic abortion, premature birth, stillbirth, and congenital arthrogryposis–hydranencephaly in cattle, sheep and goats caused by Akabane virus. *Australian Veterinary Journal*, **51**, 584–5.

Innes, J.R.M., Russell, D.S. & Wilsden, A.J. (1940) Familial cerebellar hypoplasia and degeneration in Hereford calves. *Journal of Pathology and Bacteriology*, **50**, 455–61.

Isler, C.M., Bellamy, J.E.C. & Wobeser, G.A. (1987) A neurotoxin in serum of calves with 'nervous' coccidiosis. *Canadian Journal of Veterinary Research*, **51**, 253–60.

Kimberlin, R.H. (1982) Scrapie agent: prions or virinos. *Nature*, **297**, 107–8.

Little, P.B. (1978) Identity of fluorescence in polioencephalomalacia. *Veterinary Record*, **103**, 76.

McCracken, R.M. & Dow, C. (1973) An electron microscopic study of Aujeszky's disease. *Acta Neuropathologica*, **25**, 207–19.

Menges, R.W., Harshfield, G.S. & Wenner, H.A. (1953a) Sporadic bovine encephalomyelitis. I. The natural history of the disease. *American Journal of Hygiene*, **57**, 1–14.

Menges, R.W., Harshfield, G.S. & Wenner, H.A. (1953b) Sporadic bovine encephalomyelitis. II. Studies on the pathogenesis and etiology of the disease. *Journal of the American Veterinary Medical Association*, **122**, 249–94.

Merz, P.A., Somerville, R.A., Wisniewski, H.M. & Iqbal, K. (1981) Abnormal fibrils from scrapie infected brain. *Acta Neuropathologica*, **54**, 63–74.

Morgan, K.T. (1973) An ultrastructural study of ovine polioencephalomalacia. *Journal of Pathology*, **110**, 123–30.

O'Toole, D. & Jeffrey, M. (1987) Congenital sporozoan encephalomyelitis in a calf. *Veterinary Record*, **121**, 563–6.

Padgett, G.A. (1968) The Chediak–Higashi syndrome. *Advances in Veterinary Science*, **12**, 239–84.

Palmer, A.C., Blakemore, W.F., Barlow, R.M., Fraser, J.A. & Ogden, A.C. (1972) Progressive ataxia of Charolais cattle associated with a myelin disorder. *Veterinary Record*, **91**, 592–4.

Pienaar, J.G. (1970) Electron microscopy of *Cowdria (Rickettsia) ruminantium* (Cowdry 1926) in the endothelial cells of the vertebrate host. *Onderstopoort Journal of Veterinary Research*, **37**, 67–78.

Read, W.K. & Bridges, C.H. (1969) Neuronal lipodystrophy occurrence in an inbred strain of cattle. *Veterinary Pathology*, **6**, 235–43.

Reid, H.W., Buxton, D., Pow, I. & Finlayson, J. (1984) Transmission of louping ill virus in goat milk. *Veterinary Record*, **114**, 163–5.

Richards, R.B., Edwards, J.R., Cook, R.D. & White, R. (1977) Bovine generalised glycogenosis (type II). *Neuropathology and Applied Neurobiology*, **3**, 45–56.

Saunders, L.Z., Sweet, J.D., Martin, S.M., Fox, F.H. & Fincher, M.G. (1952) Hereditary congenital ataxia in Jersey calves. *Cornell Veterinarian*, **42**, 559–91.

Stolzenberg, V. & Schonmuth, G. (1971) Experimentelle Untersuchungen uber die okonomischen Auswirkungen und die Vererbung der spastischen Parese der Hintergliedmassen. *Wissenschaft zür Humboldt Universität Berlin*, **20**, 353–70.

Stuart, L.D. & Leipold, H.W. (1985) Lesions in bovine progressive degenerative myeloencephalopathy. *Veterinary Pathology*, **22**, 13–23.

Sullivan, N.D. (1985) Cytopathology of the nervous system. In *Pathology of Domestic Animals*, 3rd edn (ed. by K.V.F. Jubb, P.C. Kennedy & N.Palmer), Vol. 1, p. 225. Academic Press, New York.

Trautwein, G., Hewicker, M., Liess, B., Orban, S. & Peters, W. (1987) Cerebellar hypoplasia and hydranencephaly in cattle associated with transplacental BVD virus infection. In *Pestivirus Infections of Ruminants* (ed. by J.W. Harkness), pp. 169–78. Commission of European Communities, Luxembourg.

Tyrrell, D.A.J. (1979) Aspects of slow and persistent virus infections. In *New Perspectives in Clinical Microbiology* 2, p. 286. Martinus Nijhoff, The Hague.

Wells, G.A.H., Scott, A.C., Johnson, C.T., Gunning, R.F., Hancock, R.D., Jeffrey, M., Dawson, M. & Bradley, R. (1987) A novel progressive spongiform encephalopathy in cattle. *Veterinary Record*, **121**, 419–20.

White, M., Whitlock, R.H. & de Lahunta, A. (1975) A cerebellar abiotrophy of calves. *Cornell Veterinarian*, **65**, 476–91.

Chapter 46: Ocular Diseases

by P.G.C. BEDFORD

Introduction

Ophthalmic disorders in cattle are more common than is generally believed, but it is only those that are of considerable economic importance that generally receive much attention. Infectious bovine keratoconjunctivitis (IBKC), variously known throughout the world as New Forest disease, pinkeye, contagious ophthalmia and blight, is undoubtedly the commonest and most important ocular disease that occurs in this species. In the USA alone it is estimated that IBKC is responsible for an annual loss in excess of £100 million, and failure to produce effective vaccines both there and in the UK means that this disease will continue to inflict severe economic loss for as long as young cattle are managed intensively. Disease of epidemic proportions occurs all the year round, and while the aetiological controversy may continue, the term IBKC generally embraces all keratoconjunctivitis of infectious nature in this species. Similarly, ocular squamous cell carcinoma of probable heritable nature in breeds with reduced palpebral pigmentation continues to account for a high carcase condemnation rate, and runs second only to lymphosarcoma in terms of condemnation for neoplastic reasons. At the other end of the scale there are many congenital, inherited and acquired defects that tend to escape diagnosis on the basis of there being no untoward effect on function, no associated discomfort or pain and no necessity to treat. Were cattle subjected to the same degree of scrutiny as the dog, then it is likely that the literature would indicate a similar incidence of disease. In one study of 500 cattle of all ages, almost 20 per cent overall demonstrated ocular anomalies of one sort or another, the incidence ranging from 3 per cent in young cattle to in excess of 70 per cent in the older individuals (Amman, 1968). Examples of this kind of survey work in cattle are few and far between, but the emergence of small animal ophthalmology as a refined discipline in today's veterinary scenario will probably stimulate further interest in animals that are primarily produced for food purposes in our society.

Anomalies of the orbit and globe

Congenital and acquired defects both occur, some congenital anomalies being inherited while others are probably environmental in origin (see also p. 150). The acquired defects are due to trauma, infection and neoplasia.

Anophthalmia

Absence of the optic vesicle means that an eye cannot develop. Histologically, primordial ectodermal and mesodermal tissues cannot be identified. The condition is rare and is often confused with the type of microphthalmia in which there has been some differentiation of the optic vesicle.

Microphthalmia

Variable degrees of development can be seen, ranging from minimal differentiation of ocular tissue to the development of a small but otherwise normal eye. Other ocular anomalies may also be present however, and persistent pupillary membrane (PPM), aniridia, cataract and neuroretinal fold and rosette formation may be seen in association with microphthalmos. Like anophthalmia, the condition is rare in cattle, but inheritance has been postulated (Gilmore, 1957), and it has been described in calves with vertebral column deformation (Leipold & Huston, 1968).

Cyclopia

The development of one eye in calves is extremely rare (Plate 46.1) but the condition has been induced teratogenically in sheep.

Strabismus

Bilateral convergent squint (esotropia) has been described as a recessively inherited defect in Jersey cattle, and it is probably inherited in Shorthorn and Friesian cattle too (Willoughby, 1968; Bedford, pers. obs.). A degree of exophthalmos may or may not be additionally present. The condition is usually noticed at four to eight weeks of age (Plate 46.2a) and the degree of esotropia (convergent squint) increases until the sixth or seventh month when only sclera presents within the palpebral fissure (Plate 46.2b). Impaired vision gives way to total blindness, and attempts at corrective surgery may be ill-perceived in the presence of possible optic nerve, central visual pathway and visual cortex anomalies.

Orbital neoplasia

Retrobulbar and periorbital lymphosarcoma can result in exophthalmos and possible squint. The lesions may be seen unilaterally or bilaterally. Squamous cell carcinoma of the membrana nictitans may invade the orbit to produce a similar clinical picture.

Anomalies of the eyelids

Congenital defects

Unlike other species congenital and inherited defects are few and far between in cattle. Eyelid colobomata and agenesis are of rare incidence. Although primary conditions in sheep, entropion and ectropion occur only as secondary defects in cattle and are associated with microphthalmia, blepharitis, keratoconjunctivitis and trauma. Correction of the cause alleviates the lid distortion except where there is palpebral or orbicularis oculi damage and where cicatrization has occurred.

Congenital supernumerary openings of the proximal part of the nasolacrimal duct and the canaliculi at the medial canthus have been described in calves, hereditary predisposition or intra-uterine dacryocystitis being the suggested possible aetiology.

Trauma

Laceration of the eyelid occurs infrequently, but when the palpebral fissure is involved repair is essential. Such wounds left to granulate or inadequately sutured may result in distortion of the margo-intermarginalis, and secondary entropion, secondary ectropion and an incomplete blink can result in conjunctival or corneal disease. Delayed closure is complicated by the problem of wound contraction. Repair is easily effected using manual restraint and local anaesthesia by infiltration; should blepharospasm be a problem then the auriculopalpebral nerve can be blocked as for disbudding and dehorning. Such wounds may require debridement, but the removal of tissue should be avoided whenever possible. The sutures are placed at two levels (Fig. 46.1). Tarsal plate and subconjunctival tissue are first repaired without penetrating the palpebral conjunctiva, and the knots are buried in the substance of the eyelid such that no suture material can cause corneal irritation. The margo-intermarginalis must be accurately reformed, the first suture ensuring precise apposition at this level. The second row of sutures involves the subcutis and skin, and single inter-

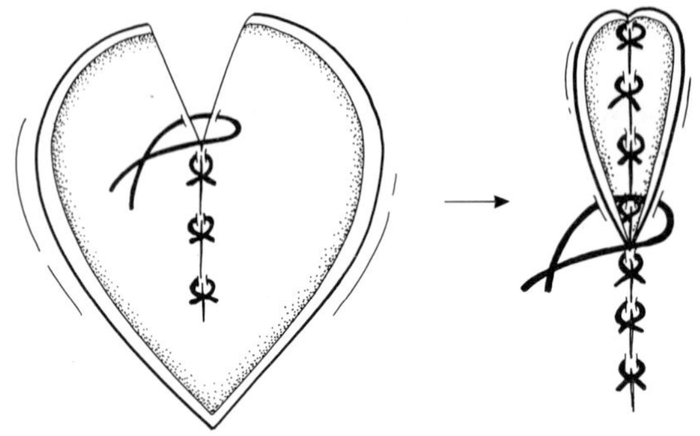

Fig. 46.1 Repair of an eyelid wound by two-layer closure. (a) Tarsal plate and subconjunctival tissue apposed; (b) subcutis and skin upposed.

rupted sutures are used to ensure accurate repair and reduce the chance of wound breakdown. Absorbable material is used for the buried sutures, and nylon is preferable for the cutaneous repair.

Diseases of the conjunctiva and cornea

The occurrence of IBKC and squamous cell carcinoma render this part of the eye important in economic terms, and so often do the disease conditions involve both structures that it is convenient to discuss the two under the same heading.

Epibulbar dermoid

Dermoid formation (choriostoma) is the result of poor differentiation of the palpebral tissue with the result that plaques of hair-bearing skin and subcutis may be found involving the lateral aspect of the globe (Plate 46.3). Both the cornea and episcleral tissues can be affected, the dermoid replacing the corneal epithelium and bulbar conjunctiva respectively. Bilateral involvement is unusual, and dermoids are only of clinical significance if they impair sight, cause trigeminal irritation and conjunctival inflammation, or they physically interfere with effective blinking and lid closure. Removal is then advocated, and topical and regional anaesthesia can be complemented by using the auriculopalpebral nerve block. The lesion must be removed in entirety to prevent recurrence. While a suprascleral lesion is easily excised, care is required with the superficial keratectomy needed to remove the corneal dermoid.

Infectious bovine keratoconjunctivitis (New Forest eye, pinkeye)

Aetiology

This disease has been recognized for at least 100 years (Billings, 1889), since when it has demonstrated both common incidence and world-wide distribution. It is highly contagious, and outbreaks of epidemic proportions can affect grazing herds during the summer and autumn months, and housed cattle the whole year round. Young animals are more severely affected, dictating possible local immunity to the disease in those previously exposed. Over the years IBKC has been attributed to several organisms (Bedford, 1976), but currently *Moraxella bovis* is still regarded by most authorities to be the cause. The root of the controversy lies in the fact that *Moraxella bovis* can be found in the normal conjunctival sac, and attempts to produce the disease using pure cultures of this bacterium have not always been successful. In addition, infectious bovine rhinotracheitis (IBR) virus, known to cause conjunctivitis in addition to rhinitis, and *Mycoplasma bovirhinitis* and *M. laidlawii* have been isolated with *Moraxella bovis* from IBKC patients. Rather than representing cause, however, these organisms may act synergistically as enhancing factors. Undoubtedly, other enhancing factors can be at work, and the increased incidence of IBKC during the warmer months has indicated that ultraviolet light, flies and dust play potentially important roles in the overall picture. Certainly flies of the *Musca* and *Stomoxys* species have been incriminated as mechanical vectors, but the occurrence of epidemic disease among winter-housed cattle suggest that flies and the other environmental factors are not essential.

Epidemiology

Variation within the clinical picture of the disease may be related to the input of the several possible enhancing factors, but may also be due to the susceptibility of the animal to infection and the type of *Moraxella bovis* present in its conjunctival sac. Older cattle are more resistant to infection, it being calves and cattle of less than two years of age that demonstrate the highest morbidity and the most severe disease. Such resistance may be the result of previous exposure, but local factors as well as antibody formation may be involved (Pugh, 1969). It has been demonstrated that two forms of the bacterium exist: a smooth non-haemolytic form that is avirulent and can usually be isolated from recovering and clinically normal carrier animals, and a rough haemolytic virulent form that causes the acute disease (Pedersen, 1973). The rough form is fimbriae for adherence (Sandhu *et al.*, 1974), and repeated passage has demonstrated its conversion into the smooth form. The presence of fimbriae would appear to be necessary for disease to occur and for immunity to develop. The difficulties experienced in the production of an effective vaccine against *Moraxella bovis* may be overcome as the result of further structural studies to determine the possible immunogenic status of the fimbriae. In the past, alteration of the surface components of bacterial cells in the preparation of vaccines may have been wholly responsible for the ineffectiveness of such vaccines. The economic importance of IBKC demands that an effective vaccine be developed, but it could be many years before the riddle is finally solved.

Signs

Epidemics occur as the result of the introduction of incubating, chronically affected or carrier animals into the herd. The presenting clinical features may vary considerably depending on the immunity of the exposed individual and the level of enhancing factors present. This variation is not only seen on a herd-to-herd basis, but between individual animals within the same herd. Both unilateral and bilateral cases will be seen; in the latter a variation in the degree of severity may be noted between the two eyes. Usually, inflammation of the bulbar and possibly the palpebral conjunctivae precedes the keratitis, but occasionally the conjunctival involvement is not seen until after corneal inflammation has made its appearance. Blepharospasm, photophobia and copious ocular discharge herald anterior segment pain, the discharge, primarily clear and thin, becoming purulent quite rapidly to mat the lashes and circumorbital hair. The conjunctiva is chemotic and swelling of the eyelids may occur. Corneal changes usually develop within 48 hours, a 3-mm wide, slightly raised area of cloudiness normally making its appearance centrally. The overlying epithelium may take up fluorescein stain, and the lesion itself may take on the yellowish hue of pyogenic necrosis. The surrounding cornea becomes oedematous and hazy, and a low-grade anterior uveitis with aqueous flare may be noticeable in some animals. Corneal vascularization from the limbal blood vessels is well established by the sixth day, the new vessels rapidly progressing towards the central lesion in the anterior stroma (Plate 46.4a). Throughout this stage of the disease the eye is extremely painful, and a bilateral involvement means that the patient is either blind or experiencing impaired vision. Inappetence, suppressed weight gain and reduced milk production are related to the severity of involvement. At this stage, and particularly in young animals, loss of epithelium and anterior stroma in the central lesion may occur, and this ulcer may rapidly enlarge to involve deeper stromal tissue. Less severe forms of the disease resolve within two to three weeks, the cornea gradually clearing from its periphery towards the centre as the vessels cease to transmit blood to the healing ulcer site. Recovery takes longer when extensive ulceration has occurred, and deep stromal scarring and keratoconus may persist. In some patients descemetocele formation may complicate deep ulcers and rupture may lead to panophthalmitis (Plate 46.4b). Blindness may result, and the eye may become glaucomatous but will eventually shrink (phthisis bulbi). The occasional death has been attributed to meningitis following presumed ascending infection of the optic nerve.

Treatment

Moraxella bovis is susceptible to most antimicrobial agents including many antiseptics, and this combined with uncertainties concerning the aetiology of the condition and a tendency for spontaneous resolution in some patients, renders the accurate assessment of any treatment difficult. It is generally agreed, however, that the earlier the treatment the less severe the disease and the greater the chance of controlling the outbreak. In the absence of isolation facilities, it is suggested that treatment of the entire herd will protect the unaffected cattle. Consideration of potential carrier status dictates the use of antibiotics in newly acquired stock before they are introduced into the herd.

Anti-microbial drugs may be administered topically, by subconjunctival injection and parenterally. The ideal therapy for a herd problem demands effective one-time dosage, and, as such, topically applied preparations, which require frequent administration to maintain therapeutically effective levels in the precorneal tear film, cannot be very effective. Their short contact time is reduced further by the presence of ocular discharge and lacrimation, and blepharospasm renders their application difficult. Currently, increased contact time as the result of specific formulation is claimed for several antibiotic preparations including cloxacillin, cephalonium and a penicillin and streptomycin combination. Subconjunctival or intrapalpebral injections of various antibiotics are used extensively as an alternative to the topical route, and long-acting ampicillin, oxytetracycline and penicillin may be used parenterally for repeated good effect. In an original study, Pedersen (1973) claimed that intravenous sulphadimidine was the treatment of choice for IBKC. He showed that although *Moraxella bovis* is present on the corneal and conjunctival surfaces, it invades the lacrimal and tarsal glands, and that any treatment must effectively penetrate these tissues. A single injection of sulphadimidine at dose rate of 100 mg/kg body weight will do this, and the drug will remain in the precorneal tear film at a therapeutically active concentration for 24 hours. It is perhaps surprising that this method of treatment is not utilized to any great extent for it seems to answer both theoretical and practical aspects of therapy. In the future other delivery systems may be evaluated, and ocular inserts that allow prolonged drug release would appear to be of potential value in this respect.

Surgery can have a part to play in the treatment of IBKC. The membrana nictitans can be used to support the severely ulcerated cornea or protect a ruptured anterior chamber, and this technique is preferred to a temporary tarsorrhaphy in which the eyelids are sutured together. Using local anaesthesia together with an auriculopalpebral nerve block to overcome any blepharospasm, the membrana nictitans and the loose bulbar conjunctiva can be apposed to cover the cornea (Fig. 46.2). Mattress sutures of non-absorbable material are used, and the cornea is left covered for two to three weeks. Should a more resilient method of repair be required then under a general anaesthetic a pedicle of bulbar conjunctiva can be sutured directly into the corneal defect (Fig. 46.3). The pedicle is separated from its bulbar conjunctival attachment three to four weeks later and the residual conjunctival tissue either sloughs or is involved in the scar. This technique offers the advantages of directly strengthening the cornea and introducing a blood supply to the ulcer site.

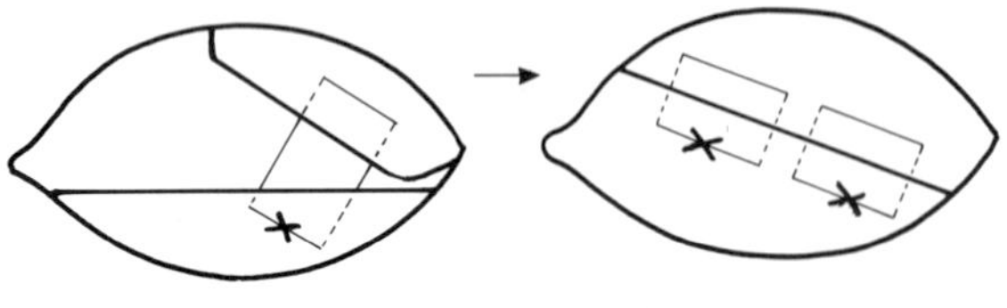

Fig. 46.2 The membrana flap. The membrana is sutured into the loose dorsal bulbar conjunctiva using two or three mattress sutures.

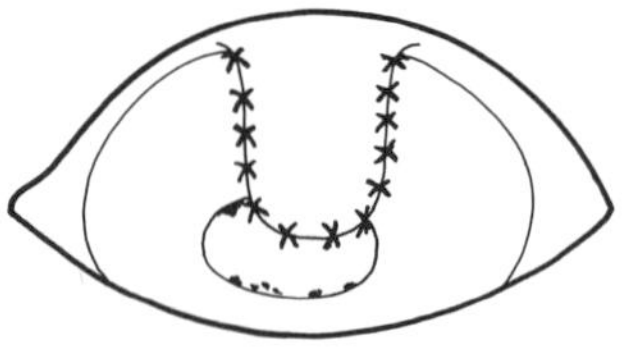

Fig. 46.3 The bulbar conjunctival pedicle flap used in the repair of deep corneal ulceration.

Infectious bovine rhinotracheitis (see also p. 256)

The role of infectious bovine rhinotracheitis virus in anterior segment disease is not fully understood. The virus is thought to enhance the effects of *Moraxella bovis* in some patients with IBKC, but it is also known to cause conjunctivitis in its own right. Respiratory disease may or may not be present, and abortion rates may be high in IBR-affected herds.

The ocular involvement may be unilateral or bilateral. Varying degrees of chemosis may be present, and a number of white plaques may be found in both the bulbar and palpebral conjunctivae. The discharge may vary from serous in early disease to a mucopurulent type later. Anterior uveitis and corneal opacity are occasional findings, and this latter should not be confused with the corneal abscess or ulcer that routinely occurs in IBKC. Confirmation of diagnosis is not always easy, for it requires virus isolation from swabs taken only in the early part of the disease. Seroconversion from negative to positive or a rising titre for IBR antibody will provide the final proof. There is no specific treatment for the condition, but antibiotics will help control any bacterial secondary infection. Normally, the disease takes three to four weeks to complete its course.

Endothelial dystrophy

Bilateral neonatal corneal oedema has been reported in several breeds including the Friesian (Deas, 1959). The oedema is uniformly present throughout the whole stroma, and its persistent nature ensures permanent impairment of sight. Treatment is not possible, but short-term clearing of the cornea can be obtained using topically applied glycerol or hypertonic saline. Signs of possible precursor or accompanying anterior uveitis and other ocular abnormalities are not present, and defective endothelial function alone is the indicated cause. The defect is considered to be inherited as a recessive trait, and affected animals and their carrier parents should be avoided in any future breeding programme.

Neoplasia

Ocular squamous cell carcinoma (SCC) or 'cancer eye' is the commonest bovine neoplasm, and its economic importance has already been stressed. Although SCC has world-wide distribution, its incidence increases in countries where cattle experience long-term exposure to intensive sunlight. The Hereford would appear the most commonly affected breed, and the tumour is rarely seen before five years of age. A presumed inherited predisposition is postulated, and genetic analysis has suggested that it is a recessive trait (Anderson & Chambers, 1957; Vogt & Anderson, 1964). However, several contributory facts seem to be involved, perhaps one of the most important being the role of melanin in palpebral, conjunctival and scleral tissues. Pigmentation is determined genetically, and undoubtedly the presence of melanin protects tissue from SCC development. Much SCC finds origin in the bulbar conjunctiva at the lateral and medial limbi, but other areas where pigmentation may be reduced (the palpebral conjunctiva, the membrana nictitans and eyelid skin) can also be affected. Other possible contributory factors are ultraviolet light, IBR virus, dust, flies and high levels of nutrition.

The indications that ultraviolet light may be an important aetiological factor are the actual tumour sites and the marked geographic variation in incidence. Squamous cell carcinoma occurs in ocular tissue where there is little or no pigment, and the bulbar conjunctiva at the lateral and medial limbi is more exposed than conjunctiva elsewhere on the globe or lining the eyelids. The incidence of ocular SCC is greater in those parts of the world with high levels of ultraviolet light, and at high altitude. The IBR virus and its inclusion bodies may be found in the neoplastic tissue (Taylor & Hanks, 1969) and it has been postulated that the virus may play a part in initiating tumour growth or be involved in the transformation of precursor lesions into carcinoma. Surprisingly, perhaps, the incidence of SCC is greater in cattle on higher levels of nutrition, but this may be associated with enhanced age changes induced by such diets (Anderson, 1970).

Several stages of development are described in SCC formation. Conjunctival plaques of hyperplastic epithelium (Plate 46.5a) or hyperkeratosis of palpebral skin represent the initial lesion. Regression may occur, but the plaques are generally replaced by papilloma formation, and this in turn is replaced by non-invasive carcinoma. Eventually, most of these carcinomas become invasive, and the whole globe can be involved (Plate 46.5b). Invasion of orbital bone can occur, and with long-standing SCC, metastasis via the lymphatics to involve the lungs, heart, liver and kidney is possible (Moulton, 1978).

Treatment is related to the extent of tumour involvement, and the possibility of metastasis may dictate a policy of early slaughter. Excision of the neoplasm, removal of the membrana nictitans, enucleation or exenteration of the orbit represent possible early treatment. Alternative techniques of cryosurgery, hyperthermia, radiation therapy and immunotherapy have all been tried with some success, again early in the course of tumour development. Small neoplasms can be excised irrespective of site, but recurrence and subsequent extension should be expected. Large lesions of the membrana nictitans may already have invaded the orbit. Premalignant lesions and small carcinomas can be destroyed using liquid nitrogen sprays, but adequate freezing demands the use of thermocouple assessment. Limbal-based lesions can be difficult to treat effectively. Again neoplastic cells can be selectively destroyed by heating tissue to 45 °C, and early SCC will respond to hyperthermic therapy. Various forms of ionizing radiation therapy have been used successfully. Beta-irradiation will destroy small lesions, and radioactive caesium, cobalt or gold implants can be similarly effective if the dose rates can be accurately calculated. Immunotherapy offers potentially effective treatment, with the parenteral use of modified or whole-cell tumour cell suspensions having demonstrated considerable promise (van Kampen *et al.*, 1973).

Diseases of the uveal tract (see also p. 150)

Both congenital and acquired disease of the uveal tract occurs in cattle, with uveitis presenting the clinician with as much difficulty in treatment as it does in the other domestic species.

Congenital anomalies

Several congenital anomalies occur in cattle, including aniridia, colobomata, polycoria, persistence of the pupillary membrane and anterior uveal cyst formation. Aniridia is seen as part of a multiocular defect syndrome in Jersey calves, in which bilateral partial absence of the iris is accompanied by microphakia or lens luxation (Saunders & Fincher, 1951). Vision can be affected to the point of blindness, and the defect is inherited as a simple recessive trait. Iris colobomata, polycoria and uveal cysts are of no clinical significance, but persistence of the pupillary membrane may be associated with lens and corneal opacities. The vascular mesoderm, which closes the fetal pupil, should be resorbed by the time of parturition, but strands of this tissue may persist to span the pupil or become adherent to the anterior lens capsule or the corneal endothelium. Cataract or corneal endothelial and deep stromal opacities mark the areas of adherence, the size of these opacities varying with the amount of the attaching remnant tissue. Heterochromia iridis, due to a reduction or absence of melanin, is seen in the colour dilute breeds, and it may occasionally be accompanied by photophobia, nystagmus and typical papillary coloboma formation.

Uveitis

Inflammation within the uveal tract occurs in association with systemic disease, corneal ulceration, keratitis, trauma and intraocular neoplasia. Anterior uveitis can accompany IBR infection, toxoplasmosis, tuberculosis and neonatal coliform septicaemia; panophthalmitis in which the whole uveal tract is involved may be seen in malignant catarrhal fever. Infectious bovine rhinotracheitis virus may be involved in IBKC and will cause conjunctivitis: occasionally there is an associated uveitis. In calves with coliform septicaemia, acute anterior uveitis characterized by episcleral congestion, miosis and hypopyon may be seen in association with septic meningitis in which paresis, ataxia and convulsions are the obvious clinical features. Occasionally, the choroid is involved, and haemorrhage and exudate will be seen in the vitreous. In peracute malignant catarrhal fever severe photophobia, marked palpebral and corneal oedema, mucopurulent discharge and panuveitis may all be seen. Anterior uveitis, choroiditis and retinitis may all be present as a result of vascular necrosis and vasculitis (Plowright, 1968). A recurrent uveitis, referred to as specific ophthalmia (Marolt *et al.*, 1963), has been described for cattle. It is similar clinically to the equine condition with corneal oedema, anterior chamber and intravitreal exudates, and retinal haemorrhage being seen in the acute stage. A viral aetiology is suggested, with IBR and other respiratory viruses isolated from affected animals.

Listeria monocytogenes has been previously associated with outbreaks of keratoconjunctivitis and uveitis in housed cattle in the UK (Morgan, 1977), but more recently this organism has been isolated from housed cattle fed on silage, presenting with anterior uveitis as the only clinical feature (Watson, 1989). The uveitis presents clinically in the same way as any other anterior segment inflammation: it is usually unilateral with marked miosis, thickening and folding of the iris, keratic precipitate (KP) and hypopyon formation and vascularization of the limbal cornea being the presenting signs (Plate 46.6). Treatment includes the use of systemic antibiosis, but subconjunctival corticosteroids and topical atropine are essential.

Neoplasia

Primary uveal tract tumours in cattle are rare, but secondary involvement with squamous cell carcinoma occurs not infrequently.

Disease of the lens

Ectopia lentis (lens luxation) occurs as part of a multiocular defect syndrome in Jersey and Friesian cattle, and cataract probably enjoys higher incidence than the literature dictates. Intraocular examinations are not commonly practised in cattle, and cataract is only diagnosed if it is large enough to be noticed, has an effect on sight or is present with other ocular anomalies.

Congenital cataract has been recorded in several breeds, and in Jersey and Friesian cattle inheritance is as a simple recessive trait (p. 150). The nuclear part of the lens is always involved, but cortical extension may severely affect vision (Plate 46.7). Nystagmoid movements of the globe may accompany the larger lesions. In both these breeds and in the Shorthorn other ocular anomalies including buphthalmia, microphakia, lens luxation and retinal detachment may accompany cataract. Cataract may follow uveitis, but the aetiology of other capsular and cortical lens opacity remains obscure (Gelatt, 1971).

The treatment of cataract is by surgery, and two techniques are possible. In young calves of several weeks of age lens discission can be successful if the attendant uveitis is minimal (Bedford, pers. obs.). The technique is a simple one in which the anterior capsule of the lens is disrupted using a Bowman's needle inserted into the anterior chamber at the dorsal limbus (Plate 46.8). Normal and cataractous lens material is released into the anterior chamber and is completely resorbed, leaving the posterior capsule *in situ* to retain the vitreous behind the pupil. Corticosteroids are used to suppress the phacoanaphylactic inflammation, but in young calves this is minimal. In older animals the uveitis renders this technique unacceptable, and extracapsular lens extraction offers the best chance of success. The anterior chamber is opened either through a corneal or limbal section, the anterior capsule removed and the cataractous material dislocated from the posterior capsule out through the section. The postoperative therapy must include corticosteroids, and, just as in other species, loss of pupil as the result of iris spasm and posterior synechiae formation is the common complication that may render the eye blind. However, the uveitis is usually controllable, and the overall prognosis for sight is good.

Disease of the retina and optic nerve

Both congenital anomaly and acquired disease can involve the bovine fundus, but as with cataract diagnosis such lesions are not normally detected unless there is an associated effect on sight or other more noticeable ocular defects are present.

Congenital defects

Papillary and peripapillary choroidal colobomata, persistence of the hyaloid artery, retinal dysplasia and maternal hypovitaminosis A induced papilloedema and optic nerve atrophy are seen in the neonate. Choroidal colobomata are reported to be commonplace but may be of no clinical significance. Typical papillary colobomata in Hereford cattle with incomplete albinism are seen bilaterally but have no noticeable effect on vision. However, the same defect in Charolais may blind the affectd animal (Plate 46.9). In both breeds the lesion is considered to be inherited, and genetic studies in the Charolais have indicated that it is a polygenic trait (Barnett & Ogden, 1972) (p. 150).

The hyaloid artery is part of the primary vitreous, but with the development of the ciliary vasculature it regresses and becomes non-functional. Unlike the dog, large remnants of this vessel can be seen commonly in cattle (Plate 46.10), but they are of no clinical importance. The vessel overlies the optic disc and extends forward from this structure into the posterior vitreous. Blood is often seen within its lumen in young calves up to eight weeks of age, and remnants of the avascular vessel will persist throughout the animal's life.

Retinal dysplasia, in which there is typical rosette formation and usually non-attachment of the neuroretina, is seen in Shorthorn cattle with hydrocephalus and multiple ocular defects, and in Herefords with microphthalmia, cerebellar hypoplasia and hydrocephalus (Blackwell *et al.*, 1959; Green & Leipold, 1974). Congenital retinal degeneration and optic nerve atrophy has been seen in association with microphthalmia, cataract and cerebellar hypoplasia in calves born of dams infected with bovine viral diarrhoea/mucosal disease. Congenital optic nerve degeneration and papilloedema can be produced by maternal hypovitaminosis A.

Inflammation

Retinal and optic nerve lesions will accompany several systemic infections including the neonatal pyosepticaemias, bovine viral diarrhoea/mucosal disease, thrombo-embolic meningo-encephalitis, toxoplasmosis, tuberculosis and rabies.

Septic chorioretinitis characterized by haemorrhages, exudate and bullous retinal detachment can accompany septicaemia in young calves caused by *Escherichia coli*, streptococci, *Pasteurella* and *Corynebacterium* infections. Maternal infection with bovine viral diarrhoea/mucosal disease can cause congenital optic neuritis among other ocular anomalies, and in thrombo-embolic meningo-encephalitis caused by *Haemophilus somnus* conjunctivitis and corneal oedema may be accompanied by retinal vasculitis and detachment. Blindness is usually due to septic thrombosis of the visual cortex. Both anterior and posterior uveitis with possible retinal involvement can occur in toxoplasmosis, and a granulomatous panuveitis with areas of retinal detachment can accompany tuberculosis. Focal retinitis has been reported in bovine rabies.

Hypovitaminosis A (see also p. 220)

Hypovitaminosis A has been described in three situations with a variability of the presenting clinical features. It occurs congenitally, and here either papilloedema and optic nerve atrophy are present. In the growing calf there is obvious papilloedema in which the disc becomes very swollen, and the resultant papillary vascular congestion may cause focal superficial haemorrhage (Plate 46.11). Optic nerve atrophy will occur if the deficiency is maintained. The papilloedema is due to compression of the optic nerve by bony overgrowth within the optic canal, and the accompanying vascular occlusion results in ischaemic necrosis of the nerve (Hayes *et al.*, 1968). Early papilloedema is reversible and optic nerve atrophy preventable if the diet is suitably adjusted. Nyctalopia due to rod degeneration also occurs. Vitamin A is essential in the formation of the visual pigment rhodopsin, and without rhodopsin the photoreceptors degenerate. This process is also reversible should vitamin A be supplemented soon enough. It is likely that the sight problems experienced by the calf are more likely to be caused by the optic nerve lesions rather than the retinal degeneration. In the adult deficient in vitamin A papilloedema is much less noticeable and optic nerve atrophy does not occur. Here the outer segment degeneration is probably more significant in terms of the effect on sight.

Male fern optic neuropathy

Permanent or transient blindness will accompany weakness, malaise and constipation in the early stages of male fern (*Dryopteris filix mas*) poisoning. The toxic effect is on the optic nerve, and varying degrees of papilloedema and associated haemorrhage are seen ophthalmoscopically. In severe cases optic nerve atrophy follows the papilloedema.

Arthrogryposis (see p. 147)

The aetiology of arthrogryposis is open to speculation, and inheritance, fetal lupin toxicosis, manganese deficiency and maternal viral infection have all been considered to be involved. Joint deformities, syringomyelia and cleft palate may be seen, and blindness is due to abnormal photoreceptor development.

Progressive retinal degeneration

A form of retinal degeneration characterized by nyctalopia, progressive pigmentation within the tapetal fundus and attenuation of the superficial retinal vasculature has been described in cattle, and compared with canine progressive retinal atrophy (PRA). It would appear to be a rare condition, and the comparison with PRA may have been somewhat overindulgent.

Glaucoma

Glaucoma is the process of ocular degeneration caused by an elevation of the intraocular fluid pressure (IOP) beyond its physiological upper limit. All bovine glaucomas are due to the impairment of aqueous drainage through a defective or diseased iridocorneal angle, and in the majority of cases the glaucoma is secondary to inflammation or neoplasia. Uveitis may result in pupillary block due to extensive posterior synechiae formation. This results in the forward displacement of the peripheral iris, the so-called iris bombé, and closure of the ciliary cleft. The presence of exudation speeds the transformation of the trabecular meshwork into an impervious physical barrier to aqueous outflow. Alternatively, these peripheral anterior synechiae or ciliary synechiae may form directly to deny bulk aqueous drainage. Tumour cells and the products of any associated inflammation will block the iridocorneal angle to produce secondary glaucoma. A primary glaucoma has been recorded in the Friesian (Carter, 1960); the condition is inherited as a dominant trait and is seen in association with cátaract formation and lens luxation.

Treatment of glaucoma in cattle is determined on the basis of whether the enlarged blind eye is of nuisance value, and enucleation may be necessary in the presence of associated corneal damage or degeneration.

References

Amman, K. (1968) Eye diseases in ruminants. In *Veterinary Encyclopaedia*, vol. II (ed. by E.A. McPherson), pp. 931–45. Medical Book Co, Copenhagen.

Anderson, D.E. (1970) Cancer eye in cattle. *Modern Veterinary Practice* **51**, 43–7.

Anderson, D.E. & Chambers, D. (1957) Genetic aspects of cancer eye in cattle. *Miscellaneous Publications of the Oklahoma Agricultural Experimental Station*, **MP48**, 28–33.

Barnett, K.C. & Ogden, A.I. (1972) Ocular colobomata in Charolais cattle. *Veterinary Record* **91**, 592.

Bedford, P.G.C. (1976) Infectious bovine keratoconjunctivitis. *Veterinary Record* **98**, 134–5.

Billings, F.S. (1889) Keratitis contagiosa in cattle. *Nebraska Agricultural Station Bulletin* **10**, 247.

Blackwell, R.L., Knox, J.H. & Cobb, E.H. (1959) A hydrocephalic lethal in Hereford cattle. *Journal of Heredity* **50**, 143–8.

Carter, A.H. (1960) An inherited blindness (cataract) in cattle. *Proceedings of the New Zealand Society for Animal Production* **20**, 108.

Cordy, D.R. (1978) Tumours of the nervous system and eye. In *Tumours in Domestic Animals*, 2nd edn (ed. by J.E. Moulton), pp. 443–53. University of California Press, Los Angeles.

Deas, D.W. (1959) A note on hereditary opacity of the diseased cornea in British Friesian cattle. *Veterinary Record* **71**, 619–20.

Gelatt, K.N. (1971) Cataracts in cattle. *Journal of the American Veterinary Medical Association* **159**, 195–200.

Gilmore, L.O. (1957) Inherited defects in cattle. *Journal of Dairy Science* **40**, 593–5.

Green, H.J. & Leipold, H.W. (1974) Hereditary internal hydrocephalus and retinal dysplasia in Shorthorn calves. *Cornell Veterinarian* **64**, 367–75.

Hayes, K.C., Nielsen, S.W. & Eaton, H.D. (1968) Pathogenesis of the optic nerve lesion in vitamin A deficient calves. *Archives of Ophthalmology* **80**, 777–87.

Leipold, H.W. & Huston, K. (1968) Congenital syndrome of anophthalmia–microphthalmia with associated defects in cattle. *Pathologia Veterinaria* **5**, 407–18.

Marolt, J., Burdnjak, Z., Vekelic, E. & Andrasic, N. (1963) Specific ophthalmia of cattle. *Zentralblatt Veterinärmedizin*. **10**, 286–294.

Morgan, J.H. (1977) Infectious keratoconjunctivitis in cattle associated with *Listeria monocytogenes*. *Veterinary Record* **100**, 113–14.

Pedersen, K.B. (1973) *Infectious keratoconjunctivitis in cattle*. PhD Thesis, Royal Veterinary College, Copenhagen, Denmark.

Plowright, W. (1968) Malignant catarrhal fever. *Journal of the American Veterinary Medical Association* **152**, 795–804.

Pugh, G.W. (1969) *Characterization of Moraxella bovis and its relationship to bovine infectious keratoconjunctivitis*. PhD Thesis, Iowa State University, Ames, Iowa.

Sandhu, T.S., White, F.H. & Simpson, C.F. (1974) Association of pili with the rough colony type of *Moraxella bovis*. *American Journal of Veterinary Research* **35**, 437–9.

Saunders, L.Z. & Fincher, M.S. (1951) Hereditary multiple eye defects in grade Jersey calves. *Cornell Veterinarian* **41**, 351–366.

Taylor, R.L. & Hanks, M.A. (1969) Viral isolations from bovine eye tumours. *American Journal of Veterinary Research* **30**, 1885–6.

van Kampen, K.R., Crisp, W.E., Martin, J.C.D. & Ellsworth, H.S. (1973) The immunologic therapy of squamous cell carcinoma. *American Journal of Obstetrics and Gynaecology*, **116**, 569–74.

Vogt, D.W. & Anderson, D.E. (1964) Studies on bovine ocular squamous cell carcinoma ('cancer eye'). XV. Heritability of susceptibility. *Journal of Heredity* **55**, 133–5.

Watson, C.L. (1989) Bovine iritis? *Veterinary Record* **124**, 411.

Willoughby, R.A. (1968) Congenital eye defects in cattle. *Modern Veterinary Practice* **49**, 36–9.

Chapter 47: Tick and Arthropod-borne Diseases

by S.M. TAYLOR, A.G. HUNTER AND A.H. ANDREWS

Tick infestations

In tropical regions ticks play an important role in causing and spreading disease. Many actively suck blood and can cause death by anaemia. Some ticks cause paralysis particularly in young animals. The life cycles vary considerably with some ticks spending all their time on a single host, others are only parasitic at certain stages and some spend each stage of the life cycle on a different host. Those spending all their time on a single host (one-host ticks) are easier to control than those on different hosts for each development stage (three-host ticks)

One-host ticks:	*Boophilus* spp.
Two-host ticks:	*Hyalomma* spp.
	Rhipicephalus bursa
	R. evertsi
Three-host ticks:	*Amblyomma* spp.
	Argaspersicus spp.
	Dermacentor spp.
	Haemaphysalis spp.
	Hyalomma spp.
	Ixodes spp.
	Rhipicephalus spp.

Ixodoidea

Their life cycle involves egg, larva, nymph and adult. Almost all ticks at each development stage require a blood meal. The unfed stage varies in its ability to survive depending on the amount of moisture present.

The engorged stage drops off the host and then does not move from where it is deposited. The group is divided into two main families, the Argasidae or soft ticks and the Ixodidae or hard ticks.

ARGASIDAE FAMILY

These have a cuticle without a hardened dorsal scutin and their mouthparts cannot be seen from above. They are mainly found in arid or semi-arid areas. When feeding they rapidly engorge with blood. They are able to survive for long periods, i.e. months or years without the presence of suitable hosts for feeding. The nymphs and adults can repeatedly feed, which allows greater capacity for transfer of infection.

There are three genera: *Argas*, *Ornithodorus* and *Otobius*.

IXODIDAE FAMILY

These have a hardened scutum that covers almost all the dorsum in adult males but only one-third of the dorsum in unfed larvae, nymphs and adult females. The mouthparts are visible. There are nymph and larval stages. All stages including the adult females only feed once. Adult males remain on the host and feed often. Up to half the engorged weight can be taken in with one feed.

The family includes one-, two- and three-host ticks and there are 10 ixodial genera of which seven have veterinary importance: *Amblyomma*, *Boophilus*, *Dermacentor*, *Haemaphysalis*, *Hyalomma*, *Ixodes* and *Rhipicephalus*.

Control

This can be directed at the ticks on or off the host. The latter is easiest to perform. When off the host control is performed it includes the use of pasture spraying with anti-tick dips, which involves keeping stock off the area for as long as possible to allow death of the ticks. It works best where the ticks are short-lived as in warm arid conditions. It is best performed by treating pastures in rotation. The effectiveness of pasture spraying depends on whether alternative hosts, either domestic or wild, are available. The practice often means underuse of pasture. However, the overuse or intensification in grazing often increases the tick population. Another method of control often underrated is that of pasture burning.

In most areas the only effective method of tick control is in the host. This is usually done by hand dressing, spraying or dipping. Hand dressing is laborious and has to be done efficiently. It can be done by the use of dusting powders, creams, pastes or in a liquid form by hand spraying, paint brushing or application by washes. In large herds sprays or dips are used. In general, dips provide a more effective overall control. Both effective spray races and dips are expensive to install. The compounds used tend to be organochlorides, organophosphates, synthetic pyrethroids and traditional compounds. The last group includes arsenic preparations such as sodium arsenite. It is cheap but has no residual effect and it can be toxic. Resistance to arsenic dips occurs in some areas. Organophosphorus dips are effective but have limited residual activity. They can be toxic especially when used by unskilled staff. Organochloride compounds are useful because they are effective and persist for several days; however, they are suspensions and so require adequate mixing, resistance has developed to them and they have a persistence in the body that can lead to a build-up of the compounds. Synthetic pyrethroids are good and relatively non-toxic but some resistance to them is developing, and occurs also when ticks are DDT resistant.

The number of dippings depends on several factors and often means the interval between dippings varies according to the season of the year. It depends on the duration of the ixodicide's activity, the toxicity of the dip, the seasonal activity of the ticks, the time the ticks spend on the host and whether it is required to control or try to eradicate the parasite. Thus one-host ticks, which remain on the host for three weeks, are far easier to deal with than three-host ticks, which only feed for a day or two. Generally, at its height, dipping will be once a week for one-host ticks and twice a week for three-host ticks. Such frequent dipping does allow tick selection for resistance. However, often where tick control is not achieved it is more likely due to not dipping frequently enough or the dip being too weak, improperly mixed or the wrong type or concentration for the stage of the tick to be killed. Where resistance does occur it can be overcome by changing the type of agent in the dip. Many farmers alternate the type of dip used on a routine basis.

Fly problems

Mosquitoes

There are many species of mosquito including *Aedes* spp., *Anopheles* spp., *Culex* spp., *Mansonia* spp. and *Psorophora* spp. They can cause problems when in large numbers due to annoyance of man and animal. Mosquitoes cause some loss of blood by feeding as well as transmitting diseases such as Rift Valley fever and probably other conditions such as lumpy skin disease and bluetongue. The mosquito life cycle is aquatic for the larva and pupa and takes 5–21 days to reach the adult stage.

Control of the insect over large areas involves drainage of still surface water. Larvae can be destroyed by treating water with oil, DDT, synthetic pyrethroid or other insecticide. Oil is easiest to use and can involve waste engine oil with kerosene or diesel oil. Applying repellants to cattle tends to be too expensive and self-applicators are often used. Otherwise, for small groups of animals the use of mosquito screens will stop contact.

Blackflies

These belong to the family Simuliidae and include blackflies, buffalo flies and sandflies. They are small (<5 mm long) and black or grey in colour. They occur in most countries and when in large numbers they are an annoyance. It is thought that there may be toxic factors in the saliva. The bites result in vesicles and these in turn can result in ulcers and secondary infection. The larvae and pupae are attached to reedy stems and branches in running water. They take about three to four weeks to pass from egg to adult. They are active during the summer months. The flies tend to gather in swarms and annoy animals. They bite the legs, belly and head, causing the animals to stamp and kick their legs. Occasionally they stampede. Cattle may wallow in mud or kick up dust to keep off the flies. Control depends on attacking the larval stages by using DDT in streams. However, rapid re-infection of the areas will occur. Treatment of the adult is difficult but a repellant such as dimethyl phthalate is helpful. Regular dipping of cattle for ticks, etc. also reduces fly levels.

Midges

These are extremely small flies (1–3 mm long) of the family Ceratopogonidae, the important genera being *Culicoides* and *Lasiohelia*. These suck the blood of animals and man. They transmit ephemeral fever, bluetongue and other pathogenic viruses. The larvae are found mainly in swamps, where they either live in wet mud or free-standing water. Some occupy more restricted habitats such as rotting vegetation. Besides acting as vectors of arboviruses they can cause hypersensitivity reactions.

Control is by draining the breeding sites. Otherwise, spraying the areas with oil or DDT gives good results. Repellants, particularly dimethyl phthalate, are effective on a short-term basis. Mosquito screens are of no use. Fires at times of biting activity will assist in herd protection.

Horseflies and deerflies

Horseflies are of the *Tabanus* spp. and are also called March flies or breeze flies. Deerflies are of the *Chrysops* spp., *Haematopota* spp. and *Pangonia* spp. They are large, brown, robust flies that bite and suck blood. They act as vectors of diseases such as anthrax, anaplasmosis and trypanosomiasis. *Haematopota* spp. are thought to help transmit summer mastitis. The eggs are laid on the leaves of plants growing close to or in water. The larval and pupal stages occur in the water or mud and the life cycle takes about four to five months to complete. The flies tend to be active during the day in summer months, particularly when it is hot and sultry, and are mainly found on the ventral abdomen and legs. Control is difficult but depends on drainage of wet areas. Breeding sites can be treated with oil or DDT. Otherwise, repellants such as dimethyl phthalate and γ-dimethyl-tolumide are useful but last only a few days. Some products are available to apply to the cows' udders.

Houseflies

The common housefly (*Musca domestica*) has a worldwide distribution. They cause worry to animals by settling on them as well as acting as vectors of diseases such as anthrax, erysipelas, brucellosis and possibly summer mastitis. They cause aggravation at wounds or other areas where there is blood, exudate, pus, etc. They cause infections by discharging some of their stomach contents, so-called vomit drop, on to the food to moisten it and often they also defaecate. This means that they are able to transfer many pathogens effectively. Eggs are laid on rotting vegetable material or faeces. The life cycle involves an egg producing a larva (a maggot), which takes about 10 days to mature, thereby completing the cycle in about 12–14 days in warm weather.

Control methods include removing all manure and organic material at least every three days. This can be stacked so as to ferment, ideally in a bunker or pit. Otherwise, it should be turned over every few days or better still treated with insecticide. Faeces can be burnt. Fly traps (Baber's) can be used to collect flies and larvae. Buildings should be kept as clean as possible and can be sprayed with insecticides, or insecticide strips can be placed in areas with little air movement. Electrocutors can be used to which the flies are attracted by an ultraviolet light. Cattle can have insecticide-impregnated ear tags but these are not too effective against the housefly.

Bush flies

These include *Musca sorbens*, *M. fergusoni*, *M. terraeregina*, *M. hilli*. They are found particularly in Australia. They tend to be found all the year round in northern Australia but only in the summer periods in the South. The flies often appear in large numbers and can be found on the lips, eyelids and other mucous membranes and by wounds. They are considered to transmit infectious bovine keratoconjunctivitis. Control is difficult but involves fly spraying cattle and buildings. A repellant such as dimethyl phthalate can be of use. Synthetic pyrethoids can be successful.

Face fly

This is *Musca autumnalis*, a small fly resembling, and slightly bigger than, the housefly, found in Europe, Asia and North America. Numbers tend to be greatest in the summer and particularly cattle outside are worried. Fresh cattle faeces are the only fly breeding grounds. Flies are particularly seen on the face around the nostrils and eyes where they feed on the secretions. They are thought to transmit infectious bovine keratoconjunctivitis. There are no wholly successful control measures although plastic insecticide-impregnated ear tags are useful and powders or cream containing organophosphorus compounds assist.

Head fly

The fly *Hydrotaea irritans* is the same size as the housefly but has an olive abdomen and yellow wing tips. It is found in Great Britain and Europe. It is a nuisance fly and does not bite although it does feed off exudate around wounds. It occurs in large swarms from July to September. The life cycle is annual and it involves periods of development in the soil. Sores on animals are made larger due to self-inflicted aggravation because of irritation. *Hydrotaea irritans* is incriminated in the transmission of summer mastitis. It is probably also concerned with infectious bovine keratoconjunctivitis. Control is difficult and involves the use of parasite sprays and dipping. Plastic insecticide-impregnated ear tags are useful.

Stable fly

The stable fly, *Stomoxys calcitrans*, is about the size of the housefly. It is grey in colour, has a sharp proboscis and when it settles it sits with its head upwards. It is a bloodsucker and feeds on the host causing great irritation. Wounds often bleed freely after the flies have fed. The eggs are laid in faeces, rotting hay or straw and the life cycle is complete in two to three weeks. The larval and pupal stages take place in organic matter. Warm damp environments encourage the flies' growth and survival. They cause considerable nuisance and worry with reduced milk and meat production and possibly anaemia. In cattle there can be a hypersensitivity of the forelimb skin, which in turn has blisters that coalesce to form bleeding sores. *Stomoxys calcitrans* can transmit anthrax. Another species, *S. nigra*, occurs in South Africa.

Control of the fly involves the frequent removal and disposal of bedding and faeces from buildings. Destruction of the flies is difficult because they feed for only a short time. It can be helped by the use of insecticide-impregnated plastic ear tags or spraying with suitable sprays, spraying of walls and shaded areas of pens.

Horn flies and buffalo flies

Horn flies include *Liperosia* or *Haematobia irritans*, *H. minuta*, and *L.* or *H. exigua*. This last is also known as the buffalo fly. The flies are greyish, smaller and less active than stable flies. At rest their wings are completely closed but are held away from the body. They thus spend more time on the host except when laying eggs, etc. Many have a limited geographical range. Thus *H. irritans* is found in the USA and Hawaii, *H. minuta* in Africa and *H. exigua* in Australia and south-west Asia. They are most common on cattle and buffalo and occur in large numbers causing much irritation. Although bloodsuckers they are not known to transmit diseases. Severe infestations lead to weakness and death. They also produce large sores.

The eggs are laid in fresh faeces and can only survive with high humidity and warm temperature. They pupate in the soil and the life cycle takes eight days to three weeks to complete. Control of the flies is difficult but removal of dung is important. The cattle and buildings should be sprayed frequently with insecticide. If tick dipping is undertaken this reduces fly numbers. The use of plastic insecticide-impregnated ear tags is helpful. Otherwise, applying DDT or other suitable spray at regular intervals will assist.

Horse louse flies

These include *Hippobasum equina*, *H. rufipes* and *H. maculata. Hippobasum equina* is the most common, is slightly larger than the housefly and is a reddish-brown, fast, glossy fly that causes problems to cattle and horses. It feeds on blood and is found on the inside of the hind legs and the perineum. The eggs are laid and develop in dry soil. They can act as mechanical vectors of disease. Plastic insecticide-impregnated ear tags are of use in control as are spraying or dipping of cattle.

Tsetse flies

The *Glossina* species are an important African fly that act as the true vector of trypanosomiasis (p. 737). They are 6–13.5 mm long, thin-bodied, yellow or brown flies. The wings are folded over each other and there is a slender proboscis. There are 20 species of *Glossina* and all are found in tropical Africa. They occur in a variety of environments but are usually found in one of three terrains: (i) forest, where they inhabit thickly wooded areas with a high humidity; (ii) riverine, where they live on the edges of forest but by streams, lakes and rivers; and (iii) savannah grasslands, where the tsetse are the most important species for spreading animal disease.

Both the male and female tsetse flies feed on blood and most of the species are attracted to certain host species. In tsetse flies the eggs hatch in the uterus and so they are larviparous. The larvae are deposited on shady dry soil and pupate there. One larva is produced every 10 days and the pupal stage lasts 28–56 days. As the adult female survives three or four months eight to twelve larvae are produced.

Control depends on surveying an area to determine the species of the tsetse fly present and their habitats. Then the possibility of control can be assessed. Methods of eradication or control are direct using insecticides to remove adult flies, removal of pupae and use of repellants on cattle. The indirect approach depends on removal of nesting sites and dry weather refuges. Insecticides including DDT and dieldrin are of long duration but have been considered by some to cause too much long-term pollution. Shorter term insecticides that are biodegradable such as synthetic pyrethroids are now favoured.

Tumbu fly

The tumbu or mango fly is *Cordylobia anthropophaga*. It infests man and animals but rarely cattle. It is about the size of a housefly and lays eggs in the soil or sand. The hatched larva attaches to the skin of a host where it produces a painful irritant swelling with a dark central hole. Once mature the larva passes out to the soil where it pupates. The adult lives on food and animal excreta. In light infestations each larva can be manually removed by covering up the airhole with liquid paraffin in Vaseline. The parasite will push its posterior abdomen out of the hole and it can then be pressed out gently. In severe infestations insecticides can be applied, such as organophosphorus compounds.

Blow flies and screw-worm flies

These result in blow fly infection or myiasis. The flies involved include several genera: *Calliphora*, *Callitroga*, *Chrysomyia*, *Lucilia* and *Sarcophaga*. Cattle are less affected than sheep. The flies are really scavengers and mainly live on dead meat. However, true screw-worm flies are only laying their eggs in fresh wounds. They are however attracted to dying flesh on live animals. Even the small wounds of ticks attract the flies. The larvae feed and grow quickly and mature in three to five days.

A local dressing of a larvicide and an antiseptic is useful after clipping away the hair. The usual compounds are organophosphates. They normally promote a complete kill in about 12 hours. All wounds should be treated with an antifly preparation. Dipping or spraying the animals with insecticides can be helpful. Otherwise, the number of flies can be reduced by trapping and quick disposal of carcasses. Chromosomal translocation of males to produce sterile or lethal mutant offspring has been tried with some success. The American screw-worm fly *Callitroga americana* has been controlled by the release of irradiated males. They mate with the females, which lay sterile eggs, thereby ultimately reducing or eliminating the fly population.

Protozoal diseases

Babesiosis

Babesiasis is caused by intraerythrocytic protozoan of the genus *Babesia* transmitted by hard ticks of the family Ixodidae. Unlike many other parasitic diseases, it affects adults more severely than young cattle in which infection is frequently subclinical. It causes fever, haemoglobinaemia, haemoglobinuria, anaemia and death.

Table 47.1 *Babesia* spp. infecting cattle

Species	Size	Climatic preference
B. bovis	Small	Tropical or subtropical
B. bigemina	Large	Tropical or subtropical
B. divergens	Small	Temperate
B. major	Large	Temperate

Aetiology and epidemiology

There are four species of *Babesia* that are the most important of those affecting cattle. These are *Babesia bovis*, *B. bigemina*, *B. divergens* and *B. major*, the first three being much more significant than the last. Two are considered 'small' *Babesia* and two 'large', and there is one large and one small species for both tropical and temperate climatic areas (Table 47.1).

The parasites are transmitted by hard ticks, which are also affected by their role as intermediate hosts in the babesial life cycle. When an infected tick attaches to the skin of cattle its mouthparts penetrate the skin and it starts to suck blood. Bloodsucking is not continuous but takes place in short periods of activity until the stage of the tick becomes fully engorged. Full engorgement for larvae requires three to five days, for nymphs five to six days and adults seven to ten days. *Babesia* spp. are not transmitted by infected ticks until the end of the engorgement period because the babesial stages in the tick have to develop and move to the salivary gland prior to becoming infective sporozoites. The sporozoites are injected into the host with saliva and then invade erythrocytes. They proceed to divide asexually in red cells forming two pear-shaped merozoites. Each erythrocyte ruptures when the merozoites leave to infect new cells. The reproduction time in erythrocytes is in the order of 12–15 hours depending on species. When sufficient multiplication has taken place for parasites to be visible in very low numbers in blood smears the animal will show a febrile reaction. The length of time required is usually approximately one to three weeks after infection, but depends on the number of *Babesia* in the infective inoculum, and in very large syringe-passed infections may be as short as two to three days. Thereafter the parasitaemia may build up and in extreme cases more than 20 per cent of erythrocytes may be infected, although the percentage infected varies with the species involved, e.g. the parasitaemia of *B. bovis* is usually less than 1 per cent in venous blood whereas *B. bigemina* and *B. divergens* on average reach 3–8 per cent. At this point the affected animal has a febrile reaction and may exhibit the characteristic haemoglobinuria that produced the colloquial term of 'redwater' for the disease, and unless treated it may die. After treatment the animal becomes a carrier of the organism and may suffer from occasional recrudescences of parasitaemia. Ticks become infected by feeding on parasitaemic cattle. Infected adult female ticks pass the infection to their eggs, the infection being termed *transovarial*, and the larvae, nymphs and adults up to the F2 generation. Some *Babesia* spp. may remain infected in the absence of feeding on carrier bovines, although for *B. bovis* infection ceases with larvae. Transmission from larva to nymph to adult is termed *transtadial* infection, and is observed with *B. bigemina* and *B. divergens*.

The epidemiology of the *Babesia* spp. is governed by the local climate and behaviour of its tick vectors. As a result they merit separate consideration as tropical or non-tropical species.

Tropical species: B. bovis *and* B. bigemina. These species are found in Australia, Africa, South and

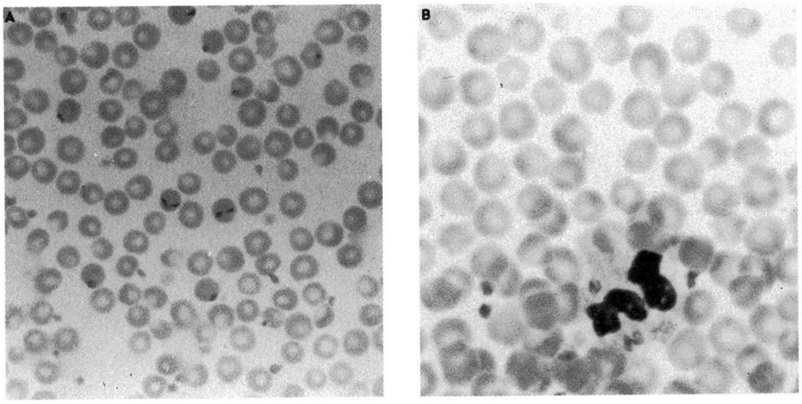

Fig. 47.1 (A) Bovine blood infected with *Babesia divergens* (× 630). (B) Bovine blood smear showing *Ehrlichia phagocytophila* in a neutrophil (× 630).

Central America, Asia and the very south of Europe. In Australia and the Americas the tick *Boophilus microplus* is the sole vector, in Africa other *Boophilus* and *Rhipicephalus* species. *Boophilus* spp. are one-host ticks, i.e. all stages of the life cycle take place on one animal, only the engorged female dropping to the ground before laying eggs. Some vectors in Africa, e.g. *R. evertsi*, are two-host, and *R. appendiculatus* a three-host tick.

Babesia bovis merozoites in erythrocytes measure 2 × 1.5 μm and those of *B. bigemina* 4.5 × 2 μm. Parasitaemia in venous blood is low with *B. bovis* but it may be high in capillaries and cause sludging of blood, which if in the brain cause early death. It also produces enzymes with severe effects on the blood coagulation system, and is generally considered the most pathogenic of the bovine *Babesia* spp.

Babesia bigemina infection results in much higher venous parasitaemia but it has few other effects other than to cause a febrile reaction and straightforward haemolytic anaemia.

Temperate species: B. divergens *and* B. major. *Babesia divergens*, the merozoites of which measure 1.5 × 0.4 μm is common in areas of permanent pasture in north-western Europe and is transmitted by the three-host tick *Ixodes ricinus*. *Babesia major* (3.2 × 1.5 μm) is found only in south-eastern England and on islands off the coast of The Netherlands, and is transmitted by *Haemaphysalis punctata*.

Babesia divergens behaves rather similarly to *B. bigemina*, i.e. it can cause a high parasitaemia, which results in fever and severe haemolytic anaemia. It has little effect on blood coagulation systems in comparison to *B. bovis*. Its epidemiology is closely bound to the ecology of its vector *I. ricinus*. In Europe, *I. ricinus* is generally active only between May and November, and in most areas has spring and autumn population increases, although in the most northerly climates it may only have one in midsummer. The ticks quest more actively in warm conditions and outbreaks of babesiasis are frequently observed two weeks after fine weather. The epidemiology of *B. major* is still only slightly investigated, but such isolations as have been reported have taken place in May and June.

Signs

Early. There is slight dullness with a pyrexia often of 40.5–41 °C (105–106 °F). The animal shows diarrhoea and because of spasm of the anal sphincter there is a narrow stream of diarrhoea (pipe-stem diarrhoea). There is also haemoglobinuria. Slight dehydration is often seen as a slightly sunken eye.

Mid. After 24–36 hours the mucous membranes tend to become pale and the pulse rate is increased. The animals tend to slow up and there is a reduction in appetite and thirst. The urine tends to become very dark in colour and reduced in quantity. The faeces may return to normal but less tends to be passed although there is still spasm of the anus.

Late. In another 24–36 hours the rectal temperature is often subnormal with the animal having blanched mucous membranes, a poor appetite and drinking little. There is marked constipation and a greatly increased heart rate.

Pregnant cows may abort following infection.

Necropsy

The carcass may be very blanched and there is sometimes jaundice. The liver is often swollen and pulpy, with the kidneys dark and enlarged. The bladder contains red–brown urine. There are ecchymotic haemorrhages under the epicardium and endocardium.

Diagnosis

Cattle suffering from babesiasis frequently have a history of recent movement to tick-infested pastures either through grazing management or after purchase, and in Europe may have suffered from tick-borne fever a week or so before babesiasis is evident. Examination of the cattle, especially the preferential feeding sites of the vector ticks will reveal evidence of recent tick bites or engorging ticks. Clinical babesiasis is unlikely to be observed in cattle less than nine months old; such cattle can be infected and show febrile reactions but the resultant parasitaemiae remains low and haemoglobinuria mild. In areas of large tick populations, most cattle are infected at an early age and become immune thereafter, the situation being described as *enzootic stability*. In the early stages of the disease, haemoglobinuria may not be present and diagnosis requires careful examination of stained blood smears. Once haemoglobinuria is present, the parasitaemia may be more obvious. Differential diagnosis requires elimination of other conditions causing haemoglobinuria, e.g. anaplasmosis (p. 737), eperythrozoonosis, leptospirosis (p. 553), postparturient and bacillary haemoglobinuria.

Treatment and control

There are two aspects to treatment: firstly, treatment with a babesicide, and secondly the need for supportive therapy such as blood transfusion and fluid replacement. There are numerous babesicides available. Quinuronium sulphate is effective at a dose of 1 ml/50 kg body weight, but is quite toxic and care is needed if treating anaemic dehydrated cattle. It is now no longer available in the UK. It is normally administered subcutaneously, frequently on the brisket to slow absorption time and remove the possibility of sloughing in more critical areas. It can cause alarming reactions of salivation, panting and collapse and adrenaline (which is the antidote) can be administered simultaneously to reduce the chances of adverse reactions. Aromatic diamidenes such as amicarbalide and diminazene aceturate are also used and are less toxic than quinuronium, but some preparations can suffer from instability of the solution. The most recently introduced treatment is imidocarb, which is given at a dose rate of 1 mg/kg body weight. Now licensed in the UK it is used widely in South America and other countries. It is highly effective and relatively non-toxic, but does have tissue residues for several weeks after its use.

It can also be used at twice the therapeutic dose as a chemoprophylactic, giving protection from infection for up to six weeks. It is used in this way to administer to cattle that will be exposed to ticks, or that have been vaccinated with live *Babesia* with the hope that cattle will become mildly affected but protected from clinical illness and immunity to further infection will be stimulated.

There have been live vaccines for *B. bovis* and *B. bigemina* available in many countries for many years notably Australia and South America. For *B. bovis* the vaccines consist of live organisms made avirulent by repeated rapid syringe-passage through splenectomized calves. In the case of *B. bigemina* rapid passage did not reduce virulence and vaccines available are either developed by 'slow' passage from recrudescences of parasitaemia or are fully virulent organisms, which are used in schemes involving infection and subsequent treatment. There are no vaccines currently available for *B. divergens*, although much research is being carried out to develop inactivated recombinant vaccines for that species and *B. bovis* and *B. bigemina*.

Blood transfusion is frequently required for severely affected adult cattle, and is normally achieved by collection of 5 l of blood from an unaffected healthy cow into a 22 per cent solution of the anticoagulant acid citrate dextrose (ACD), the mixture being immediately transfused into the recipient animal. Such single transfusions without cross-matching of blood are usually successful, but repetition can lead to problems of incompatibility of blood antigens.

Theileriosis

This comprises a group of infections caused by protozoan parasites of the genus *Theileria* (see Table 47.2)

Table 47.2 Species of the genus *Theileria* in cattle

Species	*Synonym*	*Disease*
T. annulata	*T. dispar* *T. turkeistomica*	Mediterranean coast infection
T. lawrencei	*T. bovis*	Corridor disease
T. mutans	*T. orientalis* *T. buffeli*	Benign bovine theileriasis
T. parva		East Coast fever
T. sergenti		Mediterranean coast fever (Russian)

and transmitted by ixodial ticks. They occur in a variety of ruminants and wild animals. Both members of the genus *Babesia* and the genus *Theileria* occur within red blood cells. They are collectively called piroplasms and the infections caused by the two are thus sometimes known as 'piroplasmosis'.

EAST COAST FEVER (ECF)

The disease is a major constraint for production in countries where it occurs.

Aetiology

The cause is a protozoan parasite *Theileria parva*. There is some disagreement about its classification. *Theileria lawrencei*, a parasite of buffalo, causes a high mortality in cattle, but if passaged through cattle it reverts to a parasite indistinguishable from *T. parva* and producing a syndrome similar to ECF. Thus it has been suggested that the cattle parasite should be called *T. parva parva* and that of the buffalo *T. parva lawrencei*.

Epidemiology

The disease occurs across a large area of East and Central Africa and is endemic in Burundi, Kenya,

Malawi, Sudan, Tanzania, Uganda, Zaire and Zambia. It possibly also occurs in Ethiopia and southern Somalia. It is possible to eradicate the disease and this has been done in Mozambique, South Africa, Swaziland and Zimbabwe although it can return if preventive measures are not maintained. It is a disease of cattle but can infect Indian buffalo (*Bubalus bubalis*) and African buffalo (*Syncerus caffer*). Infection is restricted to countries with a temperature and rainfall suitable to allow the survival of *Rhipicephalus appendiculatis*, a three-host tick. The tick is found from sea level to 2135 m (7000 feet) provided there is adequate vegetation and a rainfall in excess of 50 cm (20 inches). In many areas where ECF occurs rainfall is seasonal and disease follows the onset of rain and thus tick activity. In some highland areas or close to water or sea, where the rainfall is more or less constant, tick activity and ECF can occur virtually all the year round. Although *R. appendiculatis* is the main arthropod host, eight species of the genus *Rhipicephalus* and three species of the genus *Hyalomma* can be experimentally infected. In areas where there is a constant challenge then the cattle will be continually exposed to infection from the tick. If challenge is heavy then the calves die. However, those that survive are resistant to further challenge and they can thrive in these areas. In marginal areas where challenge is intermittent or seasonal then cattle previously exposed may lose or have reduced immunity. Thus if a heavy challenge occurs at the start of the rainy season the cattle are again susceptible and go down with disease. Immunity is only to challenge by a similar strain. Cattle previously exposed may be partly or totally susceptible to infection by other strains. Recovered cattle have a sterile immunity, which lasts more than three years. Levels of immunity to piroplasm antigens peak often four to six weeks after infection and persist for six months.

Life cycle

The life cycle of *T. parva* is still not completely understood but most of it is now known or extrapolated. Firstly, at the stage of introduction of infection to the cow there is the period of schizogony. Sporozoites from infected ticks are injected with saliva into the cattle while the tick feeds. There is usually a delay of three to five days after attachment before this occurs. If the tick infects a susceptible animal there is a period of five days before the parasite can be detected in the local drainage lymph node closest to the tick bite. What happens during this period is not known but it is likely that sporozoites rapidly enter target lymphocytes. By doing this the sporozoites escape the phagocytic, lytic and immunological defences of the host. Then there is a transformation of the lymphocyte to lymphoblast with larger, less dense nuclei and increased cytoplasm caused by the parasite, which in turn differentiates into a macroschizont in the cell cytoplasm. As the disease progresses the macroschizont grows to an average size of 4.8 μm. The lymphoblasts rapidly proliferate probably stimulated by the presence of the parasite, which becomes aligned along the spindle and divides by synchrony. As the infected lymphoblast divides both daughter cells are infected. Some macroschizont-infected cells degenerate releasing free macroschizonts, which invade other uninfected lymphoid cells. How this occurs is not known but it may be through membrane fusion of cells in close apposition. From about day 14 after tick attachment macroschizonts differentiate to microschizonts. The mechanism of differentiation is not known. Microschizont-infected cells then rupture and release micromerozoites (1–1.5 μm in diameter). The released micromerozoites enter erythrocytes where they form piroplasms (3–5 μm), which tend to be rod or comma-shaped. The piroplasm-infected erythrocytes are then available to infect ticks feeding on the blood of the cattle host. *Theileria parva* piroplasms rarely divide within erythrocytes, which is different from *T. mutans* and also *Babesia* spp.

Following feeding on the infected bovine the tick, usually *R. appendiculatus*, will inject piroplasm-infected blood that is around the stage of gametogamy. The tick is a three-host tick with all three stages (larva, nymph and adult) feeding on separate hosts. Infection is transitional so an infected larva can transmit infection as a nymph but not as an adult. There appears to be no transovarial transmission as occurs with *Babesia* spp. Once in the tick gut the erythrocytes lyse releasing the piroplasms, many of which are digested but some of the many forms develop into male microgametes or female microgamonts. Fusion of these by processor anisocytosis is then thought to occur to produce zygotes, which invade gut cells and thus differentiate into a motile kinete of about 19 μm. The kinete breaks out from the gut cell and enters the haemolymph. The stage of sporonts is then reached. The kinetes invade the acinar cells (usually type III acinars) of the salivary glands. The kinetes round off and nuclear division occurs to produce a sporont or primary fusion body. The sporont invaginates and forms buds. Further development is delayed until such time as the tick starts to feed in its next instar. When this occurs primary sporoblasts develop from the sporont buds and form cystomeres or secondary fission stage. There is hypertrophy of the host cell and the cell nucleus. There is then division of the primary sporoblasts to produce secondary sporoblasts or tertiary fission stage and sporozoites (1–1.5 μm) are produced. This stage is rapidly completed in three days from the onset of the tick feeding. The sporozoites are released into the salivary duct with peak sporozoite production by day 5. The host cell and nucleus degenerate and the parasite residual bodies remain. The sporozoites persist during the whole period of feeding, which may be up to 10 days for female ticks and intermittently over a long period for male ticks.

Mortality in susceptible adult cattle is 80–100 per cent with an incubation period of 10–15 days.

Signs

Peracute. There is marked pyrexia and death with swollen lymph nodes in a few days.

Acute. Usually the first sign is an enlargement of the lymph nodes for the region draining the area where the infected tick has fed. The preferred feeding sites for *R. appendiculatus* are the ears and so usually the first lymph nodes to swell are the parotids. One to two days after the swelling occurs the animal becomes pyrexic with a temperature rising to 39.5–42 °C (103–108 °F). The temperature tends to remain high until either the animal recovers or dies. Other lymph nodes begin to swell and this tends to become generalized. Some of the superficial lymph nodes such as the parotids, prescapulars and precrurals become very enlarged. Anorexia gradually develops and there is consequent loss of condition. In many cases lacrimation and nasal discharge occur. The breathing becomes rapid and dyspnoeic, and there is diarrhoea or dysentery. As the animal deteriorates and approaches death, the temperature falls and there is severe dyspnoea and recumbency. Nasal exudate pours out of the nostrils. The animal dies of asphyxiation from lung oedema. Death is usually about 18–24 days after infection but occasionally this is reduced to 14 days. The mortality tends to be near 100 per cent in susceptible animals.

Occasionally, nervous signs develop and this is known as 'turning sickness'. Foci of Koch's blue bodies are found in the cerebral tissue. The animal appears to turn often rapidly and become giddy with collapse. The less severe form involves slower turning and frequent head pressing. Both nervous forms are fatal and are considered by some to be due to a massive infection in partially immune cattle.

Chronic. This is usually seen in animals that are partially immune or are exposed for long periods to low levels of infection. It often occurs in calves in endemic areas. The lymph nodes tend to be enlarged and there is intermittent pyrexia, anorexia and loss of condition. These animals frequently recover. In cases of concurrent helminthiasis, malnutrition or other disease and a constant population of *T. parva* some animals become severely retarded and never reach their full production potential.

Pathology

The lesions will depend on the duration of signs. The most consistent finding is one of hypertrophy and hyperplasia of the lymph nodes initially, followed by lymph node oedema and some haemorrhage and necrosis later on. There is a destruction of lymphocytes leading to a destruction of lymphoid cells. Lymph node biopsy shows hypertrophy of lymphoid cells and often after the 11th day they may show macroschizonts that increase in number and size. Damaged lymphocytes are seen with free schizonts. Microschizonts are then present either intact or branching out of cells as micromerozoites. Blood examination reveals a progressive panleucopenia. A noticeable rapidly developing anaemia is only seen in the terminal stages.

The examination reveals froth at the nostrils, and the most striking feature is massive pulmonary oedema, hyperaemia and emphysema. The alveoli, bronchioles, bronchi and trachea are filled with frothy pulmonary exudate. There can also be pleural and pericardial exudate. There are excessive haemorrhages and these may be present on most serous and mucous membranes. In the abomasum the mucous membrane is red and inflamed and there may be ulceration or erosions especially in the pyloric region. In chronic cases there are ulcers in Peyer's patches. The cortex of the kidneys show haemorrhage and are often congested, and nodules of lymphoid tissue projecting from the kidney surface may be seen and are a characteristic feature when they occur. The spleen may or may not show changes and it can be enlarged or shrivelled. The liver is often enlarged with mottled grey areas. Degeneration of the organs is rapid after death.

Diagnosis

The signs are relatively specific and infection can be confirmed by the presence of piroplasms in the blood or schizonts in lymph node biopsy smears stained with giemsa. There is also panleucopenia and then anaemia.

Post-mortem findings are helpful but they are similar to those of malignant catarrhal fever. Differentiation of *T. parva* from other *Theileria* spp. depends on the acuteness of the disease, the number of piroplasms present in the blood and the number present in lymph nodes. Complement fixation, capillary titre agglutination and indirect haemagglutination tests have all been used in diagnosis but are less reliable. The indirect fluorescent antibody test (IFAT) is considered more reliable. An enzyme-linked immunosorbent assay (ELISA) test is also being increasingly used.

Treatment

There is no really effective drug for the treatment of overt clinical infection. Oxytetracycline is effective if given at the same time as infection occurs. It is also able to reduce the severity of clinical disease and appears most effective when given by injection. Chlortetracycline given at any stage of infection at a dose of 10 mg/kg body weight either parenterally or by mouth reduces the severity of parasitaemia and pyrexia.

Animals in good condition prior to infection have lower morbidity. *In vivo* and *in vitro* treatments with the naphthoquinone drug parvaquone and its derivatives have been shown selectively to kill macroschizonts and can be used in disease. A febrifugine such as halofuginone also works in theileriosis and methotrexate work *in vitro*.

Control

In endemic areas indigenous calves have a high degree of resistance to disease. However, calves of European breeds are very susceptible to infection and often die. Those that survive often succumb to further attacks. Adult cattle of any breed brought into the areas are highly susceptible to disease and probable death. The immunity is more cellular than humoral.

Thus where disease is endemic there is legislation to control ticks, to slaughter infected animals, quarantine cattle and restrict cattle movement. While it has been shown in South Africa and Zimbabwe that eradication of ECF is possible, it is expensive and in many countries the legislation is not enacted as rigorously as it might be. However, individual farmers can do much to reduce problems on their own premises by sensible cattle management and tick control. Efficient and well-maintained fencing will reduce the access of nomadic cattle or game to the farm. Areas particularly suited to ticks can also be fenced off. Grass burning, rotational grazing, alternate grazing with other species such as goats or sheep, the alternate grazing with immune cattle, or rotating land between grazing and crop all reduce the problem. Cattle should be quarantined on entry to the farm. Should disease break out its effects can be reduced by slaughtering infected cattle, stopping movement of cattle, other animals, people, hay or feed from infected areas and then creating a buffer area between the infected and clean areas.

It seems that for effective immunization of cattle against ECF it is necessary for the infection to be established in the host. Vaccination is not widely used as it often leads to unpredictable results with disease breaking out due to poor immunity or deaths due to vaccination. However, animals can be vaccinated with stabulate produced by freezing down emulsions from infected blood. After injection of the stibulate long-acting oxytetracycline is given or bupavaquone, otherwise shortacting oxytetracycline or paravaquone can be used. Cattle so treated become resistant to disease and they show little or no apparent reaction. In some cases more than one strain of *T. parva* is introduced, possibly together with a strain of *T. lawrencei*. A sporazoite vaccine is now being tried.

MEDITERRANEAN COAST FEVER

This is in many ways similar to East Coast fever but is caused by a different *Theileria* species.

Aetiology

The cause is a protozoan parasite, *Theileria annulata*. Morphologically, the parasite is similar to *T. parva* and the macroschizonts and later microschizonts are found in the lymphoid tissue. *Theileria annulata* piroplasms in the erythrocytes tend to be oval or round in shape. In Russia, there is a similar disease due to *T. sergenti*, which is different from *T. annulata* both morphologically and immunologically.

Epidemiology

The condition is found around the Mediterranean including south-eastern Europe, Russia, the Middle and Far East, India, Sri Lanka, Egypt and Sudan. Both cattle and water buffalo (*Bubalus bubalis*) are susceptible to the infection. The condition involves a development cycle in ticks of the genus *Hyalomma* and seven species are known to be vectors. The ticks involved are one-host, two-host or three-host ticks. It is believed that in most tick species there is no transovarian transmission. Thus infection is acquired in the nymph or larval stages and is transmitted in the adult. When the tick is attached to the host it must feed a considerable amount before infective stages of *T. annulata* are produced and enter the cattle. Piroplasms appear in the erythrocytes shortly after the first detection of schizonts. The intraerythrocytic form remains in the blood for many years and in natural infections they tend to have a ring or oval shape.

The disease is seasonal, depending on the activity of the ticks, which hide during the winter in crevices between rocks, walls, etc. The result is the infective adult stage being produced in late spring or early summer. Thus infection tends mainly to be seen in the summer and early autumn. Infection can also be transmitted by injecting blood or tissue from ill or recovered animals. Intra-uterine transmission has been recorded on occasion. Infection of calves in endemic areas usually produces a mild disease although up to one-quarter of calves can die.

In the Russian form involving *T. sergenti*, infection is said to be transmitted by only one species of the genus *Haemaphysalis*.

Signs

Peracute. This occurs in completely susceptible animals entering endemic areas. The animals develop marked pyrexia with anorexia, depression and weakness and they die in three or four days.

Acute. This is most commonly seen in susceptible animals moved into endemic areas and in marginal areas of tick activity. The animals develop pyrexia, which may persist for several days. It is accompanied by inappetence, lethargy, swelling of the superficial lymph nodes, oculo-nasal discharge and ruminal stasis. This is followed in a few days by anaemia with pale mucous membranes, exercise intolerance and a rapid heart rate. Later on jaundice may become apparent. Constipation is common when pyrexia first occurs but later there is diarrhoea and bloodstained faeces. The animals lose condition rapidly and about 90 per cent die over a period of eight to eighteen days after signs occur.

Subacute. There is intermittent fever for two to four weeks with moderate progressive anaemia and jaundice. Many of these animals die but some recover over a long period. Some of these cases change into a more acute phase and die.

Chronic. This is often an even more prolonged form of the subacute disease. Recovery can occur but is very protracted. However, some cases suddenly develop the more acute form and die.

Necropsy

There is a pale, anaemic carcass with the mucous and serosal membranes showing numerous petechial haemorrhages. The lymph nodes are enlarged, cystic and oedematous. The liver tends to be pale brown or yellow, enlarged and friable with an enlarged friable spleen. The kidneys tend to be pale and on occasions show pseudoinfarcts. The abomasum is red, inflamed and may show haemorrhagic ulceration. There are epicardial and endocardial haemorrhages and these may be petechial or ecchymotic. The lungs contain oedema, often red-tinged and congestion.

A lymph node smear may show schizonts present in lymphocytes but they are more common in the liver and spleen.

Diagnosis

The area, type of animals affected and signs help in diagnosis. Lymph node smears show schizonts. In some cases a liver biopsy is needed to differentiate. Serological tests used for *T. annulata* include the complement fixation test (CFT), indirect fluorescent antibody test (IFAT) and enzyme linked immunosorbent assay (ELISA).

Treatment

Many cases of *T. annulata* infection show spontaneous recovery. There have been few controlled trials of treatment. Both oxytetracycline (injection) and chlortetracycline (orally) have been claimed to give relief. However, buparvaquone is at present the best therapy.

Control

Following natural infection there exists a premunity that lasts for many years. There is no cross-immunity to other *Theileria* spp. Immunization is practised in several countries by taking blood from recently recovered cattle passaged through susceptible cattle. This is continued until no piroplasmic forms of the parasite occur. Then citrated blood is injected into susceptible stock, usually calves. Most animals show only limited reaction to such vaccination although a few die. As there are no piroplasms in the blood ticks are not infected. Immunity can then be enhanced by injecting a virulent strain. It has been possible to culture schizonts on various tissue culture cell lines and these have then been used to vaccinate susceptible cattle. They do not produce piroplasms and so the animal cannot infect ticks.

Prevention otherwise involves control of the tick and cattle movements. Cattle can be sprayed or dipped with acaricide. Some walls and buildings can be sprayed to kill off the overwintering stages. Carrier animals still contain infection in their blood and if moved to new farms or countries will take the disease with them to infect local ticks. Thus detection of carriers is of use and can be done by taking blood from the animal and injecting into susceptible cattle.

CORRIDOR DISEASE

This condition is very similar to ECF but it has a different cause.

Aetiology

It is caused by *Theileria lawrencei*, which is primarily a protozoan parasite of buffaloes. However, it is transmissible to cattle and produces a similar type of disease to ECF. The schizonts tend to be smaller and fewer in number and the piroplasms relatively rare in the blood. If *T. lawrencei* is passaged through cattle it quickly reverts to a parasite indistinguishable from ECF. It has therefore been suggested that *T. parva* is a cattle-adapted strain of *T. lawrencei*. It has also been proposed that the nomenclature for the two parasites should be *T. parva parva* and *T. parva lawrencei*.

Epidemiology

The disease has mainly been described in South Africa, Zimbabwe and Kenya. It is transmitted by the three-host tick, *R. appendiculatus* and it is possible that distribution of *T. lawrencei* is over the whole area occupied by the tick. The buffalo (*Syncerus caffer*) is considered to be the natural host and cattle brought in to the area tend to be susceptible. Those brought up in the region that survive the first few months are immune but those in marginal areas or where tick levels have only been partially introduced are not. *Theileria lawrencei* is transmissible from carrier buffaloes via ticks to cattle. It can be passed from cattle to cattle via the ticks. The recovered cattle can then act as carriers of infection. Morbidity in susceptible cattle is variable at about 60–80 per cent.

Signs

The signs are similar to those seen with *T. parva*.

Peracute. The animal develops pyrexia, lymph node enlargement and dies in a few days.

Acute. This is the most common form in susceptible cattle. There is pyrexia and swelling of the lymph node closest to the site of the infected tick bite. Other lymph nodes then start to swell and there is general dullness. There is lacrimation, nasal discharge and oedema occurs, particularly of the eyelids, face and throat. The animal becomes weak and develops diarrhoea containing blood and mucus. The respirations become laboured and dyspnoeic.

Mild. In this form there is a mild rise in temperature, swelling of the lymph nodes and some pyrexia.

Pathology

The lymph nodes are swollen and show hypertrophy and hyperplasia followed by oedema and haemorrhage. There are extensive haemorrhages on most of the serosal and mucosal surfaces. The abomasum tends to be red, inflamed and with ulcers especially of the pyloric region. The spleen may be enlarged. The kidney cortex is congested and may show nodules of lymph and tissue raised above the surface. The liver is enlarged and a mottled grey colour. The lungs are grey and contain blood and fluid with froth in the alveoli, bronchi, bronchioles and trachea. Lymph node biopsy smears show hypertrophy and hyperplasia of the node. A few lymphocytes contain schizonts and there are one or two piroplasms in the erythrocytes.

Diagnosis

The condition is similar to ECF, anaplasmosis and babesiasis and the peracute form is similar to heart-water. The signs, and area, help in diagnosis particularly of those cattle associated with buffalo. However, where *T. parva* infection is common then disease caused by *T. lawrencei* may be missed. A lymph node biopsy helps as schizonts in the lymphocytes tend to be few and small in size. Blood samples show only a few erythrocytes to contain piroplasms. There is also no marked anaemia as in anaplasmosis or babesiasis.

Treatment

Use of oxytetracycline by injection reduces the intensity and duration of signs. Similarly, chlortetracycline has an effect and can be given by mouth. The naphthoquinones, parvaquone and buparvaquone are now successfully used.

Control

Infection can be controlled by tick dipping, controlling movement of susceptible cattle, grazing tick areas with less susceptible species such as sheep or goats and ensuring no contact occurs between cattle and buffalo or other game animals. Cattle that are exposed to infection and recover are immune. However, there is not complete cross-immunity with *T. parva* infection, although it does seem that cattle previously infected with *T. parva* have a good immunity to *T. lawrencei*. When cattle are initially infected with *T. lawrencei* there is only limited resistance to *T. parva*. Stabilates of ticks infected with strains of *T. parva* have been injected into cattle followed by treatment with oxytetracycline or parvaquone, which has given some immunity to *T. lawrencei*. Some stabilates have included a *T. lawrencei* strain.

BENIGN BOVINE THIELERIOSIS

This disease tends to be less severe than ECF, Mediterranean coast fever or Corridor disease.

Aetiology

The cause is a protozoa, *Theileria mutans*, which is very similar to *T. parva*.

Epidemiology

The condition affects cattle as well as the Indian water buffalo (*Bubalus bubalis*) and the African buffalo (*Syncerus caffer*). It occurs in most parts of the world except countries north of latitude 55 °N and South America. It is thought that transmission is by a wide variety of different ticks but it has been proved to be so with *R. appendiculatus*, *R. eventsi* and *Ambylomma variegatum*. Injection of parasitized blood can produce infection. The disease is maintained by a premune state of recovered cattle, which allows continued infection of ticks. Infection often occurs with other diseases such as anaplasmosis, salmonellosis, heartwater or babesiosis.

Signs

Acute. This rarely occurs but it has been reported in Australia, India, Japan, Kenya, Korea and South Africa (where it is known as Tzaneen disease). In this case the disease involves fever with swelling of the lymph node closest to the infected tick and then more generalized lymph node swelling. There is a progressive anaemia and some of the cattle die. In Africa there is a cerebral form of the disease known as turning sickness where the animal will tend to walk in circles or head press.

Subacute. There are very few clinical signs other than a mild pyrexia with a swelling of the lymph nodes and a mild anaemia.

Pathology

In acute cases there is hyperplasia and oedema of the lymph nodes. There may be haemorrhages of the serosal and mucosal surfaces. The abomasum may be reddened and ulcerated. The kidney cortex is congested with swollen lymphoid areas. The liver is enlarged and tends to be grey in colour. The lungs contain fluid in the bronchioles, bronchi and trachea. The spleen is swollen.

Usually in the subacute form there is mild hyperplasia of lymph nodes, which contain a few schizonts. Anaemia occurs but is slight. There are only a few piroplasms in the blood and schizonts in lymph node sinuses.

Diagnosis

Diagnosis is helped by the mild nature of the signs but is not helped by the presence of only very few piroplasms in the blood or schizonts in lymph node biopsies. In addition the schizont is morphologically similar to *T. annulata* and *T. parva*. The best method of differentiation is by serology and the most effective test at present is IFAT.

Treatment

Quinoline drugs such as pamaquin are of use in the erythrocytic stage.

Control

As the disease is mild, deliberate control or eradication is not usually undertaken. However, control of ticks will result in control of disease. Cattle maintain immunity by a form of premunity with piroplasms remaining in small numbers within the blood.

Besnoitiosis

This disease was previously known as globidiosis.

Aetiology

It is due to a protozoan called *Besnoitia besnoiti*.

Epidemiology

It is mainly seen in cattle and horses as intermediate hosts in south-west Europe and in Africa. Transmission has not been elucidated but is probably via the faeces of infected cats which are the final host. Morbidity can be up to 10 per cent and recovery is often protracted.

Signs

In many animals there are no signs. In the cow there may be lesions on the teats. There is pyrexia and warm swellings develop on the ventral parts of the body resulting in reduced movement. The lymph nodes are palpably swollen and there is diarrhoea. Pulse and respiratory rates are elevated. Pregnant cattle may abort. There may be excessive lacrimation and increased nasal discharge, which is at first serous and then purulent. There are small, white, raised nodules on the conjunctiva and nasal mucosa. There then follows severe dermatitis over most of the body associated with infected cutaneous cysts.

Diagnosis

This is based on clinical signs, especially the cysts on the scleral conjunctiva, and on the geographical area, and can be confirmed by the detection of cysts containing spindle-shaped spores in scrapings of skin lesions or the conjunctiva.

Treatment

Nothing specific is available.

Control

A vaccine produced by *B. besnoiti* grown on tissue culture is effective.

Trypanosomiasis

Trypanosomes are blood-borne protozoa with flagellae. Infections are widespread in wild and domestic animals and cattle are susceptible to infection with several species, the most important of which are those cyclically transmitted by tsetse flies (*Glossina* spp.) throughout much of sub-Saharan Africa, namely *Trypanosoma congolense*, *T. vivax* and *T. brucei*. *Trypanosoma vivax* infections also occur in cattle in the absence of the tsetse fly in Central and South America and have been recorded in Mauritius. In tropical and subtropical areas other than sub-Saharan Africa, cattle are commonly infected asymptomatically with *T. evansi*.

Tsetse fly-transmitted trypanosomiases are commonly grouped together under the name 'nagana'. Their distribution lies within the tsetse fly belts of Africa, which extend from 14° N to 20° S in south-west Africa and 29° S in Mozambique, covering an area of 10 million km^2. Many species of wild animals are symptomless carriers of nagana trypanosomes and provide a sylvatic reservoir of infection in which the trypanosomes are cyclically transmitted naturally from host to host by tsetse flies. The principal carriers of these trypanosomes are wild bovids and suids, e.g. kudu, giraffe, buffalo, warthog and bushpig. Cattle, other domestic animals and man are infected when they come in contact with these wild animal carriers and are bitten by infected tsetse flies as a result.

Tsetse flies can be classified as falling into three groups, namely forest, riverine and savannah. The forest tsetse flies are found in the tropical rainforests of Central and West Africa and in scattered areas of East Afirca. Although they are efficient vectors of trypanosomes, they are of least importance as cattle rarely come in contact with them due to the lack of suitable grazing in the forest regions. Riverine tsetse flies, as their name implies, infest riverine vegetation but virtually only in river systems draining into the Atlantic Ocean. Their distribution is thus confined to Central and West Africa largely overlapping with that of forest flies. Although they are less efficient vectors of trypanosomiases than forest or savannah flies, because they infest vegetation near essential water supplies, riverine flies are important vectors of trypanosomiasis of humans (Gambian sleeping sickness) and of domestic livestock including cattle.

Savannah tsetse flies are the most important group of flies because they infest large tracts of land potentially suitable for grazing and browsing by domestic livestock. They are also efficient vectors of trypanosomes and so when cattle and other livestock encroach into tsetse-infested savannah, they are at risk of being bitten by the fly and contracting infection.

Tsetse flies become infected when they take a blood meal from an infected animal. The trypanosomes then undergo cyclical development within the alimentary system eventually developing to the infective or metacyclic forms within the fly mouthparts. These infective forms are then transmitted to another susceptible animal host via the saliva during the next fly feed(s). The development in the tsetse fly is an essential part of the life cycle and hence nagana is unique to Africa. The one exception of the nagana trypanosomes is *T. vivax* as mentioned earlier. In Central and South America it is assumed that *T. vivax* is mechanically transmitted by biting flies. This raises the possibility that it may also be transmitted mechanically in Africa, and indeed there is increasing evidence that this is the case.

Infection with *T. evansi* is also transmitted mechanically by biting flies. Infection of domestic livestock is widespread world-wide throughout the tropics and subtropics but is absent from tsetse-infested areas of Africa. It is an important pathogen of camels, horses, dogs and buffaloes but cattle, although commonly infected, rarely suffer clinical disease. However, they may be important reservoirs of infection for other more susceptible livestock.

Aetiology

Tsetse-transmitted bovine trypanosomiases are caused by *T. vivax*, *T. congolense* and *T. brucei*. All are motile, extracellular, spindle-shaped, flagellated protozoan parasites ranging from about 10 to 30 μm in length. *Trypanosoma vivax* and *T. congolense* are essentially parasites of plasma although *T. vivax* may leave the circulation in small numbers and invade extravascular tissues particularly of the heart (Losos, 1986). *Trypanosoma congolense* has a predilection for the microvasculature where it attaches to the endothelium of small blood vessels, particularly the heart and brain (Banks, 1978). *Trypanosoma brucei* as well as being a plasma parasite has a predilection for interstitial spaces and tissue fluids.

Trypanosoma evansi is related to *T. brucei* to which it is morphologically similar and has a similar infection pattern in the animal host.

Pathology

The pathogenesis of bovine trypanosomiasis is complex and not fully understood but is characterized by a chronic and progressive anaemia. Uncomplicated tsetse-transmitted infection can be considered as following a course comprised of three phases (Murray, 1978).

Phase I (fluctuating parasitaemia and fever). Following an infected tsetse fly bite, trypanosomes multiply locally causing an inflammatory reaction (chancre) within a few days at the site of the bite. Chancres are a regular feature of experimental infections, but have not been reported in natural infections. About this time, trypanosomes invade the circulation via the lymphatic system causing reaction and enlargement of locally draining lymph nodes. Trypanosomes then appear in the bloodstream, the prepatent period following initial infective tsetse bite varying with species thus:

T. congolense	12–16 days
T. vivax	8–10 days
T. brucei	5–20 days

A fluctuating but diminishing parasitaemia then develops, and parasitaemic peaks at approximately 12-day intervals are associated with febrile responses. Anaemia becomes evident early in infection and is believed to be haemolytic in the first instance but haemolysis wanes and is superseded by anaemia caused by erythrophagocytosis due to stimulation and expansion of the mononuclear phagocytic system resulting in splenomegaly.

This initial phase of fluctuating parasitaemia and fever may last from a few weeks to a few months during which cattle lose condition and, depending on the severity of infection, some may die. Cattle that survive this phase enter the second phase.

Phase II (low-grade parasitaemia and progressive anaemia). Over the next few months, infected cattle have a low fluctuating parasitaemia during which the parasites may be difficult to detect. Despite the apparent reduction in parasites, the erythrophagocytosis and anaemia continue although the spleen may return to normal size, and cattle continue to lose condition.

Phase III (apparent aparasitaemia but continuing anaemia). Cattle that survive the second phase suffer chronic disease during which the parasites apparently disappear although anaemia due to erythrophagocytosis continues. Affected animals are cachectic and normally die within six to twelve months of initial infection.

Infection at any stage may lead to congestive heart failure and death due to a combination of anaemia, circulatory failure and myocardial damage. At autopsy, post-mortem findings are not pathognomonic. They include emaciation, visceral pallor and enlargement of the heart. Cattle that die early in disease may have enlarged haemorrhagic lymph nodes and splenomegaly (Stephen, 1986).

Despite the large volume of literature on bovine trypanosomiasis, good accounts of the pathology of natural disease are scarce and the above account represents a brief synopsis of the generally accepted picture. Cattle at risk may be infected by several species and strains of trypanosomes and the pathology and clinical signs will be influenced by various factors, e.g. the age, breed and nutritional status of infected cattle, the degree of tsetse challenge and the strains and species of infective trypanosomes. Thus strains of *T. vivax* in West Africa tend to cause a more acute disease in cattle than those of East Africa, whereas strains of *T. congolense* in East Africa tend to cause a more chronic form of the disease. *Trypanosoma brucei* is the least pathogenic to cattle and normally regarded as of minor importance.

Although infection with more than one species is commonly reported in the field, virtually no studies have been done on mixed infections. Cattle infected experimentally with *T. congolense* and *T. brucei*, either simultaneously or one year apart, developed cerebral trypanosomiasis with encephalitis and associated clinical signs and both species of parasites were isolated from the cerebrospinal fluid (Masake *et al.*, 1984). The authors suggested that the higher incidence of cerebral trypanosomiasis in mixed infections than in single infections suggests an interdependence between *T. congolense* and *T. brucei* in the pathogenesis of cerebral trypanosomiasis, possibly resulting from *T. congolense*'s predilection for the brain microvasculature facilitating the entry of parasites into brain parenchymal extravascular spaces. The possibility of such interaction between different species in natural infections merits further research.

Signs

The clinical picture of cattle suffering from nagana is influenced by several factors, namely breed and health status of cattle infected, pathogenicity of infecting trypanosomes, duration of exposure to infection and level of tsetse fly challenge, which in itself is dictated by several factors. *Trypanosoma vivax* infections in cattle in West Africa are widespread and commonly produce an acute, rapidly fatal disease in which affected cattle die during the initial phase of fluctuating parasitaemia and fever. Stephen (1986) describes acute *T. vivax* infection as resembling septicaemia in which affected animals have body temperatures of 40–41 °C (104–106 °F), depression, dyspnoea, elevated pulse and respiratory rates and a jugular pulse. Less severe cases show signs of anaemia, loss of condition (see Fig. 47.2) and enlargement of superficial lymph nodes. Abortions and still-births may occur in pregnant cows.

The situation in East Africa and parts of Central Africa is different in that *T. congolense* tends to be a more serious pathogen than *T. vivax*, although this is by no means absolute as strains of *T. vivax* are known to cause an acute haemorrhagic disease in cattle in the Coast Province of Kenya (Mwongela *et al.*, 1981). *Trypanosoma congolense* in East and Central Africa tends to produce a chronic disease, although the clinical signs are essentially the same as those of *T. vivax* infection and eventual death is the usual outcome in untreated animals. In the early stages of infection appetite may be normal between periods of fever, but as the disease progresses the anaemia becomes more severe, cattle become depressed and lose bodily condition, and in the terminal stages affected cattle are too weak to rise or eat (Stephen, 1986). Superficial lymph node enlargement is not so pronounced as in *T. vivax* infections.

Trypanosoma brucei infections of cattle though common are generally regarded as of minor significance and are usually mixed with the more pathogenic *T. congolense* or *T. vivax*. Parasitaemias from *T. brucei* infections are lower than those of *T. congolense* or *T. vivax* and hence infection can be more difficult to detect, raising the possibility that disease caused by *T. brucei* infection may not always be diagnosed. A few reports of meningo-encephalitis have been recorded, and experimental infection produces a severe diffuse meningo-encephalitis resulting in depression, unsteady gait, head pressing and circling (Morrison *et al.*, 1983). There is a greater incidence of cerebral trypanosomiasis in mixed *T. congolense* and *T. brucei* infections as mentioned earlier, and the involvement of the central nervous system (CNS) in natural bovine trypanosomiasis requires investigation.

Trypanosoma vivax infections of cattle are widespread in Central and South America and the West Indies and were probably introduced with imported cattle from Africa. The importance of *T. vivax* in the New World is not clear but epidemics of serious disease have been recorded in Venezuela and Colombia (Clarkson, 1976). In general, the clinical signs appear to be the same as chronic forms of *T. vivax* infection in Africa and the swaying gait of infected emaciated cattle may be confused with the clinical signs of rabies.

Trypanosoma evansi infections of cattle, though common throughout the tropics and subtropics, rarely cause clinical disease.

Diagnosis

In tsetse-infested areas of Africa, nagana is well recognized and diagnosis is often based on a history of a chronic wasting condition of cattle in contact with the tsetse fly. Differential diagnoses are babesiosis (p. 726), anaplasmosis (p. 735), helminthiasis (Chapter 17) and any condition that causes anaemia and emaciation, notably malnutrition. Nagana can be confirmed parasitologically by demonstrating parasites in the blood of infected animals and various techniques are available (see Fig. 47.3). These techniques were reviewed by Paris *et al.* (1982) as follows.

1 Microscopic examination of stained thin blood smears. Different species of trypanosomes can be identified by this method.

2 Microscopic examination of wet blood films; this must be done at the time of sampling and cannot be used to identify different species of trypanosomes.

These techniques are not particularly sensitive and may not detect animals with low parasitaemias, such as those suffering chronic disease. More sensitive techniques are the following:

3 Microscopic examination of the buffy coat–plasma interface of haematocrit-centrifuged blood, either directly through the capillary tube glass or by breaking the capillary tube just below the buffy coat, expressing the contents of the upper part onto a slide for examination by dark-ground or phase-contrast microscopy.

4 Microscopic examination of stained de-haemoglobinized thick blood smears.

5 Subinoculation of bovine blood into laboratory rodents. This is the most sensitive technique for *T. brucei*, and is usually good for *T. congolense*, but most strains of *T. vivax* do not infect laboratory rodents.

In practice, many field programmes of monitoring cattle for infection are based on routine screening of stained thick and thin blood films; thick films are examined to detect infected animals and thin films to determine the species of the infecting trypanosomes.

Trypanosoma vivax infections in the New World may have to be differentiated from conditions causing wasting and anaemia such as anaplasmosis, babesiasis and helminthiasis and in addition, as mentioned earlier, rabies (p. 706). In general the same techniques as described can be used to confirm diagnosis.

Serological tests are not in general use for diagnosis although several are under study. Trypanosomes display the phenomenon of antigenic variation during infection in the mammalian host in which successive parasitaemic populations of trypanosomes have a different antigenic composition. Thus the host mounts successive immune responses to sequences of different antigenic populations and a test developed to detect serum antibodies to one antigenic population may not detect serum antibodies against different antigenic populations of the same strain of trypanosome. These variable antigens are confined to the surface glycoprotein coat of the parasites and although tests have been developed based on these variable antigens, they are largely confined to research in antigenic variation and have little routine diagnostic use.

Tests based on internal common somatic antigens may have potential diagnostic use as problems of cross-reactions between species become solved by monoclonal technology (Nantulya *et al.*, 1987). Of various tests developed, the IFAT and ELISA appear to have the greatest potential and the ELISA can be used to detect circulating trypanosomal antigens as well as antibodies (Rae & Luckins, 1984).

Treatment and control

Because of the phenomenon of antigenic variation, no vaccine has been developed against trypanosomiasis and is unlikely to be in the foreseeable future. In Africa this leaves tsetse control as the main method of prevention. Tsetse control programmes are widespread throughout Africa but will only be considered in summary here. Tsetse control is usually under the direction of the veterinary department and requires specialized expertise. The methods in use are as follows:

1 Application of insecticide to tsetse habitat, either on the ground by hand, or from the air by helicopters or fixed wing aircraft. This is the main method.

2 Use of fly traps. These are used extensively in francophone West Africa and Zimbabwe.

3 Removal of tsetse habitat. Tsetse flies have to rest in certain bushes and trees, which can be cleared by felling and bulldozing rendering the area unsuitable for the fly. This is expensive, however, and is now largely confined to maintaining tsetse-free barriers around areas freed of tsetse.

4 Settlement of land freed of tsetse. Housing, cropping, etc. may alter the vegetation to a form unsuitable for tsetse flies so preventing re-infestation.

5 Destruction of wild animal hosts. This is now unacceptable except in establishing animal-free corridors, possibly in conjunction with method 3.

6 Release of sterile male tsetse flies to interfere with breeding of wild tsetse populations. Because of the very low reproductive rate of tsetse flies, only small numbers of flies can be reared in colonies. Therefore this method has limited application, usually in conjunction with other methods.

Thus, the commonest form of prevention is avoidance of the fly by cattle herders who build up local knowledge on when and where pastures are safe to graze. Savannah tsetse flies retreat and disperse during the dry and rainy seasons respectively, so that certain pastures may be tsetse infested for part of the year only. In addition, grazing tends to be safest at midday when flies are least active and most dangerous around sunset when flies are most active (Pilson & Leggate, 1961).

In the absence of a vaccine, cattle can be protected prophylactically although effective prophylactics are now limited to one drug, isometamidium chloride. Isometamidium has certain disadvantages. It causes severe reactions at the site of injection, and there is considerable risk of resistance developing to the drug if cattle are exposed to infection after the active ingredient in blood has fallen to below a trypanocidal level, usually three months after injection. Thus where the risk of infection is constant, injection of the drug must be repeated at regular intervals to maintain effective levels. Despite this, under good management cattle can be efficiently reared in tsetse areas under isometamidium protection, as has been demonstrated on the Mkwaja Ranch in Tanzania over the last 30 years (Trail *et al.*, 1985).

Treatment against trypanosomiasis, in order to be effective, should be given early in the disease during the initial phase of fluctuating parasitaemia. As no new drugs have been developed against trypanosomiasis for nearly 30 years and some have been withdrawn because of resistance, treatment is now essentially limited to two compounds, diminazene aceturate and homidium (either chloride or bromide). Resistance has been recorded against both drugs and undoubtedly will be an increasing problem. As there is little likelihood of pharmaceutical companies developing new trypanocides because of the cost and uncertainty of the market, in many of the countries concerned the management of the existing drugs will require great care in the future.

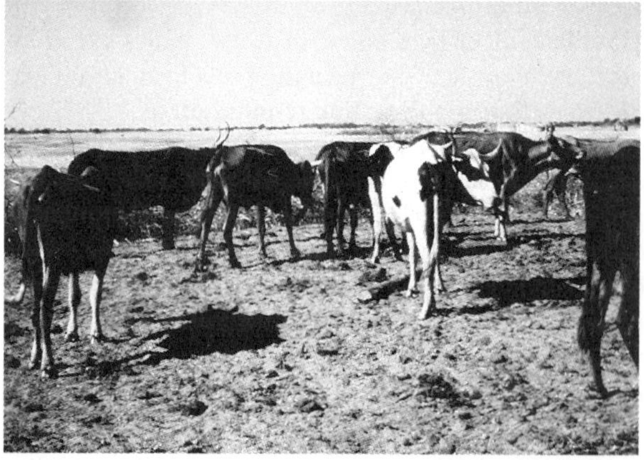

Fig. 47.2 Emaciated cattle suffering from trypanosomiasis in northern Botswana (courtesy of A.G. Hunter).

Trypanosomiasis is normally seen as a herd problem and mass chemotherapy is widely used on a herd or area basis, ideally in conjunction with some form of routine monitoring of blood smears of a percentage of cattle to indicate level of infection. Whiteside (1962) pointed out that when drugs are used regularly to treat cattle for trypanosomiasis, resistance may develop and when this occurs the drug in use must be changed to one against which there is no resistance and that should cure infections resistant to the first, i.e. a 'sanative'.

Resistance was rarely reported against diminazene, which consequently was recognized as the best sanative. The concept of 'sanative pairs' was introduced in which drug usage regimens were devised to alternate diminazene with another trypanocide to minimize the development of resistance. Thus the alternative to diminazene was used for treatment of clinical cases for as long as possible and then changed to diminazene for one year to ensure treatment of any resistant infections in circulation. Thus depending on the level of tsetse challenge the regimen shown in Table 47.3 for treatment using drugs in current use was advocated.

Table 47.3 Regimen for treatment of trypanosomiasis to minimize development of resistance

Tsetse challenge	Drug alternatives	
	Homidium	Diminazene
Very high	6 months	1 year
High	1 year	1 year
Medium	2 years	1 year
Low	As long as possible	1 year

In practice, it is virtually impossible to rear cattle in areas of very high challenge.

Because treatment is now limited to diminazene and homidium and their use must be managed very carefully, Whiteside's recommendations are possibly more valid today than when advocated nearly 30 years ago.

Diminazene aceturate is the drug of choice for treatment of *T. vivax* infections in the New World.

Use of trypanotolerant breeds of cattle

It has long been recognized that dwarf humpless breeds of cattle in West Africa have a low susceptibility to trypanosomiasis and can survive in tsetse-infested areas where zebu types or European breeds cannot. Until relatively recently these breeds were regarded as having poor productivity and of minor significance, but new research indicates this may not be the case; their potential is now under extensive investigation and the situation concerning these so-called 'trypanotolerant' breeds was recently reviewed (Hoste, 1987). Trypanotolerance has also been identified in Orma Boran cattle of East Africa (Njogu *et al.*, 1985) and the future prospects of greater utilization of breeds of cattle with natural resistance to trypanosomiasis are very real.

Rickettsial diseases

Anaplasmosis

This is an infectious and transmissible disease of cattle that is seen in most continents of the world. It is non-contagious and is transmitted by ticks.

Aetiology

The cause of the disease is an intraerythrocytic parasite, usually *Anaplasma marginale*. The red blood cells contain round inclusion bodies called anaplasma and they are peripheral in location, hence the name 'marginale'. There are three *Anaplasma* species and of the other two, *Anaplasma centrale* causes a mild condition in African cattle as does *Anaplasma caudatim*.

Anaplasma marginale when mature is 0.3–1.0 µm in diameter and more than one can be present in the same erythrocyte. The parasite transfers from cell to cell in the form of an inclusion body. This is normally oval in shape and measures 31 µm in diameter and can penetrate the red cell envelope.

A member of the genus *Paranaplasma*, *P. caudatum*, has been found in a mixed infection with *A. marginale* in cattle in the USA state of Oregon. The inclusion bodies of *A. caudatum* can be shown with special staining techniques to have unusual appendages such as rings, loops or beads in the erythrocytes. However, these are not found when deer erythrocytes are infected.

Epidemiology

The disease is particularly seen in tropical and subtropical parts of the world and it exists in some temperate areas. Africa, North, South and Central America, the Far and Middle East, India, Russia and southern Europe all have the disease present. While mainly a bovine disease, buffalo, bison, antelope, deer, gnu and wildebeeste can all be infected. All ages of cattle are susceptible but calves under six months old show few if any signs. The severity of signs depends on the age and previous exposure to infection. Generally, the older the animal at first exposure, the more severe the signs. Ticks are the natural hosts of the disease and at least 20 species have been shown to transmit infection. Little is known about the developmental life cycle in the tick although most infection is transmitted transovarially. The main genera of ticks concerned are *Argas*, *Boophilus*, *Dermacentor*, *Haemaphysalis*, *Hyalomma*, *Ixodes* and *Rhipicephalus*. Horseflies (*Tabanus* spp.) are experimentally and epizootologically the most important insect vector. They directly transmit the disease from an infected to a susceptible animal. Other arthropods that can be involved include stable flies (*Stomoxys*), deer flies (*Chrysops*), housefly (*Musca*) and mosquitoes (*Psorophora*). Cattle can be carriers of the disease as well as deer. The incubation period is usually two to six weeks but it may be up to 12 weeks.

Signs

Peracute. This usually involves cattle over three years old experiencing infection for the first time. It is most commonly seen in high-producing purebred dairy cattle and is frequently fatal. There is a pyrexia with rapid loss of milk production. Anaemia occurs with very pale mucous membranes. The breathing is rapid with excessive salivation. Some cattle show nervous signs and abnormal behaviour.

Acute. This is seen in cattle up to three years old and is occasionally found in cattle between one and two. Signs often develop unexpectedly. The animal develops a progressive pyrexia over a few days, reaching 41 °C (106 °F). There is a loss of milk yield with a progressive anaemia and weakness. In addition there is depression, inappetence, dehydration and laboured breathing. The lymph nodes tend to be enlarged. Some cattle will exhibit jaundice, there is frequent micturition of normal-coloured urine and some cows abort. Bulls may show a temporary loss of fertility. Recovery takes a period of weeks. If death occurs it is within one to four days of the onset of signs.

Chronic. The signs may follow an acute infection with gradual emaciation.

Mild. This form is mainly present in cattle infected under one year old. Signs are usually few with a mild pyrexia.

Necropsy

The main signs at post mortem are of an acute anaemia and often there is jaundice. The spleen is enlarged and the gall-bladder obstructed. The heart is usually pale and flabby and petechial haemorrhages may be present on the epicardium and pericardium. The lymph nodes are enlarged and oedematous. The blood shows a marked reduction in erythrocytes and haemoglobin. The morphology alters to include anisocytosis, poikilocytosis and often leucocytosis is present.

Diagnosis

In typical cases the signs presented plus the presence of anaplasma inclusion bodies in stained peripheral blood smears is sufficient for diagnosis. Giemsa stain is usually used but toluene blue and acridine can also be helpful. The diagnosis of carrier or chronic cases is more difficult and depends normally on complement fixation, capillary tube agglutination and agglutination tests.

Treatment

The tetracyclines, i.e. tetracycline, chlortetracycline, oxytetracycline, are the only approved drugs that are effective in treatment. Administration can be oral or parenteral. Their use in the acute phase slows down the parasitic life cycle and so reduces the crisis. Latent infections can be eliminated by tetracyclines. They act more effectively and more quickly when given by injection rather than orally. Experimentally, other compounds of the dithiosemicarbazones have been shown to be effective. It is also important to provide good management for the animals and in valuable animals blood transfusions may be necessary.

Control

The main methods of control involve reduction in the vectors of disease, which can be done by ectoparasite dipping but this does not entirely control the problem. Susceptible cattle can be separated from other carrier cattle and wild animals or carrier cattle can be detected and eliminated, although the tests used are not completely reliable. Otherwise immunization can be undertaken.

It was thought that cattle in indigenous areas do not normally show signs due to an infection immunity or premunity. However, when there is intercurrent infection or the animal is stressed in other ways then signs are evident, although it does seem that in premune animals there is also a cell-mediated immune response. Both cell-mediated and humoral responses are required to provide protective immunity to anaplasmosis. In addition, continuous antigenic response is dependent on a perpetual low-level exposure to infection. Immunity using a live laboratory attenuated *A. marginale* ovine-origin vaccine gives good protection. Inactivated *A. marginale* vaccines of bovine and ovine origin require annual boosters. Their protective effect appears to be low. Experimentally, a more effective inactivated vaccine booster has been produced. Recently, a soluble organism-free cell culture derived from *A. marginale* antigen has been developed.

Eradiction is possible where ticks can be removed. Carrier cattle can be detected by a serological test. Then the non-infected cattle need to be kept away from potential domestic or wild animal carriers. Movements of the cattle need to be controlled and it is necessary to reduce the level of biting flies. In such circumstances no live vaccination programme must be undertaken.

Tick-borne fever

Tick-borne fever is caused by the rickettsial-like organism *Ehrlichia phagocytophila*. It causes a prolonged febrile reaction, neutropenia and immunodepression in cattle in northern Europe (see Fig. 47.1b).

Aetiology and epidemiology

Ehrlichia phagocytophila is transmitted by the tick *Ixodes ricinus* during engorgement, but unlike

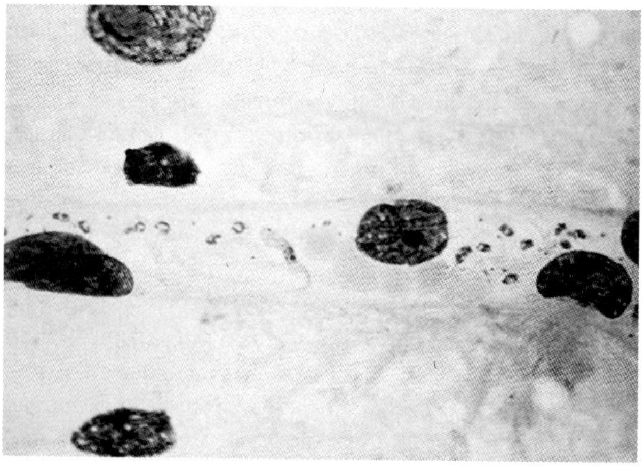

Fig. 47.3 *Trypanosoma congolense* in ox brain capillary (courtesy of CTVM Archives) (× 1000).

babesiasis, infection takes place almost immediately after ticks start to feed. The circumstances and timing of infections is dependent on the ecology of the tick, and typically takes place most often during spring or autumn tick-activity periods, but can take place at any time between April and November. Infection in ticks persists transtadially but not to the following generation of larvae.

After infection the organism enters or is phagocytosed by white blood cells, usually neutrophils but infected eosinophils and monocytes are occasionally observed. The 'elementary body' can be seen in blood smears stained with Giemsa or Leishman stains as a pale blue dot in the cytoplasm of neutrophils. It enlarges to become a morula, after which the neutrophil ruptures and the elementary bodies of which the morula is composed infect further cells (Fig. 47.1b). The disease becomes apparent five to nine days after transmission by infected ticks. The animal develops a high fever, which can persist for up to 10 days. During this period the continuous destruction of neutrophils leads to a severe neutropenia, and for as yet unknown reasons to a reduction of packed cell volume (PCV) of 30 per cent. As a result of the neutropenia the animal becomes immunodepressed and susceptible to other infections such as pneumonia, infectious pododermatitis and babesiosis due to *B. divergens*, which is frequently observed in susceptible cattle eight to twelve days after tick-borne fever. The 'parasitaemia' subsides but recrudescences occur periodically thereafter. Immunity develops slowly and persists only for a few months as cattle may be affected, albeit less severely, for some years following their infection.

Signs

Affected dairy cattle suffer an abrupt drop in milk production, which may last despite treatment for four weeks, and beef cattle lose a significant percentage of their body weight.

Diagnosis

The history is usually similar to that of cattle affected with *B. divergens*, i.e. recent purchase or movement to tick-infested pastures. Diagnosis can be confirmed by examination of blood smears for the presence of *E. phagocytophila*.

Treatment and control

Tetracyclines are the antibiotic of choice, and long-acting preparations have proved most successful. Treatment of cattle with pour-on synthetic pyrethroids has been used to prevent tick infestation, reducing the tick population for two to three weeks. It has been less successful than when used on sheep, which retain higher concentrations of the pyrethroids on skin and wool for longer than cattle. The fact that transmission of *E. phagocytophila* is transmitted early in engorgement as opposed to *B. divergens* has resulted in the observation that protection of cattle against tick-borne fever using pyrethroids is less successful than against babesiasis, as accumulation of chemicals is more likely to kill the tick before transmission.

Bovine petechial fever (Ondiri disease, ondiritis)

The condition is a rickettsial infection of ruminants but is restricted in area of occurrence.

Aetiology

The cause is a rickettsia-like organism *Cytoecetes (Ehrlichia) ondiri*. The infection initiates in the spleen, and there it parasitizes the circulating granulocytes and more rarely monocytes. The organisms are pleomorphic and occur in cytoplasmic vacuoles, particularly in neutrophils. The organisms possess a rippled cell wall and they can be small (0.2–0.4 μm) or large (1–2 μm) bodies. In some cases there are mixed groups of large and small bodies.

Epidemiology

The disease appears to be confined to the highlands of East Africa. It mainly involves cattle exotic to the region. Often very well defined areas are involved. The indigenous cattle and wild ruminants such as the bushbuck (*Tragelaphus*) and duiker (*Silvicapra* spp.) do not show clinical infection. The vegetation common to all sites is the edge of forest or thick bush. Experimentally, infection can occur in cattle, sheep, goats, impala, bushbuck, Thomson's gazelle and wildebeeste. Most of these develop latent infections. Thus carrier animals are produced from which it would seem highly likely infection could be spread by an arthropod vector. However, as yet, despite intensive investigations, the arthropod involved (probably attick) has not been detected. The incubation period is variable from four to fourteen days and in natural outbreaks disease has occurred 10 days after entering into an infected area. Mortality is around 20 per cent and occurs within a few days of onset of signs but some animals will die two or three weeks after disease develops.

Signs

Peracute. These signs are seen in recently imported exotic cattle. They develop marked pyrexia and a drop in milk yield. The signs usually coincide with a parasitaemia. After two or three days petechial haemorrhages occur on mucous membranes, and in some cases that are fatal there is general congestion, with pulmonary oedema, dullness, weakness and a staring coat. Most of the cattle collapse and die within four days.

Acute. These types tend to occur over a longer period. The temperature is high but fluctuates. There is inappetence with reduced milk yield and abortion. Although petechial haemorrhages occur in some animals on the day after the onset of fever, in most animals they have appeared by three days. The haemorrhages disappear to be replaced by fresh ones within seven to ten days. They occur on the vulva, vagina, conjunctiva, labial surface of the gums and ventral surface of the tongue. Any normal discharge and faeces may be bloodstained. In some cases a characteristic 'poached egg eye' occurs with a swollen tense eyeball with the aqueous humour containing blood, the conjunctiva swollen and haemorrhagic and the eyelid everted.

Subacute. Affected animals show a transient non-fatal condition with pyrexia and petechiation of the mucous membranes.

Inapparent. No signs are present.

Necropsy

The main findings are usually of an animal in good condition with submucosal and subserosal haemorrhages, which may be large and distributed throughout the body. There is oedema and lymphoid hyperplasia. Often there is subcutaneous and intramuscular haemorrhage and melaena. The heart shows large haemorrhages into the epicardium and endocardium. There are also haemorrhages and oedema in the respiratory tract and the mucosa and serosa of the alimentary tract. The lymph nodes show hyperplasia and oedema. Both the liver and spleen may be enlarged and show petechiae. Histologically, there is marked evidence of petechiation. Characteristically, hyperplasia of the large areas of the lymphoid sinus are seen. The rickettsiae can be found in impression smears of that surface of the spleen and liver. There is a characteristic absence of eosinophils, followed by markedly reduced numbers of lymphocytes and then neutrophils.

Diagnosis

Often, diagnosis is difficult as the condition resembles anthrax (p. 551), bracken poisoning (p. 619), arsenic poisoning (p. 613), haemorrhagic septicaemia (p. 563), heartwater, acute trypanosomiasis (p. 737) and acute theileriasis (p. 729). It is usually based on the history plus the area where it has occurred. *Ehrlichia ondiri* can be detected in blood or spleen smears stained with Giemsa where it is particularly seen in granulocytes and monocytes. Often by the time clinical signs develop the parasitaemia is low or absent. In such cases it may be necessary to collect blood in EDTA or a suspension of spleen or lung and inject this intravenously into susceptible cattle or sheep. The granulocytes and monocytes in blood smears from the recipient, stained with Giemsa, should be examined daily for 10 days after inoculation.

Treatment

The most effective time to treat is during the incubation period when tetracyclines prevent disease. Once overt signs are present double the usual therapeutic dosage of these antibiotics will reduce clinical signs and limit the parasitaemia. A single intravenous dose of alphaethoxyethylglycoxal dithiosemicarbazone at 5 mg/kg body weight will also reduce signs and the parasitaemia more effectively than tetracyclines.

Prevention and control

Eradication is impossible because wild animals act as a reservoir of infection. Clinically infected cattle are resistant to re-infection for several years but they probably carry latent infections of *E. ondiri*. Losses due to the disease can be reduced by restricting access to areas of known infection. Clearing the undergrowth and scrub aids this. If susceptible animals are to enter infected areas they should be watched daily and when infection is present a single dose of dithiosemicarbazone may then allow them to recover and become immune to infection.

Heartwater (cowdriosis or malignant rickettsia, blacklung) (see p. 707)

This is another rickettsial condition that infects both domestic and wild animals.

Aetiology

The infection is caused by the rickettsia *Cowdria ruminantium* and is transmitted by at least five species of *Amblyomma* ticks. It is first found in reticulo-endothelial cells and then parasitizes vascular endothelial cells. It is seen as close packed colonies consisting of less than 10 to many hundred cocci. The agent is pleomorphic but the rickettsia in any one group tend to be of similar size. The organism varies between groups from 0.2 μm to greater than 1.5 μm. Division is by binary fission and it produces morula-like colonies in the cytoplasm. The small granules tend to be coccoid with larger ones looking like rings, horseshoes, rods and irregular masses. It has been suggested that differences in the size and shape of the organisms are the result of a growth cycle.

Epidemiology

The disease has been reported in many African countries south of the Sahara desert. Distribution coincides with that of the *Amblyomma* ticks, which require a warm humid climate and bushy grass. Experimentally, five species of *Amblyomma* are able to transmit infection. These are three-host ticks. Transmission appears usually to be transtadial and so infected larvae are usually free from disease. Transovarian transmission can occur but is thought to be very infrequent. Infected larvae are found on non-susceptible animals but if they do become infected it can pass on to both nymph and adult stages. Infected ticks do not transmit infection immediately they become attached to the animals but a variable time after they start to feed. In many cases the level of infection is unknown as indigenous domestic and wild animals often show no signs. It is only when susceptible exotic species are introduced that infection becomes apparent. Besides cattle, sheep, goats, Asian buffalo, antelopes and deer are susceptible to infection and disease. Indigenous cattle undergo inapparent infection. Calves under three weeks old, even from susceptible stock, are difficult to infect. Heartwater can occur throughout the year but incidence declines in the dry season due to reduced tick activity. The incubation period is variable from 7 to 28 days with fever starting on average after 18 days. Mortality can be up to 60 per cent in exotic breeds but less than 5 per cent in local cattle.

Signs

Peracute. This occurs in exotic breeds introduced to the region. The animal appears clinically normal but if examined will have a marked pyrexia. It may then suddenly collapse, go into convulsions and die. Thoracic auscultation will often reveal oedema in the lungs and bronchi.

Acute. The course of infection is three to six days and consists of pyrexia (often over 41 °C, 106 °F), with nervous signs that may include ataxia, circling and abnormal posture. In other cases signs develop only to stimuli and there is then an excessive blink reflex, frequent tongue protrusion, a haggard, pained expression and muscular tremors. Pregnant cows may abort. If the condition progresses there are convulsions, paddling movements of the limbs, nystagmus, opisthotonus and chewing movements. Often a fetid profuse diarrhoea is present or there may be blood in the faeces. A mild cough may be heard. On auscultation hydrothorax, hydropericardium and lung oedema are noted.

Subacute. The signs are like those of the acute form but they are much less severe with a transient fever and sometimes diarrhoea. Disease may last for over a week and usually the animal improves gradually. A few cases progress to collapse and death. This is often the most severe form seen in indigenous cattle and those previously infected.

Inapparent. These cattle include almost all the indigenous stock as well as some of those introduced to the region. In addition they often follow cases of re-infection.

Pathology

The lesions present are very variable and not pathognomonic. In the peracute form there are few gross lesions but in some there is marked lung oedema with tracheal and bronchial froth. In the acute form there is usually ascites, hydrothorax, hydropericardium and lung oedema. The lymph nodes are often swollen. Petechial haemorrhages can occur in the heart, lungs and gastrointestinal tract. The liver is often engorged, with the gall-bladder distended. The spleen is occasionally enlarged. There may be congestion of the meningeal blood vessels.

Diagnosis

There is no completely specific method of diagnosis in the living animal. Provisional indication can be from the history and clinical signs. Lymph node material can be aspirated to examine for vacuoles containing organisms in the cytoplasm of the reticular cells. There is a method of taking brain cortex so that the capillaries of the brain can be examined for rickettsia. Blood can be obtained and injected into susceptible animals. Eosinophils also decrease in number during the course of the disease. Serum can be examined using a capillary flocculation test. Diagnosis is easier at post mortem as the organism can be discerned in brain tissue capillaries that have been fixed in methyl alcohol and stained with Giemsa.

Differential diagnosis includes anthrax (p. 551) and acute theileriosis (p. 729) in peracute cases, and in nervous cases rabies (p. 706), tetanus (p. 567), strychnine poisoning, cerebral theileriosis (p. 729), cerebral babesiosis (p. 726) and hypomagnesaemia (p. 586).

Treatment

Therapy is most effective when carried out early in disease. Tetracyclines can be used and do not interfere with development of immunity.

Control

Disease can be prevented by controlling the vector *Amblyomma* by dipping cattle at weekly intervals with reliable acaricides. However, the ticks of this genus are less susceptible than those from other genera. As the tick may transmit infection after a day on the host, better control is obtained by applying acaricide by dipping or spraying every three days. However, *Amblyomma* have in some cases shown resistance to organophosphorus, organochloride and arsenic. Care should also be taken not to introduce *Amblyomma* on infected animals or in forage to uninfected cows.

In areas where disease is endemic most cattle are immune. A carrier state develops after infection and remains for several weeks. Non-infected resistance persists a variable time lasting from a few months to several years. After this time re-infection can occur. Ideally, an effective vaccine should be used. However, at present *C. ruminantium* is difficult to culture serially or to adapt to growth in laboratory animals. One method is to inject susceptible stock intravenously with 5–10 ml of blood from an infected animal. As infected animals cannot always be available then infected blood can be stored in a freezer or liquid nitrogen provided it is frozen rapidly after addition of dimethyl sulphonate. The infection can also be retained in deep frozen brain emulsion or more recently in a supernatant of homogenized engorged *Amblyomma* ticks. The recipient animal is monitored and then treated with tetracyclines as soon as pyrexia develops. Treatment continues twice a day until the fever subsides. Pregnant cows should not be treated in this way.

Jembrana disease (Tabana disease)

Aetiology

The cause of the condition is not known but it is thought to be a rickettsial infection. Groups of small coccobacillary organisms have been found in cytoplasmic vacuoles present in circulating monocytes and in impression smears of cut organ surfaces some consider the disease may have a viral aetiology.

Epidemiology

The disease was first recognized in the Jembrana District of Bali Island, Indonesia, in 1964. Subsequently, the condition has only been detected in Indonesia. The disease is found in cattle as well as buffalo. Sheep and goats are infected with no apparent signs but pigs are refractory to infection. In cattle there is apparent age resistance to infection and cattle over two years old rarely die from the disease. Animals that recover are carriers but the duration of infection is not known. There is no direct infection from animal to animal and so it is not contagious. *Boophilus microplus*, a pantropical cattle tick, appears to be the natural vector and it is believed that infection can pass through the egg phase. The incubation period appears to be about a month to six weeks although it is considerably shorter after injection of infection. Mortality is about 25 per cent and is usually within a week of onset of signs. Some animals relapse with infection at later dates.

Signs

Invariably there is a pyrexia of about 41 °C (106 °F) with anorexia, nasal and lacrimal discharge, which can persist for one to nine days. This is soon followed by enlarged lymph nodes. Often there is excessive salivation and erosion of the oral mucosa. Petechial haemorrhages may be found on the visible mucous membranes and haemorrhage within the aqueous humour of the eye is seen. Blood tends to ooze from the skin (so-called 'blood sweating'). Diarrhoea occurs early on and persists; it is often bloodstained.

Pathology

There are widespread haemorrhages and oedema. Usually, generalized lymphadenopathy occurs with the lymph nodes being hyperplastic and often showing disorganization. Splenomegaly is common and the blood vessels show vasculitis and perivasculitis. Surrounding the blood vessels there is proliferation of lymphoreticular cells in many organs except the liver. Rickettsia-like organisms can be detected in impression smears.

Diagnosis

This is based on the area and history. Confirmation depends on the haematological changes, which include a progressive anaemia, thrombocytopenia and transient leucopenia, which particularly involves the lymphocytes. As the disease progresses 'foamy' monocytes appear and large lymphocytes with big coarse nuclei are seen. However, confirmation is difficult unless the animal dies. It is then dependent on detection of organisms in impression smears of cut organs and the vascular changes. In some cases blood is taken into EDTA from suspect cases and then injected into susceptible cattle.

Differential diagnosis includes rinderpest (p. 543), haemorrhagic septicaemia (p. 563) and plant poisonings (Chapter 41).

Treatment

Tetracycline injections during the course of the disease appear to have little effect on disease severity or duration but they do seem to reduce mortality.

Control

Not enough is known about the disease to initiate control measures. Recovered animals are often carriers of infection and so resist further challenge.

Viral diseases

Bovine ephemeral fever (BEF)

This is also known as bovine epizootic fever and three-day sickness. Although signs occur they are quite mild and seem only to affect cattle. It is caused by a rhabdovirus, which can be present in the blood where it appears to be mainly in the leucocyte–platelet fraction and is transmitted by insect vectors. At present there is only a single serological type of the virus, although in Australia several rhabdoviruses have been isolated with a distinct relationship to BEF.

The condition is present in most of Africa except possibly the North. However, the incidence varies widely between regions and countries. It is also present in Asia, Australia and New Guinea. It does not occur in North or South America. The disease is transmitted by vectors from infected host cattle, which explains the seasonality of the condition. If disease enters a new region it can cause epizootic infection with a morbidity of about 100 per cent but mortality is usually less than 1 per cent. In the enzootic areas the condition is sporadic with a morbidity of 5–10 per cent.

The cause of transmission is thought to be midges, probably of the *Culicoides* spp. and Ceratopogonidae family. Transmission is not direct between animals, indicating the need for maturation in the vector. Spread mainly depends on the number of insects infected and the direction of winds. Viral development in the insect is suspected to be cyclic. More losses occur in adult cattle although calves from three months old are susceptible. Often the disease seems to disappear only to return again as an epizootic once resistance in the cattle population is reduced.

Signs

The incubation period is two to ten days and is followed by a marked pyrexia of 40.5–41 °C (105–106 °F). This is often very transient and so is missed. Other animals have intermittent pyrexia. There is a drop in milk yield, which is the main loss caused by the disease, with anaemia, oculo-nasal discharge and increased salivation. Alimentary signs are variable and can include constipation or diarrhoea. Within four days locomotory signs appear, including muscular tremors, which then develop into stiffness and weakness. The animal often becomes lame and the hindlimbs may become stiff. Signs may resemble those of acute laminitis. Occasionally, animals show lateral recumbency.

The animal usually starts to show signs of recovery after two or three days with appetite and milk yield improving. However, the stiffness and lameness are likely to take several more days to reduce. Recovery is uneventful. Mortality is low and is usually the result of secondary infection or following aspiration pneumonia after regurgitation of ruminal contents, or following lateral recumbency. Abortion does not occur but semen quality in bulls is often affected for a period.

Necropsy

The lesions are not specific. The main sign is enlargement and oedema of all the lymph nodes. Congestion and petechial haemorrhages of the pleural membranes may occur. Other signs are usually the result of complications such as aspiration pneumonia.

Diagnosis

This depends mainly on the signs of a mild disease with pyrexia and lameness, limb stiffness and muscle tremors. There is a leucocytosis with a neutrophilia. A fluorescent antibody test will detect virus in blood. An agargel immunodiffusion test has been successfully used on serum. The virus can be isolated by serial passage in Vero or BHK cell cultures or by intracerebral injection of sucking mice.

Treatment

Treatment is symptomatic but can include antibiotics for secondary complications with the use of non-steroidal anti-inflammatory agents such as phenylbutazone or flunixin meglumine for muscle stiffness. It is best not to drench animals because of the high risk of aspiration pneumonia. Recumbent animals should be provided with adequate shade and water.

Control

Control of the insect vectors has not been attempted successfully. Immunity is long lasting after natural infection and has led to development of vaccines. Vaccines are available in Japan and South Africa. Experimentally, live cell culture vaccines in an adjuvant base have been used with success but give rise to fears of vector transmission between vaccinated and non-vaccinated stock. Control can also be by dipping cows twice weekly during the peak period of infection when conditions are wet, hot and humid.

Lumpy skin disease (LSD) (see also p. 683)

The disease, also called Knopvelsiekte, results in many pox-like skin lesions and has been associated with a virus that is serologically related to sheep pox and on tissue culture produces three different groups of virus. One, an orphan virus (Group I), is generally present on the skin of normal cattle but does not appear to cause the disease. The 'Allerton' virus (Group II) causes a condition of a mild nature and is isolated from skin nodules, saliva, nasal secretions and semen. This form appears to be identical with the bovine herpes virus 2 of bovine mammillitis. It has often given rise to the name of pseudo-lumpy skin disease (p. 689). The severe disease is caused by a 'Neethling' virus (Group III) and is found in blood, mucus, saliva and semen.

The disease is seen in most parts of Africa and is endemic in southern Africa. The virus is present on the skin even when hides are salted, in blood and in saliva and all can transmit infection.

The method of transmission has not completely been established but it is believed to be by insects, particularly mosquitoes as spread can occur without direct or indirect contact. Virus has been isolated from *Stomoxys* and *Biomyia* flies. As the saliva is infected, spread can also be by feeding at troughs or sucking milk from infected cows. Indigenous cattle are less susceptible than imported purebreds. Experimentally, giraffe and impala have been infected. All ages of stock are susceptible but calves and lactating cows are most likely to be infected. The duration of immunity is not known and appears variable. Reports suggest it to be from 11 months to five years, or even lifelong.

Morbidity rates are very variable from 5 to 80 per cent with less than 2 per cent mortality. There can be a rapid spread of the disease.

Signs

The incubation period lasts from two to five weeks in natural infection but four to fourteen days with experimental infection and is followed by a rise in temperature, which may fluctuate. In severe cases there tends to be anorexia, lacrimation and salivation. There is a clear nasal discharge, which later becomes purulent. There is then the sudden appearance of nodules, varying in number from a few to many hundreds. The nodules are firm, raised areas within the skin and vary in diameter from a few millimetres to 4–5 cm. These larger areas often have erect hair over them that exaggerates their appearance. The nodules are usually of a uniform size on individual animals and they occur over the whole body, although they are mainly found on the back, neck, brisket, legs, thighs, scrotum, udder and round the muzzle and eyes. Those on the mucosae of the muzzle, vulva, prepuce, nostrils, eyes and mouth are yellow–grey in colour and soft, and if rubbed off there is an ulcer or erosion. When the eye is affected there is keratitis and conjunctivitis. Respiratory lesions lead to dyspnoea and oral ones to salivation.

The associated lymph nodes tend to be enlarged. In some cases oedema develops. This can be of the lower limbs, brisket, udder, vulva or scrotum. The enlarged skin nodules can later ulcerate. These can then persist for several years or develop a dry surface that is lost. This becomes a deep pit, which heals by second intention. These wounds can become secondarily infected. This secondary infection can then spread to associated lymph nodes, the lungs, liver, kidney, etc. The areas of superficial oedema also remain a long time and can then slough causing suppurative areas. Involvement of the lung can lead to cicatrization and rupture of the tracheal rings several months after onset of the disease.

The disease results in a chronic loss of condition and milk yield. Secondary infection can lead to mastitis, abortion and sterility in bulls.

The 'Allerton' mild or pseudo-lumpy skin form of the disease is less severe and only lasts a few weeks. There is a mild pyrexia followed by nodule formation mainly on the head, neck and perineum. The nodules are characteristic with a hard, raised, rounded mass with a flat surface and a pit at the centre. Sometimes the skin lesions coalesce. Only the epidermis is affected, unlike the 'Neethling' form. The problem area develops into a hard, dry, necrotic lesion after a week to nine days. This is then lost over the next 10–14 days leaving a hairless area. Hair will grow again.

Necropsy

'Neethling' lesions include the whole depth of the skin producing a hard white–grey mass. The skeletal muscle may contain grey nodules. Oedema of this is seen as yellow jelly-like liquid. If the oral mucosa is affected it contains soft grey–yellow nodules with necrotic epithelium. Necrotic ulcers with surrounding inflammation can occur in the nasal cavities. In the lungs there are firm grey nodules and the whole tract may show erosions and ulcers. Pulmonary lesions may lead to oedema and a purulent pneumonia. When lymphadenitis is present the nodules are swollen, pale and oedematous. The rumen and abomasal wall can show ulcers and erosions. Microscopically, the stratum papillomis, stratum reticulis and subcutis are involved. Secondarily, the surface epithelium, hair follicles and their associated glands are infected. In the subcutaneous tissues there is oedema, fibroplasia and perivascular inflammation with mononuclear cells, which usually results in thrombosis and overlying necrosis.

Diagnosis

The rapid spread of the disease and the sudden appearance of skin nodules after pyrexia are relatively characteristic signs. However, a biopsy can be taken and inclusion bodies can be found in skin lesions and the virus can be cultured. Other diseases that may be confused are the 'Allerton' form, urticaria (p. 685), dermafophilosis (p. 688), demodicosis (p. 684), onchocerciasis (p. 754), besnoitiosis (p. 735) and severe tick and insect bites.

Treatment

There is no specific treatment but secondary infection may require the use of antibiotics or sulphonamides.

Control

Quarantine has generally not proved to be successful. In some countries a sheep pox virus tissue culture vaccine has been found to be of use. Otherwise, a vaccine produced from attenuated 'Neethling' virus on kidney tissue culture has been used successfully.

Rift Valley fever

This condition, also known as enzootic hepatitis, is a zoonosis but mainly affects sheep and cattle. Camels can be infected and also goats to a limited extent. It is caused by an insect-borne RNA virus of one main antigenic strain of the family Bunyaviridae, and genus phlebovirus. The condition is transmitted between animals by insect vectors, usually mosquitoes. The disease was first identified in the East African Rift Valley, which gave rise to its name.

The condition is only found in Africa, particularly the central and southern regions, but the mosquitoes that are responsible for transmission occur on other continents. Thus there is a possibility of spread. Disease is transmitted by various types of mosquito including *Aedes* spp. Other biting arthropods would also cause spread.

Man can be infected by contact with infected animals such as when undertaking necropsies. Infection may enter skin abrasions. The signs are of an influenza-like disease with pyrexia, severe headache, nausea, joint pains, flushing of the face, sometimes epistaxis and permanently impaired vision due to retinal haemorrhage. Death is rare but in some instances complications such as sight impairment can occur.

Usually, an epizootic outbreak occurs in cattle followed by long periods often of five years between outbreaks. The persistence of infection between epizootics is unknown but as cattle at the edge of and within forests tend to seroconvert consistently it is considered disease is maintained in wild fauna.

Disease is more common in warm wet seasons. Young animals are more severely afflicted than the adults. Mortality tends to be high in young calves, often reaching 70 per cent. In the adult, a mortality of 10 per cent can occur but the main problem is abortion.

Signs

The signs that develop depend partly on the age of the animals. They tend to be most severe in the calf where the incubation period varies from 12 hours to three days. Occasionally, death occurs within 24 hours with few characteristic signs other than collapse and colic. Others show high fever, incoordination and collapse. The rare renal form is acute and can occasionally occur in adult cattle. In this type there is pyrexia, a profuse mucopurulent discharge, vomiting and prostration. Up to 70 per cent of affected cattle can die.

In adult cattle abortion is more common than the acute form. However, up to 10 per cent can develop marked pyrexia and die. Other lesions can include erosion of the oral mucosa, and dry thickening of the unpigmented areas of the teats, udder and scrotum. Hyperaemia of the coronets also occurs.

Pathology

The main lesion is one of hepatic necrosis with white or grey foci in the subcapsular area. Other lesions are typical of septicaemia with subserous haemorrhages of the pleura, pericardium, endocardium, lymph nodes and gut. There is often also oedema, congestion or haemorrhages of the gall-bladder. Microscopically, there is focal or diffuse necrosis of the liver.

Diagnosis

The history of an outbreak is helpful in that it is in a mosquito area, there is an abortion storm plus calves becoming ill with many of them dying. Post-mortem examination of calves may show typical hepatic necrosis. There may also be evidence of human infection, and if sheep are present then again in lambs there is disease of high fever, incoordination, collapse and high mortality with abortion in ewes. Usually there is a severe leucopenia. Serological confirmation is by means of a serum neutralization or complement fixation test.

Treatment

There is no known successful treatment, although interferon is effective *in vitro* and may eventually become available.

Control

The passage from country to country is difficult to control without the exclusion of susceptible animal species. Control of the insect vectors would be uneconomic and impracticable. It is possible that humans could act as carriers. A vaccine from neurotrophic virus passage through mouse brain has been used successfully. However, it can cause abortion. In consequence, a killed vaccine produced on BHK cells has been developed. This involves two injections to produce adequate immunity. Good immunity has been produced in sheep and humans by virus grown in rhesus kidney cell cultures and then inactivated by formaldehyde. A human vaccine is now available from virus raised indiploid fetal, raised lung cells and inactivated with formalin.

Tick-borne encephalitides (flavivirus infection)

There are a series of diseases of animals resulting from tick-borne infection and characterized by nervous signs and fever (details of louping-ill are given elsewhere, see p. 703). The causes are included within a complex of flaviviruses. The infections tend to be contained in various geographical areas. As a result there are a number of diseases that are identified by the area where the disease occurs. Thus, in Europe there is Russian spring–summer encephalitis, Omsk haemorrhagic fever and Central European encephalitis. Tropical problems include Kyasamar Forest fever in India and Lanyot in Malaysia.

In almost all cases the viruses maintain their presence in ticks, small rodents and insectivores. In the endemic cases infection of wild and domestic ruminants is inapparent. However, the introduction of new ruminants can result in disease. As yet the infections of Kyasamar Forest fever, which have been found in man and horses, have not resulted in disease in native domestic cattle. Infection in cattle would be via ixodial ticks. Man can be infected by ticks or more commonly via drinking infected goat's or sheep's milk. Infections from material submitted for laboratory diagnosis also occur. Immunity following infection is good and lifelong. Colostrum results in passive immunity being conferred to the young calf.

Signs

Disease is almost always only apparent in animals introduced to the tick area. The incubation period is one or two weeks. Pyrexia suddenly occurs and is usually diphasic. It is not until the second period of temperature rise that nervous signs appear. There is then incoordination, muscle tremors, ataxia, photophobia and hypersensitivity. The nervous signs become progressively worse. There can then be a flaccid paralysis with death within a week. Those animals that recover are often subsequently debilitated.

Necropsy

There are few gross lesions. On histological examination there is necrosis of the neurones, particularly in the Purkinje layer of the motor nuclei, vestibular nuclei, cerebellum and ventral nerves of the spinal cord. Perivascular inflammation occurs throughout the white matter.

Diagnosis

The diagnosis is based on the area, presence of ticks, the signs and lesions. The virus can be isolated from the central nervous system, particularly the brain stem and spinal cord. Differential diagnoses include bovine spongiform encephalopathy (p. 708), rabies (p. 706), neuromycotoxins, plant poisoning (Chapter 41), tetanus, hypocalcaemia (p. 577) and hypomagnesaemia (p.584).

Treatment

There is no effective form of treatment.

Control

Cattle should not be introduced to endemic areas unless they are vaccinated. The vaccines available provide protection for at least a year. Control of ticks by improving grazing and reducing bracken, etc. is useful.

Tick-borne encephalitides (Near East encephalitis)

This condition is still not fully elucidated. However, there are several diseases that have been recognized for many years. The disease is endemic in some countries including Syria, Lebanon, Israel and Egypt and a similar condition is recorded in India and Russia.

In most cases the accidental infection of ruminants results in few cases of disease. Usually, the virus cycles inapparently within birds and ticks. Most clinical disease is in Equidae but occasionally problems have been recorded in sheep and cattle. The tick vector of Near East encephalitis is *Hyalomma anatolicum*. Infection passes through all stages of tick life including the egg. All infection is tick mediated and it cannot be transmitted directly between animals. Immunity follows infection in cattle but its duration is unknown.

Signs

The incubation period for the disease is unknown but may be four weeks. The severity of signs is variable and in the acute form there is a drowsiness and a pyrexia of about 40 °C (104 °F). However, in a few horses there are epileptiform fits with a progressive paralysis. Collapse and death can soon occur. In the subacute form pyrexia is usually transient and mild. Nervous signs are slight but in some cases they can persist. Inapparent infections are common.

Necropsy

The alimentary and urogenital tract of the body show mucosal congestion but there is meningeal blood vessel congestion. On histological examination there is diffuse lymphocytic infiltration, perivascular infiltration, microglial proliferation and neuronophagia and occasional rarefaction of tissues.

Diagnosis

The signs and post-mortem picture are not specific. However, cerebral injection of infected brain tissue into rabbits will aid virus identification. The major disease to be differentiated is rabies (p. 706).

Treatment

There is no effective form of treatment, only symptomatic.

Control

There are no suitable control measures that can at present be suggested.

Japanese encephalitis (flavivirus)

This is mainly a disease of man and has been given several local names including Japanese B encephalitis, Russian autumnal encephalitis and summer encephalitis. Infection of animals is often from the human source. Most disease is seen as encephalitis in horses, followed by pigs. Mosquitoes are the natural vectors. Usually, infection in cattle and other ruminants is inapparent and of little overall significance.

Other arthropod-borne diseases

There are well over 300 diseases that are arthropod transmitted. Many are of limited geographical distribution. Frequently areas do not produce overt disease. However, where signs do occur, they can be non-specific with malaise and pyrexia. Often indigenous animals and wild animals develop inapparent disease that does not cause them any hazards or reduce production. However, the introduction of new animals will frequently result in overt disease, which can reach a high morbidity level.

Akabane virus (Asian virus)

This bunyavirus is mosquito borne and related to Simbu virus. It is recorded in the Far East as well as Kenya and Australia. The condition in cattle is thought to produce arthrogryposis and hydroncephalus as well as abortion.

Bhanja virus (African virus)

This is mainly an infection of goats but it has occasionally been isolated in cattle, particularly in southern Nigeria, and has also been reported in India. Infection has been found in *Haemaphysalis* ticks. Experimentally, calves injected with Bhanja virus have developed a viraemia for several days and leucopenia.

Bunyamwera virus (African virus)

This is mainly a condition of goats but serological evidence has been found in cattle and sheep. The infection occurs throughout Africa and is considered to be mosquito borne.

Cache Valley virus (American virus)

This is found in mosquitoes in Central and North America. Disease has not been recorded but sera of cattle are often positive.

California encephalitis virus (American virus)

In America there is a high incidence of antibody in the sera of cattle. Evidence of infection can also be found in deer and horses. It is a bunyavirus transmitted by mosquitoes. The virus is the most common cause of human viral encephalitis in the USA.

Calovovirus (European virus)

This is a bunyavirus that is mosquito borne. It results in cattle infection.

Congo virus (African virus)

This is a disease of humans and also affects goats and cattle resulting in anaemia, depression and pyrexia. The virus is transmitted by *Hyalomma* ticks and infection between countries is probably accomplished by migrating birds. It is probable the condition is related to Hazna virus and others in Europe and Asia. The disease is severe in horses and is often fatal. However, in cattle and goats indigenous to Africa it results in a short period of illness that may be seen as anorexia, fever and depression.

Corriparta virus (Australian virus)

The virus is mosquito borne, particularly by *Culex* spp. The disease level is unknown but antibodies are found in the sera of cattle, horses and man as well as kangaroos and wallabies.

Dughe virus (African virus)

The virus appears to be spread by *Amblyomma variegatum* ticks, *Culicoides* and mosquitoes. It is the most frequently isolated arthropod-borne virus in Nigeria. In most cases there are no signs in cattle but calves can be infected experimentally and show a short-lasting viraemia.

Germiston virus (African virus)

This is a bunyavirus and is transmitted by mosquitoes. The virus causes infection in humans, usually in laboratories, but in cattle there are usually no signs but seroconversion. The condition is present in cattle, egrets and herons.

Harana virus (Asian virus)

The virus is transmitted by *Hyalomma* ticks and spread to other animals by migrating birds. This virus resembles, and may be identical to, Azo virus. It results in a severe infection of humans, often with haemorrhages and fever. It can be fatal. In cattle the disease is transient and usually results in anorexia, pyrexia and depression.

Ibaraki virus (Asian virus)

It is thought to be arthropod borne and is a double-stranded RNA virus. Antibody surveys show the infection to be widespread in South East Asia and the Far East. The condition is very similar to that of bluetongue. Disease is severe and only recorded in

Japan. Signs include pyrexia with oedema and haemorrhaging in the mouth, abomasum and around the horn/skin junction. Degeneration of the muscles follows. There is then dehydration and emaciation due to difficulty in swallowing. Death is commonly due to inhalation pneumonia.

Jos virus (African virus)

This unclassified virus is transmitted by *Amblyomma variegatum* ticks. The disease signs are not really known but the virus has been isolated from indigenous Nigerian cattle.

Kodam virus (African virus)

This flavivirus is found in *Rhipicephalus parvus* ticks. The signs of disease are unknown but antibody is found in cattle.

Kokobera (Australian virus)

The virus has been found in mosquitoes in Queensland. It is a flavivirus. Antibodies have been detected in sera from cattle and horses although there is no indication that the virus is a pathogen.

Kowanyama virus, Mapputta virus, Trubanaman virus (Australian viruses)

These are all found in tropical Australia and can be isolated from the *Anopheles* mosquito. Their pathogenicity is not known but antibodies are found in the sera of cattle, sheep and pigs as well as kangaroos and wallabies.

Kunjin virus (Australian virus)

This is a flavivirus found in mosquitoes in tropical Australia. There is serological evidence of infection in humans, horses, cattle and poultry. In calves experimentally infected a mild non-purulent encephalitis develops.

Kotonkan virus (African virus)

This is a rhabdovirus found in *Culicoides*. The disease resembles ephemeral fever virus. The infection is particularly present in Nigeria.

Lokern virus (American virus)

Antibodies to the bunyavirus have been found in cattle, horses and sheep. The infection is found in Californian sandflies and mosquitoes.

Middelburg virus (African virus)

While antibodies can be found in domestic cattle in South Africa, disease has not been recorded. Man is not affected. The virus is spread by *Aedes* mosquitoes.

Murray Valley encephalitis virus (Australian virus)

This is a flavivirus found in mosquitoes and wild birds. It can produce epidemics of human encephalitis in Australia and New Guinea. The infection can be detected serologically in cattle, horses, pigs and dogs. When calves are experimentally infected the disease is symptomless.

Obodhiang virus (African virus)

This is a rhabdovirus found in *Culicoides*. The disease resembles ephemeral fever. It is found in mosquitoes in Sudan and the pathogenicity is not known.

Pongola virus (African virus)

Cattle sera will show antibodies to this virus but disease is not apparent. The name also applies to infection in humans, donkeys, goats and sheep. The condition is spread by mosquitoes. The virus appears to be related to Rwamba virus.

Rwamba virus (African virus)

Cattle sera will show antibodies to this virus but disease is not apparent. The name also applies to infection in humans, donkeys, goats and sheep. The condition is spread by mosquitoes. The virus appears to be related to Pongola virus.

Sabo virus (African virus)

This virus is found in *Culicoides* in Nigeria. It is also frequently isolated from Nigerian cattle and has been isolated from goats. There is a transient fever and listlessness following infection. The virus is a member of the Simbu group of bunyaviruses.

Sango virus (African virus)

This virus is found in *Culicoides* in Nigeria. It is also frequently isolated from Nigerian cattle. There is a transient fever and listlessness following infection. The virus is a member of the Simbu group of bunyaviruses.

Shamondu virus (African virus)

This virus is found in *Culicoides* in Nigeria. It is also frequently isolated from Nigerian cattle. There is a transient fever and listlessness following infection. The virus is a member of the Simbu group of bunyaviruses.

Shuni virus (African virus)

This virus is found in *Culicoides* in Nigeria. It is also frequently isolated from Nigerian cattle and has been isolated from sheep. There is a transient fever and listlessness following infection. The virus is a member of the Simbu group of bunyaviruses.

Sindbis virus (African, Asian and Australian virus)

The life cycle is believed to involve *Culicoides*, mosquitoes and wild birds. In most cases cattle exhibit no signs but they do develop antibody titres. Infection of humans results in illness. It is a species of the alphaviruses.

Thogoto virus (African and European virus)

The virus is found in ticks in Nigeria and in *Boophilus decoloratus* ticks in Kenya. It has also been isolated in the tick *Rhipicephalus bursa* in Sicily. The infection can also involve humans and sheep. Calves when experimentally infected show viraemia and leucopenia but usually there are no other signs.

Parasites

Onchocerciosis (worm nodule disease)

Aetiology

This is a filarial infection of the genus *Onchocerca*. In cattle, *Onchocerca gibsoni* affects the subcutaneous tissues particularly the brisket and lower limbs; *O. liendis* (synonyms *O. gutturosa, O. bovis*) is found in the ligamentum nuchae, other ligaments and stifle joints; *O. ochengi* causes a dermatitis; and *O. armillata* is found in the aortic wall. The worms are thread-like and often measure 6 cm long with microfilariae 200–400 μm long.

Epidemiology

The condition occurs world-wide but is more common in the tropics and subtropics. The life cycle is indirect. Transmission is by midges (*Culicoides* spp.), sandflies and blackflies (*Simulium* spp.), which ingest microfilaria in the skin and subcutaneous tissue. They develop to the infective larval stage and then infect the final host when the vector again feeds. The larvae migrate to the predilection site where *O. gibsoni* develops into nodules and the others become enclosed in a fibrous cyst. The females produce microfilariae that remain in the skin or subcutaneous tissue.

Signs

There are few clinical signs except for the presence of nodules up to 3 cm diameter under the skin, particularly in the brisket. In *O. liendis* infections there are few signs in the ligantum nuchae but the stifle joint may be swollen. Disability can occur due to the supporting ligaments being affected. Infestation with *O. gibsoni* can result in nodules.

Pathology

There are nodules present. *Onchocerca armillata* is present in nodules in the wall of the thrombic aorta; *O. liendis* is found in the ligamentum nuchae, ligaments, stifle, the omentum, splenic ligament and capsule.

Diagnosis

The presence of infection can be detected by examining skin biopsies. Differentiation from skin tuberculosis and demodectic mange (p. 684) is necessary.

Treatment

There is no specific treatment but diethylcarbamazine citrate 4 mg/kg in the food can be helpful, otherwise ivermectin can be used.

Control

The control of insect vectors is not practicable.

Stephanofilariosis

Aetiology

This is caused by parasites of the genus *Stephanofilaria*. These include *S. assamensis*, which occurs in India and Pakistan; *S. kaeli*, found on the legs of cattle in Malaysia; *S. stilesi*, affecting the ventral surface of the body and found in many parts of Asia; and *S. dedosi*, which occurs in Indonesia affecting the head and neck. The parasites are small (2–9 mm long) and filariform in shape.

Epidemiology

The parasite occurs in cattle and buffalo in many parts of South East Asia as well as the tropics. The life cycle is indirect and involves anthomyid flies as intermediate hosts. Open skin lesions develop from which the flies feed and ingest the microfilariae. In the fly they develop to the infective larval stage and are then transmitted to the final host when the fly feeds. There appear to be more flies when conditions are moist either due to rain or presence of rivers, streams or irrigation.

Signs

There are only superficial lesions seen initially as a papular dermatitis. There is then exudate and haemorrhage lasting many months with the skin becoming thickened and dry.

Diagnosis

This is based on the lesions and recent wet weather. Scrapings or smears from skin lesions reveal adult worms and microfilariae.

Treatment

Topical application of organophosphorus compounds is effective, including trichlorophan 6 per cent and coumaphos 2 per cent.

Control

There is no effective control but in some cases fly repellents are used. However, these are expensive for routine use. In adult animals that have been repeatedly infected with *S. stilesi* there is evidence that further infestation is reduced or stops.

Thelaziosis

Aetiology

Disease is caused by infestation with spirurid nematodes of the genus *Thelazia*, in cattle by *T. rhodesii*. The worms are thin, white and can be up to 20 mm long.

Epidemiology

It occurs in the conjunctival sac of mammals in many parts of the world. In the species that have been studied the worms are viviparous and produce first-stage larvae that are infective for various Diptera including *Musca* spp. The flies act as the intermediate hosts where the parasite develops to a third-stage infective larva, which is transferred to the final host when the flies feed.

Signs

There are often no signs. Otherwise, there may be lacrimation that can be unilateral or bilateral and is often purulent. There can be conjunctivitis, keratitis, corneal opacity, ulceration, protrusion of the eyeball and photophobia. Abscesses may develop on the eyelids.

Pathology

There may be conjunctivitis, keratitis and corneal ulceration and scarring.

Diagnosis

This depends on the signs and finding the worms.

Treatment

Levamisole can be given orally at 5 mg/kg body weight or as a 1 per cent eye lotion. Otherwise, local anaesthetic can be used and the helminths removed manually. Irrigation of the unanaesthetized eye can be undertaken with 1 in 8000 aqueous iodine or 2 per cent boric acid, 3 per cent piperazine adipate or 0.2 per cent diethyl carbamazine. Ivermectin injections are useful.

Control

The condition is not usually severe and so control is not normally undertaken particularly because of the ubiquitous nature of the vector.

Other problems

Tick paralysis

Aetiology

This occurs with a number of different ticks and results in an ascending flaccid paralysis either due to acetylcholine failure at neuromuscular sites or a lack of conduction within the nerve fibres.

Epidemiology

This is seen in ticks in Australia (*Ixodes holocyclus*), North America (*Dermacentor andersoni*, *D. accidentalis*) and South Africa (*I. pilosus*, *I. rubicundus, Haemaphysalis punctata*). Most cases coincide with the peak tick populations and particularly at maximum adult activity. At times only one feeding tick may cause the problem.

Signs

The signs involve a change in temperament followed by slight incoordination. Then the animal starts to drag its hindlimbs and as the forelimbs are progressively involved it becomes recumbent. There is respiratory distress and then the animal dies of respiratory failure.

Necropsy

There are no characteristic signs at post mortem.

Diagnosis

If the ticks are removed the animal makes a recovery.

Treatment

Remove as many ticks as possible by hand. Then treat with an ixodicide.

Control

Although susceptibility decreases with age immunity varies from a few weeks to years. Prevention really involves the proper use of dips, sprays, etc.

Sweating sickness (sweetsiekte, notkalersiekte, vuursiekte, schwitzkrankheit, la dyhydrose tropicale, foma, ol macheri)

This appears to be a toxicosis with a dermatotrophic toxin related to tick infestations. Removal of the ticks results in a rapid clinical recovery. The problem is not transferred from animal to animal by the introduction of blood, saliva or tissue from ill animals. Animals appear to be susceptible or non-susceptible. In the former case cattle become ill with each exposure and can die. Only certain strains of the tick *Hyalomma truncatum*, known as the boat-legged tick, are implicated. The disease is seen in Central, East and South Africa. Although cattle are involved, particularly calves, sheep, goats, pigs and dogs are also affected. The signs vary according to individual susceptibility, age of the animal and the number of the correct strain of tick present. The inactive period is about six days but varies from four to eleven. The morbidity of the condition is very variable and mortality ranges from 30 to 70 per cent. Immediately following recovery from sweating sickness immunity persists well over a year and in some cases lasts up to four years. There appears to be no passive transfer of immunity to calves in colostrum.

Signs

Peracute. This is fatal in 48–72 hours with a sudden rise in rectal temperature, hyperaemia, anorexia, dyspnoea, hyperaesthesia of the visible mucous membranes and muscle tremors. There tends to be excessive lacrimation and nasal discharge.

Acute. This only occurs in animals under a year old and presents as a sudden rise in temperature to 40–41 °C (104–106 °F) for a period of up to eight days. The pyrexia may be continuous or intermittent and lasts longer in the latter case. The mucous membranes become hyperaemic and there is lacrimation, salivation and nasal discharge. The hair is in poor condition and wet eczematous areas develop involving the head, particularly the cheeks under the eyes, nose, ears, then the neck, abdomen and flanks, and especially the groin. In some cases the whole body may be affected, and accompanying the eczema there is hyperaesthesia, discharge and loss of the surface epithelium. Many badly affected calves show total hair loss.

Subacute. The signs are a sudden rise in temperature, but to a lesser extent and lasting only two or three days, and the mucous membranes show slight hyperaemia as can the skin.

Inapparent. These animals show few signs but there is a form of residual immunity to the problem.

Pathology

The lesions depend on the duration of the condition and any concurrent disease. There is a disseminated intravascular coagulopathy with microthrombi (Van Amstel *et al.*, 1987). The oral mucous membranes show ecchymotic dermatitis, inflammation and superficial necrosis. The nasal cavity, pharynx, larynx, oesophagus and omasum show white pseudomembranes. In the thorax there is hydrothorax, hydropericarditis with oedema and emphysema. The liver displays fatty degeneration and the abomasal, small and large intestine mucous membranes show hyperaemia.

Diagnosis

This is dependent on the area and local history of the disease and presence of *H. trunclatum* ticks on the animal. Pathological signs are helpful and there is an increased prothrombin clotting time. Peracute cases could be confused with anthrax (p. 551), babesiosis (p. 726), anaplasmosis (p. 735), heartwater (p. 744) and poisonings (Chapter 41).

Treatment

There is no specific drug that will affect sweating sickness but hyperimmune serum is useful in treatment. The inflammatory nature of the disease suggests the use of anti-inflammatory agents but corticosteroids are probably contraindicated as there are often high circulating cortisol levels in affected cattle. The use of antibiotics is indicated because of the likely immunosuppression that can occur in the presence of high cortisol levels. As there is severe intravascular coagulation the use of heparin at 10–20 iu/kg body weight may be helpful. The liver is often affected and so multivitamin injections, particularly containing cyanocobalamin, choline and methionine may be of use.

Control and prevention

Effective control of the ticks responsible with acaricides is helpful. Eradication is usually not feasible and so acaricide regimens should be designed to clear short-term infestation with the ticks insufficient to produce distress but of long enough duration to allow immunity to develop. As the tick needs to be attached to the animal for at least 7–10 days to produce disease, weekly dipping normally produces reasonable control.

Mhlosimge

This is a less important toxicosis that is transmitted by certain strains of *H. truncatum*. It affects cattle, sheep and pigs. The signs are usually milder than sweating sickness. Cattle do not die of the disease but show pyrexia and anorexia. There is no cross-immunity between sweating sickness and Mhlosimge.

Magudu

This is also a less important toxicosis transmitted by some strains of *H. truncatum*. Again the disease is non-fatal and can affect cattle, sheep and pigs. The signs are milder than those of sweating sickness, including anorexia and pyrexia. Cattle previously infected with sweating sickness are immune to Magudu.

Stomatitis–nephrosis syndrome

This condition is reported in cattle in Zimbabwe. It is a toxicosis but it is not known whether it is of the sweating sickness type or a different *Hyalomma* toxicosis.

References

Trypanosomiasis

Banks, K.L. (1978) Binding of *Trypanosoma congolense* to the walls of small blood vessels. *Journal of Protozoology*, **25**, 241–5.

Clarkson, M.J. (1976) Trypanosomiasis of domesticated animals of S. America. *Transactions of the Royal Society of Tropical Medicine and Hygiene*, **70**, 125–6.

Hoste, C. (1987) Trypanotolerant livestock and African animal trypanosomiasis. *World Animal Review*, **62**, 41–50.

Losos, G.J. (1986) Trypanosomiasis. In *Infectious Tropical Diseases of Domestic Animals*, pp. 183–318. Longman, Harlow, Essex.

Masake, R.A., Nantulya, V.M., Akol, G.W.O. & Musoke, A.J. (1984) Cerebral trypanosomiasis in cattle with mixed *T. congolense* and *T. brucei* infections. *Acta Tropica*, **41**, 237–46.

Morrison, W.I., Murray, M., Whitelaw, D.D. & Sayer, P.D. (1983) Pathology of infection with *T. brucei*: disease syndromes in dogs and cattle resulting from severe tissue damage. *Contributions to Microbiology and Immunology*, **7**, 103–19.

Murray, M. (1978) Anaemia of bovine African trypanosomiasis: an overview. In *Pathogenicity of Trypanosomes*. Proceedings of a workshop held at Nairobi, Kenya, November 1978.

Mwongela, G.N., Kovatch, R.M. & Fazil, M.A. (1981) Acute *T. vivax* infection in dairy cattle in Coast Province, Kenya. *Tropical Animal Health and Production*, **13**, 63–9.

Nantulya, V.M., Musoke, A.J., Rurangirwa, F.R., Saigar, N. & Minja, S.H. (1987) Monoclonal antibodies that distinguish *T. congolense, T. vivax* and *T. brucei. Parasite Immunology*, **9**, 421–31.

Njogu, A.R., Dolan, R.B., Wilson, A.J. & Sayer, P.P (1985) Trypanotolerance in E. African Orma Boran cattle. *Veterinary Record*, **117**, 632–6.

Paris, J., Murray, M. & McOdimba, F. (1982) A comparative evaluation of the parasitological techniques currently available for the diagnosis of African trypanosomiasis in cattle. *Acta Tropica*, **39**, 307–16.

Pilson, R.D. & Leggate, B.M. (1961) A diurnal and seasonal study of the feeding activity of *Glossina pallidipes* Aust. *Bulletin of Entomological Research*, **53**, 541–9.

Rae, P.F. & Luckins, A.G. (1984) Detection of circulating trypanosomal antigens by enzyme immunoassay. *Annals of Tropical Medicine and Parasitology*, **78**, 587–96.

Stephen, L.E. (1986) *Trypanosomiasis – A Veterinary Prospective*. Pergamon Press, Oxford.

Trail, J.C.M., Sones, K., Jibbo, J.M.C., Durkin, J., Light, D.E. & Murray, M. (1985) Productivity of Boran cattle maintained by chemoprophylaxis under trypanosomiasis risk. *ILCA Research Report* No. 9, Addis Ababa.

Whiteside, E.F. (1962) The control of cattle trypanosomiasis with drugs in Kenya: Methods and costs. *East African Agricultural and Forestry Journal*, **28**, 67–73.

Other problems

Van Amstel, S.R., Reyers, F., Oberem, P.T. & Mathee, O. (1987) Further pathological studies of the clinical pathology of sweating sickness in cattle. *Onderstepoort Journal of Veterinary Research*, **54**, 45–8.

Further Reading

Sewell, M.M.H. & Bracklesby, D.W. (1990) *Handbook on Animal Diseases in the Tropics*, 47th edn, pp. 1–385, Baillière, Tindall, London.

Chapter 48: Other Conditions

by A.H. ANDREWS

Anaphylaxis

Aetiology

Anaphylaxis is the result of antigen–antibody reaction and when severe it can cause anaphylactic shock.

Epidemiology

The condition is usually very uncommon. Most cases follow the parenteral injection of drugs or biological products such as blood. Occasionally, the problem can arise through exposure via the alimentary tract or lungs. Signs may be seen in the system exposed, or they may be generalized. Most cases follow the introduction to the blood of an antigen to which the animal has already been sensitized, but reactions can occur where the animal is not known to have been exposed previously. More anaphylactic reactions occur in some herds and families of cattle than others. Reactions are most prevalent in Channel Island breeds. Initial signs tend to be largely of a respiratory nature, but other areas affected can be the alimentary tract and skin.

Signs

Reaction can occur about 20 minutes after the introduction of the antigen. The animal exhibits pronounced dyspnoea with, on auscultation, bubbling and emphysematous sounds. Muscle tremors can occur, which causes pyrexia to 40 °C (140 °F). Other reactions include bloat, diarrhoea, increased salivation, urticaria and rhinitis. Occasionally laminitis occurs. Death is due to anoxia. Following i.v. blood transfusion, there are usually hiccoughs and then dyspnoea, muscle tremors, salivation, coughing, lacrimation and fever.

Necropsy

At necropsy usually only the lungs are involved in acute cases, with marked pulmonary oedema and vascular engorgement; some animals develop emphysema. Longer-standing cases show hyperaemia and oedema of the abomasum and small intestines.

Diagnosis

Diagnosis depends on the history of recent introduction of an antigen to which the animal may previously have been exposed. The signs are helpful, being sudden with severe dyspnoea, urticaria, etc. Haematological examination shows increased packed cell volume, leucopenia and thrombocytopenia. Biochemical changes include a hyperkalaemia and blood histamine levels are raised in some cases. Finally, there is a response to therapy.

Differential diagnoses are few because of the rapid onset but acute pneumonia could be confused, although usually there is toxaemia and lesions are more pronounced in the arterio-ventral parts of the lungs.

Treatment and control

The most effective method of treatment is an intramuscular injection of adrenaline (4–5 ml of 1 in 1000 solution) and if necessary a fifth of the dose (0.2–0.5 ml) can be given intravenously, diluted to about a 2 per cent solution. Otherwise, corticosteroids can be administered or they may be given immediately following adrenaline as they potentiate the latter's activity. Antihistamines give variable results, partly because most histamine is released early in the reaction and also there are other mediators of the anaphylactic reactions. Various other compounds have been shown to alter the reaction of mediators and these include sodium meclofenamate, acetylsalicylic acid and diethylcarbamazine.

Once a reaction has occurred in an animal, the antigen causing the problem should not be re-introduced. If a blood transfusion is given, introduce up to 200 ml in a 450 kg (990 lb) animal and wait for about 10 minutes before injecting the remainder.

Amyloidosis

Aetiology

The aetiology of amyloidosis is uncertain but it is the result of a hyperglobulinaemia, probably causing an abnormal antigen–antibody response.

Epidemiology

Is a rare condition that is not fully understood. A few cases occur as the result of repeated antigen usage in the production of hyperimmune sera. However, most animals are affected sporadically and spontaneously following prolonged suppurative infections. The origin of amyloid, which is a glycoprotein, is not certain, but is thought to be due to an abnormality of the antigen–antibody reaction. Renal amyloidosis is the most commonly recognized condition, but amyloid can also be deposited in the liver and spleen. When the main organ affected is the liver, there tends to be proteinuria. This leads to hypoproteinaemia and then oedema of the organ, resulting in marked anasarca. The diarrhoea produced is partly due to amyloid deposition and oedema of the intestinal wall. Many of the animals affected are still growing. Foci of inflammation found can include traumatic reticulo-peritonitis, traumatic pericarditis, salpingitis, mastitis, metritis (Johnson & Jamison, 1984) and nephritis.

Signs

Usually, the affected animal is thin and emaciated. In most cases there is marked anasarca with an enlarged liver palpated in the right sublumbar fossa and an enlarged kidney with loss of its lobular structure when palpated via the rectum. There is usually polydipsia and a profuse watery diarrhoea. The animals later become uraemic, recumbent and comatosed. Death occurs two to five weeks after the onset of signs. Almost all cases will eventually die unless slaughtered.

Necropsy

At necropsy there are usually one or more chronic suppurative processes present in the organs. The carcass is emaciated, usually with marked oedema. The affected organs are enlarged and pale in colour. The kidney and liver have diffuse amyloid infiltration, while in the spleen it is more localized. The amyloid can be shown by aqueous iodine staining.

Diagnosis

Diagnosis depends on signs, including an enlarged kidney, diarrhoea and oedema. There is hypoproteinaemia, proteinuria and hyperfibrinogenaemia. Blood biochemical examination shows hypomagnesaemia and at the lower end of the normal range serum calcium level. There is also a high serum urea nitrogen and high serum creatinine. The specific gravity of the urine is low and there is a prolonged bromsulphthalein (BSP) clearance test.

Differential diagnoses are few but include pyelonephritis where there is pus and haematuria, and congestive heart failure in which there is an increased heart rate, respiratory embarrassment and dyspnoea.

Treatment

No successful therapy: cattle should be slaughtered.

Congestive heart failure

Aetiology

The condition can follow diseases of the pericardium, myocardium or endocardium.

Epidemiology

It is relatively uncommon and mainly affects older cattle. Pericarditis or hydropericardium can interfere with the normal filling of the heart during diastole. Pulmonary hyperaemia, which may occur in diffuse fibrosing alveolitis, can result in right-sided congestive heart failure. In cattle, the main cause of myocardial disease is foot-and-mouth disease. Endocardial diseases are the most common and are usually due to infection or inflammation.

When extra demand is placed on the heart, or the myocardial activity is reduced, then compensation can occur by an increased heart rate, increased filling of the ventricles and improved cardiac performance. There is also dilatation and hypertrophy. Venous return increases in speed and blood distribution changes so that there is an increase in blood volume, a decrease in renal blood flow and sodium retention. Cardiac response is reduced and the animal is less able to cope with unusual exercise or other emergencies (Blood *et al.*, 1983). There is a decrease in exercise tolerance and once the compensating mechanisms have been overcome then the heart cannot cope and congestive heart failure develops. Many of the signs of cardiac insufficiency are the result of increased venous pressure. They result in congestion of organs or oedema and the decreased output produces tissue hypoxia.

Failure of the right-sided ventricle causes congestion of the major circulation with reduced blood flow through the kidney, resulting in anoxic damage to the glomeruli and venous congestion of the portal system of the liver, and eventually there is transudation into the intestinal lumen giving rise to diarrhoea. Left-sided ventricular failure results in engorgement and oedema of the lungs. Both left and right-sided failure can occur together.

Signs

Early signs are of reduced exercise tolerance with increased respiratory effort and tachypnoea following light exercise. Pulse and respiratory rates take a long time to return to normal. On percussion the heart area may be enlarged.

In left-sided failure: lungs are mainly affected so that there is a cough, tachypnoea and hyperpnoea. The heart rate is increased and a murmur may be present in the region of the aorta or left atrioventricular valve. On auscultation there are moist noises at the ventral edges of the pulmonary field and on percussion increased dullness on the lower borders of the lung. Later on there is cyanosis and dyspnoea.

In right-sided failure or cor pulmonale: appetite is poor and the animal is dull with a rapid loss of condition. There are marked areas of oedema often affecting the skin of the lower part of the body, the neck and the submandibular space. There is ascites, hydropericardium and hydrothorax. The liver may be enlarged enough to be palpated in the right sublumbar fossa. The heart rate tends to be increased and there is hyperpnoea and often slight tachypnoea. There is a marked jugular pulse. Prognosis usually poor in all cases.

Necropsy

At post-mortem examination there are abnormalities of the pericardium, myocardium or endocardium. Usually, there is pulmonary congestion and oedema. In left-sided failure there is subcutaneous oedema, hydrothorax, ascites and hydropericardium.

Diagnosis

Diagnosis is by the signs, particularly those of oedema. The heart rate is elevated and there is an increased area of cardiac dullness; abnormal heart sounds may be present, depending on the cause. Insertion of a needle into a vein shows a markedly increased venous pressure. Aspiration of fluid from oedematous areas shows it to be a transudate containing large amounts of protein. There is also a proteinuria.

Differential diagnosis

Differential diagnosis includes amyloidosis but diarrhoea tends to be marked and the kidneys are enlarged without heart abnormality. In chronic peritonitis there is often some pain and the aspirated abdominal fluid contains many leucocytes. In bladder rupture there is a normal heart and urine is present in the abdomen. In liver fibrosis the heart is normal and there is usually jaundice or photosensitization. Parasitic gastroenteritis occurs in a younger animal and there is oedema, mainly of the submandibular area, with a high faecal egg count. Fascioliasis could confuse but again there is usually only submandibular oedema and a faecal egg count. Fog fever (p. 674) could cause problems in diagnosis but usually several animals are affected quite suddenly in the autumm. Anaphylaxis is also a sudden problem with no cardiac signs.

Treatment

The primary cause should be treated as effectively as possible but with most cases the prognosis is poor. Where oedema is present it is partly due to sodium retention and so the salt intake should be kept as low as possible. Diuretics such as frusemide or hydrochlorothiazide are useful and they can be given by injection or orally. The heart can be treated to improve contractility by use of etamiphylline camsylate, theophylline or digitalis derivatives. The use of digitalis by mouth is probably of limited value because of breakdown in the rumen. Parenteral administration of digitalis extracts is little used for several reasons: intravenous use could result in toxicity whereas intramuscular administration gives variable results. Little can be done to control the congestive heart failure except to treat all infections quickly and adequately.

Diabetes mellitus

This is a very unusual condition in cattle compared with its relatively frequent occurrence in dogs and cats. However, lesions can occur in the pancreas resulting in this condition. It is usually seen in old cattle and often animals will have had other problems such as fatty liver. The signs are loss of condition with polydipsia and polyuria. There is no rise in temperature and the urine contains both ketones and glucose. Biochemical examination of the blood shows hyperglycaemia. Usually treatment is not contemplated.

Hypothermia

Aetiology

This is also called cold stress and is mainly seen in young calves in severe climatic conditions, particularly where there is wind chilling as well as a cold ambient temperature. The problem is not encountered anything like as commonly as in lambs.

Epidemiology

Exposure to cold conditions mainly occurs in calves of cows calving outside in the winter months with no shelter. It is particularly prevalent in suckler calves and occurs more frequently in countries such as Canada and Australia than say Britain. Mortality is usually higher in calves born in winter and early spring. There is a delay in the onset and rate of immunoglobulin absorption from colostrum in cold-stressed calves. Primary hypothermia with no associated disease can be seen in young calves, and secondary hypothermia with no other disease has been recorded in older calves.

Signs

The rectal temperature may be low and can be defined as a temperature less than 37 °C (98.5 °F) and there is shivering. Shivering appears to be more intense during the initial period following exposure to cold. Most calves have no problems in the cold but some are depressed and stand or walk about stiffly. A few animals may remain in sternal recumbency. The heart rate tends to be raised but respiratory rate is low.

Necropsy

At post mortem the most common lesions involve the limbs and include subcutaneous oedema and haemorrhage. Experimentally, more haemorrhages occur in the hindlimbs. Some animals show oedema of the ventral sternum. The joints may show mild to severe haemorrhage and acute synovitis. Some cases show haemorrhages of the adrenal glands and oedema of the iliac and jejunal lymph nodes.

Diagnosis

Diagnosis depends on the history and signs. Increased serum glucose and phosphorus levels occur with cooling but fall during recovery.

Treatment

Treatment is by immersion in warm water, which results in quicker rewarming than use of a heat pad or heat lamp. A hot air environment could be constructed with a straw bale shelter and a hot air heater. Control is by ensuring that adequate shelter is provided or by housing cattle during the bad weather.

Lightning strike/electrocution

Aetiology

This is exposure to high voltage electric currents, either natural or generated by man.

Epidemiology

The condition is uncommon but it is often of interest as it is one of the few problems that farmers have usually insured against. Problems arise from lightning, exposure of electrical wires or faulty wiring or earthing in farm buildings. Cases may be single or a group. In many instances, damp ground or floors help to conduct the electricity. Low voltages of 110–220 V are sufficient to kill cattle. Outside, trees such as oak, poplar, elm and conifers are all prone to lightning strike.

Signs

The signs in the severe form are such that animals die without a struggle. Burns or singeing may be seen because of the severity and often they involve the muzzle and feet. Death is usually due to paralysis of the medullary centre, accompanied in some cases by ventricular fibrillation. In the less severe form the animal becomes unconscious for a varying time and there is usually some sign of a struggle. After regaining consciousness there may be dullness, blindness, paralysis of one or more legs, and surface hyperaesthesia. The signs may persist or slowly disappear over a period of up to two weeks. If burns are present, sloughing of the skin in the area is seen. Minor problems may occur such as the animal may jump, be restless, show periodic convulsions or be knocked down.

In lightning strike the animal is usually close to a fence, barn, trees or a pond. Often there are signs of burning affecting these objects. The animal itself may show singeing of the hair or burn marks on the muzzle and feet. Half-chewed food may be present in the mouth. The animal quickly becomes distended with gas and decomposes rapidly. Blood often exudes from the nostrils, rectum and vulva. The pupils are dilated and the anus relaxed. There tend to be petechial haemorrhages throughout the body and the viscera are congested. The superficial lymph nodes are often haemorrhagic.

Diagnosis

Diagnosis depends on the history of a storm, position of the animal near trees, etc. and sudden death of a group of animals. The signs may also be helpful such as singeing of the hair, burns on the muzzle and feet and evidence of sudden death.

Differential diagnosis

Differential diagnosis includes anaphylaxis but there is marked pulmonary involvement. Acute heart failure can cause problems but there is engorgement of visceral veins and macroscopic or microscopic myocardial lesions. Brain trauma can occur but usually there is a haemorrhagic lesion of the brain. Nitrate/nitrite poisoning results in sudden death but methaemoglobin is present. Anthrax can be confused, but stained blood smears assist in determination. Bloat is a possibility but on necropsy the front part of the animal is congested, there is a distended rumen and sometimes froth present. Blackleg results in swelling of the part affected with the causal organism present.

Treatment

No treatment is usually given as often the cattle are either better or dead before any therapy can be administered. Central nervous system stimulants can be given. Artificial respiration may be helpful. Although nothing can be done about lightning strike, all electrical installations should be properly fitted and earthed.

Meloidosis

Aetiology

The cause is *Pseudomonas* (*Malleomyces*) *pseudomallei*. It can survive for long periods in the soil and water.

Epidemiology

The condition is primarily a disease of rodents but occasionally it spreads to man and farm animals such as sheep, goats, horses and pigs. It is very rare in cattle. The disease was first recognized in South East Asia but it is now seen in Australia, Malaysia, Papua New Guinea and Nigeria. Infection is passed in the faeces of rodents and is spread by ingestion of contaminated feed or water, by insect bites, wounds and possibly inhalation. Mortality is high and disease lasts about two to eight weeks.

Signs

The main signs are a marked pyrexia with anorexia and a thick yellow exudate from the eyes and nose. Nervous signs may be exhibited. Some cattle have infection without signs.

Pathology

There are multiple abscesses in many areas of the body as well as in the subcutaneous tissues and associated lymph nodes. The size of the abscesses is variable from a few millimetres to over 2.5 cm in diameter.

Diagnosis

This depends on demonstrating the causal organism by culture from pus, nasal discharges or blood.

Treatment

There is little information available on satisfactory treatment of meloidosis. Chloramphenicol is used in man and *in vitro* tests suggest oxytetracycline may be of use in animals, and perhaps novobiocin, chloramphenicol and sulphadiazine. Treatment is to be discouraged because of the possibility of spread to humans.

Control

Infected animals: slaughtered, disposed of by burning. In-contact animals slaughtered, the premises disinfected.

Mycotic diseases

Mucormycosis

Aetiology

There are various fungi of the family Mucoraceae that can cause infection, including the genera *Absidia*, *Entomophthora*, *Mortierella*, *Mucor*, *Rhizopus*.

Epidemiology

The fungi occur usually in soil and water and are often plant pathogens and food decomposers. They are opportunistic.

Signs

Infection can cause a necrotic placentitis in cattle resulting in abortion at three to seven months gestation. There is necrosis of maternal cotyledons and yellow, raised, leathery lesions on the intercotyledonary areas. Granulomatous lesions of the mesenteric and mediastinal lymph nodes can occur. Calves can develop alimentary tract lesions after prolonged antibiotic therapy. Following acidosis the ruminal wall can be invaded with *Rhizopus* spp.

Diagnosis

Hyphae are present on smears of cotyledons, fetal stomach and skin. The lymph nodes need to be examined. There may be a history of antibiotic usage and on post mortem there may be abomasal ulceration. The animal will become black tinted.

Prevention and control

As the fungi are ubiquitous it is impossible to control properly. There are no satisfactory antibiotics.

Cryptococcosis

Aetiology

The cause is *Cryptococcus* (*Saccharomyces*) *neoformans* (synonyms *C. hominis*, *Torula histolytica*).

Epidemiology

The incidence is world-wide and is high in areas of warmth and moisture.

Signs

Latent. There is a mastitis in many cases with no visible signs in the udder or milk.

Severe. The quarter(s) swells slowly and becomes firm and swollen. The subcutaneous tissue also develops oedema, which persists for several weeks. There is often some discomfort with the legs held apart. Pyrexia occurs up to 40 °C (104 °F) with anaemia. The supramammary lymph nodes are enlarged. Milk production is reduced but the milk itself shows few changes except a few flakes. Later, in persistent cases, there is a watery secretion.

Mild. A swelling of the quarter(s) is seen with little effect on the milk. Occasionally a granulomatous meningoencephalitis may develop or the nasal mucosal may show nodular lesions.

Pathology

Infection is mainly confined to the udder, although there may also be reddening and thickening of the brain tissue and oedema, and naso- or oropharyngeal nodules.

Diagnosis

Diagnosis is by direct examination of the fluids.

Prevention and control

Ensure proper disinfection.

Rhinosporidiasis

Aetiology

The causative organism is *Rhinosporidium seeberi*.

Epidemiology

The disease is distributed world-wide.

Signs

There is the formation of large polyps in the posterior nares and this interferes with respiration. The lesions are small, about 0.5–3 cm in diameter. They are soft, friable and bleed. The surface of the polyp shows many small white specks. The nasal discharge results in dyspnoea with mucopurulent and bloody discharge.

Pathology

There is a polyp of papillomatous epithelium, which is hyperplastic and contains numerous sporangia.

Diagnosis

Isolation of organism provides the diagnosis.

Treatment

Polyps are best removed surgically.

Candidiasis (moniliasis)

Aetiology

The main causal agent is *Candida albicans* but *C. tropicalis*, *C. krusei*, *C. parapsilosis* and *C. guillermondii* can also initiate disease.

Epidemiology

The organisms are world-wide and found in animal faeces.

Signs

A chronic pneumonia can occur with dyspnoea plus only a moderate fever. There is a profuse stringy salivation and brown-streaked nasal discharge. Abortion can occur and there can also be mastitis with mild transient signs that are self-terminating. Where there is severe mastitis it may follow the use of intramammary tubes. The udder is swollen and spongy and the animal's temperature is 40–41.5 °C (104–107 °F).

Diagnosis

Isolation of the organism provides the diagnosis.

Treatment and control

There is a limit to what can be done but amphotericin B can be successful. An iodine in liquid paraffin intramammary infusion can be left in the udder for 10–15 minutes, and then stripped out. This is repeated in seven days, and oral iodides may be given if necessary.

Aspergillosis

Aetiology

There are many *Aspergillus* spp. including *Aspergillus fumigatus*, *A. flavus*, *A. niger* and *A. terreus*.

Epidemiology

The organisms are widespread. Placental infection of cattle is thought to be via abomasal ulcers or from the respiratory tract. It also occurs following inhalation of spores from mouldy straw, hay and sugar-beet pulp. Outbreaks of abortions can occur following the feeding of mouldy silage.

Signs

Aspergillosis is a quite common cause of abortion with a placentitis. Abortion is in the sixth to eighth month of pregnancy. Another form is a fatal gastroenteritis with ulceration of forestomachs and oesophagus. Pulmonary aspergillosis also occurs in animals subjected to diarrhoea and poor ventilation. There is fever and dyspnoea.

Diagnosis

Examine placental direct smears for fungi. Culture stomach contents or cotyledon.

Treatment and control

Nystatin can be used in the treatment of diarrhoea. There is no effective preventive but avoid feeding mouldy silage to cows in mid to late pregnancy. Definitely mouldy straw or hay should not be used in enclosed buildings, and preferably not at all.

Histoplasmosis

Aetiology

There are two species causing infection, *Histoplasma capsulatum* and *H. duboisii*.

Epidemiology

Whereas *H. capsulatum* is found world-wide, *H. duboisii* is only found in Africa. It is a rare condition but can occur in man and other species. *Histoplasma capsulatum* is found in the soil. Infection follows inhalation of contaminated dust and entry to the lung.

Signs

Affected cattle may show chronic emaciation, dyspnoea, diarrhoea, swelling of the brisket and grinding of the teeth. At post-mortem examination there is an enlarged liver, ascites, oedematous thickening of the large intestine and interstitial emphysema. Histologically, eosinophilic round bodies can be found in endothelial cells.

Diagnosis

Diagnosis is from the signs, and samples should be taken for culture and histology.

Treatment and control

Amphotericin B given intravenously at 1 mg/kg body weight daily has been effective but a prolonged course may lead to side-effects. The imidazoles may be satisfactory.

Teat burns

Epidemiology

In parts of the world where forest and grass fires are common, burns can result in damage necessitating the slaughter of cattle. However, in other cases the animals will survive but there may be injury to the teats or udder. In such cases it is necessary to provide an accurate prognosis. Often several teats are affected.

Signs

The lesions can be assessed according to the severity of the burn (Morton *et al.*, 1987).

Mild burns are reddened with a loss of the outer, white, paper-thin tissue, which sloughs. A teat may have normal tissue interspersed with multiple small black areas over the teat surface or a uniform relatively thick black or red–brown surface layer. There may be areas of sloughing or crusts that develop in the tissue and milk is apparently normal. In all cases the teats are pliable on palpation.

Severe burns. The teats tend to be dull brown or black, dry and often are corrugated. If sloughing has occurred then a thick layer (over 1 mm thick) of tissue is sloughed. Underneath there is red haemorrhagic tissue. On palpation the teat is leather-like and lacks pliability. In some cases the teats tend to be distorted, especially in heifers.

Prognosis

With mild lesions prognosis is good. In severe lesions prognosis is variable but tends to be better in cows than heifers. Some cows only show partial return to function with reduced milk flow.

Treatment

Treatment can increase recovery. Application of 0.5 per cent cetrimide in lanolin daily is helpful. However, healing is slow, taking about 14 weeks. When the surface skin starts to peel antibiotic ointment is helpful. Teat orifice restrictions often respond to surgery.

Water availability

Water debility need not necessarily damage cattle in the dry season in semi-arid regions. Some breeds are obviously less susceptable. They are less affected when they are on pastures containing a very low crude protein level. If fed a high plane of nutrition without water, problems could arise but in practice this is unlikely to occur. The amount of water required varies but is obviously higher in a dairy cow than a beef animal. Animals are capable of being watered only once every three days if necessary but they should not have to walk more than about 2.5 km to it. If water deprivation occurs there is a reduction in milk or meat deposition. If dehydration persists there is circulatory collapse when the level of sodium reaches 170 mEq/l.

Heat stress

Acute heat stress

If the heat produced by the animal and the heat absorbed from the atmosphere is higher than the heat lost then the animal's temperature will rise. It thus develops hyperthermia and if the rise is great and sudden the animals will pant, salivate excessively, become restless and then prostrate. Problems often occur if cattle are made to walk long distances. Heat stroke can occur at a normal outside temperature if they are packed tightly in poorly ventilated vehicles travelling during the hottest parts of the day.

If action is not quick death occurs. Affected animals should be sprayed with cold water. They should be kept in the shade and attempts made to increase the air flow. Clipping the hair, particularly along the mane, withers and backbone, will assist but such animals are then susceptible to direct sunlight and so they should be kept in the shade.

Chronic heat stress

The chronic or subacute form occurs more frequently than acute heat stress. When exposed to high temperatures cattle compensate by increasing their loss of heat by panting and sweating. They can also reduce heat production by reducing food intake, drinking more and reducing activity. Cattle are able to accept high midday temperatures if the evenings and nights are cool.

In chronic heat stress there is decreased milk production, reduction in weight gain and sexual maturity. There is also some loss in fertility particularly involving spermatogenesis in the bull. When animals are affected they should be provided with shelter or otherwise given access to well-ventilated shady areas. Oestrus suppression may also occur. When cattle are grazed in very hot conditions grazing should be restricted to the evenings, nights and mornings. If necessary zero-grazing may need to be adopted. In such circumstances, where the air is hot and humid, then every attempt must be made to ensure good air flow by louvred windows, fans, etc. The cattle should receive an adequate amount of water. Feeding at night will also ensure maximum heat production is during the cool period.

Malignant catarrhal fever

Aetiology

Also known as bovine malignant catarrh and malignant head catarrh. Caused by two different agents but clinically identical. In many countries only one of the agents is present. The African strain, (alcelaphine herpes virus 1 and 2 or bovid herpes virus 3) is wildebeest-associated. The European, North American and Asian strain has not been characterized but is sheep-associated.

Epidemiology

Malignant catarrhal fever (MCF) has a sporadic worldwide distribution. It mainly affects single animals although outbreaks have occurred. The wildebeest strain is seen in Africa and in zoological gardens. The sheep-associated strain occurs when sheep associate with cattle, which are considered 'dead-end' hosts. The African form is more easily transmitted, transferred via the placenta into the foetus. Soon after birth, the wildebeest calf sheds infection which can be contracted by other species. Transmission of the sheep form is not known although cattle have usually been in contact with pregnant or lambing sheep. The virus is fragile and does not survive more than a day outside the host. There may be many distinct MCF virus forms.

The incubation period is shorter for the African form. Following infection, there is an eclipse phase of nine to seventeen days, then viraemia continues until death. After a further three to fifteen days, signs develop, followed by death five to ten days after their onset. Transmission is probably by inhalation or possibly blood transfusion.

Signs

Cases are sporadic. Animals are very ill with anorexia, pyrexia (40.5–41.5°C; 105–107°F), depression and loss of condition. An early pathognomonic sign is an intense scleral congestion with bilateral keratitis and corneal opacity starting at the edge of the sclera, causing blindness. Early lesions also involve the buccal mucosa, with reddening of the lips, gingivae and muzzle. Erosions develop, including necrosis of the tips of the labial papillae and the mouth corners.

Other signs vary. They can include nervous signs such as muscle tremors and hyperaesthesia. The superficial lymph nodes are grossly enlarged. There is profuse mucopurulent oculo-nasal discharge which can encrust around the nostrils and eyes. There is often excessive salivation, followed by dysponea and stertor due to exudate accumulation. Faeces vary between profuse diarrhoea and soft, scanty faeces. Laminitis and dermatitis can occur in the sheep-associated form.

At later stages, more prominent nervous signs may occur, such as incoordination, leg weakness and nystagmus followed finally in some by head pressing, convulsions or paralysis.

Uncommonly, a mild form occurs with mild, transient fever and some oral and nasal mucosal erosions. These animals can recover.

Necropsy

Lesions occur in many parts of the body including the respiratory, alimentary and urinary tracts. They include varying degrees of haemorrhage, hyperaemia and discrete or extensive erosions. The eyes show scleral congestion and keratitis. The lymph nodes show marked enlargement. The skin around the coronets may show lesions. Histologically, the epidermis shows extensive hydropic degeneration and vesicle formation with rupture. The dermis shows vasculitis with proliferation and necrosis and marked lymphoid cuffing.

Diagnosis

History helps with a record of other species contact and one animal affected. Nervous signs, lymph node enlargement, scleral congestion, corneal opacity, diffuse mucosal erosion are indicators. At necropsy the histological presence of vasculitis confirms diagnosis. There is leukopenia. Serological tests can be used in the African form. Viral isolation or transmission can be attempted.

Differential diagnosis

Differential diagnosis includes mucosal disease but ocular lesions are not severe and there is no lymph node enlargement. Rinderpest and foot-and-mouth disease are herd problems with no severe ocular lesions. Infectious bovine rhinotracheitis usually affects several animals, with mainly respiratory signs. Calf diphtheria does not produce ocular signs.

Treatment and control

There is no treatment or suitable vaccine. Infected animals should be separated from others. Cattle should not be grazed with sheep, particularly at the time of lambing, nor near wildebeest. Bough-in sheep should come from disease-free farms.

References

Blood, D.C., Radostits, O.M. & Henderson, J.A. (1983) *Veterinary Medicine*, 6th edn, pp. 273–5. Baillière Tindall, London.

Johnson, R. & Jamison, K. (1984) Amyloidosis in six dairy cows. *Journal of the American Veterinary Medical Association*, **185**, 1538–43.

Morton, J.M., Fitzpatrick, D.H., Morris, D.C. & White, M.B. (1987) Teat burns in dairy cattle — the prognosis and effect of treatment. *Australian Veterinary Journal*, **64**, 69–72.

Chapter 49: Welfare

by D.M. BROOM

Introduction

Most of this book is directly relevant to the improvement of cattle welfare as it refers to the treatment or prevention of disease and the welfare of animals severely affected by disease is poor. There are often links between disease and other sorts of welfare problems (Gibson, 1988) both in the consequences of disease for welfare and in the increased susceptibility of animals to disease when their welfare is poor. Many welfare problems, however, are a consequence of inadequacies of management and housing and these will be discussed in this chapter.

Welfare definition

The welfare of an individual is its state as regards its attempts to cope with its environment (Broom, 1986). When conditions are difficult, individuals use various methods to try to counteract any adverse effects of those conditions on themselves. These attempts may be unsuccessful or they may succeed but the effects of lack of success and the extent of what is done to try to cope can be measured. Hence welfare varies on a continuum from very good to very poor and it can be assessed precisely. The assessment of welfare can be carried out in a scientific way without the involvement of moral considerations. The question which is asked after the measurement is made is: How poor must the welfare be before people consider the condition or treatment to be unacceptable? A moral decision must be taken here and different people will draw the line, marking what is unacceptable, at different levels in the welfare continuum. The moral decision depends upon the availability of evidence about welfare but the process of deciding about morality and the process of assessing welfare are quite separate.

Welfare problem areas

Whilst cattle management has been changing, our knowledge of cattle physiology and behaviour has been improving. It is clear that cattle have complex regulatory processes, elaborate social structure and sophisticated learning ability (Broom, 1981; Craig, 1981; Kilgour & Dalton, 1984; Stricklin & Kautz-Scanavy, 1984; Fraser & Broom, 1990). These results have made many animal scientists reconsider the effects of conditions and procedures on farms, both in terms of their efficiency as regards production and with respect to the welfare of the animals.

The general range of welfare problem areas is the same for cattle as for other farm animals (Table 49.1). Ill-treatment refers principally to physical abuse of animals. Neglect includes failing to give food and water, or to clean out, or to treat disease, or to assist as necessary at calving. Accommodation for animals may, for example, give insufficient space, poor flooring or poor food access and conditions indoors or outdoors may lead to risk of injury (Schlichting & Smidt, 1987).

Table 49.1 Possible causes of cattle welfare problems

Ill-treatment
Neglect: calculated, accidental, or due to lack of knowledge
Inadequacies in design of housing/furniture
Inadequate management system or poor husbandry on the farm
Unnecessary or poorly executed operations on the animals
Poor conditions and procedures
During transport
At market
At slaughterhouse

Management methods and husbandry include all aspects of feeding, moving of animals, grouping, milking, serving, etc. Farm operations require some special mention, both as regards the methods used and the consequences for the animals. Methods of handling and moving animals are of importance before and after transport, at markets and at lairage as well as on the farm. There are also special problems of transport vehicle construction and usage, market accommodation and procedures, and slaughter methods. Welfare problems that should be taken into account in cattle practice have been reviewed by Broom (1988).

Welfare and production

Improved welfare often leads to improved production. If the welfare of a dairy cow is improved there is often a greater milk yield and if the welfare of very young calves is improved, the resulting increases in growth rate and survival chances lead to economic advantages for the farmer. In other situations, however, improving welfare leads to reduced profits, for example when stocking density is decreased the benefit of welfare. Modern cattle husbandry systems do lead to some welfare problems, as discussed below. A general change in cattle management methods has been an increase in production pressure. Nutritional expertise has increased to the point where animals now convert feed to meat and milk very efficiently. If animals are pushed hard energetically, there need not be welfare problems and management difficulties but these are more likely and should be taken into account when advising farmers about which system to choose.

Ill-treatment and neglect

Human actions that can lead to poor cattle welfare include ill-treatment, neglect and inadequate production systems. Ill-treatment occurs most frequently when animals are being moved around the farm, when they are being loaded into or out of vehicles, or when they are at market or lairage. Those who do ill-treat animals can be advised of likely economic effects of their actions as well as being told about the laws on the subject. Neglect includes failure to provide an adequate diet, failure to treat disease and the lack of normal husbandry procedures. The diet may be inadequate in nutrient composition or in quantity. Cattle are sometimes undernourished for a period, whilst food is scarce or expensive, with the expectation that compensatory growth will occur when more food is provided. If the undernourishment amounts to starvation and this is clear from the condition of the animal, then this is serious neglect. Lack of knowledge on the part of the farmer may result in the provision of a poor diet or in failure to treat disease. This is poor husbandry, a very important cause of welfare problems. Advice on good husbandry methods can be an important veterinary service. If animals are diseased and require treatment there is a moral obligation upon the veterinarian to treat them. In the UK, the veterinary oath, which is sworn on admission to Membership of the Royal College of Veterinary Surgeons, includes the promise that 'my constant endeavour will be to ensure the welfare of animals committed to my care'. In certain circumstances, treatment without any prospect of payment may be necessary. In other circumstances it may be best to call in the State Veterinary Service, the police, or the RSPCA, even if to do so might mean losing a client.

Housing and management

General points

Feeding of housed cattle may lead to difficulties for the animals because the acquisition of food in housing conditions is very different from that when grazing. Physical difficulties may occur, as described by Cermak (1987), but social factors are also very important. Cattle synchronize their feeding to a large extent (Benham, 1982; Potter & Broom, 1987) so where group feeding is possible, enough feeding places for each animal are required (Metz, 1983; Wierenga, 1983). Those animals that cannot find a feeding place may not get sufficient food and it is likely that there are adverse effects on their welfare. The precise effects of the frustration that occurs when food is inaccessible because of competition remain to be determined. Competitive feeding situations where there are no individual feeding places pose extra problems for cattle. The subordinate individual has to attempt to obtain food

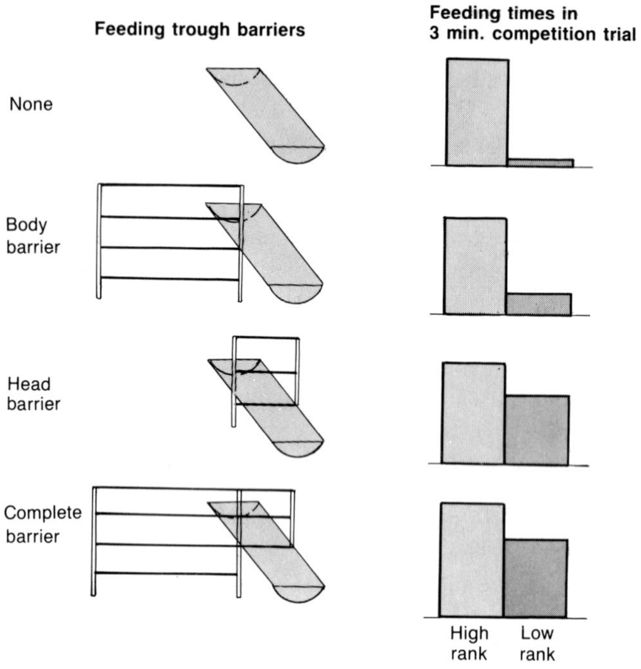

Fig. 49.1 Physical barriers affected feeding times by cows ranking high and low in a competitive order. With no barrier (a) the low ranking cows were scarcely able to feed. A body barrier (b) improved the situation slightly for the low ranking cows but a head barrier (c) and a complete barrier (d) had a much greater effect (redrawn after Craig, 1981; data from Bouissou, 1970).

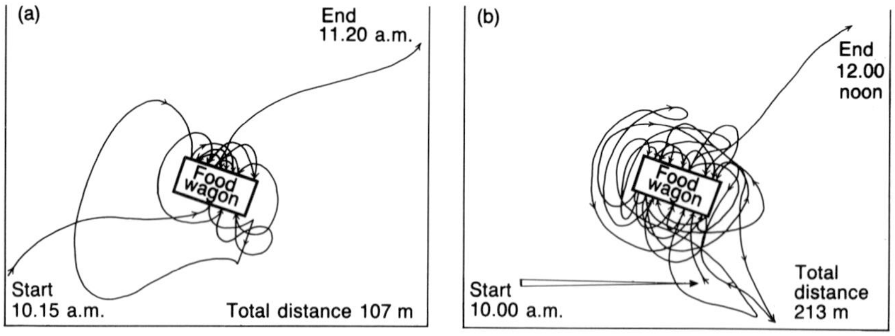

Fig. 49.2 The paths of two cows in a herd after food is provided in a food wagon are shown. Animal (a) was found to be high in a competitive order whereas animal (b), which was low in that order, walked further because of displacement at the food wagon and took longer to feed (after Broom, 1981; modified after Albright, 1969).

despite the attacks or threats of other individuals. Bouissou (1970) found that the greater the extent of the barrier between feeding places for cows, the fewer the attacks that occurred (Fig. 49.1). A trough that requires subordinate cows to come close to dominant individuals results in those subordinates walking greater distances and taking longer to obtain a meal (Albright, 1969; Fig. 49.2). Calves of low social rank obtain less of the favoured food if trough space is restricted (Broom & Leaver, 1978; Broom, 1982). In order to minimize such welfare problems, which are often associated with poor weight gain, farmers should provide feeding spaces for all individuals, preferably with barriers between the individual places. Adaptation to a single food source is possible for cattle, however, for a transponder-operated feeding stall can be quite successful (Albright, 1981), but certain individuals in a herd may have difficulties in such systems.

Another general problem for housed cattle is having to stand on floors that are wet, slippery, uneven, or hazardous because of sharp edges. Slippery slats can lead to difficulties in standing or lying (Andreae & Smidt, 1982; Fig. 49.3). These and other inadequacies of flooring can result in limb injuries, foot lameness, tail-tip necrosis and various diseases. Lameness is the greatest welfare problem of housed dairy cows and factors influencing its occurrence include floor quality and poor drainage, which results in cows standing in slurry (Wierenga & Peterse, 1987).

Calf welfare

In the first few days after birth the major calf welfare problems are enteric and respiratory diseases. The calves of dairy cows may fail to obtain sufficient colostrum for a variety of reasons (Edwards, 1982;

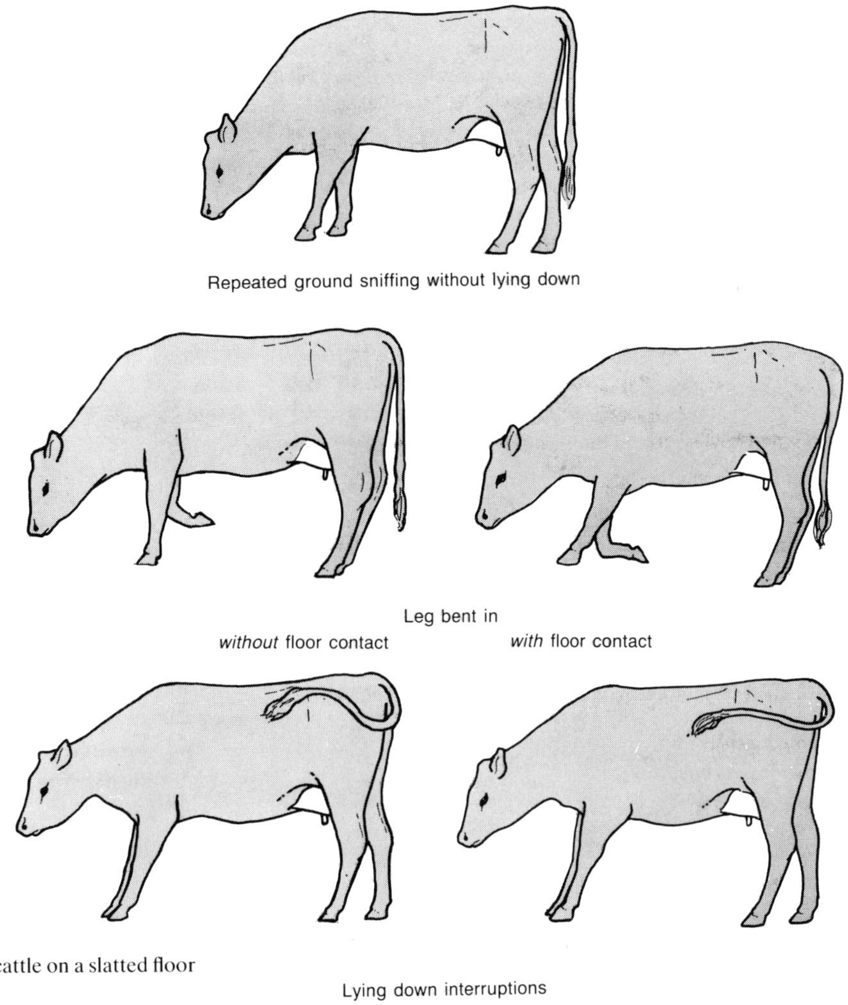

Fig. 49.3 Behavioural alterations in young cattle on a slatted floor (after Andreae & Smidt, 1982).

Edwards & Broom, 1982; Broom, 1983a). Management practices that maximize the chance that colostrum will be obtained and minimize contact with pathogens have important beneficial effects on calf welfare. If calves of dairy cows are normally left with their mother for the first 24 or 48 hours, the risk that the calf will not suckle early enough to obtain and absorb the immunoglobulin from colostrum can be minimized by the stockworker placing one of the mother's teats in the mouth of the calf as early as possible after the calf stands. Group-calving situations where several cows calve during a short period can lead to a cow's colostrum being drunk by a calf other than her own or to calves being rejected by their own mothers. Such occurrences can be prevented by providing separate calving boxes, which should ideally allow the cows some visual contact with other cows. The provision of soft bedding for the calf is also desirable and is easier where special calving accommodation is available.

Dairy calves are deprived of their mother from an early age and many are individually housed so that they are confined in a small space and deprived of all or most social contacts. In the EC, 7 million out of a total of 22 million calves per annum are reared for veal in small crates and fed on a diet with inadequate iron and roughage (Susmel, 1987). Many animals used as replacements for dairy herds are also individually housed. The welfare problems resulting from this rearing method are substantial. Calves housed for long periods in small pens (Fig. 49.4) that do not allow them to turn around are deprived in various ways. Firstly, the typical veal calf crate does not allow the animal to groom the hind part of its body. All calves do groom all of their body several times per day if given the opportunity to do so. The effects of being unable to groom a large part of the body are apparent in direct physical effects but the effects of the frustration that is likely to be associated with this inability is not known.

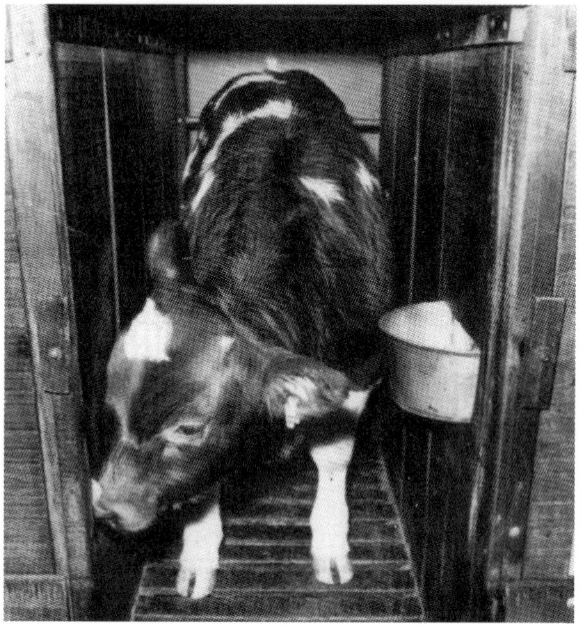

Fig. 49.4 Veal calf in crate with slatted floor. The front of the crate has been removed (after de Wilt, 1985).

The other effect on grooming when calves are housed in a small pen is that these calves show excessive amounts of grooming of those parts of the body which they can reach and this grooming often results in ingestion of much hair, with consequent formation of hair balls or bezoars in the rumen. These hair balls may on occasion block the exit from the rumen. Another restriction imposed by crates or other small pens is in the postures that can be adopted when lying. De Wilt (1985) reported that a common lying posture amongst group-housed calves involves turning the head backwards, whilst for 2–8 per cent of total lying time the hind legs are stretched out. Neither of these postures is possible in a crate so some frustration and discomfort is likely as a consequence. Stereotyped behaviours (Broom, 1983b) are shown by many crate-housed calves. Some licking is stereotyped but the commonest of such behaviours is tongue rolling. Table 49.2 shows the frequency of such behaviours in a large-scale study. Stereotyped behaviour is certainly abnormal and one of the behavioural responses to difficult conditions.

Other problems associated with close confinement include thermoregulatory difficulties and inability to escape from disturbing stimuli. In hot conditions calves stretch their limbs whilst lying but this is not possible in a small pen. An animal in a small pen may be frightened by human approach or by some sound but it is not able to avoid or retreat from the disturbing stimulus. There are no precise experimental data that allow the quantification of any adverse effects resulting from such restrictions on responses. Another major problem of individual housing is inability to show social behaviour. Young calves kept in groups interact with other calves frequently and associate closely. Individually reared calves cannot interact much with one another and long periods of social isolation lead to failure to develop normal social behaviour. When calves that were reared individually for many months were put in a social situation they failed to show some ear movements and other social signals and they did not retaliate if attacked. As a consequence they were unable to compete with animals reared in groups and they failed to grow as fast in a competitive feeding situation (Broom & Leaver, 1978; Broom, 1982).

Group housing can also lead to problems for some calves. Certain animals may show intersucking and urine drinking. This behaviour can lead to poor growth in those animals that drink urine and to soreness in the animals that are sucked. The problem is absent from many units and it is likely that current research will allow recommendations about management practices that will largely eliminate it. It is rarer in the UK, where dairy calves are usually left with the mother for 24 hours, than in countries like The Netherlands where bucket rearing from birth is common. In a study by de Wilt (1985) the use of teat buckets resulted in no preputial sucking whereas 48 per cent of calves given milk in open buckets did so but other studies in other conditions have not always given such results. Calves in groups sometimes fail to drink from teats connected to

Table 49.2 The incidence of oral stereotypies in calves kept in different conditions (per cent of time spent)

	Veal calves in crates	Veal calves in groups	Dairy calves in groups	Calves with suckler cow	Reference
Calves, 2 weeks	14	3	3	1	Webster *et al.* (1985a)
Calves, 10–14 weeks	16	4	2	0	

a milk reservoir but work by Barton (Barton, 1983; Barton & Broom, 1985) showed that in these young calves, aggressive behaviour was not the cause of this. Calves showed much social facilitation of feeding and for groups of 10 calves, the positioning of five milk supplying teats close together encouraged even the weaker calves to come to the teats and drink. Another group-housing system that can work well is an electronic feeder system triggered by transponders worn by the calves. This system facilitates rationing of milk but it allows only one calf to feed at a time. Straw-based group-housing systems are used extensively by commercial veal units in the UK and they result in low levels of disease and good economic returns (Webster *et al.*, 1986). With further refinement of management procedures such systems are likely to replace individual crate housing internationally as the normal method of calf housing.

Whether calves are kept in crates or in groups their diet has an effect on their welfare. The two commonest inadequacies are lack of iron and lack of roughage. The public demand for white veal results in many calves being fed an amount of iron that would inevitably result in their early death if they were not slaughtered whilst still young. The amount of iron needed to avoid anaemia and unnatural white meat is summarized in Fig. 49.5, which is taken from Webster *et al.* (1986). It is clear from Fig. 49.5 that some calves need more than 50 mg iron/kg dry food if they are not to be anaemic (haemoglobin <9 g/100 ml blood). As anaemia is a pathological sign it seems reasonable to assume that the welfare of anaemic calves is poor and hence that systems which produce white veal result in poor welfare for this reason as well as for other reasons stated above.

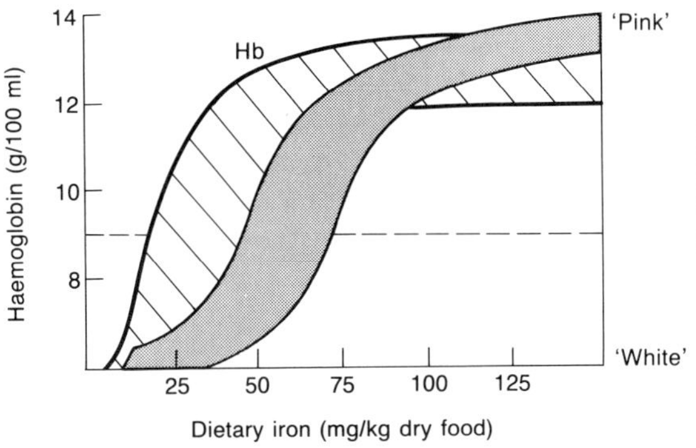

Fig. 49.5 Schematic relationships between dietary iron intake of calves and their blood haemoglobin concentration and meat colour (from Webster *et al.*, 1986).

Low roughage diets are also a consequence of white veal production. Calves are fed a diet that does not allow normal rumen development. Such conditions often result in ulceration of the abomasum. Diets that include adequate roughage have beneficial behavioural effects as well as permitting normal bodily development so all calves should be fed adequate roughage from two weeks onwards. Since white veal production is inefficient and there are inevitable welfare problems it is to be hoped that public demand for it will continue its rapid downward trend and such production systems will soon disappear.

Since young calves are so vulnerable to disease and are generally affected by adverse physical and social conditions their welfare is often poor when they are transported and taken to market. Despite this fact, a million young calves per annum are transported from France to Italy for veal production and many young calves are taken to market in the UK. The British calves should be more than a week old before marketing but many are not and even at one week the calves are ill-equipped to cope with the vicissitudes of vehicle and market conditions. In most European countries, calves are not marketed before weaning and the British practice is regarded as undesirable for production and welfare reasons. Calves should be sold from farm to farm, if movement at an early age is essential, or should be marketed after five weeks of age.

Beef cattle welfare

The housing conditions for calves destined for beef production are sometimes similar to those kept for veal production so they have similar welfare problems. Older beef animals are kept in small individual pens or are tethered in some countries and they then show much stereotyped behaviour. Riese *et al.* (1977) reported that stereotyped behaviour included tongue rolling, weaving movements and self-licking. Wierenga (1987) reported that one-third of young, individually housed bulls spent several minutes in every hour showing tongue rolling. Physiological responses to confinement also occur. Ladewig (1984) reported that tethered bulls showed more frequent episodes of high blood cortisol levels than did bulls able to interact socially in groups. Such abnormal behaviour and physiology is probably exacerbated by both social deprivation and inability to perform behaviours because of spatial restriction. Individual housing of beef animals is more frequent when they are bulls than when they are steers. In Germany 98 per cent of beef animals are bulls but in the UK 92 per cent were steers in 1987. The

UK situation is changing following the ban on growth promoters.

Fighting and mounting can lead to welfare problems when beef animals, especially bulls, are kept in groups. The most important way of minimizing such problems is to keep the animals in stable groups since social mixing leads to much fighting with consequent injuries, bruising and extreme physiological responses (Kenny & Tarrant, 1982). In stable groups, mounting may lead to more injury than does fighting (Appleby & Wood-Gush, 1986). Animals that are frequently mounted become bruised and may suffer severe leg injuries. Mounting can be greatly reduced by the use of overhead bars, which physically prevent it, or an electrified grid, which deters animals that wish to mount. The brief initial experience of an electric shock has a relatively small adverse effect on welfare as compared with the serious effects on animals that are repeatedly mounted.

The stocking density of beef animals and the flooring provided also have considerable effects on welfare. High stocking densities lead to more aggression, injury and bruising. Beef animals increase rapidly in body weight but they have little exercise if they are housed in small pens and their leg growth may not be able to keep pace with that of the rest of the body. The final weights reached are much higher now than they used to be so the legs are scarcely adequate to support the body. The consequence is cartilage damage, clear indications of limb pain and obvious difficulties in standing and lying (Dämmrich, 1987). Graf (1984) found that these problems were absent if fattening bulls were reared on deep straw and that such conditions also led to fewer behavioural problems.

Dairy cow welfare

The major welfare problems for housed dairy cows are lameness, mastitis and difficulty in gaining feeding and lying places. Most of these problems are associated with the design of the housing system but some are a consequence of poor husbandry. The causes of both lameness and mastitis are multifactorial and there is an interaction between the response of the animal to its conditions and the likelihood of clinical infection. A reduction in pathogen challenge will usually help to reduce disease incidence but changes in management methods, of the kinds that have other beneficial effects on welfare, can have an effect on minimizing disease that is as great or greater. Studies at the Institute for Animal Health, Compton have shown that there are positive correlations between lameness and mastitis incidence. High production increases the occurrence of both lameness and mastitis. Mastitis has declined in dairy herds where concentrate feeding has been introduced following the introduction of milk quotas, and in an experimental study Manson & Leaver (1986) found that the lameness incidence was higher in cows fed on a high-protein diet. The incidence of lameness can be reduced by the use of foot baths and by hoof trimming but much remains to be discovered about the conditions that lead to individuals being likely to become lame.

Space allowances are often quoted for housed dairy cows, for example Arave *et al.* (1974) quoted $2.3\,m^2$/cow, but house design and social stability must be taken into account when deciding on the best space allowance in any building. Social mixing leads to various behavioural and reproductive difficulties (Bouissou, 1976). Even when social disruption is minimal, cows need places to which to retreat so as to avoid confrontation with other individuals. Potter & Broom (1987) report that cows use cubicles and feed-barrier sections for this. If there is a shortage of feeding places, due to the highly synchronized behaviour of dairy cows (Benham, 1982; Wierenga, 1983; Potter & Broom, 1987) there are considerable effects on the cows. Metz & Mekking (1984) reported a dramatic increase in chasing and it is likely that the welfare of cows is poor when they are unable to get a feeding place because their herd mates are feeding. Narrow passageways in a cubicle house can cause problems for cows, for example Konggaard (1983) saw more contact, yielding, turning and waiting if passageways were 1.2 m wide than if they were 2 m wide. An inadequate number of cubicles, such that not all cows can lie at once, leads to more aggressive interactions and low-ranking animals having to lie in passageways where conditions are dirty and the likelihood of injury or disease is high (Kaiser & Lippitz, 1974; Friend *et al.*, 1977; Wierenga, 1987). Other welfare problems for dairy cows concern ill-treatment or neglect by the stockworker and producers when it comes to milking. The use of force is not conducive to good welfare or good milk production. Good stockworkers are consistent in their milking Parlour procedures and deal with the cows in a quiet predictable way.

Farm operations

Certain operations on cattle are performed on farms by staff with no veterinary qualification. In most cases, no anaesthetic is used. The most widespread of these operations are disbudding or dehorning, castration and various sorts of individual marking. Some of the procedures used must also cause pain to the animals but there is little precise information about this. The use of caustic materials that remain in contact with living tissue for any length of time is likely to cause severe pain and should be avoided. Any use of hot irons on living tissue must also cause pain and hot iron branding is a painful and unnecessary form of marking. Castration is often carried out by applying a rubber ring around the testicles until the tissue in them dies and it seems likely that this is also very painful for a long period. Even the ubiquitous ear notching and punching must be painful for a few days and it would be better if alternative marking methods such as freeze branding or tattooing could be used.

More extensive operations should only be carried out under anaesthetic by qualified veterinarians and should be permitted only if the animal will benefit. Farm practices that necessitate the use of operations should be avoided. An example of a problem area is the breeding of cows such that their calf cannot be born normally. No animal should be made pregnant if there is a likelihood that caesarean section or a difficult birth will occur.

Handling, transport and slaughter of cattle

Every dairy farmer has to be able to move dairy cows in milk to and from the milking parlour. If the races and collecting yards that are used or the methods of moving the animals are inadequate and disturbing to some or all of the cows, there will be welfare problems. Such welfare problems will often be associated with reduced milk yield. Cows may be reluctant to enter a milking parlour because of the behaviour of the stockworker or because of design faults in the parlour that result in uncomfortable milking stalls or stray voltages. Such problems can lead to the use of excessive force by stockworkers in the collecting yard or to forcing animals towards the parlour entrance using gates or an 'electric dog'. The 'electric dog', which is a row of electrically live wires hanging downwards and moved towards the cows in the rear of the yard, has a large adverse effect on some cows so that their milk let-down may be prevented and they may become extremely unwilling to move towards the parlour.

The problems associated with the design of races for moving cows to the milking parlour are very similar to those of designing races used for other purposes, such as movement towards vehicles prior to transport. The most extensive study of how to design good races is that of Grandin (1983). She reported that cattle often balk if they encounter dark areas or areas of extreme lighting contrast. Races with sharp angular turns in them may also pose problems for cattle that are being driven and long straight races may result in animals being either reluctant to move or moving too fast. As a consequence of these observations, Grandin recommends that races should be evenly lit, have solid walls if animals unfamiliar with them have to use them and should be gently curved rather than having sharp corners or long straights (Fig. 49.6). Other studies also suggest that if animals are being loaded into vehicles, the ramp should be long, sloping (not more than 1 in 7), should allow a good grip for the feet of the cattle and should have solid sides, and the interior of the vehicle should be well lit.

Vehicles are often not well designed as regards flooring, ventilation and ease of subdivision. Just as important as vehicle design, as regards the welfare of animals during transport, is the behaviour of the transport staff. Problems arise because of rough treatment during loading, over or under stocking of compartments on the vehicle, inconsiderate driving or leaving the animals in conditions that are too hot or too

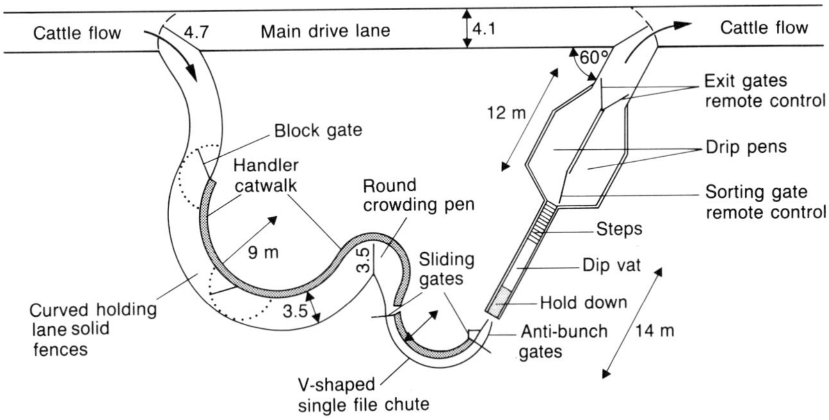

Fig. 49.6 Races for cattle should have no long straights or sharp corners so Grandin (1980) designed this race for movement to vehicles.

cold and windy for them. The other major transport problem is the effect of very long journeys, especially where there are no stops for food and water. This area has been reviewed in a Commission of the European Communities (CEC) Report (1984).

When cattle arrive at an abattoir they are often injured or bruised during unloading because of too much haste on the part of animal handlers or inadequate ramps. Grandin (1979, 1980) reported that 66 per cent of bruises of the loin area occurred during loading or unloading of trucks. At lairage, animals are often mixed with individuals that are strange to them. This causes much fighting amongst bulls and considerable emotional disturbance in other cattle. Studies of bulls by Kenny & Tarrant (1982) show that mixing at lairage causes much fighting, high levels of bruising and other injury and a great increase in the incidence of dark firm dry (DFD) meat. Both bruising and DFD meat are of economic importance as well as indicating severe welfare problems prior to slaughter.

In an efficient slaughterhouse the period during which animals are moved from pens to the point of slaughter can be very brief and the stunning and slaughter procedure itself can result in no pain for the animal. Welfare is worse if the animals are kept in a confined race for a period of more than one or two minutes before stunning, if stunning is carried out inadequately or if there is inversion before slaughter or no stunning. Poor equipment or lack of care by slaughter staff can result in extreme pain and discomfort for the animals. Extreme pain and discomfort is also inevitable if animals are not stunned, for example in the Jewish schechita or the Muslim halal ritual slaughter procedures. There is a period during which evoked potentials in the brain can still be produced after the throat is cut that may last for from a few seconds to two minutes during which the animal must be in great pain and distress. As the heart still beats after stunning and blood drains from the animal just as effectively whether or not the animal is stunned there is no logical reason why stunning should not be carried out before the throat is cut.

Welfare consequences of future developments in cattle management

Conventional methods of cattle breeding have changed the animals considerably during recent years and future changes are likely to be accelerated by new possibilities for genome manipulation. For example, selection for double muscling in beef cattle and the possibility of transferring genes that increase growth rate or modify final body form could both result in animals with larger, faster growing bodies. New growth promoters, if these are allowed to be used, could have the same effect. These techniques need not have any adverse effect on welfare but any increase in production pressure could lead to more problems. In addition, body weight increase without corresponding increase in leg size and strength could result in more lameness. Any modification of animals should be checked carefully to ensure that animals do not find it more difficult to cope with their environment. Some modifications of animals could result in improved welfare, for example if genes were implanted that increased the efficiency with which disease could be combatted by the individual.

The crossing of breeds of animals can lead to welfare problems for cows if a large breed of bull is crossed with a smaller breed of cow, resulting in increased calving difficulty. Similar problems can arise if embryo transfer is used. Multiple implantation of embryos could lead to other problems. The actual transfer of embryos could be a major operation that is traumatic for the cow but techniques which have only a minor effect are now possible. Any embryo transfer procedure should be such that cow welfare is not worse than that of cows undergoing a normal pregnancy.

A quite different development area that can have effects on welfare is the development of microprocessors and other electronic control units. Cows can already carry transponders that allow them to be fed individually and this methodology could be improved to minimize the chances that any individuals fail to obtain food. This system of feeding cows at a single or small number of feeding stalls can lead to problems because dominant individuals may attack others or deter them from feeding. Some very timid cows might be quite unwilling to approach a feeder when an aggressive individual is near it. Recent work by Wierenga & Hopster (1989) involves the use of an auditory signalling device on the cow's ear, which tells each individual when to come to feed. Animals that have already fed receive no food if they enter the feeder so this system provides a means for distributing feeding times for each individual throughout the day. Such a system should work well for all animals except for those that are stimulated to feed only when another animal is feeding. Electronic systems could also allow cattle greater control over their physical environment, for example by giving them the opportunity to regulate environmental temperature and air-flow rates. Lack of control is a major cause of welfare problems (Broom, 1985) so such possibilities could improve welfare. The development of robotics is likely to make possible in the near future the automatic milking of cows. Cows would be recognized individually on entry to a milking stall and a computer that had been preprogrammed with their udder coordinates would attach a milking machine to them. Provided that this could be done without any discomfort to the cow it could improve welfare, since the cow could come to be milked whenever she chose to do so.

Summary

The major cattle welfare problem, apart from those resulting from ill-treatment and neglect, is the close confinement in small crates of calves and fattening bulls (Broom, 1987). In veal calf management there are also adverse effects resulting from low levels of iron and roughage in the diet. Amongst dairy cows, lameness and mastitis are serious welfare problems and certain housing systems lead to injuries or other difficulties for cows. For all cattle, transport and associated handling are traumatic experiences. These may be particularly bad for young calves that are taken to market before reaching weaning age and part of the welfare problem is often increased disease incidence. Bruising and other injuries are very frequent when bulls from different social groups are mixed at any time and yet this often occurs prior to transport or at lairage. Other welfare problems during transport of any cattle are the consequences of moving casualty animals, poor loading techniques or facilities, poor vehicle design, poor driving or very long journeys. Slaughter procedures are sometimes inadequate and stunning should always be carried out prior to slaughter. Farmers should be advised to give cattle: firstly, more control over their environment, secondly, predictable but diverse surroundings, and thirdly, rapid treatment if they contract disease.

References

Albright, J.L. (1969) Social environment and growth. In *Animal Growth and Nutrition* (ed. by E.S.E. Hafez & I.A. Dyers). Lea and Febiger, Philadelphia.

Albright, J.L. (1981) Training dairy cattle. In *Dairy Sciences Handbook*, Vol. 14, pp. 363–70. Agriservices Foundation, Clovis, CA.

Andreae, U. & Smidt, D. (1982) Behavioural alterations in young cattle on slatted floors. In *Disturbed Behaviour in Farm Animals* (ed. by W. Bessei), Hohenheimer Arbeiten, Vol. 121, pp. 51–60. Eugen Ulmer, Stuttgart.

Appleby, M.C. & Wood-Gush, D.G.M. (1986) Development of behaviour in beef bulls: sexual behaviour causes more problems than aggression. *Animal Production*, **42**, 464.

Arave, C.W., Albright, J.L. & Sinclair, C.L. (1974) Behaviour, milk yield and leucocytes of dairy cows in reduced space and isolation. *Journal of Dairy Science*, **57**, 1497–1501.

Barton, M.A. (1983) Behaviour of group-reared calves fed on acid-milk replacer. *Applied Animal Ethology*, **11**, 77.

Barton, M.A. & Broom, D.M. (1985) Social factors affecting the performance of teat-fed calves. *Animal Production*, **40**, 525.

Benham, P.F.J. (1982) Synchronisation of behaviour in grazing cattle. *Applied Animal Ethology*, **8**, 403–4.

Bouissou, M.F. (1970) Role du contact physique dans la manifestation des relations hierarchiques chez les bovins: consequences pratiques. *Annales de Zootechnie*, **19**, 279–85.

Bouissou, M.F. (1976) Effet de differentes perturbations sur le nombre d'interactions sociales échargée au sein de groupes de bovins. *Biology of behaviour*, **1**, 193–8.

Broom, D.M. (1981) *Biology of Behaviour*. Cambridge University Press, Cambridge.

Broom, D.M. (1982) Husbandry methods leading to inadequate social and maternal behaviour in cattle. In *Disturbed Behaviour in Farm Animals* (ed. by W. Bessei), Hohenheimer Arbeiten, Vol. 121, pp. 42–50. Eugen Ulmer, Stuttgart.

Broom, D.M. (1983a) Cow–calf and sow–piglet behaviour in relation to colostrum ingestion. *Annales de Recherches Vétérinaires*, **14**, 342–8.

Broom, D.M. (1983b) Stereotypies as animal welfare indicators. In *Indicators Relevant to Farm Animal Welfare* (ed. by D. Smidt), Current Topics in Veterinary Medicine and Animal Science, Vol. 23, pp. 81–7. Martinus Nijhoff, The Hague.

Broom, D.M. (1985) Stress, welfare and the state of equilibrium. In *Proceedings of the 2nd European Symposium on Poultry Welfare* (ed. by R.M. Wegner), pp. 72–81. World Poultry Science Association, Celle.

Broom, D.M. (1986) Indicators of poor welfare. *British Veterinary Journal*, **142**, 524–6.

Broom, D.M. (1987) General conclusions. In *Welfare Aspects of Housing Systems for Veal Calves and Fattening Bulls* (ed. by M.C. Schlichting & D. Smidt), pp. 161–6. Commission of the European Communities, Luxembourg. EUR 10777.

Broom, D.M. (1988) Welfare considerations in cattle practice. In *Proceedings of the British Cattle Veterinary Association 1986–87* (ed. M. Vaughan), pp. 153–64. British Cattle Veterinary Association, London.

Broom, D.M. & Leaver, J.D. (1978) The effects of group-rearing or partial isolation on later social behaviour of calves. *Animal Behaviour*, **26**, 1255–63.

Cermak, J. (1987) The design of cubicles for British friesian dairy cows with reference to body weight and dimensions, spatial behaviour and upper leg lameness. In *Cattle Housing Systems, Lameness and Behaviour* (ed. by H.K. Wierenga & D.J. Peterse), Current Topics in Veterinary Medicine and Animal Science, Vol. 40, pp. 119–28. Martinus Nijhoff, Dordrecht.

Commission of the European Communities (1984) International transport of farm animals intended for slaughter. EUR 9556 EN. CEC, Luxembourg.

Craig, J.V. (1981) *Domestic Animal Behavior*. Prentice Hall, Englewood Cliffs, NJ.

Dämmrich, K. (1987) The reactions of the legs (bone; joints) to loading and its consequences for lameness. In *Cattle Housing Systems, Lameness and Behaviour* (ed. by H.K. Wierenga &

D.J. Peterse), Current Topics in Veterinary Medicine and Animal Science, Vol. 40, pp. 50–5. Martinus Nijhoff, Dordrecht.

Edwards, S.A. (1982) Factors affecting the time to first suckling in dairy calves. *Animal Production*, **34**, 339–46.

Edwards, S.A. & Broom, D.M. (1982) Behavioural interactions of dairy cows with their newborn calves and the effects of parity. *Animal Behaviour*, **30**, 525–35.

Fraser, A.F. & Broom, D.M. (1990) *Farm Animal Behaviour and Welfare*. Bailliére Tindall, London.

Friend, T.H., Polan, C.E., Gwazdauskas, F.C. & Heald, C.W. (1977) Adrenal glucocorticoid response to exogenous adrenocorticotropin mediated by density and social disruption in lactating cows. *Journal of Dairy Science*, **60**, 1958–63.

Gibson, T.E. (1988) (ed.) *Animal Disease — a Welfare Problem?* British Veterinary Association Animal Welfare Foundation, London.

Graf, B.P. (1984) *Der Einfluss unterschiedlicher Laufstall systeme auf Verhaltensmerkmale von Mastochsen*. Doktor Dissertation der Eidgenossischen Technischen Hochschule, Zürich.

Grandin, T. (1979) The effect of stress on livestock and meat quality prior to and during slaughter. *International Journal for the Study of Animal Productions*, **1**, 313–37.

Grandin, T. (1980) Observations of cattle behaviour applied to the design of cattle-handling facilities. *Applied Animal Ethology*, **6**, 19–31.

Grandin, T. (1983) Welfare requirements of handling facilities. In *Farm Animal Housing and Welfare* (ed. by S.H. Baxter, M.R. Baxter & J.A.C. MacCormack), Current Topics in Veterinary Medicine and Animal Science, Vol. 24, pp. 137–49. Martinus Nijhoff, The Hague.

Kaiser, R. & Lippitz, O. (1974) Untersuchungen zum Verhalten von Milchkuhen im Boxenlaufstall bei unterschiedlichem Tier-Liegeplatz-Verhaltniss und standig freim Zugang zur reduzierten Krippe. *Tierzucht*, **28**, 187–9.

Kenny, F.J. & Tarrant, P.V. (1982) Behaviour of cattle during transport and penning before slaughter. In *Transport of Animals Intended for Breeding, Production and Slaughter* (ed. by R. Moss), Current Topics in Veterinary Medicine and Animal Science, Vol. 18, pp. 87–102. Martinus Nijhoff, The Hague.

Kilgour, R. & Dalton, C. (1984) *Livestock Behaviour: a Practical Guide*. Granada, London.

Konggaard, S.P. (1983) Feeding conditions in relation to welfare for dairy cows in loose-housed conditions. In *Farm Animal Housing and Welfare* (ed. by S.H. Baxter, M.R. Baxter & J.A.C. MacCormack), Current Topics in Veterinary Medicine and Animal Science, Vol. 24, pp. 272–8. Martinus Nijhoff, The Hague.

Ladewig, J. (1984) The effect of behavioural stress on the episodic release and circadian variation of cortisol in bulls. In *Proceedings of the International Congress on Applied Ethology of Farm Animals* (ed. by J. Unshelm, G. van Putten & K. Zeeb), pp. 339–42. Darmstadt, KJBL.

Manson, F.J. & Leaver, J.D. (1986) Effect of hoof trimming and protein level on lameness in dairy cows. *Animal Production*, **42**, 451.

Metz, J.H.M. (1983) Food competition in cattle. In *Farm Animal Housing and Welfare* (ed. by S.H. Baxter, M.R. Baxter & J.A.C. MacCormack), Current Topics in Veterinary Medicine and Animal Science, Vol. 24, pp. 164–70. Martinus Nijhoff, The Hague.

Metz J.H.M. & Mekking, P. (1984) Crowding phenomena in dairy cows as related to available idling space in a cubicle housing system. *Applied Animal Behaviour Sciences*, **12**, 63–78.

Potter, M.J. & Broom, D.M. (1987) The behaviour and welfare of cows in relation to cubicle house design. In *Cattle Housing Systems, Lameness and Behaviour* (ed. by H.K. Wierenga & D.J. Peterse), Current Topics in Veterinary Medicine and Animal Science, Vol. 40, pp. 129–47. Martinus Nijhoff, Dordrecht.

Riese, G., Klee, G. & Sambraus, H.H. (1977) Das Verhalten von Kälbern in verschiedenen Haltungsformen. *Deutsche Tierärztliche Wochenschrift*, **84**, 388–94.

Schlichting, M.C. & Smidt, D. (eds) (1987) *Welfare Aspects of Housing Systems for Veal Calves and Fattening Bulls*. EUR 10777 EN. Commission of the European Communities, Luxembourg.

Stricklin, W.R. & Kautz-Scanavy, C.C. (1984) The role of behaviour in cattle production: a review of research. *Applied Animal Ethology*, **11**, 359–90.

Susmel, P. (1987) The veal production in the EEC countries. In *Welfare Aspects of Housing Systems for Veal Calves and Fattening Bulls* (ed. by M.C. Schlichting & D. Smidt), pp. 5–17. EUR 10777 EN. Commission of the European Communities, Luxembourg.

Webster, A.J.F., Saville, C., Church, B.M., Gnanastakthy, A. & Moss R. (1985a) The effect of different rearing conditions on the development of calf behaviour. *British Veterinary Journal*, **141**, 249–64.

Webster, A.J.F., Saville, C., Church, B.M., Gnanasakthy, A. & Moss, R. (1985b) Some effects of different rearing systems on health, cleanliness and injury in calves. *British Veterinary Journal*, **141**, 472–83.

Webster, J., Saville, C. & Welchman, D. (1986) *Improved Husbandry Systems for Veal Calves*. Farm Animal Care Trust, London.

Wierenga, H.K. (1983) The influence of space for walking and lying in a cubicle system on the behaviour of dairy cattle. In *Farm Animal Housing and Welfare* (ed. by S.H. Baxter, M.R. Baxter & S.H. MacCormack), Current Topics in Veterinary Medicine and Animal Science. Vol. 24, pp. 171–80. Martinus Nijhoff, The Hague.

Wierenga, H.K. (1987) Behavioural problems in fattening bulls. In *Welfare Aspects of Housing Systems for Veal Calves and Fattening Bulls* (ed. by M.C. Schlichting & D. Smidt), pp. 105–22. EUR 10777 EN. Commission of the European Communities, Luxembourg.

Wierenga, H.K. & Peterse, D.J. (eds) (1987) *Cattle Housing Systems, Lameness and Behaviour*. Current Topics in Veterinary Medicine and Animal Science, Vol. 40. Martinus Nijhoff, Dordrecht.

Wilt, J.G. de (1985). *Behaviour and welfare of veal calves in relation to husbandry systems*. Doctoral thesis, University of Wageningen.

Therapy and Prophylaxis

Chapter 50: Disinfection and Methods of Disease Control by Management of Animals and Buildings

by D.W.B. SAINSBURY

Introduction

Good health is the birthright of every animal. Great progress has been made towards achieving improved health in cattle but the disease pattern has changed radically in recent years. The most acute, specific, diagnosable and preventable or treatable diseases, using vaccines, sera and medicines for their control, have been largely controlled. In their place have emerged more chronic, insidious and complex diseases often caused by organisms that are the normal inhabitants of the animal body but which circumstances allow to become pathogenic. These disease conditions may be difficult to diagnose, have a large and confusing number of causal agents, create a massive morbidity and economic loss and require for their control great expertise in the exercise of husbandry, hygiene, housing and management skills rather than recourse to the use of medicines or biological products. This chapter is concerned with those underlying principles of the management, hygiene and housing of cattle that are essential to assist in the prevention and control of disease.

The essentials for good health

The size of livestock farms

From the point of view of animal health, the smaller the farm the better; nevertheless, the current trend has been towards increasing the size of units to achieve economies of scale — in manpower, buildings and services. However, in dealing with biological material, in this case cattle, there is clear evidence to show that if the farm becomes too large, efficiency generally decreases and health and productivity are adversely affected. Economic surveys have shown that very small farms as a group are generally less efficient but once the three-man unit has been reached, further improvements in performance are small or non-existent (Britton & Berkeley Hill, 1975). It is fair to say that often this knowledge goes unheeded and over-large livestock enterprises are a cause of great problems and enormous economic loss. It is, however, pertinent to emphasize that from the point of view of health it is the young immature animal which finds itself at greater risk from disease and mismanagement. Therefore, whilst there should be a limit on unit size at a reasonably low level for the young animal, it may be much higher for the adult. The main reason for this, apart from the extra vulnerability of the young animal to stress caused by bad management, is the varying immunity to infectious disease among the stock that is unavoidable on a large unit with a mixture of animals of different ages and possibly of various sources of origin. The adult presents a more stable picture in both respects, being rather more resistant to management changes or errors and very much more uniform in its disease resistance or susceptibility.

Depopulation

So far as possible the principle of periodic depopulation of a building or, preferably, even a site should be followed. The benefits of eliminating the animal hosts to disease-causing agents are well understood and the virtue of being able to clean, disinfect and fumigate a building is also accepted. Nevertheless, in practice the whole concept of the 'all-in, all-out' policy is more complex than the preceding sentences would indicate. For example, it is in the young animal that it is particularly important to consider this and far less so in the older beast, which has achieved an immunity to many of the local diseases. Much also depends on whether the herd or flock is a 'closed' one with few or no incoming animals, or an 'open' one with a constant renewal of the animal population. If the latter is the case, then the depopulation principle is of much greater importance as there is little or no opportunity for natural immunity to develop, and there is a constantly running risk, and usually a near certainty, of introducing animals that are either clinically infected or carriers of disease. Basic design specifications for such units should be quite different from those of the closed herd.

Group size

One of the principal ways of putting the housing on a firm footing is to keep the animals in groups of *minimal* size. At first sight this sounds quite an old-fashioned and even reactionary concept that may eliminate all those advantages from automation that large units can give us, but this certainly need not be the case. If groups are small it is possible easily to match the animals in them for size, weight and age. Under these circumstances it is well established that fighting and bullying are kept to a minimum, if not completely prevented.

There is yet another very important advantage in keeping animals in small groups. It is obviously good practice for a farmer to keep his livestock somewhere near the level that has been shown to be the densest possible for optimal productivity. If livestock are kept in a house at a high density it is essential that they spread across the house uniformly, so they do in actual practice occupy and use the whole area. Regrettably, this is very rarely the case in practical experience and especially so when large numbers are housed together without any subdivision at all. If the animals crowd in certain parts of the building there may be grossly overstocked floor areas. This is bad enough in itself but it has further unfortunate side-effects. If they crowd excessively in a part of the house, this part may become polluted with dung and exhalations to an abnormal and harmful degree; the humidity becomes high, proper air movement is impeded and the animals may soon become sick. Sick animals feeling cold tend to huddle together even more, so the vicious circle is perpetuated and there is seemingly no end to it unless some measures are taken to ensure a better distribution of the stock.

When animals are kept together in large numbers the effects of a fright caused by an unusual disturbance can be extremely serious. It is almost impossible to guard against all the extraneous sounds and sights that may adversely affect the stock. The best safeguard, therefore, is once again to have the animals in small groups so that the effect of a panic movement will be more limited and will never build up into highly dangerous proportions.

Housing types and systems

There are three essentially contrasting types of housing: 'climatic', giving only a cover and protection to the animals; 'controlled environment', which regulates the microclimate as completely as is required for the particular stock being housed; and the 'kennel', which is in a sense a half-way house between the other two forms and gives two environments in the one building allowing some free and appropriate choice for the animals. The methods of use of each of the types and their suitability for different countries, climatic regions and forms of livestock vary enormously and must be carefully defined.

Climatic housing (Figs 50.1 and 50.2)

The climatic house is ideal for the adult beast that has developed a large measure of adaptability to climatic stress. The house can be cheap because it is basically a cover alone but because of the lack of control of the climate the space given to the animals must be much greater, especially since there is no powered ventilation.

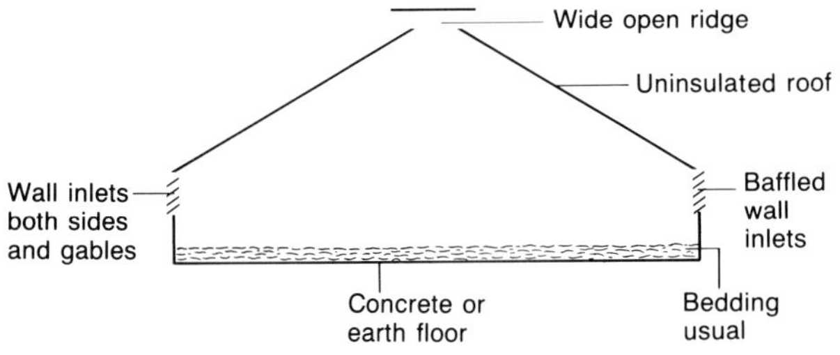

Fig. 50.1 Cross-section of 'climatic' livestock house with open ridge and baffled wall ventilators.

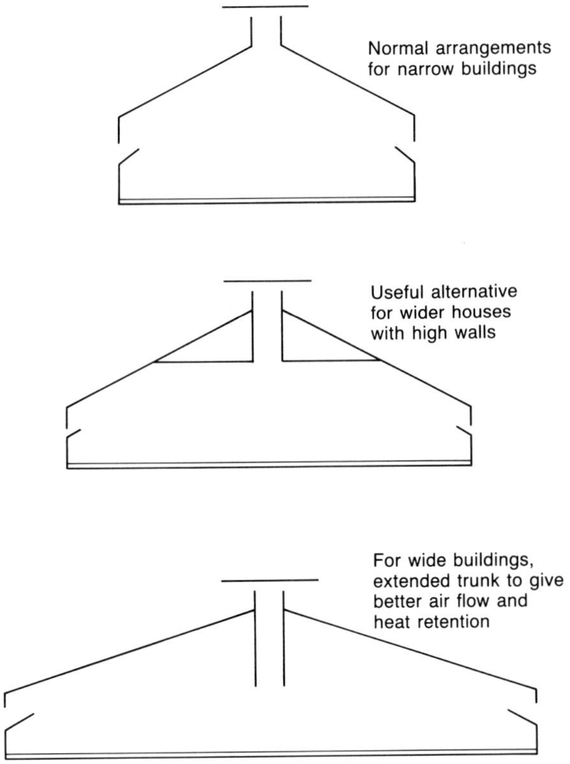

Fig. 50.2 Alternative arrangements suitable for natural ventilation of various widths of buildings and using outlet ('chimney') trunks.

In general, stocking densities tend to be half or less those in the controlled environment house. A major problem is created by agriculturists when they attempt to apply the high stocking rates that are suitable for the controlled environment house to the climatic house, as the building is unable to cope with the demands of the stock and poor productivity and high disease incidence can result. Climatic housing is usually the correct choice for cattle over about six months of age. Such housing usually requires deep bedding for its success, particularly in cooler climatic areas.

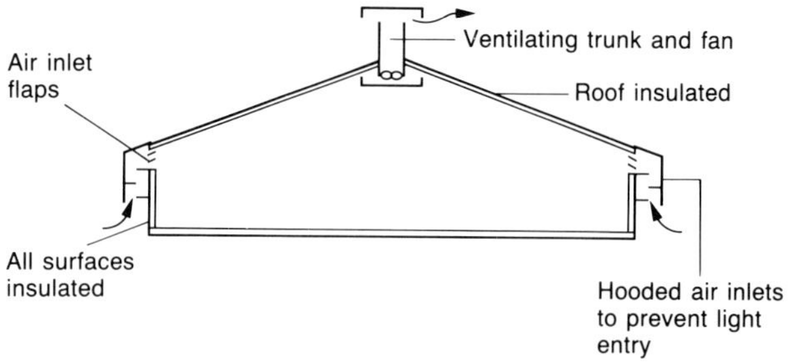

Fig. 50.3 Cross-section of a typical conventionally ventilated controlled environment house with roof fan extraction and hooded wall inlets.

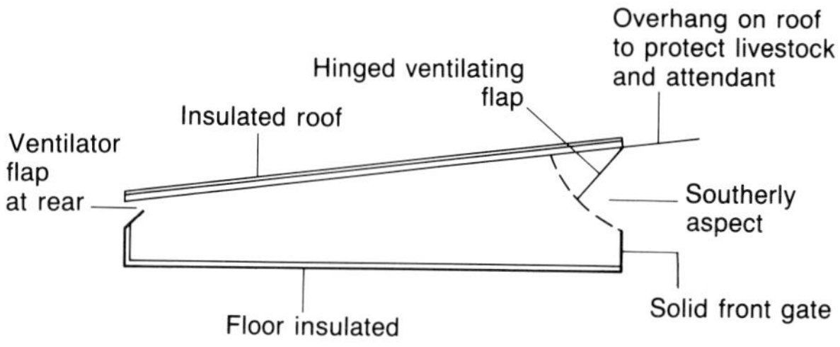

Fig. 50.4 Cross-section of a mono-pitch ('kennel') naturally ventilated stock building.

Controlled environment house (Fig. 50.3)

The controlled environment house is in great contrast. It has a limited use for cattle, being sometimes used for young calves and to a lesser extent for cattle kept on any bare surfaces, solid or slotted, without bedding. It is most economically viable with livestock that are fed largely concentrate food rather than substantial quantities of roughage, since the former is too expensive to be utilized as a form of energy. The housing is expensive and because of the cost it is usually necessary to stock the buildings as densely as possible to make them viable economically, and this can place a great strain on health control. Management to cope with their special requirements needs to be highly sophisticated and unless these criteria can be observed this is frequently the wrong type of housing to have. The rewards can be great but the dangers are greater.

'Kennel' accommodation (Fig. 50.4)

This is an increasingly popular system of accommodation that is in a way half-way between the climatic and controlled environment housing. It attempts to combine the virtues of both, but at low cost, and often succeeds. The essence of the system is that the animals are kept in pens or groups that are sufficiently small to allow them to be closely confined, at least while resting, without too great a danger from respiratory or other disease. The close confinement makes it possible to keep the groups warm and draught-free by utilizing their own body heat and by good insulation of the kennel and a limited cubic air space. This part of the accommodation is roughly a controlled environment house: the rest is the climatic house and can be justified as this is an area where the animals will be moving about freely and will not normally be inactive or lying down. It is likely to contain the dung and often the feeding and watering arrangements and so must be very adequately ventilated, usually by non-mechanical means. In harsh climatic areas it is covered; in milder regions there is no need for this and the 'yard' can, with benefit to health and productivity, be left uncovered.

It is instructive to look in some detail at the logic of the 'kennel' system.

1 The cost of the housing can be as low as any system, especially with uncovered yarding, and such buildings are also the easiest type of building for the farmer himself to erect.

2 Good health is promoted by separation of the animals into small groups. The separation of the kennels one from another should be as absolute as possible as this will limit the build-up and spread of respiratory disease. It will also be a great assistance to the health of the animals if the muck is not allowed to accumulate in the warmer or closely confined resting area. It is often possible as well, by good design, to keep the dunging areas separate so that the muck from different pens does not come together until after it is out of reach of the animals.

3 The cheapness of the housing is largely due to the fact that the environment is controlled only where it is absolutely necessary.

It is certainly a distinct virtue if the dung can be in an area where the air is moving more freely and the temperature and the humidity possibly much lower, at least in temperate climates. Feeding in an outside yard achieves this objective. Controlled environment housing is becoming more and more expensive and there is no possible justification for this control to embrace the effluent from the animals, which is not only a considerable expense but is also likely to intensify the disease risk.

Whatever the system the principal practical faults in livestock housing systems are as follows.

1 Having too close a confinement of the animals.
2 Placing too many animals in one common air space.
3 Reducing both cubic area and floor space.
4 Failing to remove muck from close proximity to the animals.
5 Transferring muck through pens, aiding the transfer of disease.
6 Failing to separate age groups.
7 Neglecting clean feeding and water arrangements.
8 Having poor or sometimes no drainage.
9 Neglecting the comfort of the stock.
10 Inefficient ventilation systems.

Table 50.1 shows the space allowances for cattle is strawed yards.

Table 50.1 A guide to space allowance for cattle at different stages of growth in strawed yards

Age	Area/animal (m^2)
Up to 14 days	0.9–1.4
14 days to 3 months	1.4–1.8
3–6 months	1.8–2.4
6–9 months	2.4–2.7
9–18 months	2.7–3.8
Adults	3.8–4.7

The environmental requirements of cattle

In most cool, temperate environments, ruminants maintain a stable body temperature by regulating evaporative loss, at little metabolic cost. Ruminants have a very marked ability to alter their zone of thermal neutrality in response to previous thermal history. Thus there are no absolute criteria for the thermal requirements of any class of ruminant livestock, except perhaps the newborn animal; they depend to a large extent on what the animal has grown accustomed to.

Some examples of the lower critical temperatures for

Table 50.2 Lower critical temperature of ruminants housed in a building with very low air movement (0.2 m/s) and in a draught (2 m/s). Source: Webster (1981)

Type of animal	Liveweight (kg)	Lower critical temperature (°C)	
		Low air speed	Draught
Calf			
Newborn	35	+9	+17
1 month old	50	0	+9
Veal	100	−14	−1
Store cattle (maintenance)	250	−32	−20
Beef cow (maintenance)	450	−17	−9
Dairy cow	500	−26	−13

cattle under conditions of varying air movements are shown in Table 50.2. This table illustrates a situation where the beasts are standing up, in a dry enclosure, under two variations in air movement (Webster, 1981).

In an unheated building at low air movement the only cattle likely to experience cold sufficient to elevate the heat production are newborn calves or young calves whose metabolic rate is low by virtue of starvation, sickness or emaciation. Such animals can undoubtedly be stressed by cold and may require special attention. Increasing air movement to 2.0 m/s, which is not uncommon in draughty buildings, increases the critical temperature in the newborn calf from +9 to +17°C. This emphasizes the necessity of ensuring that adequate ventilation for calf houses is achieved without allowing excess air movement (or 'draught') to impinge on the calves.

By one month of age the healthy calf with a good appetite has a critical temperature close to 0°C and is not likely to be stressed by cold while indoors. Well-grown veal calves by virtue of their very high energy intake and heat production are particularly tolerant to cold and by the same criteria sensitive to heat. The traditional belief that veal calves should be kept in a warm environment because they are not ruminant and are therefore somehow more sensitive to cold is unscientific and untrue.

No other class of cattle is likely to experience a systemic stress of cold when standing up in a dry enclosure unless air movement is exceptionally high. For the dairy cow, however, cold stress should not be considered as a systemic but as a local problem. Heat production in the high-yielding cow is again very high and so the critical temperature is low. Milk synthesis, however, depends on blood flow to the mammary gland, which is reduced by local cooling. The production of dairy cows has been shown to fall at temperatures below about 0°C, although it is obvious that direct chilling of the udder depends as much on the thermal properties of the floor as on the temperature.

It is worthy of stress that European cattle tend to be tolerant to cold but intolerant to heat. Their 'comfort zone' is between about 0 and 20°C. The critical temperature leading to a decline in milk yield at the higher level is approximately 21–25°C for most European cattle, including Friesians and Jerseys, but as high as 30–32°C with Brown Swiss.

The effect of high temperatures may be ameliorated in practice in a number of ways. The provision of shade makes a great difference, also of wallows and artificial showers. For example, great benefit has been found in tropical climates with cattle kept under a so-called desert-cooler consisting of a three-sided shelter open to the north, with an upper roof of aluminium, which reflects the heat rays, a ceiling underneath of three layers of old hay, and an evaporative cooler under the roof at the south end of the shelter. There are a number of highly effective methods of reducing heat stress by the use of water atomizers. In some cases atomizing units are suspended under the roof of the buildings whilst more sophisticated arrangements utilize a series of mist propagators above the stock connected by a pipe-line carrying the water. Provided the humidity of the ambient air is not too high, significant cooling effects can be achieved at a modest running cost. True refrigeration plants are very occasionally used but are rarely economic. At high temperatures farm stock also attempt to reduce their heat production by reduced feed intake. Under hot sunny conditions the temperate breeds, particularly, spend less time in grazing and, in fact, under these conditions most of the grazing will be done at night. There are very marked breed differences, as might be expected, the tropical breeds being least affected.

In loose housing systems with open fronted barns, protection from solar radiation and maximum provision of air movement represents the limit of environmental improvement. With closed buildings, such as the cowhouse, mechanical air cooling may be used and, in parts of the world where climatic temperatures warrant it, has been found worthwhile.

Environmental factors affecting susceptibility to disease

Many of the organisms that cause ill-health in intensive livestock units are normally present in the animals and their surroundings and it is environmental stress that acts as a trigger inducing their multiplication to such an extent that clinically obvious disease breaks out. There are numerous examples, such as respiratory diseases, diarrhoea and mastitis. Whilst these diseases may always become clinically obvious in the long term there may be a lengthy period beforehand when their effects are limited to poor growth or productivity and an inefficient conversion of feed by the animal. It is an essential feature of a farmer's recording system that records of productivity are kept which should allow the detection of results that are beginning to deteriorate, and this can well be a warning that urgent action is needed to stop a slide in results leading eventually to disease. Most of the conditions of this nature are insidious, chronic and difficult to diagnose by any of the popular methods that are so effective with the well-described diseases. Very limited use can be made of vaccinations or antisera, nor are antibiotics or drugs more than a short-term answer. The only effective way is to attend to the whole environment of the animal by such methods that are known to reduce the risk of disease.

It is extremely difficult to reproduce clinical disease by experimental infections even when huge doses of mixed organisms are used. Whether or not an animal becomes clinically affected depends on non-specific factors of climate, housing and husbandry, which together form the total environment that is considered in this chapter. Above all it should be made clear that the state of health of the animals can transcend all other factors in determining the economic viability of a livestock enterprise. Disease at its worst kills the animal but even in sublethal infections seriously affects productivity.

The factors influencing the dispersal, survival and deposition of airborne pathogens in farm animals have been reviewed comprehensively by Donaldson (1978). Droplet nuclei are the primary mode of spread of a variety of contagious diseases and many pathogens have been shown to have been spread in this way via the animals' breath and also from secretions and excretions of the infected animals (see p. 204).

Referring specifically to virus particles, the ambient temperature has little effect on their survival in an animal house but a general trend is that high temperatures are more harmful to their survival than low ones (Sanger, 1969). In fact it has been suggested that the inactivation of viruses immediately after exhalation and aerosol formation is dependent on the relative humidity and any temperature effect occurs secondarily (Donaldson & Ferris, 1976). The effect of relative humidity on viruses in general is that viruses with a lipoprotein envelope survive best at a low relative humidity, whereas non-enveloped viruses are unstable in dry conditions but survive best at a high relative humidity. Rhinoviruses appear to survive better at high humidities but infectious bovine rhinotracheitis (IBR) and parainfluenza 3 (PI3) viruses at low humidities. In these last examples the differences in survival time reflect the association between seasonal patterns of relative humidity and disease incidence. There is the further possibility that at high relative humidity there is accelerated sedimentation of airborne pathogens in large aerosols. *Mycoplasma* on the other hand tend to be stable at very low and at high relative humidities but sensitive to mid-range relative humidity.

So far as bacteria are concerned, a rise in temperature produces an increasing destruction of bacteria but airborne spores are highly resistant. *Escherichia coli* survives and multiplies best at about 15 °C, as also do *Mycoplasma*. Bacteria tend to be resistant to low and high relative humidity but sensitive to mid-range relative humidity but bacterial spores are resistant almost totally to relative humidity effects.

It is important to be aware that in airborne infections the size of the infecting dose will determine whether or not disease will result. Also, its severity and the likelihood of infection making headway will depend on the animal's overall resistance; for example, chilling can markedly lower an animal's resistance to inhaled pathogens by depressing lung clearance mechanisms (Whittlestone, 1976).

Systems in which the air is recirculated are being favoured as a means of reducing heating costs but in such systems some form of air cleansing, e.g. filtration, may be necessary to avoid a build-up of pathogens.

It is known from the work of Honey & McQuitty (1976) that animal buildings are often very dusty but the factors affecting dust production are ill defined. Small changes in relative humidity have been found to have significant effects on settled dust; lower humidities result in more settled dust. There is, however, mounting concern with the deleterious effect of dust on livestock health and good systems of ventilation should be able to remove it from the building in the same way and as efficiently as other environmental pollutants.

The disposal of large accumulations of animal excrement, bedding and litter is a further problem and can, in some instances, be the limiting factor in determining the size of unit. It is common practice to dilute the effluent from farm buildings into a slurry and then spray it over farmland as a fertilizer. The hazard from the dissemination of slurry-associated pathogens over a wide area in this way can be considerable, particularly in windy weather (Wray, 1975). A dairy herd of 50 cows causes a potential pollution load as large as that of a village of over 500 people, yet frequently the manure is carelessly disposed of without thought of its potential dangers to man or animal.

Intensification and immunity

There are some underlying truths in connection with disease and immunity that need to be explained as they have a close bearing on the incidence of disease and its relationship to the environment.

An animal at birth has a degree of passive immunity to local disease that is passed from the dam to the offspring, partly *in utero* and partly from the colostrum or first milk. Such immunity is, however, only practically effective to local infections to which the dam has been challenged. If the birth takes place in a 'foreign' environment, then the young may have little or no passive immunity to the infective organisms in their new local environment. In many cases the young are housed during the early stages of life in such a 'foreign' environment and it is therefore most important that the challenge of disease-causing organisms is reduced to a minimum.

Perhaps the first and foremost methods for reducing this challenge is by the processes of depopulation, and cleansing and disinfection. This can obviously be understood to be most important in the case of the younger animal, which has a poor or uncertain resistance to disease. Whilst it can never be said to be other than advantageous, it is most important on sites that have a large population of animals in an area where there are substantial numbers of animals since many diseases, especially viral ones, can pass a great distance by the airborne route. Whilst small infective particles can be carried directly by dust particles moved by the wind, other pathogens are carried indirectly by vectors, especially birds.

Disinfection

The disinfection of a building implies the elimination from the house of all micro-organisms that are capable of causing disease, thus converting the place from a potentially infective state into one that is largely free from infection. A disinfectant is the agent that is capable of achieving this and in livestock farming it is usually a chemical agent.

The processes of disinfection of a building can take place by the action of nature (natural disinfection) and by artificial means (artificial disinfection). Before discussing these processes in some detail, it should be emphasized at the outset that 'cleansing' is an essential preliminary to disinfection. Organic matter has the ability considerably to reduce the effectiveness of disinfectants so without good cleansing the action of disinfectants is often readily nullified.

Natural disinfectant agents

Most pathogenic micro-organisms do not survive long outside the animal body but unfortunately sufficient may always remain to cause renewed infection. Some vegetative bacteria and viruses can live several months if protected with organic matter and the spores of bacteria can live almost indefinitely in the soil or protected in cracks and crevices of the building. For example, *Clostridium tetani* and *Bacillus anthracis* can live many years. Even coccidial oocysts may survive for years in infected quarters.

The factors contributing towards natural destruction of microbes are nevertheless important as they do reduce the numbers and this in itself is a worthwhile aid to the artificial processes. Sunlight, heat, cold, desiccation and agitation all contribute. Sunlight is the most potent and its powers of destruction are enormous. Its efficiency is entirely due to the ultraviolet range of wavelengths. Unfortunately, these ultraviolet rays have little penetrating power and cannot pass through glass or translucent roofing sheets or through clouds of industrial haze; the value of sunlight in animal buildings is therefore wholly unreliable. Desiccation, from fresh air and wind, will also contribute to the destruction, particularly when the micro-organisms are exposed to this by prior cleansing of the building.

Another process is antibiosis; many bacteria and fungi produce substances that are antagonistic to other organisms. Penicillin and streptomycin are agents of this nature whose antibacterial action is well known. In the soil, in floors and buildings generally, pathogenic organisms will be acted upon by antibiotics produced by non-pathogenic organisms that are normal inhabitants of the soil. Warm moist conditions will assist the action of such saprophytic agents.

The action of heat

For many years heat has been used for disinfection, dry heat being used with the 'flame-gun' and moist heat in the form of the 'steam-jenny', but both tend to be inexact and uncontrolled methods of applying the agents.

Many bacterial spores can easily survive the transitory attention of the heat source and pathogenic organisms may readily be protected from the heat in cracks and crevices of the building.

Chemical disinfectants

Disinfection on the farm is generally carried out by using chemical agents. The lethal action of disinfectants is due in the main to their ability to react with the protein and, in particular, the essential enzymes of micro-organisms. Therefore, any agents that will coagulate, precipitate or otherwise denature proteins will act as general disinfectants. Among these agents are phenols, alcohols, acids, alkalis, aldehydes, halogens, chloramines and quaternary ammonium compounds, as well as heat and certain radiations.

Selective action

Many disinfectants have a selective action on different types of microbes. For example, Gram-positive and Gram-negative bacteria differ in the structure of their membranes, the latter being of a more complex nature. Micro-organisms also respond to changes in pH and as every protein has its own characteristic isoelectric point, each responds individually and will be influenced by the acidity or alkalinity of the disinfectant; for example, fungi are extremely acid-resistant, whereas viruses tend to be more susceptible to acid disinfectants, such as the iodophors. Another factor affecting the behaviour of a disinfectant is the lipoid content of the cells; in some the content is high, as in acid-fast organisms, and it will thus attract a lipophilic moiety in a disinfectant substance and dissolve it more readily, thereby increasing the germicidal activity. Some disinfectants, which are called 'broad spectrum', are almost equally active against most species of micro-organisms, while others show specificity and are only active against a restricted number of species.

Disinfection of viruses

For disinfection purposes viruses can be classified into two groups, lipophilic and hydrophilic. Lipophilic viruses have lipid envelopes, which make them sensitive to the majority of disinfectants. Most of the animal pathogenic viruses are in this group. Hydrophilic viruses are enveloped and are less sensitive to disinfectants in general. Some very important viruses are in this group and these have a tendency to become dangerously persistent on farms and in animal buildings; examples are the enteroviruses and reoviruses. Against this latter group quaternary ammonium compounds have a poor effect but are very good if associated with formaldehyde, glutaraldehyde chloramines and certain organic acids.

Dynamics of disinfection

Disinfection is not an instantaneous process; it takes place gradually. However, many more microbes are killed at the beginning of disinfection than at the end although there is an initial lag period before activity commences. The lag phase is normally only a few seconds but may be seriously prolonged if the environment is unfavourable, for example extreme cold, high humidity or excessive organic matter. An examination of the number of organisms surviving at different stages during disinfection shows that the number of bacteria killed in unit time bears a constant relationship to the number of surviving organisms. Thus, after the lag phase, destruction of the bacteria is very rapid at first but tends to slow up so that eventually destruction of all the organisms takes a considerably longer time. The usual time–survivor curve is of the sigmoid type.

The concentration of disinfectant and temperature of disinfection influence the rate of death and also alter the shape of the time–survivor curves. As the death rate is increased by using higher concentrations of disinfectant, the initial lag phase is eliminated or, in fact, is so quick that it goes undetected. The action of most disinfectants is increased, often quite markedly, as the temperature rises.

The effect of organic matter

Almost invariably when disinfection is carried out on the farm, organic matter will be present. It can be said that organic matter always interferes with the action of the disinfectant and may do so in the following ways.

1 The organic matter may protect the cell by forming a coating on it and preventing the ready access of the disinfectant.

2 The disinfectant may form an insoluble compound with the organic matter to remove it from potential activity.

3 The disinfectant may react chemically with the organic matter giving rise to a non-germicidal reaction product.

4 Particulate and colloidal matter in suspension may absorb the antibacterial agent, so that it is substantially removed from solution.

5 Fats, etc. in serum and milk may inactivate the disinfectant.

Approval of disinfectants

There is no completely satisfactory method of assessing or standardizing disinfectants and an enormous number of different techniques have been used in the past. There is also no universally effective disinfectant, so that different disinfectants are required for different purposes.

In the UK, Approvals for disinfectants are under five headings, as follows:

Group 1A are active against foot-and-mouth disease
Group 1B are active against swine vesicular disease
Group II are active against fowl pest

Group III are active against tuberculosis
Group IV are for general farm use, the test organism being *Salmonella cholerae-suis*.

The official test lays down a rigid procedure for specified reduction of the organisms in the presence of organic matter. The most recent order, The Diseases of Animals (Approved Disinfectants) (Amendment) Order 1975, specifies some 300 disinfectants in the various groups.

Disinfectants

Phenols, cresols and related compounds

The phenols, cresols and related compounds are an important group of disinfectants that were once the most popular of all such agents.

All phenols can act bactericidally or fungicidally but generally are neither sporicidal nor particularly virucidal. They have high dilution coefficients, i.e. small concentration changes give rise to large differences in their killing rates. They are always more effective as the temperature rises, and are more active as acid solutions. Organic matter can severely interfere with their efficiency and even small quantities of faeces can reduce their effectiveness to 10 per cent. There are many proprietary 'coal tar disinfectants', phenolic in nature, and in view of their inevitable low solubility in water, they are either solubilized or emulsified. The solubilized types, known as 'black fluids' are those in which the phenol fraction is dissolved in a soap base, and the emulsified types, known as 'white fluids', are those in which the phenol is emulsified into a permanent suspension with the aid of gelatin or dextrin.

In more recent years a number of synthetic phenols have been marketed. These may be a chloroxylenol, *o*-phenylphenol or one of the other diphenyl derivatives. Such preparations, in contrast to the cresols or coal tar disinfectants, are non-toxic, non-irritant and have a more pleasant colour, arising chiefly from their purer disinfectants.

Formaldehyde and glutaraldehyde

Formaldehyde is a widely used disinfectant in both the gaseous and the aqueous forms, being bactericidal, virucidal and fungicidal. In aqueous solutions, formalin, which is a solution of formaldehyde gas containing 40 g of formaldehyde in 100 ml of the solution, is widely used at 5 per cent strength as a general disinfectant, but it does need to be in contact with the surface for some time to be effective. It action is greatly affected by temperature (i.e. it has a high temperature coefficient) and the warmer it is the better, blood heat being most satisfactory. It also acts more efficiently when the surface is wet. In agricultural use formalin is largely used as a gas or an aerosol spray.

A very active complex disinfectant, which is useful against the most persistent viruses, is one containing formaldehyde, glutaraldehyde and a quaternary ammonium compound. This is active at much lower temperatures than formaldehyde.

Quaternary ammonium compounds

These are cationic neutral detergents available as aqueous solutions, powders or pastes. They are effective against a wide range of bacteria and moulds and have a high surface activity. Generally, when dissolved in water, they have a high wetting power and the ions adhere to the surfaces, giving a long-lasting residual effect. They also have low toxicity and lack odour or taste. Combined with other disinfectants they can give a wide spectrum of activity.

Oxidizing disinfectants

Hydrogen peroxide and other oxidizing agents including peracetic acid and propionic acid are emerging as increasingly popular disinfectants. At quite low concentrations they are active against bacteria, their spores, viruses and fungi. Several new proprietary forms are marketed for use in livestock buildings.

The halogens

In agriculture, chlorine is widely used for disinfecting water and in the cleansing of dairy and other farm equipment. Chlorine-releasing compounds containing up to 90 per cent available chlorine are available and have an important use in the formulation of bactericidal detergent powders of the alkaline variety. Products of this type are suitable for use in the washing down of an animal house. The inorganic chloramines, being a concentration of chlorine and ammonia, are used in water and sewage treatment; organic chloramines, such as halazone, are excellent water sanitizers.

The normal use of chlorine in cleaning milking and other utensils is to use a detergent wash with a solution containing 250–300 p.p.m. of available chlorine followed by a rinse with a weaker chlorine solution. Failure of the chlorine disinfectant is most likely due to the presence of organic matter, which does seriously interfere with its action, so that it is not normally used where much dirt is present. In favourable circumstances it is best used warm and will act quickly. Chloramines are much more active in the presence of organic matter and have found a secure place as general disinfectants.

Iodine and iodophors

Iodine is an effective germicide, although like chlorine it is much depressed by organic matter. It is effective against vegetative organisms and spores. The most widely used iodine preparations are the iodophors in which iodine is mixed with surface-active agents, which act as carriers or solubilizers for the iodine. They lack any real odour and are not irritant.

Iodophors have been used at dilutions of around 25 p.p.m. available iodine for utensils. They have built-in indicators that reveal quickly the approximate concentration of the use-dilution; a yellow tinge or pale amber colour is imparted by an iodophor even when only a few parts per million of free iodine are present in the solution. Higher concentrations give deeper shades of amber or brown to the solution. The use-dilution of 25 p.p.m. is equivalent to available chlorine concentrations up to 200 p.p.m. Iodophors are an ideal germicide to use in water utensils.

Ammonia

A 10 per cent aqueous solution of ammonia is an effective agent for the destruction of coccidial oocysts. This is the only use for ammonia as a disinfectant.

Ectoparasites

It is of great importance to control ectoparasites in and around the farm buildings. They are a nuisance both to the attendants and the animals; may be the cause of direct irritation and disease; and may indirectly spread disease, indeed any infectious agent can be carried by ectoparasitic vectors. These ectoparasites include flies (the ordinary housefly, the lesser housefly and the stable fly), mites (including red mites and northern fowl mites), ticks, lice, fleas, bugs, beetles and cockroaches.

For the control of external parasites of animals a variety of compounds are available, such as gamma-benzene hexachloride (lindane), piperoxyl-butoxide pyrethrum (pybuthrin) or O,O-dimethyldithiophosphate of diethylmercaptosuccinate (malathion) and O, O-dimethyl-O-2,4,5-trichlorphenyl phosphorathroate (fenchlorphos 12 per cent).

Recommended procedure in disinfection and disinfestation of animal buildings and equipment

Basically, two procedures should be adopted. The first is used between batches of livestock within a building in the absence of overt disease, and the second after an outbreak of a contagious and infectious disease.

Procedure of disinfection with no disease present

1 All equipment and fittings that are removable should be demounted and taken out of the building. It is advisable for them to be soaked in a bath of disinfectant where the materials are able to stand up to this treatment. Alternatively, they may be power-sprayed or steam sterilized. They should be left outside exposed to the elements and away from animals and their products as long as possible.
2 All litter should be removed (Fig. 50.5).
3 The roof and structural elements of the house should be dusted and cleaned, preferably with a vacuum cleaner.
4 The lower part of the walls and all the floors should be thoroughly cleaned, preferably using a pressure washer, with a heavy duty, wide-spectrum detergent disinfectant mixture (Fig. 50.6).
5 The surfaces must then have a disinfectant applied (Fig. 50.7) with a wide spectrum of activity, capable of killing all the pathogens that are likely to be present.
6 In some cases, if there is a heavy insect infestation, there will be a need to apply a special insecticide spray.
7 As a final measure a disinfectant is often sprayed over all the surfaces to give a residual effect. Thermal 'fogging' machines are widely used.

Procedure after contagious and infectious disease

1 The building should be closed and isolated from all visitors.
2 The bedding, litter and all areas in intimate contact with the stock should be sprayed with a strong disinfectant.
3 The litter should subsequently be removed from the building and may be burnt or buried so there is no possible contact with livestock.
4 Portable equipment and fittings should be given the same treatment as previously suggested and preferably in the house, later to be taken out and aerated.
5 Clean the floors and lower part of the walls with detergent disinfectant.
6 The house should then be treated in the same way as suggested in the previous section.
7 It may sometimes be advisable to skim off the top

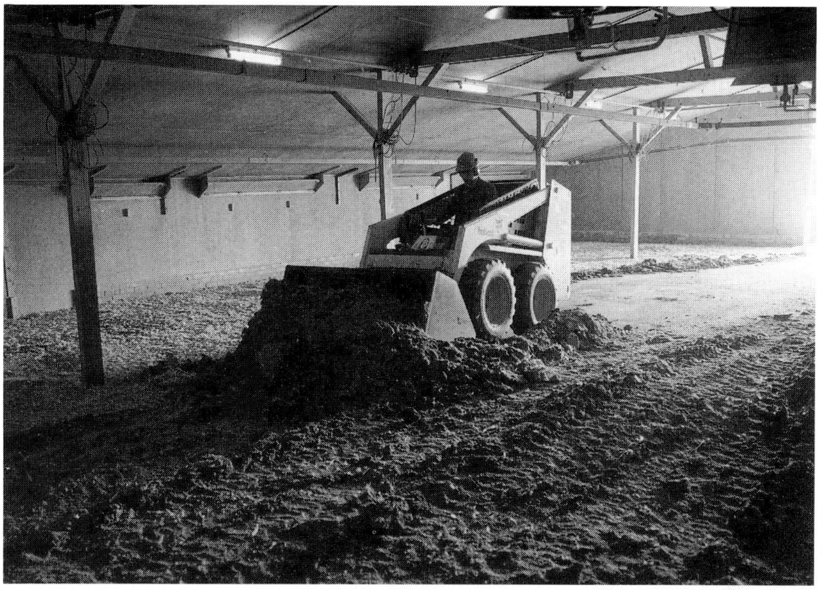

Fig. 50.5 Cleaning out the litter after removal of the animals.

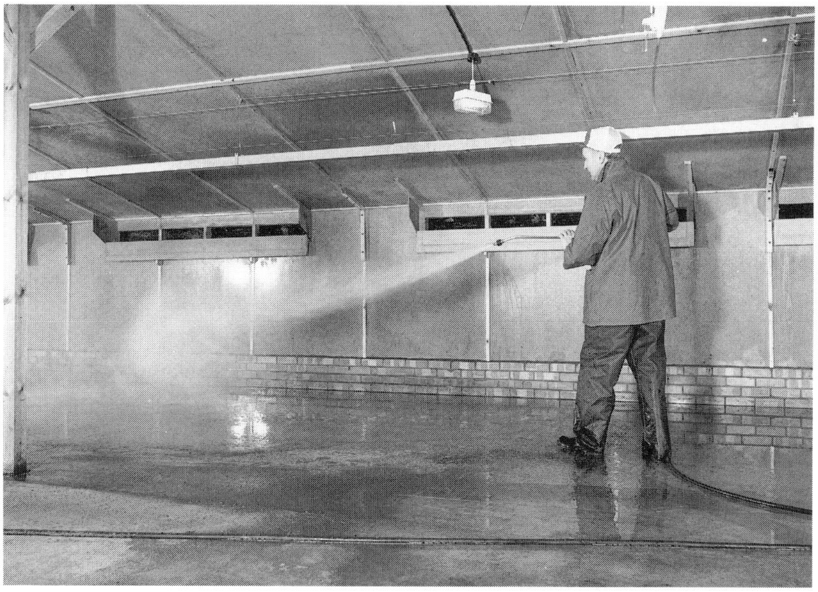

Fig. 50.6 Washing down with a pressure hose using a detergent disinfectant.

few inches of the soil around a heavily infected area.
8 The approaches to the building should be treated with disinfectant and foot-dips provided (Fig. 50.8).

Ventilation

There are few topics in animal husbandry where there have been more totally erroneous statements made than on the reasons why housed livestock require ventilation or 'air-change'. For example, for many years it was accepted that the main deleterious effects of having too little ventilation was due to the build-up of harmful concentrations of the gaseous products of respiration and in particular carbon dioxide, combined with a depletion in the oxygen content of the air. It is now known that this is far too simple and usually quite an incorrect hypothesis.

Underlying principles and calculations

In any badly under-ventilated building the stagnant air gradually becomes both warmer and more humid and

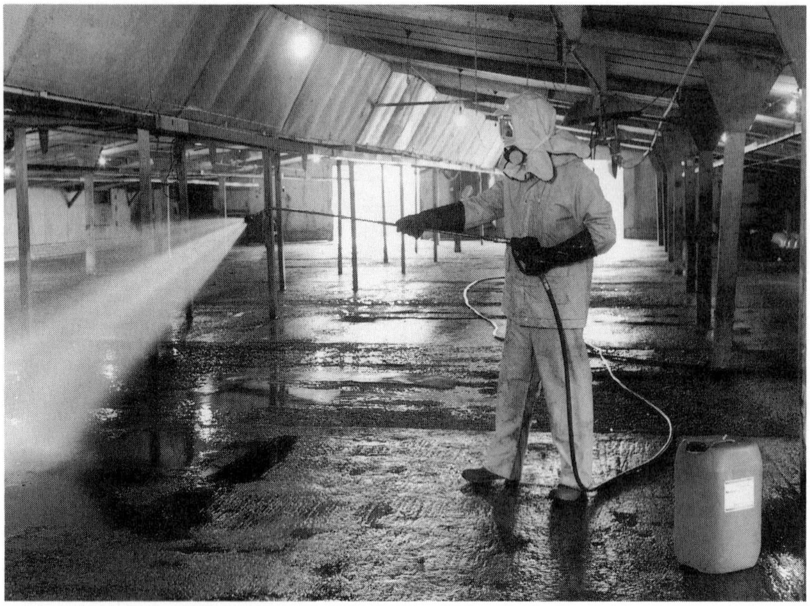

Fig. 50.7 Spraying with a disinfectant.

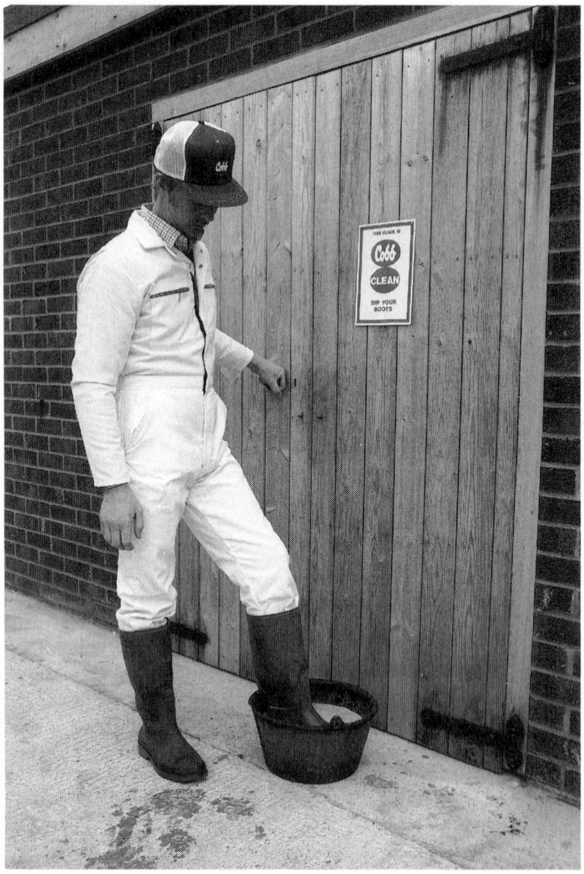

Fig. 50.8 Using protective clothing and dipping boots in disinfectant to reduce the risk of introducing infection.

there is a rising concentration of dust, other particulate matter, ammonia and other gases and any pathogenic micro-organisms the livestock may be carrying. The end result is that the animals suffer from 'heat stagnation', involving a susceptibility to chilling. Along with this will go poor productivity and a likelihood of disease, particularly respiratory, which modern experience shows to be of the greatest danger in intensive forms of housing.

In addition, in a badly ventilated building, condensation on the surface is often likely and bedding and floors may become wet and the animals uncomfortable. This will tend to exacerbate the effect of disease conditions, respiratory or enteric in nature, or infections such as mastitis.

In recent years a new hazard to livestock and their attendants has been the risk of gaseous intoxication of livestock due to the gases arising from slurry pits or channels under the animals. The risk is very great and has caused the death of many animals and several stockworkers.

The object of ventilation, therefore, is to remove the stale air in a building and replace it with fresh air and remove any danger of toxic gases. But while too little ventilation is obviously serious, so also is too much. In cold weather much valuable animal heat will be wasted. Further, over-ventilation may be synonymous with draught. Draughts are themselves responsible for causing many deaths by direct chilling and they may also act indirectly by lowering the animals' resistance to disease-producing organisms.

In planning a ventilation system allowance has to be made for all the factors that can influence the ventilation required, i.e. type, age and number of livestock, their management, the construction and locality of the house and finally the weather conditions.

Natural ventilation

If natural ventilation is to be effective, it must function well in all weathers. To try to avoid too great a dependence on external wind and weather, it is best to make use of the so-called 'stack-effect' as its foundation. The warm stale air around the body of the animal, being lighter than cold fresh air, will rise to the top of the building. Outlet ventilation is therefore provided at a suitable point or points in the ceiling or roof. The greater the difference between inside and outside temperatures, and the greater the distance between inlets and outlets, the greater the stack effect. Therefore, if an area of outlet ventilation is provided to cope with difficult conditions (i.e. a small difference between inside and outside temperatures) it can easily be restricted when temperature differences are greater or appreciable winds help in the ventilation. As mentioned, in houses where no great control is necessary, such as climatic housing for cattle, a fixed open ridge with a protective cap may be sufficient. But in other controlled-climate accommodations far more control is needed and down-draughts, which can be common with the fixed open ridge, must be avoided. Experience has shown that for the latter, good results are obtained by the use of a limited area of controlled outlet ventilation, and for this purpose a simple chimney type or insulated 'flue' is satisfactory. It is good practice to have one or a few outlets, but a much larger number of smaller air inlets as the fresh air should come in slowly all round the building, diffusely and carefully baffled. The basis of a useful inlet system consists of hopper-type windows, fitted with gussets to prevent direct draughts, serving as principal inlets, and small baffled openings between the windows which alone are left open during cold or windy weather. Since cold air coming into the building falls naturally towards the floor, there is no necessity to site inlets at floor level, where the danger of chilling draught is considerable.

The totally covered yard

In practice the following major faults are commonly found in the construction of covered yards.

1 Either there is no ridge outlet for stale air or it is inadequate.

2 Eaves openings are either absent or, where present, uncontrollable and at the mercy of the weather, causing chilling draughts in cold weather.

3 The extreme width of many yards (20 m upwards) prevents natural ventilation functioning properly. This problem is often combined with multispan construction and low eaves and roofs, so that the flow is generally impaired.

4 The gable ends are closed and sealed.

5 There is no insulation of the roof. While insulation is not usually necessary it may be a desirable 'extra' under a few circumstances, particularly where younger stock are housed or where the roof is low and natural air flow is difficult.

6 Poor drainage under or around the yard leads to excessive straw usage and contributes to the humidity of the atmosphere.

7 Bad construction of the walls leads to excessive moisture penetration at all points.

Natural ventilation works most satisfactorily on open sites; it is always useful to have it controllable but this is not usually done. An open ridge 300 mm wide, with a flat continuous top at least 150 mm above, is a simple answer to extraction in narrow yards, and a 600 mm width in yards above 14 m width.

An even more satisfactory arrangement is to have a series of chimney-type ventilators along the ridge, allowing 0.09 m^2/animal. A useful size of chimney is 1 m^2; this is sufficient for 11 animals. The throat can be controlled by a butterfly valve or hinged flap.

Alternative ways of achieving good 'top' ventilation are as follows.

1 Raised sheets, consisting of conventional steel or asbestos sheets fitted with a batten or washers raising the overlapping, allowing air to pass between the sheets.

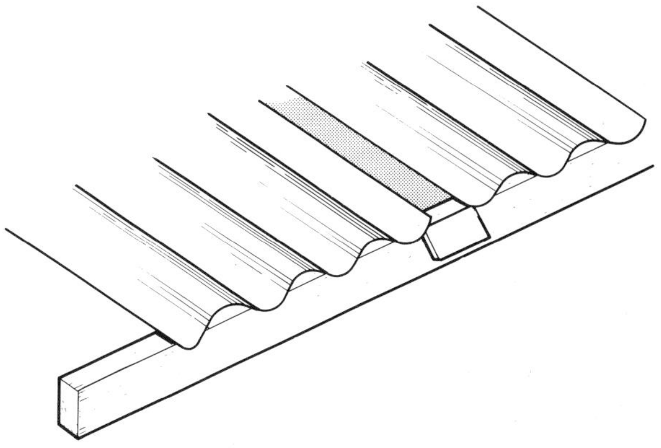

Fig. 50.9 The 'breathing' roof: ventilation achieved by leaving a gap between the roof sheets.

A spacer batten of treated timber measuring 50 × 25 mm is suitable.

2 Upturned corrugated sheeting. Conventional galvanized corrugated steel sheeting is fixed upside down with a gap between each sheet, forming a Venturi slow between each sheet. Typically, a 25 mm gap may be used, which would give 3.75 per cent opening of the roof. (Fig. 50.9).

Systems (**1**) and (**2**) are often described as 'breathing roofs'.

Mechanical ventilation

This has a place in some cattle yards as it has for other forms of intensively housed stock. With a system of chimney trunks, fans can be added as a complementary arrangement, since an extractor fan may be fitted at the base. If a 600 mm fan running at a maximum of 900 rev/min is fitted, 10 194 m^3/hour will be extracted. A maximum allowance of 510 m^3/hour per beast (or approximately 0.42 m^3/hour per kg body weight) is found satisfactory, so that one fan will serve approximately 30 beef animals to slaughter.

Automatic or semi-automatic control can be achieved if a proportion (one-half to two-thirds) of the fans are put on thermostatic control, with a thermostat that is easily seen and adjusted. Fans thus operated should have automatic antiback-draught flaps fitted to prevent down-draughts when they are switched off. All fans should be speed controlled. Alternatively, a system of variable fan speed on a motorized thermostat or electronic control will give full automation on all fans.

Fan ventilation halves the number of roof outlets that need to be installed. The total capital cost of a fan-operated system will hardly be more than £30 per animal-place, an economical cost for automatic environmental control. Running costs may be a rather more daunting charge.

The main use of fan ventilation in cattle yards is in those cases where extremely high stocking rates are used, as with slatted floor units, or where the topography of the site or restriction of wind around the building makes natural flow all but impossible.

The inlet of fresh air is no less important, and it has been found satisfactory to provide inward-opening hopper flaps along both side walls, bottom-hung and 700–900 mm deep, with gussets and variable control through casement stays or remote control from the feeding passage. Alternatively, the hoppers may be controlled from the ends with horticultural glasshouse type fittings. It is preferable if the inlets are not closer than 600 mm to the eaves, to prevent incoming air

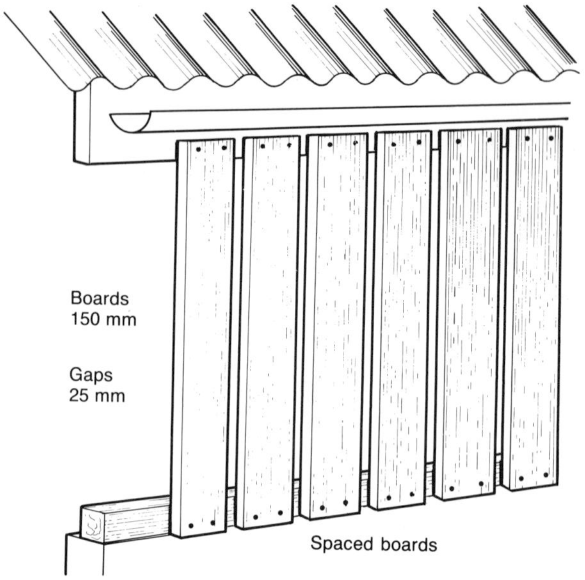

Fig. 50.10 Wall ventilation with spaced boarding.

'bouncing' off exposed purlins and causing an irritating down-draught on the animals. The flaps should be made so that they can be removed or hinged down flat in the summer; they should extend along at least one-half and preferably two-thirds of the wall length.

With wide-span yards over 21 m, slatted boarding (100 mm boards and 12 mm gaps or 150 mm boards and 25 mm gaps) should be fitted at the gable ends and part of this area made as hinged doors that can be opened in the summer. This is normally not necessary, however, in narrow-span yards. In addition, there are a number of other excellent techniques for achieving good inlet ventilation for cattle and other yards.

'Space-boarding' is excellent all around a yard — at the gable ends and along the walls above 'animal height'. It gives an opening area of about 20 per cent of the total but is uncontrollable; an alternative is to have an adjustable system with fixed outer slats and inner sliding slats. There are also various other arrangements, such as the Ventair steel sheet with patented louvres (13 per cent open); slatted hardboard with slats 5 × 25 mm giving 30 per cent opening; Netlon polypropylene mesh (45 per cent open); Ventrex steel sheet with louvres (0.7 per cent open); and a common device of a space left between the outer sheet and the wall, giving a baffled protected inlet.

It is in no way suggested that the systems outlined are the only satisfactory methods of ventilating intensive cattle yards. For example, other mechanical means have been used, often with equal success. These do, however, often need more careful designing and management to prevent draughts and to give adequate control. The systems suggested are logical and generally understood and easily controlled by the stockworker. Mechanical assistance with the designs shown are complementary to natural flow and indeed may be used as an additional stage in the development and improvement of a design. Draughts are least likely where there is the fullest control of the system. Ventilation continues to function at a reduced rate in the event of power failure with the system advocated, since natural stack-effect ventilation takes over from the fans to tide the stock over this period.

If the trend towards high stocking rates continues it is inevitable that the farmer will turn increasingly to thermal insulation of the surfaces, especially the roof. Farmers who have used insulation of the roof have recorded considerable benefits in terms of liveweight gain and food conversion efficiency, but above all because it helps also to solve environmental problems. A popular way of arranging the insulation is by using two skins of metal or fibre-cement sheeting for the roof separated by a vapour-sealed layer of mineral wool or glass wool. For the latter, a 50 mm thickness is minimal but 100 mm is very much better. A cheap treatment for an existing uninsulated building is to build a false ceiling of wire mesh supporting vapour-sealed insulation. It is an economical way of insulating the building, though somewhat temporary. It must be emphasized that individual attention does need to be given to each yard according to the site and locality. It is one of the advantages of fan ventilation that with mechanical ventilation this statement is much less true. The use of fans partially rules out the dependence on site and weather. It is generally better to have yards in exposed positions because it is easier to restrict the open area if too much air comes in than to open-up the ventilation space in a sheltered site. Sometimes the proximity of other buildings makes it impossible to increase the airflow at all.

Livestock yards are now often made very wide, of the order of 40–50 m. These are invariably the most difficult units to ventilate. From the point of view of ventilation it is desirable to limit the span to some 30 m. Indeed, if the trend towards the use of thermal insulation continues, views on what constitutes an adequate cubic area may change. In an uninsulated yard a large cubic area helps to buffer the outside weather extremes. But in an insulated construction, the roofing area must be reduced to a minimum to cut costs and more economical dimensions would be a height of 3.6 m to eaves with a maximum yard span of 21 m. These recommendations widely used and required for cattle buildings apply, with only minor modifications, to climatic yard accommodation generally, including that for pigs, sheep and turkeys.

Open-fronted yards and kennels

A fundamentally different approach to climatic housing is the 'lean-to' or open-fronted yard, often called the mono-pitch building. This is attractive in several respects and continues to gain in popularity as an alternative to the span roof yard. For a start it is usually cheaper. Also, by its very nature, it is impossible to make it very wide — a depth of 10 m being about the limit — so the enormous problems of ventilation created by wide spans are avoided and stock concentrations in one air-space are limited. Best of all, such a system gives cheap isolation of groups by carrying vertical partitions to the roof and if necessary supporting it every 3–6 m. With an open-fronted design animals have a choice of environment, as they can go towards the lower back part in colder conditions to keep warm, or come to the front for sunlight and more fresh air in warmer weather. Control of airflow can be by simple hinged flaps on the front and kennels can be incorporated if desired. It is most desirable that open-fronted yards in the northern hemisphere face in a southerly direction only; it is preferable not to face two rows together, since there is a risk of the passage-way between becoming a wind tunnel, and in this situation one side at least will face north or east and so may get little sun and indeed suffer from distinctly cooler conditions.

Dangers from gases in farm buildings

Problems associated with gases in and around the livestock farm have been highlighted recently, particularly in association with gas effusion from slurry channels under perforated floors, but it would be wrong to regard these as the only dangers. While there have been numerous fatalities of livestock recorded, and indeed in man, due to gas intoxication, there is also mounting evidence that there may be concentrations of gases in many livestock buildings that may affect production adversely by reducing feed consumption, lowering growth rates and the animals' susceptibility to invasion by pathogenic micro-organisms.

The most serious incidence of gas intoxication arises from areas of manure storage in slurry pits or channels under the stock, usually but not always associated with forms of perforated floors. The greatest risk arises when the manure is agitated for any reason, usually when it is removed. There is also an ever-present danger if a mechanical system of ventilation fails and this is the only method of moving air in the house. Several cases of poisoning have been reported when sluice-gates are opened at the end of slurry channels and the movement of the liquid manure has forced gas up at one end of the building.

High concentrations of gases, chiefly ammonia, may also arise from built-up litter in animal housing. The danger has undoubtedly been exacerbated within more recent years owing to the mistaken insistence of maintaining relatively high house temperatures in order to reduce food costs. The farmer has often attempted to achieve such temperatures by restricting ventilation and in the absence of good thermal insulation of the house surfaces, so that the result may often be generally harmful if not actually dangerous.

References

Britton, D.K. & Berkeley Hill (1975) *Size and Efficiency in Farming*, pp. 132–47. Saxon House Studies, Farnborough.

Donaldson, A.I. (1978) Factors influencing the dispersal, survival and deposition of airborne pathogens of farm animals. *Veterinary Bulletin*, **48**, 83–94.

Donaldson, A.I. & Ferris, N.P. (1976) The survival of some airborne animal viruses in relation to relative humidity. *Veterinary Microbiology*, **1**, 413–20.

Honey, H.F. & McQuitty, J.B. (1976) *Dust in the Animal Environment*. Department of Agricultural Engineering, University of Alberta, Canada.

Sanger, J.R. (1969) Influence of relative humidity on the survival of some airborne viruses. *Applied Microbiology*, **15**, 35–42.

Webster, A.J.F. (1981) Optimal housing criteria for ruminants. In *Environmental Aspects of Housing for Animal Production* (ed. by J.A. Clark) pp. 217–32. Butterworth, London.

Whittlestone, P. (1976) Effect of climatic conditions on enzootic pneumonia in pigs. *International Journal of Biometeorology*, **20**, 42–8.

Wray, C. (1975) Survival and spread of pathogenic bacteria of veterinary importance within the environment. *Veterinary Bulletin*, **45**, 543–57.

Chapter 51: Immunological Fundamentals

by W.P.H. DUFFUS

Introduction

What does the word 'immune' mean? The derivation of the word stems from 'exempt from burden'. In reality the word was coined to explain what we now term immunological memory. Populations, both human and domestic stock, suffered and continue to suffer from epidemic disease; the old observation was that individuals recovering from a clinical syndrome were 'exempt' at the appearance of the next epidemic.

This ability of the vertebrate immune system to 'remember' a previous exposure to a foreign or non-self material is at the very heart of preventive medicine. The response is normally termed an *adaptive immune response*. This is in contrast to the *innate immune response* which covers the mechanisms pre-existing within an individual. The division between these two main areas of the immune system is not absolute; there is much interaction and interdependence between effector mechanisms in both camps. What do we mean by effector mechanisms? The term usefully describes the sharp end of the immune response: the antibody that actually causes the destruction of a bacteria, the cell that actually destroys another, but potentially malignant, cell.

There are three other broad concepts to consider at an early stage. First, the immune response can itself be harmful. The millions of individuals suffering from allergy will know this fact only too well. The second main concept is one of specificity/recognition. The immune system is exquisitively specific and has the ability to recognize millions of different combinations of molecules that make up the myriad of different types of 'non-self' material that individuals are exposed to constantly. These are termed *antigens*, each site on the antigen that retains the ability to be recognized by the immune system being termed an *epitope*. Note the use of the word 'non-self'; this is a useful term as 'self' means the immune system has lost the ability to recognize that particular antigen within an individual and therefore the latter remains free of potentially harmful effector mechanisms. Unfortunately this protection can break down leading to an increasing plethora of autoimmune disease. The third main concept is the division of both the acquired and innate immune response into *cellular* (e.g. lymphocyte, etc.) and *humoral* (e.g. antibody, etc.) components.

A study of immunology as it relates to bovine medicine is artificially skewed towards two of the four main areas that cause sickness/death: injury and infection. The other two main areas are degenerative disease and cancer but these are problems of the older individual, subsequently defence mechanisms against these latter two are not as important within a population, such as cattle, with a fast turnover of generations.

The majority of the mechanisms, both cellular and humoral, that make up the ruminant immune system are common to all mammals. The highly developed mammalian immune system is the culmination of evolutionary pressures with effector mechanisms that are traceable in the lower animal kingdom. However, there are aspects of this mammalian immune system that are specifically enhanced and specialized within ruminants (such as the passive transfer of lactogenic antibody). These differences will be discussed within the relevant sections. An important conceptual point to get across early on is one of balance between two conflicting points of view. On one side is the animal trying to preserve its integrity against a variety of potential pathogens by utilizing the effector mechanisms themselves comprising the innate and adaptive immune response. On the other side are the organisms that are trying to survive in the face of these mechanisms, relying on a fast turnover of generations and natural selection. This balance is at the heart of almost all host–pathogen interrelationships. With cattle and intensive husbandry we are tilting this balance in favour of the organism and allowing them to replicate and cause diseases such as mastitis, enzootic pneumonia, etc. Intensive husbandry is here to stay for production reasons and we will have to turn to artificial means to restore the balance. This scenario will involve research to ascertain which 'batch' of effector mechanisms is applicable to a particular pathogen, and then how can we artificially boost this immunity.

Innate immunity

These immune mechanisms pre-exist in an individual and are not improved by repeated infection. Like acquired immunity they can be divided up into humoral and cellular components.

Humoral

COMPLEMENT

The word 'complement' is a collective term for 15 or so plasma proteins (enzymes) which can be activated sequentially into functional units that then have three major effects.

1 Production of peptides which are active in inflammatory processes.

2 Production of C3b which, by its ability to 'opsonize' micro-organisms or other particulate matter, is a powerful incentive for phagocytosis.

3 Attachment to cell membranes to create lysis and destruction of the target.

After immunoglobulins, albumin and transferrin, C3 is the most abundant of bovine serum proteins (in excess of 1 mg/ml).

How is complement activated? The combination of immunoglobulin with antigen will often cause activation, but enzymes such as trypsin and bacterial components such as endotoxin will all activate complement. The normal route of activation by such agents is termed the *classical pathway* and as far as the antibody–antigen reaction is concerned it relies on the availability of the Fc portion of the antibody molecule. In the cow it used to be thought that of the two major subclasses of IgG (IgG_1 and IgG_2) only IgG_1 could fix complement by this route. Recent research using a homologous bovine IgG_2/complement system, has clearly shown that both subclasses can fix complement. Another pathway of complement activation is via the *alternative route*. This is a more primitive pathway and does not require the Fc portion of the antibody and can indeed be activated by antibodies such as IgA which is not effective by the classical route. Certain isolates of *E. coli* and virus-infected cells can all set the alternative pathway going, an important point in assessing complement as a defence mechanism.

LYSOZYME AND OTHER SERUM PROTEINS

Lysozyme, a protein with a molecular weight of approximately 14 000, is highly active against bacteria and is found in many biological fluids and is sometimes called the 'natural antibiotic'. It is not often realized that Fleming discovered both penicillin and lysozyme!

Neutrophils can be stimulated to produce lactoferrin. This protein works by competing with bacteria for the available iron molecules. Milk contains approximately 6 mg/ml.

Acute phase proteins appear within hours of tissue damage or infection. The best known one is C reactive protein which binds to phosphorylcholine on the surface of certain bacteria thus promoting phagocytosis by complement fixation.

INTERFERON (IFN)

These glycoproteins are a family of cell-regulating proteins produced by many cell types in response to stimuli. Although viruses are well known as interferon (IFN) inducers, others include endotoxin, bacteria and a variety of other antigenic stimuli. Interferons are classified as follows.

1 IFN-α is produced by leucocytes.

2 IFN-β is produced by fibroblasts.

3 IFN-γ is produced by T lymphocytes.

Interferon offers a rapid protection to viral infection. It induces an anti-viral state in cells by firstly triggering a receptor (IFN-αβ share a receptor, IFN-γ remains separate). This stimulates the cell itself to produce proteins to block the transcription of viruses, so protecting them from infection.

Interferon can be produced within hours of stimulation and the antiviral state can last several days. Interferon also has a number of other effects both on the immune system (such as stimulation of cytotoxicity and increased expression of major histocompalability complex (MHC) products), as well as other functions such as cell division.

All three types of bovine IFN have now been genetically engineered and are being investigated for their potential as therapeutic agents. There may well be a role in diseases such as enzootic calf pneumonia.

Cellular

PHAGOCYTIC CELLS

These include neutrophils, macrophages and other cells of the reticuloendothelial system. Free-living bacteria are fairly easy to kill without antibody or complement, but bacterial pathogens such as streptococci with large capsules can alter the surface tension between the phagocyte and the bacteria so preventing phagocytosis. It is for this reason that specific antibody and/or complement is needed to 'coat' or 'opsonize' the bacteria, altering the surface tension and allowing phagocytosis to proceed. Bovine neutrophils and macrophages/monocytes have C3 and Fc membrane receptors. Cattle have unusually high numbers of monocytes in circulation.

The phagocytic cells have several agents such as acid hydrolases, peroxidase and cationic proteins which can kill micro-organisms after phagocytosis. The cationic proteins come into play first when the pH goes up and in fact these mechanisms are now thought to be at least or even more important than the traditional peroxidase-dependent pathways involving H_2O_2.

Several pathogens such as *Brucella abortus*, *Salmonella* spp., *Listeria* spp. and *Mycobacterium* spp. can live intracellularly and thus pose a problem for the immune system. The solution is by activation of the macrophage, usually by specific protein messengers released especially by T lymphocytes, called cytokines. Activated macrophages are basically a lot 'meaner', more efficient and, for example, contain more lysosomes; they are quite capable of dealing with these more awkward pathogens.

We must also consider another vital, indeed pivotal, role for macrophages. This is one we term *antigen presentation*. These antigen presenting cells (APCs) are found throughout lymphoid tissue, the archetypal one being the Langerhans' cell in the skin. Other specialized APCs are found in the gut, respiratory tract and mammary gland. These cells basically phagocytose the antigen, process it and then deliver it as a neat package to lymphocytes of the immune system. They combine this 'antigen presentation' with MHC products on their membrane and by the release of a soluble mediator such as interleukin-1 (IL-1).

NATURAL KILLER (NK) CELLS

It is only in the last five years or so that natural killer or NK cells have come into their own. They are basically lymphocytes with a separate lineage from T and B lymphocytes. The geneaology of NK cells remains unclear, they share membrane determinants with both monocytes and lymphocytes. They have Fc receptors and are quite large cells, often with noticeable granules. Two fascinating things about NK cells is that: (i) they pre-exist within individuals and do not require antigenic stimulation; (ii) they can kill innumerable targets from virus-infected cells to tumour cells without the need for antibody. Therefore, they could operate a type of 'policing' role within the body, ready to destroy spontaneous tumour cells when they arise or help clear up virus infections. Cattle have NK cells, although the term almost certainly covers a heterogeneous population. Natural killer cells can easily be recruited (stimulated by cytokines such as IFN and IL-2). Interestingly in cattle, NK activity is quite low in stock reared outside in extensive systems but is often very high in intensive systems. Whether this is caused by the greater prevalence of microbial infection in such individuals is not clear.

Natural killer activity can also be down-regulated by agents such as prostaglandins. Do NK cells have any *in vivo* relevance? They certainly will kill virus-infected cells such as IBR-infected fibroblasts and tumour cells, but the real clinical relevance requires further research.

Acquired immunity

Humoral

Acquired humoral immunity is mediated through immunoglobulin, or antibodies as they are commonly known. These are a group of glycoproteins that have combinations of incredible variety and specificity. The basic units are two identical polypeptide chains, termed light chains, linked to two further identical polypeptide chains, heavy chain, by several disulphide bonds (Fig. 51.1).

The Fc portion of the molecule is responsible for linking to the Fc receptor on leucocytes, while the other end, Fab, carries the actual antigen-combining site itself. This latter site is also called the hypervariable

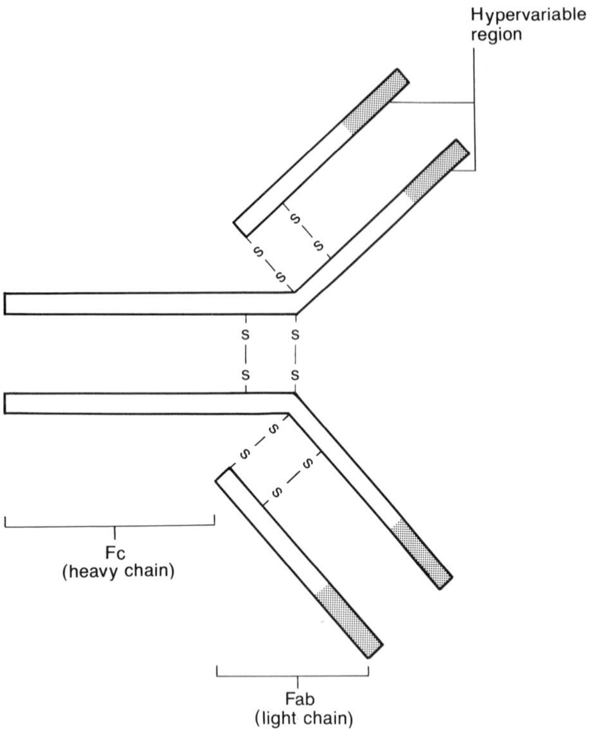

Fig. 51.1 Basic structure of an antibody.

Table 51.1 Descriptions used for immunoglobulins

Class	Five major classes are distinguished in mammals: IgM, IgG, IgA, IgE and IgD. These are distinguished in structure and major variations within the heavy chains.
Subclass	Several of the individual classes are further split into subclasses, e.g. IgG_1 and IgG_2. These are very similar in structure, but vary in the amino acid sequence of the heavy chain.
Allotype	This is a term used to refer to genetic variation within a given animal species involving alleles at a given locus; the variants normally occur within heavy chains. Allotypes in domestic animals could well be linked to disease resistance/production efficiency.
Idiotype	This term describes the product of a single clone of B cells, a unique antibody with a unique antigen combining site. Monoclonal antibodies consist of a single idiotype.

region simply because it is the variation in amino acid sequence in this region that produces the incredible diversity of antibodies.

An explanation of the plethora of titles that accompany a description of immunoglobulins is given in Table 51.1.

IgM

IgM has five of the basic units forming a pentamer structure and represents an early stage in the evolution of antibodies. All vertebrates (with the exception of cyclostomes such as the lamprey) have an IgM closely resembling that of mammalian IgM except for the number of units polymerized into the complete molecule. The level of IgM in normal cattle is in the range of 2–3 mg/ml from the age of 4 months. Levels of IgM in calves is complicated by the amount absorbed in colostrum. The actual amount in bovine colostrum is about 6 mg/ml which drops to approximately 0.1 mg/ml in milk. Interestingly the bovine fetus is quite capable of producing IgM from about the third or fourth month of gestation.

It is, of course, well established that in a primary immune response the major antibody produced early on is IgM. What is not so well recognized is that certain antigens can bypass many of the normal T cell interactions and stimulate B cells directly. Such antigens, including bacterial lipopolysaccharides, normally stimulate only IgM production. The efficacy of specific IgM should not be underestimated. Not only is IgM highly efficient at aggregating antigen, it can bind with the secretory component (see below under IgA) and act as a protective antibody at mucosal surfaces. In diseases, such as *Escherichia coli* enteritis in calves, IgM has been shown to be a major protective mechanism.

In cattle suffering from infection with trypanosomes, IgM levels can rise in serum to over 20 mg/ml, although the majority of this overproduction is not particularly useful against the trypanosomes. On the other hand, in bovine leukaemia IgM levels can fall quite dramatically.

IgG

IgG predominates over other immunoglobulin classes in serum and contributes in excess of 85 per cent of all circulating immunoglobulins. Its structure is based on the usual immunoglobulin model, and it has molecular weight of approximately 180 000.

IgG occurs in two subclasses: IgG_1 and IgG_2. Adult serum contains approximately 11 mg/ml of IgG_1 and 9 mg/ml IgG_2. In colostrum the figure is well in excess of 50mg/ml IgG_1 and 3 mg/ml IgG_2; this reflects the incredible selective concentration of IgG_1 in colostrum (more details are given in the section Maternal immunity, p. 803). Twenty-four hours after successful suckling the calf has approximately 20 mg/ml IgG_1 and 1 mg/ml IgG_2, underlining the obvious and often reiterated importance of successful colostral transfer.

As mentioned above, both subclasses can fix bovine complement; IgG_1 somewhat more so than IgG_2. As for their reaction with leucocytes exhibiting Fc receptors, a somewhat paradoxical situation exists. In experiments involving freshly purified monocytes or neutrophils, IgG_2 was always much more efficient at mediating phagocytosis or antibody-dependent cell-mediated cytotoxicity (ADCC). Yet IgG_1 is the predominant subclass that the calf receives from the dam.

In the cow and calf IgG_1 has a highly significant presence at the mucosal surfaces. While IgA is the predominant immunoglobulin in nasal secretions in the adult, IgG_1 is the predominant immunoglobulin in the calf up to at least the 6th week of life. In the lower respiratory tract, for instance the broncho-alveolar secretions, IgG_1 becomes the dominant immunoglobulin in all ages. Even infections at mucosal surfaces will produce high levels of circulating and specific IgG_1 equal to those achieved by intramuscular injection. When one considers that the main site of the IgG_1 synthesis is in the respiratory tract mucosa, it underlines the important potential of this immunoglobulin subclass in local defence mechanisms.

IgA

IgA is recognized as a major immunoglobulin associated with mucosal surfaces. It is basically a dimer (consisting of two of the basic units) joined by another molecule called the J chain (molecular weight of approximately 15 000). This structure is combined with a secretory component (molecular weight of approximately 60 000) to form secretory IgA or SIgA for short.

Individuals with mucosal surfaces have to have a selective system that can decide which antigen to ignore and which to respond to. It is not in the animal's interest to respond to dietary antigens, although of course this can occur leading to disease. Conversely the mucosal immune system must be able to respond quickly and effectively against a pathogen. One of the most important mechanisms in this decision-making process are distinctive epithelial cells called 'M cells' that overlie Peyers patches and other mucosal lymphoid aggregates. These cells have a tubulovesicular system with pits in the lumen surface and cytoplasmic processes on the opposite surface enfolding lymphocytes and other mononuclear cells. These cells can actively 'sample' the micro-environment within the lumen and pass information on to the proactive cells of the lymphoid system.

The stimulation and subsequent expansion of the plasma cells that are responding to a particular antigen takes place within the local lymphoid tissue itself. These IgA-producing cells migrate to the submucosa where they assemble and secrete the complete dimer and J chain. The epithelial cells on the microvilli have a receptor for IgA on their internal side that is probably the secretory component itself. The whole molecule, now the complete SIgA, is transported across the cell in endocytic vesicles and discharged into the mucus itself. This process can also take place in the liver where hepatocytes can make secretory component; therefore bile has high levels of SIgA.

What is the function of the secretory component? It can be found free within normal gut contents or saliva, with large amounts in the newborn calf when very little IgA is being produced. It seems to increase the resistance of the complete SIgA to proteolytic enzymes, although there is little evidence for any direct antipathogenic role. One of its major roles may be to help anchor the SIgA on the mucous layer on top of the epithelium, creating a high concentration of antibody activity at this crucial site.

The IgA part of the SIgA is not particularly effective at 'traditional' roles of antibody such as opsonization, aggregation and complement fixation. Its major, and highly successful role, is simply to block adherence. Micro-organisms *must* attach before penetration of mucosal barriers, e.g. the filamentous K antigen of *E. coli*. So by a simple steric hindrance such microbes are unable to attach and are excreted.

This local stimulation does underline the necessity to consider vaccination via a local mucosal route when dealing with diseases where a major defence mechanism involves secretory immunoglobulin. Many of the currently successful vaccines are given via the mucosal route and even more are under active research.

Another property of IgA lies in the dimer itself rather than the complete SIgA, or as one famous immunologist put it 'IgA can be more important beyond its laudable but essentially unglamorous role in intestinal sanitation'. Thus, if a dietary or microbial antigen penetrates the mucosal barrier, a high-affinity IgA attaches to it. There is no complement fixation or inflammatory process, so the whole complex is carried off in the blood to the liver where the IgA dimer reacts with the secretory component on hepatocytes with subsequent release into bile.

IgE

This immunoglobulin was first described for humans in the mid 1960s, and is sometimes called the reaginic antibody. It is, of course, associated with immediate hypersensitivity reactions. The structure of IgE is based on the usual immunoglobulin model but has a higher molecular weight than IgG (196 000 as compared with 180 000). This is due to an additional structure in the heavy chain, which is thought to help in the high affinity this immunoglobulin has for Fc receptors on mast cells. IgE normally exists in very low concentrations in serum (e.g. 20–400 ng/ml in dogs). Reliable and specific reagents are not yet available for the cow but by sensitive *in vivo* tests like the passive cutaneous anaphylaxis (PCA) test, potent IgE-like activity can be demonstrated in cattle.

The antigens that can elicit a specific IgE response are called allergens. The allergens are processed in the normal way and plasma cells in lymph nodes local to the area through which the allergen gained access, produce the specific anti-allergen IgE. Mast cell precursors also migrate to the lymph node and they take up the IgE via their Fc receptors. The mast cells now coated with the IgE migrate back to areas underlying the skin and/or mucosal surfaces. When the allergen again gains access it reacts with the IgE and this causes the mast cell to release the contents of its granules, a whole range of pharmacologically active substances. These latter include 5-hydroxytryptamine, histamine, prostaglandins and cytokines such as eosinophil chemotactic factor. The outcome is smooth muscle contraction, increased permeability of capillaries and, through the chemotactic agents, migration of leucocytes. In fact the latter function is a component of the mechanisms that 'dampen down' the reaction: eosinophils contain many factors such as phospholipase D and histaminase that will inactivate the products of the mast cells.

Although such IgE reactions are considered a real clinical nuisance both by humans and their animals, there must have been an evolutionary advantage to develop and then retain this hypersensitivity reaction. One clue for this is a possible mechanism against parasites, especially intestinal nematodes. Although there is a lot of experimental evidence in rodents, using parasites such as *Nippostrongylus brasiliensis*, there is some evidence for nematodes of ruminants such as *Haemonchus*. The antiparasite mechanism works by antigens secreted by the nematode (often those associated with their mouth parts) being recognized as allergens by the host. This results in suitably and specifically sensitized mast cells migrating back to the gut. When the worm feeds again the freshly released allergens activate the mast cells. The resultant smooth muscle contractions, and increase in permeability allowing through other factors such as IgG, and the possible direct action of the mast cell mediators themselves, causes a mass expulsion of the worms. Prostaglandin might be one of the important effector mechanisms. A lot of research needs to be done to extend our knowledge of this intriguing immunoglobulin before it could be confidently stated that it is a main mediator of intestinal immunity.

IgD

A brief and quite basic chapter such as this cannot go into details of this immunoglobulin which, although presumed to occur in the cow, has yet to be convincingly demonstrated. IgD is linked to B lymphocytes and appears on the surface of B cells after the initial expression of IgM. The IgD will co-express with IgM and subsequently other immunoglobulin classes. The IgD is lost when the B cells respond to antigen by differentiating into immunoglobulin-producing plasma cells or memory B cells. The exact role of IgD remains unclear.

Cell-mediated immunity

This is an often used 'catch-all' phrase that by strict definition could cover most of the immune system. Early on in fetal development the ubiquitous haemopoietic stem cells produce two distinct progenitors: a common myeloid and a common lymphoid. It is the eventual offspring of the latter cell population that are often considered to constitute cell-mediated immunity.

The lymphoid progenitors produce several different populations of lymphocytes. The rapid development of monoclonal antibodies has meant a highly specific and accurate assessment of these lymphocyte subpopulations. These are in today's parlance called CD (or cluster determinant) markers, each CD classification describing an identifiable membrane molecule which helps identify subpopulations. The major groups of lymphocytes to consider are:

1 T lymphocytes, especially the major subsets coded for by the CD4 (T helper) and CD8 (T cytotoxic) markers.

2 B lymphocytes; lymphocytes involved in delayed-type hypersensitivity.

3 An increasingly well-researched group of lymphocytes lacking the classical T and B cell markers.

The average human adult has about 10^{12} lymphoid cells, representing approximately 20 per cent of all leucocytes.

T lymphocytes

The thymus is central to immunological function. The T-cell precursors migrate there from the bone marrow via the blood. The thymus extends a complicated but highly effective 'education' of these immature T cells, after acting through a cascade of thymic-derived hormones such as thymosin and thymopoietin. The precursor T lymphocytes undergo about eight to ten cell divisions before they leave the thymus. A lot of the cells die within the thymus (maybe up to 90 per cent) and it would be a neat solution to claim that this is how the host rids itself of all potential self-reactive lymphocytes. Unfortunately there is much conflicting evidence as to how exactly the thymus does its job.

What is certain is that when the lymphocytes eventually leave the thymus they can be classified as CD4+ve or CD8+ve cells, two populations that are mutually exclusive in peripheral blood. The lymphocytes have an amazing ability to migrate from blood to secondary lymphoid tissue (within lymph nodes, spleen, gut, skin, respiratory tract, etc.) and often back again to blood. This thorough 'mixing and movement' of lymphocytes is essential for them firstly to respond to antigen when it first appears, and then to be able to contact other cells with a view to initiating and finally curtailing an immune response. T lymphocytes tend to mass into their own areas within secondary lymphoid tissues, quite distinct from B lymphocytes.

CD4 T cells are often called 'helper T cells', which does underlie their important role. The antigen-presenting cells or APCs are responsible for the initial processing and presentation of antigen to the CD4 cells. The latter then further present the antigen to other lymphocytes such as the CD8 population and B lymphocytes. The whole business of presentation is not only dependent on cytokines such as Il-1 and Il-2 but it is also MHC-restricted at the class II level. Crucial to the immune reaction is the T-cell receptor (TCR). The identification of the TCR remained a mystery until a few years ago when the TCR was shown to consist of two chains which clearly belong to the immunoglobulin supergene family. This structure is closely linked to another CD marker: CD3. The human immunodeficiency virus (HIV) preferentially binds to CD4 cells and it is the gradual destruction of this population that is an important factor in the marked immunosuppression that is such a feature of HIV infection.

The CD8 population is also MHC restricted but at the MHC class I level. This is useful as a major function of CD8 cells is cytotoxicity. Like other T cells, CD8 cells are highly specific for antigen, and for cytotoxicity to occur the CD8 cell needs to recognize antigen and MHC. As most body cells express MHC class I then any cell expressing say a virus antigen could be attacked and destroyed by the appropriate CD8 effector cell. In cattle diseases such as *Theileria parva* or IBR infection, these CD8 effector cells, or cytotoxic T lymphocytes (CTL), have been shown to be important.

A single CTL can kill several individual target cells and there is evidence that in virus infection, for example, recognition and then destruction of the target cell can occur before fully infectious virus is assembled inside the cell. The molecular basis behind the actual destruction itself remains poorly understood. Certainly it is vital to have the all-important recognition and close contact. The killing probably involves the release of more than one soluble 'mediators'.

B lymphocytes

B cells develop initially in the fetal liver but production then shifts to the bone marrow. The pre-B cell has IgM heavy chains within the cytoplasm. On a commitment to B cell lineage the B cell acquires surface IgM, the initial antigen receptor. A second phase of development allows the B cells to express immunoglobulins of a different class or subclass (plus IgD). On meeting its pre-ordained antigen the B cell retains only the immunoglobulin it is programmed actually to produce and then enter the terminal stage of immunoglobulin-secreting plasma cells. A proportion of the antigen-specific cells remain as an enlarged population of memory cells.

Although B and plasma cells produce the immunoglobulins, they are under the tight control of the CD4 helper T cells for the majority of antibodies; a proportion of T-independent antigens can avoid this control but at a cost of only IgM production and no immunological memory.

Maternal immunity

This is an important area for cattle. In the harsh economics of farm animal practice, death in the neonate is a major problem, and the passive protection provided by the mother is vital. Ruminants have five tissue layers between maternal and fetal circulation, so there is little or no transfer of immunoglobulin during pregnancy.

In bovine colostrum the level of IgG is up to a massive 75 mg/ml with 4 mg/ml IgA and 6 mg/ml IgM. Why does the neonate actually need all this antibody? The newly born calf has a somewhat limited capacity to mount a fully effective immune response. It can produce IgM and some IgG_1 at birth; from 36 hours old it will start producing a lot of IgG_1 at a rate of approximately 1 g/day (depending on antigenic challenge). From one to two weeks SIgA starts production and it is several weeks before IgG_2 production starts in earnest.

The neonate is thus basically immunocompetent but has not 'tuned' its immune system to deal with the environment, and it is in this period of tuning and massive primary antibody responses that the neonate needs passive protection. How does this concentration of immunoglobulin in the bovine colostrum occur? The major constituent of the immunoglobulins in colostrum is IgG_1 which is *selectively* transferred from serum. For example, a sheep can produce up to 2500 g of colostrum in the first 48 hours after parturition of which 90 g will be IgG_1. When one considers that the concentration of IgG_1 in her own serum is probably less than 0.015 g/ml, it is a major transfer. This transfer of IgG_1 occurs via receptors on the heavy chain which binds to the acinar epithelial cells. This receptor interaction is under hormonal control and only occurs during late pregnancy. There is no such selective concentration for the much smaller amounts of IgG_2, IgM and IgA.

The specificity of the immunoglobulins is also of obvious importance, not only reflecting the micro-environment of the dam herself, but also as a result of a deliberate immunization policy. The neonatal calf has a greatly increased intestinal permeability due to specialized epithelial cells capable of pinocytosis. These cells are activated by the presence of macromolecules and eventually slough off after relasing their contents into the circulation. This spontaneous closure starts in the calf at 12 hours postparturition with a mean complete closure time of approximately 30 hours. Degradation of this colostrum in the neonatal calf is minimal because it contains a trypsin inhibitor, and pancreatic activity itself is low. Abomasal pH is between 6 and 7 due to the delayed development of parietal cells, but by 36 hours postparturition the pH has dropped to between pH 3.0 and 4.0, and pepsin is then active. A final point concerning immunoglobulin in colostrum/milk is that in some diseases in cattle, such as rotavirus in calves, the passive protection is better obtained by the *ingested* immunoglobulin rather than systemic immunoglobulin being re-excreted into the gut. Therefore, it would make more sense to feed diluted colostrum from vaccinated dams during the first week of life rather than relying totally on the protection acquired passively during the first 24 hours of life.

As well as the immunoglobulins in colostrum there is a high concentration of other effector proteins such as lactoferrin. In addition, there are leucocytes, with the macrophage and other mononuclear cells predominant in the resting mammary gland and at parturition. During lactation, however, the predominant leucocyte is the neutrophil, possibly reflecting the constant, although usually non-clinical, bacterial presence. The importance of leucocytes in mammary secretions is as yet unclear for the neonate, but of obvious use for the mammary gland itself; the area of local and effective immunity in the working mammary gland will continue to be a goal for researchers.

Homeostasis and stress

In any book involving diseases of cattle, environmental stress must be a major consideration. Every living organism in an effort to cope with its environment attempts to reach *homeostasis* which can be defined as the steady state achieved by the optimum action of physiological regulation. Stress can be achieved by changes in the animal's environment such as restraint, handling, housing, weather, etc. Although there are many definitions of stress, one of the most useful is 'the cumulative response of an animal resulting from interaction with its environment via receptors'.

This is therefore an adaptive response and is primarily directed at coping with changes in the environment and, perhaps most importantly it is to a large extent an *automatic* response. The response is switched on in three main areas.

1 A voluntary motor response, which operates via the lower brain centre → spinal cord → peripheral nerves and results in fight/flight, etc.

2 The adrenal medulla. This works via the autonomic nervous system and adrenal medulla releasing catecholamines, inducing the alarm reaction.

3 The hypothalamus, which is probably the most important for cattle.

This latter mechanism involves the neuroendocrine system, with the hypothalamic stimulating adenohypophysis, which in turn stimulates (via ACTH) the adrenal cortex, which releases cortisol. The latter hormone has an alarmingly high number of effects such as vasoconstriction in skin and intestine, vasodilatation in muscles, raising blood glucose, raising pain threshold, reducing secretions, etc. The integrity of lysosomal membranes is enhanced by cortisol, so although phagocytosis of bacteria and other particulate matter still occurs, it is more difficult for the enzymes to be released from the lysosomes into the phagosomes. Clinically this can manifest itself as muscle weakness, trembling, impaired immune response, poor wound healing, weight loss, etc. Cortisol normally inhibits the production of adrenocorticotrophic hormone (ACTH) in a feedback mechanism; however, this latter mechanism can be overridden by highly stressful conditions.

Summing up this section: the body attempts to respond to stress by a variety of means to restore homeostasis. These responses evolved to occur in an open environment where the individual can move, seek shelter, etc. But in a crowded calf pen there is no escape, the stress conditions remain with the inevitable consequences.

Chapter 52: Vaccines and Vaccination of Cattle

by I.D. BAKER

There are many vaccines available for use in cattle in the UK and world-wide. This chapter is an attempt to summarize some of those available.

Definitions

A *vaccine* is a suspension of attenuated or killed micro-organisms administered for the prevention, amelioration or treatment of infectious diseases.

Vaccination is the introduction of a vaccine into the body to produce immunity to a specific disease. The vaccine may be administered by subcutaneous, intradermal or intramuscular injection, by mouth, by inhalation or by scarification.

There are various types of vaccine. An *attenuated vaccine* is a vaccine prepared from live micro-organisms that have lost their virulence but retained their ability to induce protective immunity.

An *autogenous vaccine* is a vaccine prepared from cultures of material derived from a lesion of the animal to be vaccinated.

A *toxoid* is a toxin that has been treated by heat or chemical agents to destroy its deleterious properties without destroying its abilities to stimulate the formation of antibody.

A *serovaccine* is a combination of an antisera with a vaccine to produce passive and active immunity.

Anthrax (see p. 551)

Many types of vaccine are available internationally but only one is available in the UK. This is a live vaccine prepared from a suspension of living spores of an uncapsulated avirulent strain of *Bacillus anthracis*. The vaccine can be kept for long periods.

Vaccines have been produced by overcoming virulence using saponins or saturated saline to delay absorption (Carbozo vaccines). In Britain the Stern vaccine provides an avirulent strain.

Dosage and administration

A dose of 1 ml is given by subcutaneous injection. This confers an immunity in seven to ten days that lasts nine months. Annual booster doses are recommended except in areas of increased risk when they should be given at six-monthly intervals.

Contraindications

The use of antibiotics should be avoided from shortly before to 14 days after vaccination to avoid any interference in the production of immunity. Animals in the last stages of pregnancy should not be vaccinated unless there is a serious risk of infection.

Table 52.1 *Clostridium* spp. and disease syndromes in cattle

Causative organism	Disease
Cl. chauvoei	Blackleg
	Postparturient gangrene
Cl. septicum	Braxy
Cl. novyi type B	Black disease
Cl. haemolyticum type D	Bacillary haemoglobinuria
Cl. tetani	Tetanus
Cl. botulinum	Botulism
Cl. perfringens (*welchii*)	Enterotoxaemia
Mixed species of *Clostridium*	Gas gangrene

There may be a slight reaction at the site of injection and animals may have a slight pyrexia for one to two days and milk yield may be depressed. These side-effects will subside.

Empty or part-filled vials must be destroyed by incineration.

Other vaccines

Another vaccine incapable of producing disease is a cell-free filtrate of a culture of a non-encapsulated spore-forming strain of *B. anthracis*. This requires two injections to produce immunity but is long lasting.

Clostridial disease (see Chapter 38)

The clostridial organisms are common and responsible for many serious diseases in cattle (Table 52.1).

Vaccines against these disease are available individually, e.g. blackleg and tetanus, but they are often combined as polyvalent vaccines. In general, the vaccines are prepared from formalin-killed cells adsorbed on to aluminium hydroxidè producing a toxoid. Vaccines for *Cl. chauvoei* are often a mixture of formalin-killed cells and a purified toxoid.

Dosage and adminstration

Usually 2 ml is given by subcutaneous injection. The initial course is two inoculations separated by four to six weeks followed by an annual booster unless there is great risk when it should be every six months.

Specific vaccines

Blackleg. If this disease is identified at pasture then cattle should be removed from the pasture until the vaccination course is complete. Some veterinarians give a concurrent dose of long-acting procaine penicillin at the same time as the initial vaccination to avoid further disease outbreaks during the period of developing immunity.

Tetanus immunity usually lasts for three years following an initial course of vaccination and one annual booster.

For especially valuable animals there is a tetanus vaccine that carries a minimum risk of hypersensitivity; whilst primarily designed for horses it can be used in cattle. It is prepared from purified tetanus toxin converted to toxoid by treatment with formalin and then adsorbed on to aluminium phosphate.

A polyvalent vaccine that is commonly available contains the following organisms: *Cl. chauvoei, Cl. septicum, Cl. novyi, Cl. haemolyticum* and *Cl. tetani*. It seems eminently sensible to use a polyvalent vaccine such as this instead of an individual vaccine since all these diseases occur commonly.

Botulism vaccination is practised in enzootic areas with either a combined *Cl. botulinum* types C–O or a type-specific toxoid vaccine.

Salmonellosis (see Chapter 13)

Many species of *Salmonella* can cause disease in cattle, e.g. *S. dublin*, *S. typhimurium*, *S. newport*, *S. arizona*. The two commonest species in the UK are *S. typhimurium* and *S. dublin* and these can be endemic in a herd. The so-called exotic species are not usually endemic.

Both live and killed vaccines to *S. dublin* and *S. typhimurium* are available, as are serovaccines. In field experience live vaccines appear to be more effective.

SALMONELLA DUBLIN VACCINE

A live vaccine prepared from an avirulent strain (H.W.S.51). The vaccine is freeze dried and reconstituted immediately before use. This vaccine has been removed from use at present.

Dosage and administration

A dose of 1 ml is given subcutaneously. When possible calves should be vaccinated one week before exposure to disease. If this is not possible calves should be vaccinated as soon as possible even if they are infected before they arrive on the premises. A high level of immunity is produced in seven days.

The vaccine is equally effective in adult animals when the disease is endemic in the herd with cows showing signs of infection, i.e. diarrhoea and abortion. It also produces good cross-immunity to *S. typhimurium*.

Contraindications

Sterile syringes and needles must be used. Disinfectants or surgical spirit must not be used in association with the vaccine since small traces may inactivate the vaccine. Simultaneous administration of antibiotics or sulphonamides may also inactivate the vaccine. When such drugs have to be used this effect is minimized by using oral preparations that are not absorbed from the intestinal tract, e.g. neomycin, streptomycin or framycetin. Unhealthy or colostrum-deprived calves must not be vaccinated. In the field, part-used vials should be destroyed safely by incineration.

Side-effects

There may be a slight local reaction at the site of inoculation, which will subside. Rarely, some animals show a hypersensitivity reaction to the vaccine. This shows as respiratory distress within approximately 1 hour of injection. Deaths have been reported but prompt treatment with adrenaline usually relieves this reaction.

KILLED VACCINES

Killed vaccines containing strains of both *S. dublin* and *S. typhimurium* are available. These products also contain serotypes to *Escherichia coli* and Roberts type 1, 2, 3 and 4 of *Pasteurella multocida*.

Dosage and administration

Calves are given 2 ml subcutaneously to be repeated after 14–21 days. Adult cattle are given 5 ml subcutaneously to be repeated after 21 days. Pregnant cows should be vaccinated six and three weeks before calving. This will then confer passive immunity to the calves via the colostrum. Annual booster doses are recommended, to be given approximately three weeks before calving.

Risks

A small number of animals may not show an adequate response to vaccination. Ideally, healthy animals should be vaccinated. Adequate immune levels will not be reached until two weeks after the second injection. Avoid stress when vaccinating pregnant cows or abortion or metabolic disease may occur.

SEROVACCINES

Commercial serovaccines are available containing mixed antisera to *S. dublin* and *S. typhimurium* together with polyvalent strains of *E. coli* and *P. multocida*. These are designed to give passive immunity to calves for prophylaxis and treatment as active immunization.

Dosage and administration

For prophylaxis in calves up to 20 ml is given subcutaneously and repeated at 10–14 day intervals during the period of risk. For therapy up to 40 ml is given subcutaneously and repeated at 24 hours if required. In the author's experience these products are not always cost-effective.

Neonatal calf diarrhoea (see Chapter 12)

The causes of neonatal calf diarrhoea are complex and multifactorial. Certain bacteria and viruses, fungi and protozoa, are associated with the condition, e.g. *E. coli*, *Salmonella* spp., rotavirus, coronavirus, and there are vaccines and serovaccines available.

Escherichia coli. Pathogenic infections of *E. coli* are most common in the first four days of life, certain strains being more pathogenic than others, e.g. K99, and specific vaccines are available.

The vaccination of pregnant cows with *E. coli* K99 antigens is very successful in preventing colibacillosis in young calves especially if the vaccine contains K99 pilus antigen and K99 capsular antigen. Calf protection does of course depend upon the passive immunity conferred by the intake of adequate colostrum.

The oral immunization of young calves using heat-inactivated *E. coli* has shown some beneficial results but more work is needed.

The *in utero* vaccination of the fetus has been achieved experimentally with some success but this is not a practical method at present.

Viral diarrhoea. Rotavirus and coronavirus are the two viruses most commonly isolated in outbreaks of viral diarrhoea. Both viruses are primary pathogens but can also occur with secondary involvement. A vaccine is available against rotavirus, which also includes *E. coli* K99 antigen (see p. 162).

The vaccine

The main vaccine available is a white oily emulsion containing inactivated bovine rotavirus and *E. coli* K99 antigens adsorbed on to aluminium hydroxide gel and emulsified in a light mineral oil.

Dosage and administration

Cows and heifers are given 1 ml of the vaccine by intramuscular injection, the recommended site being the side of the neck. A single dose is given from 12 to 14 weeks before the expected calving date. This stimulates the production of antibodies, which are then passed to the calves via the colostrum and milk. Each calf must receive adequate colostrum within the first 6 hours of life and then continue to receive colostrum and/or milk from vaccinated cows for the duration of the critical period. This occurs naturally with suckled calves. However, in the dairy herd the first six to eight milkings from vaccinated cows should be pooled and retained and then fed to calves at a rate of 2.5–3.5 l/day, according to size, for the first 14 days of life. The best results are achieved if all the cows in a herd are vaccinated; in this way infection and the level of excretion is kept to a minimum.

Contraindications

Only healthy animals should be vaccinated. Partly-used vials of vaccine should be discarded.

Side-effects

Occasionally, there is a reaction at the site of injection. Hypersensitivity reactions may occur.

Comments

The K99 antigen enables *E. coli* to adhere to the calf's small intestine where rapid bacterial multiplication causes the production of toxins that cause the diarrhoea. Calf diarrhoea is a complex disease syndrome of which *E. coli* and rotavirus are two of the major components and vaccination with this vaccine certainly helps in the control of the condition.

Serovaccines

Commercial serovaccines containing mixed antisera to *E. coli*, *S. dublin* and *S. typhimurium* are available and details of their use can be found under Salmonellosis.

Respiratory disease (see Chapter 15)

ENZOOTIC PNEUMONIA

This is a multifactorial disease associated with environmental *Mycoplasma*, viral and bacterial elements. In practice the parainfluenza 3 (PI3) virus is usually involved and vaccination with PI3 vaccine can be very successful. Much work still continues world-wide against the calf pneumonia complex.

The PI3 virus vaccine is a freeze-dried preparation containing live PI3 virus strain RLB103ts.

Dosage and administration

The vaccine is administered intranasally. The calf is held with its head inclined upwards and the whole 2 ml dose is instilled into one nostril using a special applicator that is provided. A short time is allowed for the vaccine to flow out into the upper respiratory tract. A single dose only is necessary for calves of 12 weeks of age or older but in young calves two doses should be given at three weeks and ten weeks old. Vaccination can commence at a week old. Calves that have received corticosteroid therapy should not be vaccinated for at least one month after the last treatment. Usually there are no side-effects.

The RLB103ts strain of PI3 virus is temperature specific and will not replicate in the higher temperatures of the inner tissues.

The vaccine can be used in animals of any age. In cases of severe challenge calves as young as one week can be treated and the vaccine can be used in the face of active infection as a therapeutic agent.

RESPIRATORY SYNCYTIAL VIRUS (RSV)

This is a freeze-dried preparation containing living bovine RSV. It is used when RSV has been shown or is suspected of causing disease.

Dosage and administration

A dose of 2 ml of the reconstituted vaccine is given by intramuscular injection. Two doses separated by three weeks are given to calves over four months of age. Younger calves require three inoculations with two doses at three-week intervals and the third dose at four months old.

Animal receiving corticosteroid treatment should not be vaccinated until one month after last treatment. If there is any allergic reaction then appropriate antihistamine therapy should be given.

INFECTIOUS BOVINE RHINOTRACHEITIS (IBR)

Like PI3 vaccine this is a freeze-dried preparation containing living IBR virus (bovine herpes 1).

It is used for the protection of all ages of cattle against infection with IBR. One product is also recommended for the protection of cows against abortion caused by IBR. Whilst the vaccine affords good protection against IBR it will not protect cattle incubating the disease.

Animals may remain serologically positive after vaccination. This must be considered when the animal's disease status is considered in the future, for example with export animals and with the MAFF Cattle Health Scheme.

Dosage and administration

As with PI3 vaccine, the animal is restrained with head elevated slightly and the vaccine is given intranasally using the specific applicator.

The dose is 2 ml of the reconstituted vaccine. Animals on corticosteroid treatment should not be vaccinated for at least one month after the last treatment. Cattle can be vaccinated at any age but, if under three months, a second application should be given. Annual vaccination is recommended.

MULTIFACTORIAL BOVINE PNEUMONIA VACCINE

A multifactorial pneumonia vaccine is available containing inactivated strains of IBR virus, bovine PI3 virus, bovine virus diarrhoea (BVD) virus, bovine adenovirus 3, and bovine reovirus 1.

Dosage and administration

A dose of 2 ml is given by intramuscular injection on the three-dose schedule: at four weeks, six weeks and twelve weeks of age with a single annual booster if necessary.

The vaccine is included for completeness but its efficacy, in the opinion of the author, is doubtful.

Parasitic bronchitis (see pp. 236–238)

There is a very successful oral vaccine available. It is a live vaccine consisting of an aqueous suspension of third-stage infective larvae of *Dictyocaulus viviparus* partially inactivated by exposure to ionizing radiation. Each dose contains at least 1000 irradiated larvae.

Administration

Each dose comes in a bottle that should be shaken well and the contents then given orally. Calves should be at least eight weeks old when dosed and a second dose is given four weeks after the first. Calves should not be exposed to any potential source of lungworm infection for at least two weeks after the second dose.

During the following grazing season exposure to lungworm infection reinforces this initial immunity. Vaccinated stock should not be grazed with unvaccinated animals or follow behind unvaccinated stock in a grazing system since any increase in pasture lungworm burden may cause a vaccine breakdown.

Only healthy calves should be vaccinated. Careful consideration should be given to calves suffering from any respiratory disease before dosing. It is advisable not to use any other live vaccine for a period of two weeks either side of vaccination.

The use of anthelmintics should be avoided for at least two weeks after the second dose, particularly the use of sustained-release boluses. Similarly, the use of ivermectin must be avoided for four weeks before and ten days after the dosing regimen is complete. The routine use of other anthelmintics and parasiticides must also be avoided for seven days before and at least ten days after treatment. This is due to the residual effects of modern anthelmintics.

Following vaccination it is not uncommon for there to be transient periods of coughing. This occurs after some seven to ten days. Indeed on rare occasions vaccination can initiate an outbreak of calf pneumonia by activating latent infection.

It has been suggested that where ivermectin is used to control both lungworm and gastrointestinal worms in a control programme then cattle may enter the second grazing year with no immunity to lungworm. In this case vaccination against lungworm may be carried out before the second grazing season. This is a suggestion only as, at present, no trial work on this has been carried out.

Transit fever (see p. 253)

The exact aetiology of this disease is not firmly established. *Pasteurella haemolytica* serotype I is most frequently isolated from the diseased tissues but the role of viruses as an initiating factor cannot be ruled out. Consequently, vaccination is not a very successful prophylaxis and there are little data to support their effective use in North American feedlot units.

Formalin-killed vaccines containing *P. multocida*

strains Roberts type 1, 2, 3 and 4 and *P. haemolytica* are available.

Dosage and administration

A 2 ml dose is given subcutaneously; two doses are given at two to three week intervals.

Contraindications

A few cattle in any group may fail to respond to vaccination. Satisfactory immunity does not occur when animals are unhealthy, have intercurrent disease or have a poor nutritional status. Occasionally hypersensitivity reactions may occur.

Haemophilus somnus infection
(see pp. 203, 215)

Haemophilus somnus is considered by many to be the aetiological agent of *Haemophilus* septicaemia in cattle. The disease is recognized in the USA and also in the UK and Europe.

A vaccine is available in America. It is a killed bacterin containing whole bacteria adhered on to an aluminium hydroxide adjuvant.

It is given by subcutaneous injection and two doses are given at a two to three week interval. Immunity is not long-lasting. Various vaccination programmes have been tried in feedlot conditions and its efficacy is difficult to evaluate. Some success is claimed for protection in the face of an outbreak.

No claims are made on the efficacy of the vaccine in the reproductive form of the disease.

Johne's disease (see pp. 664–665)

Vaccines are available for the control of the disease. Two vaccines are commonly available. The Vallee vaccine, which contains live *Mycobacterium paratuberculosis* organisms in a paraffin oil/pumice stone vehicle, and the Sigurdsson killed vaccine.

In the UK only the live vaccine is available and its use is strictly controlled by the Ministry of Agriculture, Fisheries and Food. Control is necessary because the vaccine causes interference in the interpretation of the tuberculin test. It causes a positive reaction to tuberculin particularly to the avian component. Obviously, it also causes a positive reaction to the Johne's intradermal test where it is used.

Dosage and administration

Individual 2 ml doses are given by subcutaneous injection usually in the dewlap. The vaccine is only given to calves that are under one month of age. The dewlap is used as an injection site because the vaccine usually produces a localized reaction. The vaccine has a very short shelf-life of 14 days.

Bovine viral diarrhoea (see pp. 660–663)

In the UK there is no effective vaccine available and caution will be needed before live virus vaccines are introduced. Vaccination at weaning may be effective but it is almost impossible to evaluate the efficacy in animals of this age. If vaccination is undertaken it should be in breeding females before they are pregnant and that are immunocompetent. Both modified live and inactivated vaccines have been used. Whilst the inactivated vaccines are safe, there is evidence from Europe and the USA that has shown that live vaccines which originate from cytopathic BVD virus can precipitate mucosal disease.

Rinderpest (see pp. 543–546)

Vaccination against this disease is common practice in areas where it is endemic. There are several good vaccines available and in theory complete eradication is possible with a vaccination programme.

Tissue culture vaccine

Attenuated vaccines manufactured from cell culture have largely replaced other attenuated vaccines. They are safe and effective and produce a long-lasting immunity suitable for all cattle.

Goat-adapted vaccine

An attenuated vaccine that produces life-long immunity. It is useful for Zebu-type cattle. It is a fairly virulent vaccine, which produces severe generalized reactions in susceptible stock. The signs seen are severe gastroenteritis with high temperatures and loss of milk.

Rabbit-adapted vaccine

This vaccine produces a good immunity that lasts for two years. It can be attenuated to a point where it will not cause severe side reactions but then is not effective in Zebu-type cattle.

Chicken embryo vaccine

A cheap, stable and safe vaccine that is unfortunately difficult to manufacture and produces variable degrees of immunity.

Measles vaccine

Measles, rinderpest and distemper are antigenically related and human measles vaccine will produce good immunity to rinderpest in all ages of cattle. It is especially useful in very young calves, which can be vaccinated at an earlier age than with normal vaccines. Measles vaccine is not affected by the calf's colostral immunity.

Contagious bovine pleuropneumonia (CBPP)
(see pp. 669–670)

A highly infectious disease causing septicaemia with localization in the lungs and pleura. It is common in many countries of the world.

Control by vaccination is possible and several vaccines are available. They are all live vaccines and are considered by some people to be responsible for some spread of the disease.

The vaccines available include the following.

1 Pleural exudate from natural cases. This is not a satisfactory vaccine since it can cause severe reactions and spreads natural disease.

2 Vaccines produced from culturing the organism, *Mycoplasma mycoides* var. *mycoides*.

3 Vaccines produced by attenuating the organism in avian egg cultures.

Administration

Vaccination in the tail is the route of administration using a high pressure syringe. Severe reactions can occur both generalized and localized in the tail. Intranasal vaccination is now being developed with some satisfactory results. Antimycoplasmal drugs should not be used during vaccination as they will possibly reduce the immune response. However, if the side-effects are very severe then treatment may be essential.

The immunity to the vaccine varies from six to ten months for some of the cultured broth vaccines to three to four years for the avian egg attenuated vaccines. All vaccines against CBPP are light susceptible and should therefore be stored in the dark.

Leptospirosis (see pp. 477, 570–571)

Leptospira serotypes are found in all farm animals and are an important zoonosis. In cattle the important serotype is *Leptospira interrogans* serovar *hardjo* where it is responsible for abortion and for the milk drop syndrome. A vaccine is available.

The vaccine is prepared from formalin-killed cultures of *L. interrogans* serovar *hardjo*, which is grown in a synthetic medium free of all proteins with potash alum as an adjuvant. It is a fluid vaccine with a precipitate that resuspends on shaking.

Dosage and administration

A dose of 2 ml of vaccine is given by subcutaneous injection and the recommended site of inoculation is the side of the neck or over the chest wall.

Initially, the vaccination course consists of two injections at an interval of at least four, and not more than, six weeks. This course can be given at any time but ideally should be completed before the main period of disease transmission, before service in the case of heifers. A single annual booster is recommended.

Calves can be vaccinated but if they are less than five months old then a further initial course must be given at five months as maternal antibodies may interfere with their immune response.

Contraindications

The usual contraindications apply, i.e. using sterile syringes and needles, and disposing of part-used containers of vaccine, which may become accidentally contaminated during use.

Cattle that have been vaccinated may be positive to diagnostic tests for *Leptospira*. This may be important and must be remembered where cattle are due to be exported or when considering national health schemes.

Vaccinated cattle may still be carriers of leptospires as a result of prevaccination infection and as such are still a zoonotic risk.

Brucellosis (see pp. 476–477)

Abortion and infertility in cattle caused by *Brucella abortus* can be very successfully controlled by vaccination. There are two vaccines available, strain 19 (S19) and strain 45/20 (45/20). Once eradication is in progress the use of either is limited or prohibited.

STRAIN 19 VACCINE

S19 is a live vaccine and is presented in freeze-dried form, which is reconstituted with diluent immediately prior to use.

Dosage and administration

The dosage is 5 ml given subcutaneously. It can be given to any age of stock from two months of age onwards. The ideal time is in calves from two to six months of age; at this time it confers a good immunity for approximately seven years.

Inoculation of adult cattle is very successful in controlling severe outbreaks of abortion. In an infected herd the incidence of abortion will begin to subside 40–60 days after vaccination and most herds will be free of infection within two years.

Bulls should not be vaccinated with S19; it does not seem to protect them from infection and has been known to be responsible for the development of an orchitis with *Brucella abortus* S19 present in the semen.

Side-effects

Vaccination reactions. Localized swellings at the site of injection can occur, especially in adult cattle. These reactions are sterile, do not rupture and persist for many months as fibrous nodules. Generalized systemic reactions can also occur with high temperatures and loss of milk in lactating cows. Heavily pregnant cows have been known to abort and should not be vaccinated. Idiopathic gonitis (p. 386) may be caused by vaccination.

Serological reactions. Following vaccination the serological titres can remain very high for a long period of time and therefore they can interfere with the interpretation of serological testing in an eradication programme. The complement fixation test becomes negative sooner than the serum agglutination test and can be used to identify a postvaccinal reaction from an infected cow.

Zoonotic risk. The vaccine is live and accidental injection into cattle handlers and veterinary surgeons can cause severe illness (undulant fever) and so great care must be taken when handling the vaccine.

STRAIN 45/20 VACCINE

Strain 45/20 is a killed vaccine.

Dosage and administration

Two inoculations are given by subcutaneous injection to animals over six months of age. There are often large localized reactions at the site of injection.

Although said to be non-agglutinogenic there is usually a rise in serum titres but these are such that they never reach inconclusive levels.

Brucellosis has been eradicated from many countries by a programme of initial vaccination followed some years later by serological screening.

Foot-and-mouth disease (see pp. 536–542)

This is an acute and very contagious viral disease. There are three major strains of causative virus (enterovirus), namely A, O and C and there are several serologically distinct subgroups. In Africa there are three further strains SAT1, SAT2 and SAT3 and an Asian strain ASIA1.

Vaccines are available and many cattle in the world are regularly vaccinated. The vaccine most commonly used is a killed trivalent vaccine containing strains A, O and C but because of the increase in new virulent substrains vaccines are often produced from locally isolated virus.

The virus is produced in tissue culture on bovine tongue epithelia or more commonly now on baby hamster kidney cells and inactivated using formalin and other agents.

A single dose gives an immunity in seven to twenty-one days and which lasts six to eight months. Young stock should be vaccinated every six months from four to six months of age if they come from vaccinated cows, due to maternal colostral immunity.

Live vaccines are available but not in common use since there is a narrow safety margin between loss of virulence and loss of immunogenicity.

Vaccination programmes

These need to be planned with specific local knowledge. In parts of Europe, adult stock tend to be vaccinated annually and young stock every six months, whereas in South America all cattle are inoculated every four months.

Where an outbreak of foot-and-mouth disease occurs within a disease-free area a ring vaccination policy can be employed to prevent spread. Frontier vaccination can be used to produce a buffer zone between an infected and a non-infected area.

Disadvantages of vaccination

1 Symptomless carriers can occur especially where the disease is very common. This carrier state can last up to six months.
2 Small numbers of animals can show anaphylactic reactions when given repeated vaccinations.

3 Some bacterial contamination while vaccinating can cause abortion or premature births in cows vaccinated in the last four months of pregnancy.

Louping-ill (see pp. 703–704)

A vaccine is available for use in cattle in tick-infested areas where louping-ill is a problem. It is an inactivated tissue culture vaccine prepared from the arbovirus and is a thick oily emulsion.

Dosage and administration

A dose of 2 ml is given subcutaneously. Because of the thickness of the vaccine, prewarming can facilitate its use. This prewarming must not exceed 37 °C for 30 minutes because the vaccine is heat labile.

Initially, two inoculations are given not less than three weeks and not more than six months apart, with annual boosters. The initial course should be completed at least two weeks before exposure and in pregnant cows before the last month of pregnancy.

Accidental injection of the vaccine into the operator can cause severe localized reactions and immediate medical attention should be sought.

The oily vehicle can sometimes cause localized vaccination reactions, which may persist for some time.

Papillomatosis (warts) (see pp. 684–685)

Autogenous vaccines can be prepared for the treatment of warts in individual animals. In the author's opinion their efficacy is doubtful as warts have a tendency to regress spontaneously.

Individual vaccines can be prepared by removing 5 g of the lesion from the animal, grinding it up and extracting the virus using glycerine. After sterilization the autogenous vaccine is administered to the affected animal in two doses one month apart.

Erysipelas (see pp. 213, 384)

Erysipelas is a rare disease of cattle but has been associated with clinical arthritis of calves and isolated on post mortem from adults. In an outbreak of disease vaccination is possible using the available porcine vaccines. The vaccine is killed and produced from cultures of *Erysipelothrix insidiosa* inactivated with formalin and adsorbed on the aluminium hydroxide gel.

Dosage

A dose of 2 ml is given by subcutaneous injection. Two doses are given separated by two to six weeks. If pregnant cows are vaccinated, with a second dose being given three weeks before the expected calving date, then there is good passive immunity in the calves via the colostrum.

Further reading

Blood, D.C. & Studdert, V.P. (1988) *Baillière's Comprehensive Veterinary Dictionary*, pp. 1–1124. Baillière Tindall, London.

Blood, D.C. & Radostits, O.M. (1983) *Veterinary Medicine*, 7th edn. Baillière Tindall, London.

Brownlie, J. (1985) Clinical aspects of the bovine viral diarrhoea–mucosal disease complex in cattle. *In Practice*, **7**, 195–202.

National Organization for Animal Health. (1990–91) *Compendium of Data Sheets for Veterinary Products*, Noah. Enfield, pp. 1–695.

Chapter 53: Anthelmintics

by M.A. TAYLOR

Introduction

The control of parasitic helminths in both domestic animals and man relies heavily on the use of anthelmintic drugs. For the purposes of this chapter, the internal parasites (endoparasites) of cattle can be divided into three main groups: roundworms (nematodes), which parasitize the abomasum, intestines and lungs; the flukes (trematodes), which parasitize the rumen, intestines and liver; and the tapeworms (cestodes), which parasitize the intestines.

Anthelmintics have been in use from the days of early man when it was first recognized that certain disease conditions were associated with parasitic helminth infections. Up to 1938, before the discovery of phenothiazine, few useful drugs existed for the treatment of nematode infections. Since then, and particularly over the last 20 years, considerable advances have been made in the development of safer and more effective drugs. Potentially toxic chemicals in use less than half a century ago have been superseded by modern highly effective anthelmintics with higher safety margins and ease of application. The introduction of thiabendazole in 1961, the first of the benzimidazoles, saw the beginning of broad-spectrum anthelmintic therapy that has led to the development of drugs with broad-spectrum activity against gastrointestinal nematodes, lungworms, tapeworms and liver fluke. The discovery of the avermectins in 1976, followed by the introduction of ivermectin with its endectocide activity, i.e. activity against endo- and ectoparasites, has taken the stage one step further.

Classification of anthelmintics

Anthelmintics can be classified into several groups on the basis of their mode of action, range of activity against different parasites or their chemical structure. A classification of anthelmintics, based on their chemical structures, is given in Table 53.1.

Benzimidazoles and probenzimidazoles

Most anthelmintics available for cattle belong to a group of chemicals referred to as the benzimidazoles. Thiabendazole was the first to be introduced in 1961 and was followed by parbendazole (1967), oxibendazole (1973), fenbendazole (1974), oxfendazole (1975), albendazole (1976), triclabendazole (1981) and ricobendazole (1987).

Three other chemicals, febantel, netobimin and thiophanate, usually referred to as probenzimidazoles, are also included in this group because they are metabolized in the body by *in vivo* ruminal and hepatic pathways to a variety of benzimidazole compounds.

Table 53.1 Classification of anthelmintics

Range chemical group	Gut worms	Lung worms	Tapeworms	Liver fluke	Ectoparasites
Broad spectrum					
Benzimidazole and probenzimidazoles	+	+	±	±	−
Imidazothiazoles	+	+	−	−	−
Tetrahydropyrimidines	+	−	−	−	−
Avermectins	+	+	−	−	+
Narrow spectrum					
Salicylanilides and substituted phenols	±	−	±	+	±
Diphenoxyalkyl ethers	−	−	−	+	−
Organophosphates	+	−	−	−	+
Chlorinated hydrocarbons	−	−	−	+	−
Piperazines	±	±	−	−	−
Others	−	−	+	−	−

Netobimin is particularly interesting because, as an ionic salt, it shows good solubility in water, which offers flexibility for its administration.

The benzimidazole group is derived from substitution of various side chains and radicals on the parent benzimidazole nucleus giving rise to individual members of the group. Modification of a particular benzimidazole can affect the pharmacokinetic behaviour of the drug through changes in relative insolubility, slow elimination and persistent circulation of the parent drug and/or active metabolites. Thus, greater efficacy and wider spectrum of activity of the most recently introduced benzimidazoles appears to be due to the relative insolubility of these chemicals, which affects the absorption, transport, passage along the gastrointestinal tract and metabolism within the host, and ultimately the final excretion of the anthelmintic compound from the host. The longer the persistence in the animal body, the more effective the anthelmintic appears to be.

Benzimidazoles are highly effective against most of the gastrointestinal worms of cattle. The range of activity of the more recently introduced compounds also includes lungworms, tapeworms and, with some, liver fluke. All of the benzimidazoles and probenzimidazoles are ovicidal. Triclabendazole is the exception in that it lacks any activity against gastrointestinal worms, lungworms and tapeworms, but it is highly effective against immature and adult liver fluke.

This group of chemicals are amongst the least toxic of all the anthelmintics available. However, several members of the group have been found to be teratogenic in cattle (parbendazole, oxfendazole, albendazole and netobimin); therefore these have limitations on their use in pregnant animals.

Benzimidazoles are virtually insoluble in water and are therefore generally available in suspension, for oral dosing. Oxfendazole is available either incorporated in pulse-release devices or for injection via an intraruminal injector. Albendazole is available in a sustained-release device in some countries. Netobimin can be solubilized and administered via drinking water. Fenbendazole can also be incorporated into drinking water using specialized metering equipment.

Following drenching, the drug usually passes to the rumen, which acts as a reservoir, allowing gradual release and absorption of the drug into the bloodstream. Thereafter, concentrations of the principal circulatory metabolites (Fig. 53.1) can be found in the plasma from where they are extensively recycled between the circulation and the gut wall, down the whole length of the intestinal tract. Nematodes attached to the gut wall may be more exposed to the recycled drug than to drug present in the digested food passing down the intestinal tract.

Host physiological factors may affect the efficacy of benzimidazoles administered orally. The oral administration of anthelmintic solutions may result in closure of the oesophageal groove in some animals, with subsequent bypass of the rumen and delivery of the anthelmintic to the abomasum. From here absorption, metabolism and excretion of the drug may be rapid resulting in reduced exposure of the parasite to the drug, and lowered efficacy. In some disease and nutritional states, the pH of the abomasum may be altered. This may not only reduce exposure of parasites in the abomasum to some of the anthelmintics, but it may also reduce solubilization of relatively insoluble drugs and thus reduce absorption.

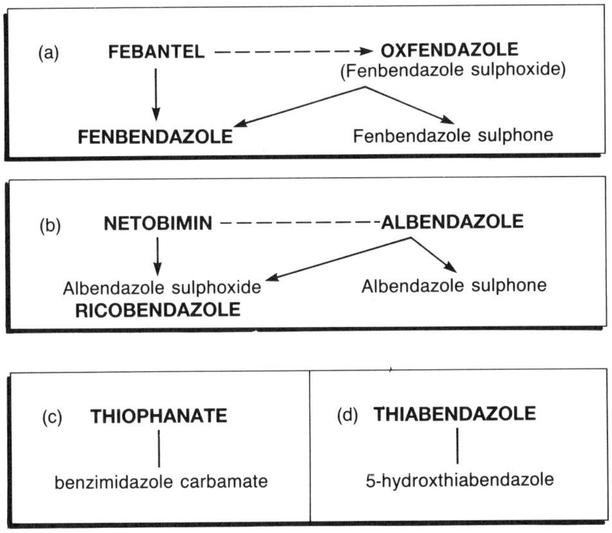

Fig. 53.1 *In vivo* metabolic pathways of the common benzimidazole and probenzimidazole anthelmintics in cattle.

Mode of action

The mode of action of this group of anthelmintics appears to be a direct effect on the uptake and metabolism of carbohydrates within the parasite by binding to tubulin, a constituent protein present in microtubules and in plasma and mitochondrial membranes. The resulting metabolic effects of the tubulin-binding properties of the benzimidazole anthelmintics includes inhibition of glucose uptake, protein secretion and microtubule (MT) production. There is also a reduction in enzyme activity such as acetylcholinesterase secretion, and carbohydrate catabolism by the fumarate reductase system. The overall effect is a 'starvation' of the parasite (Fig. 53.2).

The mode of action of triclabendazole, on *Fasciola hepatica*, is at present unknown. It appears to have no

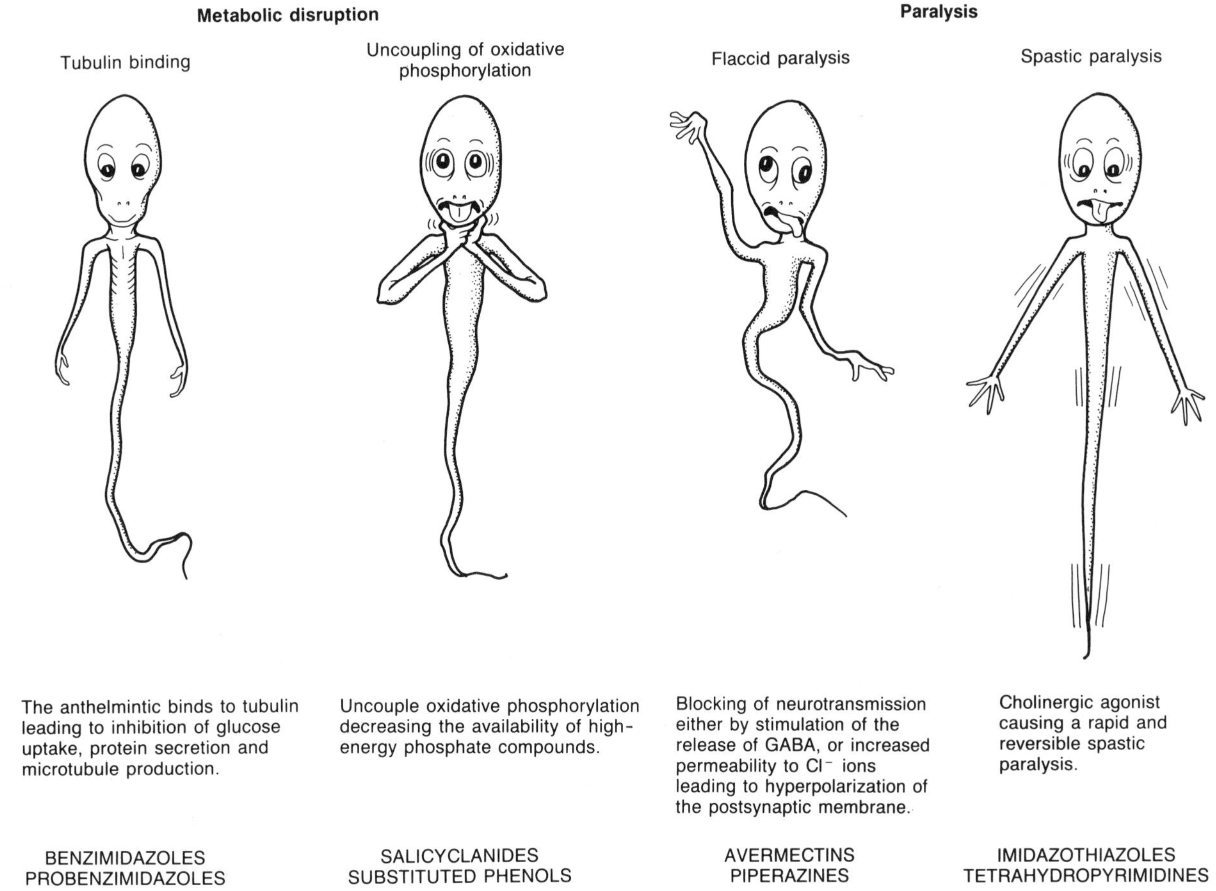

Metabolic disruption
Paralysis
Tubulin binding
Uncoupling of oxidative phosphorylation
Flaccid paralysis
Spastic paralysis
The anthelmintic binds to tubulin leading to inhibition of glucose uptake, protein secretion and microtubule production.
Uncouple oxidative phosphorylation decreasing the availability of high-energy phosphate compounds.
Blocking of neurotransmission either by stimulation of the release of GABA, or increased permeability to Cl⁻ ions leading to hyperpolarization of the postsynaptic membrane.
Cholinergic agonist causing a rapid and reversible spastic paralysis.
BENZIMIDAZOLES
PROBENZIMIDAZOLES
SALICYCLANIDES
SUBSTITUTED PHENOLS
AVERMECTINS
PIPERAZINES
IMIDAZOTHIAZOLES
TETRAHYDROPYRIMIDINES

Fig. 53.2 Anthelmintic modes of action.

tubulin-binding properties, unlike other members of this group, and it must therefore act along alternative pathways.

Imidazothiazoles

The two drugs in this chemical group that are used as anthelmintics are tetramisole and levamisole. Tetramisole is a racemic mixture of dextro and levo forms. Levamisole is the levo-isomer and it is with this form that anthelmintic potency resides. It is used at half the dose rate of tetramisole, and with twice the safety index.

Levamisole has good activity against a range of adult and developing larval stages of gastrointestinal nematodes of cattle, but not against arrested larvae. It is also highly effective against lungworms. Unlike the benzimidazoles it is not ovicidal. Levamisole is non-teratogenic and therefore safe to use in pregnant animals. The therapeutic index in relation to other anthelmintics is, however, low. Animals given levamisole may be frisky for a few minutes after receiving the recommended therapeutic dose. Toxic signs, due to a stimulant effect on nerve ganglia, may manifest as salivation, bradycardia, muscular tremors and in extreme cases death from respiratory failure. Injectable levamisole may cause inflammation at the site of injection.

Levamisole is available as oral drench, in feed, injectable and pour-on preparations. A levamisole sustained-release bolus is also available in certain countries.

Pharmacokinetics

Levamisole is rapidly absorbed and excreted, most of the dose being removed within 24 hours. Because of the mode of action of these compounds nematode paralysis occurs quickly and removal of the worms is rapid. Unlike the benzimidazoles it is therefore not as essential to maintain high drug levels over a protracted period.

Mode of action

Levamisole appears to act as a cholinergic agonist at the neuromuscular junction causing a rapid, reversible spastic paralysis (Fig. 53.2). In addition, in high concentrations, it has been shown to affect nematode metabolism by inhibition of the fumarate reductase system. The extent to which this contributes to overall anthelmintic efficacy is unknown. In addition to its anthelmintic properties, levamisole has been shown to stimulate the mammalian immune system by increasing cellular activity. The relationship between the immunostimulatory and nematocidal properties of levamisole are unknown.

Tetrahydropyrimidines

Pyrantel and morantel are the only members of this group available for cattle. Morantel, as its tartrate salt, is the more potent and the most widely available in the form of a sustained-release bolus. Neither drug is particularly toxic and can be used safely in pregnant and young animals.

Pharmacokinetics and mode of action

The pharmacokinetics and mode of action of this group of chemicals are similar to that of levamisole. They act as nerve ganglion stimulants, causing a spastic reversible paralysis of the worms that results in rapid expulsion from the host.

Avermectins

At present ivermectin is the only commercially available derivative of this group and is a macrocyclic lactone produced by an actinomycete, *Streptomyces avermilitis*. It shows high activity against nematodes and some ectoparasites, but has no effect against trematodes and cestodes. In cattle the route of administration is by subcutaneous injection or by pour-on. A drench formulation is available in New Zealand. It is highly effective against adult and larval stages of abomasal parasites and lungworms, including arrested *Ostertagia ostertagi*, but appears to have variable efficacy against some intestinal species, notably *Nematodirus helvetianus*. It is also reported to be active against the eyeworm, *Thelazia rhodesii*, and the filarial parasite, *Parafilaria bovicola*. Ectoparasiticidal activity includes warbles, lice, mange mites and ticks in cattle.

After parenteral or topical treatment, ivermectin persists in the tissues, being temporarily sequestered in lipid and liver, and provides protection against the development of certain immature stages of nematodes for at least two weeks after a single administration. This, as will be discussed later, reduces the need to place cattle on parasite-free pasture immediately after treatment, and also reduces the frequency of treatments needed.

Pharmacokinetics

Ivermectin is absorbed systemically following oral, subcutaneous or dermal administration, but is absorbed to a greater degree, and has a longer half-life, when given subcutaneously or dermally. A temporary depot appears to occur in the fat and liver, from which there is a slow release. Excretion, of the unaltered molecule, is mainly in the faeces with less than 2 per cent excreted in the urine. The reduced absorption and bioavailability of ivermectin when given orally in cattle may be due to its metabolism in the rumen.

Mode of action

The mode of action of ivermectin in nematodes and arthropods is thought to be mediated by action on gamma-aminobutyric acid (GABA) neurotransmission at two or more sites. In nematodes, ivermectin blocks interneuronal stimulation of excitatory motor neurones leading to a 'flaccid' paralysis (Fig. 53.2). It appears to achieve this by stimulating release of GABA from nerve endings and to enhance the binding of GABA to its receptor on the postsynaptic membrane of an excitatory motor neurone. The enhanced GABA binding results in an increased flow of Cl^- ions into the cell leading to hyperpolarization (Fig. 53.3). In mammals GABA neurotransmission is confined to the central nervous system; the lack of effect of avermectin on the mammalian nervous system at therapeutic concentrations is probably because, being a large molecule, it does not readily cross the blood–brain barrier.

Piperazines

Diethylcarbamazine is still marketed in certain parts of the world for the treatment of lungworm infections in cattle and sheep. It is primarily active against immature lungworms. Because it has to be given over a period of three days to achieve its effect, more modern anthelmintics such as the benzimidazoles, levamisole and ivermectin have tended to replace it. It is also active against microfilariae, the mode of action being incompletely understood, but it is thought to enhance phagocytosis of the microfilariae by the host immune system. The action of diethylcarbamazine on immature lungworm larvae is thought to be a 'flaccid' paralysis due to hyperpolarization of neuronal postsynaptic membranes resulting from an increase in flow of Cl^- ions into the cell. This mode of action, similar to the GABA agonist action of piperazine, is probably unrelated to its antifilarial action.

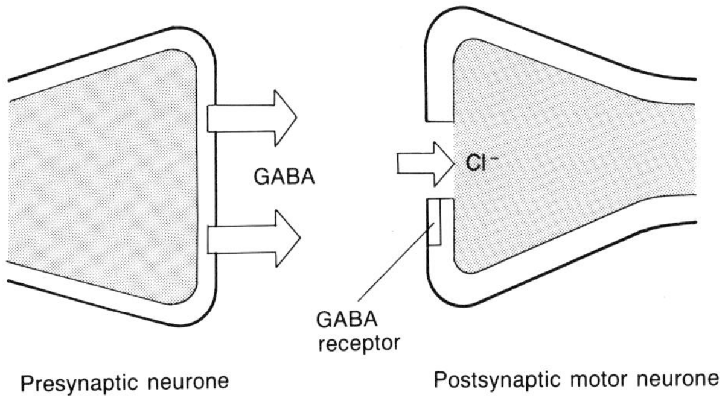

Fig. 53.3 Mode of action of ivermectin at the nematode synapse.

Organophosphates

Several organophosphorus compounds have been marketed for use in cattle, and are still available in a limited number of countries. They are usually effective against adult species of gastrointestinal nematodes but not against arrested larvae and lungworms.

The mode of action of organophosphates is to cause phosphorylation of the enzyme acetylcholinesterase, which is involved in regulating the concentration of the neurotransmitter, acetylcholine, at neuromuscular junctions. As a result of this inhibition, neuromuscular transmission may be interrupted, leading to paralysis of the worms (Fig. 53.2).

Phosphorylation of acetylcholinesterase and other enzymes can occur in higher vertebrates as well, which accounts for host toxicity seen at higher dose rates. Typical cholinergic signs include salivation, miosis, diarrhoea, muscle fasciculations and respiratory embarrassment. Toxic clinical signs can be treated with atropine (see p. 612).

Salicylanilides and substituted phenols

With the exception of niclosamide, the salicylanilides and substituted phenols are usually marketed as flukicides, being highly effective against adult and to a lesser extent immature *F. hepatica*. Some also possess activity against blood-sucking nematodes such as *Haemonchus*. Most are given orally to cattle; nitroxynil is usually given by subcutaneous injection.

The salicylanilides, substituted phenols and bisphenols can be regarded as close analogues and include the bromsalans, clioxanide, oxyclozanide, brotianide, rafoxanide and closantel (salicylanilides), nitroxynil (substituted phenol), bithionol, hexachlorophene and niclofolan (bisphenols). Niclosamide (salicylanilide) is highly effective against tapeworms and possibly against immature paramphistomes.

Pharmacokinetics

Salicylanilides and substituted phenols appear to be extensively bound to plasma proteins (>99 per cent), which may explain their high efficacy against blood-ingesting parasites. Fasciolicidal activity is dependent on the extent to which they persist in the plasma. Rafoxanide and closantel have long plasma half-lives when compared with oxyclozanide. Evidence suggests that the apparent efficacy of these drugs, against immature *F. hepatica*, may be due more to their persistence in the plasma, and the effect they have on maturing adult flukes when they reach the bile ducts, rather than effect on the immature stages themselves. Young flukes probably ingest mainly liver cells, which contain little anthelmintic. As they grow and migrate through the liver they cause extensive haemorrhage and come into contact with anthelmintic. Finally, when they reach the bile ducts they are in contact with even greater concentrations of anthelmintic, as the bile ducts are important in the excretion of these compounds as evidenced by the high proportion of these and their metabolites excreted in the faeces rather than the urine.

Mode of action

Salicylanilides and substituted phenols uncouple oxidative phosphorylation and therefore decrease the availability of high-energy phosphate compounds such as adenosine triphosphate (ATP) and reduced nicotinamide-adenine-dinucleotide (NADH) in the mitochondria. They have been shown to inhibit succinate dehydrogenase activity and the fumarate reductase system, which is associated with oxidative phosphorylation (Fig. 53.2). Because of the long half-life of the plasma protein-bound molecules, the parasites experience prolonged exposure to the drugs (as with the benzimidazoles but in a different manner), which reduces the energy available to the parasites.

Plasma binding reduces incorporation of the drugs into host tissues and accounts for the selective parasite toxicity. Looseness of faeces and slight loss of appetite may be seen in some animals after treatment at recommended dose rates. High doses may cause blindness and symptoms of uncoupled oxidative phosphorylation, i.e. hyperventilation, hyperthermia, convulsions, tachycardia and ultimately death.

Clorsulon

The sulphonamide, clorsulon, is available as an injectable solution in cattle, and is highly effective against against 8-week-old immature and adult *F. hepatica*. It has been shown to inhibit the glycolytic enzyme phosphoglyceromutase in *F. hepatica* by competition with 3-phosphoglycerate and 2,3-diphosphoglycerate.

Chemotherapy of parasitic gastroenteritis in cattle

Anthelmintics for the treatment and control of parasitic gastroenteritis (PGE) (p. 231) in cattle comprise the benzimidazoles, probenzimidazoles, levamisole, morantel and ivermectin. Their activities have been described under the respective chemical groups, and are summarized in Table 53.2. All are highly effective against the adult and developing larval stages of the common gastrointestinal nematodes. Their activities against arrested fourth-stage larvae vary. At recommended dose rates, fenbendazole, oxfendazole, albendazole, ricobendazole and ivermectin are more effective against arrested fourth-stage larvae of *Ostertagia ostertagi* than other anthelmintics. The activities of the probenzimidazoles, netobimin, febantel and thiophanate, against arrested larvae is also high if the dose rate is either increased or administered over several days.

In selecting an anthelmintic for parasitic gastroenteritis in calves in the summer months, there is little to choose between any of the anthelmintics available. For the treatment of type II ostertagiasis (p. 233), or for treating animals on housing in autumn to prevent disease in late winter or early spring, it is advisable to use a product that has high efficacy against arrested larvae. An anthelmintic that lacks such efficacy may necessitate repeated treatment for it will only remove adult worms and developing larvae leaving arrested larvae to resume development and cause damage to the abomasal wall.

Control of parasitic gastroenteritis using anthelmintics

Traditionally, attempts at chemotherapeutic control of parasitic gastroenteritis in cattle have involved the routine application of anthelmintics at times designated by the farm management system. Epidemiological knowledge has played little part in such methods of control, they have done little to prevent infection, and have been used mainly in the treatment of animals once infection has occurred.

Table 53.2 Activities of anthelmintic chemicals (at manufacturers' recommended dose rates) against stomach and intestinal worms, lungworms and tapeworms in cattle

Chemical group	Drug	Recommended dose rate (mg/kg)	Gutworms	Lungworms	Tapeworms	Liver fluke	Comments
Benzimidazoles	Thiabendazole	66	+	–	–	–	110 mg/kg in severe infections
	Parbendazole	20	+	N/A	–	–	30 mg/kg in severe infections
	Oxibendazole	10	+	N/A	+	–	
	Fenbendazole	7·5	+	+	+	–	
	Oxfendazole	4·5	+	+	+	–	
	Albendazole	7·5	+	+	+	±	10 mg/kg for liver fluke
	Ricobendazole	7·5	+	+	+	–	
Probenzimidazoles	Febantel	7·5	+	+	–	–	
	Netobimin	7·5	+	+	+	±	20 mg/kg for arrested larvae. Do not give during first 7 weeks of pregnancy
	Thiophanate	66	+	–	–	–	132 mg/kg in severe infections. Give over 5 days for arrested larvae at 20 mg/kg
Imidazothiazoles	Levamisole	7·5	+	+	–	–	
Tetrahydropyrimidines	Morantel	–	+	–	–	–	Sustained-release devices only
Avermectins	Ivermectin	0.2	+	+	–	–	See note below
Piperazines	Diethylcarbamazine	55	–	±	–	–	Immature lungworm. Dose over 3 days

Note: ivermectin is active against eyeworms, warbles, mites on beef and non-lactating dairy cattle. At recommended dose rates it provides persistent activity against *Ostertagia ostertagi* and *Cooperia* spp. for seven days and against *Dictyocaulus viviparus* for 14 days after treatment. Do not give to cows in last 28 days of pregnancy.
+, active against a particular parasite category.
–, not active against a particular parasite category.
N/A, insufficient evidence available.

Integrated systems of grazing management and parasite control, or 'clean grazing' systems, aim to withhold susceptible grazing animals from heavily infested grazing and rely very little on anthelmintic usage. However, they require effective pasture management for their success. The two strategies available for controlling parasitic gastroenteritis in first-year calves in temperate climates are the *preventative* strategy, where clean grazing in the form of new leys are provided at the start of the grazing season; and the *evasive* strategy, where clean grazing in the form of aftermath is provided in the second half of the grazing season.

On farms where such control methods are not feasible, similar control can be achieved by the use of anthelmintics during the early part of the grazing season as a means of reducing pasture contamination for the remainder of the grazing season. Anthelmintic suppression of pasture contamination is continued until the early summer by which time the overwintering infection has declined to low levels, thus effectively rendering the pasture 'safe' for the remainder of the grazing season. This can be achieved by dosing first-year calves every three weeks from the date of turnout, until the overwintering infection has died out, usually by mid June in temperate countries. This treatment interval approximates the prepatent period of most of the important nematode parasites of cattle. Where ivermectin is used, the treatment interval can be extended by at least seven days because of its persistent activity in cattle. For this reason the recommended dosing interval for the use of ivermectin in controlling gastrointestinal nematodes is three, eight and thirteen weeks after turnout.

Anthelmintic delivery systems

The advent of novel methods of presentation of anthelmintics and anthelmintics with greater persistence in the body has meant that strategic control of parasitic gastroenteritis in calves can be achieved with the minimal handling of stock. The use of pour-on levamisole and ivermectin preparations, and the oxfendazole intraruminal injector, are convenient to use, less traumatic to both animal and handler, and gaining widespread acceptance. The latter method avoids the possibility of ruminal bypass of orally administered drug, which as discussed earlier can affect the pharmacokinetic behaviour of the relatively insoluble benzimidazoles. The major disadvantage of strategic single-dose treatments is the labour costs in gathering and handling the cattle.

The most important developments of the last few years have been, and for the foreseeable future are likely to be, in the development of controlled release systems.

INTRARUMINAL DEVICES

Intraruminal devices represent a new approach to administering anthelmintics for the control of parasitic helminths. The reticulo-rumen provides an ideal site for the location of these devices, which can release anthelmintic over an extended period either continuously (sustained-release devices, SRD), or at pulsed intervals (pulse-release devices, PRD). Ruminal retention is achieved either on the basis of density or the variable geometric configuration of the device. Several devices are available for cattle: morantel sustained-release devices (MSRD); a levamisole sustained-release bolus (LSRB) available in certain countries; and pulse-release devices containing oxfendazole.

Sustained-release devices

Sustained-release devices for mineral or trace element supplementation have been used for a number of years, but it is only recently that the technology has been applied to the delivery of anthelmintic drugs. Available devices are designed to deliver a constant rate of anthelmintic over a period of time.

The 'Paratect' bolus consists of a metal cylinder, with permeable ends, containing the anthelmintic morantel tartrate in a slow dissolving vehicle. The 'Paratect' Flex bolus is a trilaminate sheet consisting of a central lamina of a morantel tartrate/ethylene vinyl acetate matrix coated on both sides with a thin impermeable layer of ethylene vinyl acetate. A symmetrical pattern of circular perforations is punched through the three layers and, when the device is in the rumen, morantel is released from the uncoated edges of the perforations and the perimeter of the device. For oral administration, the device is rolled up and sealed with tape, and plugged at each end so that it resembles a solid cylinder. Once in the rumen the device unrolls so that it cannot be regurgitated.

The 'Chronomintic' bolus consists of a compressed PVC matrix containing levamisole encased in an outer impermeable shell. Anthelmintic is released from the internal surface area through a single outer pore.

These devices, after lodging in the forestomachs, are designed to release anthelmintic over a 90-day period, creating an environment toxic to any worms ingested over this period. If animals are given one of these devices on turnout in late spring, most of the worms ingested as overwintered infective larvae will be killed before they can develop into adult worms and contaminate the pasture. The result is that the pasture remains comparatively free of infective larvae during the second half of the grazing season (Fig. 53.4). If the animals have to be moved to contaminated pasture in the second half of the grazing season, or after the life expectancy of the bolus has passed, these benefits will be lost. With these systems, the dose/weight ratio reduces as the animal grows and the release rates decline with time. Both of these factors may result in considerable selection pressure for resistance and since these systems are recommended as a form of clean grazing system, the build-up of resistant over susceptible species could occur rapidly. For reasons that will be discussed later, resistance problems are much rarer in cattle than in sheep or goats, so that in practice, the situation may be overstated.

Another limiting factor in the use of these bolus systems is that they are dependent on the date of turnout in attaining maximum benefits. Where turnout is early, overwintering larvae may still be present on the pasture beyond the life expectancy of the bolus. Where this occurs, the effect of the bolus is to delay build-up of pasture infectivity with the result that calves either experience sufficient challenge to develop clin-

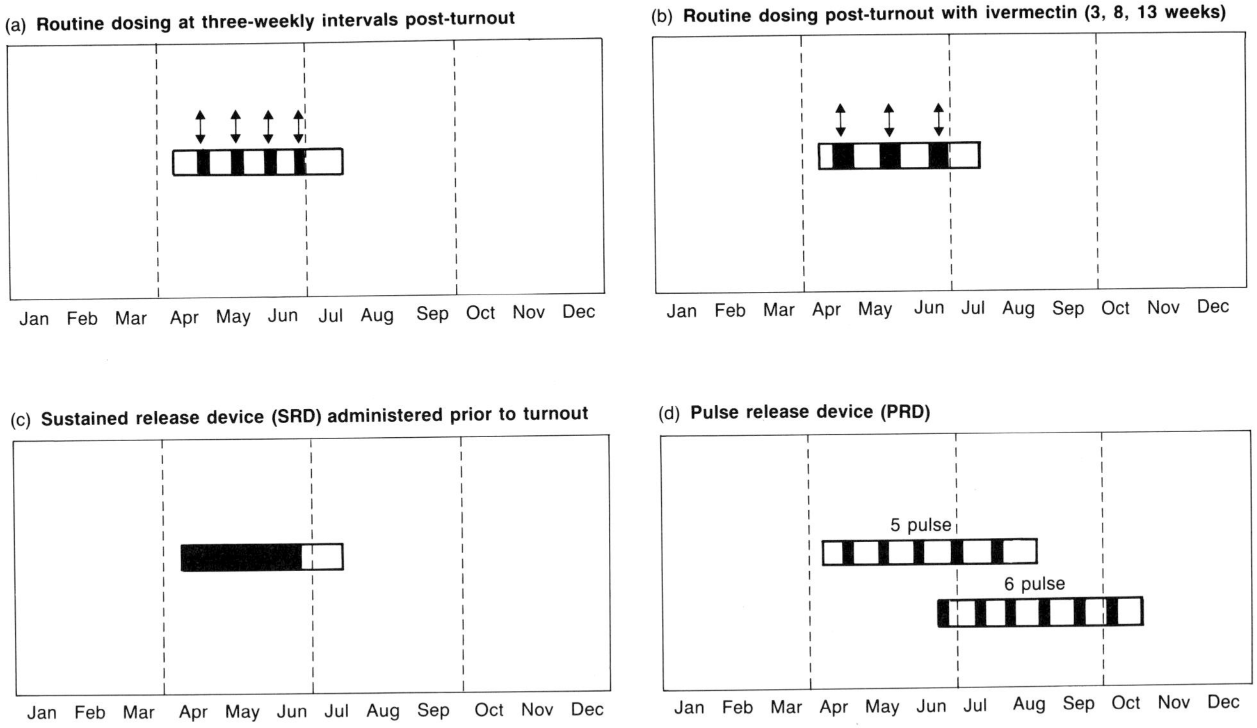

Fig. 53.4 Strategic use of anthelmintics for controlling parasitic gastroenteritis in first-year calves.

ical disease in the autumn or, alternatively, they acquire large numbers of arrested larvae that may cause clinical disease in the spring. In this situation calves may either require dosing in the autumn while still at grass, or on housing to remove arrested burdens.

Pulse-release devices

Bioengineering advances have resulted in the development of a pulse-release system for use in worm control of cattle. The oxfendazole pulse-release bolus consists of a cylindrical bolus with a central alloy core on which sit five annular anthelmintic tablets separated by washers. Dissolution of the central core results in release of the anthelmintic tablet at timed intervals over a 130-day period. Further modification has seen the introduction of a six-pulse bolus or front-end bolus suitable for larger cattle and which delivers six doses of anthelmintic over a four-month period. Devices of this nature are subject to some variation in release intervals dependent on factors such as diet, rumen pH and gut motility, so that release may vary by a few days either side of the optimum.

A novel development from this type of corrosion-based pulse-release system is the electronic bolus based on microchip technology. As well as offering the potential of multiple anthelmintic therapy, the system could be used to pulse release other drugs such as growth promoters and mineral supplements.

Anthelmintic resistance

Although widely reported in sheep, anthelmintic resistance appears less of a problem in cattle. This may be a reflection of the relative frequency of treatment and also differences in parasite population dynamics between the two hosts. It may also reflect the prolonged survivability of free-living larval stages within the bovine faecal pat, thus ensuring a supply of susceptible worms.

To date only a few cases of anthelmintic resistance in cattle nematodes have been reported. Oxfendazole-resistant *Trichostrongylus axei* in Australia, and oxfendazole-resistant *Cooperia oncophora* in New Zealand, are the only reports of benzimidazole resistance. Levamisole resistance has been suspected in *O. ostertagi* in Belgium and the USA. Differences in resistance to morantel were noted in *O. ostertagi* in the cattle in The Netherlands.

The effects of intraruminal devices on the development of resistance, given the selection pressures they exert, are not yet apparent. Until the inheritance of anthelmintic resistance is understood, this will remain a matter for speculation.

Chemotherapy of parasitic bronchitis

(see pp. 236–238)

The anthelmintics fenbendazole, oxfendazole, albendazole, febantel, netobimin, levamisole and ivermectin are all highly effective against adult and developing fourth-stage larvae of *Dictyocaulus viviparus* (Table 53.2). Diethylcarbamazine is primarily active against immature larvae if given over a three-day period. Some degree of control of parasitic bronchitis in calves can be achieved by early season suppression of pasture contamination, in much the same way as for the control of parasitic gastroenteritis. However, the epidemiology of lungworm infection is complex and still not fully understood, and it is the opinion of the author that the vaccination of calves with an irradiated larval vaccine is the most reliable form of control.

Chemotherapy of trematode infections in cattle

Fasciolioasis

Table 53.3 shows the comparative efficacy of currently used and recently developed drugs against *F. hepatica* (p. 238). All have good efficacy against adult fluke and are therefore suitable for the treatment of chronic fascioliasis in cattle. Where acute fascioliasis is suspected, triclabendazole is the drug of choice, because of its high efficacy against immature stages.

Where cattle are housed in the winter months, dosing with triclabendazole on housing should remove burdens of adult and immature fluke. Further treatment should then be unnecessary. When one of the other flukicides is used, a second dose at turnout may be necessary to remove any fluke missed by the first treatment. Where animals were housed for at least eight weeks prior to the first treatment, the second dose should be unnecessary.

In outwintered stock, two doses of anthelmintic may be necessary: the first in early winter, to remove adult and immature fluke burdens acquired from the autumnal flush of pasture metacercariae; the second in early spring to prevent heavy pasture contamination and infection of the snail intermediate host.

Other *Fasciola* spp.

The drugs and dose rates given for the treatment of *F. hepatica* are generally applicable for the treatment of *F. gigantica*. *Fascioloides magna*, a parasite of deer that can affect cattle, appears susceptible to several flukicidal drugs, although some of the more recently introduced anthelmintics have yet to be tested. From the limited information available on the chemotherapy of paramphistomes in cattle, oxyclozanide alone, or

Table 53.3 Activities of anthelmintic chemicals (at manufacturers' recommended dose rates) against liver fluke in cattle

Chemical group	Drug	Recommended dose rate (mg/kg)	Active against			Comments
			Adult	6–12 week	1–6 week	
Salicylanilides	Rafoxanide	7.5 (drench) 3 (injection)	+	+	–	
	Closantel	NR	+	+	±	Available for cattle in some countries
	Oxyclozanide	10	+	–	–	Some activity against tapeworm segments
Substituted phenols	Nitroxynil	10	+	+	–	Also active against blood nematodes
	Bithionol	30	+	–	–	Also has anticestodal activity
	Niclofan	3	+	–	–	
Benzimidazoles	Albendazole	10	+	–	–	Also active against nematodes and cestodes
	Triclabendazole	12	+	+	+	Do not give to dairy cows within 7 days of calving
Probenzimidazoles	Netobimin	20	+	–	–	Do not administer to cattle in the first 7 weeks of pregnancy
Sulphonamide	Clorsulon	7	+	+	±	

NR, no recommended dose rate.

in combination with levamisole, appears to give the greatest control of both ruminal and intestinal forms. Other newer compounds, as yet untried, may prove to be more effective.

Schistosomes

In contrast to the chemotherapy of schistosomes in humans, little information is available on the treatment of schistosomiasis in cattle. The most promising compound for the treatment of human schistosomiasis is praziquantel, and this may prove to be the drug of choice in ruminants also.

Chemotherapy of cestode infections in cattle

Adult stages of tapeworms parasitizing cattle are usually of little consequence. Several of the benzimidazoles used in the treatment of gastrointestinal nematodes are also effective against cestodes (Table 53.2). Several of the flukicidal drugs also have cestocidal activity (Table 53.3). Larval stages of cestodes affecting cattle, notably *Echinococcus* spp. and *Taenia saginata*, are generally refractory to treatment with anthelmintics. However, praziquantel has been shown to have activity against the intermediate stages of both these parasites, although the cost of treatment may preclude its use.

Further reading

Anderson, N. (1985) Controlled release technology for the control of helminths in ruminants. *Veterinary Parasitology*, **18**, 59–66.

Armour, J., Bairden, K., Pirie, H.M. & Ryan, W.G. (1987) Control of parasitic bronchitis and gastroenteritis by strategic prophylaxis with ivermectin. *Veterinary Record*, **121**, 5–8.

Barth, D. (1987) Treatment of inhibited *Dictyocaulus viviparus* in cattle with ivermectin. *Veterinary Parasitology*, **25**, 61–6.

Bennett, D.G. (1986) Clinical pharmacology of ivermectin. *Journal of the American Veterinary Medical Association*, **189**, 100–4.

Boersma, J.H. (1985) Chemotherapy of gastrointestinal nematodiasis in ruminants. In *Chemotherapy of Gastrointestinal Helminths* (ed. by H. vanden Bossche, D. Thienpont & P.G. Jannsens), Handbook of Experimental Pharmacology vol. 77, pp. 407–42. Springer-Verlag, Berlin.

Boray, J.C. (1986) Trematode infections of domestic animals. In *Chemotherapy of Parasitic Diseases* (ed. by W.C. Campbell & R.S. Rew), pp. 401–25. Plenum Press, New York.

Caldow, G.L., Taylor, M.A. & Hunt, K. (1989) Comparison of two early season anthelmintic programmes on a commercial beef farm. *Veterinary Record*, **124**, 111–14.

Campbell, W.C. (1985) Ivermectin: An update. *Parasitology Today*, **1**, 10–16.

Craig, T.M. & Huey, R.L. (1984) Efficacy of triclabendazole against *Fasciola hepatica* and *Fascioloides magna* in naturally infected calves. *American Journal of Veterinary Research*, **46**, 1644–5.

Donald, A.D. (1985) New methods of drug application for control of helminths. *Veterinary Parasitology*, **18**, 121–37.

Eagleson, J.S. & Bowie, J.Y. (1986) Oxfendazole resistance in *Trichostrongylus axei* in cattle in Australia. *Veterinary Record*, **119**, 604.

Egerton, J.R., Suhayda, D. & Eary, C.H. (1986) Prophylaxis of nematode infections in cattle with an indwelling ruminoreticular ivermectin sustained release bolus. *Veterinary Parasitology*, **22**, 67–75.

Eysker, M. (1986) The prophylactic effect of ivermectin treatment of calves, three weeks after turnout, on gastro-intestinal helminthiasis. *Veterinary Parasitology*, **22**, 95–103.

Geerts, S., Brandt, J., Kumar, V. & Biesemans, L. (1987) Suspected resistance of *Ostertagia ostertagi* in cattle to levamisole. *Veterinary Parasitology*, **23**, 77–82.

Grimshaw, W.T.R., Weatherley, A.J. & Jones, R.M. (1989) Evaluation of the morantel sustained release trilaminate in the control of parasitic gastroenteritis in first season grazing cattle.

Jacobs, D.E., Fox, M.T. & Ryan, W.G. (1987) Early season parasitic gastroenteritis in calves and its prevention with ivermectin. *Veterinary Record*, **120**, 29–31.

Jacobs, D.E., Thomas, J.G., Foster, J., Fox, M.T. & Oakley, G.A. (1987) Oxfendazole pulse release intraruminal devices and bovine parasitic bronchitis: Comparison of two control strategies in a field experiment. *Veterinary Record*, **121**, 221–4.

Jones, R.M. (1983) Therapeutic and prophylactic efficacy of morantel when administered directly into the rumen of cattle on a continuous basis. *Veterinary Parasitology*, **12**, 223–32.

Prichard, R.K. (1985) Interaction of host physiology and efficacy of antiparasitic drugs. *Veterinary Parasitology*, **18**, 103–10.

Prichard, R.K. (1986) Anthelmintics for cattle. *Veterinary Clinics of North America: Food Animal Practices*, **2**, 489–501.

Prichard, R.K., Hennessy, D.R. & Steel, J.W. (1978) Prolonged administration: A new concept for increasing the spectrum and effectiveness of anthelmintics. *Veterinary Parasitology*, **4**, 309–15.

Prichard, R.K., Hennessy, D.R., Steel, J.W. & Lacey, E. (1985) Metabolic concentrations in plasma following treatment of cattle with five metabolites. *Research in Veterinary Science*, **39**, 173–8.

Rew, R.S. & Fetterer, R.H. (1986) Mode of action of antinematocidal drugs. In *Chemotherapy of Parasitic Diseases* (ed. by W.C. Campbell & R.S. Rew), pp. 321–37. Plenum Press, New York.

Schulman, M.D. & Valentino, D. (1982) Purification, characterisation and inhibition by MK-401 of *Fasciola hepatica* phosphoglyceromutase. *Molecular and Biochemical Parasitology*, **5**, 321–32.

Seibert, B.P., Guerrero, J., Newcomb, K.M., Ruth, D.T. & Swites, B.J. (1986) Seasonal comparisons of anthelmintic activity of levamisole pour-on in cattle in the USA. *Veterinary Record*, **118**, 40–2.

Taylor, M.A. (1987) Liver fluke treatment. *In Practice*, **9**, 163–6.

Taylor, S.M., Mallon, T.R. & Kenny, J. (1985) Comparison of early season suppressive anthelmintic prophylactic methods for parasitic gastroenteritis and bronchitis in calves. *Veterinary Record*, **117**, 521–4.

Yazwinski, T.A., Featherstone, H., Presson, B.L., Greenway, T.E., Pote, L.M. & Holtzen, H. (1985) Efficacy of injectable chlorsulon in the treatment of immature bovine *Fasciola hepatica* infections. *AgriPractice*, **6**, 6–8.

Chapter 54: Antimicrobial Agents

by A.H. ANDREWS

Introduction

The choice of a suitable antimicrobial agent is very difficult. It first depends on deciding whether the problem encountered is an infection and even then whether it warrants such therapy. The site of infection needs to be located and the type of microbe established. Then the *in vitro* antimicrobial sensitivity of the organism and the minimal inhibitory concentration need to be determined. The likely ability to penetrate the area, the action of the antibiotic in the local environment and the maintenance of an effective concentration at the area must be considered. The selection also has to include the possibility of any potential toxic side-effects as well as the meat and milk withholding times. Once all these factors have been taken into consideration, the drug to be used, its dosage, route and frequency of administration can be determined. All the above, however, has to be undertaken on an economic basis.

There are various ways of defining antimicrobial preparations. Chemotherapy can be defined as the use in the treatment of a disease of pure chemicals that have a special antagonistic effect(s) on the organism causing the disease.

Antibiotics are complex organic chemicals synthesized by micro-organisms during their growth and which, in minute quantities, have a detrimental effect on other organisms. These chemical compounds are the metabolic products of bacteria and fungi. Most commonly, antibiotics are effective against bacteria but some have activity against viruses, *Rickettsia*, *Mycoplasma*, fungi and helminths (see Table 54.1).

Identification of the causal agent

Some decisions regarding therapy can only be made once a diagnosis is reached. Clinical examination is used to identify the nature of the infection, its site and possible cause. The signs of some diseases are so clear-cut that diagnosis is easy to establish and the organism is readily identifiable, e.g. wooden tongue, actinomycosis. In such cases the choice of drug is easy to make as well as its dosage, rate and duration of treatment. The likely outcome of therapy can also be predicted with some confidence. However, in many cases the disease signs are not clear-cut, the area of infection is difficult to localize or the sensitivity pattern of the organism is irregular. In such cases the identification of the causal agent is important not only for treatment of the individual animal affected but also for possible future action on a herd basis. However, in many situations, the site of infection and the cause of the condition are not known. In such instances laboratory diagnosis, other than haematological examination to indicate that an infection is present, is of no value. Therapy in these cases usually involves the use of one or more antimicrobial agents to ensure a broad

Table 54.1 Non-antibacterial activity of some antibiotics

Mycoplasma	Chlortetracycline, doxycycline, erythromycin, lincomycin, methacycline, oleandomycin, oxytetracycline, spiramycin, tetracycline, tylosin
Rickettsia	Chloramphenicol, chlortetracycline, doxycycline, methacycline, oxytetracycline, tetracycline
Protozoa	Monensin
Fungi	
Candida albicans	Amphotericin, nystatin
Dermatophytes	Griseofulvin, natamycin
Ectoparasites and endoparasites	Ivermectin

spectrum of activity. Subsequent progress will depend on evaluation of the effect of the chosen treatment.

Sampling

Wherever possible sampling should be undertaken to try to determine the causal organism. This will be considered academic by many but if it is looked at objectively it has much to commend it. At the first examination and, hopefully, before any therapy has been initiated is the best time to obtain samples to establish the likely cause of the problem. In addition, the cost of micro-organism determination is usually less, or at least no more, than the cost of appropriate therapy. In almost all cases the value of the individual animal will be sufficient to make it worthwhile and this is multiplied many times when problems are encountered on a herd basis. There is virtually no justification for not sampling problems of a herd nature when infections are suspected. In addition, the treatment of chronic conditions or those that have responded poorly is important. Besides positively determining the cause, sampling may help to eliminate other potential agents.

The method of sampling is important in that it should involve fresh clinical cases rather than those of a chronic nature. The sample should be taken from as near the inflamed area as possible. This is difficult with problems such as salmonellosis, as organisms in the faeces may be diluted by those further down the gut, which in themselves may be much faster growing. Sampling of pneumonias is always difficult as the organisms present in the upper respiratory tract may be unrepresentative of those in the lung.

Direct examination of the sample after staining is of use as in some circumstances organisms will not subsequently grow. Rapid staining methods are now available and these allow the shape of the organism and whether it is Gram-positive or Gram-negative to be determined. This in turn can be useful in making a quick decision about the drug most likely to be effective.

Sensitivity testing

Identification of the causal organism allows a decision to be made as to whether or not to test for antimicrobial sensitivity. In many cases there is no need to undertake this. Thus organisms of *Clostridium* spp. are sensitive to high doses of penicillin G. However, in cases involving *Escherichia coli* and *Salmonella typhimurium* there will be considerable variations in the sensitivity pattern, bearing in mind the origin of the organism.

The Kirby–Bauer disc sensitivity test is that most commonly used for *in vitro* testing. The aim is to determine if an organism is likely to be affected by specific antimicrobial agents at the usual therapeutic levels. While the drug concentration reflects levels achieved in the plasma, it does not take into account quantities in various tissues such as the brain or udder. The test organism is usually classified as sensitive, intermediate or resistant to the specific antimicrobial agent. The test was produced for use in human medicine where it provides a quantitative assessment. However, in animals it is a useful guide. Quantitative tests involve determining the minimal inhibitory concentration and usually consist of tube sensitivity tests. In general, an organism sensitive *in vitro* may be sensitive *in vivo*, but one resistant *in vitro* is also likely to be resistant *in vivo*.

Penetration

The ability of a drug to penetrate the infected area needs to be considered (see Table 54.2). Penetration depends on the degree of the pathological process as is seen with abscess or thrombus formation. It also depends on the tissue involved and whether there are natural limits to penetration such as in the brain or in milk. The location of the organism is also important, i.e. whether it is intracellular or extracellular.

The ability of an antimicrobial drug to cross biological membranes depends on many factors. These include protein binding, lipid solubility, pH of the drug

Table 54.2 Drugs with reasonable penetration of various fluids and tissues

Bile	Erythromycin
Bone	Chlortetracycline, doxycycline, fucidin, lincomycin, methacycline, oxytetracycline, tetracycline
Cerebrospinal fluid	Chloramphenicol, sulphonamides, trimethoprim and sulphonamides
Eye	Amoxycillin, ampicillin, cephalexin, cephaloridine, cephalothin, chloramphenicol, lincomycin
Milk	Benzylpenicillin, erythromycin, lincomycin (but toxic), oleandomycin, penethamate, spiramycin, tylosin
Prostate	Erythromycin, trimethoprim
Serosal fluids	Chloramphenicol, dihydrostreptomycin, erythromycin, framycetin, gentamicin, kanamycin, lincomycin, neomycin, paramomycin, streptomycin

in relation to environmental pH, molecular size and in some cases specific cellular transport mechanisms. Antibiotic is absorbed into the circulation, partly becoming bound to plasma protein. Binding varies, e.g. from less than 50 per cent with amoxycillin, streptomycin or oxytetracycline to more than 80 per cent with cloxacillin or erythromycin. Binding is readily reversible and the bound fraction is in equilibrium with the unbound (active) form. Protein binding can be a disadvantage, as with sulphonamides, which are highly protein bound. As purulent fluids often contain much protein, sulphonamides can be relatively inactive.

Water-soluble drugs are useful for extracellular organisms and where intracellular organisms have a high turnover rate, usually in the lysis of cells and release of the organisms into fluids containing the antimicrobial agent. Lipid solubility does have advantages for organisms that spend most of their time within cells or behind tissue barriers. Inflammation can also alter penetration of drugs. Thus penetration of the central nervous system by many drugs is minimal in the healthy animal although penicillin G and other antibiotics can enter during inflammation. However, the effect of inflammation on the penetration of many drugs is unknown. Thus it can be the local environment in which the organism is present that is important. Most antimicrobial agents do maintain their activity; however, aminoglycosides are more active in aerobic conditions with a slightly alkaline pH. As such conditions do not exist around staphylococcal abscesses this group of drugs is relatively inactive in such circumstances. Activity of antibacterial agent in urine is often influenced by the pH (see Table 54.3.) The problem of sulphonamides and pus has already been mentioned. Some antibiotics do have more effect on anaerobic bacteria then others under such conditions (see Table 54.4).

Antibiotic resistance

The advent of antimicrobial drugs has resulted in the emergence of resistance to these drugs (see Table 54.4). The use of antibiotics in therapeutic concentration results in an alteration of the microflora within the host. There is a tendency for a loss of the sensitive strains with the resistant ones remaining. This selection

Table 54.3 Antibacterial drug activity in urine. Urinary infections are relatively uncommon in cattle but can lead to therapeutic problems

Not affected by urine pH	Most active in alkaline urine	Most active in acid urine
Cephalexin	Colistin	Carbenicillin
Cephaloridine	Dihydrostreptomycin	Chlortetracycline
Cephalothin	Erythromycin	Doxycycline
Chloramphenicol	Framycetin	Methacycline
Nalidixic acid	Gentamicin	Nitrofurantoin
Sulphonamides	Kanamycin	Oxytetracycline
Trimethoprim and sulphonamides	Neomycin	Penicillin G
	Paramomycin	Tetracycline
	Polymyxin B	*Acidification*
	Streptomycin	D-Methionine (oral)
	Alkalinization	Ascorbic acid (oral)
	Sodium bicarbonate (oral)	

Table 54.4 Antibiotics effective *in vitro* against anaerobic bacteria

High efficacy	Moderate efficacy	Low efficacy
Amoxycillin	Chlortetracycline	Dihydrostreptomycin
Ampicillin	Erythromycin	Framycetin
Carbenicillin	Oxytetracycline	Gentamicin
Chloramphenicol	Procaine penicillin G	Kanamycin
Clindamycin		Neomycin
Metronidazole	Tetracycline	Paramomycin
		Streptomycin

Table 54.5 Penicillinase (β-lactamase) active antimicrobials

Penicillins	Cloxacillin, methicillin
Cephalosporins	Cefoperazone, cephalexin, cephalonium, cephaloridine, cephalothin
Aminoglycosides	Amikacin, framycetin, gentamicin, kanamycin, neomycin, paramomycin
Macrolides	Erythromycin, oleandomycin, spiramycin, tylosin
Nitrofurans	Furazolidone, nitrofurantoin, nitrofurazone
Others	Bacitracin, chloramphenicol, lincomycin, novobiocin, sulphonamide and trimethoprim, vancomycin

allows multiplication of resistant strains within the less competitive environment. The resistant organisms can remain in the animal and also contaminate the environment, thereby allowing passage to other animals. The prevalence of the resistant organisms tends to reduce the longer the period since the drug was used.

Spontaneous mutation of organisms can occur but it is probably only of limited importance in practice. However, transferable drug resistance is of significance. This resistance, as determined in the form of plasmids or transposons, is transferred to susceptible strains. Plasmids are extrachromosomal genetic material that can replicate independently of the chromosome. These plasmids can be transferred by conjugation within or between bacterial species and they can also act as vectors for transposons. This allows the transfer of single or multiple antibiotic resistance and has produced many of the resistant bacteria found in enteric calf infections including both *E. coli* and *S. typhimurium* as well as in *Staphylococcus aureus* and some *Pasteurella* spp. infections. In some countries the use of chloramphenicol in food animals is restricted because of the usage in humans.

Dosage

When an antimicrobial agent is selected it must be in a high enough concentration and used for a long enough period to result in contact with the organism and its consequent demise. Various factors influence this, including the dose, formulation and rate of administration. Doses are usually based on body weight. The recommended dose usually provides good blood and tissue levels that are effective against most susceptible organisms, with minimal side-effects. In most cases the recommended dose is the minimal dose. This is particularly so for farm animals where both the interval between therapy and the suggested dose level tend to be lower than for man or small animals due to cost.

Less susceptible organisms require higher levels to ensure success. Increasing the dose needs to be considered carefully, but it is of little danger if the drug has a low toxicity. However, when the antimicrobial agent is of high toxicity any increase in dosage should be undertaken with caution. Different dosages may also influence the drug withdrawal time. It should be remembered that when different companies produce the same antibiotic it may well contain different amounts of the drug and the vehicle in which it is presented may vary.

Route of administration

The choice of administration route depends on the speed with which infection has to be counteracted as well as the volume to be given, ease of administration, etc. The principal routes used are given in Table 54.6.

Duration of therapy

In general terms, most injections are used for three to five days and for at least one day after normality is reached. However, there is a tendency not to treat for long enough in chronic conditions such as some cases of chronic joint or thoracic infections when therapy should be continued for at least 10–14 days. If it was a human or small animal there would often be no dispute about such a length of therapy. Many antibacterial preparations are now available that can be injected at extended intervals to provide adequate drug concentrations for several days. However, in some cases the duration of effective therapy can be overestimated.

Table 54.6 Routes of administration of antimicrobial drugs

Intravenous (i.v.): always give slowly

Advantages
- Rapid high blood and tissue levels, therefore, useful for septicaemias
- Always higher circulating levels than i.m. or oral
- Increased levels at areas where levels usually low, e.g. necrotic areas, chronic abscesses
- Useful for large volumes
- Useful for painful injections
- Useful for irritant injections
- Only method of obtaining accurate blood and tissue levels

Disadvantages
- Acute toxic reactions more common
- Specific formulations necessary
- Requires good technique
- Perivascular and intravascular thrombosis can occur

Intramuscular (i.m.)

Advantages
- Most common route
- Only 20 ml per injection site
- Peak blood and tissue levels within 2 hours
- Slightly less irritant injections than those given i.v. can be given by deep i.m. injection
- Allows a reasonable level to be maintained over a period of time

Disadvantages
- Muscle damage
- Try not to do within 3 weeks of slaughter
- Severe reactions to some drugs
- Some injections painful
- Accurate blood and tissue levels not obtained

Intraperitoneal (i.p.)

Advantages
- Speed of absorption similar to i.m. injection
- Usually well absorbed
- Useful for peritonitis
- Useful if very toxic
- Useful for irritant drugs
- Useful in severe respiratory distress (especially tetracyclines)
- Large volumes can be given

Disadvantages
- Possible sepsis
- Accurate blood and tissue levels not obtained

Subcutaneous (s.c.)

Advantages
- Little used for antimicrobials except sulphonamides
- Large volumes can be given
- Less irritant than i.m.

Disadvantages
- May provoke marked fluid reaction
- Only slowly absorbed
- Speed of absorption less than i.m.

Intra-articular
- Increased level in joint
- Must be sterile technique

Intrapleural
- Increased level in thorax
- Must be non-irritant
- Must be a sterile technique

Subconjunctival
- Useful for ocular conditions
- Must be non-irritant
- Must be sterile technique

Oral (water or feed)

Advantages
- Easiest method of administration
- Can be undertaken by owner

Disadvantages
- Blood and tissue levels less than for comparable parenteral dose
- Higher doses usually used
- Absorption is variable (depends on gut motility, type of feed, volume of feed, drug binding, e.g. calcium, kaolin impair absorption of tetracycline, oxytetracycline, chlortetracycline, methacycline doxycycline, ampicillin, lincomycin)
- Blood levels do not peak for 12–18 hours
- Antibiotics may influence normal ruminal flora
- Some antibiotics not absorbed, e.g. streptomycin, dihydrostreptomycin, neomycin, framycetin, phthalylsulphathiazole
- Some antibiotics destroyed, e.g. benzylpenicillin

Topical
- Ointments, powders, aerosol sprays

Ophthalmic preparations
- Ointments and drops. Limited retention at site except some special preparations

Aural preparations
- Drops and ointments

Intramammary (use aseptic technique)

Advantages
- Convenient
- Good efficacy

Disadvantages
- Often diffusion reduced by blocked lactiferous ducts, etc.
- Used for clinical treatment
- Dry-cow therapy used for subclinical mastitis and prophylaxis
- If intramammary tube used in one quarter all milk should be withheld

Spectrum of drug activity

Antibacterial drugs vary in their degree of activity against various classes of organism. They are usually considered narrow spectrum if they are only active against bacteria, but broad spectrum if they also have activity against *Mycoplasma*, *Rickettsia* and *Chlamydia*. The antibacterial activity of drugs can also vary (see Table 54.7): some have a narrow spectrum, only inhibiting either Gram-negative or Gram-positive organisms; others have most activity against Gram-positive organisms but will inhibit some Gram-negative agents. However, some have a broad spectrum inhibiting both Gram-positive and Gram-negative bacteria.

Bacteriostatic or bactericidal activity

At times it is important to know the activity of a drug. Some drugs are bactericidal, e.g. penicillin, aminoglycosides, while others are bacteriostatic and require the animal's own defence mechanism to help in the organisms' removal (Table 54.8). These definitions are only relative and some agents are bactericidal in high concentrations but only bacteriostatic at low levels.

Drug combinations

These are frequently used in veterinary practice but are often best avoided. They are of use where infection is due to mixed organisms. They can be helpful where synergism has been shown with the combination, e.g. penicillin and aminoglycosides, or trimethoprim and sulphonamides. Although the bacteriostatic or bactericidal nature of many drugs is dependent on the concentration used, it is still a good ploy to combine antibiotics with a similar activity. This is of particular importance when treating immunocompromised animals. Besides the broader spectrum of activity attained with some combinations, cost may be less and in some cases there may be a reduction in toxicity.

When using combinations it is best to give each drug individually at the correct dose with an interval between administrations. When two drugs are com-

Table 54.7 Antibacterial activity other than for anaerobic bacteria

Gram-positive bacteria	Gram-negative bacteria	Broad spectrum: Gram-positive and Gram-negative bacteria
Penicillins	*Penicillins*	*Penicillins*
Cloxacillin	Carbenicillin	Amoxycillin
Methacillin		Ampicillin
Penicillin G	*Polymyxins*	Clavulanic acid and amoxycillin
Penicillin V	Colistin	
	Polymyxin B	*Sulphonamides*
Macrolides		Many forms
Erythromycin	*Aminoglycosides*	
Oleandomycin	Amikacin	*Tetracyclines*
Spiramycin	Dihydrostreptomycin	Chlortetracycline
Tylosin	Framycetin	Doxycycline
	Gentamicin	Methacycline
Others	Kanamycin	Oxytetracycline
Bacitracin	Neomycin	Tetracycline
Lincomycin	Paramomycin	
Novobiocin	Streptomycin	*Cephalosporins*
Tiamulin		Cephalexin
Vancomycin	*Others*	Cephaloridine
	Apramycin	Cephalothin
	Spectinomycin	
		Nitrofurans
		Furazolidone
		Nitrofurantoin
		Nitrofurazone
		Others
		Chloramphenicol
		Halquinol
		Sulphonamide and trimethoprim

Table 54.8 Bactericidal and bacteriostatic drugs

Bactericidal	Bacteriostatic
Penicillins	Halquinol
Amoxycillin	Novobiocin (high concentration)
Ampicillin	Spectinomycin (occasionally)
Carbenicillin	Sulphonamide and trimethoprim
Cloxacillin	Vancomycin
Methicillin	*Macrolides*
Penicillin G (benzylpenicillin)	Carbomycin
Penicillin V (phenoxypenicillin)	Erythromycin (low concentration)
Macrolides	Oleandomycin
Erythromycin (high concentration)	Spiramycin
Nitrofurans	Tilmicosin
Furazolidone (high concentration)	Tylosin
Nitrofurantoin (high concentration)	*Sulphonamides*
Nitrofurazone (high concentration)	All types
Cephalosporins	*Nitrofurans*
Ceftiofur	Furazolidone (low concentration)
Cephalexin	Nitrofurantoin (low concentration)
Cephaloridine	Nitrofurazone (low concentration)
Cephalothin	*Tetracyclines*
Polymyxins	Chlortetracycline
Colistin	Doxycycline
Polymyxin B	Methacycline
Aminoglycosides	Oxytetracycline
Amikacin	Tetracycline, etc.
Dihydrostreptomycin	*Others*
Framycetin	Apramycin
Gentamicin	Chloramphenicol
Kanamycin	Clindamycin
Neomycin	Lincomycin
Paramomycin	Novobiocin (low concentration)
Streptomycin, etc.	Spectinomycin (usually)
Others	Tiamulin
Bacitracin	Trimethoprim
Panfloxacin	

Whether a drug is bactericidal or bacteriostatic needs to be known as problems can occur with combinations.

bined in commercial preparations then the dosage of each is fixed regardless of the needs of the particular situation or the interval between doses. Care should be taken in the choice of antimicrobial agent when used in combination with corticosteroids.

Cost

This is a major drawback in that often the best therapy cannot be instituted because of the expense. Repeat doses also cause problems especially as oral therapy is not often advisable in ruminants. The problem can be overcome by long-acting preparations or providing combination injections for the farmer or stockworker to administer. It must be remembered there is an indirect cost, particularly to the dairy farmer, in the length of time the milk has to be withheld after the end of treatment. The beef farmer encounters a similar problem regarding meat withdrawal time but to a lesser extent.

Toxicity

Except where there is routine usage of antimicrobial drugs in adult animals, few problems of toxicity arise. Some of the more common are given in Table 54.9.

Table 54.9 Toxicity of antimicrobiol drugs

Penicillins	Very low toxicity, hypersensitivity. Occasional severe adverse reactions
Sulphonamides	Toxicity rare, rapid intravenous injection causes collapse and respiratory distress
Macrolides	Pain and reaction following s.c. or i.m. injections. Crystalluria not a problem in large animals. Erythromycin and tylosin irritant following injection
Lincomycin	Diarrhoea, reduced milk production (oral)
Aminoglycosides	Ototoxicity (unlikely), cardiovascular damage, hypotension (for toxic and shocked animals), renal toxicity
Tetracyclines	Acute collapse syndrome (i.v.). Alimentary tract dysfunction (if oral). Deposition in bone and teeth
Chloramphenicol	Little toxicity. Superinfection (oral)
Polymyxyn B Colistin	Usually only used topically as toxic shock and death can occur following parenteral use
Nitrofurans	Acute — nervous signs Chronic — haemorrhagic syndrome

Drug withdrawal times

Following use of an antimicrobial agent there is now usually a period between finishing therapy and the use of the milk or the slaughter of the animal for meat. Milk or meat containing antibiotics can present a public health risk. There is the possibility of allergy to penicillins or other antibacterials following medical prescription. Documented cases are rare and are now almost non-existent in countries with adequate antibiotic testing. Where they have occurred they involved usage of milk. Another possible hazard is drug resistance in humans but adequate documented evidence for the occurrence of this following consumption of milk or meat is still required. The main effect of antibiotics in milk is a commercial one in that it can affect the starter cultures for cheese or yoghurt.

Various factors influence the withdrawal time and these include the drug dose rate, age, disease, duration and role of therapy. The injection site will obviously contain higher levels than other sites. Depending on how the drug is metabolized, the kidney and liver may have higher levels than other tissues. In all cases it is the duty of the veterinary surgeon to ensure that any withdrawal time is observed and that the owner of the animal is made aware of this. It is always best to write the time down either on the drug vial if doses are to be provided for administration by the farmer, or on an invoice or note to the farmer. Where a withdrawal time is not known then the manufacturer or distributor of the drug should be contacted. However, in general, when no withholding time is stated then milk must be discarded for seven days and cattle may not be slaughtered for human consumption for 28 days. In the USA veterinarians can obtain information on withdrawal times and residues by contacting the Food Animal Residue Avoidance Data book (FARAD).

Frequency of dosing

The frequency of administering therapeutic preparations varies. Some compounds are placed in slow-release boluses to facilitate this. The rate of absorption also varies between different preparations, dependent on the particle size; thus those with micronized particles are rapidly absorbed. The form of the antibiotic will also influence the level of activity. Thus with penicillin, benzylpenicillin is rapidly absorbed (in minutes) to reach peak levels but only persists for about 6 hours. However, procaine benzylpenicillin reaches a maximum level in 2–4 hours and persists for 24 hours, benethamine benzylpenicillin has a slow absorption (6–24 hours) and may be effective for three to four days, and benzathine benzylpenicillin is slowly ab-

Table 54.10 Advantages and disadvantages of slow-release antibiotic preparations

Advantages
Often used in prophylaxis
Postoperatively
Post calving where there has been intervention
Dry-cow therapy: most remain about 3–4 weeks in udder but some persist six weeks or longer
Less stress to animal
Reduced handling
Less pain to animal
Convenience
Disadvantages
Animals may not be examined as regularly as when injected often
Thus animal less monitored
Usually tissue and blood levels lower than routine injections
Increased withholding time for milk or injection-to-slaughter time

sorbed over 6–24 hours and is often effective for four to seven days.

The advantages and disadvantages of slow-release antibiotic preparations are given in Table 54.10.

Possible antibacterial therapy for cattle

A survey of some cf the drugs used in the treatment of cattle is given in Table 54.11. It is emphasized that this list is not complete.

Table 54.11 Possible antibacterial therapy for infections in cattle

Calves	
Diarrhoea (acute)	Amoxycillin, ampicillin, chloramphenicol chlortetracycline, clavulanic acid and amoxycillin, framycetin, neomycin, oxytetracycline, trimethoprim and sulphonamide
Diarrhoea (subacute)	Neomycin, nitrofurazone, oxytetracycline, sulphonamides
Joint ill	Lincomycin, oxytetracycline
Meningitis	Chloramphenicol, trimethoprim and sulphonamide
Navel ill	Amoxycillin, ampicillin, clavulanic acid and amoxycillin, oxytetracycline, trimethoprim and sulphonamide
Pneumonia	Amoxycillin, ampicillin, ceftiofur, clavulanic acid and amoxycillin, danfloxacin oxytetracycline, penicillin and streptomycin, tilmicosin, tylosin
Ringworm	Griseofulvin, natamycin
Salmonella spp.	Amoxycillin, ampicillin, apramycin, chloramphenicol, clavulanic acid and amoxycillin, neomycin, nitrofurazone, trimethoprim and sulphonamide
Septicaemia	Amoxycillin, ampicillin, chloramphenicol, clavulanic acid and amoxycillin, trimethoprim and sulphonamide
Older cattle — injections	
Actinomycosis	Amoxycillin, cephalexin, oxytetracycline, penicillin, sulphonamides
Anthrax	Amoxycillin, oxytetracycline, penicillin and streptomycin
Blackleg	Benzylpenicillin
Clostridial infections	Oxytetracycline, pencillin
Diarrhoea (acute)	Sulphonamide
Infectious bovine keratoconjunctivitis	Chloramphenicol, oxytetracycline
Leptospirosis	Oxytetracycline, streptomycin
Mastitis (peracute) (parenteral)	Amoxycillin, ampicillin, cephalexin, oxytetracycline, trimethoprim and sulphonamide
Metritis	Amoxycillin, cephalexin, clavulanic acid and amoxycillin, oxytetracycline
Peritonitis	Sulphonamides, trimethoprim and sulphonamides
Pneumonia (acute)	Amoxycillin, oxytetracycline, trimethoprim and sulphonamide
Pneumonia (subacute)	Amoxycillin, ampicillin, oxytetracycline, penicillin and streptomycin, trimethoprim and sulphonamide
Pyelonephritis	Procaine penicillin
Salmonella spp.	Amoxycillin, ampicillin, chloramphenicol, neomycin, trimethoprim and sulphonamide
Tetanus	Benzyl and procaine penicillin
Wooden tongue	Amoxycillin, oxytetracycline, penicillin and streptomycin, sulphonamide

Note: Not all these drugs are registered for the species or for the use suggested.

Chapter 55: Antimicrobial Therapy of Mastitis

by J.W. TYLER AND J.D. BAGGOT

General considerations

Mastitis is the single most common disease of the adult dairy cow, accounting for 38 per cent of all morbidity. Additionally, 70 per cent of affected cattle will be culled and 1 per cent die as a consequence of the mastitis (United States Department of Agriculture, 1988). One-quarter of all clinical disease-related economic losses are directly attributed to mastitis (United States Department of Agriculture, 1988). Decreases in milk yield caused by subclinical mastitis are responsible for even greater economic losses (Janzen, 1970; Fetrow, 1981; Tyler *et al.*, 1989). Efficacious, economical treatment of mastitis is therefore an important component of livestock medicine.

The most frequent causes of mastitis are *Staphylococcus aureus*, *Streptococcus agalactiae, Strep. uberis, Strep. dysgalactiae, Escherichia coli, Enterobacter* sp., *Pseudomonas* sp., *Klebsiella* sp., *Actinomyces (Corynebacterium) pyogenes* and *Mycoplasma* sp. (see Chapters 21, 22). Differences in climate, management, and national or regional regulatory efforts result in patterns of disease that vary markedly. Surveys conducted in the USA report higher prevalences of *Staph. aureus* and *Step. agalactiae* infections than observed in Britain. One American source has stated that *Staph. aureus* and *Strep. agalactiae* are isolated from 90 per cent of infected quarters (Jarrett, 1981). The arid southwestern regions of North America have repeatedly identified prevalences of intramammary *Mycoplasma* sp. infections exceeding those observed in other parts of the world (Jasper *et al.*, 1966; Jasper, 1980; Thurmond *et al.*, 1989). A representative study conducted in Canada reported the following prevalences of various mastitis pathogens (per cent cows, per cent quarters); *Staph. aureus* (12 per cent, 8 per cent), *Strep. agalactiae* (6.6 per cent, 4.1 per cent), and other streptococci (8.8 per cent, 4.5 per cent) (Brooks *et al.*, 1982).

Laboratory testing is an integral part of treatment and control programmes and identification of the causal agents will have a direct bearing on subsequent therapeutic decisions. Several handbooks are available to assist the identification of mastitis pathogens (National Mastitis Council Research Committee, 1981). Although limited in distribution the monograph *Laboratory Procedures for the Evaluation of Milk Quality*, edited by Thurmond, is one of the most complete references available (Thurmond, 1986).

Antimicrobial resistance

Although useful, antibiotic sensitivity testing does not guarantee the efficacy of any antibiotic. Generally, the major streptococcal pathogens of the bovine mammary gland are sensitive (>90 per cent) to penicillin, ampicillin, cephalothin and erythromycin (Prescott & Baggot, 1988). Actual cure rates will vary with clinical and lactation status. Sensitivity patterns for the two most common Gram-negative intramammary pathogens, *E. coli* and *Klebsiella* sp., are reported in Table 55.1 and may be used to guide the choice of an antibiotic when treating peracute mastitis (Davidson, 1980; Prescott & Baggot, 1988). One should be cautioned that sensitivity patterns will vary locally with antibiotic use. Historical susceptibility information drawn from individual farms will likely prove more useful. Table 55.2 reports *in vitro* sensitivity and *in vivo* cure rates

Table 55.1 Antibiotic sensitivities of selected Gram-negative bacteria isolated from cattle with clinical mastitis (reported as per cent of isolates sensitive)

	Davidson (1980)		Prescott (1985)*	
	E. coli	*Klebsiella*	*E. coli*	*Klebsiella*
Gentamicin	99	99	99–100	100
Polymyxin	–[†]	–	100	100
Chloramphenicol	76	93	68–99	67–100
Cephalothin	60	77	60–73	82–83
Tetracycline	68	63	23	42–54
Ampicillin	64	12	35	0
Erythromycin	–	–	39	25
Lincomycin	–	–	29	17
Furizolidone	–	–	92–98	25–92
Neomycin	85	91	56–70	33–90
Streptomycin	67	47	73	77
Penicillin	6	1	0	0
Triple Sulfa	–	–	5	33

* Compiled from several sources.
[†] Tests not performed.

Table 55.2 Antibiotic sensitivities and bacteriological cure rates based on cultures four weeks following treatment for *Staphylococcus aureus* following intramammary treatment with various antibiotics (adapted from Le Loudec, 1978 and Prescott, 1988)

Drug	% sensitive	Cure rates (%)	
		Lactation	Dry period
Penicillin	26–47	32	52
Cloxicillin*	99	41	76
Cephalosporins	95–100	72	60
Neomycin	96–99	27	51
Tetracycline	69–97	54	–
Tylosin	–[†]	55	–
Erythromycin	83–92	63	73
Spiramycin	–	70	40
Rifamycin	78	66	–
Penicillin–streptomycin	–	39	79
Penicillin–neomycin	–	96	–
Penicillin–novobiocin	–	–	73

* Sensitivity to methicillin reported.
[†] Values not reported.

with respect to *Staph. aureus* for several commonly used antimicrobial agents (Le Loudec, 1978). It should be noted that the percentage of sensitive isolates uniformly and greatly exceeds cure rates. The absence of *in vitro* activity may suggest a lack of efficacy while sensitivity infers, but does not guarantee, efficacy.

Pharmacology of the mammary gland

Severe mastitis is usually treated systemically, although intramammary therapy will often be used adjunctively. Drugs are transferred from the general circulation to the mammary gland by passive diffusion (Baggot, 1977; Ziv, 1980a–d). Consequently, non-ionized lipid-soluble agents that are not extensively bound to plasma proteins more readily reach the mammary gland. Because milk is weakly acidic (pH 6.4–6.8), drugs that are weak bases (trimethoprim, macrolides, lincosamides) are preferentially concentrated by ion trapping (Ziv, 1980a–d; Prescott & Baggot, 1988). The low degree of lipid solubility of aminoglycosides and polymyxin B limits their passage into milk. In cases of clinical mastitis, the pH of milk increases, approaching that of plasma. Under these circumstances weak acids (sulphonamides, penicillins, cephalosporins, rifampin), although typically not concentrated in milk, may reach effective concentrations (Ziv, 1980a–d; Prescott & Baggot, 1988). However, this is not a consistent property. Lipophilic drugs of various pharmacological classes will also be concentrated in milk.

The ideal antibiotic for systemic antimicrobial therapy of acute mastitis would have the following properties (adapted from Ziv, 1980a–d).

1 Low minimum inhibitory concentration (MIC) with respect to the known or suspected cause of mastitis.
2 Rapid absorption if administered intramuscularly or orally.
3 High bioavailability.
4 Weakly basic, permitting concentration in milk by ion trapping.
5 Lipophilic.
6 Low binding to plasma proteins.
7 Half-lives consistent with treatment intervals ⩾12 hours.
8 Minimal host toxicity at effective doses.
9 Short slaughter and milk withdrawal times.

Based on pharmacokinetic properties and anticipated sensitivities one can choose an antibiotic for use in the initial treatment of mastitis. Macrolide antibiotics would probably be the best choice for streptococcal and staphylococcal infections, followed by tetracyclines (Prescott & Baggot, 1988). Several antimicrobial agents, including aminoglycosides, chloramphenicol, polymyxin B, and trimethoprim–sulpha have pharmacological properties and sensitivity patterns consistent with systemic treatment of Gram-negative mastitis (Prescott & Baggot, 1980). Unfortunately, cost, toxicities, residues, and regulatory concerns preclude their widespread use. These problems may be resolved as new generations of antibiotic become available to the practitioner.

Intramammary administration is the preferred route in the treatment of mild clinical or subclinical mastitis. The same properties governing the transfer of antibiotic from the systemic circulation to the milk will determine the behaviour of a drug following intramammary administration. Weakly basic or drugs with low lipid solubility tend to remain in the mammary gland following treatment (Ziv, 1980a–d). Intramammary administration permits delivery of antibiotic directly to the mammary gland, a site where the drug's inherent physicochemical properties often preclude effective parenteral treatment. Penicillin derivatives, which are poorly transferred to the mammary gland, have demonstrated efficacy in the intramammary treatment of *Strep. agalactiae*. Intramammary infusions are available in single-use syringes. Lactating-cow products are generally designed for rapid clearance and, consequently, shorter milk withholding periods. Antibiotics with extensive tissue binding (polymyxin B and aminoglycosides) will have extended milk withholding periods (Prescott & Baggot, 1988). Dry-cow formulations are designed to produce extended duration of effective drug concentrations. Consequently, a large amount of drug in the product, oil or repository vehicles, and benzathine salts, are common constituents of dry-cow products.

Benefits of antimicrobial therapy of mastitis

Rather than provide actual monetary values and costs, the following section is an attempt to provide items to be considered (Janzen, 1970; Fetrow, 1981). The values and costs associated with agricultural products and veterinary services are not readily interpretable across international boundaries.

Salvage of peracute cases

Appropriate therapy, including with antimicrobial agents, may reduce the mortality associated with peracute mastitis. The value of a cull cow, as well as humane considerations, dictate timely appropriate intervention. Even following the loss of productive capacity, the value of cull cows can be applied toward replacement purchases and cannot be neglected as a benefit of therapy.

Prevention of irreversible parenchymal loss

Left untreated many intramammary infections are followed by chronic inflammatory responses. Functional secretory components are replaced by fibrous connective tissue. The affected quarter may become entirely non-functional or blind. Effective treatment can prevent or reduce the severity of these changes. The effect of halting these changes on productive longevity is of unknown magnitude, but probably important. When mature cattle are sold as replacements, buyers should avoid at all costs blind quartered cattle, although they are heavily discounted.

Improved milk quality

Subclinical mastitis has documented effects on the quality of dairy products. Milk from infected cattle is less palatable, has a shorter shelf-life, and produces lower yields of processed dairy products. Consequently, cooperatives, commercial concerns, and regulatory agencies often impose penalties, based on the somatic cell and bacteria counts of bulk tank milk. The most severe penalty arises with milk that is deemed unfit for human consumption and discarded. Although treatment of clinical mastitis may not effect a microbiological cure, macroscopic milk quality will return to normal more quickly following treatment. This return to saleable production is an important benefit of treatment.

Increased milk production

The single largest cost associated with intramammary infection is the reduced milk yield associated with subclinical infections. One recent study observed a 3 kg reduction in daily milk yield in cattle with somatic cell counts as low as 665 000 cells/ml (Tyler *et al.*, 1989). Less substantive data are available relative to the benefits of antimicrobial therapy during lactation. At least in the case of *Strep. agalactiae* infections, increases in milk production may offset treatment and milk discard costs in the early period of lactation (Janzen, 1970; Fetrow, 1981).

Effective microbiological cures, eliminating reservoirs of infection

A very real, but often overlooked, benefit of antimicrobial therapy relates not to the individual cow but to the overall herd health status. Each infected cow may represent not only an individual with suboptimal health and production, but also a reservoir of infection. Each infected cow thus poses a threat to the productive capacity of non-infected cattle. *Streptococcus agalactiae* is an obligate parasite of the mammary gland. *Staphylococcus aureus* and *Mycoplasma* sp., although not obligate parasites of the mammary gland, are transmitted primarily from cow to cow (Tyler *et al.*, 1989). Identification followed by treatment, isolation, or eradication can markedly reduce numbers of new infections if coupled with appropriate hygienic measures. Coliform infections arise primarily from environmental sources (Eberhart *et al.*, 1979; Eberhart, 1984). Elimination of any single infection will not alter the incidence of new infections. *Streptococcus* spp. (non-*agalactiae*) and *Staphylococcus* spp. (non-*aureus*) may both be transmitted to a non-infected gland either from an infected gland or a non-mammary source. Consequently, microbiological cures of infected glands will reduce, but not eliminate, new infections (McDonald, 1984).

Costs associated with antimicrobial therapy of mastitis

Drug and veterinary services

These costs will not be detailed, but should be considered when evaluating the costs associated with treatment.

Discarded milk

Available intramammary antibiotic preparations have recommended milk withholding periods (discard times) that vary from 36 to 96 hours. When treating subclinical mastitis cattle are typically infused at two consecutive milkings. Cattle with clinical mastitis are often treated four times at 12 or 24 hour intervals. The antibiotic-contaminated, and hence discarded, milk may total as much as 400 kg in a high-producing cow. The decision to undertake treatment cannot be taken lightly. Dry-cow therapy is particularly cost-effective because it does not require milk discarding.

Slaughter withdrawal times

Both systemic and local (intramammary) antibiotic preparations have slaughter withdrawal times. Treated individuals cannot be marketed for salvage purposes, regardless of the success of treatment.

Risks of new infections/altered host defences

Intramammary infusion of antibiotics is far from being an innocuous procedure. Infusion procedure may remove the keratin lining of the streak canal, an important barrier to intramammary infections (see p. 284). The antibiotics and vehicles used in the formulation of intramammary products have been demonstrated to impair the function of milk phagocytic cells (Lintner & Eberhart, 1990a,b). Strict sanitation must be practised to prevent the accidental introduction of micro-organisms at the time of treatment. Only commercially available formulations of known efficacy and guaranteed safety are suitable for intramammary therapy. Special care must be exercised when large numbers of cattle are being treated on a single occasion. Explosive outbreaks of peracute and often fatal mastitis have been known to follow either poor hygiene during insertion or use of a contaminated product.

Therapy of specific mastitis syndromes

Mastitis can be subdivided into three overlapping categories based on the source or reservoir of infection. These differences will dictate alternate treatment strategies. In the first category are *Staph. aureus, Strep. agalactiae* and *Mycoplasma* sp. organisms which tend to behave primarily as parasites of the mammary gland (McDonald, 1984). The second category contains those organisms which, although transmitted from cow to cow, have significant reservoirs either in non-mammary host tissues or the environment. Streptococci (excluding *Strep. agalactiae*) and coagulase-negative staphylococci are representative of this category (McDonald, 1984). The last category contains organisms that act as opportunistic or coincidental pathogens. The Gram-negative infection is the classic representative of this group (Eberhart *et al.*, 1979).

Antimicrobial therapy of mastitis should only be undertaken when the practitioner can answer yes to one of the following questions. Will therapy alter the prognosis of clinical disease? Will therapy increase the productivity of the individual treated? Will individual therapy remove a source of infectious micro-organisms and, consequently, reduce the incidence of mastitis? Antibiotic use is otherwise counterproductive.

Streptococcus agalactiae (see p. 296)

Antibiotic therapy for mastitis caused by *Strep. agalactiae* will include intramammary treatment of dry cows and lactating cows, both clinical and subclinical. Clinical signs are restricted to the mammary gland and extensive systemic therapy is not indicated on either medical or economic considerations. *Streptococcus agalactiae* is usually sensitive to most available intramammary antibiotics, including penicillins, cephalosporins, tetracyclines and macrolides (Prescott & Baggot, 1988). Cure rates greater than 90 per cent are commonly achieved by either lactating or dry-cow therapy. Costs associated with lactating-cow therapy, microbiological testing, drug purchases, and milk discards, are often offset by increased milk production. Cows in the latter half of lactation will probably not have production increased in sufficient magnitude to offset these costs. A benefit of lactating-cow therapy is the elimination of infected glands as sources of new infections. Recognition of an infected herd is often followed by whole-herd cultures of composite milk samples and intramammary treatment of infected cows two to three times at 12 hour intervals. Strict hygienic precautions should be followed, both at the time of sample collection and at the time of treatment to prevent iatrogenic infections. Follow-up cultures may be performed in two to three weeks. Cows that fail to respond are retreated or culled at this time. Extensive treatment of subclinical lactating cows should not be undertaken until any errors in premilking hygiene, teat dipping and dry therapy are corrected. Alternatively, less ambitious programmes involving only teat disinfection and dry-cow therapy will gradually reduce prevalence in the herd over a period of two to three years (McDonald, 1984).

Streptococcus dysgalactiae (p. 296)

Antibiotic therapy and expected responses will be similar to those seen with *Strep. agalactiae* (see Table 55.3) (Prescott & Baggot, 1988). Comprehensive culture and treatment of subclinical cases is rarely undertaken because the organism is less infectious and, consequently, tends not to create as severe a herd problem, and the presence of extramammary reservoirs (tonsils and reproductive tracts) precludes eradication efforts. Treatment of clinical cases, routine dry-cow treatment and milking hygiene, including germicidal teat dips, will control this infection in most herds (McDonald, 1984).

Table 55.3 Bacteriological cure rates for selected Gram-positive intramammary infections using cloxicillin (adapted from Dodd, 1978)

Bacteria	Lactation		At drying off
	Clinical	Subclinical	
Streptococcus agalactiae	85	>90	>95
Staphylococcus aureus	25	40	65
Streptococcus dysgalactiae	90	>90	>95
Streptococcus uberis	70	85	85

Streptococcus uberis (p. 297)

Antibiotic therapy for this organism is restricted to clinical cases and dry-cow therapy. *Streptococcus uberis* not only has extramammary host reservoirs, tonsils, gastrointestinal and reproductive tract, but also exists free living in the environment (McDonald, 1984). Consequently, case finding and treatment programmes will not be successful in eradicating the organism. Many infections occur in the latter part of the dry period (McDonald, 1984). Consequently, the use of a specially formulated product that produces high intramammary antibiotic concentrations over an extended time interval is critical in the prevention of new infections. Treatment of lactating, subclinical and clinical, and dry cow infections, is helpful in reducing prevalence, but is less successful than in the case of *Strep. agalactiae* and *Strep. dysgalactiae* (Dodd, 1976).

Staphylococcus aureus (p. 296)

This organism is highly resistant to intramammary antimicrobial therapy (see Table 55.3) (Dodd, 1976). Bacteriological cures are not the expected outcome of therapy. Lactational therapy should be restricted to clinical cases, and even then the only goal is to hasten a return to saleable milk production. Although extramammary reservoirs of infection exist, the principal mode of spread is from cow to cow at milking. Routine dry-cow treatment coupled with hygienic measures will reduce and, in some cases, lead to eradication over a period of several years (McDonald, 1984).

Coliform mastitis (p. 247)

Therapy of coliform mastitis is largely restricted to clinical cases. Subclinical Gram-negative infections are usually self-limiting and, consequently, therapeutic intervention is contraindicated. Current dry-cow infusions will have minimal impact on the incidence of recent Gram-negative infections in the early postcalving period (Eberhart *et al.*, 1979). The treatment of clinical cases will largely be dictated by the severity of clinical signs, coupled with economic constraints. Frequent stripping of the affected quarter following the administration of oxytocin is probably the most important, yet most often neglected, component of therapy. Evacuation of the udder serves to remove both bacterial endotoxins and inflammatory host mediators, thus markedly ameliorating the severity of clinical signs. Gentamicin, amikacin, polymyxin B, chloramphenicol and potentiated sulphonamides have minimal inhibitory concentration (MIC) and distribution properties suitable for treatment of coliform mastitis (Table 55.1). Local regulations may severely restrict or ban the use of these antimicrobial agents. In addition to antibiotics, intravenous fluids and non-steroidal anti-inflammatory agents are useful adjuncts to therapy. Successful treatment of peracute cases probably hinges more upon early recognition and intervention than the choice of antimicrobial agent. Systemic therapy of coliform mastitis poses several problems and at the present time available antibiotics all have significant drawbacks.

Most of the drugs with suitable Gram-negative spectra are not approved for use in food-producing animals. In the USA and in some other countries, drugs approved for systemic use in lactating dairy cattle are restricted to sulphonamides, penicillin, penicillin–dihydrostreptomycin, ampicillin and erythromycin. None of these drugs can be used with a high degree of confidence to treat peracute coliform mastitis (see Table 55.2).

Microbiological cultures and sensitivity testing do not provide a clear-cut solution. Gram-negative mastitis is caused by environmental opportunists rather than specific contagious pathogens (Eberhart *et al.*, 1979). The responsible bacteria typically are not passed from one infected cow to another, but enter the streak canal following faecal contamination of bedding or the mammary gland (Eberhart, 1984). Consequently, the antibiogram from any clinical isolate need not relate in a meaningful fashion to the herd history, either in terms of causal agent or antibiotic sensitivity. By the time appropriate microbiological tests can be performed, therapeutic decisions will have been made and the patient will often have either succumbed or recovered. The exception to this rule will be the rare herd outbreak of Gram-negative mastitis caused by a point source of infection. Examples would be massive bacterial overgrowth of teat dips, wash water, or bedding. In these circumstances antibiotic sensitivities may prove helpful.

When the veterinarian, in consultation with the client, initiates treatment and decides to use antibiotics in an unapproved dose, route of administration or species, a commitment must be made to ensure these compounds do not enter the human food chain. The extended withdrawal times associated with off-label aminoglycoside or chloramphenicol use virtually eliminate slaughter as a salvage procedure should the response to treatment be unsatisfactory.

Mycoplasma mastitis (p. 298)

At this time no drugs have demonstrated satisfactory efficacy in the treatment of *Mycoplasma* mastitis (Bushnell, 1984). *In vitro* sensitivity testing results do not correlate with *in vivo* efficacy (Jasper *et al.*, 1966). Control strategies will centre on strict hygiene and either isolation or culling of infected cattle following identification of the pathogenic micro-organism by microbiological testing (Bushnell, 1984). Administration of antibiotic will result in unnecessary milk discards time and eliminate the option of eradication by culling of infected cattle for slaughter.

References

Baggot, J.D. (1977) *Principles of Drug Disposition in Domestic Animals*, p. 10. W.B. Saunders, Philadelphia.

Brooks, B.W., Barnum, D.A. & Meek, A.H. (1982) A survey of mastitis in selected Ontario dairy herds. *Canadian Veterinary Journal*, **23**, 156–9.

Bushnell, R.B. (1984) *Mycoplasma* mastitis. *Veterinary Clinics of North America: Large Animal Practice*, **6**, 301–12.

Davidson, J.N. (1980) Antibiotic resistance patterns of bovine mastitis pathogens. In *Proceedings of the National Mastitis Council*, p. 181 Washington, DC.

Dodd, F.A. (1976) The role of therapy in a control system. *Proceedings No. 28 of Post-graduate Committee in Veterinary Science*. 280 Pitt Street, Sydney, Australia.

Eberhart, R.J, Natzke, R.P., Newbould, F.H.S., Nonnecke, B. & Thompson, P. (1979) Coliform mastitis — A review. *Journal of Dairy Science*, **62**, 1–22.

Eberhart, R.J. (1984) Coliform mastitis. *Veterinary of Clinics of North America: Large Animal Practice*, **6**, 287–300.

Fetrow, J. (1981) Subclinical mastitis: biology and economics. *Compendium of Continuing Education for the Practising Veterinarian*, **2**, S223–8.

Janzen, J.J. (1970) Economic losses resulting from mastitis: a review. *Journal of Dairy Science*, **53**, 1151–61.

Jarrett, J.A. (1981) Mastitis in dairy cows. *Veterinary Clinics of North America*: *Large Animal Practice*, **3**, 447–54.

Jasper, D.E., Jain, N.C. & Brazil L.H. (1966) Clinical and laboratory observations on bovine mastitis due to *Mycoplasma*. *Journal of the American Veterinary Medical Association*, **148**, 1017–29.

Jasper, D.E. (1980) Prevalence of *Mycoplasma* mastitis in Western states. *California Veterinarian*, **34**, 24–6.

Le Louedec, C. (1978) Efficacités des antibiotiques contre les mammites bovines staphylococciques et streptococciques. *Annales de Recherches Veterinaires*, **9**, 63.

Lintner, T.J. & Eberhart, R.J. (1990a) Effects of bovine mammary secretion during the early nonlactating period and antibiotics on polymorphonuclear neutrophil function and morphology. *American Journal of Veterinary Research*, **51**, 524–32.

Lintner, T.J. & Eberhart, R.J. (1990b) Effects of antibiotics on phagocyte recruitment, function, and morphology in the bovine mammary gland during the early lactating period. *American Journal of Veterinary Research*, **51**, 533–42.

McDonald, J.S. (1984) Streptococcal and staphylococcal mastitis. *Veterinary Clinics of North America: Large Animal Practice*, **6**, 269–85.

National Mastitis Council Research Committee. (1981) *Microbiologic Procedures for Use in the Diagnosis of Bovine Mastitis*, 2nd edn. Washington, DC.

Prescott, J.F. & Baggot, J.D. (1988) Bovine mastitis. In *Antimicrobial Therapy in Veterinary Medicine*, pp. 321–31. Blackwell Scientific Publications, Boston.

Thurmond, M.C. (ed.) (1986) *Laboratory Procedures for the Examination of Milk Quality*, 2nd edn. Published by the author.

Thurmond, M.C., Tyler, J.W., Luiz, D.M. *et al.* (1989) The effect of pre-enrichment on recovery of *Streptococcus agalactiae*, *Staphylococcus aureus*, and *Mycoplasma* from bovine milk. *Epidemiology and Infection*, **103**, 465–74.

Tyler, J.W., Thurmond, M.C. & Lasslo, L. (1989) Relationship between test-day measures of somatic cell count and milk production in California dairy cows. *Canadian Journal of Veterinary Research*, **53**, 182–7.

United States Department of Agriculture, Animal and Plant Health Inspection Service Veterinary Services (1988) *National Animal Health Monitoring System. California Report: Summary of Round 2.*

Ziv, G. (1980a) Drug selection and use in mastitis: systemic vs local drug therapy. *Journal of the American Veterinary Medical Association*, **176**, 1109–15.

Ziv, G. (1980b) Practical pharmacokinetic aspects of mastitis therapy — 1: Parenteral treatment. *Veterinary Medicine and Small Animal Clinician*, **75**, 277–90.

Ziv, G. (1980c) Practical pharmacokinetic aspects of mastitis therapy — 2: Practical and therapeutic applications. *Veterinary Medicine and Small Animal Clinician*, **75**, 469–74.

Ziv, G. (1980d) Practical pharmacokinetic aspects of mastitis therapy — 3: Intramammary treatment. *Veterinary Medicine and Small Animal Clinician*, **75**, 657–70.

Chapter 56: Inflammation and Anti-inflammatory Drugs

by P. LEES AND S.A. MAY

The nature of inflammation

Inflammation (from the Latin *inflammare*, to burn) is common to many diseases involving injury to living tissues. Inflammation is, in fact, the basis of most pathology. Acute or chronic inflammation occurs as a consequence of chemical, physical or microbiological damage to tissues. Acute inflammation has been described as the response of the living microcirculation and its contents to injury. In this definition the words deserving particular emphasis are living, microcirculation and contents. It is important to recognize that necrotic tissue cannot undergo acute inflammation. Only living tissue can respond to damage in a manner intended to protect the body from the stimulus by first localizing and subsequently destroying it. A range of defence mechanisms including the immune system may be utilized. If the inflammation is caused by micro-organisms, tissue damage may proceed as far as host cell death. As with dead tissue, an avascular tissue like cartilage, although in some circumstances it may degrade, cannot respond to injury by mounting an acute inflammatory response.

The microcirculation therefore plays a crucial role in tissue response to injury. Blood vessels dilate and initially local blood flow increases. Vascular endothelial cells change their shape, with the formation of inter-endothelial cell gaps, through which plasma leaks. This leads to the formation of protein-containing exudate (oedema fluid) in the interstitial compartment. At this stage blood flow slows and eventually becomes static. As well as plasma, the contents of the microcirculation include the cellular elements of blood. The phagocytic leucocytes (neutrophils and monocytes) emigrate from the circulation in the inflammatory process and engulf the tissue irritant in the inflammatory exudate. The initial step is margination and adherence of leucocytes to the vascular endothelial wall, followed by pavementing, the process whereby the cells roll along the wall to interendothelial cell gaps. Passage through the wall and directional movement to the site of injury occurs by the process of diapedesis. Neutrophils are the first cell type to enter the lesion, followed after several hours by mononuclear phagocytes. Other circulating cells (platelets, eosinophils and basophils) may also migrate to the extravascular space.

The pain component of inflammation arises from sensitization of nociceptive (pain) receptors to the actions of released chemicals (Ferreira, 1983). Inflammation, if associated with infection, may be accompanied by fever, as the result of resetting of the 'thermostat' in the hypothalamus. These changes at whole animal level comprise Celsus' four classical signs of inflammation, *rubor et tumor cum calore et dolore*. To these Virchow added a fifth sign, *functio laesa* (loss of function) some centuries later. The essential features of the acute inflammatory process are outlined in Fig. 56.1.

The suffix '-itis' is appended to the name of the affected tissue to describe organ-based inflammation in the conditions of mastitis, bursitis, colitis, cystitis, metritis, arthritis, tendonitis, laminitis and many others.

The outcome of acute inflammation may be resolution or repair and hence restoration of normal tissue function. However, if the stimulus persists, tissue destruction may occur with fibrous tissue formation and the occurrence of chronic inflammation, with local proliferation of connective tissue and mononuclear

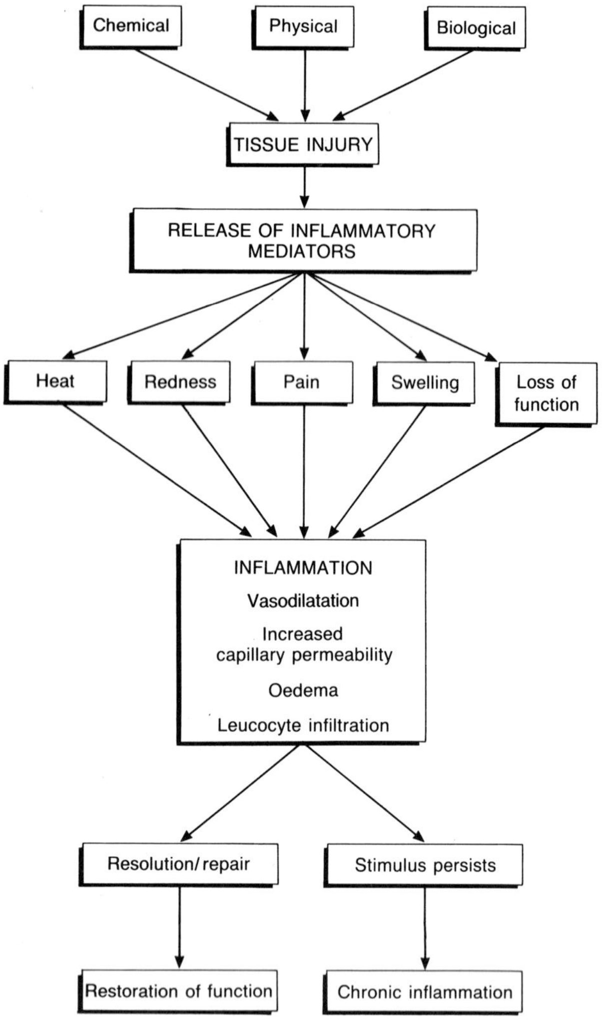

Fig. 56.1 The inflammatory process.

cell accumulation. The granulation tissue in chronic inflammation comprises highly vascularized connective tissue. In some forms of chronic inflammation lymphocytes are present suggesting an immune response superimposed on the inflammatory response.

Mediators and modulators of inflammation

The characteristic pathophysiological changes of acute and chronic inflammation are produced by the action of chemicals either released from cells such as mast cells, macrophages and fibroblasts or formed by *de novo* synthesis (Davies *et al.*, 1984). If there is an immune basis to the inflammatory response, lymphocytes are also involved. Those mediators like histamine that act directly to produce microvascular changes or like bradykinin to cause pain are called mediators or, if their role has not been firmly established, putative mediators.

The number of putative mediators identified is considerable. Moreover, there are some species differences in mediators, so that 5-HT is probably an acute inflammatory mediator in rodents only, for example. Some mediators, such as complement fragments C5a and C3a, not only act directly on the microcirculation but also cause mast cell degranulation, leading to histamine release and hence reinforcement of the inflammatory response. In addition, there is a sequential release of mediators, such that histamine, 5-HT and bradykinin are involved in the early part of the acute phase, whereas lysosomal and other proteolytic enzymes are involved subsequently. Much is now known about acute inflammatory mediators; information on the mediators responsible for the transition to, and the subsequent persistence of, chronic inflammation is more sparse. Examples of mediators inducing vascular leakage are bradykinin, histamine, platelet activating factor (PAF), which act directly, and leukotriene B_4 (LTB_4) and complement fragment C5a, which exert their effect through neutrophil-dependent mechanisms (Williams, 1983). Mediators of cell migration and accumulation include C5a, PAF, prostaglandin E_2 (PGE_2), LTB_4 and interleukin-1 (IL-1), whilst mediators responsible for producing tissue damage include the neutral proteases and the highly reactive oxygen (free) radicals, notably the hydroxyl radical.

Mediator interactions are complex, and there are compounds whose principal role is to interact synergistically with inflammatory mediators. For example, the vasodilator prostanoid PGE_2 enhances markedly both the pain produced by kinins such as bradykinin and the increased vascular permeability produced by simple amines like histamine (Davies *et al.*, 1984). Those compounds that amplify the actions of others are described as modulators of inflammation. The properties and sources of some important mediators and modulators of inflammation and joint disease are described in Table 56.1. It should be noted that the list is not comprehensive!

The eicosanoid group of mediators and modulators are particularly important to a consideration of the two important anti-inflammatory drug groups in cattle medicine, steroids and non-steroidal anti-inflammatory drugs (NSAIDs). Eicosanoids are formed from the 20-carbon unsaturated fatty acid substrate arachidonic acid (Willoughby, 1968). Arachidonic acid is released from an esterified form in which it is bound as a natural component of the phospholipid of cell membranes. The release is catalysed by phospholipase A_2, an acylhydrolase enzyme that is activated by tissue injury. Arachidonic acid may act as a substrate for two enzyme groups, the cyclo-oxygenases and lipoxygenases. Cyclo-oxygenases catalyse the production of prostanoids (PGE_2) and prostacyclin (PGI_2) and thromboxane A_2 (TXA_2) from the cyclic endoperoxides PGG_2 and PGH_2 (Fig. 56.2). Lipoxygenases, on the other hand, are responsible for the synthesis of hydroxyeicosatetraenoic acids (HETEs) and the leukotriene mediators (Fig. 56.2). The importance of the arachidonic acid pathway in inflammation in general, and in veterinary therapeutics in particular, lies in the fact that the extensively used groups of anti-inflammatory drugs, steroids and NSAIDs probably act at least partially by inhibiting enzymes in the arachidonic acid pathway (Fig. 56.2) (Higgs *et al*, 1981).

Classification of anti-inflammatory drugs

In view of the complexity of the inflammatory process and the involvement of many mediators and modulators in determining the outcome and time course of inflammatory reactions, it is inevitable that those anti-inflammatory drugs with restricted activity against a single mediator have only limited clinical effectiveness. With currently available drugs, it is easier to inhibit the pain, increased blood flow and oedema associated with acute inflammation than it is to suppress chronic

Table 56.1 Mediators and modulators of acute and chronic inflammation

Putative mediator/modulator	Properties and source
Histamine	An amine produced from histidine by decarboxylation. Stored in mast cells, basophils and platelets. Mast cell degranulation leads to release into extracellular environment in immune and non-immune inflammation. Causes vasodilatation and increased permeability of small postcapillary venules. Local administration causes pain and itching
5-Hydroxytryptamine (serotonin)	Another simple amine stored in platelets and mast cells. Increases permeability of small venules in rodents but probably at most a minor mediator in other species
Bradykinin	A peptide containing nine amino acids. Synthesized from plasma kinins *de novo*, i.e. not stored but produced afresh by inflammatory stimulus. Produces vasodilatation, increased vascular permeability and pain
Complement system	Several complement components including C3a, C5a, C8, C9 exert pro-inflammatory actions, e.g. vasodilatation, increased vascular permeability, mast cell degranulation, leucocyte chemotaxis and cytolysis
Eicosanoids	
PGE_2	Derived from cell membrane phospholipid, following release of the precursor arachidonic acid. Produces prolonged dilatation of small arterioles and potentiates the increased vascular permeability and pain produced by other mediators like histamine and bradykinin
PGI_2	A potent dilator of small arterioles. Possesses similar properties to PGE_2 but with shorter duration of action
LTB_4	Potent chemoattractant for polymorphonuclear leucocytes and mononuclear cells. Enhances vascular permeability produced by other mediators such as PGE_2, PGI_2 and bradykinin
Lipoxin A	Produced from cell membrane phospholipid by polymorphonuclear leucoctyes. Stimulates leucocytes to generate superoxide radical and causes release of lysosomal enzymes
Platelet activating factor (PAF)	An ether-linked analogue of phosphatidylcholine. Derived from cell membrane phospholipid. Produces platelet and neutrophil aggregation, bronchoconstriction, vasodilatation, increased capillary permeability and chemotaxis
Interleukins and other cytokines, e.g. IL-1	Produced by macrophages, chondrocytes and synovial cells. Chemotactic for leucocytes and possess mitogenic and pyretic properties. Stimulates release of PGE_2 and collagenase by chondrocytes, synovial cells and dermal fibroblasts. Possibly involved in cartilage breakdown
Enzymes	Lysosomal enzymes such as lysozyme and acid phosphatase concerned with lysis of foreign and host cells in acute and chronic inflammation. Non-lysosomal metalloproteinases such as stromelysin concerned with proteoglycan breakdown in arthritis

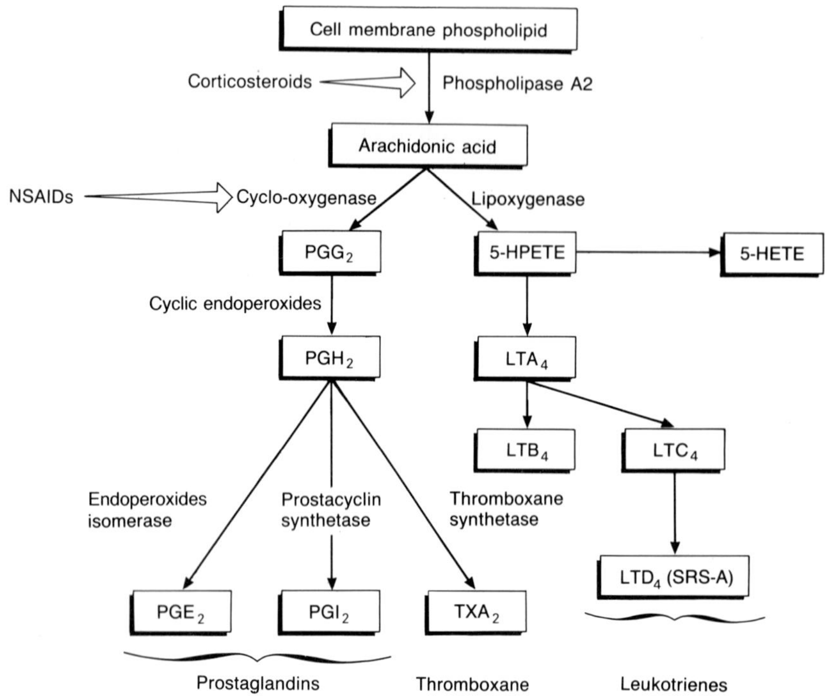

Fig. 56.2 The arachidonic acid cascade illustrating pathways of generation of eicosanoids and proposed sites of action of steroid and non-steroidal anti-inflammatory drugs.

inflammation or the cartilage breakdown that characterizes degenerative joint disease. However, there have been some interesting recent advances in the latter field.

Table 56.2 gives a general classification of drugs that either possess anti-inflammatory properties or that have been used to treat various joint diseases. There are additional drugs, like the phenothiazine and α_2-agonist sedatives, which possess anti-inflammatory properties but these are not used clinically for this purpose and are therefore excluded from this account.

The limited efficacy of drugs that are antagonists for histamine (H_1-receptor blockers) is probably due to the limited role of this mediator except for the early phase of acute inflammation.

Drugs that inhibit cyclo-oxygenase are the classical aspirin-like drugs collectively known as NSAIDs (Higgs *et al.*, 1980, 1981). The first compound of this class in clinical use was salicylate, derived initially from the bark of willow and poplar trees. Extracts of willow bark were used as early as the first century AD in man for the therapy of gout and colic. Aspirin was the first synthetic NSAID; it is the acetyl derivative of salicylate and was introduced into clinical medicine by Hoffman in 1895.

More recently introduced are the drugs that inhibit both lipoxygenase and cyclo-oxygenase enzymes, so-called dual inhibitors (Higgs *et al*, 1979). By inhibiting the synthesis of HETE compounds and leukotrienes such as LTB_4 as well as prostanoids like PGE_2, these experimental and novel compounds may provide the basis for the introduction of agents with a broader spectrum of activity than cyclo-oxygenase inhibitors. They may be of use in immune-based diseases such as asthma, chronic obstructive pulmonary disease and insect bite allergies. However, no compounds of this class are as yet in veterinary use.

Corticosteroids are the anti-inflammatory agents that provide a greater control of all elements of both acute and chronic inflammation than any other drug class. They exert membrane-stabilizing properties on lysosomal and cell membranes. Through this and other actions they suppress the release of inflammatory mediators and act to preserve cell integrity. The precise mode of action is unknown. It may be attributable partly to their action on the cell nucleus to promote, by protein transcription, the synthesis of a group of endogenous polypeptides with antiphospholipase activity, the lipocortins (Fig. 56.2).

Of other drug classes listed in Table 56.2 several, including immune stimulants, disease modifying agents and cytotoxic agents, have been used extensively to treat rheumatoid arthritis in man. All of these classes of agent slow the progressive degenerative changes in cartilage and the soft tissue inflammation in this disease. Some have also been used for similar therapy in veterinary medicine, notably in the dog, but their use has been limited by several factors such as slow onset of action, and some potentially severe side-effects have prevented extensive veterinary use. They are not used in cattle medicine and are included here only for the sake of completion.

Table 56.2 Classification of anti-inflammatory drugs and drugs used in the treatment of joint disease

Drug class	Examples	General properties
Antihistamines	Tripellenamine, mepyramine diphenhydramine	Classical H_1-receptor antagonists. Produce some suppression of acute inflammation but limited to early phase of acute inflammation
Antiserotonergic drugs	Lysergic acid diethylamide	Similar to antihistamines. Probably effective only in rodents. Newer more specific drugs block 5-HT receptor subtypes. Influence of 5-HT_2 blockers on tendon healing under evaluation
Cyclo-oxygenase inhibitors	Aspirin, phenylbutazone, flunixin, naproxen, meclofenamate, carprofen	Provide analgesia in inflammatory pain and some suppression of vascular changes in inflammation. Little or no effect on leucocyte migration. Gastrointestinal ulceration common and blood dyscrasias, hepatotoxicity and renotoxicity may arise occasionally
Dual inhibitors of cyclo-oxygenase/lipoxygenase	BW755C, BW540C	Inhibit most changes in acute inflammation but side-effects and low potency have limited their clinical value
Corticosteroids	Hydrocortisone, cortisone, dexamethasone, betamethasone, prednisolone, prednisone, fluamcinolone	Suppress all components of acute and chronic inflammation but side-effects associated with medium- to long-term use (adrenal atrophy, immune suppression, decreased bone strength. Cushinoid symptoms, delayed wound healing, muscle wastage, etc.)
Disease modifying agents	Penicillamine, gold salts	Retard the degenerative changes in immune-based arthritides. Very slow onset of effects (several weeks). Potentially severe side-effects, little veterinary use
Immune stimulants	Levamisole	Raise immune status in immune comprised animals and have been used in rheumatoid arthritis. Slow onset of action
Cytotoxic agents	Cyclophosphamide, chlorambucil	Used in rheumatoid arthritis. Immune suppression and other toxic effects to rapidly dividing cells limit clinical value
Free radical scavengers	Orgotein, copper-containing compounds, DMSO	Possess superoxide dismutase activity. Scavenge toxic free radicals, e.g. superoxide, hydroxyl
Miscellaneous	Hyaluronic acid, polysulphated glycosaminoglycan, pentosan sulphate	Mode of action unclear. Inhibit proteolytic enzymes, e.g. stromelysin. Administration by intra-articular injection may be required for some drugs

Other drugs used in the therapy of joint disease, especially in the horse, are the free radical scavengers orgotein and dimethyl sulphoxide (DMSO) and drugs with uncertain mechanisms of action, hyaluronic acid and chondroprotective agents. Again, the use of these compounds in cattle medicine has been very restricted to date.

Non-steroidal anti-inflammatory agents

Classification and mechanism of action

The very many organic acid drugs in this important group of compounds can be divided into two subclasses, carboxylic acids (R–COOH) and enolic acids (R–COH) (Table 56.3). Further subdivisions, on the basis of chemical structure, can be made. For example, the main enolic acid groups are pyrazolone derivatives such as phenylbutazone and oxicams like piroxicam. Carboxylic acids also comprise several groups as listed in Table 56.3.

Most NSAIDs possess three principal types of pharmacological activity: a peripheral anti-inflammatory action (which includes a peripheral analgesic component) and central antipyretic and analgesic actions (Table 56.4). Some differences between drugs have been reported for the three types of activity. For example, phenylbutazone is effective as a peripheral anti-inflammatory agent but is probably a weak central analgesic, whereas isopyrin seems to be an effective central analgesic but a fairly weak anti-inflammatory agent. Paracetamol on the other hand possesses weak peripheral actions and therefore does not produce significant gastrointestinal irritation. However, it is a relatively weak anti-inflammatory drug and is prin-

Table 56.3 Chemical classification of NSAIDs

Primary classification	*Secondary classification (continued)*
Carboxylic acids	Aminonicotinic acids
Enolic acids	Flunixin
	Clonixin
Secondary classification	
	Quinolines
Salicylates	Cinchophen
Sodium salicylate	
Acetylsalicylic acid	Indolines
	Indomethacin
Propionic acids	
Naproxen	Phenylacetic acids
Ibuprofen	Paracetamol
Flurbiprofen	
Carprofen	Pyrazolones
	Phenylbutazone
Anthranilic acids	Oxyphenbutazone
Meclofenamic acid	Dipyrone
Mefenamic acid	Isopyrin
Flufenamic acid	
	Oxicams
	Piroxicam
	Miloxicam
	Tenoxicam

cipally a centrally acting analgesic (Lees *et al.*, 1991; McKellar *et al.*, 1991).

As discussed above an important action of NSAIDs, underlying their therapeutic uses, is inhibition of cyclo-oxygenase and consequent inhibition of production of the eicosanoids, which produce hyperalgesia, inflammation, pyrexia and platelet coagulation (Fig. 56.2). Differences in relative potency between drugs for these activities are probably due to tissue differences in enzyme structure, i.e. to the existence of isoenzymes. The existence of cyclo-oxygenase isoenzymes may also explain species differences in plasma concentrations required for efficacy. Plasma phenylbutazone concentrations required for treating arthritis in man are of the order of 100–150 μg/ml, whereas therapeutic concentrations in the horse are of the order of 10–30 μg/ml (Gerring *et al.*, 1981).

While most NSAIDs very effectively inhibit cyclo-oxygenase, other actions both on the arachidonic acid pathway and on other unrelated enzymes may contribute to their actions. For example, some evidence indicates that phenylbutazone blocks the more distal enzyme, endoperoxide isomerase (Fig. 56.2). Moreover, some fenamate derivatives inhibit some (but not all) actions of prostaglandins in addition to blocking their synthesis. High doses of most NSAIDs also block lipoxygenase, and thus suppress HETE and leukotriene synthesis. However, it is doubtful whether this action contributes significantly to the clinical efficacy of most NSAIDs. Finally, some NSAIDs (carprofen is one example) though relatively weak cyclo-oxygenase inhibitors are nevertheless effective anti-inflammatory agents and this suggests that the principal mechanism of action of at least some drugs is due to some other (unknown) effect.

In general, NSAIDs do not, at clinical dose rates, affect all components of the inflammatory response. They do not affect cellular events or minimize tissue damage, although high doses of some drugs do possess free radical scavenging properties and tissue healing mechanisms are not impaired.

Actions and interactions of NSAIDs and general uses

The analgesic action of NSAIDs on the central nervous system (CNS) is weaker than that provided by narcotic analgesic drugs of the morphine type. To what extent the central analgesic effect accounts for the clinical efficacy of NSAIDs is unclear but it is probably of limited importance for most drugs. The more important peripheral analgesic effect is thought to be due to blockade of synthesis of the prostanoid PGE_2, which exerts its hyperalgesic action through synergism with pain-inducing mediators like bradykinin (Ferreira, 1983). Suppression of the pain produced by tissue damage is a major use of NSAIDs, together with suppression of the acute inflammation associated with tissue trauma. Postsurgical use of NSAIDs to provide analgesia and to reduce oedematous swelling that can lead to wound breakdown is increasing. These drugs are clearly of value in the former circumstance but the doses required for anti-oedematous actions are generally higher and less well established in veterinary medicine. Intravenous administration of those NSAIDs available as solutions, usually either flunixin or phenylbutazone, is used to obtain effective analgesia in equine patients with spasmodic colic (Vernimb and Hennesey, 1977). The clinician must remember that the suppression of clinical signs by these drugs may render diagnosis of the subject's condition difficult.

NSAIDs have been used increasingly to treat acute inflammatory conditions caused by microbial diseases both alone and combined with antibacterial agents. Thus, duration of scouring is reduced and mortality is lowered in young calves and piglets with gastrointestinal infections (Jones *et al.*, 1977). In addition, the severe and acute pulmonary oedema associated with pneumonia in calves is suppressed. There are available combination products of NSAIDs plus antibacterial drugs such as flunixin and oxytetracycline (Anderson, 1989). Further evaluation of NSAIDs in acute life-

Table 56.4 Principal therapeutic and toxic effects of NSAIDs

Site of action	Pharmacological or toxicological action/therapeutic use
Therapeutic effects	
CNS	Antipyretic. Lowering of body temperature in patients with fever but not in normothermic subjects. Action on temperature regulating centre in hypothalamus
	Analgesic. Mechanisms poorly understood but action weak in comparison with morphine-like drugs
Peripheral	Anti-inflammatory in acute inflammation and analgesic against inflammatory, but not against non-inflammatory, pain
	Antithrombotic through inhibition of platelet cyclo-oxygenase and hence platelet release of the pro-aggregatory eicosanoid TXA_2. Aspirin, an irreversible inhibitor of cyclo-oxygenase, especially useful
	Anti-endotoxin. Some effects of endotoxin due to release of eicosanoids, synthesis being inhibited by NSAIDs
Toxic effects	
Gastrointestinal tract	Ulcerogenic following parenteral as well as oral administration. Blood or plasma loss. Melaena. Emesis in simple-stomached animals only
Kidney	Nephropathies such as renal papillary necrosis
Liver	Both cholestatic and parenchymal cell toxicity
Blood cells and cardiovascular system	Various dyscrasias including aplastic and haemolytic anaemias and agranulocytosis described. Methaemoglobinaemia, hypoprothrombinaemia and prolongation of bleeding time. Small vein phlebopathy. Alteration of acid–base and electrolyte balance
Skin	Urticaria, erythema
Fetus	Teratogenic and embryopathic effects with some drugs. Delayed gestation at term

threatening gastrointestinal and respiratory infections is needed, since some of the reports have reached conflicting conclusions.

Endotoxic shock may result from a number of disease states when endotoxin derived from Gram-negative bacterial cell walls is released into the circulatory system. This may occur, for example, in cases of equine colic, acute and peracute mastitis and in septic peritonitis. Some of the ensuing effects on cardiovascular function and the respiratory system together with metabolic and gastrointestinal changes are produced by the release of eicosanoids such as PGI_2 and TXA_2. Hence, the pathophysiological changes associated with endotoxaemia are generally suppressed, though rarely abolished, by NSAIDs such as flunixin. This is particularly so when, in experimental circumstances, the drugs are administered prior to the onset of endotoxaemia. However, the effectiveness of these drugs once shock is established is likely to be less than when pretreatment is possible. The clinical value of NSAIDs therefore remains to be established.

Prostaglandin E_2 is a pyretic agent released as a result of the action of endogenous pyrogens such as IL-I. The local release of PGE_2 in the anterior hypothalamus leads to resetting of the thermoregulatory centre. The NSAID inhibition of PGE_2 synthesis accounts for their antipyretic action when infections are accompanied by fever. The reduction in body temperature gives symptomatic relief in such patients. However, NSAIDs may theoretically influence adversely viral diseases, since the production and release of interferons are increased in pyrexia. In spite of this, NSAIDs have been used in the treatment of respiratory disease produced by parainfluenza type 3 (PI3) virus in calves and in the therapy of acute interstitial pneumonia caused by *Ascaris suum* in pigs (Selman *et al.*, 1984, 1988). Both the anti-inflammatory action in the lungs and the central antipyretic action may underlie the therapeutic response in these diseases.

Aspirin differs from other NSAIDs in that its inhibitory action on cyclo-oxygenase is irreversible (Lees *et al.*, 1987). It covalently acetylates the enzyme, which is, in consequence, permanently inhibited. In most body cells new cyclo-oxygenase enzyme can be synthesized in the cell nucleus. As aspirin concentration falls the cell's ability to form the products of cyclo-oxygenase metabolism is restored. However, the platelet is one cell that cannot do this. The platelet is anuclear and the enzyme is thus inactivated permanently, i.e. for the lifespan of the platelet. Partial inhibition may persist for several days since platelets are replaced at the rate of approximately 10 per cent per day. Longer inhibition can occur if significant amounts of aspirin penetrate to the developing megakaryocytes in bone marrow.

This action of aspirin explains its use in preventing clot formation in humans who may be prone to thrombo-embolic diseases. It is of interest that low doses of aspirin are preferred in these subjects, because inhibition of synthesis of PGI_2, an endogenous anti-aggregatory agent released from endothelial cells, by high aspirin doses could offset blockade of synthesis of TXA_2 by platelets. Low aspirin doses, administered once daily or every second day, very effectively inhibit platelet cyclo-oxygenase, without seriously impairing cyclo-oxygenase in endothelial cells. The full potential for the antithrombotic action of aspirin in veterinary medicine has not yet been fully explored, although it is recommended for use in prevention of aortic embolism in cats and may be of value in conditions such as laminitis, navicular disease and disseminated intravascular coagulation.

The use of two or more NSAIDs in combination generally has no clear advantages over the administration of a single drug at a higher dose rate. Most NSAIDs probably act by the same mechanisms, and they are likely to be additive in their toxic as well as their therapeutic effects. However, there are potential advantages with some combinations. The enolic acid NSAIDs, phenylbutazone and isopyrin, have been widely used in a single combination product. Phenylbutazone may be a more potent anti-inflammatory drug, whereas isopyrin is a more effective analgesic. As well as these differences in drug actions, there is a pharmacokinetic interaction between these two agents. The half-life of each drug is greater when given together than when they are administered singly.

Pharmacokinetics of NSAIDs

The pH of fluids within the gastrointestinal tract vares but at all sites it is usually more acidic than plasma. In the stomach of monogastric species, fluid pH can be as low as 1.0. This marked difference from plasma increses, by the mechanism of ionic trapping, the rate at which NSAIDs are absorbed. Being weak organic acids they are relatively less ionized in gastrointestinal tract liquor than in plasma and this facilitates absorption. A similar mechanism, enhancing NSAID absorption, will operate in ruminants in the reticulum and rumen, where liquor pH is also acid relative to plasma. However, the normal pH, approximately 4–5, is less acid than the gastric juice of monogastric species. Moreover, other factors are involved in determining rates of absorption. Low drug solubility in acidic conditions for some NSAIDs, such as aspirin, can lead to precipitation in the stomach and this prolongs and slows absorption and may also increase local irritation. Diet can also be an important factor in horses and ruminants, since some NSAIDs may be adsorbed on to hay. Such binding to feed, with subsequent release of the drug by fermentative digestion within the large intestine of the horse, has been suggested as a cause of the ulcerogenic action of phenylbutazone in the distal parts of the gastrointestinal tract (Lees and Higgins, 1985; Maitho *et al.*, 1986). In spite of these factors, absorption of most NSAIDs is generally good after oral dosing in all species and bioavailability generally exceeds 50 per cent. Figure 56.3 illustrates the absorption patterns for a single dose rate (4.4 mg/kg) of phenylbutazone administered orally to adult cattle with free access to hay (a), horses with free access to hay (b) and horses deprived of access to hay for a few hours before and after dosing (c). Two points to note are first the delayed absorption in horses with access to hay (as a consequence of binding to feed) but no comparable effect in cattle. This probably reflects both the much greater volume of ruminal liquor than exists in the equine gastrointestinal tract and the greater fluid : solid ratio of ruminal liquor, leading to less drug binding to feed. Secondly, the higher plasma drug concentration and its greater persistence in cattle is explained by the markedly slower clearance of the drug in cattle compared with horses. The elimination half-life is of the order of 40–60 hours in cattle and 4–6 hours in the horse (Table 56).

Another factor that may potentially markedly influence NSAID absorption following oral dosing in ruminants is operation of the oesophageal groove reflex. Closure of the groove can direct orally administered substances directly to the abomasum and this will generally speed absorption into plasma, since dilution within the vast fluid volume in the rumen inevitably spreads the time course of absorption. Double peaks in the plasma concentration–time curve of the NSAID, meclofenamate, after oral dosing in sheep have been attributed to an initial rapid absorption phase from the abomasum and slower subsequent absorption from the rumen–reticulum of that fraction of the administered

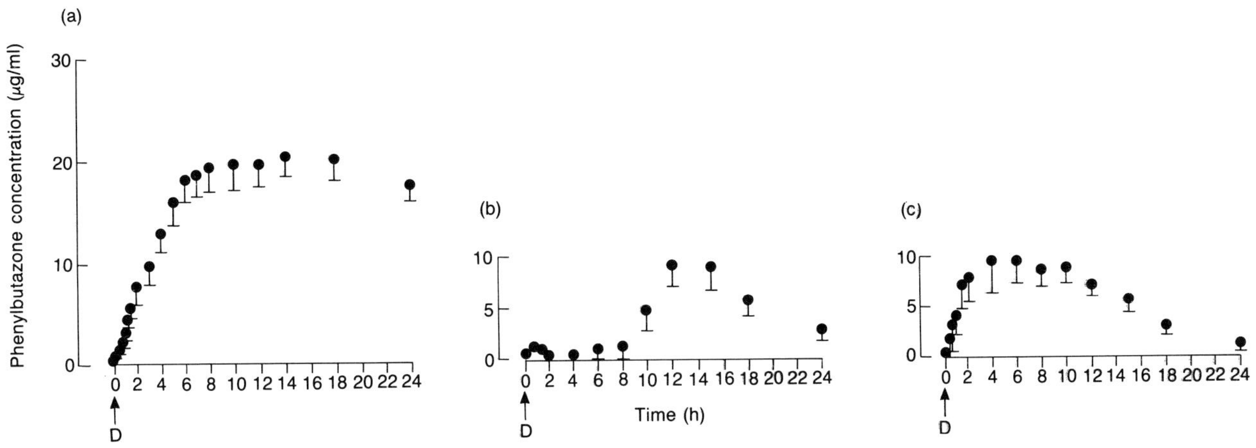

Fig. 56.3 Absorption of phenylbutazone following the oral administration of 4.4 mg/kg body weight (a) to adult cattle with free access to hay; (b) to horses with free access to hay; and (c) to horses deprived of access to feed for a few hours before and after dosing. Each point is the mean ± SEM for six animals. Data reproduced with permission from Maitho *et al.* (1986) and Lees *et al.* (1988). D, time of dosing

dose which enters the rumen (Marriner and Bogan, 1979). A similar mechanism of oesophageal closure does not seem to operate for oral phenylbutazone in adult cattle (Lees *et al.*, 1988). Further studies are required to determine to what extent species, drug substance, drug formulation and age determine operation of the oesophageal groove reflex. The total quantity of phenylbutazone absorbed in adult cattle (relative to intravenous dosing) is fairly high, the bioavailability being of the order of 60 per cent.

NSAIDs are usually administered orally, but some drugs are available commercially as solutions or as powders for dissolving prior to use by intravenous administration, e.g. phenylbutazone, aspirin, dipyrone, isopyrin, flunixin. Some NSAIDs are very irritant to tissues when injected perivascularly but flunixin, which is used as the meglumine salt, can be given intramuscularly when absorption is very rapid and tissue irritation is not great. Maximal concentrations are attained within 5–15 minutes of administration (Fig. 56.4). For all practical purposes plasma concentrations of flunixin following intramuscular dosing may be regarded as similar to those attained after intravenous administration. In contrast, plasma concentrations rise much more slowly with intramuscularly administered phenylbutazone in cattle and peak concentrations are reached only after 10–12 hours (Fig. 56.5). This difference between phenylbutazone and flunixin meglumine, which may seem surprising for two agents with such similar actions, is due to the high water solubility of the latter, probably with little or no precipitation at the injection site. Phenylbutazone, on the other hand, is believed to precipitate at the site of injection to give a depot of drug for subsequent absorption and, in all probability, some degree of irritation. In spite of the slowed absorption of phenylbutazone from intramuscular sites, total absorption is high, with bioavailability approaching 100 per cent (Fig. 56.5).

Profound species differences in pharmacokinetic parameters, including elimination half-life, have been described for many NSAIDs. Some of the published data are presented in Table 56.5. In consequence there are significant differences in dosing schedules between species. Since aspirin is rapidly de-acetylated to salicylate and the elimination half-life of the parent compound is only 8–12 minutes, most of the therapeutic activity (with the exception of the antithrombotic action) is due to salicylate. The half-life of salicylate is short in such species as man, horse and cow, intermediate in the dog and long in the cat. In the cow, the longer half-life after oral compared with intravenous dosing (Table 56.5) is attributable to continued absorption in the elimination phase. Careful selection of aspirin dosage is required in the cat, since the half-life is dose dependent in this species increasing with the administered dose.

Dose-dependent pharmacokinetics, which is due in most instances to drug saturation of hepatic metabolizing enzymes, has been described for other NSAIDs in addition to aspirin. This can cause difficulties in the establishment of dosing schedules that are both efficacious and safe. Thus, the relatively narrow safety margin of certain drugs in some species (phenylbutazone in the horse is an example) is at least partly due to increased half-life when doses are increased. In the horse, phenylbutazone can be used safely for

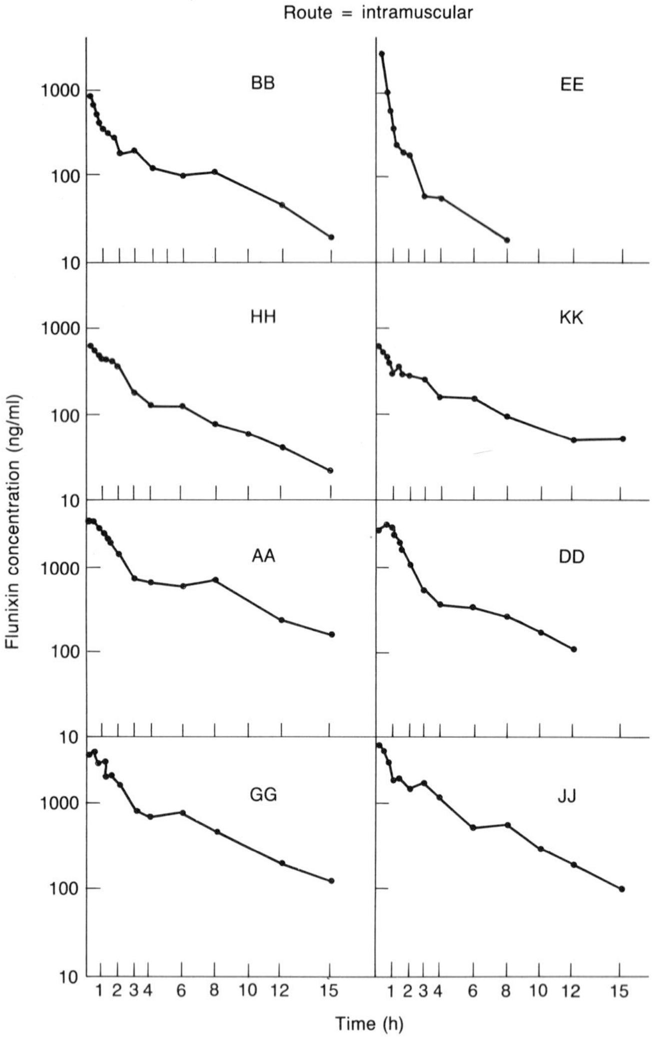

Fig. 56.4 Plasma concentration–time curves for eight calves receiving flunixin meglumine by intramuscular injection at two dose rates: 2.2 mg/kg body weight (BB, EE, HH, KK) and 8.8 mg/kg body weight (AA, DD, GG, JJ) (P. Lees, S.A. May & D. White, unpublished data).

long periods but only when administered doses do not exceed recommended levels.

As well as species differences in pharmacokinetics, the possibility of breed differences should be noted. This has been described for naproxen in dogs; the half-life of this drug in beagles is approximately half that in mongrels (Table 56.5). Whether similar differences occur for any NSAIDs in other species including cattle is not known, but such information is clearly important to the rational setting of efficacious and safe dosage schedules.

A further factor relevant to the activity of some NSAIDs is the formation *in vivo* of active metabolites. The conversion of aspirin to salicylate has been discussed. Another example is the hydroxylation of phenylbutazone in several positions. One such metabolite, oxyphenbutazone, is of similar potency to phenylbutazone; and is formed in the liver in quantities that are sufficient to contribute about one-fifth of the overall activity.

A number of pharmacokinetic interactions between NSAIDs are potentially important to their therapeutic use. One known example involves isopyrin and phenylbutazone in the horse. The elimination half-life is longer for both drugs when they are administered in a commercially available combination product. Whether a similar interaction occurs in cattle is not known, although this combination product is indicated for use in cattle.

Age may also affect NSAID pharmacokinetics. In general, both urinary excretion and hepatic biotransformation of drugs are less efficient in very young animals, aged less than two to six weeks depending on species. Aged animals may also metabolize and excrete NSAIDs less readily than young adults. There is some evidence in support of this for phenylbutazone in the

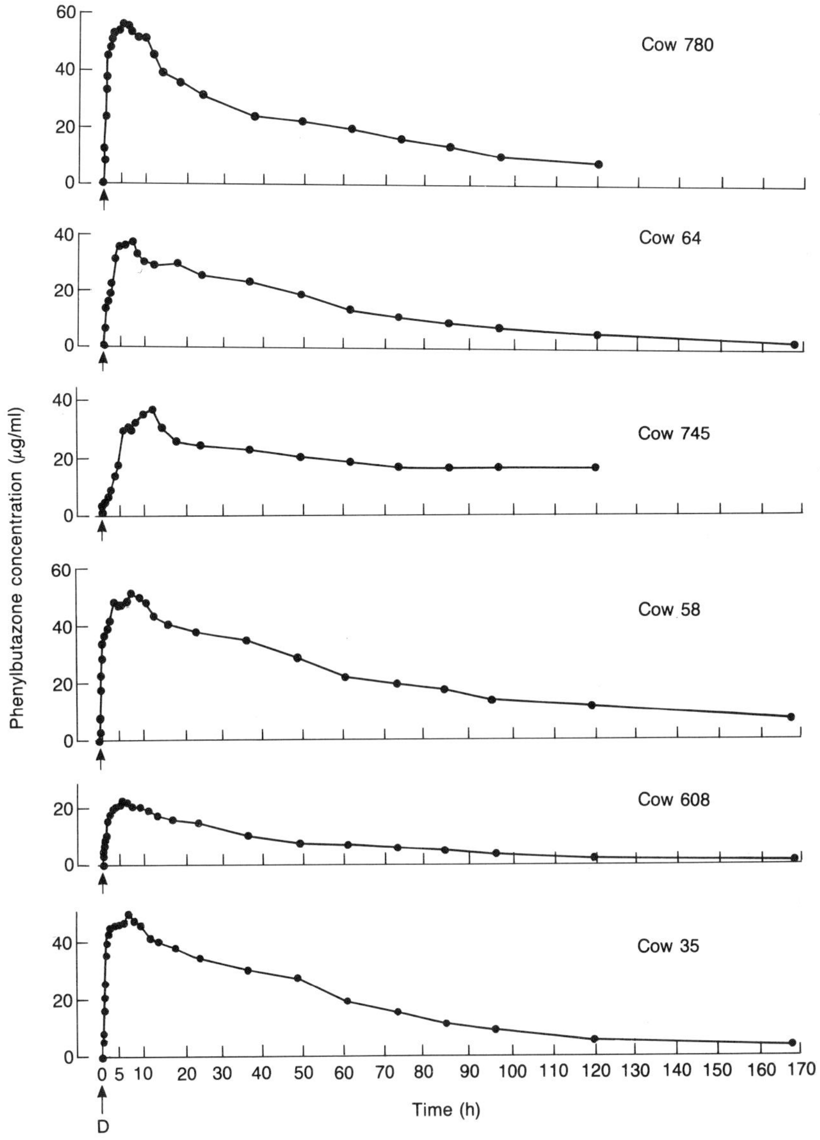

Fig. 56.5 Plasma concentration–time curves for six calves receiving phenylbutazne by intramuscular injection at a dose rate 4.4 mg/kg body weight. Data reproduced with permission from Lees *et al.* (1988). D = time of dosing.

Table 56.5 Elimination half-life (hours) of NSAIDs in five species

Drug	Human	Horse	Cow	Dog	Cat
Aspirin (salicylate)*	2–5	1–3	0.5 (i.v.) 3.7 (oral)	8	22–45†
Phenylbutazone	72	4–8†	35–60	2.5–6†	–
Naproxen	12–15	4–5	–	35–74‡	–
Flunixin	–	1.6–2.5	8	3.7	–
Meclofenamate	–	0.9 (i.v.) 2.6–8.0 (oral)†	–	–	–
Indomethacin	2	–	–	0.3	–
Miloxicam	20–50†	2.7	13	12–36†	–

* Aspirin is rapidly de-acetylated *in vivo* and most of the analgesic and anti-inflammatory activity is due to salicylate.
† Dose-dependent pharmacokinetics.
‡ Breed-dependent pharmacokinetics.

horse (Lees *et al.*, 1985), but there are no definitive studies in this field in those species, including cattle, of major veterinary interest. Reduced capacity to metabolize drugs in the liver is likely to be of greater significance than any decreased renal excretory capacity in the case of NSAIDs, since virtually all (salicylate is an exception) are highly bound (greater than 98 per cent) to plasma protein. Consequently, less than 2 per cent of the drug in plasma is available for excretion in urine by glomerular filtration. This small fraction is readily excreted in the urine of herbivores, since it is 'trapped' in ionized form in the alkaline urine, i.e. tubular re-absorption is limited or absent. Nevertheless, only a very small proportion of the administered dose will be removed from the body by urinary excretion of parent drug. Reduced dosage or longer intervals between doses are probably required in both young and old animals.

Limited and indirect evidence indicates that at least some NSAIDs are excreted by active secretion in bile, in cattle, possibly with subsequent re-absorption to create an enterohepatic shunt. This is suggested, for example, by the 'kink' in the plasma concentration–time curve that occurs consistently following the administration of flunixin intravenously and intramuscularly to calves (Fig. 56.4). Studies of bile : plasma concentration ratio are required to investigate this possibility further.

Knowledge of the pharmacokinetics of particular NSAIDs cannot be transposed between species since interspecies differences are marked. Hence, the only drug that can currently be recommended with confidence for use in the cat is aspirin. Similarly, pharmacokinetic data in cattle are available for only three NSAIDs, aspirin, phenylbutazone and flunixin. Even when basic pharmacokinetic data are available, it is not possible to define dosage schedules with such data alone for two reasons. First, different plasma and tissue concentrations of NSAIDs are likely to be required for the various therapeutic effects of analgesic, anti-inflammatory, antipyretic and antithrombotic actions. Secondly, the pharmacological actions may be longer for NSAIDs than might be predicted from plasma clearance data. Recent studies from our laboratory have shown that relatively prolonged inhibition of production of the inflammatory and hyperalgesic mediator, PGE_2, is produced by therapeutic doses of flunixin administered intramuscularly to calves (Fig. 56.6; P. Lees, S.A. May & D. White, unpublished data). In the same study it was found that, whilst penetration of the drug into tissue cage fluid was poor, passage into acute inflammatory exudate was good and clearance from the latter fluid was slow, i.e. there was a strong tendency for flunixin to accumulate. The very high degree of binding to plasma protein of flunixin probably explains both the relatively high concentration in inflammatory exudate, into which plasma protein passes readily, and the low concentration in interstitial fluid into which it does not. Similar considerations probably apply to most other NSAIDs, since almost all are highly bound to plasma protein, but actual data in cattle are lacking.

Side-effects and toxicity of NSAIDs

At high dose rates NSAIDs may affect a number of biochemical pathways. However, with clinical doses the toxic effects of most drugs, like the therapeutic effects, are probably caused primarily by inhibition of cyclo-oxygenase. There are exceptions, however. Carprofen, a recently introduced NSAID of the propionic acid class, is a relatively weak inhibitor of cyclo-oxygenase but it is an effective anti-inflammatory agent.

The NSAID side-effect reported most commonly is irritation leading potentially to ulceration of the gastro-intestinal mucosa. All NSAIDs produce this effect at high dose rates and with most drugs some gastric

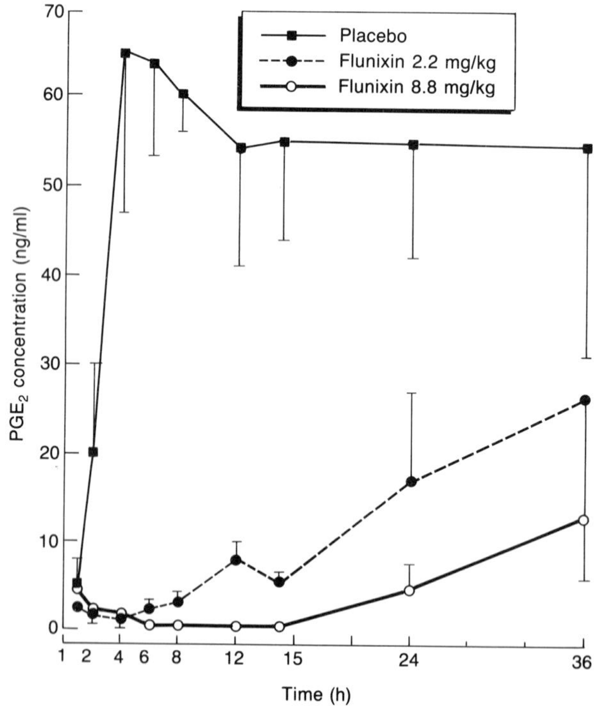

Fig. 56.6 Influence of two dose rates of flunixin (2.2 and 8.8 mg/kg body weight) administered intramuscularly to calves on the generation of the pro-inflammatory mediator, PGE_2, in carrageenan-induced inflammatory exudate. Each point is the mean ± SEM for six animals (P. Lees, S.A. May & D. White, unpublished data).

irritation is associated with oral dosing with therapeutic dose levels. The mechanism of action may involve back-diffusion of acid, although ulceration is not restricted to the stomach; it may occur throughout the gastrointestinal tract and it may accompany intravenous as well as oral dosing. The vasodilator eicosanoid, PGI_2, generated in the cyclo-oxygenase pathway may be a local hormone controlling blood flow to the gastrointestinal mucosa. By inhibiting the synthesis of PGI_2 NSAIDs may produce ischaemia and hence hypoxia of the mucosal surface. This may be the mechanism that causes erosion and hence ulceration of the gastrointestinal tract mucosa.

The ratio of doses of NSAIDs producing ulcerogenicity relative to anti-inflammatory and analgesic activities seems to be low for some drugs, e.g. aspirin, intermediate for others such as naproxen and phenylbutazone and high for some agents, e.g. salicylate. It is, however, not really possible to draw general conclusions concerning particular NSAIDs since many factors have been claimed to influence their ulcerogenicity (Rainsford, 1977). These include species, age, sex and the animal's nutritional status. Moreover, high drug concentrations in bile for some NSAIDs may explain lesions occurring in distal regions of the gut. The latter mechanism may account, for example, for the greater ulcerogenic effect of indomethacin in the dog than in most other species that have a less effective enterohepatic circulation for this drug. When severe, the gastrointestinal ulceration induced by NSAIDs can lead to plasma protein-losing enteropathy or to blood losses into the gastrointestinal tract and melaena. For example, high doses of phenylbutazone administered to the horse can quickly lead to significant plasma loss, haemoconcentration and death only a few days after the commencement of therapy, from hypovolaemic shock. The horse may be particularly susceptible to this effect of phenylbutazone (Lees and Higgins, 1985).

Useful data on the ulcerogenic actions of particular NSAIDs in cattle and any relationship to age, dose administered and route of administration are generally lacking. However, there is no reason to suppose that ruminant species are not susceptible to the ulcerogenic action of these drugs and some evidence for such an effect has been provided from the use of flurbiprofen in goats. Attempts have been made to reduce the degree of gastrointestinal tract irritation by the use of slow-release formulations, enteric coating and water-soluble salts. These approaches have not been entirely successful, although lysine acetylsalicylate, which is a soluble salt of aspirin that does not precipitate out of solution at the acid pH that prevails in the stomach, seems to cause less vomiting and anorexia in dogs. It is also not markedly irritant when given intramuscularly. The use of such approaches in cattle does not seem to have been described in the literature.

Non-steroidal anti-inflammatory drugs may be nephrotoxic. At high dose rates they may produce tubular nephritis. Renal papillary necrosis has also been reported in man. In horses papillary necrosis has been described in animals that received clinical doses of NSAIDs. However, this occurred only when horses on NSAID therapy also had restricted access to water. Retention of fluid leading to oedema are commonly reported side-effects of NSAIDs in humans. Oedema seems uncommon and transient in animals, but has been described in horses receiving phenylbutazone (Lees *et al.*, 1983). Cholestatic and parenchymal hepatotoxicity have also been reported in animals. Since most NSAIDs are metabolized in the liver, any toxicity to parenchymal cells might, potentially, lead to a cycle of drug cumulation and toxicity. Again, evidence for drug-induced hepatotoxicity has been described for horses receiving a high dose rate of phenylbutazone, but whether similar effects occur in cattle has not been reported.

A number of blood dyscrasias have been reported in human subjects treated with NSAIDs, generally over long periods. Similar blood cell effects in dogs, cats and horses have been described. However, the data available are limited and it has not been established whether particular drugs or certain species are especially implicated. With the use of clinical dose rates of NSAIDs, the incidence of blood dyscrasias in animals seems to be low.

At high dose rates some NSAIDs, notably aspirin and particularly when administered for long periods, impair platelet aggregation and thereby affect blood clotting. Potentially, this may lead to internal or external bleeding. Another problem of impaired clotting, through an indirect mechanism, may occur when NSAIDs are used together with anticlotting drugs of the coumarin group. For example, the combination of phenylbutazone and warfarin has been used in the therapy of navicular disease in the horse. Both drugs are very highly bound to plasma protein and competition for binding sites may lead to displacement of warfarin by phenylbutazone. The resulting high unbound concentration of warfarin in plasma can enhance anticlotting activity and lead to haemorrhage.

Both cardiovascular and respiratory effects result when very high doses of NSAIDs are administered but acute cardiovascular/respiratory effects do not generally occur with normal dose rates. The general side-effects of NSAIDs are described in Table 56.4.

Residues

Published data on NSAID and NSAID metabolite residues in cattle are sparse. However, it has been shown that tissue concentrations of meclofenamate and phenylbutazone are lower than corresponding concentrations in plasma, and for the latter drug plasma and tissue concentrations decrease in parallel. In view of the long half-life of phenylbutazone in cattle, it is not surprising that the drug and its metabolites, oxyphenbutazone and γ-hydroxyphenylbutazone, can be detected in urine for several days after dosing. Theoretically, the passage of NSAIDs into milk in healthy cattle will be severely limited by the more acid pH of urine relative to plasma and by the high degree of drug binding to plasma protein. In practice, this has been found to be the case for one drug, phenylbutazone (milk concentration about 1 per cent of plasma concentration) and will almost certainly apply to others. Milk from treated animals is therefore unlikely to present a hazard when consumed by most humans. In mastitis, however, the pH of milk is less acid and the 'blood–milk' barrier is much more permeable, so that much higher NSAID concentrations in milk will occur.

Steroids

Classification and general properties

Three classes of steroid hormone are secreted by the adrenal cortex into the peripheral circulation: sex steroids (generally in small quantities only), mineralocorticoids and glucocorticoids. The latter two groups together comprise the corticosteroid hormones. The mineralocorticoids, secreted by the zona glomerulosa and zona fasciculata include aldosterone. Their principal endocrinological actions are exerted on electrolyte and water balance. They promote sodium and chloride retention and potassium loss by their actions on the renal distal tubule and on parts of the gastrointestinal tract, notably the large intestine. Sodium retention is accompanied by osmotically obliged water. When administered as drugs or secreted in excessive amounts in some disease states, aldosterone and related compounds cause oedema. Glucocorticoids influence lipid, carbohydrate and protein metabolism and some exert weak mineralocorticoid effects also. The principal glucocorticoid hormone secreted by the zona fasciculata and zona reticularis in most species is cortisol (hydrocortisone).

The main veterinary use of glucocorticoids derives from the fact that they are potent anti-inflammatory agents. Cortisol itself is used as an anti-inflammatory agent, being administered systemically or applied locally. In addition, a number of synthetic steroids with much greater glucocorticoid potency than cortisol and with the advantage of reduced mineralocorticoid potency are available for clinical use. For example, prednisone and prednisolone are some four to five times more potent than cortisol as glucocorticoids, but they possess slightly weaker mineralocorticoid activities. Unwanted side-effects on water and electrolyte balance are therefore less likely when prednisone and prednisolone are used at equieffective dose rates to hydrocortisone. The relative potencies of a number of corticosteroids in producing glucocorticoid and mineralocorticoid effects (in arbitrary units, cortisol = 1) have been reported by Keen (1987) and are presented in Table 56.6. It will be seen that methylprednisolone and triamcinolone are about five times as potent as cortisol as glucocorticoids, and both have little or no mineralocorticoid activity. For dexamethasone and betamethasone effects on electrolyte balance are also slight, but these drugs are 25–30 times as potent as cortisol and glucocorticoids. In contrast, the synthetic corticosteroid deoxycorticosterone acetate (DOCA) is a potent mineralocorticoid with negligible glucocorticoid activity.

Anti-inflammatory potency of corticosteroids closely parallels glucocorticoid activity. Clinically, this is most important since it means that whilst mineralocorticoid activity can be divorced from anti-inflammatory activity, glucocorticoid effects cannot and this dictates the side-effects associated with clinical usage. An appreciation of the general actions of glucocorticoids will therefore assist an understanding of these potential side-effects, which are described in a subsequent section of this chapter. Glucocorticoids are gluconeogenic, promoting the release of amino acids from skin, muscle and connective tissue, and they subsequently increase the conversion of amino acids to glucose. Glucocorticoids produce hyperglycaemia in many species, especially in ruminants, and they promote the storage of glucose as liver glycogen, although both uptake and utilization of glucose by other tissue is reduced. In general, rates of lipolysis are increased, leading to fatty acid and glycerol release from adipose tissue. Subsequently, the glycerol may be converted to glucose. Calcium metabolism is altered by glucocorticoids in several ways. First, calcium absorption from the intestines is decreased and renal excretion is increased. Secondly, there is increased parathormone secretion and a resulting osteoclast stimulation whilst osteoblast activity is inhibited. These actions together promote calcium mobilization from bone, and bone strength is reduced. Glucocorticoids cause diuresis by dilating glomerular afferent arterioles and thus increas-

Table 56.6 Relative potencies and biological half-lives of some corticosteroids used in veterinary practice (from Keen, 1987)

	Relative potency (hydrocortisone = 1.0)		Biological half-life (h)
	Glucocorticoid*	Sodium retaining	
Hydrocortisone (cortisol)	1	1	8–12
Cortisone[†]	0.8	0.8	
Prednisolone	5	0.8	
Prednisone[†]	4	0.8	12–36
Methylprednisolone	5	Minimal	
Triamcinolone	5	None	24–48
Dexamethasone	30	Minimal	
Betamethasone	25	Negligible	36–54
Flumethasone	100	Negligible	
Desoxycorticosterone	Negligible	50	8–12
Fludrocortisone	15	100	

* Closely paralleled by anti-inflammatory and HPA-suppressant activity.
[†] Inactive until converted to active drug in the body.

ing glomerular filtration rate and also by depressing tubular water re-absorption in the distal nephron.

The main action of glucocorticoids on blood is to promote leucophilia, principally reflecting an increased number of circulating neutrophils. However, circulating lymphocyte and eosinophil numbers are reduced. In addition, glucocorticoids are depressant to lymphoid tissue. For example, in some species (rabbit, mouse) high doses reduce thymus weight, and reduction in the size of the spleen and lymph nodes occurs. Immunosuppression by glucocorticoids is reflected in a number of ways, principally by a reduction in cell-mediated immunity and, usually at higher dose rates, by suppression of antibody production. The latter effect can occur in some species with low steroid doses.

The secretion of mineralocorticoid hormones is regulated in a number of ways, but the principal mechanism involves the renal release of renin from the juxtaglomerular apparatus and subsequent conversion of angiotensin I to angiotensin II, which acts on the adrenal cortex zona glomerulosa cells. Glucocorticoid secretion from the zona fasciculata, on the other hand, is increased in response to stress, but there is also a basal level of secretion that is subject to a diurnal rhythm. In the dog, cortisol secretion peaks during the day, usually late morning, whilst in nocturnal species, like the cat, peak levels occur at night. The regulatory control involves secretion of adrenocorticotrophic hormone (ACTH) from the anterior pituitary, which in turn is regulated by the release of corticotrophin-releasing factor from the hypothalamus (Fig. 56.7). There is a negative feedback of cortisol on this system, and high levels of glucocorticoid drugs in the circulation similarly suppress ACTH secretion. Long-term suppression induced by steroid drugs leads not only to inhibition of cortisol secretion, but also to reduced cell function to the point of adrenal atrophy.

Mechanism of action

The precise mode of action of steroids is not known, although unlike NSAIDs they generally suppress all components of acute and chronic inflammation. Indeed, steroids are the anti-inflammatory drugs 'par excellence' and it is unlikely that compounds with such potent and comprehensive actions act through any one mechanism. Steroids inhibit the vascular dilatation in the microcirculation, the increased capillary and small vein permeability and they thereby lessen oedema. Steroids also inhibit hyperalgesia and fibrin deposition. The extravascular migration of polymorphonuclear leucocytes initially, and subsequent movement of monocytes, are reduced. In addition, phagocytic activity of leucocytes is depressed. In the repair stage of the inflammatory response and in chronic inflammation, proliferation and the deposition of collagen are suppressed. In consequence, wound healing and cicatrization are delayed. Glucocorticoids also decrease the production of inflammatory complement components, reduce lymphocyte accumulation and decrease production of IL-2 and other lymphokines from lymphocytes.

Glucocorticoids exert a stabilizing action on all biological membranes. Cell, mitochondrial and lysosomal membranes are affected and this suppresses the synthesis or release of acute inflammatory mediators such as PGE_2 and histamine, and subsequently the tissue breakdown arising from the effects of released lysosomal and non-lysosomal enzymes is suppressed.

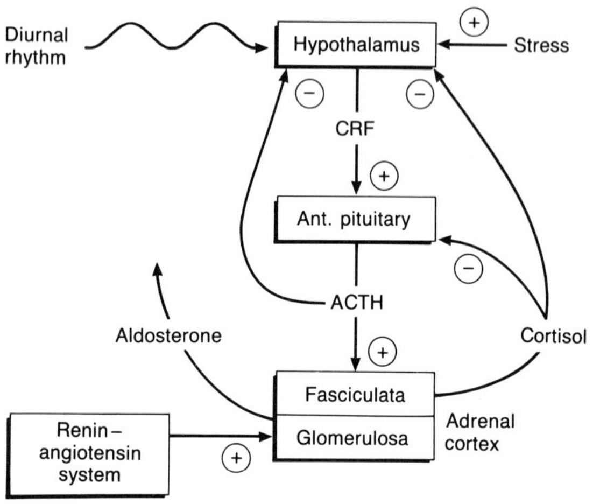

Fig. 56.7 Pathways of mechanisms of control of secretion of adrenal steroids.

However, these actions, though relevant to the anti-inflammatory effects of steroids, do not explain how they act at the molecular level.

Many studies have shown that one biochemical pathway inhibited by glucocorticoids is the arachidonic acid cascade. Arachidonic acid is released from its esterified form from the phospholipid component of cell membranes by the action of phospholipase A_2 (Fig. 56.2). Anti-inflammatory steroids inhibit this enzyme indirectly by promoting the synthesis of a family of endogenous polypeptides, the lipocortins, which possess antiphospholipase activity. This indirect mechanism of action may account for the lag period of 1–5 hours between steroid administration and the biological response. Because of this delay, it follows that any relationship between effect achieved and plasma or tissue drug concentration will be complex. Drug effects will generally outlast the period for which they can be detected in biological fluids. This may explain why dexamethasone, which has an elimination half-life of approximately 1 hour in horses and 2.5 hours in cattle (Toutain *et al.*, 1982), possesses a 'biological' half-life of 36–54 hours (Table 56.6).

As discussed earlier, arachidonic acid may act as a substrate for two enzymes, cyclo-oxygenase and lipoxygenase. Through the production of lipocortins and consequential blockade of phospholipase A_2 steroids can be expected to block the synthesis of cyclo-oxygenase-derived inflammatory mediators, including PGE_2 and PGI_2, and lipoxygenase-derived HETE and leukotriene compounds. As discussed earlier, one of these, LTB_4, is a potent chemotactic agent for neutrophils and the peptidoleukotrienes, LTC_4 and LTD_4, are believed to be important mediators of allergic airway diseases. They may be involved in such conditions as fog fever in cattle and chronic obstructive pulmonary disease in horses. The evidence that anti-inflammatory steroids act solely, or even principally, through the production of lipocortins and blockade of eicosanoid synthetic pathways is, however, controversial (Lane *et al.*, 1990). High doses certainly do affect eicosanoid synthesis, but whether doses used in veterinary therapy effectively do so is far less certain.

Administration and pharmacokinetics of steroids

The application of steroids topically to skin and mucous membranes, e.g. the eye, is commonly used in veterinary practice. It provides high drug concentrations at required sites of action and at the same time minimizes the risks of inducing systemic side-effects, although some systemic absorption is likely. In addition, most steroids are readily absorbed from the gastrointestinal tract, so that licking sites of drug application can lead to significant absorption from the gut, resulting in some systemic effects. In some topical products local activity is high, but systemic absorption from the site of application is low and systemic side-effects are thus unlikely. Betamethasone-17-valerate and beclomethasone dipropionate are examples of esters with activity restricted to local sites.

Oral corticosteroid administration is a frequently used route for medium or long-term therapy. There are unavoidable potential risks of significant suppression of the hypothalamic–pituitary adrenal axis (HPA) when long-term treatment is employed and ways of reducing this to a minimum have been sought. A short-acting preparation administered at twice the recommended dose rate on alternate days instead of normal dosing once per day has been proposed on the assumption that HPA suppression will decline on the non-treatment days. The therapeutic effects, on the other hand, may persist since steroid biological half-life is generally much longer than the pharmacokinetic half-life (Table 56.6). Another approach has been to recommend drug dosing in the morning in the dog and in the evening in the cat. Then, maximum circulating concentrations of drug can be expected to coincide with peak circulating concentrations of endogenous cortisol. This, in theory, will produce HPA suppression for the minimum time over each period of 24 hours.

Corticosteroids are frequently administered parenterally and generally this will give less variable plasma concentrations than oral dosing for short- or medium-term therapy. Water-soluble formulations include succinates, phosphates and *m*-sulphobenzoates. They may be administered intravenously or intramuscularly. Pharmacokinetic properties have been reported for commonly used corticosteroids. Thus, with intravenous dosing the half-life of dexamethasone ranges from 290–335 minutes in the cow, 53 minutes in the horse to 110–130 minutes in the dog (Toutain *et al.*, 1982).

The water-soluble short-acting esters are rapidly absorbed from intramuscular injection sites, to give an onset and duration of action almost as quick and of fairly similar duration to intravenous administration. In addition, water-insoluble esters providing longer duration of action, from 2 to 14 days, are available. These suspensions, providing a depot at the injection site, include acetate, undecanoate, pivalate and phenylpropionate esters. Some very insoluble esters, e.g. acetonide and adamantoate, provide effective concentrations over several weeks, and the use of these esters involves undesirable but unavoidable HPA axis suppression.

Intra-articular injection, for the treatment of joint diseases, is another route employed. Intra-articular dosing reduces but does not prevent the risks of systemic side-effects, since some formulations are rapidly absorbed. Long-acting formulations maintaining local concentrations for several days are sometimes used. A careful aseptic technique is required with all intra-articular injections. Steroids are used in this way to suppress soft tissue inflammation, reduce stiffness and pain, and allow more joint movement. Disadvantages are that they suppress natural repair processes, and they may induce osteoporosis and osseus metaplasia. Steroids are chondrodepressant and can lead to 'steroid arthropathy'.

Some steroids are prodrugs, requiring metabolic conversion in the body. This is true of cortisone and prednisone which are converted, respectively, to cortisol and prednisolone. Such drugs may be used for systemic therapy, but they are not applied locally.

Side-effects of steroids

The side-effects of those steroids with mineralocorticoid activity, e.g. prednisolone and prednisone, include sodium and water retention and resulting oedema, and hydrogen and potassium loss leading to hypokalaemia and metabolic alkalosis. Effects arising from glucocorticoid action on the kidney include a transient polyuria and a compensatory polydipsia. Hyperglycaemia possibly leading to glucosuria also occurs. Protein catabolism with long-term therapy causes muscle wasting and in the short term may delay wound healing. The lipolytic action of glucocorticoids is associated with redistribution of body fat with the characteristic 'moonface' appearance in man and pendulous abdomen in animals. With prolonged treatment changes in calcium metabolism can lead to osteoporosis and bone fractures. Gastrointestinal side-effects include reduced motility, thinning of the gastric mucosa and reduced mucus production. However, unlike NSAIDs, glucocorticoids are not normally regarded ulcerogenic. Nevertheless, colonic perforatium in corticosteroid — treated dogs has been described (Toombs *et al.*, 1986). The immunosuppressant actions involve a reduction in cell-mediated immunity, suppression of lymphoid tissue and lymphocyte movement and activity and, possibly, reduced antibody production.

When long- or medium-term steroid therapy is terminated, the HPA axis suppression present during therapy is restored only over several weeks, and animals are susceptible to stress during this period. Stepwise reduction in steroid dose rate and increasing the inter-dose interval may be helpful in assisting restoration of HPA axis function.

General uses of steroids

Anti-inflammatory steroids are widely used for the therapy of immune and non-immune inflammatory conditions. Allergic and non-allergic eczemas respond to steroid therapy, and steroids are used in the treatment of inflammatory conditions of the eye and the ear. In dogs and cats, steroids have been used to terminate the itch–scratch cycle in non-specific dermatoses. Steroids have been used extensively in the therapy of anaphylactic, endotoxic and haemorrhagic shock but there are several disadvantages. The slow onset of action of steroids has been discussed earlier, and very large doses are required, making therapy in cattle and other large animal subjects often impractical and/or prohibitively expensive. Administration should be by intravenous injection since absorption from intramuscular and subcutaneous sites in shocked patients would be slow.

In inflammatory conditions associated with bacterial infections, steroids are commonly administered with appropriate antibacterial agents. However, the immunosuppressant actions are very undesirable and some authorities believe that such combinations are not justified. Where antimicrobial cover cannot be provided, as in many viral infections, corticosteroid therapy is generally totally contraindicated.

There are a number of musculoskeletal conditions for which steroids may be indicated, including traumatic arthritis, osteoarthritis, myositis, eosinophilic myositis, tendonitis and bursitis. In joint diseases steroids provide relief through their analgesic and anti-inflammatory actions. However, they suppress natural repair mechanisms and repeated injections or long-acting formulations may produce degenerative changes in cartilage (steroid arthropathy). For this reason, glucocorticoid use in all forms of arthritis is increasingly controversial, and they are definitely contraindicated in septic arthritis. Similarly, in patients with laminitis steroids have fewer and fewer advocates. If they are used treatment should be limited to the initial 24-hour period after the appearance of signs. Otherwise steroids may exacerbate the condition.

A number of respiratory conditions, both allergic and non-allergic, have been treated with systemic steroids. They include acute respiratory distress syndrome in cattle and chronic obstructive pulmonary disease in horses. In these conditions steroids are most useful when disease symptoms are severe; high doses of water-soluble formulations are administered intravenously. Other indications for steroid therapy are ulcerative colitis, cerebral oedema and autoimmune haemolytic anaemia.

In view of the potentially serious side-effects of steroids, guidelines in their use have been recommended, and a number of contraindications may be stated.

Guidelines

1 Because animals vary in their response, which depends on disease severity, dosing schedules should be established for individual subjects.
2 Single large doses of steroids or short-term therapy are unlikely to produce serious side-effects.
3 Both incidence and severity of side-effects generally increase with the duration of treatment.
4 Corticosteroid treatment is almost always symptomatic and is usually not curative.
5 Cessation of therapy abruptly after a prolonged course of treatment may reveal a serious degree of adrenal insufficiency.
6 The immunosuppressant actions of corticosteroids may increase the risk of serious infection in the absence of antimicrobial therapy.

Contraindications

1 Glucocorticoids are insulin antagonists and may, therefore, exacerbate or precipitate diabetes mellitus. They should not generally be used in diabetic patients.
2 Steroids should not be used in acute infections because of their immunosuppressant actions and if used in non-acute bacterial infections, they should be used in combination with bactericidal antibiotics.
3 Steroids are generally contraindicated in viral infections, in late pregnancy, since they may induce parturition, and in subjects with corneal ulcers.
4 Administration by intra-articular injection should be avoided when there is sepsis in or close to the joint, in the presence of intra-articular fracture, when the articular cartilage is damaged, when extensive degenerative bony lesions are present, if previous injections were ineffective and when there is any likelihood that the treated joint will be overexercised.

Therapy with anti-inflammatory drugs

Respiratory diseases

Acute and sometimes overwhelming life-threatening inflammatory conditions occur in cattle and it is possible that the use of anti-inflammatory drugs, especially non-immunosuppressant agents, will reduce morbidity and mortality in such cases. Acute calf pneumonias of viral or bacterial origin and those of mixed aetiology, for example, have been shown to respond to flunixin treatment. Although such treatment is symptomatic it can be effective in life-threatening pneumonias. Selman and co-workers have shown that flunixin reduced significantly lung consolidation scores in calves infected experimentally with PI3 virus (Selmon *et al.*, 1984). Flunixin also reduced lung lesions, post-mortem lung weights (reflecting an anti-oedematous action) and clinical symptoms of the disease in an experimental bovine pasteurellosis model based upon challenge with *Pasteurella haemolytica* A1. *However*, the benefits of flunixin therapy were apparent not when the drug was used alone but in combination with oxytetracycline (Selman, 1988). The additional benefits provided by the combination over oxytetracycline by itself comprised a lower body temperature, decreased respiratory rate and improved food intake. Anderson (1989) has confirmed the benefits of a flunixin/oxytetracycline product in comparison with oxytetracycline alone in field cases of pneumonia, with treatment daily for three days. Reduction in coughing, return to normal food intake and weight gain were improved more with the combination product and there were fewer relapses. The precise way in which flunixin acts in these subjects is unclear, but it seems likely that the anti-inflammatory action (reduced pulmonary oedema) will improve pulmonary function and respiratory gas exchange while the antipyretic action may improve the clinical status to the point where animals wish to eat and drink, In this way nutritional and fluid requirements will be maintained. Species such as cattle, which rely principally on respiration for temperature regulation, may be under particular stress from infections causing pyrexia. The antipyretic actions of NSAIDs may be particularly useful in such species. Flunixin is also a potent analgesic (against inflammatory pain) and when pain is a significant element in cattle pneumonias, this analgesic action of flunixin is likely to contribute to the improved clinical status.

Ingestion of 3-methylindole (3MI) in cattle produces a chemical toxicosis characterized by respiratory signs and pulmonary lesions (congestion, oedema, interstitial emphysema) that are indistinguishable from naturally occurring acute bovine pulmonary emphysema (fog fever). Intoxication with 3MI is accepted as a valid model of the natural disease. Selman and co-workers have shown that parenteral flunixin (2.2 mg/kg) markedly reduces respiratory rate and the extent of lung lesions assessed by lung weights and both pathological and histopathological examinations. Flunixin resulted in a prompt return to normal of demeanour and respiratory rate, and it reduced the degree and severity of alveolar epithelial hyperplasia.

Acute interstitial pneumonia in calves, induced experimentally with *Ascaris suum* eggs, has been treated with the NSAIDs aspirin (100 or 250 mg/kg orally twice daily) or meclofenamate (5 mg/kg orally once daily). Whereas antihistamines and antiserotonergic drugs provided no clinical improvement, aspirin gave good symptomatic control, reducing or abolishing the characteristic 'setback', but meclofenamate was less effective at the dose levels used. The actions of aspirin were manifested through effects on heart rate, respiration, feed intake and weight gain. However, reductions in pathological changes were minimal.

Mastitis and endotoxaemia

Mastitis in cattle may also benefit from NSAID treatment. The main indication is likely to be in acute and peracute cases in which *Escherichia coli* or similar endotoxin release has occurred. Thus, within the udder, the endotoxin-induced increases in prostaglandin and thromboxane concentrations were significantly reduced by systemic flunixin therapy (1.1 mg/kg at 8-hour intervals for seven doses) (Anderson *et al.*, 1986a) and clinical signs of both udder inflammation and depression as well as pyrexia were suppressed (Anderson *et al.*, 1986b). The enhanced phagocytosis of staphylococci, which occurs in milk neutrophils harvested from endotoxin-inoculated quarters, was not affected by flunixin treatment. However, flunixin did suppress significantly the increased whey IgG_1 and IgM concentrations produced by endotoxin inoculation (Anderson *et al.*, 1986c). The local effects of systemically administered flunixin may seem surprising when the high degree of binding to plasma protein and its acidic nature are considered; these properties should severely limit penetration across the blood–milk barrier. However, in the acutely inflamed udder blood flow is increased, and milk pH will be much closer to plasma pH than in non-mastitic milk and the permeability of the blood–milk barrier will be increased. Probably of even greater significance in peracute cases will be antagonism of the acute systemic effects of endotoxin by NSAIDs, since these are mediated in part through activation of the arachidonic acid cascade with release of prostaglandins and thromboxanes. Clinically, Anderson *et al.*, (1986b) have also demonstrated improvements, including reduction in rectal temperature, in mastitic cows with coliform mastitis.

Flunixin in combination with oxytetracycline has also been evaluated in cases of peracute mastitis in comparison with the antibiotic alone and clinical appraisal suggested that the combination product gave better results (Christie, 1988). Further and more detailed studies are required to confirm this evaluation.

Carprofen has also been evaluated in cows with endotoxin-induced mastitis, at a dose rate of 0.7 mg/kg. Clearance of the drug was slower, elimination half-life longer and penetration into milk greater in endotoxaemic compared with normal cows. In the mastitic animals carprofen reduced heart rate, rectal temperature and quarter swelling significantly and usage in field cases is awaited with interest (Lohuis, 1991).

Whether systemically administered NSAIDs are beneficial or harmful in clinical cases of mastitis that are not so severe as to be classified as acute or peracute is unknown. However, Pyorala and co-workers (1988) examined the influence of phenylbutazone (10 mg/kg) and flunixin (2.2 mg/kg) administered intravenously in cases of subclinical chronic mastitis. Neither drug influenced bacterial growth, somatic cell count or the levels of inflammatory markers (*N*-acetyl-β-D-glucosaminidase activity and trypsin-inhibitory capacity).

There have been few attempts to administer NSAIDs locally by intramammary infusion to establish if their analgesic and anti-inflammatory effects are of value in providing symptomatic relief in any form of mastitis. No doubt such use has been precluded by the irritant properties of many NSAIDs. One NSAID, ibuprofen, has been administered locally into udders of cows with induced endotoxin mastitis. The drug attenuated reduction in milk yield when compared both with control cows and steroid-treated cows (DeGraves 1991).

Steroids with anti-inflammatory actions, such as prednisolone, have been used extensively for the therapy of clinical bovine mastitis. Corticosteroids are incorporated in a number of products containing also one or more antibiotics and used to treat clinical cases during lactation. The popularity of such products is indicated by volume usage; in the UK at the present time the three most widely used lactating-cow intramammary products all contain an anti-inflammatory steroid. The value of steroids in such products is unclear, and in view of their potential immunosuppressant actions such usage has been questioned. One suggestion has been that the main value of steroids is not to influence the disease, but merely to suppress the irritancy that inevitably accompanies intramammary infusions, and which varies in degree with the product formulation/excipients. However, studies have been undertaken comparing intramammary antibiotic products with and without steroids in bovine models of mastitis induced by *E. coli* endotoxin, *Streptococcus uberis* and *Staphylococcus aureus* (Bywater *et al.*, 1988). Signs of inflammation (swelling, milk consistency) were reduced, but leucocyte infiltration was not impaired. Further studies in this field, for example to establish that the phagocytic capacity of infiltrating neutrophils and immune protective mechanisms are not impaired, would provide confirmation of the value of steroids in some forms of mastitis. In acute and peracute mastitis the slow onset of action of steroids is likely severely to limit their value, but in the *Strep. uberis* model mentioned above, benefit was obtained when treatment was administered 16–18 hours after challenge (Bywater, personal communication).

In summary, it seems at least possible that the anti-endotoxaemic effects of systemically administered NSAIDs may be of value (together with other supportive therapy, including fluids and systemic antibiotic administration) in cases of acute and peracute mastitis, whereas reduced swelling and pain provided by intramammary infusion of steroid/antibiotic products may assist recovery in less severe clinical mastitis. The latter proposal is compatible with the suggestion of Sandholm and co-workers (1990) that inflammatory changes in the mastitic gland seem to improve the nutrition and favour the growth of bacteria. However, further studies are urgently needed to examine these proposals concerning steroids and NSAIDs.

Steroids have also been used, usually systemically, to counteract the life-threatening symptoms of endotoxic shock in cattle, commonly together with large volumes of fluids. In addition to their anti-endotoxaemic effects, steroids promote gluconeogenesis and this may contribute to the therapeutic response. The disadvantages of steroids are the large doses required and consequential high cost of treatment and the latent period prior to onset of action. This can be minimized by the use of water-soluble steroids.

Hypersensitivity reactions

Anaphylaxis can be inhibited both *in vivo* and *in vitro* in cattle by the NSAIDs, sodium meclofenamate and aspirin, and the actions of these drugs in acute interstitial pneumonia has been described above.

Arthritis and joint diseases

In contrast to the horse and dog, long-term therapy of joint diseases in cattle is not commonly undertaken. This in part relates to economic factors, in part to drug and drug metabolite residue problems in milk and edible tissues, and in part to the lack of knowledge of drug pharmacokinetics linked to dosage regimens that are known to be effective and safe. Such dosage regimens have not been established, and one standard text refers to treatment of degenerative arthritis, coxitis, hip dysplasia and gonitis with the comment 'none is possible'. However, some joint diseases of cattle have been treated with phenylbutazone or corticosteroids but there is, as stated, an urgent need to establish rational dosage schedules. Whether the chondroprotective class of agents, which includes PSGAG and pentosan sulphate, is likely to be used in future is not clear. Some increase in therapy in this field can be anticipated.

Foot-and-mouth disease

This contagious viral disease is characterized by fever and vesicular eruption in the mouth and on the feet. The use of NSAIDs might be of value as adjunctive therapy and one agent, flunixin, has been studied. Artificially infected cattle showed clinical improvement, indicated by lowered body temperature and increased weight gain, whilst antibody titres were not affected.

Conclusions

It seems likely that both steroids and NSAIDs, judiciously used, may be of value in a number of cattle diseases in which inflammation or endotoxaemia is a major component. However, much further work is needed if such prospects are to be realized.

References

Anderson, D.B. (1989) Utilisation de la flunixine dans les maladies respiratoires. *L'Action Veterinaire*. Suppl. 1092, 22–7.

Anderson, K.L., Kindah, H., Smith, A.R., Davis, L.E. & Gustafsson, B.K. (1986a) Endotoxin-induced bovine mastitis: arachidonic acid metabolites in milk and plasma and effect of flunixin meglumine. *American Journal of Veterinary Research*, **47**, 1373–7.

Anderson, K.L., Smith, A.R., Shanks, R.D., Davis, L.E. & Gustafsson, B.K. (1986b) Efficacy of flunixin meglumine for the treatment of endotoxin-induced bovine mastitis. *American Journal of Veterinary Research*, **47**, 1366–72.

Anderson, K.L., Smith, A.R., Shanks, R.D., Whitmore, H.L., Davis, L.E. & Gustafsson, B.K. (1986c) Endotoxin-induced bovine mastitis: immunoglobulins, phagocytosis and effect of flunixin meglumine. *American Journal of Veterinary Research*, **47**, 2405–10.

Bywater, R.J., Godinho, K. & Buswell, J.F. (1988) Effects of prednisolone on experimentally induced mastitis treated with amoxycillin and clavulanic acid. *15th World Buiatric Congress*, Spain. (abstract).

Christie, H. (1988) The veterinary uses of a non-steroidal anti-inflammatory agent: flunixin meglumine. *British Veterinary Journal*, Suppl. No. 1., **8**.

Davies, P., Bailey, P.J. & Goldenberg, M. (1984) The role of arachidonic acid oxygenation products in pain and inflammation. *Annual Review Immunological*, **2**, 235–57.

DeGraves, F.J. & Anderson, K.L. (1991) Ibuprofen treatment of endotoxin-induced coliform mastitis. *Proceedings of International Congress of Mastitis*, Ghent, Belgium.

Ferreira, S.H. (1983) Prostaglandins: peripheral and central analgesia. In: *Advances in Pain Research and Therapy* (ed. J.L. Bonica), Raven Press, New York.

Gerring, E.L., Lees, P. & Taylor, J.B. (1981) Pharmacokinetics of phenylbutazone and its metabolites in the horse. *Equine Veterinary Journal*, **13**, 152–7.

Higgs, G.A., Flower, R.J. & Vane, J.R. (1979) A new approach to anti-inflammatory drugs. *Biochemical Pharmacology*, **28**, 1959–61.

Higgs, G.A., Moncada, S. & Vane, J.R. (1980) The mode of action of anti-inflammatory drugs which prevent the peroxidation of arachidonic acid. *Clinics in Rheumatic Diseases*, **6**, 675–93.

Higgs, G.A., Palmer, R.M.J., Eakins, K.E. & Moncada, S. (1981) Arachidonic acid metabolism as a source of inflammatory mediators and its inhibition as a mechanism of action of anti-inflammatory drugs. *Molecular Aspects of Medicine*, **4**, 275–301.

Jones, E.W., Hamm, D., Cooley, L. & Bush, L. (1977) Diarrhoeal diseases of the calf: observations on treatment and prevention. *New Z. Vet. J.*, **25**, 312–16.

Keen, P.M. (1987) Uses and abuses of corticosteroids. In: *The Veterinary Annual, 27th issue* (Eds. C.S.G. Grunsell, F.W.G. Hill and M.E. Raw). Scietechnica, Bristol. p. 45–62.

Lane, P., Lees, P. & Fink, J. (1990) Action of dexamethasone in an equine model of acute non-immune inflammation. *Research Veterinary Science*, **48**, 87–95.

Lees, P. & Higgins, A.J. (1985) Clinical pharmacology and therapeutic uses of non-steroidal anti-inflammatory drugs in the horse. *Equine Veterinary Journal*, **17**, 83–96.

Lees, P., Maitho, T.E. & Taylor, J.B. (1985) Pharmacokinetics of phenylbutazone in young and old ponies. *Veterinary Record.*, **116**, 229–32.

Lees, P., Ewins, C.P., Taylor, J.B.O. & Sedgwick, A.D. (1987) Serum thromboxane in the horse and its inhibition by aspirin, phenylbutazone and flunixin. *British Veterinary Journal*, **143**, 462–76.

Lees, P. Ayliffe, T., Maitho, T.E. & Taylor J.B.O. (1988) Pharmacokinetics, metabolism and excretion of phenylbutazone in cattle following intravenous, intramuscular and oral administration *Research Veterinary Science*, **44**, 57–67.

Lees, P. *et al.* (1983) Biochemical and haematological effects of recommended dosage with phenylbutazone in horses. *Equine Veterinary Journal*, **15**, 158–67.

Lees, P., May, S.A. & McKellar, Q.A. (1991) Pharmacology and therapeutics of non-steroidal anti-inflammatory drugs in the dog and cat: 1 General Pharmacology. *Journal Small Animal Pract*, **32**, 183–93.

Lohuis, J.A.C.M. *et al.* (1991) Pharmacodynamics and pharmacokinetics of carprofen, a non-steroidal anti-inflammatory drug in healthy cows and cows with *E. coli*-endotoxin-induced mastitis. *Journal Veterinary Pharmacol. Ther.*, (in press).

Marriner, S. & Bogan J.A. (1979) The influence of the rumen on the absorption of drugs; study using meclofenamic acid administered by various routes to sheep and cattle. *Journal Veterinary Pharmacol. Ther.*, **2**, 109–15.

Maitho, T.E., Lees, P. & Taylor, J.B. (1986) Absorption and pharmacokinetics of phenylbutazone in Welsh Mountain ponies. *Journal Veterinary Pharmacol. Ther.*, **9**, 26–39.

McKellar, Q.A., May, S.A. & Lees, P. (1991) Pharmacology and therapeutics of non-steroidal anti-inflammatory drugs in the dog and cat: 2 Individual agents. *Journal Small Animal Pract.*, **32**, 225–35.

Pyorala, S., Patila, J. & Sandholm, M. (1988) Phenylbutazone and flunixin meglumine fail to show beneficial effects on bovine subclinical mastitis. *Acta. Veterinary Scandinavica*, **29**, 501–3.

Rainsford, K.D., (1977) The comparative gastric ulcerogenic activities of non-steroid anti-inflammatory drugs. Agents and Actions. **7**, 573–7.

Sandholm, M., Kaartinen, L. & Pyorala, S. (1990) Bovine mastitis — why does antibiotic therapy not always work? An overview. *Journal Veterinary Pharmacol. Ther.*, **13**, 248–60.

Selman, I.E., Allan, E.M., Gibbs, M.A., Wiseman, A. & Young, W.B. (1984) Effect of anti-prostaglandin therapy in experimental parainfluenza type 3 pneumonia in weaned conventional calves. *Veterinary Record* **115**, 101–5.

Selman, I.E. (1988) The veterinary uses of a non-steroidal anti-inflammatory agent: flunixin meglumine. *British Veterinary Journal*, Suppl. No. 1. 4–6.

Toutain, P.L., Brandon, R.A., Alvinerie, M., Garcia-Villar, R. & Ruckebusch, Y. (1982) Dexamethasone in cattle: pharmacokinetics and action on the adrenal gland. *Journal Veterinary Pharmacol. Ther.*, **5**, 33–43.

Toombs, J.P., Collins, L.G., Graves, G.M. Crowe, D.T. and Caywood, D.D. (1986) Colonic perforation in corticosteroid-treated dogs. *Journal American Veterinary Medical Association*, **188**, 145–50.

Vernimb, G.D. and Hennessey, D.W. (1977) Clinical studies on flunixin meglumine in the treatment of equine colic. *Journal Equine Medical Surg.* **1**, 111–16.

Williams, T.J. (1983) Prostaglandin E_2, prostaglandin I and the vascular changes of inflammation. *British Journal Pharmacol.*, **65**, 517–24.

Willoughby, D.A. (1968) Effects of prostaglandins F2α and PGE_1 on vascular permeability. *Journal Pathological Bact.*, **96**, 381–87.

Chapter 57: Production Enhancers

by A.R. PETERS

Bovine somatotrophin

The onset and maintenance of milk production is controlled by a complex of hormones including ovarian steroids, corticosteroids, thyroid hormones, insulin, prolactin and growth hormone (somatotrophin). Once established milk secretion is normally maintained for about 300 days in domestic cows. Peak production is usually achieved after about six weeks and then yield gradually declines over the next eight to nine months before 'drying-off' in preparation for the next parturition and lactation. Somatotrophin (ST) from the anterior pituitary gland has been shown to be the major hormonal limiting factor to milk production, particularly after peak lactation has been reached. Consequently, there has been considerable interest in using exogenous bovine ST (BST) to increase milk production in commercial dairy herds.

The BST used to stimulate milk yield is a recombinant-DNA-derived protein molecule resembling natural pituitary material. A number of slightly different variants have been produced, differing only in a few amino acid residues at the N terminus of the molecule. The galactopoietic effect of ST has been well known since the 1940s but commercial exploitation has had to await development of the technology required for bulk manufacture. Commercial products have now been developed that require repeated injection at frequencies varying from daily to monthly. A considerable volume of data has now been published on the use of BST although much still remains the confidential property of the pharmaceutical companies.

Pituitary BST consists of 191 amino acids and is involved in the control of a number of metabolic processes including cell division, bone growth, protein synthesis, lipolysis and the inhibition of glucose transport into cells (the diabetogenic effect) (Johnson & Hart, 1986). Most commercial interest has concentrated so far on the ability of BST to stimulate milk yield.

Trial results

Despite the slight variations in the amino acid composition of different commercial STs, their galactopoietic activity is assumed to be similar. However, doses and injection frequency will probably vary between products. Peel *et al.* (1989) have recently published a comprehensive review of trials on over 600 cows using the Monsanto product Sometribove. Results of trials are reported in four American states, France, West Germany, The Netherlands and the UK. Treated cows were injected with 500 mg BST at two-weekly intervals. Mean responses in terms of fat-corrected milk yield between weeks 9 and 41 of lactation in the different trials varied from 2.2 to 5.2 kg/cow per day increase in production. Data for the first 84 days of treatment are shown in Table 57.1. In these trials cows were usually fed concentrates calculated on the basis of yield plus *ad libitum* access to forage. In a winter trial where all cows received 7.9 kg/day concentrates irrespective of yield, production was increased by 4.8 kg/cow per day (Furniss *et al.*, 1988). Silage intake of treated cows increased only slightly suggesting that cows were utilizing body reserves for much of the additional milk. After turnout in the spring, when concentrate feeding was stopped, the treated cows maintained an increase in production of 4.5 kg/day and restored body reserves so that body weights of treated and control groups were similar at the end of lactation. However, in studies where body

Table 57.1 The effect of formulated sometribove on 3.5 per cent fat-corrected milk production (FCM), energy balance (EB) and reproductive performance during the first 84 days of treatment (after Peel *et al.*, 1989)

Site	Dose n (mg)	*n*	3.5% FCM (kg/cow per day)	Diff. FCM (kg/cow per day)	EB (Mcal/day)	Change in EB (Mcal/day)	Service per conception	Conception rate (%)	Days open
Arizona	0	41	31.6		7.3		1.8	88	79
	500	40	35.8*	4.2	4.6*	−2.7	1.9	78	98*
New York	0	42	31.4		0.9		2.0	88	87
	500	42	34.5*	3.1	−0.2*	−1.1	2.3	83	98
Missouri	0	63	30.4		8.1		2.3	95	82
	500	63	36.2*	5.8	4.8*	−3.3	2.0	79*	77
Utah	0	36	29.8		7.2		2.7	83	126
	500	37	33.1*	3.3	5.2*	−2.0	2.3	76	119
France	0	28	28.8		2.4		1.8	82	87
	500	30	33.3*	4.5	0.7*	−1.7	1.9	80	94
Germany	0	30	27.3		1.7		2.1	83	101
	500	30	32.1*	4.8	0.2*	−1.5	2.4	80	105
Netherlands	0	32	31.9		4.1		1.6	84	104
	500	32	37.5*	5.6	1.7*	−2.4	2.4	84	127
UK	0	45	25.1		4.3		2.0	96	91
	500	45	30.2*	5.1	0.7*	−3.6	2.5	91	117*

Values are on a net energy basis at all sites except UK where values are on a metabolizable energy basis.
* Different from the control ($P < 0.05$).

condition was monitored, treated cows tended to be in a slightly lower condition than controls. There are no consistent reports of any significant changes in milk composition following BST treatment.

Typically, the milk production response is greatest during the first three months of treatment and then declines towards the end of lactation. Dry matter intake gradually increases during BST treatment to peak at around 10 weeks. Overall, feed conversion efficiency improves by 2–9 per cent with the largest improvements occurring early in the treatment period.

Health aspects

The likely effects of BST on the cow's general health and welfare are clearly of great importance in determining the acceptability of such a product. Most studies published have shown no significant effects on the health of BST-treated animals (e.g. Whitaker *et al.*, 1988). However, results on the prevalence of mastitis have been somewhat equivocal with higher prevalence in treated cows in some studies, including higher somatic cell counts in non-mastitic cows in some trials (Peel *et al.*, 1989). However, a mechanism by which BST might increase the incidence of mastitis remains unexplained and indeed there have been counter claims of beneficial effects of BST on mastitis (Burveneich, pers. comm.).

Treatment with BST resulted in longer (average 12 days) calving-to-conception intervals than in control animals and conception rates tended to be lower by about 6 per cent (see Table 57.1; Peel *et al.*, 1989). However, the authors claim that much of this effect could be explained on the basis of the higher milk yield *per se* rather than by a direct hormonal effect of BST. There are also indications that any effect on fertility is minimized if BST treatment is not started until after conception.

Whitaker *et al.* (1989) studied several biochemical parameters in treated cows (see Table 57.2). Plasma β-hydroxybutyrate concentrations were increased in treated cows as were glucose and inorganic phosphate levels. Urea nitrogen and albumin were decreased but other metabolites were not affected. The changes in β-hydroxybutyrate reflect the change in energy demand of treated cows and the glucose concentrations are consistent with diabetogenic effects of the hormone.

Peel *et al.* (1989) reported the results of a series of toxicological experiments where BST was administered at a dose rate higher than the therapeutic dose. In the most extreme case cows were given two injections of 15 g BST at an interval of seven days. There was a

Table 57.2 Concentrations (mg/100 ml) of blood constituents in BST treated cows (147 samples) and heifers (96 samples) and control cows (118 samples) and heifers (92 samples) (used with permission of Whitaker *et al.*, 1989)

Plasma constituent	Cows Sometribove	Control	Heifers Sometribove	Control
β-hydroxybutyrate	18.2	15.5**	17.0	15.7
Log β-hydroxybutyrate	1.21	1.16*	1.19	1.16
Glucose	62.3	59.8*	63.3	59.3***
Urea nitrogen	20.0	21.7***	20.0	22.2***
Albumin	3554	3637*	3415	3419
Globulin	4159	4189	3902	4066
Magnesium	2.41	2.45	2.44	2.49
Inorganic phosphate	6.2	5.7**	7.0	6.1***

* $P<0.05$, ** $P<0.01$, *** $P<0.001$.

short-term increase in milk yield but no ill effects were observed and there were no detectable abnormalities at post mortem.

A long-term toxicity study was also carried out where cows received 600, 1800 or 3000 mg BST at 14-day intervals for two successive lactations. In the first year fat-corrected milk yield increases were between 8.0 and 9.5 kg/day and there were similar increases in those cows that continued into the second lactation. The improvement in feed efficiency varied between 7 and 25 per cent. No significant differences in mastitis, somatic cell counts or minor illnesses were reported. Conception rates were reduced in treated cows although numbers were too small to evaluate statistically. There were no differences in ease of calving, incidence of milk fever, retained placenta or cystic ovaries among the various treatment groups. There was no evidence of subclinical ketosis as determined by β-hydroxybutyrate concentrations in plasma. Changes in non-esterified fatty acids and blood urea nitrogen were transient and returned to normal as the treated cows adjusted their feed intake. Blood concentrations of somatotrophin, glucose and insulin were elevated in a dose-dependent manner. There were no significant changes in adrenocorticotrophic hormone (ACTH), prolactin, thyroid-stimulating hormone, luteinizing hormone, follicle-stimulating hormone, cortisol, progesterone or oestradiol-17β concentrations. Thyroxine but not tri-iodothyronine concentrations were elevated. Occasional differences in calcium, phosphorus and magnesium were recorded that were apparently related to changes in milk production.

Mode of action of BST

The exact mode of action of BST in stimulating milk yield is not very well understood. Fullerton *et al.* (1989) found that mammary blood flow increased as did cardiac output. The haematocrit of treated animals decreased suggesting an increase in plasma volume. Glucose and acetate, important substrates for milk synthesis, were taken up in greater quantities by the mammary gland as a consequence of both increased blood flow and greater extraction by the gland. This and similar studies in other ruminant species suggest that BST exerts its effects at several different points. There is substantial evidence from both *in vitro* and *in vivo* studies that the hormone does not exert a direct effect on mammary tissue. Treatment with BST causes increased circulating concentrations of insulin-like growth factor 1 (IGF1) from the liver and it has been suggested that this hormone is responsible for at least some of the effects, since specific IGF receptors are present on mammary epithelial cells.

Regulatory and political aspects

Bovine somatotrophin is one of the first of a series of products to be derived from recombinant-DNA technology. It is also a product designed specifically for performance enhancement rather than improvement of animal health. It has thus already proved controversial for two reasons.

1 It is considered by some to be a similar issue to that of steroid hormone growth promoters, already banned in EC countries following several years of acrimonious debate.

2 There is a general concern among some consumer organizations that the products of new biotechology are being marketed too rapidly, before the full implications of their use are understood.

It is apparent that this debate will continue to develop on both sides of the Atlantic.

Under Directive EC 87/22 it is necessary for veterinary products derived from biotechnology to be scrutinized by the EC Committee on Veterinary Medicinal Products before they can be approved for use in any member state. It is known that several companies have submitted applications under this procedure.

The registration of animal health products in the EC and many other countries is dependent on the demonstration of safety, pharmaceutical quality and efficacy alone. However, the registration laws are currently under review and there have been proposals for further critieria to be added including that of 'need' of 'socio-economic impact'. The impetus for such a change has largely resulted from the BST issue. For the moment a moratorium on the licensing of BST products has been declared for an 18-month period while the European Commission decides on the acceptability of this and related products.

Anabolic agents

For many centuries man has employed the technique of surgical castration to control the behaviour and influence the growth and carcass characteristics of male animals used for meat, particularly for cattle, sheep and pigs. However, in the last half century the use of breeds with faster growth rates and the development of intensive systems of rearing of these improved stock has resulted, in some countries, in a selective decrease in the castration of males, particularly for the production of fat lamb, pork and bacon, and intensive beef and veal production. The situation for beef and veal in selected countries of the EC is shown in Table 57.3. In Denmark, the Federal Republic of Germany and Italy, the majority of male cattle used for beef meat are not castrated. However, in countries such as the UK and Ireland, where pastoral beef and sheep systems prevail and where, from the point of animal and human welfare, leaving bulls intact is not widely feasible, castration of males remains the preferred method of husbandry. In these countries particularly, as well as in the USA, the availability of anabolic agents that can be administered to offset the decreased growth rate and decreased efficiency of feed conversion usually associated with castration of males was therefore of considerable economic importance. Initially, there was common usage of the synthetic stilbene derivatives, e.g. stilboestrol, hexoestrol, dinoestrol. However, these products are now widely banned because of potential carcinogenic activity.

In the EC, Directive 81/602 banned the use of stilbenes but permitted the continued use of the three natural steroids, oestradiol-17β, testosterone and progesterone and the xenobiotic compounds, trenbolone and zeranol (see Fig. 57.1). Following several years of intense debate all these substances were banned for use in the EC by Directive 85/649. The exact motives for the ban are still unclear to outside observers but centred around overproduction of beef, imports from third countries and consumer safety. However, the five compounds above are still widely used in many other countries of the world.

The compounds

Oestradiol-17β is the major physiologically active oestrogen. It is produced by ovarian follicles in the female and high plasma concentrations cause the behavioural pattern of oestrus around the time of ovulation.

Progesterone is produced by the corpus luteum, which persists during gestation in the pregnant animal or until just before the next ovulation in the non-pregnant animal. Progesterone temporarily suppresses uterine activity and pituitary gonadotrophin release and is the major hormone involved in the maintenance of pregnancy. Perhaps the main action of progesterone

Table 57.3 Categories of beef and veal production in EC countries (% by weight)

	Cows	Bulls	Steers	Heifers	Veal
Belgium/Luxembourg	29	32	9	20	11
Denmark	40	47	1	10	1
West Germany	30	51	2	13	4
France	35	12	18	14	21
Ireland	21	1	53	25	<1
Italy	26	48	5	7	14
Netherlands	42	15	1	11	31
UK	22	2	52	23	1

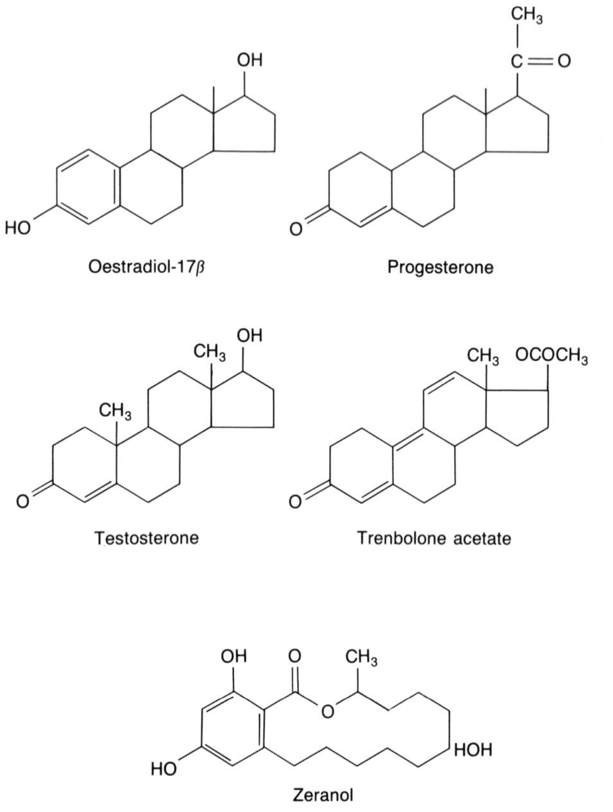

Fig. 57.1 Molecular structure of steroid and related compounds formerly permitted for use as growth promoters in the EC.

in this context is to suppress sexual activity when used in females. Also, synthetic progestagens, e.g. melengoestrol acetate, are used for this purpose in some countries. These synthetic analogues have the advantage of being orally active and can therefore be administered in feed. This is common practice to suppress oestrous activity thereby impairing growth rates and reducing disruptive behaviour in heifers in feedlots.

Testosterone is the major steroid hormone produced by the Leydig (interstitial) cells of the testis and is responsible for the development and maintenance of the male sexual characteristics.

Trenbolone acetate is a steroid synthesized by Roussel-Uclaf and is a potent androgen and analogue of testosterone.

Zeranol is a derivative of zearalenone, a natural metabolite of the mould *Giberella zeae* and is now synthesized by a multistep fermentation process.

Products commercially available. The products formerly available in the UK are shown in Table 57.4 and were all in subcutaneous implant form. All were of prescription-only status immediately prior to the ban. Hoechst-Roussel has also recently introduced a combination product, trenbolone–oestradiol-17β, known

Table 57.4 Hormonal products formerly available for growth promotion in UK

Product name	Active principle	Pharmaceutical company	Class of stock	Withdrawal period (days)
Compudose	Oestradiol	Elanco	Steers	0
Finaplix	Trenbolone acetate	Hoechst	Steers, heifers, cull cows	60
Ralgro	Zeranol	Crown Chemical Company	Cattle (unspecified)	70
Synovex S	Oestradiol + progesterone	Syntex	Steers	0
Synovex H	Testosterone + oestradiol	Syntex	Heifers	0
Implixa-BM	Oestradiol + progesterone	Hoechst	Male veal calves	90
Implixa-BF	Testosterone + oestradiol	Hoechst	Female veal calves	90

Table 57.5 Estimated growth response to anabolic implants over 100–120-day periods in kilograms (of expected increased liveweight over controls)

	Expected increased liveweight (kg) over controls			
	Steers	Heifers	Cull cows	Bulls
Finishing phase				
Ralgro	12	8	8	6
Ralgro plus Finaplix*	19			
Compudose	18			
Compudose plus Finaplix	27			
Finaplix	8	9	14–38	
Synovex H		13–19		
Synovex S	24			
Growing and finishing				
Ralgro, Ralgro†	20	15		
Ralgro, Ralgro plus Finaplix	27	17		
Ralgro, Ralgro, Ralgro	26	20		
Ralgro, Ralgro, Ralgro plus Finaplix	33			
Compudose	25			
Compudose plus Finaplix	33			

* 'Plus' indicates simultaneous implantation of two different implants.
† Commas indicate sequential implantation at intervals of 80–100 days.

as Revalor. These products are available in similar forms in other countries together with some other generic-type products.

Mode of action of anabolic steroids

The compounds listed above, with the exception of progesterone, may be subdivided into two categories based on their hormonal action, i.e. oestrogenic (oestradiol-17β, zeranol) or androgenic (testosterone, trenbolone).

Androgens exert a direct effect on the muscle cell after binding to specific intracellular receptors. They may also exert indirect effects by modifying the secretion of the endogenous hormones that control metabolism.

Oestrogens appear to act primarily via the metabolic hormones. They increase the secretion of growth hormone from the anterior pituitary gland and probably insulin and thyroid hormones also.

The net effect of all these steroids is to increase protein accretion (accumulation) inside the muscle cell. In the case of trenbolone at least, this seems to be brought about by decreasing the natural rate of protein catabolism (breakdown) rather than increasing the rate of synthesis.

The overall effect is to increase the rate of daily liveweight gain, the feed conversion efficiency and the proportion of lean meat in the carcass.

The growth promoting effect

It is difficult to be precise about the magnitude of growth responses, since they are dependent on a variety of factors, including breed, sex and management. An additional complicating factor is the possible implanting programmes that may be adopted by the beef producer. However, some average expected liveweight responses to various regimens are given as examples in Table 57.5. The values in this table are drawn from various published sources and are intended as an approximate guide only.

1 Growth responses are likely to be greatest in steers and less in intact animals (bulls and heifers). Generally, younger and lighter cattle show a smaller response than older and heavier cattle.

2 Androgenic agents are more effective in females and oestrogens are more effective in males. However, in steers there is a synergistic effect of combined oestrogens and androgens and some studies have shown liveweight gains in steers receiving both to be equivalent to those of intact bulls.

3 The response obtained will depend on the management/feeding system. There is evidence that

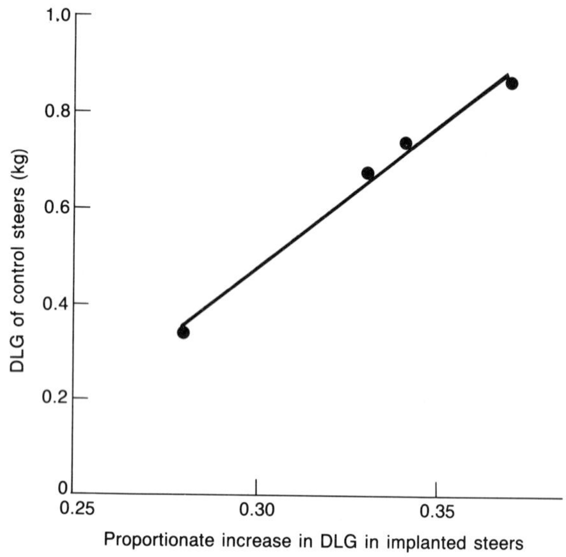

Fig. 57.2 Relationship between daily liveweight gain and proportionate increase in liveweight gain in anabolic-treated steers. Note that the better the basal performance of the control animals the greater is the response to hormonal treatment.

greater benefit will be obtained in cattle already growing at a high rate, e.g. intensively as opposed to semi-intensively reared steers. The relationship between initial liveweight gain and response is shown in Fig. 57.2. Therefore, the type of management system practised should be borne in mind when designing implanting programmes.

4 Repeat implantation of anabolic agents is sometimes practised. The withdrawal period of the product should be allowed to lapse before re-implantation and advice should always be sought from the pharmaceutical company concerned before giving recommendations to clients.

Growth responses to repeat implants are likely to be progressively reduced. For example, the total response to one, two or three sequential Ralgro implants in steers was of the order of 12, 20 and 26 kg in studies carried out by the East of Scotland College of Agriculture.

5 There is limited information on the combined use of in-feed growth promoters and hormone implants but most evidence suggests that their effects are additive.

An important aspect of the activity of anabolic agents is their effect on carcass composition. In steers the proportion of fat between muscles (intermuscular) and also abdominal fat (retroperitoneal and perinephric) is decreased. One would normally expect subcutaneous fat to be reduced also but this may be dependent on the time at which the animals are slaughtered, i.e. the earlier they are slaughtered the less fat they will be. Anabolic agents have also been shown to improve carcass conformation or shape and this was a particularly important feature in the UK where a considerable quantity of beef is produced from animals that are a byproduct of the dairy industry. Extreme dairy-type cattle, e.g. Holstein-Friesian, do not have good conformation for beef production and this could be considerably improved by the use of hormone implants.

In bulls also conformation is improved and most of the extra meat is deposited in the forequarter area. Anabolics are also of use in the improvement of beefing quality of heifers and culled cows.

Side-effects of hormone implants

Any side-effects of hormonal growth promoters are usually related to their effects on the reproductive system.

In heifers, the side-effects reported include an increased bulling behaviour, raised tailhead and udder development. There is evidence that ovarian function is impaired for a period, depending on the nature of the steroid used.

In steers, there have been reports of an increase in bulling behaviour and mammary development. If immature intact animals are implanted there is often a delay in the onset of puberty. It is generally recommended that hormonal growth promoters are not used in animals intended for future breeding.

Safety of growth promoters to the consumer

Since the growth promoter implants have potent hormonal activity it is important that they present no risk to the meat consumer. Concerns over consumer safety arise from the possibility of side-effects on human reproductive function and sexual characteristics, and the association of reproductive hormones with cancer. The three natural steroids, testosterone, oestradiol-17β and progesterone, are present naturally in humans and intact animals, in concentrations that are orders of magnitude higher than any possible intake likely to be achieved from eating meat from implanted animals. The increase in amounts taken in from correctly implanted animals is negligible. Furthermore, the anabolic agents have a low oral activity and are rapidly metabolized and excreted by the enterohepatic system. Implantation in the ear, a non-edible part of the carcass, and strict observance of withdrawal periods, will prevent the intake of significant amounts of the anabolic agent by the consumer. For these reasons various international committees on toxicology of residues in animals have considered it unnecessary to establish residue tolerances for these compounds. On the basis of recent extensive toxicological evaluation of zeranol and trenbolone residue tolerances have been recommended for these compounds (Lamming *et al.*, 1987) and these values are similar to those adopted by the FAO/WHO and FDA. These tolerance values enable regulatory authorities to set an appropriate withdrawal of these products and therefore prescribe their safe use in food animals.

At the time of writing there is clear international political disagreement as to the use of these products, with a blanket ban in the EC but widespread approval and use in other parts of the world. One would envisage that ultimately there must be international agreement or at least compromise but there are few signs of this at the present time.

β-Agonists as repartitioning agents

The rate of liveweight gain and feed conversion efficiency have long been major determinants of efficiency in animal production systems. However, for a number of reasons, carcass composition has become an increasingly important issue.

Firstly, the process of fat deposition in animals is less efficient in energy terms than the deposition of muscle protein, and thus requires more energy per unit weight in the form of feed. Secondly, the population of the wealthy countries has become more health conscious, particularly in the light of the decreased necessity for manual labour and hence decreased calorific requirements, and the associations between high intakes of animal fat, human obesity, cardiovascular disease and premature death. Thirdly, fat is regarded by many consumers as a waste product: its production therefore incurs unnecessary cost.

Thus the development of products that will reduce carcass fatness is consistent with current consumer preference and with medical advice favouring the consumption of leaner meat. The steroid hormones helped to fulfil this role to some extent, at least in beef, but since their ban in EC countries alternative methods of controlling carcass fatness have been sought.

Fat is deposited in spherical cells known as adipocytes. Adipocytes are found in large numbers together, known as adipose tissue. Fat itself is formed largely of triglyceride, each molecule consisting of three fatty acid molecules and glycerol. The process of fat breakdown, or lipolysis, consists of the breakdown of triglyceride molecules to liberate free fatty acids. This results in a decrease in fat stores inside the adipocytes and consequently a decrease in the size of the cells and hence the whole adipose tissue.

Fat synthesis or production (lipogenesis) consists of assembly of the triglyceride molecules from fatty acids and glycerol. The β-agonists inhibit the process of lipogenesis and stimulate lipolysis at the level of the fat cell by binding to specialized receptor sites on the adipocyte surface and stimulating a train of biochemical events involving the production of cyclic adenosine monophosphate (cyclic-AMP).

The protein yield of a carcass is most important since it is the major component of the muscle cells that are consumed. Protein undergoes a continual cycle of synthesis and degradation. In degradation the protein molecules are broken down to form the constituent amino acids.

It has been known for many years that a group of compounds related chemically to the natural hormone adrenaline stimulate lipolysis in adipose tissue resulting in the release of free fatty acids. They also have a positive effect on nitrogen retention within the animal resulting in increased rates of protein accumulation particularly within skeletal muscle.

Adrenaline belongs to a class of compounds known as the catecholamines and these are associated with the activity of the sympathetic branch of the autonomic nervous system. Activation of the sympathetic system involves an increase in heart rate, blood flow to skeletal muscle and diversion of blood supply from non-essential organs and functions, thus mobilizing energy. Synthetic catecholamine derivatives such as the β-agnoists, e.g. clenbuterol, have been shown to reduce fat deposition and increase protein deposition in sheep, cattle, pigs and poultry.

Timmermann (1987) has recently written an excellent review of the pharmacology of β-agonists so only a brief summary is given here. As so often happens when novel mechanisms or compounds are discovered classification is necessarily based on information at that time. As knowledge develops then the classifications used are found to have exceptions and anomalies. β-Agonists are a good example of such problems.

Adrenergic hormones and drugs act partially on their target cells by binding to receptor molecules located on the cell surface. Such a mechanism of action is common to many hormonal compounds. After receptor binding takes place this active complex then stimulates other actions inside the cell. Adrenergic receptors were originally classified as to whether the drug caused contraction (α) or relaxation (β) of involuntary or smooth muscle. The β-receptors were further classified as to whether a tissue responds at all to β-type drugs, as some adrenergic drugs affect involuntary muscle in some tissues but not in others. As a result, cardiac and internal smooth muscle receptors are classified as β_1 and bronchial and uterine smooth muscle are classified as β_2. The β_2-receptors are also found on skeletal (voluntary) muscle cells and on adipocytes, and thus it is the β_2-agonists that are primarily involved in carcass repartitioning. However, as already suggested, the above classification is not absolute and there is some overlap in the affinity of specific β-agonists between β_1 and β_2-receptors. While the relevance of this may not be immediately apparent it gives us some clue to the reason for certain side-effects observed with some of these compounds. Cell surface β-receptor function is mediated in the cell by the second messenger adenyl cyclase system. Several β_2-stimulants are already used in human and veterinary medicine for therapeutic purposes, e.g. salbutamol as an anti-asthmatic and clenbuterol as a uterine relaxant and bronchodilator. The β_1-agonists are also used sometimes to treat cardiac failure. Carcass repartitioning effects in animals generally require larger doses of β-agonists than human therapeutic applications (see Timmerman, 1987).

Chemical structure

The β-agonists are substituted catecholamines derived from adrenaline and noradrenaline (Fig. 57.3). Although no products are yet commercially available for this purpose the compounds of major interest for repartitioning over recent years have been clenbuterol, cimaterol, salbutamol (GAH 034), ractopamine and various other analogues produced by several companies. Most of these compounds are active both orally and by injection but most recent trials have used oral administration. The concentrations in feed have varied from 0.25 to approximately 12.0 mg/kg depending on the analogue and target species, equivalent to doses of 20–200 μg/kg body weight daily.

The duration of treatment with β-agonists varies between studies but it is necessary to treat animals daily for periods of at least several weeks in order to achieve maximum effects.

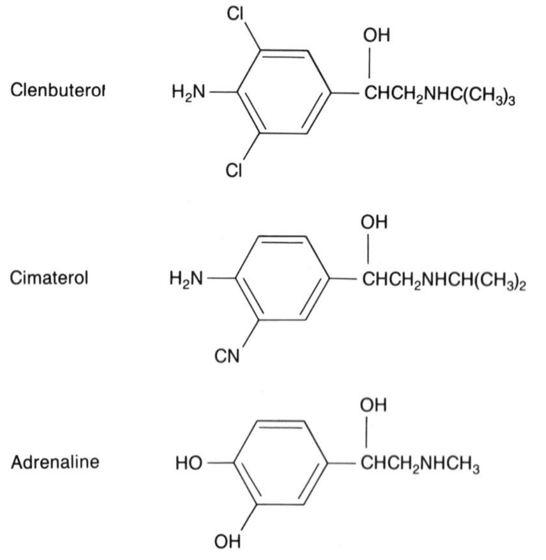

Fig. 57.3 The structural relationship of some β-agonists to adrenaline.

Mechanisms of action

Receptors for β_2-type compounds are present on the cell surface of both skeletal muscle and adipocytes although other mechanisms may also be involved (see below). It is clear that the effects on fat and muscle are brought about by at least two distinct biochemical mechanisms. The fat-reducing effect is thought to include effects both on lipogenesis and lipolysis. In other words, β-agonist treatment may reduce the rate of fat production but also increase the rate of fat breakdown. Either or both of these processes may be affected and there are likely to be differences between compounds, tissues and animal species. The most consistent evidence seems to be that β-agonists primarily increase the rate of lipolysis.

The effects of β-agonists on muscle cells result in hypertrophy or an increase in size of the cells. This seems to be brought about largely by reducing the rate of protein breakdown rather than by stimulating protein synthesis. There is also evidence of selectivity for certain muscle cell types in that the so-called type II fast conducting fibres are most affected.

Increases in the rate of blood flow to peripheral tissues occur during β-agonist treatment particularly to the hindquarters, and the rate of uptake of substrate chemicals from the blood is enhanced. However, the effects on blood flow, at least in muscle, appear to be temporary and therefore cannot explain the persistent anabolic effects on muscle. However, blood flow is increased for more prolonged periods in fat tissue, at least in experimental studies on rats.

β-Agonist compounds are also known to influence the release of other hormones, e.g. insulin, growth hormone, thyroid hormones and corticosteroids. This is suggestive of an indirect role for these hormones in the action of β-agonists since these hormones are all normally involved in the control of muscle and fat

Table 57.6 Percentage improvement in animal performance after treatment with β-agonists. Values were obtained as approximate averages from the available literature

Measurement	Cattle	Sheep	Pigs	Poultry
Liveweight gain	+5	+15	+5	+2
Feed intake	−9	−2	−3	−1.5
Food efficiency	+15	+15	+6	+2
Dressing percentage	+6	+6	+1.5	+1
Kidney fat	−35	−30	−15	–
Carcass lean	+15	+10	+7	+2
Carcass fat	−30	−25	−25	−7
Area of longissimus dorsi	+40	+25	+8.5	–

metabolism. However, such a mechanism for the action of β-agonists has not been elucidated. This area has recently been reviewed by Buttery & Dawson (1987).

Efficacy of β-agonists

There are many reports on the effects of β-agonists on the carcass composition of several species. The literature is confusing owing to the wide variety of doses and types of animals and husbandry systems used. However, some general conclusions can be drawn. The average values for live performance and carcass effects have been estimated approximately from the literature for cattle, sheep, pigs and poultry and are presented in Table 57.6.

Effects in cattle

Most work has been carried out in steers, although the effects in entire bulls and heifers seem to be similar. The effects on liveweight have been inconsistent, varying from zero to 40 per cent increases. In those studies where there was a positive effect on liveweight gain, the effect appears to decrease as the treatment continues. The effects on feed intake have varied, with the intake having been decreased in several studies but unaffected in others. However, the improvements in feed conversion efficiency, dressing percentage (killing-out percentage) and carcass weight have been more uniform: carcass weight and dressing percentage have been increased by about 7 per cent. The reduction in fatness is clearly dose dependent, and subcutaneous abdominal and intermuscular fat deposits are reduced. Moloney (1988) has used data from steers treated with the Merck analogue L644,969 to calculate the efficiency of weight gain of lean meat. Treated steers gained 60 kg of lean meat in 84 days compared with 34 kg in control animals. The feed required to produce 1 kg lean meat was 9.4 kg and 19.6 kg in the treated and control animals respectively. The improvement in the efficiency of treated animals in putting on lean meat was, therefore, remarkable.

Notwithstanding their great potential for reducing fatness in cattle, most commercial interest in β-agonists to date has been in pigs. This is important for two reasons.

1 There is considerable scope for reduction of fatness in pigmeat in certain countries, e.g. in the EC, carcasses are graded and producers are paid on the basis of the thickness of backfat.

2 Fattening pigs are by and large reared intensively, which makes them a cost-effective and convenient proposition for the use of such agents.

Meat quality

There have been numerous studies of the effects of β-agonists on live performance and carcass composition, but there have been few published studies on meat quality. β-Agonists affect the composition of the carcass and meat quality could clearly be changed. The measurement of the resistance of meat to shear forces has been negatively correlated with tenderness as assessed by trained taste panellists. The resistance to shear forces of meat from β-agonist-treated animals has been shown to be higher than that from control animals. However, this change does not appear to be directly due to the change in fat content but rather there may be other effects, for example on collagen.

Warriss & Kestin (1988) studied the effects of clenbuterol and cimaterol on the quality of sheep meat. Catecholamines are known to stimulate glycogenolysis in muscle and this can lead to reduced acidification after death. This effect occurred in the longissimus dorsi muscle of sheep. Consequently, there was less drip loss during storage but the meat tended to look darker and duller with reduced lightness and saturation values. Intramuscular fat content and haem pigmentation were also reduced. The authors suggested that the higher pH would increase the likelihood of early spoilage, that the effects on colour might make the meat less attractive, and that the reduced fat could affect its organoleptic qualities, such as juiciness, after cooking.

The cardiovascular system

Since adrenaline and related compounds are involved in the sympathetic nervous system, which controls cardiovascular function, there have been a number of studies on the effects of β-agonists on the cardiovascular system of animals. Clenbuterol treatment of sheep and calves produces an immediate decrease in blood pressure and an increase in heart rate; however, the measurements return to normal within 72 hours despite continued β-agonist treatment.

Because of possible effects on the cardiovascular system concern has been expressed on the likely effects of β-agonists and the welfare of treated animals, particularly pigs prone to stress sensitivity. However, there is little evidence to suggest that β-agonists exacerbate such conditions.

Withdrawal periods

EC directives require withdrawal periods to be specified for all licensed products used in food animals, in order to prevent harmful residues. The withdrawal of cimaterol from treated pigs has resulted in a rapid compensatory deposition of fat. In cimaterol-treated sheep, the carcass improvements persisted for three weeks after the drug was withdrawn but, although muscle hypertrophy was maintained, the reduction in carcass fat was abolished within 28 days. Similarly, the treatment of broilers with cimaterol for 14 days, followed by seven days withdrawal, has resulted in the loss of most of the beneficial effects. If these reversal effects are confirmed then products are needed that require a very short withdrawal period. However, β-agonists in general are eliminated from the body or metabolized quite rapidly and it is unlikely that withdrawal periods would have to be set in excess of a few days. However, this would clearly depend on companies being able to provide satisfactory toxicity and other safety data to the licensing authorities.

References

Buttery, P.J. & Dawson, J.M. (1987) The mode of action of beta-agonists as manipulators of carcass composition. In *Beta-agonists and their Effects on Animal Growth Ca,cass Quality* (ed. by J.P. Hanrahan), pp. 29–43. Elsevier Applied Science, London.

Fullerton, F.M., Fleet, I.R., Heap, R.B., Hart, I.C. & Mepham, T.B. (1989) Cardiovascular responses and mammary substrate uptake in Jersey cows treated with pituitary-derived growth hormone during late lactation. *Journal of Dairy Research*, **56**, 27–35.

Furniss, S.J., Stroud, A.J., Brown, A.C.G. & Smith, G. (1988) Milk production, food intakes and weight change of autumn-calving, flat-rate fed dairy cows given 2-weekly injections of recombinantly derived bovine somatotrophin (BST). *Animal Production*, **46**, 483–527.

Johnson, I.D. & Hart, I.C. (1986) Manipulation of milk yield with growth hormone. In *Recent Advances in Animal Nutrition* (ed. by W.Haresign & D.J.A. Cole), pp. 105–23. Butterworths, London.

Lamming, G.E., Ballarini, G., Baulieu, E.E., Brookes, P., Elias, P.S., Ferrando, R., Galli, C.L., Heitzman, R.J., Hoffman, B., Karg, H., Meyer, H.H.D., Michel, G., Poulsen, E., Rico, A., Van Leeuwen, F.X.R. & White, D.S. (1987) Scientific report on anabolic agents in animal products. *Veterinary Record*, **121**, 389–92.

Moloney, A. (1988) Application of beta agonists in ruminants explored. *Feedstuffs*, July **11**, 13–26.

Peel, C.J., Eppard, P.J. & Hard, D.L. (1989) Evaluation of sometribove (methionyl bovine somatotrophin) in toxicology and clinical trials in Europe and the United States. In *Biotechnology in Growth Regulation* (ed. by R.B. Heap, C.G. Prosser & G.E. Lamming), pp. 107–16. Butterworths, London.

Peters, A.R. (1985) Correct use of growth promoting implants. *In Practice*, **7**, 14–20.

Timmerman, H. (1987) β-adrenergics: physiology, pharmacology, applications, structures and structure–activity relationships. In *Beta-agonists and their Effects on Animal Growth and Carcass Quality* (ed. by J.P. Hanrahan), pp. 13–28. Elsevier Applied Science, London.

Warriss, P.D. & Kestin, S.C. (1988) Beta-agonists improve the carcass but may reduce meat quality in sheep. *Animal Production*, **46**, 502.

Whitaker, D.A., Smith, E.J., Kelly, J.M. & Hodgson-Jones, L.S. (1988) Health, welfare and fertility implications of the use of bovine somatotrophin in dairy cattle. *Veterinary Record*, **122**, 503–5.

Whitaker, D.A., Smith, E.J. & Kelly, J.M. (1989) Milk production, weight changes and blood biochemical measurements in dairy cattle receiving recombinant bovine somatotrophin. *Veterinary Record*, **124**, 83–6.

Chapter 58: Pharmacological Manipulation of Reproduction

by A.R. PETERS

This chapter aims to cover the zootechnical manipulation of reproduction in cattle where this is not covered in the chapters on general fertility. The discussion includes control of the oestrous cycle, induction and postponement of parturition and the establishment and maintenance of pregnancy.

Control of the oestrous cycle

The control of the oestrous cycle is dependent on manipulation of the hormonal events occurring during the normal ovarian/oestrous cycle. The overriding event controlling the development of an ovarian follicle to the point of ovulation in the cyclic cow is believed to be the process of luteolysis or decrease in progesterone secretion occurring between days 17 and 18 of the normal cycle (see Fig. 58.1). This fall in peripheral progesterone concentrations may be manipulated artificially in two ways.

1 By the artificial induction of premature luteolysis using luteolytic agents, e.g. the prostaglandins.

2 By the simulation of corpus luteum function, by administration of progesterone (or one of its synthetic derivatives) for a number of days, followed by abrupt withdrawal.

The two methods will now be discussed in greater detail.

Induction of luteolysis

The most potent luteolytic agents available are derivatives of prostaglandin $F_{2\alpha}$ ($PGF_{2\alpha}$). Injection of exogenous $PGF_{2\alpha}$ or one of its analogues during the mid-luteal phase of the cycle results in a premature luteolysis and consequential fall in peripheral progesterone concentrations. This is followed by a rise in secretion of gonadotrophins and eventual ovulation. The fall in progesterone concentrations is rapid, invariably reaching basal levels within 30 hours of injection. There are now several commercial analogues of $PGF_{2\alpha}$. As an example those currently on sale in the UK are shown in Table 58.1. They are all closely related to the natural PGF_{α}.

Prostaglandins have been used to control the oestrous cycle in several different ways. Some possible methods are shown below.

1 Following rectal examination, to inject only those cows with a corpus luteum. These cows should then show oestrus and ovulate three to five days later. This method has the disadvantage that it is time-consuming and that rectal palpation involves added expense. The results also depend on the accuracy of the rectal palpation.

2 To observe all cattle for oestrus for a seven-day period, serving any that show oestrus. The rest are injected with prostaglandin on the following day and may be inseminated either once or twice at fixed times or at observed oestrus. The reason for the initial seven-day observation period is that there is a period of about seven days in the cycle (day 18 to day 0 and day 1 to day

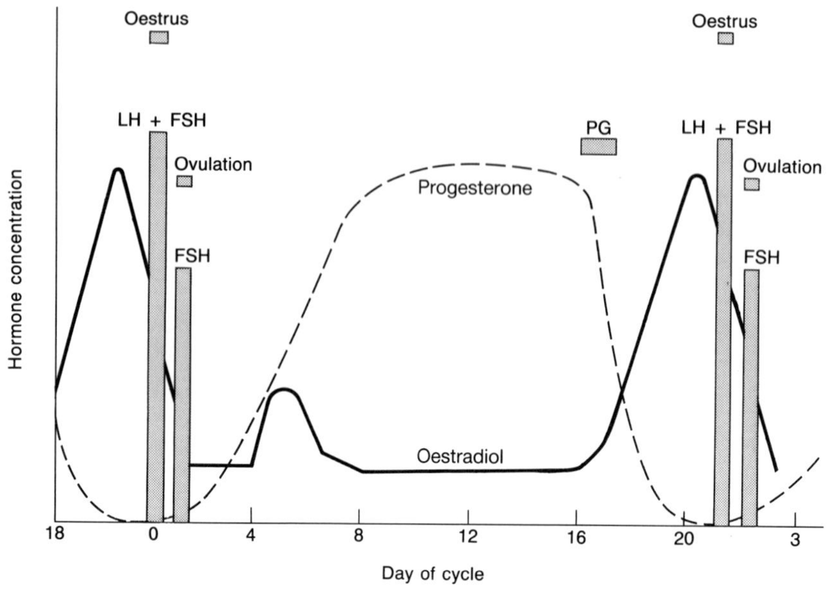

Fig. 58.1 Changes in blood plasma hormone concentrations during the bovine oestrous cycle (schematic): —— oestradiol; ---- progesterone.

Table 58.1 Prostaglandin analogues available in the UK (1990)

Trade name	Active component	Distributor	Route of injection	Dose rate (mg)	Insemination timing recommendations (hours)	
					Double	Single
Alphacept	Alfaprostol	Smith Kline Beechman	i.m.	1.5 mg/100 kg	Observed heat only	
Estrumate	Cloprostenol	Upjohn	i.m.	0.5	72, 96	72–84
Lutalyse	Dinoprost tromethamine (THAM salt)		i.m.	25.0	72, 90	78
Prosolvin	Luprostiol	Intervet	i.m.	15.0	72, 96	72
Synchrocept B	Fenprostalene	Syntex	s.c.	1.0	72, 96	No recommendation

4) when the animal is unresponsive to prostaglandin, i.e. when no corpus luteum is present. After seven days, those originally between days 18 and 0 will have shown heat and been served, while those that were between days 1 and 4 will now be between days 8 and 11, i.e. in the mid-luteal phase, and therefore responsive to prostaglandin.

3 The two injection plus two insemination method. The so-called 'two plus two' technique was designed to synchronize groups of animals cycling at random without prior knowledge of their precise ovarian status. All cattle are injected on day 1 of treatment and the injection repeated 11 days later. Artificial insemination (AI) is then carried out usually three and four days later.

The principle of this regimen is illustrated in Fig. 58.2. At the time of the first injection some animals will be responsive to the prostaglandin, i.e. between days 5 and 17 of the cycle. These will undergo luteolysis in response to the injection and will ovulate some four days or so later. At the time of the second injection (11 days later) these cows will be on about day 8 and 15 of the next cycle (Fig. 58.2). The cows that were not responsive to the first injection, i.e. those between days 18 and 4 of the cycle would be between days 8 and 15 at the time of the second injection. Therefore, all animals are theoretically in the responsive mid-luteal phase at the time of the second injection. The technique is popular and quite successful in synchronizing cycles in heifers (Cooper, 1974) and has resulted in pregnancy rates equivalent to control animals. However, pregnancy rates achieved with this technique in adult cows

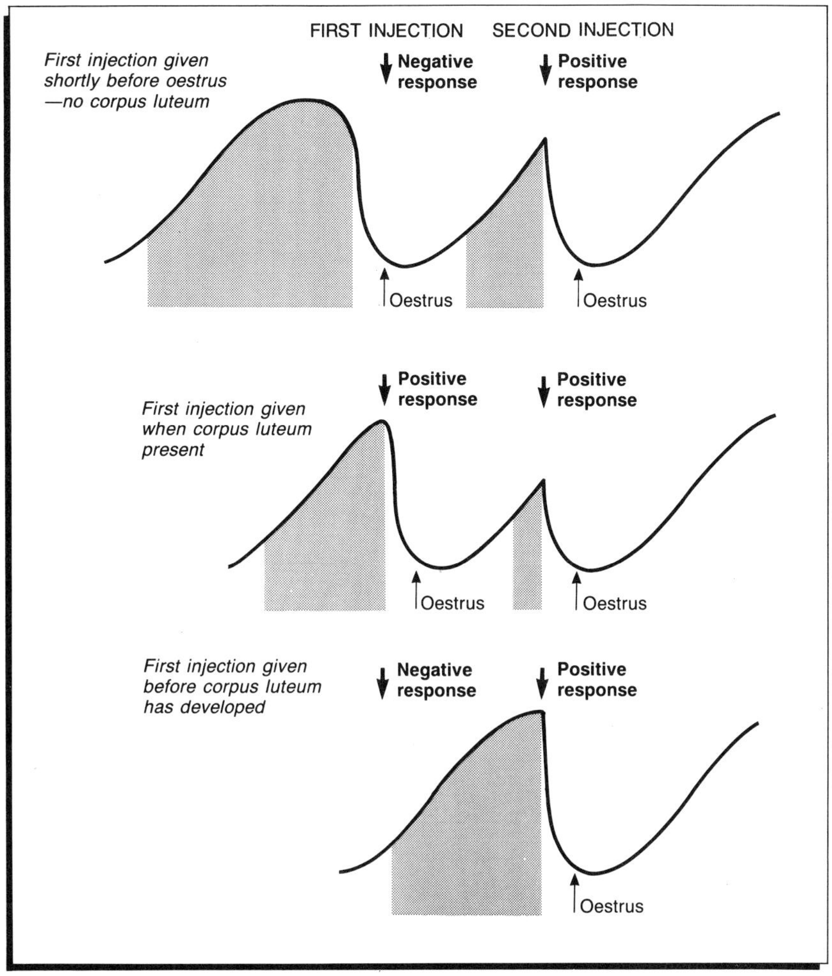

Fig. 58.2 The effect on progesterone concentrations of giving two injections of prostaglandin 11 days apart. (By permission from MAFF (1984) Dairy Herd Fertility. Reference book 259, p. 46, HMSO.)

have not always been consistent and reasons for this are discussed later.

4 A further method of using prostaglandins and that has been quite popular is the so-called '1½ method'. Cows are injected with prostaglandin and those that show oestrus are inseminated. Those that have not been seen in oestrus are injected again 11 days after the first injection and may be inseminated either at a fixed time(s) or at observed oestrus. Although requiring further effort in terms of oestrus detection, this method tends to give better results than the 'two plus two' regimen and is perhaps the current method of choice. Its main advantage however, is the reduction in cost by the reduction of both the number of treatments used and number of inseminations per cow.

Use of progestagens

The second method of controlling the cycle is to simulate the function of the corpus luteum by the administration of progesterone or one of its derivatives. In this method, gonadotrophin release, and hence ovarian follicular maturation, is suppressed until progesterone withdrawal. If a group of cows is treated with progesterone and then it is withdrawn from all cows simultaneously, this will theoretically synchronize ovulation in the group.

In order to synchronize a group of randomly cycling cows effectively, it is necessary to treat them with progesterone for a period equivalent to the length of the natural luteal phase, i.e. at least 16 days. This is due to the fact that exogenous progesterone has little or no effect on the lifespan of the natural corpus luteum and therefore in some cases the natural corpus luteum might outlive a short-term progesterone treatment, resulting in a failure of synchrony. However, it has been shown that long-term progesterone treatments (18–21 days) result in poor pregnancy rates and it is thought that this is due to adverse changes in the intra-uterine environment that inhibit sperm transport.

Shorter term progesterone treatments (seven to twelve days) generally result in more acceptable pregnancy rates. Unfortunately, short-term progesterone treatment does not control the cycle adequately since, if treatment is started early in the cycle, the natural corpus luteum may outlast the progesterone treatment. Therefore, it is necessary to incorporate a luteolytic agent with short-term progesterone treatments in order to eliminate any existing corpus luteum.

Progestagens (progesterone-like compounds) can be administered in the feed, by injection or by implant. Treatment in feed requires that the compound is 'orally active', i.e. it is absorbed into the systemic circulation unchanged Progesterone itself is relatively inactive orally and thus synthetic analogues, e.g. medroxyprogesterone acetate (MPA), melengoestrol acetate (MGA), were developed for this purpose. However, this route of administration presents problems of controlled dosing and the possibility of tissue or milk residues particularly in dairy cows. Therefore, such techniques are not favoured in the UK for oestrus control in cattle; however, they are used widely in the the USA and other countries particularly in heifers.

Progestagens can be given by injection, but repeated treatments may be necessary and the rate of absorption may be too imprecise to allow synchronized withdrawal of the compound. Implants are the most suitable method of administration of progestagens since withdrawal can then be precisely controlled by implant removal.

The progesterone-releasing intravaginal device (PRID)

The PRID (Sanofi Ltd) is a specialized form of implant in that it is inserted into and held within the cow's vagina for a period of seven to twelve days. The PRID consists of a stainless steel coil covered by a layer of grey inert silastic (Fig. 58.3) in which 1.55 mg progesterone is impregnated. A red gelatin capsule containing 10 mg oestradiol benzoate is attached to the inner surface of the coil. The PRID is inserted into the vagina by means of a speculum and is left in place for up to 12 days.

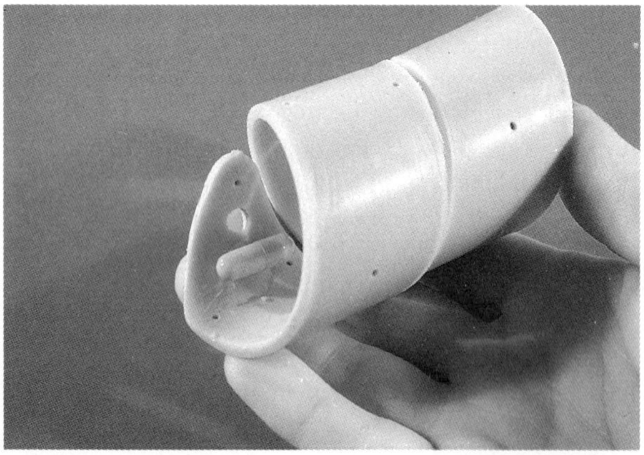

Fig. 58.3 A progesterone-releasing intravaginal device (PRID).

The oestradiol benzoate in the gelatin capsule is rapidly absorbed through the vaginal wall into the systemic circulation and is intended to act as a luteolytic agent. The progesterone is released from the elastomer for a longer period, i.e. until removal of the device. Removal is effected by pulling on the string, which is left protruding from the vulva after coil insertion. Removal of the device after seven to twelve days causes peripheral plasma progesterone concentrations to fall, thus simulating natural luteolysis. Consequently, the cow should show oestrus 48–72 hours later and fixed-time AI may be used at these times. The PRID contains natural progesterone and therefore its effects can be monitored by measuring progesterone concentrations in the blood plasma or milk of the animal.

A controlled intravaginal delivery device (CIDR) developed in New Zealand for the administration of progesterone is becoming available in a number of countries. It is anticipated that its effects are similar to those of the PRID.

Norgestomet

Norgestomet, 17α-acetoxy-β-methyl-19-nor-preg-4-ene,20-dione (Synchromate B), is commercially available in several countries. It is an example of a synthetic analogue of progesterone and consists of an impregnated silastic subcutaneous implant.

The implant is inserted subcutaneously behind the ear for a period of nine days during which time the progesterone is absorbed into the blood circulation. The implant is removed by making a small scalpel incision in the skin of the ear over the implant. At the time of the implantation an intramuscular injection of 5 mg oestradiol valerate is given as luteolysin, in combination with an initial injection of 3 mg norgestomet.

Factors affecting pregnancy rate after controlled ovulation

It cannot be overemphasized that in order to maximize results obtained with pharmacological control of the oestrous cycle, nutritional status and general management must be of a high standard. The efficacy of the pharmacological control of ovulation can be considered as two components.

1 The degree of synchrony obtained following treatment. This may be defined as the proportion of animals beginning to show oestrus or ovulating within a specified time period after the end of hormonal treatment. For the present purposes the target of synchrony is for the maximum number of animals to show oestrus within approximately 48 hours of progesterone withdrawal or 72 hours after prostaglandin injection (or to ovulate approximately 24 hours later in each case).

2 Reproductive performance, which may be expressed, for example, as the pregnancy rate achieved after treatment.

Obviously in some circumstances the pregnancy rate may be highly dependent on the degree of synchrony, particularly if fixed-time AI is used. For example, if there is a poor degree of synchrony there will be a wide variation in the timing of ovulation between cows or, more correctly, a proportion of cows will ovulate beyond the specified period referred to above. Therefore, the pregnancy following fixed-time AI may be poor.

In view of the natural variation in timing of the behavioural and ovarian events around natural oestrus, it is perhaps not surprising that even after hormone treatments there is still considerable variation in the timing of responses between animals. Hence where fixed-time AI is used, two inseminations are usually recommended in order to maximize the probability of conception. In addition, other problems occur that appear to be specific to the particular compounds used and these are described below.

Failure of synchrony after prostaglandins

Three major circumstances in which asynchrony can arise have been reported in the literature (Jackson *et al.*, 1979; Baishya *et al.*, 1980; Peters *et al.*, 1980).

Failure of complete luteolysis

This has occurred in 10 per cent or more of cows treated with prostaglandins. It takes the form either of complete lack of effect on progesterone concentrations or, for example, a fall to 50 per cent of preinjection levels, followed by luteal recovery usually within 24–48 hours. Causes of luteolytic failure are not clear but may be related to several factors including the following.

1 Non-responsiveness of some corpora lutea even in the appropriate phase of the cycle.

2 Treatment too early in the luteal phase.

3 Incorrect injection site or technique: in the case of intramuscular injections, occasionally the material may be injected accidentally into fat or ligamentous tissue.

4 Short half-life of the exogenous prostaglandin in the animal.

The extent of these various problems is not known and it must be admitted that all are to some extent speculative.

Long follicular phases after injection

In up to 20 per cent of cows injected with prostaglandin, although luteolysis appears to occur normally, progesterone concentrations remain low for an unusually long period and this may be associated with the delay in the timing of oestrus and ovulation. However, extended follicular phases (longer than eight days) also occur in about 17 per cent of untreated dairy cows. Thus it is likely that this phenomenon is related to an aberration in the adult cow's ovarian cycle. The problem has not been reported in heifers and certainly the cycles of adult cows would appear to be less uniform than those of heifers.

Acyclic cows

The ovary can only respond to prostaglandin if there is a functional corpus luteum. Therefore, cows not undergoing ovarian activity do not respond. The proportion of cows in this state will vary from herd to herd and the average stage after calving, but it is generally regarded as a more serious problem in suckling beef cows. For this reason it is recommended by some pharmaceutical companies that prostaglandins are not used before day 42 after calving.

Failure of synchrony after progestagens

There are two major circumstances in which asynchrony may arise following progestagen treatment.

Ineffectiveness of the luteolytic agent

As discussed above, oestradiol is often used as a luteolytic agent, along with progestagen treatments. If, for example, a nine-day progestagen treatment is started, without a luteolytic agent, between day 9 of one cycle and day 1 of the next, then these animals should synchronize adequately, since the end of treatment either coincides with or occurs after luteolysis, or the progesterone blocks ovulation. However, if treatment is started between days 2 and 8, then the corpus luteum will outlive the progestagen treatment. Hence it is for cows in the early stages of the cycle that the luteolysin is required. If it is assumed that the group of cows is cycling at random, then one would expect about 70 per cent of them to ovulate to within a day or two of each other. This degree of synchronization has been reported in practice (e.g. Drew *et al.*, 1979). More direct evidence using the Synchromate B package (norgestomet) has shown that oestradiol is not always an effective luteolytic agent nor does it prevent formation of the corpus luteum when administered early in the cycle (Peters, 1984).

Failure to maintain high blood concentration of progesterone

It has been shown that in some circumstances progesterone concentrations in the cow may fall before withdrawal of the progesterone source (Roche & Ireland, 1981). Obviously this could result in oestrus and ovulation occurring before removal of the device. This premature fall has occurred particularly with the intravaginal method of administration. It is thought to be related to progesterone-induced changes in absorption across the vaginal wall rather than to exhaustion of progesterone in the device.

Possible methods of overcoming problems of asynchrony

Failure to undergo complete luteolysis

An alternative to the use of oestradiol as a luteolytic agent in combination with progestagens is to use prostaglandin. Whilst problems of prostaglandin usage have been referred to above, they are clearly far more potent luteolytic agents than oestradiol. Prostaglandin is injected usually on the day before progestagen withdrawal. Various studies have shown that such combinations give well-synchronized oestrus and endocrine responses (Beal, 1983; Peters, 1984). However, there have been few reports where fixed-time AI has been used (Smith *et al.*, 1984). Unfortunately, such a treatment combination would obviously add further expense to a controlled breeding programme.

Prolonged follicular phases

Since it is apparent that a delay in oestrus and ovulation is associated with this phenomenon, a logical approach might be to attempt artificially to induce ovulation at a standard time after prostaglandin treatment. Experiments have been carried out where a single injection of gonadotrophin-releasing hormone (GnRH) is administered approximately 60 hours after prostaglandin injection (Coulson *et al.*, 1980). This has the effect of inducing a preovulatory-type LH surge, normally responsible for ovulation. However, there is a lack of controlled experimental data on the effect of GnRH treatment in this situation on the timing of ovulation and subsequent fertility.

Acyclic cows

This problem may be due to ineffective management in that either the cows are being treated too early after calving or that nutritional management is, and has been, inadequate (see Chapter 7). Assuming these problems are not present, then acyclicity may be overcome in a proportion of cows by the use of progestagens as opposed to prostaglandins.

Premature fall in progesterone concentrations (PRID)

This can be best avoided by minimizing the length of the treatment period. However, it is inadvisable to reduce the length of treatment below seven days, since this would result in inadequate synchronization.

Effect of the length of progestagen treatment on pregnancy rate

The deleterious effects of long-term progestagen treatment on fertility have already been discussed. However, there is some evidence that even short-term treatments can cause reduced fertility particularly where the treatment is started during the late luteal phase of the cycle. It is possible that this occurs because the animal is exposed to an uninterrupted long-term progestagen treatment, albeit a combination of endogenous and exogenous sources.

Field evaluation of oestrous synchronization techniques

Many field trials have been carried out to assess the effect of the various treatments on reproductive performance. These will not be discussed in detail here but they may be summarized as follows.

1 In adult cows the calving rate of control groups to single AI at observed oestrus is of the order of 50 per cent. Most studies report equivalent rates in treated cows.

2 Fertility results are often up to 20 per cent better in heifers than in cows.

3 In general, single fixed-time AI might be expected to result in 10–15 per cent lower pregnancy rates than two fixed-time AIs. However, Young & Henderson

Table 58.2 Effect of cloprostenol treatment of cyclic cows that had not been observed in oestrus by day 50 after calving (from Ball, 1982)

Treatment	Time of insemination	No. of cows	Calving-to-conception interval (days)
None until 90 days after calving	Observed oestrus	166	107.4
Cloprostenol*	Observed oestrus	61	98.1
Cloprostenol*	2 and 3 days after injection	75	104.0

* 0.5 mg cloprostenol (Estrumate, ICI) was injected intramuscularly 10–14 days after ovulation had occurred as judged from three times weekly milk progesterone measurements.

(1981) have claimed similar conception rates following either one or two fixed-time AIs after prostaglandin treatment.

4 It is clear that the best reproductive performance is achieved when oestrous cycle control is combined with insemination at observed oestrus. In that situation the reproductive performance of treated cows may often be higher than that of controls. This may happen particularly in a herd where the efficiency of oestrous detection is normally low. Following a synchronization treatment, it is to be expected that the vast majority of cows should show oestrus within 10 days after treatment. Therefore, the effect of treatment in this situation is to concentrate the occurrence of oestrous periods, so that detection efficiency can be increased over a relatively short time. Results of a recent study of use of the prostaglandin analogue cloprostenol with either fixed-time AI or observed oestrus are shown in Table 58.2 and illustrate the advantage of insemination at observed oestrus.

Following retrospective analysis of data from 17 published trials McIntosh *et al.* (1984) concluded that prostaglandin treatment combined with insemination at observed oestrus improved conception rates over controls by an average of 7 per cent.

Pharmacological induction of parturition

Many attempts have been made to induce parturition artificially in the final days of gestation. These methods have used exogenous hormones to simulate the mechanisms involved in the normal parturition process. These have included the use of corticosteroids, oestrogens and prostaglandins since these are all involved in the endocrine pathway (see Fig. 58.4).

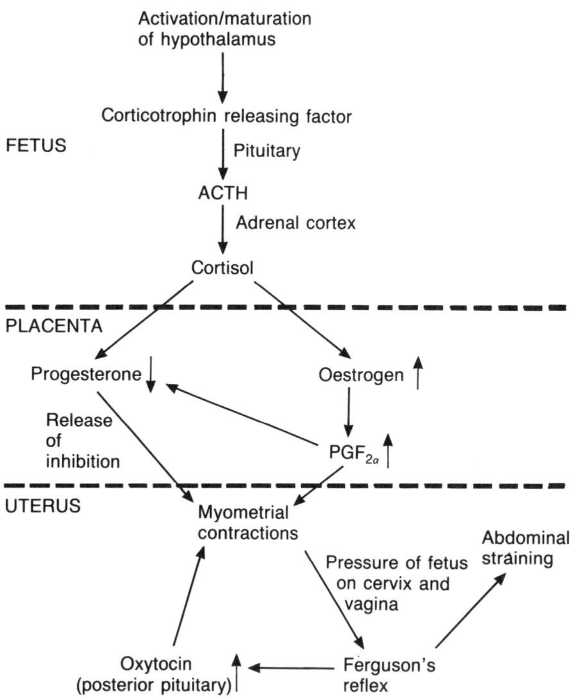

Fig. 58.4 The endocrine pathways controlling the induction of parturition.

There are several justifiable indications for the induction of parturition in cows. Firstly, in countries such as New Zealand, where a tight seasonal calving pattern is often required, this is considered to be an important aid to optimum management and utilization of feed resources. Secondly, cows can be induced to calve at a time when supervision is most readily available. Thirdly, if it is suspected that a high calf birth weight might result in dystokia early induction may alleviate the problem.

Methods of induction of parturition

Corticosteroids

There is now a considerable body of information on the effects of corticosteroids on the pregnant cow. Parturition can be induced quite reliably from about day 255 of pregnancy onwards by a single injection of a synthetic glucocorticoid, such as dexamethasone, betamethasone or flumethasone. It is assumed that such therapy simulates the effect of the fetal adrenal cortex.

Induction of parturition using corticosteroids is an important part of management in many New Zealand dairy herds and considerable experience of the technique has been gained (Welch *et al.*, 1979). Both short- and long-acting formulations have been used.

Short-acting formulations, generally in the form of a soluble ester of the steroid, usually result in parturition two to three days later. Although the calves are usually viable, this method has been associated with a high rate of retention of the fetal membranes. Thus use of long-acting corticosteroid formulations, for example a concentrated suspension of 'betamethasone alcohol' (MacDiarmid, 1979) resulted in a more protracted response, up to two weeks in some cases, and a high incidence of calf mortality.

Oestrogens

There is no clear evidence that exogenous oestrogen is effective in inducing parturition in cows although in one trial cited by First (1979) treatment with oestradiol-17β before corticosteroid treatment shortened the time to delivery and reduced the variation between cows.

Prostaglandins

Prostaglandins, both $PGF_{2\alpha}$ and synthetic analogues, may be used to induce parturition in cows, although treatment before day 270 of gestation is not recommended. Parturition usually occurs between one and eight days after injection but at an average of three days. A higher incidence of retained placenta may be expected.

A recent study under UK conditions (Murray *et al.*, 1984) used a treatment regimen whereby cows were injected with 20 mg dexamethasone and those that had not calved 10 days later received an injection of 0.5 mg cloprostenol (an analogue of $PGF_{2\alpha}$). Although there was a high incidence of retained placenta, this did not affect subsequent reproductive performance. It was concluded that provided management was organized adequately to supervise parturition and take care of the newborn calves then this procedure could be carried out to advantage.

A characteristic of early studies on the pharmacological induction of parturition was the high rate of calf mortality and post-calving problems, particularly retained placenta. An important determinant of the incidence of retained placenta appears to be the oestrogen status of the cow at the time of induction. As discussed above, oestrogen concentrations rise during late pregnancy, hence the oestrogen status may simply be a reflection of the proximity of term or 'readiness to calve'. From an exhaustive review of the available literature, First (1979) concluded that if induction is carried out when oestrogen levels are elevated, both glucocorticoids and prostaglandins are effective. However, glucocorticoids were the most appropriate treatment if induction was to be attempted earlier. The earlier that interference is attempted the higher the probability of calf mortality, retained placenta and other related problems.

Delay of parturition

It is now possible to delay parturition for several hours by pharmacological means. This is usually carried out so that supervision for calving can be more conveniently and readily available. Injection of the potent adrenergic drug, clenbuterol, inhibits myometrial contractions, thus slowing down the first stage of labour. However, if treatment is started after second-stage labour has already commenced, it would have little effect.

Establishment of pregnancy

The ability to conceive is clearly vital in determining reproductive performance. A low pregnancy rate to first service is a major cause of poor reproductive performance. In the absence of specific infectious disease it has been shown that the major problem here, at least in cattle, is early embryonic death (Sreenan & Diskin, 1986), normally occurring before day 25 after service. The exact cause(s) of embryonic death is unknown but it is circumstantially related to premature regression of the corpus luteum. In other words the corpus luteum is normally maintained for the whole of gestation and early embryonic mortality is associated with its early loss. This results in a decrease in progesterone concentrations allowing the animal to return to oestrus, probably at the normal time.

Before examining methods of reducing embryo mortality it would be useful to provide a brief review of new findings in relation to the establishment of pregnancy. In the non-pregnant animal $PGF_{2\alpha}$ secreted by the endometrium causes regression of the corpus luteum. This is illustrated in Fig. 58.5. There is evidence that oestradiol-17β from developing ovarian follicles stimulates the synthesis of receptors for oxytocin on endometrial cells. Oxytocin, now known to be of luteal origin (see Wathes, 1984) binds to these receptors thereby stimulating the synthesis and secretion of $PGF_{2\alpha}$. In early pregnancy of a normal ruminant a protein of molecular weight of approximately 18 000 is secreted by the embryo that has an antiluteolytic effect. This has been termed ovine or bovine trophoblast protein 1 (e.g. oTP-1). Stewart *et al.* (1989) recently showed that the amino acid sequence of oTP1

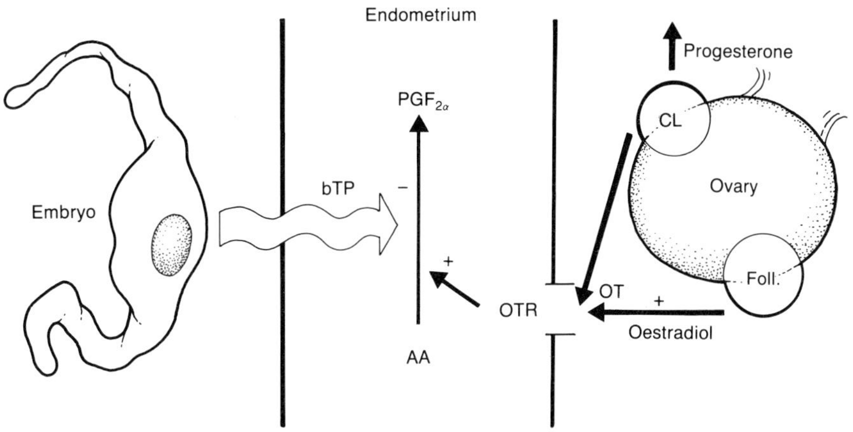

Fig. 58.5 Possible endocrine relationship between the early embryo, endometrium and ovary. bTP, bovine trophoblast protein; AA, arachidonic acid; OT, oxytocin; OTR, oxytocin receptor; CL, corpus luteum; Foll, follicle.

is 70.3 per cent similar to bovine α_2-interferon. Further studies have shown that oTP-1 and bTP-1 bind to receptors on the endometrium, and intra-uterine infusion of trophoblast proteins or recombinant interferon can extend the length of the luteal phase in non-pregnant animals (Stewart *et al.*, 1989; Thatcher *et al.*, 1989). This work has led to the tentative conclusion that some embryo mortality may be caused by a failure of some embryos to produce sufficient trophoblast protein. These early results clearly offer the exciting possibility of using recombinant trophoblast protein to prevent or reduce embryo mortality in domestic animals.

A number of methods have been used in the field to improve pregnancy rates in cattle. Diskin and Sreenan (1986) reviewed literature on comparisons of progesterone concentrations in pregnant and non-conceiving cows before and after insemination and concluded that the data were conflicting and inconclusive in all respects. Similarly, progesterone supplementation during early pregnancy has given equivocal results but does seem to be effective where control pregnancy rates are particularly low, i.e. 40 per cent or below.

It has been common veterinary practice for many year to inject cows at the time of service with a 'holding' injection using either human chorionic gonadotrophin (HCG) (luteinizing hormone (LH)-like) or GnRH to stimulate endogenous LH release. The exact physiological rationale for this has not always been clear since such treatment could potentially have at least two effects. Firstly, there is a widely held belief that under some circumstances ovulation may be delayed relative to the timing of oestrus. Administration of GnRH will result in preovulatory gonadotrophin release and subsequent ovulation. Secondly, LH is considered to be the major luteotrophic hormone at least during the first few days of pregnancy. Therefore, GnRH-induced LH release may facilitate the development and maintenance of the corpus luteum in the postovulatory period.

Numerous trials have been carried out where either HCG (LH) or GnRH has been given on the day of service but the results are generally equivocal since some results have shown good responses and others show no differences from control animals. This could be for one or more of the following reasons.

1 Poor design of trials, particularly inadequate number of animals per group. This is a common problem where fertility rates are being studied. Due to the fact that pregnancy rate is a discrete variable and that rates are very different between farms, very large numbers (several hundred per group) may be required to establish statistically significant differences between groups where there are differences of only a few percentage points.

2 The actual cause of pregnancy failure may differ widely between farms and therefore one may be attempting to rectify many different primary problems by the use of such a treatment. The primary cause is often impossible to diagnose at least at that time.

3 Thus it is probably a fair summary to state that the best results for the improvement of pregnancy rates have been achieved where the control or background fertility of the herd is poor; although there are some exceptions to this.

A somewhat different approach was used by MacMillan *et al.* (1986), to attempt to support the corpus luteum when it becomes susceptible to the luteolytic mechanism, i.e. approaching day 16 after oestrus in the cow. Treated cows (approximately 225)

Table 58.3 Pregnancy rate (per cent) to first insemination with 10 μg buserelin injected between days 11 and 13 after insemination (from MacMillan *et al.*, 1986)

Trial	Treated	Control
A	75.4	62.2
B	67.5	57.8
Overall	72.4*	60.9

* = $p < 0.01$.

Table 58.4 Pregnancy rates (per cent) to second insemination (from MacMillan *et al.*, 1986)

Trial	Treated	Control
A	78.6	69.0
B	94.7	70.8
Overall	85.1*	69.5

* = $p < 0.05$.

received a single injection of 10 μg buserelin (synthetic analogue of GnRH) on day 11, 12 or 13 after AI. Treated and control cows were palpated at six to nine weeks to determine pregnancy status. Cows returning to service were re-inseminated. Pregnancy rates at six to nine weeks were 72.5 per cent and 60.9 per cent for the treated and control cows respectively (see Table 58.3). Of those cows returning to service the pregnancy rates to second service were 85.1 per cent and 69.5 per cent for treated and control (see Table 58.4). The differences between groups were highly significant on both occasions.

Thatcher *et al.* (1989) have suggested that buserelin acts in these situations by disrupting normal waves of ovarian follicular growth and oestradiol secretion during this period, resulting in a failure of the luteolytic mechanism (see Fig. 58.5). It is also possible that accessory corpora lutea are formed, which may boost progesterone production.

References

Baishya, N., Ball, P.J.H. Leaver, J.D. & Pope, G.S. (1980) Fertility of lactating dairy cows inseminated after treatment with cloprostenol. *British Veterinary Journal*, **136**, 227–39.

Ball, P.J.H. (1982) Milk progesterone profiles in relation to dairy fertility. *British Veterinary Journal*, **138**, 546–51.

Beal, W.E. (1983) A note on synchronisation of oestrus in post-partum cows with prostaglandin $F_{2\alpha}$ and a progesterone-releasing device. *Animal Production*, **37**, 305–8.

Cooper, M.J. (1974) Control of oestrous cycles of heifers with a synthetic prostaglandin analogue. *Veterinary Record*, **95**, 200–3.

Coulson, A., Noakes, D.E., Hamer, J. & Cockrill, T. (1980) Effect of gonadotrophin releasing hormone on levels of luteinising hormone in cattle synchronised with dinoprost. *Veterinary Record*, **107**, 108–9.

Diskin, M.G. & Sreenan, J.M. (1986) Progesterone and embryo survival in the cow. In *Embryonic Mortality in Farm Animals* (ed. by J.M. Sreenan & M.G. Diskin), pp. 142–55. Martinus Nijhoff, Dordrecht.

Drew, S.B., Wishart, D.R. & Young, I.M. (1979) Fertility of Norgestomet treated suckler cows. *Veterinary Record*, **104**, 523–5.

First, N.D. (1979) Mechanisms controlling parturition in farm animals. In *Animal Reproduction* (ed. by H.W. Hawk), Beltsville Symposia in Agricultural Research No. 3, pp. 215–57. John Wiley & Sons, New York.

Jackson, P.S., Johnson, C.T., Bulman, D.C. & Holdsworth, R.J. (1979) A study of cloprostenol-induced oestrus and spontaneous oestrus by means of the milk progesterone assay. *British Veterinary Journal*, **135**, 378–90.

MacDiarmid, S.D. (1979) Betamethasone for the induction of parturition on dairy cows: a comparison of formulation. *New Zealand Veterinary Journal*, **28**, 61–4.

McIntosh, D.A.D. Lewis, J.A. & Hammond, D. (1984) Conception rates in dairy cattle treated with cloprostenol. *Veterinary Record*, **115**, 129–30.

MacMilllan, K.L., Taufa, V.K. & Day, A.M. (1986) Effects of an agonist of gonadotrophin releasing hormone in cattle: III. Pregnancy rates after a post-insemination injection during metoestrus or dioestrus. *Animal Reproduction Science*, **11**, 1–10.

Murray, R.D. Nutter, W.T., Wilman, S. & Harker, D.B. (1984) Induction of parturition using dexamethasone and cloprostenol. Economic performance and disease incidence after treatment. *Veterinary Record*, **115**, 296–330.

Peters, A.R. (1984) Plasma progesterone and gonadotrophin concentrations following Norgestomet treatment with and without cloprostenol in beef cows. *Veterinary Record*, **115**, 164–6.

Peters, A.R., Riley, G.M., Rahim, S.E.A. & Lowman, B.G. (1980) Milk progesterone profiles and the double injection of cloprostenol in post-partum beef cows. *Veterinary Record*, **107**, 174–7.

Roche, J.F. & Ireland, J.J. (1981) Effect of exogenous progesterone on time of occurrence of the LH surge in heifers. *Journal of Animal Science*, **52**, 580–6.

Smith, R.D. Pomerantz, A.J., Beal, W.E., McCann, J.P., Pilbeam, T.E. & Hansel, W. (1984) Insemination of Holstein heifers at a preset time after oestrous cycle synchronisation using progesterone and prostaglandin. *Journal of Animal Science*, **58**, 792–800.

Sreenan, J.M. & Diskin, M.J. (1986) The extent and timing of embryonic mortality. In *Embryonic Mortality in Farm Animals* (ed. by J.M. Sreenan & M.G. Diskin), pp. 1–11. Martinus Nijhoff, Dordrecht.

Stewart, H.J. Flint, A.P.F., Lamming, G.E., McCann, S.H.E. & Parkinson, T.J. (1989) Antiluteolytic effects of blastocyst-secreted interferon investigated *in-vitro* and *in-vivo* in the sheep. *Journal of Reproduction and Fertility*, suppl. 37, 127–38.

Thatcher, W.W., MacMillan, K.L., Hansen, P.J. & Drost, M. (1989) Concepts for regulation of corpus luteum function by the conceptus and ovarian follicles to improve fertility. *Theriogenology*, **31**, 149–64.

Wathes, D.C. (1984) Possible actions of gonadal oxytocin and vasopressin. *Journal of Reproduction and Fertility*, **71**, 315–45.

Welch, R.A.S., Day, A.M., Duganzich, D.M. & Featherstone, P. (1979) Induced calving: a comparison of treatment regimes. *New Zealand Veterinary Journal*, **27**, 190–4.

Young, I.M. & Henderson, D.C. (1981) Evaluation of single and double insemination regimes as methods of shortening calving intervals in dairy cows treated with dinoprost. *Veterinary Record*, **109**, 446–9.

Chapter 59: Alternative Medicine

by C.E.I. DAY

Introduction

All forms of alternative medicine have received a high degree of interest in latter years. The reasons for this are many. It is part of the trend towards environmental consciousness (the so-called 'Green' movement), awareness of the importance and mechanisms of health and how medical systems impinge on this and, lastly, the realization of the vital role that diet plays in health and the effect of additives and residues on the value of food items.

Alternative medicine is relevant to this in that it provides, as is suggested by the epithet, an alternative to what has become the accepted system of medicine, modern conventional drug medicine. There are many so-called systems of alternative medicine (sometimes now called complementary medicine in an attempt to attenuate the overtones of conflict embodied in the word alternative). The wide range of such systems can present a baffling array to the casual observer, but they are united in several respects being:

1 natural, relying on no man-made chemicals for their effect;
2 able to work with and through the body's own mechanisms, stimulating the 'vital force' or 'life energy';
3 holistic, embracing the concept of mind and body as a whole in harmony with the environment; and
4 environmentally and dietarily appropriate since they give rise to no tissue residues in animals so treated.

There are two main systems of alternative medicine that have been developed and refined in the field of bovine medicine and that have become partially accepted by the conventional 'scientific' community. These are *homoeopathy* and *acupuncture* and of these the one used to the greater extent is homoeopathy. It lends itself more easily to rapid, less specialized treatments and is applicable to herd medicine. The title 'alternative' is more appropriate than 'complementary' in that each is a complete system of medicine in its own right, demanding a full understanding of its principles and practice for its true value to be manifested. The following is a brief introduction of concepts followed by more medical detail.

Homoeopathy

Introduction

Founded by a German physician, Hahnemann, in the latter part of the eighteenth century (1790), homoeopathy is a system of medicine embodying the principle *'similia similibus curentur'* meaning 'let like be cured by like'. This classical slogan is often enough in itself to deter the casual student since it constitutes an entirely opposite stratagem to that of conventional 'school medicine'. It is hoped the reader will keep an open mind and form opinions after searching and objective study into the relative merits of each strategy and the part each system may play in the overall fight against disease. The provision of an objective study requires some comparisons with the 'known' to be made, so as to shed light on the 'unknown' which homoeopathy represents.

The principle of like curing like is elevated from the status of an amusing idea or the product of a fertile imagination by the fact that it exploits a *natural law (The Law of Similars)*. It was not an invention therefore that occurred in 1790 but a discovery. Hahnemann hit on his discovery as a result of objective testing of the effects of Cinchona bark (the parent material of quinine and an accepted cure for malaria even today. He dosed a healthy person (namely himself) in order to try to discover the mode of action of Cinchona bark as he could not accept the current eighteenth-century explanation for its activity. What happened must have been a great shock to his system for he developed symptoms quite indistinguishable from malaria. Cause and effect he objectively established by alternately withholding and restarting the administration of the substance. This led him to formulate his hypothesis: '*To cure mildly, rapidly, certainly and permanently, choose in every case of disease, a medicine which can itself produce an affection similar to that sought to be cured*' (quotation from *Organon der Heilkunst* by Hahnemann 1790, translation by Boericke & Dudgeon). Having carried out tests (Prüfungen in German, which became translated as 'provings') on healthy volunteers with many substances, he started to use this system of medicine on his patients. He soon found that his crude substances evoked quite serious 'aggravations' in his patients so he proceeded to dilute the remedies. This led to the second great stumbling block for the modern conventionally trained observer in that his commonly used dilutions exceeded those that could reasonably be expected to contain even a single molecule of the original substance. His dilutions, called 'potencies', were often to the extent of 30c and beyond (i.e. 1/100 thirty times diluted) giving rise to a dilution of 10^{-60} (at 10^{-23} Avogadro's hypothesis suggests it is unlikely a fluid will carry a molecule over to the next stage). What Hahnemann found with his serial dilution and succussion method (succussion is the violent shaking of the solution at each stage of dilution) was that the toxic power of the substance was reduced at each stage (understandable) but the curative power was increased (not so readily acceptable). It is a fact of life that this phenomenon exists and that science has not yet found the way to explain it. It therefore remains, unexplained, to puzzle the reader and, in so many cases, act as a complete blockade to further enquiry.

That Hahnemann went on to cure all but two (one of them being a very old man) out of 180 typhus patients under his care after the battle of Leipzig in 1812 was a testimony to its efficacy. This result could hardly be said (statistically) to differ from 100 per cent success and occurred over a century before the advent of antibiosis! One of Hahnemann's disciples also recorded an astounding success rate against cholera in Raab in Hungary. He lost six of his 154 patients (3.9 per cent) compared with the other physicians in the town who lost between them 820 out of 1501 (54.6 per cent).

These two reports furnished the first clinical trial data available and certainly give cause for inquiry. In more modern times, and in a veterinary context, clinical trials have revealed good results in many fields, e.g. Caulophyllum and its use in controlling porcine stillbirths (Day, 1984a), bovine mastitis prevention studies (Day, 1986), bovine dystokia prevention (Day, 1985), reduction of calf rearing losses (Mahe, 1987) and control of canine kennel cough (Day, 1987a).

Principles

A more detailed approach to veterinary homoeopathy is provided by Day (1984b, 1987b).

HOW TO CURE

Hahnemann's four steps to cure (a word he used very objectively to indicate a removal of symptoms/signs with no further need for therapy to maintain that healthy state) were: (i) know the remedies, (ii) know the disease, (iii) match the remedy to the disease, and (iv) remove the obstacles to recovery. Our objective in veterinary medicine is to *cure* disease wherever possible, and it is difficult to argue with Hahnemann's four steps.

Know the remedies

A knowledge of the provings of each remedy is the basis of this stage. Obtaining this knowledge requires dedication. The remedies are written up in books of Materia Medica (e.g. Boericke, 1972; Clarke, 1982; Macleod, 1983), which may run into several volumes. These books give an account of the properties of the remedies in terms of source, general properties, 'provings' and clinical findings with applications. This represents a huge body of knowledge on each remedy's known ('proven' by Hahnemannian tests) capabilities in very fine detail and for each part of the body and mind, and its assumed capabilities (from clinical data).

It is fair to say that despite our pharmacological knowledge of modern drugs there is not the equivalent amount of knowledge of their actions in the body and, for the most part, very little is known of a drug's possible actions apart from the major primary and local effects. It may also be fair to say that not enough pharmacodynamic studies have been made of homoeopathic remedy actions but if research is never directed this way then the information will never accrue.

Not even the most learned homoeopath has a *full* knowledge of even the major remedies (let alone the several thousand available), since there is so much detail. However, a basic knowledge of major remedies is essential as well as superficial knowledge of minor remedies. Obtaining the necessary knowledge discourages many would-be practitioners.

Know the disease

Since each set of symptoms and signs in each individual suffering disease is a product of the individual's own reaction to a disease influence, then each disease occurrence encountered is a *unique* incident (Fig. 59.1).

Knowledge of each disease incident must depend therefore on one's ability to discern as much as possible of its aetiology in broad terms and on one's ability to read the symptoms/signs shown by the organism, i.e. its reaction to the disease influence. A detailed effort must therefore be made in history taking and in clinical examination. The findings can be grouped as follows.

1 *Aetiological* influences.
2 *Generals*. Symptoms/signs/properties of the whole body, e.g. build, disposition, response to environment, response to food, response to climate, etc.
3 *Mentals*. Symptoms/signs relating to the mind, e.g. demeanour, behaviour, character, responses to various mental stimuli.
4 *Particulars*. The symptoms/signs displayed by each part of the body in fine detail (the gleanings of a very thorough clinical examination). Also any 'modalities' shown by these signs, e.g. worse when cold and wet, worse after food, better after exercise, etc.

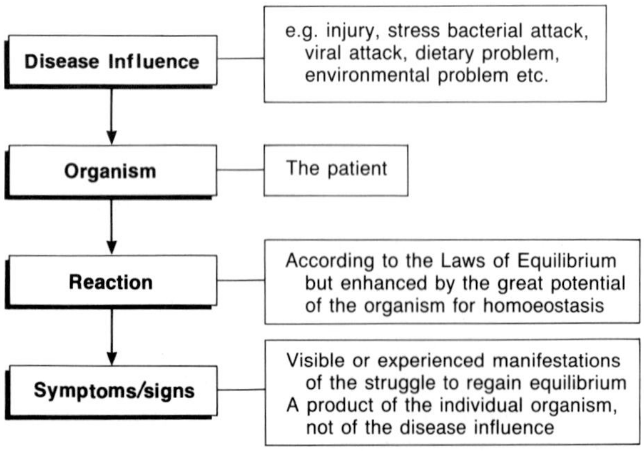

Fig. 59.1 A disease event in an animal.

Match the remedy to the disease

The detailed history taking plus clinical examination and knowledge contained in Materia Medica each constitute a picture that can be cross-matched but this is often a daunting task. As each disease incident is considered to be a unique event and several thousand possible remedies exist, the task may appear impossible. However, once a basic knowledge of a good number of remedies is obtained then the ability of the human brain to 'compute' at high speed makes the task achievable in an acceptable number of cases for the conscientious student after several years of practice and study. There are also books to aid the process, which are basically computers in print. These are called Repertories (Boericke, 1972; Kent, 1986) and are basically lists of symptoms (in human terms) listed under generals, mentals and particulars (for each part of the body). Several remedies are then suggested that are able to cause the precise symptoms sought and which may therefore be applicable in the particular patient. If one lists enough symptoms and looks up each in the Repertory the highest scoring remedy (in theoretical terms at least) is the ideal choice. A resort to the Materia Medica will help to confirm or negate this choice. Obviously, this is a fairly long-winded process and, though helpful in difficult cases, it is not applicable to rapid selection of remedies on-farm. Thus a basic remedy knowledge is required together with an effort to think rapidly in 'picture' format. No equivalent veterinary Repertory exists although, in slightly differing form, it can be found in books by MacLeod (1981, 1983), Brock & Nielsen (1986) and Day (1984b, 1987b). Each work gives an easily assimilated guide to remedy choices under given conditions, but (therefore?) is less accurate. Computer programs are being developed for this type of work but again are not applicable to on-farm use with presently available technology.

Remove the obstacles to recovery

Even in the late twentieth century the insight of Hahnemann in the eighteenth century is remarkable.

The single most exceptional example of futuristic perspicacity is in the concept of removal of obstacles to recovery. In trying to observe this fourth provision for cure not only must there be obvious remedial efforts such as splinting/fixing of fractures, dietary investigation/correction, removal of an obstructive foreign body from the bowel, etc. but also in the herd context, the myriad parameters (environmental, management, dietary, etc.) affecting herd health must be considered. The idea that herd factors are important has been practised by forward-thinking veterinarians for *only the last thirty or so years*. However, Hahnemann made clear provision for it 200 years ago! Sadly, however, the most stringent efforts to improve the husbandry of modern cattle farms will never provide ideal environmental and nutritional conditions for the animals although some measures can approach the ideal. Thus, in modern dairy cattle practice, one is presented with an imperfectly fulfilled provision for real cure (Hahnemann's definition). This explains the need for repeated or possibly continuous medication on intensive farms but this must not be an excuse for lack of effort. The unattainability of perfection must not be an excuse for failure to achieve the best conditions possible and removal, to a maximum possible extent, of the obstacles to recovery.

CONVERSION TO VETERINARY APPLICATION

Homoeopathic medicine was developed *in* humans *for* humans and presents some difficulties in conversion to veterinary practice. The difficulties can be summarized as:

1 lack of speech in animal patients;
2 interspecies differences in reaction to remedies;
3 lack of family history; and
4 intensivism in farm management.

Hahnemann (1814) did however advocate use in animals and so veterinary homoeopathy has a long tradition.

Lack of speech

The lack of speech in animal patients leads to loss of a large range of symptoms of value to the prescriber in human medicine. The ability to detail *mental symptoms and feelings* is lost but much of what is needed can be discerned from the demeanour and behaviour of the patient. However, the finer details of how the mind is affected by the disease influence or why it responds in the way it does cannot be determined. Only the end result of behaviour is seen rather than the mental processes behind that behaviour. Since the mental symptoms of disease are a sure guide to the unique individual response to disease a large proportion of diagnostic (remedy-selecting) parameters is therefore lost. However, deductions about mental symptoms from the external behavioural signs can provide an invaluable guide to the sensitive observer. Lack of speech also deprives us of the enormous field of subjective symptoms. Thus, the adjectives used by human patients to describe pain symptoms are legion. They are again an expression of the individuality of each disease incident and are therefore invaluable. Descriptions of pain such as 'tearing', 'cutting', 'burning ', 'aching', etc. are all lost in veterinary medicine. Also, hidden among these symptoms is the headache in its many forms. We can rarely diagnose headache in animals let alone describe it. However, approximately 100 pages of Kent's Repertory (1986) are devoted to headache!

Interspecies difference

It is not unreasonable to suppose that different species of animals will react differently to remedies when compared with *human* reactions. Also there will be differences *between* the individual domestic species. To reconstruct the painstaking 'provings' of Hahnemann and followers for each remedy for each species would involve several laboratories for many generations with an enormous usage of laboratory animals. Despite the obvious existence of such a problem, as shown by the varying toxicology and pharmacology known in different species for many poisons (Garner, 1967), drugs (Daykin, 1960) and foods, homoeopathy is largely transferable *en bloc*! This is a fortunate fact but one that should never be taken for granted. Thus the astute practitioner of the art will need to be aware of the possibility of failure due to species difference, and will use pharmacological and toxicological knowledge to advantage.

Lack of family history

Although not strictly applicable to units where pedigree breeding and recording has gone on down the years, the lack of family history, particularly in terms of disease, of bovine patients will lead to loss of some accuracy in prescribing. Known line susceptibilities are an important factor in choosing remedies in such conditions as cancer, mastitis, lameness, etc. but the loss of some of this material is not likely to be as deleterious as the lack of speech and interspecies differences.

Intensive farming

This factor has been discussed previously (see. p. 889).

Application

Disease can affect an animal to a greater or lesser depth and therefore so can the so-called remedies of homoeopathy since they are also disease-producing agents when administered to a healthy body. These different levels of prescribing can be classified as:

1 pathological;
2 local;
3 organ-specific;
4 constitutional;
5 facultative/regulatory;
6 detoxifying;
7 historical;
8 specific; and
9 preventive.

Pathological

To prescribe at the pathological level one needs to be satisfied that the disease influence has evoked an acute and easily identifiable disease process that could be easily matched to the actions of a particular remedy. The effects of *traumatic injury*, for instance, are very well covered by the properties of arnica, the administration of which, as rapidly as possible after the traumatic insult, will swiftly and effectively initiate a healing process that will reduce the pain, shock, haemorrhage, tissue fluid accumulation and resultant tissue damage that normally follows trauma. The net result is a happier patient, less distortion at the site of injury and, more importantly, less disturbance to the circulation in the area. Therefore there is more effective and rapid restoration of normal tissue integrity and structure. The fact that one remedy covers this process is very convenient for the prescriber and very helpful to the patient. It removes the need to apply the rigours of the homoeopathic method in times of emergency and this pathological level of prescribing provides a simple proving ground for homoeopathy to the sceptic and a useful starting point for learning the first steps of the homoeopathic method. Other commonly used remedy/pathological indication pairings are:

Hypericum:	injury to areas rich in nerve endings, e.g. digit, tail, etc., injury to nerves, painful grazes, photosensitization
Ledum:	puncture wounds
Aconitum:	sudden shock to the mind or body
Calendula:	open wound – promotes healing and disinfection

Local

One would apply this level of prescribing when the nature of the disease is acute and fairly superficial to an otherwise healthy animal. Examples of this are acute onset mastitis (see p. 296) resulting from a chill, where aconitum is useful, New Forest eye infection (see p. 714), where mercurius corrosivus may be effective, and foul-in-the-foot infection (see p. 356), where hepar sulphuris could be the correct remedy. To prescribe effectively for these conditions one only needs to take note of the local presenting signs and match these to a remedy. One does not need, again, to delve into the deeper homoeopathic method, discussed in previous pages, in order to achieve a good result. However, ensure that the disease is not chronic in nature or an acute exacerbation of an underlying chronic disorder. If this should prove to be the case satisfactory results will not follow and one would need to apply the constitutional approach.

Organ-specific

Organ-specific remedies may be used when one organ is particularly embarrassed in an illness. Some remedies have a particular affinity for specific organs or tissues and the most important are:

Rhus toxicodendron:	muscles
Ruta graveolens:	tendons, ligaments, joint capsules, periosteum
Hypericum:	nerve fibres
Symphytum:	bone
Nux vomica:	liver
Flor de piedra:	liver
Lycopodium:	liver
Berberis:	liver, kidney
Kali chlor:	kidney
Digitalis:	heart

Constitutional

The concept of a constitution embodies everything that is unique to an individual organism. It embraces the idea of the 'programmed' nature of each body's response to a disease influence. Response to disease is programmed by a number of factors: genetic make-up inherited from the parents, *in utero* influences during pregnancy, the birth process, postnatal influences, influences during the growing period and influences during adulthood. In the farm context, one can see how breeding, pregnancy, calving, rearing and general management and dietary regimens can affect the make-up of an adult cow. By reading the response pattern of the animal in the face of disease or situations, and by studying her conformation and behaviour, one can formulate an idea of her 'constitutional type'. This whole picture can be matched to a whole remedy picture as previously discussed. Not many remedies have a combination of wide and deep enough effects on the body to rank as constitutional remedies and, in the world of cattle, the major nine examples can be listed, conveniently classified into three groups.

Aurum Pulsatilla Sepia	Corresponding to a great many cows that suffer typically female or hormonal problems as a rule
Antimonium crudum Nux vomica Lycopodium	As a rule fitting those cattle that suffer digestive problems
Calcarea carbonica Calcarea phosphorica Phosphorus	As a rule matching those cows suffering from lactation-induced disorders

These generalizations are too sweeping to be strictly followed but the pictures of the remedies listed above are suitable to be grouped in the way shown. These are 'big' remedies (Hahnemann's so-called polycrests) and have effects on all parts of the body. They therefore cannot be purely type-cast in the roles shown above. These are only trends in the relevant animal's disease response patterns. The major remedies will be discussed later (see pp. 893–895).

When confronted by a patient affected by *chronic* disease, no real cure can follow treatment unless this method of prescribing is followed. The organism has learnt, in the case of chronic disease, to live in a state of uneasy harmony with the disease. The animal is therefore unable to regain health, often lost a long time previous to therapy, unless the deep, powerful and most appropriate stimulus of true holistic homoeopathy is prescribed.

Facultative/regulatory

The facultative level of prescribing exploits the ability of certain potentized substances to facilitate metabolism with respect to those substances. Examples are the use of potencies of the various calcium salts to facilitate metabolism with respect to calcium, magnesium phosphorica will help magnesium metabolism, and cuprum will assist copper metabolism. It is well known that so-called mineral deficiencies are rarely absolute deficiencies but more often a malfunction of the relevant absorptive, metabolic and eliminative processes for that mineral. Excesses and deficiencies can both be helped by such methods. In the case of hormone disturbances, potentized hormone may help regulate and balance the body.

Detoxifying

The detoxifying method of prescribing echoes very closely preceding remarks. Should a specific substance be causing a toxic effect, e.g. alkaloids, metals, chemicals, etc., then the body's natural ability to break down and/or eliminate such toxins will be enhanced by administration of the specific substance, or a close relative, in potency (dilution). Examples are the use of plumbum in cases of lead toxicity, coumarin or melilotus in cases of warfarin toxicity, opium or nux vomica in cases of anaesthetic toxicity or even carbohydrate overdose in the ruminant. Such methods have often been shown to produce very unexpected results even in extreme cases of toxicity.

Historical

The historical method of prescribing utilizes the body's ability to respond to an appropriate curative homoeopathic stimulus, long after the initial disease-producing influence has subsided, should the body still be suffering from the effects of that influence. Examples are: using arnica long after an initial injury, should the body still be suffering disease from that injury; using aconitum long after a mental or physical shock if the body is still suffering effects or fears produced by that shock; using a 'specific' remedy (see below) long after a specific infectious disease has passed its acute phase, should the body still be suffering effects from that disease.

All that is necessary to utilize this method is to detect, in a chronic disease situation, a facet of the history that leads one to believe that the chronic disease has its origins in a specific historic incident and then treat that incident as if it was in the here and now even if it occurred years previously.

Specific

The specific method of prescribing would be used in an acute disease context where a known specific infectious disease agent is involved. Generally speaking this method of treatment would imply use of nosodes (remedies made from disease material), e.g. mastitis nosode in cases of mastitis (see Chapter 21), infectious bovine rhinotracheitis (IBR) nosode in cases of IBR (see p. 256), bovine virus diarrhoea (BVD) nosode in cases of BVD (see p. 660), or salmonella nosode in cases of salmonellosis. In the acute phase of an infectious disease it may be dangerous to use the nosode in an attempt to produce a cure and it is usually reserved for use during the recovery phase of the disease in order to prevent any tendency for the disease to become chronic. During the acute phase it is always better to select a remedy for cure according to the law of Similars in the usual way. This implies that, in each case of specific disease, there will be no remedy specific to the disease but a whole host of possible remedies that need to be suited to each patient. Having said this, it is possible that baptisia could be specific to salmonellosis (Chapter 13), mercurius cyanatus to calf diphtheria (see p. 214), mercurius corrosivus to New Forest eye or even borax to foot-and-mouth disease (see Chapter 37c) (where it is permitted to treat this disease!).

Preventive

In herd medicine it is very important to apply preventive principles to minimize or obviate the risk of spread of a known or predicted infectious disease within the herd. This is the basis of effective veterinary involvement on the modern bovine farm unit. In an individual animal context it is important to prevent disease occurring in the face of a predicted challenge or disease-producting event.

The greatest demands on the veterinarian using homoeopathy are on a herd basis. Where infectious disease has either entered the herd, in which case the healthy individuals must be protected; or is threatening the herd, in which case the whole herd must be protected, one would select for prevention a specific remedy. This would generally be a *nosode* (see Specific prescribing, p. 891) although it could be any remedy from the homoeopathic Materia Medica that the prescriber feels specific enough to a certain disease (see Specific prescribing, p. 891). In conventional medicine one would be reaching for a vaccine in this context, but in the case of many infectious diseases no effective vaccine is available or no vaccine exists at all, e.g. BVD in Britain. Nosodes may be considered as vaccines, if it helps the reader to understand the principle of their application in this context. However, they do not produce any antibody response in the treated animal due to the extreme dilutions in which they are usually used (30c). These nosodes do not carry the potential hazards that vaccination sometimes can, e.g. strain 19 *Brucella abortus* vaccine (Day, 1986, 1987b).

These preventive remedies, in order to be swiftly and easily applied to the whole group at risk, may be administered via the drinking water. Water troughs should be as clean as possible and should be large enough or well-enough supplied with water so as not to run dry on the day of dosing. The quantity of remedy used does not appear to be very critical but an easy guide is to use 5 ml per drinking trough unless it is unusually large or small. Frequency of dosing would depend upon the estimated properties of the challenge. In an enzootic disease situation within the herd the frequency would be selected corresponding to the estimated violence and virulence of the disease and the animals' estimated ability to withstand it. At times of high risk when the disease agent is perhaps given the upper hand by management factors or climate or the animal is compromised by similar factors, then one would dose more frequently. In the case of *risk* from epizootic disease, i.e. new to the herd, dosing could be more sporadic.

The second sphere of use of the preventive technique is in the case of the individual animal threatened by a predictable disease challenge. Thus with impending parturition caulophyllum could be used to help prevent problems (Day, 1985, 1987b), or for an anticipated stressful journey aconitum could be used in advance of the challenge. Incidentally, aconitum can be used on a herd basis to prevent the production losses consequent on herd stress, such as the periodic tuberculin test.

Thus application of the homoeopathic method has come a long way since it was first devised in humans some 200 years ago. Although the real and in-depth diagnostic and prescribing processes may daunt the novice, the different levels at which the method can be applied provide scope for even the newly initiated and hesitant prescriber to test the principle of homoeopathy and its efficacy without being committed to long-term study or expensive stocks of medicines.

Materia medica

There follows a brief summary of the properties of some of the most commonly used remedies in a farm context, and some of their possible clinical applications. This is not intended to be an exhaustive source on the subject but an introduction to these 30 useful remedies. Fuller works on this material can be found in the Further reading section. Remedies are presented in alphabetical order for simplicity and not in order of importance or grouped according to possible application. The way in which these remedies are presented shows the emphasis placed on the 'picture' presented by the disease rather than the *name*, of the disease. Remedies are taken from the plant kingdom, animal kingdom and minerals and are available in tablet, pillule, crystal, powder, tincture, injection, cream, ointment or lotion forms; 30c is a useful potency for beginners.

Aconitum napellus

A remedy suitable for use in cases of sudden shock (physical or mental in nature), sudden-onset fevers, disorders from chilling and cold winds, and in cases of profuse bright red haemorrhage.

Affected animals tend to shudder in response to fear or shock, display a rapid pulse, run a fever and suffer conjunctivitis with fluid lacrimation and nasal discharge.

Antimonium tartaricum

A remedy particularly suited to respiratory signs. Indications are mucoid rattly breathing or coughing, frothy saliva and a tendency to cyanosis. Animals display minimal thirst and a rapid weak pulse. Cold, damp weather aggravates the condition and affected animals are unwilling to lie on their sides. This remedy is one of several useful pneumonia remedies and should be considered in cases of fog fever.

Apis mellifica

Useful in cases characterized by oedema. Urine retention, pulmonary oedema, oedematous swellings of vulva/perineum or udder, ascites, cystic ovaries, etc. may all respond if concomitant signs agree. The patient is usually thirstless and prefers open cool air. Cold bathing of affected areas produces comfort.

Arnica montana

A remedy useful in all conditions arising from trauma. Bruising, haematoma formation, pain, swelling, shock and even resultant local infection will respond to treatment. Patients often display a fear of being touched.

Arsenicum album

This remedy is a polycrest and therefore of constitutional importance. Restlessness, chilliness and thirst characterize the patient. The remedy can be useful, on a more local basis, in cases of diarrhoea, dehydration and collapse if concomitant signs agree. Diarrhoea is usually profuse, watery and offensive smelling.

Belladonna (atropa)

A 'fever' remedy, this is useful in cases where there is an acute febrile or inflammatory state characterized by heat, redness, swelling, fullness and pain. The pulse may be full and bounding. There are often delirious or convulsive signs too. The animal is usually thirsty and displays a dilated pupil.

Bryonia alba

This remedy has an affinity for serous membranes. All conditions are worsened by movement so the animal is unwilling to move. Affected animals are thirsty for long cold drinks. Guided by these three points one may prescribe confidently in cases of pneumonia, mastitis, arthritis, peritonitis, etc. The pneumonic calf will stand still, despite its fear, and tend to lie on its affected side to prevent movement. The mastitic cow would rather allow herself and her hot swollen painful udder to be examined than move away.

Calcarea carbonica

Another polycrest this remedy has constitutional applications. Disorders of production are an indication, e.g. fertility, lameness, mastitis. The animal has a heavy skeletal structure, large limbs, large joints and large feet. It usually has a good condition score and is generally peaceful but dominant. Movements tend to be unhurried. The appetite is very good and, if a milking cow, the milk yield is high. The animal is susceptible to chilling and usually shows catarrhal-type responses from the mucous membranes.

Calcarea phosphorica

Another polycrest, this remedy is suited to similar conditions to *calcarea carbonica* and the typical animal is similar although lighter in skeletal structure, quicker in movement and responses, difficult to handle and more fearful.

Carbo vegetabilis

Abdominal distension by gas, flatus, flatulent colic, weakness of circulation and musculature, poor resistance to infection and even collapse characterize this remedy. Its main application is in the treatment of the cold collapsed individual where its results can be spectacular.

Caulophyllum thalyctroides

One of the North American Indians' so-called 'squaw-root' remedies it has great application in all disorders of labour at any stage (Day, 1984a, 1985). It also has an effect on shifting lamenesses particularly if the origin is in the small joints.

Colocynthis (cucumis)

This remedy is of particular use in colic. The abdomen is distended and the back arched. Animals will roll and kick at the belly in cramp-like paroxysms.

Hepar sulphuris

If any homoeopathic remedy could be said to fill the role of antibiotics in septic conditions then this is the one. Suppurative processes in their early stages respond well. There is always great sensitivity to pain and relief from warm applications. Pain is aggravated by the least touch. Joint ill and navel ill usually respond.

Hypericum

Injury to nerves or areas rich in nerve endings is an indication for this remedy. It has a very rapid healing effect on the pain and damage. Not surprisingly the lesions and pain of photosensitization also respond well.

Lycopodium clavatum

A polycrest, this remedy has an application constitutionally. With an affinity for the liver the remedy is often used in this context. Possible digestive disturbance, dry withered appearance to the skin, tendency to flatus, abdominal distension, liver dysfunction, dyspnoea, tachypnoea, movement of the nostrils with every breath and an overall anxiety distinguish this animal type in disease. Problems are often right-sided and the animal prefers warmer water to drink (if offered).

Mercurius cyanatus

A thirsty patient with a paradoxically wet mouth and possibly even drooling saliva may require a mercury-type remedy. *Mercurius cyanatus* patients display offensive breath, offensive-smelling ulceration of mouth and throat and swollen glands. The picture fits that of calf diphtheria.

Mercurius solubilis

As with all mercury remedies there is a tendency to thirst, profuse salivation, offensive breath, to swollen glands in the throat and ulceration of mouth, bowel or teats. Ulcers will discharge pus. If there is diarrhoea there will also be a degree of tenesmus. Since the remedy is a polycrest it has constitutional applications and the preceding disease tendencies in a dominant, usually heavy, animal are an indication for its use.

Nux vomica

As a polycrest it has wide application in a constitutional context in the bovine. Patients tend to be quick in movements and reactions, bad tempered and thin. They suffer digestive complaints, characterized by cessation of rumen function and a tendency to constipation, having hard knotty stools. Complaints following from overeating of concentrate will respond well. Conditions tend to be worse in the morning and worse for disturbance or chilling (Mahe, 1987).

Phosphoric acid

In common with all the acids, phosphoric acid is indicated in cases of general weakness. More specifically there is debility, dehydration, pale flatulent painless diarrhoea with a dry mouth, thirst and possibly a degree of jaundice.

Phosphorus

Because of its extent of action it is a polycrest and therefore of great value in a constitutional context. Phosphorus conditions are characterized by sudden onset and their serious nature, e.g. sudden-onset pneumonia, sudden haemorrhages, hepatitis, haematogenous jaundice, etc. The phosphorus animal is also sudden in temperament, being averse to separation from the rest of the herd and apt to panic. The type is of lean build and averse to handling. Conditions are worse for touch and change of weather.

Phytolacca americana

This is the remedy above all others with a reputation in mastitis. This reputation can lead to overuse in this context as it will only produce results when used in the correct homoeopathic context. Lymph glands and mammary glands become indurated swollen and painful. There is usually heat too. Milk becomes thickened, stringy and yellowish. Cold wet weather aggravates.

Pulsatilla nigricans

A common constitutional type in the bovine particularly in the case of heifers. The type is shy, feminine in appearance, suffers catarrhal complaints and has little thirst. Breeding problems respond well if it is used in the correct constitutional context. Catarrhal syndromes of respiratory tract, udder, reproductive tract, etc. are typical. The animal prefers fresh open air and conditions are aggravated by warm stuffy atmospheres and in the evening.

Pyrogenium

Fevers particularly of a septic nature respond well to this remedy especially if pulse and temperature are not in agreement. There is a tendency to toxaemia, offensive secretions, dark blood and offensive dark septic lesions.

Rhus toxicodendron

American poison ivy produces, and therefore is able to help, severe pruritic conditions, rheumatic or arthritic stiffness and pains with great thirst and an aggravation from cold wet or damp conditions. Skin lesions are often vesicular in nature resembling cowpox lesions. Musculoskeletal problems are characterized by an aggravation from moving from rest with a subsequent 'loosening' and easing of the stiffness and pain. Diarrhoea displays dysentery and tenesmus.

Ruta graveolens

With an affinity for fibrous structural tissues such as ligaments, tendons, joint capsules and periosteum, this remedy is a powerful aid in the treatment of sprains and other damage to such tissues and regions of the body.

Sabina (juniperus)

Sabina's main sphere of activity is the uterus, where bloody discharges and lack of tone may respond. It is not indicated where sepsis exists. Retained fetal membranes may also be expelled under its influence.

Sepia

A polycrest, sepia has great value as a bovine constitutional remedy. It is predominantly a female remedy. Lack of tone and lack of tautness typify the conditions and constitutional type suited by this remedy. The animal takes on a worn-out, tired, sagging appearance and so also do individual body regions, e.g. uterus/perineum, limbs, udder, etc. Venous congestion and tendency to prolapse are also characteristic. Fertility problems may respond if constitutional aspects agree.

Silicea

Better known for its ability to stimulate expulsion of foreign bodies from the tissues or awaken chronic low-grade inflammatory lesions, *silicea* is also a great constitutional remedy. Structural weakness and distortion, whether of skeleton or feet, with a poor immune response typify the animal able to respond to the remedy.

Thuja occidentalis

The reputation of this remedy rests mostly on its action on papillomatous lesions, especially when they occur on neck or abdomen. Ill-effects of vaccination also may respond. The constitutional and other effects of the remedy are not so important in cattle work.

Urtica urens

The lesions of nettle rash are well known to everyone and the pain that follows. Apart from these properties the remedy has the ability, in high potency, to promote milk flow and, in low potency, to induce suppression. This power gives the remedy great value in bovine medicine. Lesions respond favourably to warm applications and negatively to cold applications, so too does the mastitis helped by *urtica*.

It is hoped that the foregoing brief account of 30 remedies will allow a start to be made in homoeopathic prescribing. It cannot be expected that, in so few pages, it will provide a comprehensive knowledge of the remedies. The reader must also realize that these few remedies, although forming a good nucleus of prescribing material, actually represent only a fraction of what is available. For each condition or syndrome mentioned, a great many other remedies have a potential value should they prove to be 'similar' to the problem.

Prescribing guide

There follows a small vade-mecum showing some indicated remedies that may prove effective in the named syndrome. Please be reminded that true homoeopathy does not rely on the *name* of a condition for remedy selection but the similarity between disease picture and remedy picture on as many counts as possible. The following list only serves as a pointer to some commonly indicated remedies and final selection between those remedies mentioned (and many not mentioned) rests with the prescriber. All the remedies mentioned below appear in the preceding section so that there is a brief guide to help selection of the most relevant remedy. (Remedies may be given orally, by injection, topically or orally via the drinking water.)

Acetonaemia (p. 590)	*Lycopodium, nux vomica*
Arthritis (pp. 363–386)	*Bryonia, caulophyllum, phytolacca, rhustox, ruta graveolens*
Bloat (p. 637)	*Carbo veg., lycopodium, nux vomica*
Calf diphtheria (p. 214)	*Mercurius cy.*
Constipation	*Nux vomica, sepia*
Convulsions	*Belladonna, nux vomica*
Dystokia (Day, 1984a, 1985)	*Caulophyllum, pulsatilla*
Fever	*Aconitum, belladonna, pyrogenium*
Foul-in-the-foot (p. 356)	*Hepar sulphuris*
Haemorrhage	*Aconitum, arnica, phosphorus*
Infertility	*Apis mell., aurum, pulsatilla, sepia*
Injury (Chapter 33)	*Aconitum, arnica, calendula, hypericum, ledum, rhus tox., ruta grav., symphytum*
Joint ill (p. 213)	*Hepar sulphuris*
Ketosis (p. 590)	See Acetonaemia
Mastitis (Day, 1986) (Chapter 21)	*Aconitum, belladonna, bryonia, carbo veg., hepar sulphuris, mercurius sol., phytolacca, silicea, urtica*
Metritis (Chapter 31)	*Caulophyllum, pulsatilla, pyrogenium, sabina, sepia*
Navel ill (p. 213)	*Hepar sulphuris, silicea*
Papillomatosis (p. 684)	*Thuja*
Placenta (retained) (Chapter 31)	*Caulophyllum, sabina, sepia*
Pneumonia (Chapter 15)	*Aconitum, antimonium tart., bryonia, lycopodium, phosphorus, pyrogenium*

This list is far from complete and is aimed at providing, an insight and a starting platform for deeper homoeopathic prescribing and learning.

Having read this guide to the principles of homoeopathy and tried out some of the methods and suggestions contained in this chapter it is hoped that the reader will go on to further study and venture into more ambitious prescribing from a position of confidence. Books giving a greater depth of homoeopathic knowledge are listed in the Further reading section and courses in Britain on veterinary homoeopathy are conducted in London under the auspices of the Faculty of Homoeopathy in Great Ormond Street.

Acupuncture

Acupuncture is a science of energy medicine having its origins in ancient China anything up to 4000 years ago. The oldest medical textbook known, the Huang Ti Nei Jing Su Wen (Veith, 1972), may have originally been written anything up to 1000 BC. Its origins are confused since it has undergone many alterations and commentaries since it was first written. (In fact the Su Wen was possibly a later addition to a scaled down Nei Jing.) This book has formed the basis of Traditional Chinese Medicine theory down the centuries but there have been myriad adaptations and variations applied since its inception, giving rise to Chinese medicine as we know it today. Acupuncture is but a component of this, herbalism also forming an integral part, along with moxibustion (the application of heat).

The Chinese have long treated animals with acupuncture so our veterinary use of this in the West is no new thing. In the UK, acupuncture is much more widely used on dogs and cats than in horses, and more in horses than in cattle. This is more a function of the pattern of specialization in the veterinary profession, and that more interest has been shown by those in small animal practice, than a reflection of the efficacy and value of acupuncture in cattle. The species responds very well to the methods but chronic disease is less a feature of bovine medicine than in the other species. This means that the call for a specialist second opinion is less utilized. The scope is reduced since the species is kept more for financial (productivity) reasons than emotional reasons or for its ability to perform competitively.

Acupuncture is a system of *internal* medicine devised in ancient times purely from the *outside* of the body. The human body was not to be violated in life or in death so post-mortem examinations and anatomical or physiological studies were not performed. The basis of the system is the relationship of points on the surface of the body to internal organs and their integrated functions. The mechanism of the relationship is not clear to Western science and is unquestioned in the East, where such a different philosophy of life and living pertains as to be incomparable. Clearly, as far as some of the points are concerned, there is a cutaneous–visceral reflex at work but this does not explain the mechanism of acupuncture any more than does the discovery of the release of endorphins in response to treatments. Our Western way of looking at life leads to a linear thought process, trying to establish 'cause and effect', and an attempt to classify and compartmentalize that does not sit well with an oriental philosophy and method.

The Chinese discovered, empirically, a collection of points (some 700 forming the basis of the system) that related to bodily function and to disease patterns or pictures. In order to explain the indisputable facts and verifiable correlations so discovered they wove a web of philosophical concepts in harmony, of course, with their philosophy of life (so turning an empirical art into a science). In ancient China, and still today, medical lore, religion and their way of life are inextricably entangled and form a unity not found in any comparable form in Western culture, where it seems that all three tend to be separate. This chapter does not argue which view is the more correct, valid or healthy but merely presents comparisons.

The philosophical lattice work is not there to confuse the would-be student but to explain and elucidate the empirical findings. This is not apparent to the sceptical Western observer who will undoubtedly find the concepts not only confusing but amphigoric. Atavism and Taoism are indigenous to the oriental way of thinking and are totally foreign to us. However, acupuncture was devised in the East and developed in the light of oriental concepts. It must be taken or left at present until some more readily assimilable theory is formulated that works as well as the original. This is not in the offing. It is hoped that by presenting a rapid overview of the theory it will not confuse the reader but will serve to give an introduction to the theory and method of acupuncture and encourage the diligent to look further into the subject.

Theory

The theory of the science of acupuncture is based on concepts of energy and forces rooted in Taoist philosophy. In this there exists no linear thinking, no cause and effect. The order and pattern of life (and therefore disease, which is a part of life) and the universe are governed by principles of inevitability. Concepts are not placed one under the other in a deductive sequence or subsumption but side by side in a picture, events following each other not by cause and effect but by a kind of inductance. Light does not cause darkness and vice versa, one becomes or leads to the other inevitably. Similarly, the concept of light cannot exist without darkness nor the concept of good without that of evil. The two forces that maintain the universe and the life in it are called Yin and Yang and represent philosophical polarities. They are aligned to other pairings of polarities, ranging over the whole of our existence, respectively: dark and light, cold and hot, female and male, low and high, sluggish and fast, lower and upper, night and day, soft and hard, earth and heaven, light and heavy, passive and active, inside and outside, empty and full, water and fire, weak and strong, under- and overactivity, humble and exalted, front and back (more logical in quadruped terms than in the human biped, i.e. ventral and dorsal), etc. It should be becoming clear that these two polarities act simultaneously within the universe (and its microcosm the body) and antagonistically. There is however no absolute in life and so with Yin and Yang. Nothing is all Yin, nothing is all Yang. Within Yin there is Yang and within Yang there is Yin and so on *ad infinitum*. Zou Yen, the philosopher of the third century BC, observed: 'Heaven is high, the earth is low, and thus they are fixed. As the high and low are thus made clear, the honourable and humble have their place accordingly. As activity and tranquility have their constancy the strong and weak are thus differentiated . . . . Cold and hot season take their turn . . . and Heaven knows the great beginning, and Earth acts to bring things to completion. Heaven is Yang and Earth is Yin' (Kaptchuk, 1983). Thus are embodied the consistencies and (apparent) inconsistencies of the oriental approach and there is no way to determine the beginning or end. The classic 'chicken and egg' situation holds.

Yin and Yang act together and antagonistically within the body and are components of the life energy — Qi. This energy is said to circulate continuously and rhythmically (on a diurnal cycle) through 12 paired (left and right) channels. These channels are often also called meridians. The complete balance and harmony of Yin and Yang within the body and the even and regular circulation of energy within the channels maintains perfect health. The converse applies: an imbalance of Yin and Yang and an interrupted flow of energy will imply disease. Thus disease tends to be more Yin or more Yang *relative* to the state of health. This can occur as a relative deficiency of one or the other, or as an excess of one or the other. Each would produce an apparent excess of one over the other.

The channels are related to organ function thus the 12 have names indicating their relationships. The organs to which they relate are said to be Yin or Yang in nature and, needless to say, there are six Yin and six Yang organs/channels (Table 59.1). The Yin organs are the solid Tsang organs, the Yang organs are the hollow or Fu organs. Each Tsang organ is related to a Fu organ, e.g. kidney is related to bladder.

The energy flow pattern follows a Yin–Yang–Yang–Yin cycle repeated three times. So we then are able to draw a flow chart built from the preceding lists (Fig. 59.2).

On the body these are represented in diagrammatic and simplified form in Figs 59.3–59.6. Routes of meridians and point locations thereupon are approximate guides. Accurate point location requires reference to more substantial works; titles can be found in the Further reading section. Owing to the loss of digits on the bovine limb (compared with the human five per limb) the distal sections of some meridians are open to interpretation (Fig. 59.7).

Table 59.1 The organs relating to Yin and Yang

Yin	Yang
Heart	Small intestine
Kidney	Bladder
Pericardium	Triple Heater
Liver	Gall-bladder
Lung	Large intestine
Spleen/pancreas	Stomach

Having said that the channels are each related to an organ the reader is probably wondering about the Triple Heater. This 'organ' represents thorax, abdomen and lower abdomen (pelvic), and therefore takes in the functions of respiration, digestion and the urogenital system.

There are two other (Extraordinary) vessels or meridians, which are of similar importance to the six pairs and these are the Conception Vessel and the Governor Vessel. These follow, respectively, the ventral and dorsal midlines. The energy flows from anus to mouth in both and therefore the vessels are not 'paired'. They differ also from the other meridians in that they lack special tonification and sedation points, etc. as described later for the other meridians, and are not an integral part of the diurnal energy circulation system. The Governor Vessel is dorsal and therefore Yang, the conception vessel is ventral and therefore Yin (see Fig. 59.6).

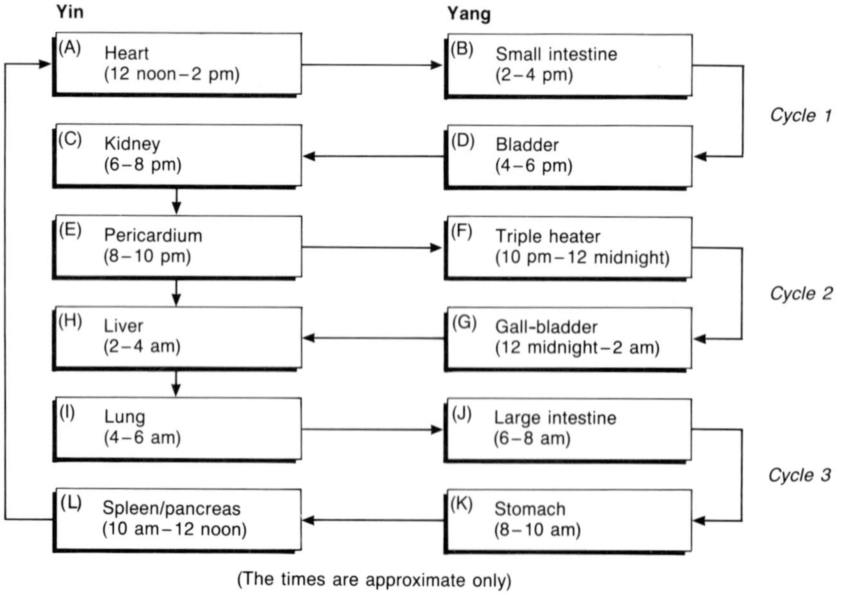

Fig. 59.2 An energy flow chart for the Yin–Yang–Yang–Yin cycle.

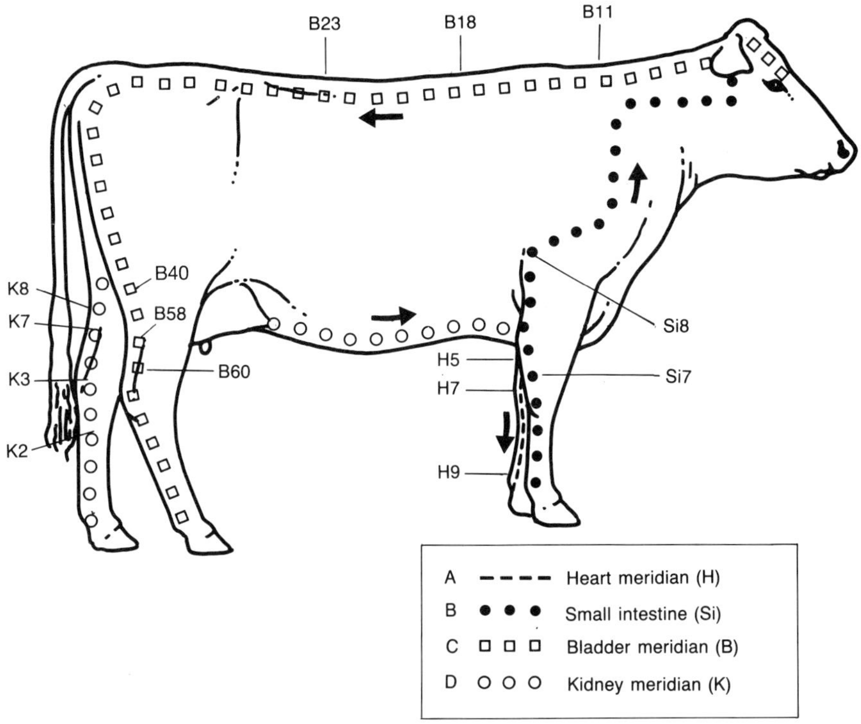

Fig. 59.3 Cycle of the energy flow chart for Yin–Yang–Yang–Yin.

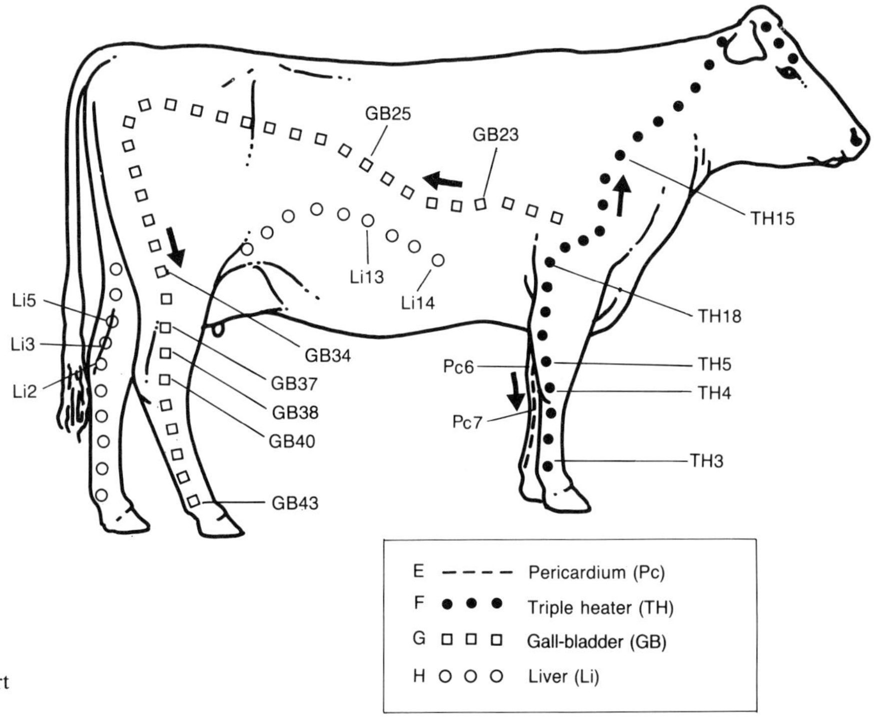

Fig. 59.4 Cycle 2 of the energy flow chart for Yin–Yang–Yang–Yin cycle.

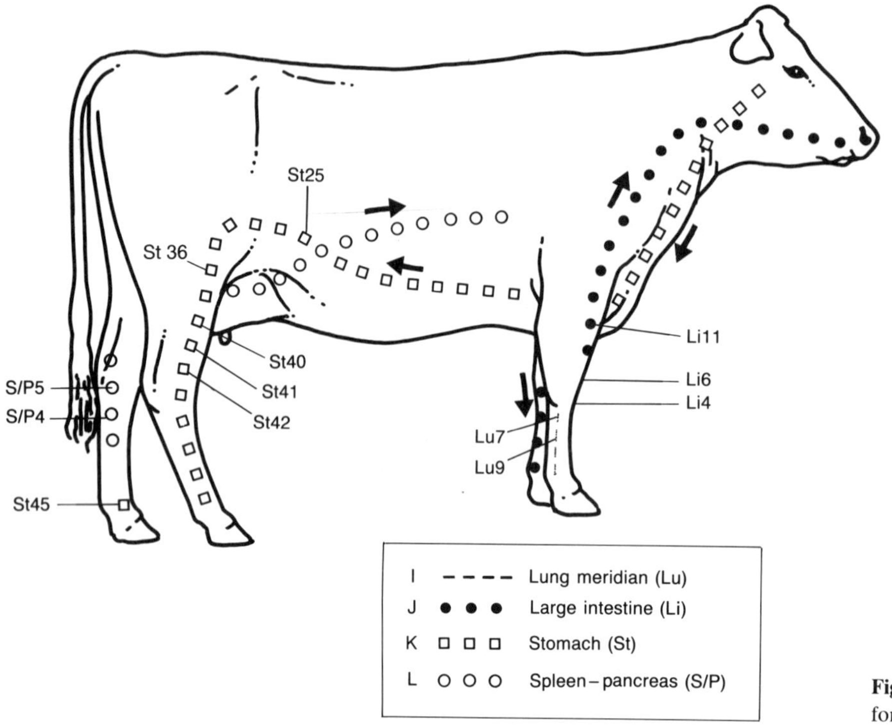

Fig. 59.5 Cycle 3 of the energy flow chart for the Yin–Yang–Yang–Yin cycle.

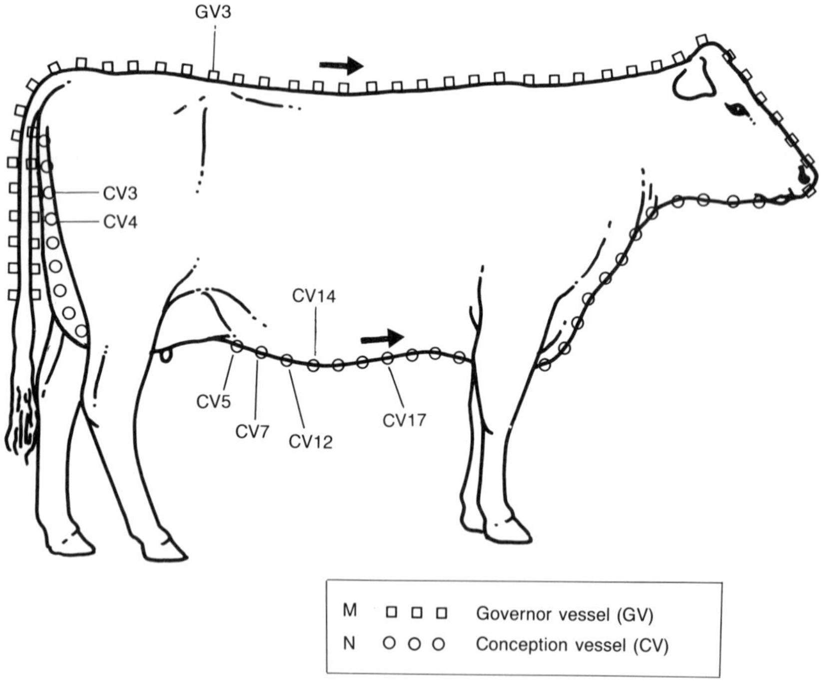

Fig. 59.6 The two extraordinary (unpaired) meridians (Governor vessel and Conception vessel).

The circulation of the energy is allowed to occur through the 12 seemingly disconnected channels, with apparent open circuits at each end, by means of the deep connections creating continuity proximally and 'secondary vessels' at the extremities.

The opposing forces of Yin and Yang are constantly at work in the body and are supposed to be in total balance flowing evenly through the 'channels' that the meridians represent. In fact it is better to picture a constant strife between Yin and Yang with alternating conquest and defeat but, in a state of health, with a balanced result throughout the 'championship'.

Anything that leads to an uneven 'contest', with one or other side in the ascendancy on balance, will lead to disease. The Chinese called such adverse forces the 'Pernicious Influences'. These are wind, cold, heat/fire, dampness, dryness and summer heat. They also believed disease could originate under the influence of emotions (joy, anger, sadness, grief, pensiveness, fear and fright), way of life (departure from Tao — 'the way'), diet, sexual activity and physical activity. They also recognized factors that did not fit into these categories, e.g. burns, bites, stings, trauma, etc.

Diagnosis

Diagnosis of the nature of disorders in the body in terms of the information given in the preceding pages was by pulse diagnosis in the human wrist (Fig. 59.7). Kothbauer & Meng (1983) give a method using the caudal artery in the bovine (Fig. 59.8) but this is sadly a long way from the complex and refined method developed for the human. Overall impressions only can be gained by this method. Inference can be made from the signs of disease displayed as to the nature of pernicious influence and which meridians are the key to the treatment (Kaptchuk, 1983). This requires a great deal of further reading if the reader is to develop these skills

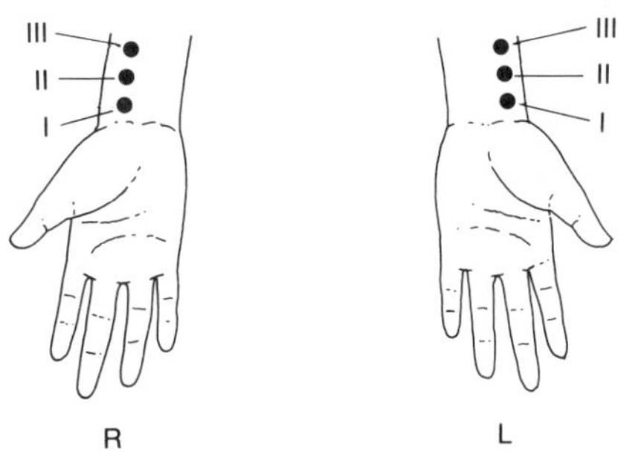

Fig. 59.7 Pulse positions on the human wrists. Each position has a deep and superficial pulse.

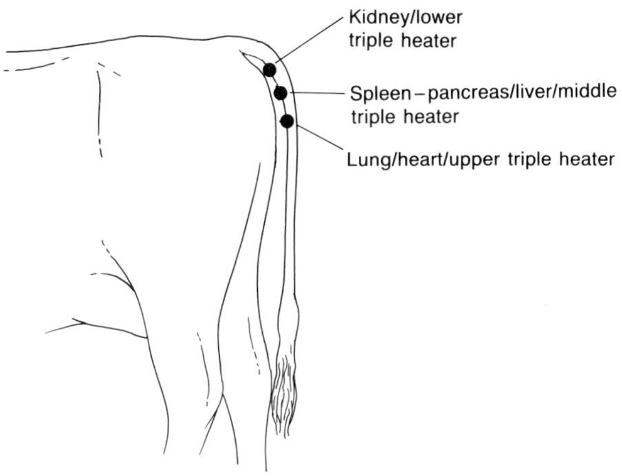

Fig. 59.8 Pulse diagnosis in the bovine (according to Kothbauer & Meng, 1983).

and is too large a subject for this small treatise but help can be derived from the following charts of relationships (Table 59.2).

The Five Number system was very important to the Chinese and here we can see the concept of the 'Five Elements' too. In this concept there are cycles of creation and destruction.

Water destroys Fire but creates Wood
Wood destroys Earth but creates Fire
Fire destroys Metal but creates Earth
Earth destroys Water but creates Metal
Metal destroys Wood but creates Water

The organs and function of the body are related, for example:

The Kidneys are connected to the Bones and rule over the Spleen
The Heart is connected with the Pulse and rules over the Kidneys

These connections are not so far-fetched even in modern Western terms!

What has been described, although briefly, is an attempt on the part of the ancients to explain the rhythm and dynamics of life and disease, albeit often by metaphor, which can be offputting to the Western mind. The explanation does seem to embrace the reality of the integrity of the whole body both in anatomy and function and its relationship to the outside world. Disease does not come in tidy parcels, affecting only one part of the body in a single way, but in complex patterns of whole body dysfunction. The philosophy behind Traditional Chinese Medicine embraces this idea very satisfactorily.

Table 59.2 Pernicious influences on disease

	Yang	Yang		Yin	Yin
Season	Spring	Summer	Late summer	Autumn	Winter
Climate	Wind	Heat	Dampness	Dryness	Cold
Direction	East	South	Centre	West	North
Organs (Tsang)	Liver	Heart	Spleen	Lungs	Kidneys
Organs (Fu)	Gall-bladder	Small intestines	Stomach	Large intestines	Triple Heater and bladder
Orifices	Eyes	Ears	Nose	Mouth	Urogenital orifices
Tissues	Ligaments	Arteries	Muscles	Skin and hair	Bones
Elements	Wood	Fire	Earth	Metal	Water
Odour	Rancid	Scorched	Fragrant	Rotten	Putrid
Emotions	Anger	Joy	Sympathy	Grief	Fear
Fluids	Tears	Perspiration	Saliva	Mucus	Spittle

Treatment (Plates 59.1 and 59.2)

Treatment of the body in Traditional Chinese Medicine, whether by herbs, moxibustion or needles (this treatise really only deals with needles) attempts to restore the balance in the constant conflict between Yin and Yang. Moxibustion is the application of heat to specific points of the body to supply heat energy to the system. Usually, *Artemisia vulgaris* herb is used as a 'wool', sometimes without herbs. Heat is applied directly to the area or a few millimetres above it. Needles can also be inserted at the point and heated. There are many different categories of points that can be utilized in acupuncture prescriptions in an attempt to restore this balance.

The points

Locus-Dolendi needling is the use of points of local pain directly related to the site of injury or illness. The effect is not very long-lasting but provides relief from pain in local conditions. It requires little knowledge on the part of the prescriber but should probably be reserved for locomotor pain or injury.

Master points relate to individual organs or tissues and can be used regardless of the nature of pathology or dysfunction which that target suffers. These master points will usually be sensitive to stimulus when there is a dysfunction or injury in the influenced organ/tissue. Effects of using this method of prescribing alone will lead to disappointment. There is no deep and lasting influence on disease if the prescriber sticks to this elementary process. The master point of the musculature, for instance, is Gall Bladder 34.

Symptomatic points have an influence over certain specific functions. For instance, Bladder 31 influences female hormonal function very strongly and can be used in a prescription when such problems predominate (Plate 59.1). The action of these points is usually fairly narrow so, again, prescriptions based on these alone are unlikely to be far-reaching. Both symptomatic and master points may also be used in reverse as diagnostic tools.

Pilot points are used properly to redistribute or balance the Yin–Yang conflict. Main points are the *Tonification points*, which increase energy in an energy-deficient meridian (gold needles are often used) and *Sedation points* decrease energy in overactive meridians (silver needles are often used). Each meridian has one of each of these.

The Source point on each meridian acts as an adjuvant to one or other of the two above-mentioned points. The metal used is selected according to which function it is wished to augment.

The Passage points, situated on each meridian, will help to shunt energy from the meridian in question to its partner. Energy usually flows 'downhill'.

The Alarm point may or may not lie on the meridian to which it relates but may be used for diagnosis or treatment if sensitive.

The Associated points, lying on the Bladder meridian, are also of value diagnostically or therapeutically and relate to specific organs and meridians. For example, the Associated point for the spleen/pancreas is Bladder 20, for the stomach it is Bladder 21.

Table 59.3 Useful points

Heart (H) meridian
5. Passage point
7. Sedation point and Source point
(9.) Tonification point (open to interpretation)

Small intestine (SI) meridian (open to interpretation)
(3.) Tonification point
(4.) Source point
7. Passage point
8. Sedation point

Bladder (B) meridian
11. Bone disorders
13. Associated point lung
14. Associated point pericardium
15. Associated point heart
18. Associated point liver
19. Associated point gall-bladder
20. Associated point spleen/pancreas
21. Associated point stomach and Master point stomach
22. Associated point Triple Heater
23. Associated point kidney
25. Associated point large intestine
27. Associated point small intestine
28. Associated point bladder
31. Master point female hormones
58 Passage point
60 Master point for pain
(640) Source point (open to interpretation)
(650) Sedation point (open to interpretation)
(670) Tonification point (open to interpretation)

Kidney (K) meridian
1/2. Sedation point
3. Source point
4. Passage point
7. Tonification point
8. Master point blood
(11.) Alarm point pericardium (not clearly identifiable in bovine) (in groin)

Pericardium (P) meridian
1. Alarm point pericardium (lateral thorax in posterior axilla)
6. Passage point
7. Sedation point and Source point
(9.) Tonification point (anterolateral of second digit)

Triple Heater (TH) meridian
3. Tonification point
4. Source point
5. Passage point
10. Sedation point
15. Master point for forelimbs

Gall-Bladder (GB) meridian
23. Alarm point for gall-bladder
25. Alarm point for kidney (caudal to last rib)
34. Master point of muscles
37. Passage point
38. Sedation point
40. Source point
43. Tonification point

Liver (Li) meridian
2. Sedation point (medial hock)
3. Source point (medial hock)
5. Passage point (postero-medial tibia)
8. Tonification point (postero-medial stifle joint)
13. Alarm point for spleen pancreas (caudal to last rib)
14. Alarm point of the liver

Lung (Lu) meridian
1. Alarm point for lung (between shoulder joint and third rib on chest wall)
5. Sedation point (medial elbow)
7. Passage point
9. Tonification point and Source point
(11.) Master point for the throat (not clearly identifiable in the bovine)

Large Intestine (LI) meridian
(1.) Master point for teeth (open to interpretation)
(2/3) Sedation points (open to interpretation)
4. Source point (medial carpus)
6. Passage point (medial carpus)
11. Tonification point

Stomach (St) meridian
25. Alarm point for large intestine
40. Passage point
41. Tonification point
42. Source point
45. Sedation point

Spleen Pancreas (S/P) meridian
(2.) Tonification point (open to interpretation)
(3.) Source point (open to interpretation)
4. Passage point (anteromedial tarsus)
5. Master point for connective tissue and Sedation point (anteromedial tarsus)

Conception Vessel (CV) (Fig. 59.6)
3. Alarm point for the bladder
4. Alarm point for small intestine
5. Alarm point for Triple Heater
7. Alarm point for lower Triple Heater
12. Alarm point for stomach and Alarm point for middle Triple Heater (caudal to xiphoid, cranial to navel)
14. Alarm point for the heart (caudal to xiphoid)
17. Alarm point for upper Triple Heater (on sternum, rib 7)

Governor Vessel (GV) (Fig. 59.6)
No Main or Special points.

It is helpful to list here some useful points for earlier selection by the beginner; see Table 59.3 and refer to Figs 59.2–59.5.

Table 59.3 is clearly by no means comprehensive (as can be seen from the numeration) but represents a useful reference list for the main functional points. For more comprehensive point descriptions the reader is referred to much fuller works on acupuncture therapy. Their location, as shown on Figs 59.3–59.6, is a synthesis of information from personal experience and the work of Klide & Kung (1977), Lewith (1982), Kothbauer & Meng (1983), Bishchko (1983), Gilchrist (1984) and Janssens (1984) in order to maintain a standard nomenclature that prevents confusion.

Use of these points

The meridians are interconnected energetically in various 'rules' of therapy. Treatment strategies may be based on these relationships. Again the Chinese show their proclivity towards metaphorical description. The first relationship is based upon the human system of pulse diagnosis and relates to the position of pulse-taking in the human wrist (Table 59.3; see also Fig. 59.7).

1 The 'Husband–Wife' rule relates meridians sharing the same positions on either wrist. Tonifying one will sedate its partner and vice versa. They oppose each other.

2 The 'Mother–Son' rule relates to the sequence of the meridians in the circadian rhythm. A meridian preceding that in question is its Mother and that succeeding is its Son. It is logical to assume that the Mother is ready to give energy, the Son receive it. Tonifying the meridian in question *and* its Mother will produce extra effects. Similarly, sedating both the meridian in question and its Son will increase the effects of sedation. Passage points may be used instead when the meridians in question are partners.

3 The 'Midday–Midnight' rule relates meridians most active in a similar time period, a.m. and p.m. One will be Yin and one Yang, e.g. lung (Yin), 4 a.m. to 6 a.m., bladder (Yang), 4 p.m. to 6 p.m. Tonifying a meridian in its active time will sedate its opposite number.

These three rules should always be borne in mind because, even if it is not the intention of the prescriber, the rule will operate on stimulation of the relevant points with appropriate needles. Using the three rules together can achieve a rapid restoration of harmony within the body. The system of acupuncture thus used is not only complete but also quite simple to apply providing infinite combinations of therapy. It is sad that pulse diagnosis is not so refined in animals but the relationships of the meridians are still valid and so too is the correspondence of disease patterns with Yin and Yang effects from the pernicious influences and other origins of disharmony. Conclusions about meridian malfunction are inferred from the disease patterns displayed by the patient and by the demonstrable point sensitivities.

Technique of needling and treatment

Steel, gold or silver needles are selected according to the effect required. They should be inserted confidently into the skin as near to the centre of the point as possible. Depth of insertion is generally up to 1 cm. During a treatment the body 'reacts' with the needles in a way that has not been defined physiologically or anatomically during this time, the needles, are firmly held by the tissues. When a treatment is over, perhaps between 5 and 20 minutes later, the needles may be removed with ease.

After treatment there may be a 'slump' in the patient's apparent energy for the next 24 hours. The author has observed this less in cattle than in other species. Treatments may be repeated at intervals of several days to several weeks but a useful guide for an initial course of therapy is a three to fourteen day interval for three or four treatments. If no improve-

Table 59.4 The relationships based on the human pulse system

Position	Right		Left	
	Superficial	Deep	Deep	Superficial
III	Large intestine	Lung	Heart	Small intestine
II	Stomach	Spleen/pancreas	Liver	Gall-bladder
I	Triple Heater	Pericardium	Kidney	Bladder
	(Yang)	(Yin)	(Yin)	(Yang)

ment is noted in this period, it is possibly a sign of a poor prognosis. After a good initial result, treatment may need repeating at longer intervals (say six monthly) in chronic conditions.

Conclusion

It is to be hoped that the reader, having studied this chapter or one or other part of it, will have experienced adequate stimulation to take a deeper look into either system of medicine (see Further reading section) and have gleaned sufficient information to take the first steps in applying the therapies. What should be clear is that either system of medicine is a very large and complex subject. Should the reader wish to go further it must be said that a great deal of motivation and dedication will be required. If this chapter has provided the motivation, that is good. If not, then it should at least serve to dispel some of the mists of ignorance and suspicion that enshroud the art and science of both homoeopathy and acupuncture. Those who choose to apply themselves to diligent study and to professional application of these methods will be able to enjoy a life full of surprises and rewards commensurate with effort, but will not have chosen an easy option.

References and further reading

Bischko, J. (1983) *Einführung in die Akupunktur*, 13th edn. Karl F. Haug, Heidelberg.

Boericke, W. (1972) *Materia Medica with Repertory*. Boericke & Runyon, Philadelphia.

Brock, K. & Nielsen, J. (1986) *Veterinaer Homøopati*. DSR Forlag, København.

Clarke, J.H. (1982) *Dictionary of Materia Medica*, 3rd edn, Vols 1, 2 and 3. Health Science Press, Saffron Walden.

Day, C.E.I. (1984a) Control of stillbirths using homoeopathy. *Veterinary Record*, **114**, 216.

Day, C.E.I. (1984b) *The Homoeopathic Treatment of Small Animals, Principles and Practice*. Wigmores, London (to be republished by C.W. Daniel, Saffron Walden).

Day, C.E.I. (1985) Dystocia Prevention. Proceedings of LMHI Congress, Lyon.

Day, C.E.I. (1986) Clinical trials in bovine mastitis using nosodes for prevention. *International Journal for Veterinary Homoeopathy*, **1**, 11.

Day, C.E.I. (1987a) Isopathic prevention of kennel cough. *International Journal for Veterinary Homoeopathy*, **2**, 57.

Day, C.E.I. (1987b) *A Guide to the Homoeopathic Treatment of Beef and Dairy Cattle*. Beaconsfield Publ. Ltd, Beaconsfield.

Daykin, P.W. (1960) *Veterinary Applied Pharmacology and Therapeutics*. Baillière, Tindall & Cassell, London.

Garner, R.J. (1967) *Veterinary Toxicology*, (revised by E.S.C. Clarke & M.L. Clarke). Baillière, Tindall & Cassell, London.

Gilchrist, D. (1984) *Greyhound Acupuncture*. Pro-Prom Pty Ltd, Mareeba.

Hahnemann, C.F.S. (c1814) Unpublished Homöopatische Heilkunde der Hausthiere, Leipziger Universitätsbibliothek.

Hahnemann, C.F.S. (1833/42) *The Organon of Medicine*, 5th/6th edn (translated by Boericke & Dudgeon). B. Jain, New Delhi.

Janssens, L.A.A. (1984) *Acupuncture Points and Meridians in the Dog*. Blondiau Print, Beersel.

Kaptchuk, T.J. (1983) *Chinese Medicine*. Rider, Melbourne.

Kent, J.T. (1986) *Repertory of the Homoeopathic Materia Medica*. Homoeopathic Book Service, London.

Klide, A.M. & Kung, S.H. (1977) *Veterinary Acupuncture*. University of Pennsylvania Press.

Kothbauer, O. & Meng, A. (1983) *Grundlagen der Veterinär — Akupunktur*. Verlag Welsermühl, Wels.

Lewith, G.T. (1982) *Acupuncture, its Place in Western Medical Science*. Thorsons, Wellingborough.

MacLeod, G. (1981) *The Treatment of Cattle by Homoeopathy*. Health Science, Press, Saffron Walden.

MacLeod, G. (1983) *A Veterinary Materia Medica and Clinical Repertory*. C.W. Daniel, Saffron Walden.

Mahe, F. (1987) Evaluation of the effect of a collective homoeopathic cure on morbidity and the butchering qualities in fattening calves. *International Journal for Veterinary Homoeopathy*, **2**, 13.

Veith, I. (1972) *The Yellow Emperor's Classic of Internal Medicine*. University of California Press, Los Angeles.

Chapter 60: Injection Damage

by J.H. PRATT

Introduction

The faulty administration of veterinary medicines by injection can give rise to complaints from meat wholesalers and retailers and on occasions from consumers. The lesion resulting from the injection of a drug may be aesthetically repugnant to the consumer and commercially unacceptable in the case of abscessation or fibrosis in muscle tissue to the wholesaler, the retailing butcher and the supermarket outlet.

Damage produced by injection

Abscesses deep in the gluteal region of cattle are reported since the site is frequently used for intramuscular injection of drugs. Damage in this area reduces the value of a relatively expensive part of the carcass. Abscessation may render the entire limb unsuitable for human consumption. Intravenous injections can result in haematoma formation and abscess production. In some cases this is due to irritant substances invading the perivascular tissue rather than being delivered properly into the bloodstream. In addition, the deep injection of an irritant substance causing a localized reaction within muscle tissue may elude detection at meat inspection and even later in the cutting premises. The damage may not be revealed until further butchering procedures are performed on the beef in the processing plant or retail shop by which time it may prove difficult to trace the animal back to the farm of origin. Indeed, in countries where complex marketing arrangements exist, the tracing of animals back through marketing chains may prove impossible until unique individual identification of the live animal and the resultant carcass and cuts becomes feasible in all stock. Such an achievement would constitute a major contribution to future meat quality standards.

Where the farm of origin can be determined, advice on proper injection techniques can be given thereby improving the welfare interests of the animal and enhancing the future profitability of the producer. Losses incurred by the abattoir through the downgrading of affected cuts of beef from incorrect injection procedures would also be reduced.

It is to be regretted that in Britain the use of data collected in the abattoir has not been exploited to its full potential. Such information can play a significant role in future preventive veterinary medicine strategies and in the depiction of regional and national animal disease patterns.

The losses incurred by the meat industry through poor injection technique are spasmodic but nevertheless can be substantial. There are, unfortunately, no reliable figures in UK meat inspection records for condemnation of meat for abscessation due to faulty injection procedures alone. However, on occasions a number of animals within one consignment of cattle exhibit deep muscle fibrosis consistent with damage from injected material, necessitating the rejection of 1.5–2 kg of a high-priced cut of meat. These lesions are formed in the same anatomical area in a number of animals within a group from the same unit. The similarity in age, character and distribution of these lesions suggests a common cause, the introduction of foreign material by injection. Both injectable nemicides and substances used in the regulation of bovine reproduction, e.g. some prostaglandins, may have been responsible for such damage encountered in recent years in this country.

The leather industry also suffers financial loss, as injection damage due to scarring and abscessation can

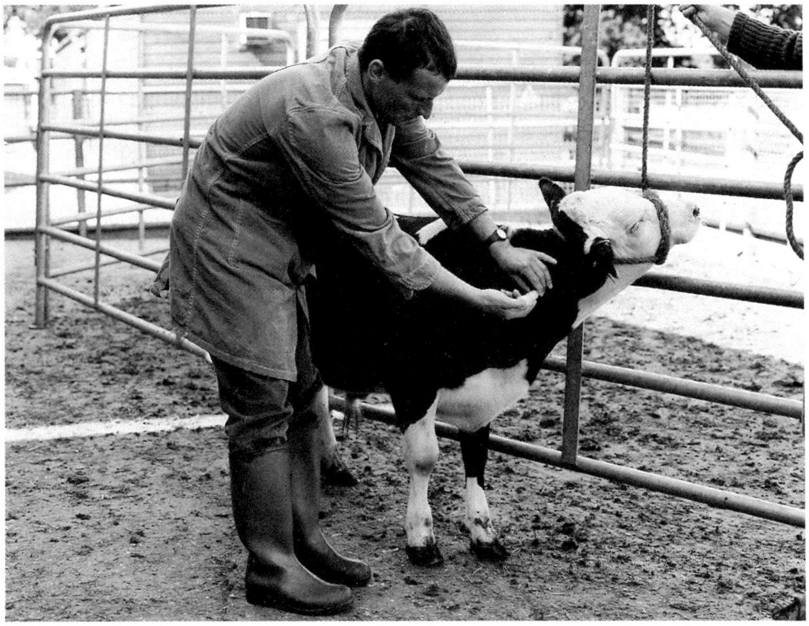

Fig. 60.1 A growing calf being injected into the neck muscle.

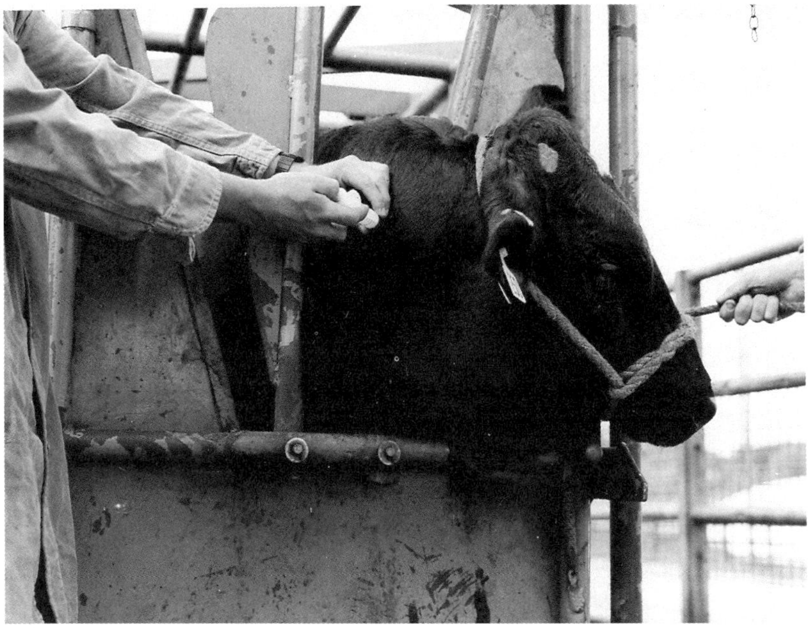

Fig. 60.2 A bull adequately restrained before introducing an injection into the neck muscles.

reduce the value of the hide, particularly if the lesion is in a position that prevents the optimal use of the complete hide for large leather or suede items of clothing and upholstery.

Intramuscular injection sites

Alternative siting of injections to that of the gluteal region is therefore desirable. The middle third of the neck, about one-third of the way down from the top, is recommended (see Figs 60.1 and 60.2); this in itself does not reduce the incidence of abscessation or muscle scarring following the injection of drugs but trimming of this less expensive area reduces blemishing of the carcass. This area also tends to be cleaner than the hindquarters and so it is less likely that infection will be introduced with injection.

The factors contributing to muscle damage and

abscess formation must therefore be identified to allow the formulation of advice for veterinarians and animal owners to reduce such damage.

The efficiency of the host animal's inflammatory response in removing the foreign protein and devitalized tissue together with the persistence of the stimulus determine the size and progression of the abscess formation. In mild cases no abscess may form, but scar tissue will mark the tissue damage. When an abscess has been formed and the inflammatory stimulus removed the abscess may persist for a prolonged period before resolving to scar tissue.

Methods of introducing contamination

The introduction of foreign protein may occur in a variety of ways.

Contamination of injected drugs is most likely to occur prior to administration as a result of poor hygienic procedures employed. To obviate contamination of the contents of a bottle or vial a separate sterile needle to that used for injection must remain attached to the container and used only to refill the syringe. In multiple dosing an automatic injection mechanism avoids this requirement and results in a smoother and more efficient operation. The manufacturer's storage instructions should be followed; unused vaccine should be discarded. When therapeutic agents such as antibiotics are used they should be used up as quickly as possible after opening.

Contamination of needle or syringe. Ideally, a sterile needle should be used for every injection but in practical situations this is often not feasible; however, in special circumstances this approach may be applicable on veterinary advice in certain herds to avoid transfer of specific viral and other infections such as enzootic bovine leukosis (EBL). It is good practice, however, to change needles and syringes regularly, i.e. after every 10–15 cattle, when groups of animals are injected and in any event when contamination of the equipment occurs or is suspected or the needle is in any way damaged.

Punching a fragment of host skin. The introduction of host tissue along with the injection material is most likely to occur when damaged needles are used. The regular changing of needles will reduce the chances of this occurring. When needle damage has obviously occurred a replacement is necessary in order to avoid possible injury to the animal and to maintain good meat hygiene and quality standards.

Irritant injections. The introduction of an irritant substance that devitalizes tissue locally can be responsible for direct or indirect damage to muscle tissue. Examples used in veterinary medicine are: basic and acidic compounds, such as the sulphonamide drugs and spectinomycin; hypertoxic preparations, e.g. long-acting oxytetracycline; and adjuvants, e.g. aluminium hydroxide, saponin.

Vasoactive substances, e.g. local anaesthetic preparations containing adrenaline and some synthetic prostaglandins, lead to ischaemic necrosis.

Contaminated skin. Pathogenic bacteria may be introduced not only when injecting cattle with a contaminated drug or when the needle or syringe is dirty but when the skin surface is not clean; the introduction of pathogens from the site of injection will occur in a proportion of cattle treated. It is therefore incumbent upon the veterinarian and the stock owner to employ hygienic injection procedures at all times using sterile equipment and uncontaminated injectable materials. Preparation of the injection site is an integral part of this hygienic approach; the avoidance of contaminated sites of injection is essential. A clean site should be chosen. If not available an area should be cleaned, or if necessary clipped and cleaned.

There are now available multidose syringes with special sterilization caps to reduce the possibility of infections. Caps can also be placed on the tops of therapeutic agents.

The recommended route of administration and the injection technique outlined in the manufacturer's instructions must be followed. The incorrect route can lead to tissue damage, e.g. drugs recommended for subcutaneous administration must not be given by the intramuscular route or intraperitoneally unless specifically indicated.

Proper restraint of the animal will lessen the likelihood of tissue damage and allow hygienic procedures to be followed. The injection of a fractious or nervous animal can lead to unnecessary suffering and damage to the animal, not to say injury to the operator also. Furthermore, struggling while injecting an animal may preclude the proper administration of the medicine with less than the prescribed dose deposited at the recommended site, the remainder forming a depot with ensuing damage. Thus all animals should be adequately restrained (see Figs 60.1 and 60.2).

Index